T0328333

THE BIOLOGY AND IDENTIFICATION OF THE COCCIDIA (APICOMPLEXA) OF CARNIVORES OF THE WORLD

THE BIOLOGY AND IDENTIFICATION OF THE COCCIDIA (APICOMPLEXA) OF CARNIVORES OF THE WORLD

DONALD W. DUSZYNSKI

Department of Biology, University of New Mexico, Albuquerque, NM, USA

JANA KVIČEROVÁ

*Department of Parasitology, Faculty of Science, University of South Bohemia,
České Budějovice, Czech Republic*

R. SCOTT SEVILLE

Professor of Zoology and Physiology, University of Wyoming at Casper, WY, USA

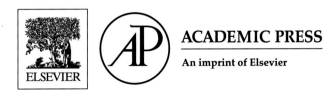

ACADEMIC PRESS

An imprint of Elsevier

ELSEVIER

Academic Press is an imprint of Elsevier
125 London Wall, London EC2Y 5AS, United Kingdom
525 B Street, Suite 1650, San Diego, CA 92101, United States
50 Hampshire Street, 5th Floor, Cambridge, MA 02139, United States
The Boulevard, Langford Lane, Kidlington, Oxford OX5 1GB, United Kingdom

Copyright © 2018 Donald W. Duszynski published by Elsevier Inc. All rights reserved.

No part of this publication may be reproduced or transmitted in any form or by any means, electronic or mechanical, including photocopying, recording, or any information storage and retrieval system, without permission in writing from the publisher. Details on how to seek permission, further information about the Publisher's permissions policies and our arrangements with organizations such as the Copyright Clearance Center and the Copyright Licensing Agency, can be found at our website: www.elsevier.com/permissions.

This book and the individual contributions contained in it are protected under copyright by the Publisher (other than as may be noted herein).

Notices
Knowledge and best practice in this field are constantly changing. As new research and experience broaden our understanding, changes in research methods, professional practices, or medical treatment may become necessary.

Practitioners and researchers must always rely on their own experience and knowledge in evaluating and using any information, methods, compounds, or experiments described herein. In using such information or methods they should be mindful of their own safety and the safety of others, including parties for whom they have a professional responsibility.

To the fullest extent of the law, neither the Publisher nor the authors, contributors, or editors, assume any liability for any injury and/or damage to persons or property as a matter of products liability, negligence or otherwise, or from any use or operation of any methods, products, instructions, or ideas contained in the material herein.

Library of Congress Cataloging-in-Publication Data
A catalog record for this book is available from the Library of Congress

British Library Cataloguing-in-Publication Data
A catalogue record for this book is available from the British Library

ISBN: 978-0-12-811349-3

For information on all Academic Press publications visit our website at
https://www.elsevier.com/books-and-journals

**Working together
to grow libraries in
developing countries**

www.elsevier.com • www.bookaid.org

Publisher: John Fedor
Acquisition Editor: Linda Versteeg-Buschman
Editorial Project Manager: Pat Gonzalez
Production Project Manager: Mohanapriyan Rajendran
Cover Designer: Mark Rogers

Typeset by TNQ Technologies

Contents

7. Eimeriidae in the Caniformia Families Odobenidae, Otariidae, and Phocidae

8. Eimeriidae in the Caniformia Family Procyonidae

9. Eimeriidae in the Caniformia Family Ursidae

10. Eimeriidae in the Feliformia Family Felidae

15. Sarcocystidae: Sarcocystinae in the Carnivora

16. Sarcocystidae: Toxoplasmatinae in the Carnivora

17. Cryptosporidiidae in the Carnivora

20. Discussion, Summary and Conclusions

APPENDICES

Preface and Acknowledgments

In 1992–93, the National Science Foundation announced its initiative, Partnerships for Establishing Expertise in Taxonomy (PEET), to support research that targeted groups of poorly known organisms and "to encourage the training of new generations of taxonomists and to translate current expertise into electronic databases and other formats with broad accessibility to the scientific community." In 1995, DWD was fortunate to be in the first cohort of PEET recipients and began working on "The Coccidia of the World (DBS/DEB-9521687);" this contribution by Drs. Kvičerová and Seville and me is an extension of that program, as is the Coccidia of the World online database (http://biology.unm.edu/coccidia/home.html), and a number of revisionary taxonomic works that include marmotine squirrels (Wilber et al., 1998); primates and tree shrews (Duszynski et al., 1999); insectivores (Duszynski and Upton, 2000); *Eimeria* and *Cryptosporidium* in wild mammals (Duszynski and Upton, 2001), bats (Duszynski, 2002); amphibians (Duszynski et al., 2007); snakes (Duszynski and Upton, 2010); rabbits (Duszynski and Couch, 2013); turtles (Duszynski and Morrow, 2014); marsupials (Duszynski, 2016); and our current treatise revising the Norman Levine and Virginia Ivens contribution on the Coccidian Parasites of Carnivores (1981).

We could not have completed this effort and want to acknowledge our gratitude to the following friends, colleagues, and agencies: Lee Couch, wife (of DWD) and friend to all, retired teacher of medical microbiology for 25+ years at the University of New Mexico, current Secretary–Treasurer of the American Society of Parasitology, and current Emergency Medical Technician of the Year (2012, 2014, 2016) of Sandoval County, New Mexico, for her expertise and help scanning, adjusting, and archiving all the line drawings and photomicrographs used in the species descriptions in this book. Special thanks are due Dr. Norman D. Levine (deceased) who, many years ago after his retirement from the University of Illinois, sent DWD substantial portions of his personal reprint library. To Dr. Geru Tao (Sarah), National Animal Protozoa Laboratory, College of Veterinary Medicine, China Agricultural University, Beijing, China PRC for her friendship, support, and kindness during a 2016 lecture tour in China (DWD), and for her help with several Chinese translations. To Dr. Hidetoshi Ota, PhD, FLS, Director and Professor, Institute of Natural and Environmental Sciences, University of Hyogo, and Head, Phylogeny and Systematics Section, Museum of Nature and Human Activities, Yayoigaoka 6, Sanda, Hyogo 669-1546, Japan for his decades-long friendship and for his help with certain Japanese translations. To Dr. J.P. Dubey, USDA, ARS, APDL, BARC-East Bldg 1001, Beltsville, MD 20705, for his longtime friendship to us all, for his unwavering and steadfast support with literature retrieval and for sharing prepublication manuscript copies of his two most recent books, *Sarcocystosis of Animals and Humans*, second ed. (Dubey, J.P., Calero-Bernal, R., Rosenthal, B.M., Speer, C.A., Fayer, R., 2016. CRC Press, Taylor & Francis Group, Boca Raton, Florida, 481 p.) and *Neosporosis in Animals* (Dubey, J.P., Hemphill, A., Calero-Bernal, R., Schares, G., 2017. CRC Press, Inc., Taylor & Francis Group, Boca Raton, Florida, 529 p.). To Dr. Lada Hofmannová, DVM, PhD,

Faculty of Veterinary Medicine, University of Veterinary and Pharmaceutical Sciences Brno, Brno, Czech Republic for help with providing full texts of some scientific publications. We thank our families for inexhaustible patience and support, and we are most grateful for financial support, in part, for Dr. R. Scott Seville during the writing of this book, by a grant from the National Institute of General Medical Sciences (2P20GM103432) from the National Institutes of Health. The content is solely the responsibility of the authors and does not necessarily represent the official views of the National Institutes of Health.

Finally, we are grateful to and appreciate the help and the work of the professional staff at Elsevier, especially to Linda Versteeg, Senior Acquisitions Editor, Fundamental Life Sciences, Microbiology, Immunology, Virology, and Parasitology, Elsevier/Academic Press, Radarweg 291043 NX Amsterdam, The Netherlands; to Pat Gonzalez, Editorial Project Manager, Animal and Plant Sciences, 525 B Street, Suite 1800, San Diego, CA 92101 USA; and to Mohanapriyan (Monu) Rajendran, Senior Project Manager, Reference Content Production, Elsevier/Academic Press, Radarweg 29, 1043 NX Amsterdam, The Netherlands.

Donald W. Duszynski, PhD
Placitas, NM, United States

R. Scott Seville, PhD
Casper, WY, United States

Jana Kvičerová, DVM PhD
České Budějovice, Czech Republic

Introduction

This book summarizes several important groups of pervasive protist parasites (Apicomplexa: Conoidasida) that infect the most iconic order of mammals, the Carnivora. We intend this work to be a comprehensive, if not *the most* comprehensive, treatise describing the structural and biological knowledge of all known, named, and some unnamed, species within the Coccidia. These parasites are common in carnivores and are now represented by about 201 named and 483 unnamed species that fit taxonomically into 12 genera in 4 families that include Adeleidae Mesnil, 1903 (*Hepatozoon*, 6 named species); Cryptosporidiidae Léger, 1911 (*Cryptosporidium*, 10 named spp.), Eimeriidae Minchin, 1903 (*Caryospora, Eimeria, Isospora*, 47 named spp.), and Sarcocystidae (subfamilies Cystoisosporinae Frenkel et al., 1987) (*Cystoisospora*, 50 named spp.), Sarcocystinae, Poche, 1913 (*Sarcocystis, Frenkelia*, 78 named spp.), and Toxoplasmatinae Biocca, 1957 (*Besnoitia, Hammondia, Neospora, Toxoplasma*, 10 named spp.). An overview of the general biology, taxonomy, life cycles, and relative numbers of species of *Eimeria* and *Cryptosporidium* species from wild mammals was published almost two decades ago (Duszynski and Upton, 2001), and monographic works or books on the coccidia of certain selected vertebrate groups also are available; these include amphibians (Duszynski et al., 2007); bats (Duszynski, 2002); insectivores (Duszynski and Upton, 2000); marmotine squirrels in the Rodentia (Wilber et al., 1998); primates and Scandentia (Duszynski et al., 1999); snakes (Duszynski and Upton, 2010); rabbits (Duszynski and Couch, 2013); turtles (Duszynski and Morrow, 2014); and marsupials (Duszynski, 2016).

The last review of the coccidia of carnivores was by Levine and Ivens (1981), and over the ensuing 37 years our knowledge about the general biology, taxonomy, life cycles, and biodiversity of both these hosts and their apicomplexan parasites has increased dramatically. In particular, advances in survey techniques, access to remote locations and rare species, advances in technology that minimally includes new molecular techniques with quick and inexpensive gene sequencing, and the ready availability of scientific information on the worldwide web have added greatly to the depth of discovery of these fascinating parasite species and their hosts, and the speed at which our knowledge of them has accumulated. We hope this book is a timely and a useful resource for a variety of individuals, including biology teachers, parasitologists, veterinarians, medical practitioners, conservation biologists, zoo and laboratory personnel, college and university professors, and anyone with an interest in carnivores, biodiversity, and global

© 2018 Donald W. Duszynski published by Elsevier Inc. All rights reserved.

medical/veterinary health issues, to name just a few.

The order Carnivora comprises a diverse group of species, which are hosts to a fascinating diversity of apicomplexan parasites (Williams and Thorne, 1996). According to Wozencraft (2005), the order is composed of two major lineages (suborders), Feliformia Kretzoi, 1945, and Caniformia Kretzoi, 1938. Feliformia has 121 extant species consisting of 6 families: Felidae Fischer de Waldheim, 1817 (all cats, 40 species), Viverridae Gray, 1821 (civets, genets, 35 species), Eupleridae Chenu, 1850 (8 species of Madagascar carnivores, e.g., fossa), Nandiniidae Pocock, 1929 (African palm civet, monotypic), Herpestidae Bonaparte, 1845 (mongooses, meerkat, 33 species), and Hyaenidae Gray, 1821 (hyenas, aardwolf, 4 species); the Caniformia lineage is somewhat larger with 165 species identified as 9 family lineages that include the Canidae Fisher, 1817 (dogs, foxes, 35 species), Ursidae Fischer de Waldheim, 1817 (bears, 8 species), Otariidae Gray, 1825 (eared seals, sea lions, 16 species), Odobenidae Allen, 1880 (walrus, monotypic), Phocidae Gray, 1821 (earless seals, 19 species), Mustelidae Fischer, 1817 (badgers, weasels, ferrets, 59 species), Mephitidae Bonaparte, 1845 (skunks, 12 species), Procyonidae Gray, 1825 (raccoons, coatis, 14 species), and the monotypic Ailuridae Gray, 1843 (red panda).

Originally, the coccidia were placed taxonomically into the protozoan phylum Sporozoa Leuckart, 1879, which historically served as a catch-all category for any protist that was not an amoeba, a ciliate, or a flagellate; thus, it contained many organisms that did not have "spores" in their life cycle and many groups, such as the myxo- and microsporidians, which were not closely related to the more traditional sporozoans, such as malaria and intestinal coccidia. Many readers will remember the protozoan class Sporozoa from basic biology courses, some of which—unfortunately—still utilize this category today in introducing the Kingdom Protozoa. As our knowledge increased this name became unsuitable, unwieldy, and in fact did not represent the true evolutionary relationships between the organisms included therein. The phylum Apicomplexa Levine, 1970, was created to provide a descriptive name that was better suited to the organisms contained within it. For historical perspective, it is important to recall that it was not possible to create the name for, and classify organisms within, this phylum until after the advent of the transmission electron microscope (TEM). The widespread use of the TEM for biological specimens, beginning in the 1950s and continuing throughout the 1960s and 1970s, examining the fine structure of "zoites" belonging to many different protists, revealed a suite of common, shared structures (e.g., polar ring, conoid, rhoptries, etc.) at the more pointed end (now termed anterior) of certain life stages; these structures, in whatever combination, were termed the apical complex. When protozoologists sought a more unifying and, hopefully, more phylogenetically relevant term, Dr. Norman D. Levine, from the University of Illinois, came up with "Apicomplexa."

Within the Apicomplexa, the class Conoidasida Levine, 1988 (organisms with all organelles of the apical complex present), has two principal lineages: the gregarines and the coccidia. Within the coccidia, the order Eucoccidiorida Léger and Duboscq, 1910, is characterized by organisms in which **merogony**, **gamogony**, and **sporogony** are sequential life cycle stages, and they are found in both invertebrates and vertebrates (Lee et al., 2000; Perkins et al., 2000). There are two suborders in the Eucoccidia: Adeleorina Léger, 1911, and Eimeriorina Léger, 1911. Species within the Eimeriorina differ in two biologically significant ways from those in the Adeleorina: (1) their macro- and microgametocytes develop independently (i.e., without syzygy); and (2) their microgametocytes typically produce many microgametes versus the small number of microgametes produced by microgametocytes of adeleids (Upton, 2000). As we noted above, coccidians from the Eimeriorina and Adeleorina are commonly found within species of the Carnivora that have been examined for them, and these are the subjects of this book.

Historically, the taxonomy and identification of coccidian parasites was based primarily on studying the morphology of oocysts found in the feces. Morphology of sporulated oocysts is still a useful taxonomic tool, as evidenced by the large number of species descriptions in the literature for *Caryospora*, *Eimeria*, *Isospora*, and *Isospora*-like species from carnivores, and as is reflected in this book. Thus, we have tried to present a robust accounting of all apicomplexan species with species descriptions primarily consisting of oocyst morphology data, which occur naturally in carnivores, and use their gastrointestinal or urinary tracts to discharge these resistant propagules. However, morphology alone is not sufficient to identify many coccidian species, especially those in genera such as *Besnoitia*, *Cryptosporidium*, *Cystoisospora*, *Neospora*, and *Sarcocystis*, which have species with oocysts and sporocysts, respectively, which are very small and have only a limited number of mensural characters. Thus, identifications ideally should be supplemented by multiple data sets with information collected from, but not limited to, location of sporulation (endogenous vs. exogenous), length of time needed for exogenous sporulation at a constant temperature, morphology and timing of some or all of the developmental stages in their endogenous life cycle (e.g., merogony, gamogony), length of prepatent and patent periods, host-specificity as determined via cross-transmission experiments, observations on histological changes, and pathology due to asexual and sexual endogenous development, and others, to clarify and compliment the complex taxonomy of these parasites. In addition, with advances in DNA/RNA technologies, sequence data are increasingly required as a component of contemporary species descriptions, and they are employed to conduct phylogenetic analyses to more robustly assign a parasite to a group, genus, or even species (e.g., see Merino et al., 2008, 2009, 2010). Thus, molecular tools to ensure accurate species identifications are becoming part of one's common taxonomic practice to better understand the host–parasite associations of these species and genera. Molecular data alone, however, are not sufficient for a species description and name, although their use as a critical tool can help sort out complicated and associated taxonomic problems. For example, molecular methods were employed to differentiate between the *Isospora* species that possess sporocysts with, and those without, Stieda bodies (SBs); evidence has accumulated that those with SBs share a phylogenetic origin with the eimeriid coccidia, whereas those without SBs are best placed in the *Cystoisospora* (Carreno and Barta, 1999). Molecular techniques also have helped resurrect some genera (Modrý, 2001) and have allowed proper phylogenetic assignment when data were limited because, perhaps, only endogenous developmental stages were known (Garner et al., 2006). Tenter et al. (2002) proposed that an improved classification system for parasitic protists was both needed and required, and that molecular data must be included to supplement morphological and biological information. Such combined data sets will enable more robust phylogenetic inferences to be made and will result in a more stable taxonomy for the coccidia. Numerous examples in this book affirm we are moving in the right direction.

In reviewing and compiling the vast literature pertaining to the coccidia in carnivores, it has become clear that, as for previous host groups we have studied, the taxonomic state of affairs for carnivores is sometimes confusing because many previous investigators either have not provided adequate descriptions and/or have not adhered to accepted practices for identifying and naming new species (or higher taxa) of coccidia. We hope this book helps to clear some of this confusion and will serve as a useful resource, with both up-to-date and the most complete taxonomic information available.

We also strongly encourage investigators planning to engage in taxonomic research on the coccidia in Carnivora, or any host taxon, that this can be an enriching experience of discovery and learning, but we caution that certain rules should be adhered to. For colleagues who have cause to propose a new species or higher taxon name, we encourage them to evaluate both the formal requirements of the International Rules of Zoological Nomenclature (Ride et al., 1999), and the specific scientific reasons why they believe the description of new taxa (genera, species) are needed. When creating a new genus, the criteria should be established as to how and why this suite of characters differs from already existing genera within the familial lineage, and a formal, detailed definition of the new genus should be presented that convincingly differentiates it from existing, presumably closely related genera. Do the editors of biological research journals really embrace and understand the use of the internationally accepted rules of properly naming new genera and species, or do they even know these rules exist? Unfortunately, the answer seems to end up on the negative side of that fulcrum. We should remember that taxonomy and nomenclature are instruments to prevent confusion, not to produce confusion, and the complete scientific name acts as the anchor for that species being described, whether parasite or host. Of course, we need to expect that the application of new technologies/methods/tools will lead to new results, and more knowledge, possibly demonstrating so far unknown differences in organisms, which were thought to be well-known (e.g., sporocysts with SBs vs. those without). The question is which differences are essential or useful for strain, species, genus, or family discrimination? It is nonsense to discriminate species or genera and give them new names before they are investigated and compared with already existing ones.

Members within the Carnivora, as a host group, are important in many contexts due to the deep emotional and high economic status they share as both wild (iconic carnivores such as polar bears, cute ones such as sea otters) and domesticated (pet and laboratory dogs and cats) animals, which engage humans in so many different ways. Both domesticated and increasingly nondomesticated carnivore species are kept in captivity for educational and recreational purposes such as pets, fur production, scientific research (food additives, chemotherapeutics), and as research models in captive breeding programs for endangered species recovery programs. Additionally, many injured wild and domestic carnivores undergo rehabilitation in wildlife centers and/or veterinary clinics worldwide. The infectious disease burdens carried by captive carnivores are influenced by a myriad of factors, including, but not limited to, length of time since the animal was removed from the wild, degree of adjustment to captivity, the quality and dedication of husbandry management techniques and caregivers involved, specific species needs that may be known (or not), and their proximity to other species with which they may exchange parasitic pathogens (Williams and Thorne, 1996). The sources of various infectious agents for captive carnivores can be highly varied, including the kind and quality of their food and water, utensils and bowls used in feeding, contaminated clothing of handlers, the handlers themselves, contact with individuals of the same, related, or distant species, access to invertebrates that might act as mechanical carriers of transmission stages, and many others.

Wild carnivore species and populations are experiencing serious impacts from increasing contact with human populations and with those of their domestic pets, some of which have increased the opportunity for contact with potentially pathogenic coccidian species that will become serious veterinary issues for wild Carnivora species (see Chapter 14).

Habitat disturbance and loss result in reduced numbers of endemic carnivores, loss of home range, and increased population densities. This has two important consequences. First, reduced populations suffer from reduced genetic diversity (population bottleneck), which can result in increased susceptibility to infectious and parasitic diseases. Second, when animals are forced into smaller suitable habitat space, it increases their population density, which enhances disease transmission. Wild carnivores also compete directly with humans, and/or other species introduced by humans (e.g., domestic cats, dogs) for food, which further stresses wild animals resulting in increased susceptibility to disease. Climate change is an additive impact to habitat and can cause animals to move to new areas where they may overlap with species that can expose them to novel infectious agents. Environmental pollution and contamination also are hazards to wild carnivores, as keystone predators, because toxic industrial chemicals, and biological waste from domestic and captive animals as sources of novel or infectious agents, can accumulate along the food chain in the bodies of the prey consumed by carnivores. Regardless of whether they are wild, captive, or domestic, all carnivores display a wide spectrum of disease susceptibility, and our understanding of these disease agents, how to identify them, what their life histories are, and how to treat them once carnivores become infected with them, is appallingly incomplete at present. This seems especially true for parasitic protists that infect carnivores, especially members of the Apicomplexa, most of which have direct hand-to-mouth life cycles and highly resistant infection propagules they discharge into the environment, both of which facilitate the ease of transmission and infection.

Only Levine and Ivens (1981) attempted to catalog the apicomplexan parasites of carnivores known to that time, and they provided a brief, relatively superficial, series of known species descriptions, and line drawings of sporulated oocysts. In their (1981) monograph, they found coccidia in about 50 carnivore species in 28 genera, and they (1981) included 102 named coccidian species in 5 genera. They pointed out,

however, that their named species included "quite a number of dubious species of parasites." At the time of their work, only the domestic dog and cat had been well studied at all, and parasitologists were just beginning to understand the life cycle complexities of some of these apicomplexans. For example, although the genera had been named, the phylogenetic arrangement of the sarcocystid coccidians (*Besnoitia*, *Sarcocystis*, *Hammondia*, *Toxoplasma*, etc.) was unknown; *Neospora* from dogs, the cause of limb paralysis and abortion in cattle was neither known nor was the fact that sporocysts of *S. neurona* from opossums and cats could cause fatal myeloencephalitis in horses; and the name *Cystoisospora* had not yet been widely accepted nor was it completely understood that coccidian species with *Isospora*-like oocysts that lacked SBs could infect multiple hosts with tissue stages that later could be infective to carnivores that consumed them. We document apicomplexans in 13 families, in 70 genera, and in 134 carnivore species. The number of coccidians in carnivores is also greatly increased and, as reported herein, more than doubles the numbers reported by Levine and Ivens (1981) (206 apicomplexan species in 11 parasite genera). Additionally, we also know, and are able to discuss, a great deal more about the biology and interrelationships of both these parasites and their hosts.

Since Levine and Ivens (1981), it was generally accepted that very few bacterial and parasitic pathogens were significant in captive populations of carnivores, and that if good husbandry, therapy, vaccines, and quarantine protocols were in place it would minimize the risk of disease in them (Williams and Thorne, 1996). Even though this dogma proved to be short-sighted and felonious, following Levine and Ivens (1981) there seemed to be no attempt to look further at this subject; thus, we have attempted to address that void in this treatise.

As a quick overview of the contents of this book, Chapter 2 presents a short account of the evolution of the order Carnivora. Beginning in

Chapter 3 we systematically present species descriptions and details of all published information for all known coccidia in the Eimeriidae (*Caryospora*, *Eimeria*, and *Isospora*) from all carnivore families. Thus, Chapter 3 covers these parasites in the family Ailuridae; Chapter 4 in the Canidae; Chapter 5 in Mephitidae; Chapter 6 in Mustelidae; Chapter 7 in Odobenidae, Otariidae, and Phocidae; Chapter 8 in Procyonidae; Chapter 9 in Ursidae; Chapter 10 in Felidae; Chapter 11 in Herpestidae; and Chapter 12 in the Eupleridae, Hyaenidae, Nandiniidae, and Viverridae. Then our focus on organization changes a little in Chapter 13, which presents basic taxonomic and biological information on the six *Hepatozoon* (Adeleorina) species reported to infect six different carnivore families. Chapter 14 provides a review of published information on the coccidian parasites of carnivores in the family Sarcocystidae, subfamily Cystoisosporinae (*Cystoisospora* species). Chapters 15 and 16 provide similar reviews for the Sarcocystid subfamilies Sarcocystinae (*Sarcocystis*, *Frenkelia* species), and Toxoplasmatinae (*Besnoitia*, *Hammondia*, *Neospora*, *Toxoplasma* species), respectively. Chapter 17 covers the *Cryptosporidium* species now known to infect carnivores and is the last of our descriptive chapters. Chapter 18 is presented to give a current overview of known treatments and drug therapy for various coccidiosis in carnivores, from a veterinary perspective. Chapter 19 summarizes the nearly 500 notations by investigators, who have surveyed carnivores mostly for intestinal/fecal stages of coccidians, but never attempted identification beyond genus names, and sometimes not even beyond very generalized descriptive terms (e.g., coccidian); also in Chapter 19, we provide the rationale for assigning some of the "named" species reported in the literature to *species inquirendae*, *nomen nudum*, or *nomen nuda* because their descriptions are insufficient, or they may be parasites of canid prey, not the predator. Chapter 20 is a brief overview or our summary and conclusions.

In the chapters of this book, we use the standardized abbreviations of Wilber et al. (1998) to describe various oocyst structures: length (L), width (W), and their ratio (L/W), micropyle (M), oocyst residuum (OR), polar granule (PG), sporocyst (SP) L and W and their L/W ratio, Stieda body (SB), substieda body (SSB), parastieda body (PSB), sporocyst residuum (SR), sporozoite (SZ), refractile body (RB), and nucleus (N). Other abbreviations used, as well as some terms that may be unfamiliar, are **bolded** in the text and definitions are found in the Glossary and Abbreviation section. All measurements given in the chapters are in micrometers (μm) unless otherwise indicated (sometimes using mm) for larger structures such as muscle sarcocysts in tissue.

Review of Carnivore Evolution

REVIEW OF CARNIVORE EVOLUTION

To provide context to the following chapters detailing the biology and biodiversity of the coccidia in the mammalian order Carnivora, this chapter provides a brief outline of the evolution of carnivores, including a timeline of major events up to the present-day global extinction crisis. In addition to providing the evolutionary context for the host taxon, host evolution is important in understanding the major forces that drive parasite and coccidian evolution and generate biodiversity, primarily parasite–host coevolution and parasite–host switching. In the former case, new parasite species arise via tracking of host species. As the host diverges and undergoes speciation over evolutionary time, the parasite species likewise diverges and speciates. Thus, the host and parasite phylogenies are in near alignment when layered over one another. Host switching occurs when a parasite species colonizes a new host (usually closely related), when ranges of the hosts overlap, providing opportunity for a parasite to colonize a novel host in space and time (Brooks and Hoberg, 2007; Poulin, 2007). At present, our understanding of the evolutionary forces driving coccidian diversity in mammals, and carnivores specifically, is limited. Ideally, future studies on carnivores and their coccidia should yield more

details regarding forces driving the diversity of coccidia in carnivores, much like the work of Kvičerová and Hypša (2013), who studied host specificity, phylogenetic conservativeness, and species origin of *Eimeria* spp. in rodents. They found that the distribution of eimerian species from different hosts indicates that the clustering of species is influenced by their host specificity but does not arise from parasite–host cospeciation. Rather, while some clusters are specific to a particular host group, relationships within these clusters do not reflect host phylogeny but indicate host specificity of *Eimeria* in rodents is due to adaptive and not cophylogenetic processes.

WHAT ARE THE CARNIVORES?

For the purpose of this book, carnivores are members of the mammalian order Carnivora, which includes common wild species such as lions, tigers, bears, wolves, and raccoons and a variety of important domestic species including dogs and cats. With 15 families, 10 subfamilies, 126 genera, and approximately 286 species, the Carnivora represents a medium-sized order within the taxonomic class Mammalia. The carnivores are notable for the charismatic appeal of many of their species, which is reflected in carnivore characterizations in the popular media,

© 2018 Donald W. Duszynski published by Elsevier Inc. All rights reserved.

their large representation in zoological park exhibits, and the large diversity of species and life histories found within the order. Carnivores include many of the world's key predators (cheetah, leopard, lion, tiger, hyena, bear, sea lion, seal, and wolf), many of which are of conservation concern, and a number of pet species (dog, cat, ferret). Including tropical, temperate, arctic, terrestrial, and aquatic species, the Carnivora is one of only a few mammalian orders that occur naturally in the Old and New Worlds and on all continents. The Carnivora also has among its species one of the largest size and weight spans of any mammalian order ranging from the polar bear (*Ursus maritimus*), with adult males weighing from 400–600 or even up to 1000 kg, and having a nose-to-tail length of 2.4–2.6 m, to the least weasel (*Mustela nivalis*) weighing as little as 25 g and no longer than 26 cm long. (Wund and Myers, 2005; Vaughn et al., 2011; Wilson and Reeder, 2017).

Carnivora means "meat eater" and most members of this order are predators and/or scavengers. However, some species including raccoons, civets, jackals, badgers, bears, and others supplement their diet with honey, roots, seeds, and/or other plant parts and products. In addition, some species do not eat meat at all, including tropical fruit-eating coatis and kinkajous and the bamboo-eating pandas. As primarily flesh-eaters, carnivore species are distinguished by characteristics reflecting adaptation to a predatory, meat-eating life history, and the defining characteristics of the group includes enlarged canine teeth, the presence of three pairs of incisors in each jaw (with rare exceptions), and the shape and/or absence of some molar teeth. Except in bears and pinnipeds, the last premolar of the upper jaw and the first molar of the lower jaw, called carnassial teeth, are sharp and articulate when the animal chews, like the blades of a scissor, to cut food into smaller pieces. Molars farther back in the jaw are usually either missing or highly reduced. In addition, unlike other mammals, carnivores cannot move

their jaws from side-to-side (Wund and Myers, 2005; Vaughn et al., 2011).

CARNIVORE EVOLUTION

There is an extensive body of literature focused on the evolution of mammals and individual mammalian orders, including the Carnivora. Nonetheless there is debate regarding details of some relationships among different taxa and the divergence times for a number of mammal groups. Central to the resolution of remaining issues is the increasing use and accuracy of estimating relationships and divergence times using molecular data and differences in carefully-selected DNA/RNA sequences. Here we present a general account of mammal and carnivore evolutions and note the unresolved relationships and dates for important events. Much of the outline of mammal and carnivore evolutions, and their confidence intervals (CIs) for specific events presented below, was acquired using the TimeTree.org web resource (http://timetree.org/) (Hedges et al., 2006; Kumar et al., 2017). TimeTree is a web-based public knowledge-base for information on the tree-of-life and its evolutionary timescale that provides phylogenies and molecular time estimates based on extensive surveys and syntheses of published scientific research papers (for a detailed description of the methodology, see Hedges et al., 2015). In our discussion that follows, estimates for events and time CIs were calculated by TimeTree using ≥5 molecular time estimates from the scientific literature to calculate an average time estimate and a t-distribution that is used to calculate a CI for the time estimate.

The earliest mammals are thought to have evolved from **synapsid reptiles**, and mammal-like synapsids appeared in the fossil record during the mid-Triassic with the lineage leading to mammals appearing in the Lower Jurassic, 177 million years ago (MYA) (CI = 163–191 MYA). They were warm-blooded, egg-laying species much like contemporary monotremes (subclass

Prototheria; order Monotremata) (platypus and echidna). Sometime during the Upper Jurassic, 159 (150–167) MYA, ancestral mammals split into the lineages that gave rise to the metatherian (marsupial) and eutherian (placental) mammals. The Carnivora is classified in the mammalian infraclass Eutheria that comprises all placental mammals. Although species ancestral to both the Eutheria and Metatheria were present during the Jurassic, it is not completely resolved whether true placental mammals evolved before or after the Cretaceous–Paleogene extinction event (KPg) 65–66 MYA (Kemp, 2005; Vaughn et al., 2011). O'Leary et al. (2013) used phenomic characters from fossil and living species, and molecular sequence data, to generate a phylogenetic tree that, when calibrated with fossils, shows that placental orders originated after the KPg boundary. The only stem lineage to placental mammals that crossed the KPg boundary, and then speciated in the early Paleocene, is slightly younger than the KPg boundary, ~36 million years younger than molecular clock-based mean estimates reported in earlier studies. Meredith et al. (2011) reported an analysis of relations, divergence times, and diversification patterns among 97%–99% of mammalian families generating a molecular supermatrix that included 164 mammals, 5 outgroups, and 26 gene fragments. They proposed that both the Cretaceous Terrestrial Revolution (i.e., the intense diversification of angiosperms, insects, reptiles, birds, and mammals) during the mid- to late-Cretaceous (80–125 MYA) and the KPg mass extinction (65–66 MYA) were keys to the early diversification and radiation of mammals. The former increased ecospace diversity, and the mass extinction made more ecospace available for mammals. TimeTree.org, based on the synthesis of a number of different published studies, places the origins of most mammalian orders within the CI of the KPg mass extinction at 65 MYA.

Approximately 105 (100–111) MYA, during the Lower Cretaceous, the Eutheria diverged into the clade Boreoeutheria and a second group that further diversified into a collection of mammalian orders including the Cingulata (armadillos), Hyracoidea (hyraxes), Macroscelidea (elephant-, jumping-shrews), Pilosa (anteaters, sloths), Proboscidea (elephants), Sirenia (sea cows, manatees, dugongs), and Tubulidentata (aardvarks) (Fig. 2.1). During the Upper Cretaceous, 96 (91–102) MYA, the Boreoeutheria diverged into the superorders Laurasiatheria and Euarchontoglires, with the latter diversifying into the orders Dermoptera (colugos), Lagomorpha (rabbits, hares), Primates (monkeys, gorillas), Rodentia (rodents), and Scandentia (tree shrews). The Luarasiatheria then diverged during the Upper Cretaceous, 89 (83–96) MYA, into the insectivores and the taxon that radiated ~79 (73–84) MYA into lineages that gave rise to the orders Carnivora, Cetacea (whales), Chiroptera (bats), Pholidota (pangolins), and Perissodactyla (horses). Springer et al. (2011) noted the first fossil occurrences of the Laurasiatheria were exclusively found in regions associated with the supercontinent Laurasia, the northern of the two continents (the other being Gondwana) that were part of the Pangea supercontinent, 175–335 MYA. Laurasia split from Gondwana, 175–215 MYA. Their reconstructions provided support for Eurasia, but not North America, as the ancestral area for these clades, including the Carnivora. Current thinking regarding carnivore relationships to other extant mammalian orders is that they are most closely related to the Pholidota (family Manidae, the pangolins) and more distantly related to either the Chiroptera (bats) (Meredith et al., 2011) or the Perrisodactyla (horses, tapirs, and rhinos) (Gatesy et al., 2016). TimeTree estimates the Carnivora species diverged from their closest relatives (pangolins) ~75 (70–79) MYA.

From fossil evidence, early Paleogene mammals were small-sized (?) insectivores and omnivores, but there were several new groups with medium-sized (5–40 kg) and large (>40 kg) members. The most abundant Paleogene mammals

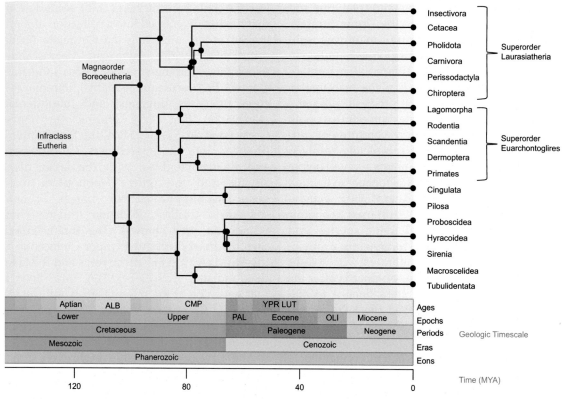

FIGURE 2.1   Hypothesized phylogeny for evolution of extant mammalian orders. *Modified from TimeTree.org with permission.* *ALB*, Albian; *CMP*, Campanian; *LUT*, Lutetian; *OLI*, Oligocene; *PAL*, Paleocene; *YPR*, Ypresian.

were the "condylarths" that included the first ecologically carnivorous, placental mammals in the form of actocyonids and mesonychids. Other new placental orders were the specialized herbivorous taeniodonts, tillodonts, and pantodonts, all of which were possibly derived from Cretaceous palaeoryctidans. The arboreal plesiadapiforms, possibly the stem primates, and the earliest Carnivora were mainly small but included some cat-sized animals. During the Paleocene, two carnivorous orders appeared in the fossil record, the Creodonta is now considered archaic because it did not survive beyond the Miocene and the Carnivora, which eventually radiated to become the dominant terrestrial carnivores of today (Fig. 2.2). The possibility of a sister group relationship between Carnivora and Creodonta is not likely. Both creodonts and

carnivores possess the specialized, shearing carnassial teeth located in the postcanine dentition, although the actual teeth involved differ from group to group. In the Carnivora the major carnassials are the upper fourth premolar and lower first molar (M1). In Creodonta, the tendency was for some shearing along the entire molar row but most apparent on either the upper M1 and lower second molar (M2) or the upper M2 and lower third molar. Rather than being due to shared ancestry, it is believed that the differences provide evidence of convergent evolution of specialized carnassial teeth (Kemp, 2005).

Following the KPg and throughout the Cenozoic, mammals including different carnivore lineages underwent extensive radiation. The extinction of dinosaurs eliminated many

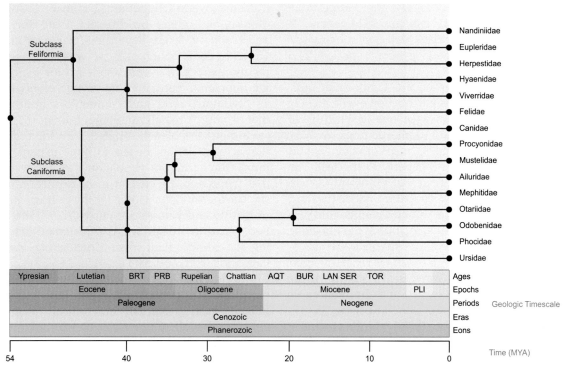

FIGURE 2.2 Hypothesized phylogeny for extant carnivore families. *Modified from TimeTree.org with permission.* AQT, Aquitanian; *BRT*, Bartonian; *BUR*, Burdigalian; *LAN*, Langhian; *PRB*, Priabonian; *SER*, Serravallian; *TOR*, Tortonian.

impediments to mammalian diversification, and mammals could diversify to fill empty herbivore and carnivore niches and nocturnal mammals could become active diurnally. Beginning in the Mesozoic, the breakup of the supercontinent Pangea, and the drifting of continents, created new continents with new and varying connections and separations resulting in dispersal, altered climatic conditions, increased landscape diversity, and geographic isolation of populations leading to conditions ideal for allopatric speciation. In addition, geologic processes driving continental mountain building (Andes, Himalayas, Sierras, Rocky Mountains) with the above processes created greater landscape and climatic diversity including expanded grassland and savanna ecosystems (Strickberger, 1996). Combined with the availability of ecological

niches previously occupied by the nonavian Dinosauria, conditions were created that, by the mid-Miocene, ~20 MYA, with the splitting of the lineage leading to the Otariidae (eared seals) and Odobenidae (walruses), all 15 extant carnivore families were present.

At the start of the Paleogene, 54 (52–57) MYA, the ancestral carnivore lineage split into two groups, one of which gave rise to the suborder Feliformia and the second the Caniformia (Fig. 2.2). Approximately 47 (41–53) MYA, the Feliformia split into two lineages, one of which diverged into the monotypic family Nandiniidae (African palm civet) and the second into the Felidae (cats; 2 subfamilies, 14 genera, 40 species) and Viverridae (civets, genets; 4 subfamilies, 15 genera, 35 species), 40 (33–46) MYA; the Hyaenidae (hyenas; 3 genera,

4 species), 33 (28–39) MYA; the Herpestidae (mongoose, meerkat, kusimanses; 14 genera, 33 species); and Eupleridae (Malagasy mongoose/euplerid; 2 subfamilies, 7 genera, 8 species), 24.6 (19.7–29.4) MYA.

The second suborder, the Caniformia, radiated following the KPg extinction event, 46 (42–49) MYA, into two lineages, one of which gave rise to modern canids (domestic dogs, wolves, foxes, jackals, dingoes, many extinct/extant dog-like carnivores; 13 genera, 35 species). The second lineage diverged ~40 (37–43) MYA into three clades. The first led to the Ursidae (bears; 5 genera, 8 species). The second diverged into pinnipeds (seal-like canids) including the Phocidae (true seals; 13 genera, 19 species) ~26 (23.1–28.9) MYA; and 19.5 (16.8–22.1) MYA, it diverged into the Otariidae (eared seals, sea lions, fur seals; 7 genera, 16 species) and the monotypic Odobenidae (walruses). The third clade, 35 (33–37) MYA, diverged into the Mephitidae (skunks; 4 genera, 12 species); 34 (31–37) MYA, it diverged into the monotypic Ailuridae (red panda); and 29.3 (27.5–31.1) MYA, it diverged into the Mustelidae (badger, ferret, marten, mink, otter, stout, weasel, wolverine; 22 genera, 59 species) and the Procyonidae (coatis, raccoons, kinkajous, olingos, olinguitos, ringtails, cacomisties; 6 genera, 14 species).

By the beginning of the Pleistocene, approximately 2 MYA, many mammals and carnivores were present in their current forms. During the Pleistocene, at least seven different glaciations or "Ice Ages" at different times covered up to one-third of the Earth's surface. These major climatic events drove the evolution of a number of mammals toward large size, including woolly mammoths and rhinoceroses, giant deer and cattle, and a number of carnivores including large cave bears and saber-toothed tigers.

During the late Pleistocene, ~11,000 YA, many large species including carnivores went extinct in North American and other continents. A number of hypotheses have been proposed to explain these extinctions including predation by humans (overkill hypothesis), climate change, disease, and others (Strickberger, 1996; Burney and Flannery, 2005). Regardless of which individual or combination of forces was responsible for the extinction events, evidence for increasing interaction between humans and carnivores as predators, prey, and competitors indicates that at approximately this time, human dispersal around the planet, coupled with increasing human population, began to have a negative impact on carnivore populations and diversity that persists in the current mass extinction crisis. The International Union for the Conservation of Nature and Natural Resources (2017) identified 84 carnivore species as threatened including six extinct (giant fossa, *Cryptoprocta spelea*; Falklands wolf, *Dusicyon australis*; *Dusicyon avis*; Caribbean monk seal, *Neomonachus tropicalis*; sea mink, *Neovison macrodon*; and Japanese sea lion, *Zalophus japonicus*), four critically endangered (red wolf, *Canis rufus*; European mink, *Mustela lutreola*; pygmy raccoon, *Procyon pygmaeus*; and Malabar civet, *Viverra civettina*), 32 endangered, and 42 vulnerable species (http://www.iucnredlist.org/). The fact that many carnivores are at risk has direct implications for our knowledge of the biodiversity of carnivore coccidian parasites. Several authors have noted that the impacts of climate change and the global extinction crisis extend beyond the charismatic megafauna, including many iconic carnivores, and they include the parasite species dependent on specific host species that will decline and become extinct along with their hosts (Brooks and Hoberg, 2007; Carlson et al., 2017). Although the focus thus far has been primarily on metazoan parasites including ticks and helminths, the same concepts apply to host-specific protozoan parasites including the coccidia. Thus, the comprehensive taxonomic survey presented in this book serves as a baseline for the future study of coccidian biodiversity in a race against the loss of host species that will diminish the opportunity to build a comprehensive knowledge base for carnivore coccidia.

Eimeriidae in the Caniformia Family Ailuridae

EIMERIIDAE IN THE AILURIDAE GRAY, 1843

INTRODUCTION

Ailuridae Gray, 1843, is a **monotypic** family consisting of a single genus with one species, the red (or lesser) panda, *Ailurus fulgens* F.G. Cuvier, 1825, and its fossil relatives. According to Wilson and Reeder (http://vertebrates.si.edu/msw/mswCFApp/msw/index.cfm), this extant species has two subspecies, *A. f. fulgens* and *A. f. refulgens*, in the Himalayas and south-central and western China, respectively.

Red pandas are found only in high (2,200–4,800 m), isolated temperate forests of the Himalayan mountain chain of Nepal, India, Bhutan, and Burma and isolated mountain ranges in Sichuan, Yunnan (south-central), and Tibet (western) provinces of China (Yang and Wang, 2000; Lan et al., 2012). These are subalpine, broad-leaf deciduous habitats where climatic zones provide moist, well-drained soil suitable for bamboo growth, the main dietary staple of this panda (Roberts and Gittleman, 1984). Seasonal fruits, berries, mushrooms, other leafy vegetation, and opportunistic animal protein complete

the panda's diet (Reid et al., 1991; Eriksson et al., 2010). Red pandas are active in the wild both day and night, primarily during **crepuscular** hours, and they are active one-third to one-half of their diurnal time (Yonzon and Hunter, 1991).

Cuvier (1825) first described *Ailurus* to be a member of the raccoon family (Procyonidae Gray, 1825) because of its unique facial markings and colored ringed tail, and it also has been assigned to the bear family (Ursidae Fischer de Waldheim, 1817) (Mayr, 1986). Today, molecular studies place the red panda into its own family more closely related to the raccoons (*Procyon lotor* [L., 1758]) and skunks (Mephitidae Bonaparte, 1845) but not to bears (Zhang and Ryder, 1993; Slattery and O'Brien, 1995; Su et al., 2001). The fossil record, however, indicates that the red panda diverged from its common ancestor with bears about 40 million years ago (Mayr, 1986). This species has no close living relatives as far as mammalogists are able to determine (Roberts and Gittleman, 1984).

This endangered species is listed both on the International Union for the Conservation of Nature and Natural Resources Red List and the Convention on International Traffic in Endangered Species, with Class 2 protections

© 2018 Donald W. Duszynski published by Elsevier Inc. All rights reserved.

in China, where it is endemic and where populations continue to decline due to habitat loss, habitat fragmentation, and poaching for the fur trade (Qin Qin et al., 2007), and the ever increasing populations of domesticated carnivores such as dogs and cats (see Discussion section).

SPECIES DESCRIPTIONS

GENUS *AILURUS* F.G. CUVIER, 1825 (MONOTYPIC)

EIMERIA AILURI AGRAWAL, AHLUWALIA, BHATIA, AND CHAUHAN, 1981

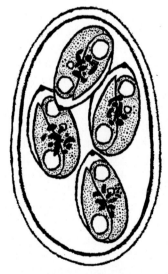

FIGURE 3.1 Original line drawing of the sporulated oocyst of *Eimeria ailuri*. *Modified from Figure 5, Agrawal et al. (1981), Indian Journal of Animal Science 51 (1–6), 125–128.*

Type host: *Ailurus fulgens* F.G. Cuvier, 1825, Red Panda.

Type locality: Asia: India, Uttar Pradesh, Lucknow, Lucknow Zoo (Prince of Wales Zoological Gardens).

Other hosts: None to date.

Geographic distribution: Asia: India.

Description of sporulated oocyst: Oocyst shape: ellipsoidal to slightly elongate-ovoidal; number of walls, 2; wall characteristics: outer is light greenish, whereas the inner is dark brown, total thickness ~1.5; L×W: 23.8×13.3 (22–27×12–16); L/W ratio: 1.8 (1.7–1.9); M, OR, PG: all absent. Distinctive features of oocyst: smooth, transparent outer wall with a thinner, dark inner wall and lack of M, OR, and PG.

Description of sporocyst and sporozoites: Sporocyst shape: ovoidal; L×W: 7.9×5.1 (7–10×4–6); L/W ratio: 1.5; SB: inconspicuous at pointed end of sporocyst; SSB, PSB: both absent; SR: present; SR characteristics: "an aggregation of dark granules in the center;" SZ: sausage-shaped, 7.6×2.9 (6.5–9×2–4), with one end broader and the other end pointed; RB: 1, present at broader end. Distinctive features of sporocyst: very small size containing SZ that is exactly the same length as sporocyst (line drawing).

Prevalence: Unknown; no mention was made as to how many type hosts were examined or infected.

Sporulation: Exogenous. Oocysts were sporulated at "room temperature" in Petri dishes, in 2.5% aqueous potassium dichromate ($K_2Cr_2O_7$) solution, but the time was not given.

Prepatent and patent periods: Unknown, oocysts were collected from the feces.

Site of infection: Unknown.

Endogenous stages: Unknown.

Cross-transmission: None to date.

Pathology: Unknown.

Materials deposited: None.

Remarks: Agrawal et al. (1981) provided the first and only description of a coccidian oocyst from the red panda. The only other mention of this eimerian was by Chaudhuri and Das (1992) when they used *E. ailuri* as an example of a host-specific coccidian, but with no evidence of any kind to support their statement. To our knowledge, there are no other intestinal coccidia described from the red panda.

DISCUSSION AND SUMMARY

The future of the red panda depends, in part, on the development and enforcement of successful husbandry practices, successful captive breeding and health programs, and on the implementation of protective measures against infectious diseases. At the end of 2008, there were 762 documented red pandas living in 252 zoos worldwide, in countries where records are available. Of these, 230 pandas lived in 98 zoos in Europe, 167 in 70 zoos in North America, and 43 in 12 zoos in Australia/New Zealand (Eriksson et al., 2010). Unfortunately, captive breeding success in zoos has been relatively poor with low reproductive success and high infant mortality. To compound their plight, captive animals face numerous stressors such as adverse sounds, restricted movement, forced proximity to humans and other species, unnatural diet and/or reduced foraging opportunities, compromised expression of their natural behaviors, and increased exposure to disease agents that are not present in their natural habitats (Eriksson et al., 2010).

The rapid rise in populations of domestic carnivores, especially dogs and cats, increases the potential for exposure of captive and free-ranging pandas to cat and dog diseases and enhances conditions for the emergence of new pathogens (Qin Qin et al., 2007). Red pandas are known to be highly susceptible to canine distemper virus (Montali et al., 1983; Qin Qin et al., 2007) and to a number of protist and helminth disease-causing organisms from domesticated companion animals. These include *Toxoplasma gondii* (cats), *Neospora caninum* (dogs), and heartworm infections with *Dirofilaria immitis* (dogs), to name a few (Lan et al., 2012). In addition, ascarid nematodes such as *Baylisascaris ailuri* (Yang and Wang, 2000; Xie et al., 2011) and several genera of metastrongylid nematodes such as *Angiostrongylus vasorum* (Patterson-Kane et al., 2009; Bertelsen et al., 2010) have been strongly implicated in inducing pneumonia and visceral, ocular, and neural larval migrans in these pandas. All have been documented to cause other pathological conditions and death in pandas and offer the potential for significant degradation of red panda populations.

Finally, limited habitats, whether natural or human made, can dramatically increase the concentration and transmission of direct life cycle parasites such as the coccidia, but as we have seen above, we know virtually nothing about their occurrence, biology, and diversity in red pandas. The only coccidian species described to date, *E. ailuri*, is from a red panda in a zoo in India. There are no survey studies for coccidia, to our knowledge, from red pandas in any of their natural habitats, which is truly a shame because noninvasive collections of feces are so easy and cost-effective to do. Clearly, there is still a lot of work to do and a lot of knowledge to be learned.

Eimeriidae in the Caniformia Family Canidae

EIMERIIDAE IN THE CANIDAE FISCHER, 1817

INTRODUCTION

The Canidae is one of the most specialized carnivore groups and includes dogs, wolves, coyotes, jackals, and foxes, comprising 13 genera (9 are monotypic) with 35 species (Wilson and Reeder, 2005). They have relatively long legs adapted for running, especially their foot segment that allows them to stand on the bottom of their toes in what is called a digitigrade posture (Findley, 1987). Other distinguishing features include a relatively long, bushy tail, an elongate muzzle, large pointed (erect) ears, and lithe, muscular, deep-chested bodies. Living canid groups were once divided, mainly on their dentition, into three subgroups (Caninae, Simocyoninae, and Otocyoninae), but, as molecular and other data became more readily available, these artificial divisions were not warranted.

The Eimeriidae coccidia described from Canidae present us with three conundrums. First, there is a genus of eimeriid coccidia, *Caryospora* that is composed of 83 named species, with the majority from snakes (55) and birds of prey (23) and the remainder from lizards (3), a turtle (1), and a rodent (1) *as their definitive hosts* (unpublished personal data). Since 1982 there has accumulated a small, but growing body of evidence that at least one snake *Caryospora* species is capable of infecting mammals, including and especially canids, and completing its life cycle in nonintestinal locations; and it can be debilitating and sometimes fatal.

Second, although there are eight *Eimeria* species described from eight canid species, our view, and the view of most of our colleagues, is that none of these are valid species but are instead unsporulated oocysts of prey species just passing through the canid's gut after ingesting that prey. Our reasons for doubting these species are that there are no life cycles, good cross-transmission studies, or any detailed studies on endogenous developmental stages from any canid *Eimeria* species. Thus, the *Eimeria* species currently described from all Canidae are likely spurious parasites.

Finally, Carreno et al. (1998) and Franzen et al. (2000) used analysis of the 18S rRNA gene to show that some *Cystoisospora* (formerly *Isospora*) species were more closely related to *Neospora*, *Sarcocystis*, and *Toxoplasma* species and belonged

17

© 2018 Donald W. Duszynski published by Elsevier Inc. All rights reserved.

in the Sarcocystidae rather than the Eimeriidae, an idea initially proposed by Frenkel (1977), who erected the genus *Cystoisospora* to include those mammalian *Isospora* species with no Stieda body complex in their sporocysts. Barta et al. (2005) examined the morphology of the sporocysts along with the available molecular data and assigned all *Isospora*-like species that sporulated outside their host and produced sporocysts without Stieda bodies (from mammals) to the *Cystoisospora*, and assigned all such oocysts from birds, which had Stieda (and often substieda) bodies on their sporocysts, to the genus *Isospora* (see Chapter 14 for more information). Accordingly, we have reviewed the literature on *Isospora* species that do not have a Stieda body on their sporocysts, reported from the Canidae (this chapter) and other carnivores (Chapters 5–12), and we have reassigned them to the genus *Cystoisospora*, if this had already not been done by others.

Thus, the third part of our conundrum is that all *Isospora* species known from canids that have been studied in detail have certain unique traits that distinguish them. First, they lack a SB complex; second, they have a heteroxenous life cycle with secondary hosts that harbor certain asexual, monozoic tissue cyst stages (Dubey and Frenkel, 1972b) typically found in mesenteric lymph nodes of intermediate/paratenic hosts (e.g., rodents); and third, some are now known to have extraintestinal stages (Dubey, 1975b, 1978a,b; Rommel and Zielasko, 1981) that can occur in the tissues (mesenteric lymph nodes, liver, spleen, lungs, brain, musculature) of cats and dogs (definitive hosts) when they are fed sporulated oocysts. To reiterate, these *Cystoisospora* species oocysts are identical to those of *Isospora* except for their ability to infect additional host species (Fayer and Dubey, 1987), and they all have sporocysts that lack any remnant of a Stieda body complex. As molecular sequencing evidence has accumulated, we see that Frenkel (1977) was correct in separating heteroxenous isosporans into *Cystoisospora* species,

and Frenkel et al. (1987) later provided us with an important conceptual basis for thinking about all these "isosporans" by pointing out, "How we classify the heretofore unthought of cycles and stages is a scientific problem of taxonomy rather than of nomenclature." Thus, there are 14 *Isospora* species described from nine canid species, and all except one (*I. fennechi*) have oocysts that do not have a SB complex; these all have been assigned to the *Cystoisospora* (see Chapter 14). We also think that *I. fennechi* is a spurious finding of oocysts from a prey item of the fennec fox.

SPECIES DESCRIPTIONS

GENUS CANIS L., 1758 (6 SPECIES)

CARYOSPORA BIGENETICA WACHA AND CHRISTIANSEN, 1982

Type host: *Crotalus horridus* L., 1758, Timber or Cane-brake Rattlesnake.

Type locality: North America: USA: Iowa, Madison County.

Other Viperidae hosts: See Duszynski and Upton (2010).

Secondary hosts: *Canis lupus familiaris* (syn. *C. familiaris*), Domestic Dog (experimental and natural); *Capra hircus* L., 1758, Domestic Goat; *Mus musculus* L., 1766, House Mouse (experimental); *Microtus arvalis* (Pallas, 1778), Common Vole; *Meriones unguiculatus* (Milne-Edwards, 1867), Gerbil; *Sigmodon hispidus* Say and Ord, 1825, Hispid Cotton Rat; *Sus scrofa* L., 1758, Domestic Pig.

Geographic distribution: North America: USA: Alabama, Arkansas, Georgia, Iowa, Missouri, New Jersey, Texas; Eastern Europe: Czech Republic (zoo animal).

Description of sporulated oocyst: Oocyst shape: spheroidal; number of walls, 2; wall characteristics: ~1 thick, outer wall is mammillated, ~⅔ of

(A) (B)

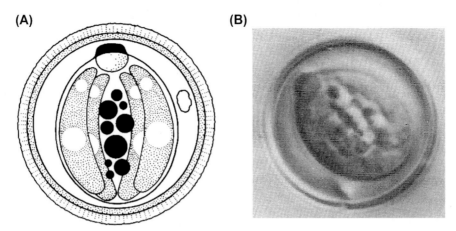

FIGURE 4.1 (A) Line drawing of the sporulated oocyst of *Caryospora bigenetica*. (B) Original photomicrograph of *C. bigenetica* sporulated oocyst. *(A) From Duszynski, D.W., Upton, S.J., 2010. The biology of the coccidia (Apicomplexa) of snakes of the world. A Scholarly Handbook for Identification and Treatment. CreateSpace Independent Publishing Platform, USA, p. 422. ISBN: 1448617995. (B) From Dr. S.J. Upton's (deceased) personal collection, with permission of copyright holder.*

total thickness, appears striated in optical cross section, stippled in tangential section; L×W (n=50): 13.2 (11–15.5); L/W ratio: 1.0; M and OR: both absent; PG: one to two present, ~1.5, usually attached to inner wall of oocyst. Distinctive features of oocyst: one to two PGs attached to inner surface of oocyst wall.

Description of sporocyst and sporozoites: Sporocyst shape: ellipsoidal, ovoidal, or pyriform; L×W (n=50): 10.1×7.7 (8–11.5×6.5–9); L/W ratio: 1.3; SB: distinct, discoidal, of uniform thickness, 1.6 wide×0.9 high (1–2×0.75–1.0); SSB: same width as SB (Wacha and Christiansen, 1982) or 2.6 wide×1.6 high (2.5–3×1–2) (Koudela, 1993); PSB: absent; SR: present as a cluster of several spheroidal bodies, approximately one to two; SZ: lanceolate, 9.4×2.0 (8.5–10×2) (Koudela, 1993) or ~8.9×2.0 (Wacha and Christiansen, 1982), each SZ with two RBs, one anterior and one posterior. Distinctive features of sporocyst: both discoidal SB and SSB present and SZ with two prominent RBs.

Prevalence: Oocysts have been found in many viperid snake species (see Duszynski and Upton, 2010).

Sporulation: Exogenous, sporulation occurred in 5–6 days when snake feces with oocysts were left in 2.5% potassium dichromate ($K_2Cr_2O_7$) solution at 22–25°C (Duszynski and Upton, 2010).

Prepatent and patent periods: See Duszynski and Upton (2010).

Site of infection, definitive snake hosts: Epithelial cells of the duodenum and jejunum in viperid hosts.

Site of infection, secondary hosts: A wide variety of dermal tissues, especially the connective tissues of the cheek, jaws, snout, eyelids, bases of the ears, tongue, nose, neck, scrotum, legs, and footpads.

Endogenous stages, definitive hosts: See Duszynski and Upton (2010).

Endogenous stages, secondary hosts: Various asexual (meronts) and sexual (gamonts) stages have been reported from the connective tissues of the cheek, nose, tongue, scrotum, dermis, and hypodermis of experimental lab mice (Wacha and Christiansen, 1982). Upton and Barnard (1988) described three generations (types I, II, III) of meronts, micro- and macrogametocytes, unsporulated and sporulated oocysts and caryocysts, and free SZ in mouse tissues during experimental infections (Duszynski and Upton, 2010, for details). Dubey et al. (1990a) found numerous developmental stages of a *Caryospora* species in skin and lymph nodes of a 2-month-old dog, including meronts up to 20 long, with up to 25 merozoites, gamonts, both unsporulated and sporulated oocysts, and caryocysts up to 18 long, with 1–3 SZ, in macrophages, connective tissue cells, and various other host cells. All developmental stages reacted positively with anti–*C. bigenetica* serum in an immunoperoxidase test. Koudela (1993) found young sexual stages, sporulated oocysts, and caryocysts in the dermal tissues of all rodents and pigs that he inoculated orally, either with oocysts or with homogenized dermal tissues containing oocysts and caryocysts.

Cross-transmission: Can be transmitted from viperid snake to viperid snake via infected lab mice (Wacha and Christiansen, 1982), but transfer via sporulated oocyst from snake to snake is not yet documented.

Pathology: Apparently there is no discernible pathology in snake definitive hosts, but all secondary hosts inoculated with sufficient numbers of sporulated oocysts develop clinical signs of dermal coccidiosis including swelling of infected tissues, reduced activity, and anorexia. Lethargy, coma, and death can also occur.

Materials deposited: Syntypes of sporulated oocysts are in the US National Parasite Collection, Nos. 76935, 76951, 76952.

Remarks: Shelton et al. (1968) may have been the first to document a dermal *Caryospora* infection in dogs when they described subcutaneous nodules and a nonfebrile wasting illness in a 6-month-old border collie in Missouri, USA (see Chapter 19). Tissue sections prepared for LM with H&E showed trophozoites, meronts with mature merozoites, and micro- and macrogametocytes in the same host cell. Levine and Ivens (1981) thought that these meronts appeared to be more like *Besnoitia* than any other genus, but

they were unaware, at the time, that *C. bigenetica* from rattlesnakes could produce similar infections in some mammals. Sangster et al. (1985) reported a similar dermal infection in a 6-month-old female hound in Georgia, USA, which exhibited anorexia, lethargy, and bilateral mucopurulent nasal and ocular discharges. Ultrastructural (TEM) examination showed that the various developmental stages of the parasite occurred in fibroblasts within parasitophorous vacuoles. Both asexual and sexual stages seen had structural characteristics of coccidia including subpellicular microtubules, rhoptries, micronemes, conoid, and anterior and apical rings. Sangster et al. (1985) had read the report of Wacha and Christiansen (1982), and it suggested to them that their infected dog was infected by a coccidium with a heteroxenous life cycle, similar to the cycle Wacha and Christiansen (1982) had reported.

Later, Sundermann (1988) and Sundermann et al. (1990) published two almost identical abstracts of work they presented at annual scientific meetings, on dermal coccidiosis in dogs infected with *C. bigenetica*. In both abstracts, they reported inducing dermal coccidiosis in 3/4 (75%) 9-week-old dogs by inoculating them with 1×10^6 sporulated oocysts obtained from rattlesnakes; three of the dogs received intramuscular injections of methylprednisolone (MPN) and all three displayed clinical signs of dermal coccidiosis 10 days post-inoculation. On necropsy, numerous caryocysts were present in the eyelid, muzzle, footpad, and abdominal skin. The dog that received oocysts but no MPN injection remained healthy, and no coccidial stages were seen in histological sections of the dermis. Unfortunately, this work was never published in peer-reviewed journals, to our knowledge. Given Sundermann's work, and the documentation of endogenous developmental stages in many canine tissues by Dubey et al. (1990a) and Koudela (1993) reported above, it seems to us that this condition is of clinical significance to the practicing veterinarian and there is a lot of work yet to be done on this topic.

EIMERIA AUREI BHATIA, CHAUHAN, AGRAWAL, AND AHLUWALIA, 1979

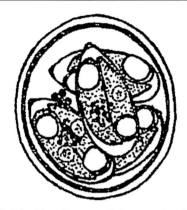

FIGURE 4.2 Line drawing of the sporulated oocyst of *Eimeria aurei*. From Bhatia, B.B., Chauhan, P.P.S., Agrawal, R.D., Ahluwalia, S.S., 1979. Eimeria aurei *n. sp. from jackal. Indian Journal of Parasitology 3 (1), 49–50, with permission from the editor and permission of the copyright holder.*

Type host: *Canis aureus naria* Wroughton, 1916, Golden Jackal.

Type locality: Asia: India: Uttar Pradesh, Mathura District.

Other hosts: None to date.

Geographic distribution: Asia: India.

Description of sporulated oocyst: Oocyst shape: subspheroidal; number of walls, 2; wall characteristics: thin, smooth, ~1 thick, consisting of an inner dark brown and an outer straw-colored layer; L×W: 16.3×14.7 (15–17×13–15); L/W ratio: 1.1; M and OR: both absent, PG: present as one or more dark particles. Distinctive features of oocyst: nearly spheroidal shape, wall with a dark brown inner layer, and one or more PGs of dark particles.

Description of sporocyst and sporozoites: Sporocyst shape: elongate-ellipsoidal, pointed at one end and rounded at the other (line drawing); L×W: 10.2×5.7 (9–11×5–7); L/W ratio: 1.8; SB: distinct and obvious as a dark thickening at the pointed end of sporocyst; SSB and PSB: both absent (line drawing); SR: present as an irregular to round mass of coarse granules; SZ: banana-shaped, slightly pointed at one end,

9.0×2.6, each with a large RB at more rounded end. Distinctive features of sporocyst: elongate-ellipsoidal shape with a dark, thickened SB at the pointed end of SP.

Prevalence: Found in the viscera of 1/2 (50%) golden jackals examined.

Sporulation: Exogenous, sporulation was reported to occur in 3 days when feces were left in 2.5% potassium dichromate ($K_2Cr_2O_7$) solution at 37°C (Bhatia et al., 1979).

Prepatent and patent periods: Unknown.

Site of infection: Unknown, oocysts found in the feces.

Endogenous stages: Unknown.

Cross-transmission: None to date.

Pathology: Unknown.

Materials deposited: None.

Remarks: Levine and Ivens (1981) were unaware of the paper by Bhatia et al. (1979), which mentioned looking at both fecal material and the intestinal scrapings of the two jackal viscera they examined; in their abbreviated report they made no mention of seeing or describing any endogenous stages. Chaudhuri and Das (1992) said they found *E. aurei* in a golden jackal in the Zoological Gardens of Alipore, Calcutta, India, but provided no evidence or other documentation. To our knowledge there are no endogenous developmental stages ever documented for this or any other *Eimeria* species from canids or felids. Thus, we believe that this form and the other *Eimeria* species listed below are pseudoparasites, a view shared by many others (see Gherman and Mihalca, 2017); we include these descriptions here only for historical record keeping.

EIMERIA CANIS WENYON, 1923

Type host: *Canis lupus familiaris* (syn. *C. familiaris*), L., 1758, Domestic Dog.

Type locality: Europe: United Kingdom: London.

Other hosts: *Canis latrans* Say, 1823, Coyote; *Canis lupus dingo* Meyer, 1793, Dingo; *Felis catus* L., 1758, Domestic Cat (?).

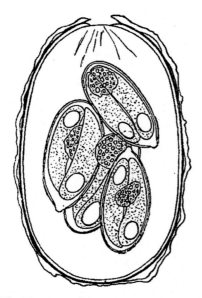

FIGURE 4.3 Original line drawing of the large form sporulated oocyst of *Eimeria canis* with its rough outer wall intact. *Modified from Fig. 4, Levine, N.D., Ivens, V., 1981. The Coccidian Parasites (Protozoa, Apicomplexa) of Carnivores, Illinois Biological Monograph No. 51. University of Illinois Press, Urbana, Illinois, USA, 249 p. The University of Illinois Press, Urbana, Illinois, has released the copyright.*

Geographic distribution: Worldwide (if it exists).

Description of sporulated oocyst: Oocyst shape: ovoidal to ellipsoidal; number of walls, 2; wall characteristics: rough, colorless, pink or red; L × W: 18–45 × 11–28 (means not given); L/W ratio: unknown; M: present as an opening in the rough outer layer (or not); OR: present as a spheroidal mass of large granules and appears to be membrane-bounded (line drawings), PG: apparently absent (line drawings) but not mentioned in original description. Distinctive features of oocyst: very rough outer wall that detaches easily, the presence of a M and a membrane-bounded OR.

Description of sporocyst and sporozoites: Sporocyst shape: elongate-ellipsoidal, slightly pointed at one end (line drawings); L × W: 9.0 × 7.1 (7–12 × 7–8); L/W ratio: 1.3; SB: present as a nipple-like structure at pointed end of sporocyst (line drawing); SSB and PSB: both

absent (line drawing); SR: present as a compact mass of granules, usually tucked between SZ; SZ: banana-shaped, slightly pointed at one end, 9.5 × 2.5 (9–11 × 2.5), and with one RB at more rounded end. Distinctive features of sporocyst: elongate-ellipsoidal shape, with nipple-like SB.

Prevalence: Wenyon (1923) reported this from 3/3 domestic dog feces in London, England. Mimioğlu et al. (1960) said they found *E. canis* in 1/50 (2%) dogs in Ankara, Turkey. Levine and Ivens (1981) stated that the prevalence is unknown but very uncommon and that this is likely not a real parasite of dogs.

Sporulation: Exogenous, 1–4 days (Wenyon, 1923).

Prepatent and patent periods: Unknown.

Site of infection: Unknown, oocysts found in the feces.

Endogenous stages: Unknown.

Cross-transmission: None to date.

Pathology: Unknown.

Materials deposited: None.

Remarks: Wenyon (1923) named and partially described this form from dog scat found on the streets of London, as first reported by Brown and Stammers (1922); in his initial description he remarked that in many respects the oocysts resembled a mixture of *Eimeria stiedae* and *Eimeria perforans* oocysts from rabbits. Wenyon (1923) also reported that the "oocyst wall was enclosed by an irregular thick membrane which gradually peeled off during the development outside the body." Nieschulz (1924a) measured some oocysts he said belonged to *E. canis* and reported the size as 17–32 × 12–20. Skidmore and McGrath (1933) said they found *E. canis* oocysts in a 3-month-old Boston terrier in Lincoln, Nebraska, USA; their oocysts were L × W (n = 35): 28.8 × 16.2 (24–34 × 16–19); L/W ratio: 1.8, with four SP that measured L × W (n = 15): 9.4 × 7.3 (6–12 × 6–7.5); L/W ratio: 1.3; SZ were 9.5 × 2.5. Their oocysts had a M, but no other mensural information was given nor was a line drawing or photomicrograph provided. Goodrich (1944) thought that *E. canis* reported from dogs was a rabbit coccidium that dogs had eaten, with the oocysts passing through their gut unaltered. Bearup (1954) said that he found oocysts of *E. canis* in 1/4 (25%) dingoes in Sydney, Australia, and that the oocysts were unsporulated when first examined; he described the oocysts as ovoidal, with a prominent M, and they measured L×W: 32×22 (30–35×19–29). No other information was given. Choquette and Gelinas (1950) said they found oocysts of *E. canis* in 26/155 (17%) dogs from which at least one fecal sample was collected, but they neither provided a line drawing or photomicrograph nor did they give any additional mensural information about the parasite. Mimioğlu et al. (1960) said they found oocysts of *E. canis* in 1/39 (2%) domestic dogs they examined in Ankara, Turkey. Dubey et al. (1978a) found *Eimeria* sp. oocysts in the feces of 15/169 (9%) adult coyotes in Montana, USA; probably they were also seeing oocysts that originated in prey animals that coyotes had eaten. Skofitsch et al. (1983) took measurements of oocysts they found in dogs that were L×W: 37.5×23.9 and presented photomicrographs of five sporulated oocysts (their Figs. 2–6); however, their oocysts are clearly oocysts of rabbit coccidia. Levine and Ivens (1981) pointed out that, "It is far from certain that this is a valid species," and we agree completely. We include this species description here only for historical purpose, and we are convinced that this "species" along with all other *Eimeria* described from dogs are oocysts from prey animals.

ISOSPORA ARCTOPITHECI RODHAIN, 1933

Synonym: *Isospora scorzai* Arcay-de-Peraza, 1967.

Type host: *Callithrix penicillata* (I. Geoffroy, 1812) (syn. *Hapale penicilatus*), Black Tufted-ear Marmoset.

Other hosts: Hendricks (1974, 1977) said that he found this species in five carnivore genera/species, as definitive hosts, including: *Canis lupus familiaris* (syn. *C. familiaris*), L., 1758, Domestic Dog (Canidae); *Eira barbara* (L., 1758), Tayra (Mustelidae); *Nasua nasua* (L., 1766), South American Coati, and *Potos flavus* (Schreber, 1774), Kinkajou (both Procyonidae); *Felis catus* L., 1758, Domestic Cat (Felidae).

Remarks: This species name has been emended to *Cystoisospora arctopitheci* N. Comb. (see Chapter 14, Sarcocystidae: Cystoisosporinae).

ISOSPORA BABIENSIS DE MOURA COSTA, 1956 EMEND. LEVINE, 1978

Synonyms: Small *Isospora bigemina* (Stiles, 1891) Lühe, 1906 of *auctores*; [non] *Isospora bigemina* (Stiles, 1891) Lühe, 1906; *Isospora bigemina* Stiles, 1891 var. *babiensis* de Moura Costa, 1956; *Isospora wallacei* Dubey, 1976; *Isospora heydorni* Tadros and Laarman, 1976; *Hammondia heydorni* (Tadros and Laarman, 1976) Dubey, 1977c.

Type host: *Canis lupus familiaris* (syn. *C. familiaris*), L., 1758, Domestic Dog.

Other definitive hosts: *Vulpes vulpes* (L., 1758), (syn. *Vulpes fulvus* (Desmarest, 1820)), Red or Silver Fox; *Canis lupus dingo* Meyer 1753, Dingo.

Geographic distribution: Probably worldwide. Levine and Ivens (1981) pointed out that it is impossible to say for certain where *I. babiensis* has been found because it has often been reported as *I. bigemina*, which is now known to refer both to *I. babiensis* and to several species of *Sarcocystis* (see Levine, 1977). It is known that *I. babiensis* has been reported in canids in Brazil (de Moura Costa, 1956), Bulgaria (Golemansky and Ridzhakov, 1975), England (Wenyon and Sheather, 1925; Wenyon, 1926c), Germany (Heydorn, 1973), The Netherlands (Tadros and Laarman, 1976), Russia (? Yakimoff and Matschoulsky, 1935), and the USA: Illinois (Levine and Ivens, 1965), Maryland (Fayer, 1974), Colorado (Gassner, 1940), and Iowa (Lee, 1934).

Remarks: Initially, on reading the literature, we were inclined to emend this form to *Cystoisospora babiensis*. However, the more recent evidence points to the fact that this form is now best called *H. heydorni* (Tadros and Laarman, 1976) Dubey, 1977c, a name that was established and accepted, before Levine (1978) renamed the small race of *I. bigemina* to be *I. babiensis*, based on the paper by de Moura Costa (1956), who reported oocysts that measured 13 × 11 (12.3–13.6 × 10.7–12.3) in one dog and 11.4–13.6 × 10.7–12.3 in a second dog from Bahia, Brazil, and had named the parasite, *I. bigemina* var. *bahiensis*. Levine (1978) should not have made this designation because the name *H. heydorni* (Tadros and Laarman, 1976) Dubey, 1977c, had priority (see Chapter 16).

ISOSPORA BURROWSI
TRAYSER AND TODD, 1978

Type host: *Canis lupus familiaris* (syn. *C. familiaris*), L., 1758, Domestic Dog.

Other definitive hosts: None to date.

Remarks: This species name has been emended to *Cystoisospora burrowsi* N. Comb. (see Chapter 14, Sarcocystidae: Cystoisosporinae).

ISOSPORA CANIS NEMESÉRI, 1959

Synonyms: *Diplospora bigemina* Wasielewsky, 1904, from the dog, *pro parte*; *Isospora felis* (Wasielewsky, 1904) Wenyon, 1923, of *auctores*, from the domestic dog; *Isospora bigemina* (Stiles, 1891) Lühe, 1906, of *auctores*, *pro parte*; *Levinea canis* (Neméseri, 1959) Dubey, 1977c; *Isospora canis* Neméseri, 1959.

Type host: *Canis lupus familiaris* (syn. *C. familiaris*), L., 1758, Domestic Dog.

Other definitive hosts: *Vulpes vulpes* (L., 1758), (syn. *Vulpes fulvus* (Desmarest, 1820)), Red or Silver Fox; *Canis latrans* Say, 1823, Coyote; *Canis aureus* L., 1758, Golden Jackal.

Remarks: This species name has been emended to *Cystoisospora canis* N. Comb. (see Chapter 14, Sarcocystidae: Cystoisosporinae).

ISOSPORA DUTOITI
YAKIMOFF, MATIKASCHWILI,
AND RASTEGAÏEFF, 1933a

Synonym: *Eimeria dutoiti* Yakimoff, Matikaschwili, and Rastegaïeff, 1933a, *lapsus calami*.

Type host: *Canis aureus* L., 1758, Golden Jackal.

Remarks: This species name has been emended to *Cystoisospora dutoiti* N. Comb. (see Chapter 14, Sarcocystidae: Cystoisosporinae).

ISOSPORA NEORIVOLTA
DUBEY AND MAHRT, 1978

Synonym: *Isospora rivolta* (Grassi, 1879) Wenyon, 1923, of Mahrt (1967).

Type host: *Canis lupus familiaris* (syn. *C. familiaris*), L., 1758, Domestic Dog.

Other hosts: None to date.

Remarks: This species name has been emended to *Cystoisospora neorivolta* N. Comb. (see Chapter 14, Sarcocystidae: Cystoisosporinae).

ISOSPORA OHIOENSIS
DUBEY, 1975c

Synonym: *Diplospora bigemina* Wasielewski, 1904, from the dog, *pro parte*; *Isospora rivolta* (Grassi, 1879) Wenyon, 1923, of *auctores*, from the domestic dog; *Lucetina rivolta* (Grassi, 1879) Henry and Leblois, 1926, from the domestic dog; *Levinea ohioensis* (Dubey, 1975c) Dubey, 1977c.

Type host: *Canis lupus familiaris* (syn. *C. familiaris*), L., 1758, Domestic Dog.

Other hosts: *Canis latrans* Say, 1823, Coyote; *Canis lupus dingo* Meyer, 1793, Dingo (?); *Vulpes vulpes* (L., 1758), (syn. *Vulpes vulgaris* Oken, 1816), Red or Silver Fox (?); *Nyctereutes procyonoides ussuriensis* Matschie, 1907, Raccoon Dog.

Remarks: This species name was appropriately emended to *Cystoisospora ohioensis* (Dubey, 1975c) Frenkel, 1977 (see Chapter 14, Sarcocystidae: Cystoisosporinae).

ISOSPORA THEILERI YAKIMOFF AND LEWKOWITSCH, 1932

Type host: *Canis aureus* L., 1758, Golden Jackal.
Other hosts: None to date.
Remarks: This species name has been emended to *Cystoisospora theileri* N. Comb. (see Chapter 14, Sarcocystidae: Cystoisosporinae).

GENUS *VULPES* FRISCH, 1775 (12 SPECIES)

EIMERIA ADLERI YAKIMOFF AND GOUSSEFF, 1936

Type host: *Vulpes vulpes* (L., 1758), (syn. *Vulpes fulvus* (Desmarest, 1820)), Red or Silver Fox.
Type locality: Asia: Kazakhstan (former USSR).
Other hosts: None to date.

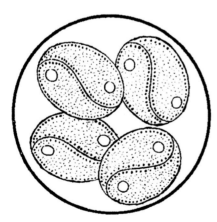

FIGURE 4.4 Original line drawing of the sporulated oocyst of *Eimeria adleri*. *Modified from Fig. 8, Levine, N.D., Ivens, V., 1981. The Coccidian Parasites (Protozoa, Apicomplexa) of Carnivores, Illinois Biological Monograph No. 51. University of Illinois Press, Urbana, Illinois, USA, 249 p. The University of Illinois Press, Urbana, Illinois, has released the copyright.*

Geographic distribution: Asia: Kazakhstan (former USSR).
Description of sporulated oocyst: Oocyst shape: spheroidal; number of walls, 1; wall characteristics: smooth, transparent, yellowish green, ~1.2–1.4 thick; L×W: 18–25; L/W ratio: 1.0; M, OR, PG: all absent. Distinctive features of oocyst: spheroidal with a thin, transparent wall and lacking M, OR, and PG.
Description of sporocyst and sporozoites: Sporocyst shape: broadly ovoidal to ellipsoidal; L×W: 9–16×8–10 (means not given); L/W ratio: unknown; SB, SSB, PSB, SR: all absent; SZ: comma-shaped, 9×4 (6–11×4–5), with one clear RB at the rounded end. Distinctive features of sporocyst: small size, with SB, SSB, PSB, and SR all absent.
Prevalence: Unknown.
Sporulation: Exogenous. Sporulation was reported to be 4 days at 25°C, when oocysts were placed in 2% aqueous potassium dichromate ($K_2Cr_2O_7$) solution (Svanbaev, 1960).
Prepatent and patent periods: Unknown.
Site of infection: Unknown.
Endogenous stages: Unknown.
Cross-transmission: None to date.
Pathology: Unknown.
Materials deposited: None.
Remarks: Yakimoff and Gousseff (1936) said that they found this species in the red fox in Kazakhstan, but the description they gave was minimal by any standard, even in 1936. Litvenkova (1969) also reported it from the fox in Belarus. Not much else is known about this form, and we suspect that there are no real eimerians that parasitize canids, but we include it here for completeness.

EIMERIA BAKANENSIS SVANBAEV AND RACHMATULLINA, 1971

Type host: *Vulpes vulpes* (L., 1758), (syn. *Vulpes vulgaris* Oken, 1816), Red or Silver Fox.
Type locality: Asia: Kazakhstan (former USSR), Alma-Ata Region.
Other hosts: *Mustela erminae* L., 1758, Ermine.

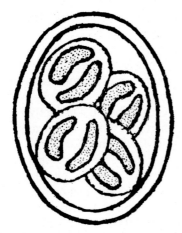

FIGURE 4.5 Original line drawing of the sporulated oocyst of *Eimeria bakanensis. Modified from Svanbaev, S.K., Rachmatullina, N.K., 1971. The question on coccidia from fur-bearing animals in Kazachstan. Akademia Nauk Kazakhskoi SSR, Trudy Instituta Zoologii 31, 165–170 (in Russian).*

Geographic distribution: Asia: Kazakhstan (former USSR).

Description of sporulated oocyst: Oocyst shape: ovoidal; number of walls, 2; wall characteristics: outer is light gray, thin, but the inner layer is clearly visible; L×W: 14.0×11.2 (11–17×8–11); L/W ratio: 1.4 (1.2–1.7); M, OR, PG: all absent. Distinctive features of oocyst: very small size, thin wall, and lacking M, OR, and PG.

Description of sporocyst and sporozoites: Sporocyst shape: spheroidal; L×W: 4.0–5.6 wide; L/W ratio: 1.0; SB, SSB, PSB: all absent (as per line drawing and not mentioned in the description); SR: absent; SZ: bean-shaped, but neither RBs nor N were visible. Distinctive features of sporocyst: small size, with SB, SSB, PSB, and SR all absent.

Prevalence: Svanbaev and Rachmatullina (1971) mentioned that 25/85 (29%) common foxes they examined were positive for coccidia. They went on to say that *Isospora vulpis* Galli-Valerio, 1931 was found in 6/85 (7%) foxes, and *E. vulpis* Galli-Valerio, 1929b was found in 19/85 (22%) common foxes, but they did not say how many of the foxes were found with *E. bakanensis*. However, Nukerbaeva and Svanbaev (1977)

made reference to this species again, saying they recovered it from 14% of the ermines (*Mustela erminae* L., 1758) they examined.

Sporulation: Exogenous.
Prepatent and patent periods: Unknown.
Site of infection: Unknown.
Endogenous stages: Unknown.
Cross-transmission: None to date.
Pathology: Unknown.
Materials deposited: None.

Remarks: Neither Levine and Ivens (1981) nor Pellérdy (1974a) mentions this species or makes reference to it. Oocysts from the ermine (Nukerbaeva and Svanbaev, 1977) were 11.2–12.6×8.4–9.8.

EIMERIA HEISSINI
SVANBAEV, 1956

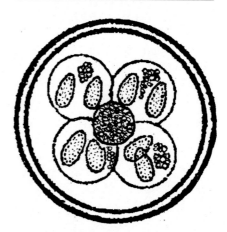

FIGURE 4.6 Original line drawing of the sporulated oocyst of *Eimeria heissini. Modified from Fig. 20, Levine, N.D., Ivens, V., 1981. The Coccidian Parasites (Protozoa, Apicomplexa) of Carnivores, Illinois Biological Monograph No. 51. University of Illinois Press, Urbana, Illinois, USA, 249 p. The University of Illinois Press, Urbana, Illinois, has released the copyright.*

Type host: *Vulpes corsac* (L., 1768), Corsac Fox.
Type locality: Asia: Kazakhstan (former USSR)
Other hosts: None to date.
Geographic distribution: Asia: Kazakhstan (former USSR).

Description of sporulated oocyst: Oocyst shape: spheroidal; number of walls, 2; wall characteristics: colorless, smooth, ~1 thick; L×W: 20.4 (range not given); L/W ratio: 1.0; M and PG: both absent, but a distinct OR is present in the middle of the oocyst between SPs. Distinctive features of oocyst: small spheroidal form, with a distinct OR, while lacking M and PG.

Description of sporocyst and sporozoites: Sporocyst shape: spheroidal; L×W: 7.8 wide; L/W ratio: 1.0; SB, SSB, PSB: all absent (from the line drawing and not mentioned in the description); SR: present as an irregular mass of small granules (line drawing); SZ: ovoidal, 4.7×3.1, but neither RBs nor N were visible. Distinctive features of sporocyst: small size, with SB, SSB, PSB, and SR all absent.

Prevalence: Svanbaev (1956) found this species in the only fox he examined.

Sporulation: Exogenous. Oocysts sporulated in 3–4 days in potassium dichromate ($K_2Cr_2O_7$) solution when stored at 20–25°C (Svanbaev, 1956).

Prepatent and patent periods: Unknown.

Site of infection: Unknown.

Endogenous stages: Unknown.

Cross-transmission: None to date.

Pathology: Unknown.

Materials deposited: None.

Remarks: This species has not been reported since its original description and, likely, the oocysts described represent a spurious finding when passing through the gut from an animal the fox ate.

EIMERIA LI
GOLEMANSKY, 1975a

Type host: *Vulpes vulpes* (L., 1758), (syn. *Vulpes vulgaris* Oken, 1816), Red or Silver Fox.

Type locality: Eastern Europe: Bulgaria.

Other hosts: None to date.

Geographic distribution: Eastern Europe: Bulgaria.

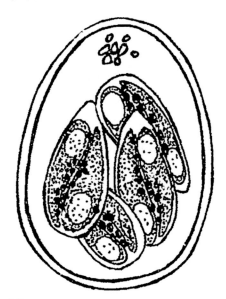

FIGURE 4.7 Original line drawing of the sporulated oocyst of *Eimeria li*. Modified Fig. 23, from Levine, N.D., Ivens, V., 1981. The Coccidian Parasites (Protozoa, Apicomplexa) of Carnivores, Illinois Biological Monograph No. 51. University of Illinois Press, Urbana, Illinois, USA, 249 p. The University of Illinois Press, Urbana, Illinois, has released the copyright.

Description of sporulated oocyst: Oocyst shape: ovoidal; number of walls, 2; wall characteristics: outer layer is smooth, yellowish, and lighter and thicker than inner layer, total wall thickness: 2.5; L×W: 31×23 (29–33×22–25), L/W ratio: 1.3; M, OR: absent; PG: present as a cluster of two to six PGs near the more pointed end of the oocyst. Distinctive features of oocyst: ovoidal shape, lacking M and OR, but with an accumulation of two to six PGs at more pointed end of oocyst.

Description of sporocyst and sporozoites: Sporocyst shape: elongate ovoidal with one end distinctly pointed; L×W: 16×8 (14–18×6–10); L/W ratio: 2.0; SB: described as absent, but his line drawing showed a distinctly pointed end on each SP that can only be an SB; SSB and PSB: both absent; SR: present as large granules scattered between the SZ (line drawing); SZ: banana-shaped, 12×3, with one end distinctly pointed and the other distinctly rounded; one RB at the more rounded end of SZ. Distinctive features of sporocyst: distinctly pointed at one end and large L/W ratio of 2.0.

Prevalence: Golemansky and Ridzhakov (1975) and Golemansky (1986) said that they found this species in 2/146 (1%) red foxes, and both foxes were <1-month-old.

Sporulation: Exogenous. Oocysts were reported to sporulate in 86 hours when kept in 3% potassium dichromate ($K_2Cr_2O_7$) solution at 23°C.

Prepatent and patent periods: Unknown.

Site of infection: Unknown; oocysts were recovered from feces.

Endogenous stages: Unknown.

Cross-transmission: None to date.

Pathology: Unknown.

Materials deposited: None.

Remarks: The original description was modest/marginal, but Golemansky (1975a) did provide a line drawing and four photomicrographs of sporulated oocysts.

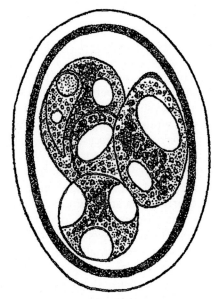

FIGURE 4.8   Line drawing of the sporulated oocyst of *Eimeria lomarii. Modified from Dubey, J.P., 1963b. Observations on coccidian oocysts from the Indian fox (Vulpes bengalensis). Indian Journal of Microbiology 3 (1), 143–146, with permission of the editor and of the copyright holder.*

EIMERIA LOMARII DUBEY, 1963b

Type host: *Vulpes bengalensis* (Shaw, 1800), Bengal Fox.

Type locality: Asia: India: Uttar Pradesh, near Mathura.

Other hosts: None to date.

Geographic distribution: Asia: India.

Description of sporulated oocyst: Oocyst shape: ellipsoidal; number of walls, 2; wall characteristics: outer wall is thicker, greyish, smooth and inner wall is darker with a "shining contour," 1–2 thick; L×W (n=25): 24–29×19–22 (means not given); L/W ratio: 1.1–1.3; M, OR, PG: all absent. Distinctive features of oocyst: ellipsoidal form with a darker, thick inner wall, while lacking M, OR, and PG.

Description of sporocyst and sporozoites: Sporocyst shape: broadly ovoidal; L×W (n=25): 11–14×8–10 (means not given); L/W ratio: unknown; SB: vestigial, visible as a small thickening at narrower end of SP; SSB and PSB: both absent; SR: present as an irregular mass of small granules distributed throughout SP; SZ: comma-shaped, 8–10×2–3, with a central N and a RB at broader end. Distinctive features of sporocyst: ellipsoidal, with a small SB, lacking SSB and PSB and having a SR distributed throughout the SP.

Prevalence: Dubey (1963b) found this species in 4/4 (100%) foxes he examined.

Sporulation: Exogenous. Oocysts sporulated in 4 days.

Prepatent and patent periods: Unknown.

Site of infection: Unknown; oocysts were recovered from feces taken from the intestine.

Endogenous stages: Unknown.

Cross-transmission: None to date.

Pathology: Unknown.

Materials deposited: None.

Remarks: Dubey (1963b) determined that this form could not be assigned to any of the four eimerians known up to the time he described it. Its sporulated oocysts differed from those of *Eimeria hessini*, which has round oocysts, from those of *Eimeria adleri* by lacking an OR, from those of *Eimeria mesnili*, which are distinctly ovoidal, smaller, and have a distinct M, and from those of *E. vulpis*, which are distinctly ovoidal and have smaller sporocysts. This species has not been reported since its original description.

EIMERIA MACROTIS MAYBERRY, BRISTOL, DUSZYNSKI, AND REID, 1980

Type host: *Vulpes macrotis neomexicanus* Merriam, 1902, New Mexico Kit Fox.

Type locality: North America: USA: New Mexico, White Sands National Monument.

Other hosts: None to date.

Geographic distribution: North America: USA: New Mexico.

Description of sporulated oocyst: Oocyst shape: ellipsoidal; number of walls, 2; wall characteristics: outer wall is thicker, transparent, smooth and inner wall is darker, thin; L×W (n=25): 31.6×19.1 (28–37×17–21); L/W ratio: 1.65 (1.2–2.1); M and

OR: both absent; PG: one to two always present. Distinctive features of oocyst: elongate-ellipsoidal shape, L/W ratio >1.6, lack of M and OR, but presence of one to two PG.

Description of sporocyst and sporozoites: Sporocyst shape: spheroidal; L×W (n=25): 9.6×9.1 (9–11×8–10); L/W ratio: 1.0 (1.0–1.3); SB, SSB, PSB: all absent; SR: present as lipid-like body between SZ; SZ: sausage-shaped, with a tiny RB at each end. Distinctive features of sporocyst: lacking an SB, a lipid-like SR, and two tiny RBs in the SZ.

Prevalence: Mayberry et al. (1980) found this species in 3/19 (16%) kit foxes they examined.

Sporulation: Exogenous; 70%–80% of the oocysts had sporulated after 3 days when maintained in 2.5% aqueous potassium dichromate ($K_2Cr_2O_7$) solution.

Prepatent and patent periods: Unknown.

Site of infection: Unknown; oocysts were recovered from feces taken from the intestine.

Endogenous stages: Unknown.

Cross-transmission: None to date.

Pathology: Unknown.

Materials deposited: None.

(A)   **(B)**

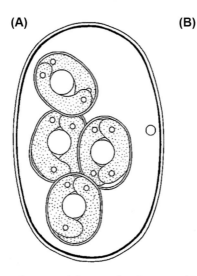
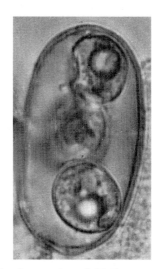

FIGURE 4.9   (A) Line drawing of the sporulated oocyst of *Eimeria macrotis*, and (B) Photomicrograph of a sporulated oocyst. *Both from Mayberry, L.F., Bristol, J.R., Duszynski, D.W., Reid, W.H., 1980. Eimeria macrotis sp. n. from Vulpes macrotis neomexicanus Merriam, 1902. Zeitschrift für Parasitenkunde 61, 197–200, with permission of all the authors and Springer Science and Business Media, copyright holder of Parasitology Research (formerly Zeitschrift für Parasitenkunde).*

Remarks: In hindsight, these oocysts look like lizard eimerian oocysts and could have been passing through the intestine of the foxes having eaten common, local desert lizards.

ISOSPORA BURIATICA YAKIMOFF AND MATSCHOULSKY, 1940

Type host: *Vulpes corsac* (L., 1768), Corsac Fox.
Remarks: This species name has been emended to *Cystoisospora buriatica* N. Comb. (see Chapter 14, Sarcocystidae: Cystoisosporinae).

ISOSPORA CANIVELOCIS WEIDMAN, 1915 EMEND. WENYON, 1923

Synonyms: *Coccidium bigeminum* var. *canivelocis* Weidman, 1915; *Isospora bigemina* var. *canivelocis* (Weidman, 1915) Mesnil, 1916; *Isospora canivecolis* (sic) (Weidman, 1915) Wenyon, 1923; *Isospora canivelocis* (Weidman, 1915) Wenyon, 1923, of *auctores*; *Lucetina canivelocis* (Weidman, 1915) Henry and Leblois, 1926.
Type host: *Vulpes velox* (Say, 1823), Swift Fox.
Remarks: This species name has been emended to *Cystoisospora canivelocis* N. Comb. (see Chapter 14, Sarcocystidae: Cystoisosporinae).

ISOSPORA FENNECHI PRASAD, 1961a

Type host: *Vulpes* (syn. *Fennecus*) *zerda* (Zimmermann, 1780), Fennec Fox.
Type locality: Europe: United Kingdom: London, London Zoo, captive animal that originally came from Africa.
Other hosts: None to date.
Geographic distribution: Africa (?); Europe: United Kingdom.
Description of sporulated oocyst: Oocyst shape: variable, from subspheroidal to ovoidal to

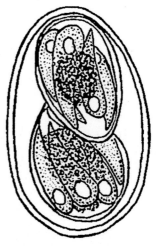

FIGURE 4.10 Original line drawing of the sporulated oocyst of *Eimeria fennechi*. *Modified from Fig. 10, Levine, N.D., Ivens, V., 1981. The Coccidian Parasites (Protozoa, Apicomplexa) of Carnivores, Illinois Biological Monograph No. 51. University of Illinois Press, Urbana, Illinois, USA, 249 p. The University of Illinois Press, Urbana, Illinois, has released the copyright.*

ellipsoidal; number of walls, 2; wall characteristics: smooth, thin, of uniform thickness; L×W (n=100): 27.5×17.2 (24.5–30.5×15–19.5); L/W ratio: 1.5 (1.5–1.6); M, OR, PG: all absent. Distinctive features of oocyst: ellipsoidal form, with a thin, smooth wall, and lacking M, OR, and PG.

Description of sporocyst and sporozoites: Sporocyst shape: ovoidal; L×W (n=100): 15–16.5×10–11.5 (means not given); L/W ratio: unknown; SB: Prasad (1961a) said that there was "no polar cap ('Stieda body') seen," but Levine and Ivens (1981) thought that Prasad's (1961a) line drawing showed a vestigial SB at the slightly pointed end of the SP, and we are inclined to agree with their view; SSB and PSB: both absent; SR: present, consisting of granular material and a few refractile bodies that stand out prominently in SP; SZ: club-shaped, 14×5, but with no visible details. Distinctive features of sporocyst: egg-shaped, with a small, almost vestigial SB but lacking SSB and PSB, and having a prominent SR of granules.

Prevalence: Found in the only fox examined by Prasad (1961a).

Sporulation: Mostly exogenous. Prasad (1961a) said that oocysts found in the feces already had two sporoblasts and then needed only 24 hours to sporulate.

Prepatent and patent periods: Unknown.

Site of infection: Unknown; oocysts were recovered from feces.

Endogenous stages: Unknown.

Cross-transmission: Prasad (1961a) could not infect two puppies with sporulated oocysts of this species.

Pathology: Unknown.

Materials deposited: None.

Remarks: The existence of this organism as a distinct species infecting foxes, or any other canids, is questionable. It has not been found/reported by anyone since its initial discovery. We regard it as a spurious finding and it easily could have been noted as a *species inquirenda* (Chapter 19), but we list it here only for historic record keeping.

ISOSPORA PAVLODARICA NUKERBAEVA AND SVANBAEV, 1973

Type host: *Vulpes vulpes* (L., 1758) (syn. *Vulpes fulvus* (Desmarest, 1820)), Red or Silver Fox.

Remarks: This species name has been emended to *Cystoisospora pavlodarica* N. Comb. (see Chapter 14, Sarcocystidae: Cystoisosporinae).

ISOSPORA TRIFFITTI NUKERBAEVA AND SVANBAEV, 1973

Type host: *Vulpes* (syn. *Alopex*) *lagopus* (L., 1758), Blue or Arctic Fox.

Type locality: Asia: Kazakhstan (former USSR).

Remarks: This species name has been emended to *Cystoisospora triffitti* N. Comb. (see Chapter 14, Sarcocystidae: Cystoisosporinae).

ISOSPORA VULPINA NIESCHULZ AND BOS, 1933

Type host: *Vulpes vulpes* (L., 1758) (syn. *Vulpes fulvus* (Desmarest, 1820)), Red or Silver Fox.

Remarks: This species name, already emended by Frenkel (1977), and the description have been moved to Chapter 14 (Sarcocystidae: Cystoisosporinae).

DISCUSSION AND SUMMARY

We know of no eimeriid coccidia described from the 16 species in these 10 genera in the Canidae: *Atelocynus* Cabrera, 1940 (monotypic); *Cerdocyon* C.E.H. Smith, 1839 (monotypic); *Chrysocyon* C.E.H. Smith, 1839 (monotypic); *Cuon* Hodgson, 1838 (monotypic); *Dusicyon* C.E.H. Smith, 1839 (monotypic); *Lycalopex* Burmeister, 1854 (6 species); *Lycaon* Brookes, 1827 (monotypic); *Otocyon* Müller, 1836 (monotypic); *Speothos* Lund, 1836 (monotypic); and *Urocyon* Baird, 1857 (2 species). In addition, only three of the six extant *Canis* species, the only *Nyctereutes* species, and only 5 of the 12 *Vulpes* species have been found to harbor enteric coccidian species. Thus, only 3/13 (23%) genera and only 9/35 (26%) species in the Canidae have been examined for eimeriid coccidia. And, of course, there are questions about the validity of some of these (the *Eimeria* species), as detailed in the above descriptions.

Eight *Eimeria* species have been found in canine feces, two from *Canis* and six from *Vulpes* species. However, we concur with Dubey (1976) and many others that these oocysts found in fecal samples all represent **spurious** findings resulting from the sampled dogs/foxes having eaten infected animal carcasses or feces from infected animals. Unsporulated and sporulated oocysts of *Eimeria* species can pass unchanged and unharmed through the canid intestinal tract, and attempts to infect lab-reared dogs with *Eimeria* species recovered in their feces have been unsuccessful (e.g., Prasad, 1961a; Streitel and Dubey, 1976). To our knowledge, the only valid coccidia passing infective propagules in the feces, after undergoing some development in the dog intestine, are *Cystoisospora* (Chapter 14), *Neospora* (Chapter 16), and *Sarcocystis* (Chapter 15) species. In addition, *Caryospora* species are capable of infecting mammals, including canids, as their secondary hosts. In these hosts, however, they undergo all their developmental stages: merogony, gamogony, fertilization, and sporulation, but the sporulated oocysts and/or their specialized caryocysts must be eaten by the appropriate serpent or raptor to complete the life cycle.

Eimeriidae in the Caniformia Family Mephitidae

EIMERIIDAE IN THE MEPHITIDAE BONAPARTE, 1845

INTRODUCTION

The Mephitidae Bonaparte, 1845, is a family of carnivores with 4 genera and 12 species. Levine and Ivens (1981) listed the skunks as a subfamily (Mephitinae) within the Mustelidae, using the taxonomy for carnivores at that time, as set forth in Walker et al. (1975). However, both mitochondrial and nuclear sequence data have consistently demonstrated that skunks and stink badgers (*Mydaus*) descended from a common ancestor, do not lie within the mustelid group, and should be recognized as their own family, Mephitidae. The family is most closely related to the Ailuridae (red pandas), Mustelidae (weasels, badgers, otters, martens, mink, wolverines, etc.), and Procyonidae (raccoons, coatis, ringtails, kinkajous, cacomistles, etc.) having split from its most recent common ancestor 35 (33–37) million years ago (MYA). Approximately 19.6 (14.1–25) MYA, this ancestral group diverged into two lineages, one directly giving rise to the stink badgers (*Mydaus*), found only on the islands of Indonesia and the Philippines in Southeast Asia. The second lineage diverged 11.4 (5.5–16)

MYA, with one branch leading to hog-nosed skunks (*Conepatus*) and the second diverging 9.6 (5–14.2) MYA, to give rise to *Mephitis* (stripped, hooded skunks) and *Spilogale* (spotted skunks). These latter three genera only occur in the New World, from southern Canada, through central South America, to Argentina (http://timetree.org/) (Hedges et al., 2006; Kumar et al., 2017).

Skunks are primarily omnivores, eating vegetation, insects, and other small invertebrates, as well as smaller vertebrates such as snakes, birds, and rodents. During the day, stink badgers and skunks shelter themselves in burrows, which they dig themselves, or use those of other mammals such as badgers and marmots. All these species are nocturnal and can be found in woodlands, deserts, grasslands, agricultural areas, open fields, and rocky mountain areas, but they are not found in dense forests or wetlands. Some, such as *Spilogale* species, are agile climbers and may be found in trees, either searching for food or avoiding predators. Skunks typically have conspicuous patterns of black and white stripes or spots that vary within and among species, and which serve as a warning signal (**aposematic coloration**) to potential predators to stay away, because they have very well-developed anal scent glands that produce noxious odors to deter their enemies. The product(s) of

33

© 2018 Donald W. Duszynski published by Elsevier Inc. All rights reserved.

the scent glands, secreted through nipples near the anus, can be projected from 1 to 6m toward threatening animals (Nowak, 1991; Vaughn et al., 2011). *Conepatus* species (hog-nosed skunks) are the largest skunks, whereas *Spilogale* species (spotted skunks) are the smallest skunks, and *Mephitis* species are intermediate in size. All skunks have short limbs and robust claws that are well-suited to digging, and these allow them to find food in the soil as well as excavate their dens (Wund, 2005; Vaughn et al., 2011).

Numerous kinds of parasites have been documented from skunks including lice, fleas, ticks, flatworms (trematodes, cestodes), nematodes, acanthocephala (Samuel et al., 2001), and even a number of tissue-inhabiting apicomplexan species (see Chapters 14–16) (Dubey and Beattie, 1988; Dubey et al., 2015a,b,c, 2017b,c), but virtually nothing is known about the eimeriid parasites from these 12 species except for the forms described below.

SPECIES DESCRIPTIONS

GENUS *MEPHITIS* É. GEOFFROY SAINT-HILAIRE AND F.G. CUVIER, 1795 (2 SPECIES)

EIMERIA MEPHITIDIS ANDREWS, 1928

Type host: *Mephitis mephitis* (Schreber, 1776) (syn. *Mephitis hudsonica* Richardson, 1829), Striped Skunk.

Type locality: North America: USA: Ohio, from an animal supply house.

Other hosts: *Spilogale putorius* (L., 1758), Eastern Spotted Skunk.

Geographic distribution: North America: USA: Ohio.

Description of sporulated oocyst: Oocyst shape: varied from broadly ovoidal to spheroidal; number of walls, 2; wall characteristics: smooth; total thickness: ~1.0; L×W (n=50): 20.7×19.2

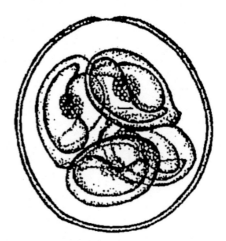

FIGURE 5.1   Line drawing of the sporulated oocyst of *Eimeria mephitidis*. *Fig. 2, from Andrews, J., 1928. New species of coccidia from the skunk and prairie dog. Journal of Parasitology 14 (1), 143–145, copyright by Allen Press publisher, with permission.*

(17–25×16–22); L/W ratio: 1.1 (1.0–1.1); M: present, difficult to see unless oocysts are properly oriented, ~1.5 wide, circular, penetrating one end of the oocyst; OR and PG: both absent. Distinctive features of oocyst: smooth, transparent bilayered wall with a small, circular M, and lacking OR and PG.

Description of sporocyst and sporozoites: Sporocyst shape: ovoidal; L×W: 10–12×7–9 (means not given); L/W ratio: ~1.4 (extrapolated from ranges); SB: present as a nipple-like structure ("rostrum") at pointed end of sporocyst (line drawing); SSB and PSB: both absent; SR: present; SR characteristics: roughly spheroidal aggregation of granules in the center of SP; SZ: sickle-shaped ("falcated"), 10–14×4–5 (means not given), with one end broad and the other end pointed; SZ lie lengthwise in SP, one on either side of the SR; RB and N were not visible in living specimens (Andrews, 1928). Distinctive features of sporocyst: sickle-shaped SZs that are slightly longer than the SP, lying on each side of the SR (line drawing).

Prevalence: Andrews (1928) reported that both skunks he examined were infected. Lesmeister et al. (2008) said they found oocysts, which they identified as *E. mephitidis*, in the feces of 22/29 (76%) spotted skunks, *S. putorius*, in western Arkansas, USA.

Sporulation: Unknown. Oocysts were passed unsporulated in the feces and Andrews (1928) said, "development took place readily in moist feces at room temperature, so that after a few days, individuals could be found with four sporoblasts or with completely formed sporocysts and sporozoites."

Prepatent and patent periods: Unknown, oocysts were collected from the feces.

Site of infection: Unknown. Andrews (1928) said, "no schizogonic stages could be found, though the intestines were carefully searched."

Endogenous stages: Unknown.

Cross-transmission: None to date.

Pathology: Unknown.

Materials deposited: None.

Remarks: Andrews (1928) collected two "common skunks of North America" from an animal supply house in Ohio, USA, found oocysts in the feces of both and, based on his observations, he named this species. Yakimoff and Matikaschwili (1932) examined the feces of 13 *M. hudsonica* (=*M. mephitis*) in Voronezh, Russia, found oocysts of an *Eimeria* species, and thought they found *E. mephitidis*. However, their measurements, description, and line drawing of a sporulated oocyst clearly distinguished their form from those seen by Andrews (1928). These differences motivated Levine and Ivens (1981) to name the form described by Yakimoff and Matikaschwili (1932) as *E. voronezbensis*, which we have included here. Lesmeister et al. (2008) found oocysts, which they identified as *E. mephitidis*, in the feces of 22/29 (76%) *S. putorius* in western Arkansas, USA. Unfortunately, they neither measured nor photographed their oocysts; however, if their identification was correct, it suggests that *E. mephitidis* may be a common inhabitant of skunk intestines. This also suggests that there is still some very good and needed work to be done in this area.

EIMERIA VORONEZBENSIS LEVINE AND IVENS, 1981

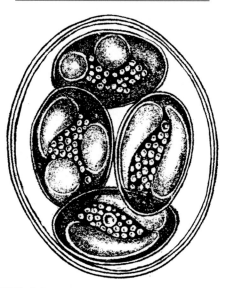

FIGURE 5.2 Original line drawing of the sporulated oocyst of *Eimeria voronezbensis*. Modified Fig. 86, from Levine, N.D., Ivens, V., 1981. The Coccidian Parasites (Protozoa, Apicomplexa) of Carnivores, Illinois Biological Monograph No. 51. University of Illinois Press, Urbana, Illinois, USA, p. 249. The University of Illinois Press has released the copyright.

Synonym: *Eimeria mephitidis* Andrews (1928) of Yakimoff and Matikaschwili (1932).

Type host: *Mephitis mephitis* (Schreber, 1776) (syn. *Mephitis hudsonica* Richardson, 1829), Striped Skunk.

Type locality: Asia: Russia (former USSR): Voronezh Oblast, on a fur farm of raccoons.

Other hosts: None to date.

Geographic distribution: Asia: Russia (former USSR): Voronezh Oblast.

Description of sporulated oocyst: Oocyst shape: varied from distinctly ovoidal (rare) to almost spheroidal; number of walls, 2–3 (line drawing with two); wall characteristics: smooth, total thickness of ~1.0; L×W (subspheroidal to "oviform" to ovoidal, n=57): 23×20.5 (17–27×15–23), whereas spheroidal oocysts (n=41) were 21.8 (25.2×18.0); L/W ratio: 1.0–1.1; M, OR, PG: all absent. Distinctive features of oocyst: smooth, transparent bilayered wall, without M, OR, and PG.

Description of sporocyst and sporozoites: Sporocyst shape: slightly ovoidal to ellipsoidal (line drawing); L×W: 9–12×7–8 (means not given); L/W ratio: unknown; SB, SSB, PSB: all absent; SR: present; SR characteristics: large spheroidal granules aggregated loosely in the center of SP between SZ; SZ: elongate pear-shaped, and slightly bent (line drawing), 6.5–7.0×2.0–2.7 (means not given), with one end broad and the other end pointed; SZ lie lengthwise in SP, one on either side of the SR; RB and N were not visible. Distinctive features of sporocyst: elongate pear-shaped SZ, almost as long as the SP, lying on each side of the elongate mass of SR granules (line drawing).

Prevalence: Yakimoff and Matikaschwili (1932) reported 10/13 (77%) skunks they examined to be infected with oocysts of this species.

Sporulation: Unknown, but Yakimoff and Matikaschwili (1932) said oocysts collected from a "whelp" that was infected with oocysts from skunks sporulated in 2.5% potassium dichromate ($K_2Cr_2O_7$) after 24 hours (see below, *Cross-transmission*).

Prepatent and patent periods: Unknown, but oocysts were first seen in the feces of the whelp infected with oocysts from skunks on the ninth day post-inoculation (DPI), and continued to 13 DPI, but not thereafter. Thus, prepatency may be 9 days and patency only 5 days.

Site of infection: Unknown. Yakimoff and Matikaschwili (1932) did not examine the intestines of their 10 infected skunks, nor of their experimentally-infected whelp.

Endogenous stages: Unknown.

Cross-transmission: Yakimoff and Matikaschwili (1932) took sporulated oocysts from infected *M. mephitis* and fed them to "a whelp," which was presumably uninfected because it had been "several times looked over." Levine and Ivens (1981) said the whelp was "presumably a dog, but possibly a skunk or raccoon." We presume that development of this eimerian could be done in a juvenile striped skunk, but not in a dog or raccoon.

Pathology: Unknown.

Materials deposited: None.

Remarks: This "species" has not been reported from skunks since the report by Yakimoff and Matikaschwili (1932).

GENUS *SPILOGALE* GRAY, 1865 (4 SPECIES)

ISOSPORA SENGERI LEVINE AND IVENS, 1964

Type host: *Spilogale putorius ambarvalis* (Bangs, 1898), Eastern Spotted Skunk.

Remarks: Levine and Ivens (1964) described this species from the eastern spotted skunk. As explained briefly in Chapter 4, and in detail in Chapter 14, the placement of *Isospora*-like coccidians having sporulated oocysts with two sporocysts, each with four sporozoites, has been controversial almost since the genus *Isospora* was first proposed by Schneider (1881). However, based on molecular and life history evidence, all the known *Isospora* species from carnivores, in which their sporocysts lack a SB, now belong in the *Cystoisospora* because of their unusual heteroxenous life histories and molecular affinities with the Sarcocystidae (Carreno and Barta, 1999; Franzen et al., 2000; Barta et al., 2005; Samarasinghe et al., 2008). To reiterate briefly, it now seems clear that isosporans reported from vertebrates comprise a **paraphyletic** clade that is divisible into at least two groupings: (1) *Isospora* species that have sporocysts with a SB are more closely related to the monoxenous Eimeriidae (e.g., *Eimeria*) and occur mostly in birds; and (2) *Isospora* that have sporocysts without a SB are most closely associated with the "tissue coccidia" in the Sarcocystidae, and are found in mammals. Such oocysts (sporocysts without SB) infecting mammals can be further divided into two additional types: (1) larger forms with distinct oocyst walls that most often maintain their integrity in their passage through the gastrointestinal tract and have **exogenous** sporulation. These *Isospora*-like species should be transferred to *Cystoisospora*, as first proposed by Frenkel (1977), and others (Frenkel and Smith, 2003; Barta et al., 2005). And (2) smaller forms with very thin, membranous walls that sporulate **endogenously** and hold their sporocysts tightly together or rupture easily, releasing their sporocysts after being released from their host cell and/or in transit through the gastrointestinal tract. These *Isospora*-like species should be transferred to *Sarcocystis* Lankester, 1882. Thus, we have transferred and emended *I. sengeri* into *Cystoisospora* (see Chapter 14, Sarcocystinae in the Carnivora).

ISOSPORA SPILOGALES LEVINE AND IVENS, 1964

Type host: *Spilogale putorius ambarvalis* (Bangs, 1898), Eastern Spotted Skunk.

Remarks: Given the arguments noted above, we have transferred and emended *I. spilogales* into *Cystoisospora* (see Chapter 14).

DISCUSSION AND SUMMARY

This small family of carnivores has only 12 species placed into 4 genera. Two of these genera, *Conepatus* Gray, 1837 (4 species) and *Mydaus* F.G. Cuvier, 1821 (2 species) have not been examined for eimeriid coccidia; in addition, only one of two *Mephitis* and one of four *Spilogale* species have been examined for coccidia, and these only in small numbers, and each in a limited locality. Thus, only 2/4 (50%) of the genera and only 2/12 (17%) of extant skunks have been studied in this manner. Obviously, there is still a lot of work to be done.

Only two *Eimeria* species have been described from 1/12 (8%) species of Mephitidae, both from the striped skunk, *M. mephitis*. Interestingly, both reports are from animals in captive conditions. *Eimeria mephitidis* was described from two skunks at an animal supply house in Ohio, USA (Andrews, 1928) and *E. voronezbensis* from skunks collected at a raccoon fur farm in Russia (Yakimoff and Matikaschwili, 1932). The possible significance of the captive condition was not explored in either case, although Yakimoff and Matikaschwili (1932) attempted cross-transmission to a "whelp" (dog? raccoon? skunk?), but with questionable results.

It is possible that these two cases are unique and, for whatever reason, these are spurious infections, and one or both of these eimerians do not actually occur in wild host populations. For *E. voronezbensis*, 10/13 (77%) skunks were positive, suggesting this species readily infects skunks. Andrews (1928) found both of two skunks positive for *E. mephitidis* so the case for spurious infection is stronger, but not certain.

Two *Cystoisospora* species have been described from the eastern spotted skunk, *S. putorius*, and all the information we have on these species is given in Chapter 14. However, the finding of only these four coccidian organisms in skunks still demonstrates loud and clear, the paucity of our knowledge on this subject; that is, 10/12 (83%) of the species in this family have never been examined for coccidia. We know nothing about the geographic distribution, location of endogenous development, cross-transmission, pathology, or details of the endogenous stages for the two known eimerians, and neither has any "types" deposited in accredited museums. Fortunately, unlike other carnivore families where there are significant numbers of species that are of conservation concern, only 2 of 12 species in the Mephitidae are classified as vulnerable by the International Union for Conservation of Nature and Natural Resources (http://www.iucnredlist.org/); these are the eastern spotted skunk (*S. putorius*) and the pygmy spotted skunk (*S. pygmaea*), both have decreasing populations. Thus, there are still ample host populations and opportunity to add to our knowledge of the diversity and biology of coccidians infecting this host family.

Finally, this chapter concludes with just a comment about skunk biology and threats from human populations. Skunks are **altricial,** born without fur and with their eyes closed, and they cannot use their stink glands until they are at least 1-week-old. Thus, they are defenseless and must rely on their mother to protect them from predators during their first year of life, when they suffer their highest mortality (50%–70%) from predations and diseases. When not in their burrows, they are relatively conspicuous and rely on their warning coloration to deter predators; nonetheless, all skunk species are susceptible to attack by coyotes, foxes, pumas, badgers, lynx, eagles, and owls. Humans, however, are *the most significant threat* to skunks, both through deliberate killing and/or killing them accidentally on roads and highways. Skunks are not typically aggressive toward each other, or toward other species, and they generally live 5–7 years in the wild and can live up to 10 years in captivity. Many skunk species consume large quantities of insects and rodents, lending a positive impact in their respective communities, but they can transmit distemper, and rabies which is a significant problem for them. In the midwestern United States, striped skunks are more commonly afflicted with rabies than are domestic dogs (Nowak, 1991).

6

Eimeriidae in the Caniformia Family Mustelidae

EIMERIIDAE IN THE MUSTELIDAE FISCHER, 1817

INTRODUCTION

The Mustelidae is the most species-rich family within the Carnivora with 59 species placed into 22 genera. Extant mustelids display extensive morphological and ecological diversity, with various lineages having evolved into an array of adaptive zones including fossorial (badgers), semiarboreal (martens), and semiaquatic (otters), and diets that vary from fish (otters) to small mammals/rodents (weasels). The members of this family are widely distributed with multiple genera found on different continents, and this eco-morphological complexity has made constructing taxonomic schemes for the group quite challenging. At one extreme, Pocock (1921) divided the extant mustelids into 15 subfamilies that were based on descriptive analyses of external characters. At the other extreme, the latest classification scheme (Wilson and Reeder, 2005) places these 22 genera/59 species into two subfamilies. The first, Lutrinae Bonaparte, 1838, recognized the uniqueness of otters, as had the molecular work of others (Koepfli and Wayne, 1998; Marmi et al., 2004; Sato et al., 2004). The second, acknowledged the

paraphyletic nature of the Mustelinae Fischer, 1817. Koepfli et al. (2008) constructed a generic-level phylogeny of the family using a data matrix of ~12,000 base pairs of mitochondrial and nuclear DNA from 22 gene segments. Their analysis indicated that most of the extant diversity of mustelids originated in Eurasia and later colonized Africa, North and South America on multiple occasions (Koepfli et al., 2008).

Mustelids are most closely related to the Procyonidae, diverging from their most recent shared ancestor approximately 29 (27.5–31) million years ago (MYA). The extant lineages within the Mustelidae presented below differ from that given by Wilson and Reeder (2005) because it is based on some of the more recent molecular work of mammalogists and evolutionary biologists. Within the family, the Taxidiinae (badger) is the most ancient subfamily diverging from the main mustelid lineage about 21 (18–24) MYA. Later, approximately 19 (13–30) MYA, the subfamily Melinae diverged from the mustelid line and splits into the genera *Meles* (Eurasian/European badger) and *Arctonyx* (hog badger) about 5 (3–6) MYA. Finally, the remaining lineage diverged into two lineages, ~17.5 (13–21) MYA, and each of them diverged into two subfamilies; one splits into the subfamilies Helictidinae (ferret badgers) and Martinae

© 2018 Donald W. Duszynski published by Elsevier Inc. All rights reserved.

(martens, fisher, wolverine), and the second into the Lutrinae (otters) and Mustelinae (weasels, tayra, minks, polecats) (Hedges et al., 2006; Kumar and Hedges, 2011; Yu et al., 2011; Kumar et al., 2017).

SPECIES DESCRIPTIONS

SUBFAMILY LUTRINAE BONAPARTE, 1838

GENUS *LUTRA* BRISSON, 1762 (3 SPECIES)

ISOSPORA LUTRAE TORRES, MODRÝ, FERNÁNDEZ, ŠLAPETA, AND KOUDELA, 2000

Type host: *Lutra lutra* (L., 1758), European Otter.
Remarks: Torres et al. (2000) described and named *Isospora lutrae* from *Lutra lutra* (L., 1758), the European otter, in Spain. Later that year, von Cord Gottschalk (2000), apparently unaware of the paper by Torres et al. (2000), published another new species description of an *Isospora*-like oocyst, which he also named *Isospora lutrae*, from *L. lutra* in Germany. Based on the morphology of their sporulated oocysts, these two "species" are clearly different. In Chapter 4, we discussed the appropriate placement of *Isospora*-like oocysts, having sporocysts without Stieda bodies, into the genus *Cystoisospora* within the Sarcocystidae, while leaving those with Stieda bodies within the Eimeriidae. Our decision for making such name changes here is based on independent phylogenetic analyses, repeated by several authors, all with the same results (Carreno and Barta, 1999; Franzen et al., 2000; Barta et al., 2005; Samarasinghe et al., 2008). We believe such results are robust and clearly support transferring *Isospora*-like oocysts having sporocysts without SBs to the Cystoisosporinae; thus, this species name has been emended to *Cystoisospora lutrae* (Chapter 14, Sarcocystidae: Cystoisosporinae).

ISOSPORA LUTRAE VON CORD GOTTSCHALK, 2000

Type host: *Lutra lutra* (L., 1758), European Otter.
Remarks: This species name has been emended to *Cystoisospora gottschalki* and because the name *C. lutrae* has priority, we give this species a new name (Chapter 14, Sarcocystidae: Cystoisosporinae).

SUBFAMILY MUSTELINAE FISCHER, 1817

GENUS *EIRA* C.E.H. SMITH, 1842 (MONOTYPIC)

EIMERIA IRARA CARINI AND FONSECA, 1938

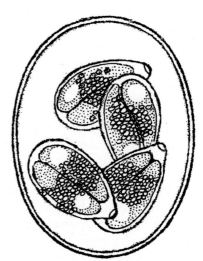

FIGURE 6.1   Original line drawing of the sporulated oocyst of *Eimeria irara*. *Modified from Fig. 17, Levine, N.D., Ivens, V., 1981. The Coccidian Parasites (Protozoa, Apicomplexa) of Carnivores, Illinois Biological Monograph No. 51. University of Illinois Press, Urbana, Illinois, USA, 249 p. The University of Illinois Press, Urbana, Illinois, USA has released the copyright.*

Type host: *Eira barbara* (L., 1758) (syns. *Eirara* Lund, 1839; *Eraria* Gray, 1843; *Galera* Gray, 1843; *Tayra* Palmer, 1904), Tayra.
Type locality: South America: Brazil.

Other hosts: None to date.

Geographic distribution: South America: Brazil.

Description of sporulated oocyst: Oocyst shape: ovoidal; number of walls, 1 (line drawing); wall characteristics: smooth, colorless; L×W: 21–25×18–20 (means not given); L/W ratio: 1.3 (calculated from original line drawing); M, OR, PG: all absent. Distinctive features of oocyst: smooth, transparent bilayered wall and lacking M, OR and PG.

Description of sporocyst and sporozoites: Sporocyst shape: ellipsoidal; L×W: 10–12×6.5 (means not given); L/W ratio: ~1.8 (calculated from line drawing); SB: present as a small nipple-like structure at pointed end of sporocyst (line drawing); SSB, PSB: both absent; SR: present; SR characteristics: irregular aggregation of small granules clustered in the center of SP; SZ: banana-shaped, with one end broader than the other and they lie lengthwise in SP; each SZ has a large RB at the broader end (line drawing). Distinctive features of sporocyst: small ellipsoidal body with a small, but distinct SB.

Prevalence: Carini and Fonseca (1938) apparently examined only one tayra, which they found to be passing unsporulated oocysts.

Sporulation: Exogenous. Oocysts sporulated in 2 days when feces were placed into potassium "bichromate" solution (Carini and Fonseca, 1938).

Prepatent and patent periods: Unknown, oocysts were collected from the feces.

Site of infection: Unknown.

Endogenous stages: Unknown.

Cross-transmission: None to date.

Pathology: Unknown.

Materials deposited: None.

Remarks: Carini and Fonseca's (1938) description is grossly inadequate by present-day standards, and this form has not been seen by others since its original description. The oocysts they described may well have originated in a prey animal consumed by the tayra, an opportunistic omnivore that consumes rodents and other small mammals.

ISOSPORA ARCTOPITHECI RODHAIN, 1933

Synonym: *Isospora scorzai* Arcay-de-Peraza, 1967.

Type host: *Callithrix penicillata* (I. Geoffroy, 1812) (syn. *Hapale penicillatus*), Black Tufted-ear Marmoset.

Other hosts: Hendricks (1974, 1977) reported that he experimentally infected five carnivore genera/species demonstrating their suitability as definitive hosts including *Canis familiaris* L., 1758, Domestic Dog (Canidae); **Eira barbara** (L., 1758), Tayra (Mustelidae); *Nasua nasua* (L., 1766), South American Coati and *Potos flavus* (Schreber, 1774), Kinkajou, (both Procyonidae); *Felis catus* L., 1758, Domestic Cat (Felidae).

Remarks: This species name has been emended to *Cystoisospora arctopitheci* N. Comb. (see Chapter 14, Sarcocystidae: Cystoisosporinae).

GENUS *ICTONYX* KAUP, 1835 (2 SPECIES)

ISOSPORA AFRICANA PRASAD, 1961b

Type host: *Ictonyx* (syn. *Poecilictis*) *libyca alexandrae* Setzer, 1959, Saharan Striped Polecat.

Remarks: This species name has been emended to *Cystoisospora africana* N. Comb. (see Chapter 14, Sarcocystidae: Cystoisosporinae).

ISOSPORA HOOGSTRAALI PRASAD, 1961b

Type host: *Ictonyx* (syn. *Poecilictis*) *libyca alexandrae* Setzer, 1959, Saharan Striped Polecat.

Remarks: This species name has been emended to *Cystoisospora hoogstraali* N. Comb. (see Chapter 14, Sarcocystidae: Cystoisosporinae).

ISOSPORA ZORILLAE (PRASAD, 1961b) EMEND. PELLÉRDY, 1963

Synonym: *Isospora bigemina* var. *zorillae* Prasad, 1961b.

Type host: *Ictonyx* (syn. *Poecilictis*) *libyca alexandrae* Setzer, 1959, Saharan Striped Polecat.

Remarks: This species name has been emended to *Cystoisospora zorillae* N. Comb. (see Chapter 14, Sarcocystidae: Cystoisosporinae).

GENUS *MARTES* PINEL, 1792 (8 SPECIES)

EIMERIA SABLII NUKERBAEVA, 1981a

Figure For the only known image of *E. sablii*, see the photomicrograph, Fig. "6," in Nukerbaeva (1981a), which we were unable to reproduce.

Type host: *Martes zibellina* (L., 1758), Sable.

Type locality: Asia: Siberia (former USSR).

Other hosts: None to date.

Geographic distribution: Asia: Siberia (former USSR).

Description of sporulated oocyst: Oocyst shape: spheroidal or subspheroidal; number of walls, 2; wall characteristics: outer is smooth; L × W: 12.6 × 11.2 (subspheroidal) or 11.2 (spheroidal); L/W ratio: 1.0–1.1; M, OR: both absent; it was neither stated if a PG was present or not nor could we determine its presence or absence from the published photomicrograph. Distinctive features of oocyst: smooth bilayered wall and lacking M, OR, and PG (?).

Description of sporocyst and sporozoites: Sporocyst shape: ovoidal, slightly tapering at one pole; L × W: 5.6 × 4.2; L/W ratio: 1.3; SB: present at slightly pointed tip of SP; SSB, PSB: both absent, apparently; SR: present; SR characteristics: small granules; SZ: described only as "elongate" and neither RB nor N were mentioned. Distinctive

features of sporocyst: slightly pointed at one end and presence of a small SB.

Prevalence: Nukerbaeva (1981a) found 24/320 (7.5%) sables in the Altai Region of Siberia infected with oocysts of one to three coccidian species but neglected to mention how many of the 24 sables were infected with which species. She did say, however, "infection was higher in summer (15%) compared with spring (5%)."

Sporulation: Exogenous. Oocysts in 2% potassium dichromate ($K_2Cr_2O_7$) solution sporulated in 72 hours (Nukerbaeva, 1981a).

Prepatent and patent periods: Prepatent period was 5 days; patent period is unknown, but at least 4 days.

Site of infection: Described only as "gut" by Nukerbaeva (1981a).

Endogenous stages: Unknown.

Cross-transmission: Nukerbaeva (1981a) used a mixture of $5–7 × 10^3$ oocysts of *E. sibirica* and *E. sablii* from a sable and was able to infect another sable in which oocysts were discharged 5–8 days postinoculation (PI). She also infected two minks (presumably *Neovison vison*, but the species was not stated) with oocysts of *E. sablii*, but they did not discharge oocysts. However, she did not state how long PI she continued to examine the animals for oocysts in their feces.

Pathology: Unknown.

Materials deposited: None.

Remarks: The description of this "species" provided by Nukerbaeva (1981a) is marginal, even when the most lenient descriptive criteria are applied. The only reason we include it here is that she provided a *tiny* (1 cm) photomicrograph, which we are unable to reproduce because of its poor quality, but which is certainly an *Eimeria* oocyst. Nukerbaeva (1981a) stated that the *E. sablii* oocysts she saw and described were identical with those of *E. furonis* described previously by Hoare (1927) from polecats and by Nukerbaeva and Svanbaev (1973) in minks. To clarify this morphological dilemma, Nukerbaeva (1981a) did cross-infections with oocysts of various *Eimeria* species found/ collected from both mink and sable hosts. Based on her negative cross-transmission results with *E. vison*, *E. furonis*, and *I.* (=C.) *laidlawi* from minks into sables, and of *E. sibirica*, *E. sablii*, and *I.* (=C.) *martesii* from sables into minks, she concluded that "the coccidia of minks and sables, regardless their morphological identity, differ from each other physiologically," and "these parasites are strictly host-specific and are not able to develop in other animals." We believe this understates the problem, and Nukerbaeva's (1981a) morphological dilemma cannot be solved until some investigator(s) begin to amplify genomic DNA from each *Eimeria* "species" and generate sequences that can be used to assess their phylogenetic positions relative to each other and to other *Eimeria* sequences in GenBank.

EIMERIA SIBIRICA YAKIMOFF AND TERWINSKY, 1931

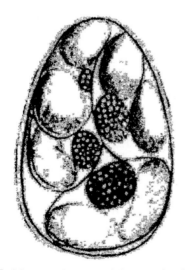

FIGURE 6.2   Line drawing of the sporulated oocyst of *Eimeria sibirica. Modified from Fig. 4, Yakimoff, W.L., Gousseff, W.F.F. 1934. Coccidia of martins and sables. Journal of Parasitology 20 (4), 251–252, with permission of Allen Press, Inc., Lawrence, Kansas, USA, copyright holder.*

Type host: *Martes zibellina* (L., 1758), Sable.
Type locality: Asia: Siberia (former USSR): Baku, Azerbaijan Zoo.

Other hosts: *Martes martes* (L., 1758), European Pine Marten.
Geographic distribution: Asia: Siberia (former USSR).
Description of sporulated oocyst: Oocyst shape: ellipsoidal to elongate-ovoidal; number of walls, 2 (described as double contoured); wall characteristics: outer is smooth, colorless; L × W (n = 100): 24.5 × 19.0 (21–28 × 17–21); L/W ratio: 1.3 (Yakimoff and Terwinsky, 1930, from the sable) or L × W (n = 101): 21.6 × 18.0 (20–31 × 16–20); L/W 1.2 (Yakimoff and Gousseff, 1934, from the marten); M, OR, PG: all absent. Distinctive features of oocyst: smooth, transparent bilayered wall, and lacking M, OR, and PG.
Description of sporocyst and sporozoites: Sporocyst shape: elongate-ovoidal (line drawing, Yakimoff and Gousseff, 1934); L × W: length not given, 7.2 wide; L/W ratio: unknown; SB, SSB, PSB: all absent; SR: present; SR characteristics: spheroidal aggregation of small granules clustered in the center of SP; SZ: sausage-shaped, ~12.6 × 6.0, with one end slightly broader than the other; neither RB nor N were visible. Distinctive features of sporocyst: very thin wall, presence of a distinct SR, and absence of SB, SSB, PSB.
Prevalence: Yakimoff and Terwinsky (1931) apparently examined a number of sables, but said only that they found 40% of the fur animals examined (using saturated salt flotation of fecal material) to have "coccidiosis (sic)." They also mentioned that a "puppy separated from its mother, born in captivity, already had oocysts in its feces but was in a good state of health." Yakimoff and Gousseff (1934) examined only one marten (*M. martes*) and one sable (*M. zibellina*), both had oocysts, and both animals were from the Zoological Garden in Baku, Azerbaijan. Nukerbaeva (1981a) found 24/320 (7.5%) sables in the Altai Region of Siberia infected with one to three coccidian species but neglected to mention which of the 24 sables was infected with which species. She did say, however, "infection was higher in summer (15%) compared with spring (5%)."

Sporulation: Exogenous. Oocysts in 5% potassium dichromate ($K_2Cr_2O_7$) solution at 16°C reached the four-sporoblast stage in 24 hours, and 73% of them contained four sporoblasts in 48 hours. "Later, spores and sporozoites developed" (Yakimoff and Gousseff, 1934). Nukerbaeva (1981a) said oocysts sporulated in 56–72 hours.

Prepatent and patent periods: Unknown.

Site of infection: Unknown. Oocysts were recovered in feces and intestinal contents.

Endogenous stages: Unknown.

Cross-transmission: Nukerbaeva (1981a) used a mixture of $5–7 \times 10^3$ oocysts of *E. sibirica* and *E. sablii* from a sable and was able to infect another sable in which oocysts, presumably of both species, were discharged 5–8 days PI. She also infected two minks (presumably, *N. vison*, but the species was not stated) with oocysts of *E. siberica*, but they did not discharge oocysts. However, she did not state how long PI she continued to examine the animals for oocysts in their feces.

Pathology: Yakimoff and Terwinsky (1930) said, "Purely by accident, we obtained interestingly ill sables (*Martes zibellina zibellina* Gmel, 1760, and *M. z. genisseesis* Ogn, 1925) in May, 1930, which were delivered to the Novosibirsk breeding center immediately after their collection." With no other evidence, they attributed this illness to finding oocysts in their feces and "both sables died very quickly."

Materials deposited: None.

Remarks: The description(s) of this "species" gets a bit convoluted. Yakimoff and Terwinsky (1930) first named this species but described only the unsporulated oocyst because they could not get the oocysts to sporulate beyond the four-sporoblast stage, therefore making it a *species inquirenda*, with no type illustration. They also said the oocysts they saw and measured were "strictly ovoidal" in shape. According to Pellérdy (1974a) and Levine and Ivens (1981), they may have published another paper on this parasite (Yakimoff and Terwinsky, 1931) but, like them, we cannot locate that

manuscript. Later, Yakimoff and Gousseff (1934) examined two mustelids, a sable and a marten, from the Zoological Gardens in Baku (Azerbaijan; Transcaucase) in Siberia. In their 1934 paper, they mentioned the earlier and badly incomplete description of Yakimoff and Terwinsky (1931), but said the paper was published in 1930, and the oocysts they described (as *E. sibirica*) were "oval, had a double-contoured membrane, and were 40 in diameter" (both statements being contrary to their published paper!). In their 1934 publication, which described oocysts from the feces of one marten and one sable from the same Zoo, they said that oocysts from the sable were L×W (n=50): 21.6×18.0 ($18–25 \times 16–20$), L/W ratio 1.2, and concluded, "The coccidia from this sable with those previously described as *E. sibirica* reveals no differences." Their (unstated) implication was that the oocysts from both the marten and the sable represented the same *Eimeria* species. However, the Yakimoff and Gousseff (1934) form should likely be considered a *species inquirenda* (see Chapter 19).

Nukerbaeva (1981a) examined 320 sables on an animal farm, "Lesnoi," in the Altai Region, in the spring and summer, 1979, and "redescribed" *E. sibirica*, saying the oocysts were light brown, had a bilayered wall ~1.5 thick, were ovoidal in shape, L×W: $22.4 \times 16.8–18.2$, no M or OR, and sporocysts were, L×W: $9.6–11.2 \times 5.6–7.2$, with a SR of fine granules. She provided one poor-quality photomicrograph of a sporulated oocyst, but we were not able to reproduce it here. Prior to Nukerbaeva's paper (1981a), neither of the morphotypes described by Yakimoff and Terwinsky (1930, 1931) and Yakimoff and Gousseff (1934) had been reported in the nearly 50 years since they were first named.

Nukerbaeva (1981a) stated that the *E. siberica* oocysts she saw and described were identical with the oocysts of *E. vison* described previously by Kingscote (1935) from mink. To clarify this morphological dilemma, she did cross-infections between oocysts of various *Eimeria* species found/collected from both minks and sable hosts. Based on her negative cross-transmission results with *E. vison, E. furonis,* and *I.* (=*C.*) *laidlawi* from minks into sables, and of *E. sibirica, E. sablii,* and *I.* (=*C.*) *martesii* from sables into minks, she concluded that "the coccidia of minks and sables, regardless their morphological identity, differ from each other physiologically," and "these parasites are strictly host-specific and are not able to develop in other animals." Once again, only sequencing the genes of these look-alike "species" can begin to resolve this issue.

ISOSPORA MARTESSII NUKERBAEVA (1981a)

Type host: *Martes zibellina* (L., 1758), Sable.
Remarks: This species name has been emended to *Cystoisospora martessii* N. Comb. (see Chapter 14, Sarcocystidae: Cystoisosporinae).

GENUS *MELES* BRISSON, 1762 (3 SPECIES)

EIMERIA MELIS KOTLÁN AND POSPESCH, 1933

Type host: *Meles meles* (L., 1758) (syn. *Meles taxus* Boddaert, 1785), European Badger.
Type locality: Eastern Europe: Hungary: Budapest, Zoological Gardens.
Other hosts: *Neovison vison* (Schreber, 1777) (syns. *Mustela vison* (Schreber, 1777); *Lutreola vison*, Wagner, 1841), American Mink (?).
Geographic distribution: Middle East: Israel (?); Eastern Europe: Hungary; Europe: Germany (?), the United Kingdom (UK).
Description of sporulated oocyst: Oocyst shape: most are symmetrically ovoidal (Kotlán and Pospesch, 1933) or ellipsoidal (Anwar et al.,

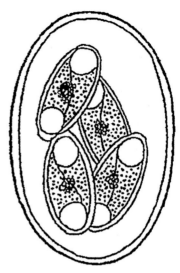

FIGURE 6.3 Original line drawing of the sporulated oocyst of *Eimeria melis. Modified from Fig. 4I, Ryšavý, B.B., 1954. Příspěvek k poznání kokcidií našich i dovezených obratlovců (Contribution to the knowledge of our and imported vertebrates). Ceskoslovenska Parasitologie 1, 131–174, with permission of the Editor-in-Chief and copyright holder, Folia Parasitologica (formerly Ceskoslovenska Parasitologie).*

2000); number of walls, 2, ~1.2 thick; wall characteristics: outer is smooth, colorless; L×W: 17–24×13–17 (means not given); L/W ratio: unknown (Kotlán and Pospesch, 1933) or L×W (n=50): 20.0×15.7 (16–23×13–19); L/W ratio: 1.3 (1.1–1.5) (Anwar et al., 2000); M, OR: both absent; PG: present, but very small (1.4×0.4) (Anwar et al., 2000). Distinctive features of oocyst: Kotlán and Pospesch (1933) said that an OR is present at first but disappears during sporulation and M and PG are both absent, whereas Anwar et al. (2000) said a small PG is present.

Description of sporocyst and sporozoites: Sporocyst shape: more or less fusiform or spindle-shaped; L×W: not given; L/W ratio: unknown (Kotlán and Pospesch, 1933); or ovoidal; L×W (n=50): 11.9×6.5 (10–14×5–8); L/W ratio: 1.8 (1.6–2.4) (Anwar et al., 2000); SB: present (see Figs. 1 and 3, Kotlán and Pospesch, 1933), small; SSB, PSB: both absent; SR: present; SR characteristics: a small, compact body in young sporocysts that "soon loses its definitive contours;" SZ: 9.0×3.2 (8–9×3–4), with a spheroidal RB, 3.6×2.0, at its more rounded end. Distinctive features of sporocyst: small SB and presence of a small, compact SR that disintegrates when mature (Kotlán and Pospesch, 1933) or disappears in a few days after sporulation (Pellérdy, 1965).

Prevalence: Kotlán and Pospesch (1933) found this eimerian in 2/4 (50%) adult badgers at the Zoological Gardens, Budapest, Hungary; both badgers, which were concurrently infected with a *Lucetina* species (later named *Cystoisospora melis*), died. Ryšavý (1954) examined two European badgers and presumably both of them were infected. Zimmerman (1959) said he found this species in 40/190 (21%) mink (?) in Germany. Anwar et al. (2000) examined badgers from Wytham Woods, Oxfordshire, the United Kingdom and found 115/259 (44%) to be infected with this species and 51/115 (44%) also were concurrently infected with *I.* (=*C.*) *melis*. There was no detectable difference in the prevalence rate between males and females as adults and cubs.

Sporulation: Exogenous. Oocysts sporulated in 2–4 days (Kotlán and Pospesch, 1933) or 72 hours at 25±2°C when placed in Petri dishes containing a thin layer of 2.5% aqueous potassium dichromate ($K_2Cr_2O_7$) solution (Anwar et al., 2000).

Prepatent and patent periods: Prepatent period is 4 days.

Site of infection: Ryšavý (1954) said he found some developmental stages of this species in the intestine.

Endogenous stages: Ryšavý (1954) reported young meronts that were, L×W: 21.6×14.4, and a spheroidal macrogametocyte, with coarse dark spots (wall-forming bodies?), which was, L×W: 19.8×14.4.

Cross-transmission: Kotlán and Pospesch (1933) transmitted sporulated oocysts of *E. melis*, from the intestine of a badger that had died at the zoo, to a young, wild, recently captured *M. meles*

that they observed to shed only *Isospora*-like oocysts "within a couple of days." Unsporulated oocysts of *E. melis* appeared in the feces on day 5 PI and "on the seventh day after the administration of the infective material the faeces of the experimental animal contained large numbers of oocysts belonging to *Eimeria* and… (the) diplosporid Coccidia of the same type as that present prior to the artificial infection." Kotlán and Pospesch (1933) also attempted to transmit oocysts of *E. melis* to young cats but with negative results.

Pathology: The preliminary report by Anwar et al. (2000) on infections in the United Kingdom indicated a potential for *E. melis* to be pathogenic in badger cubs. Badger cubs raised in captivity have been documented to suffer diarrheal enteritis leading to morbidity and mortality (Rewell, 1948; Ratcliffe, 1974; Neal, 1977), symptoms consistent with coccidiosis, although intestinal coccidia have never been directly linked to these conditions in badgers. However, the preliminary epidemiological study by Anwar et al. (2000), and the follow-up population study between 1992 and 1995 by Newman et al. (2001), led the latter to conclude that heavy infection by *E. melis* in badger cubs in the Wyndham Woods was significantly associated with reduced survival. Cubs with high levels of *E. melis* had diarrheal enteritis with a swollen abdomen and discharged soft dark feces (Newman et al., 2001; and see *Remarks*, below).

Materials deposited: None.

Remarks: On the one hand, this species was poorly and inadequately described and probably should have been relegated to a *species inquirenda*, but Kotlán and Pospesch (1933) did publish three photomicrographs of sporulated oocysts (poor quality that we are not able to reproduce here), which lent credibility to its existence. On the other hand, in spite of its initial poor description, it has been reported on, and studied more, than any other eimeriid coccidian from mustelids. Ryšavý (1954) surveyed endemic and imported (zoo) vertebrates in the Czech Republic for coccidia and found this species only in the European badger (*M. meles*) around Karlštejn. The oocysts he saw were L×W: 17.6×15.8 (18–25×14–20); L/W ratio 1.1; with a very thin wall; M, OR: both absent; PG: sometimes present as small bodies; sporocysts were ellipsoidal, slightly pointed at one end (line drawing) and measured, L×W: 7.2×4.3; L/W ratio 1.7; SB: present, very small (line drawing), but SSB, PSB: both absent; SR: present as a congregation of small granules in the center of SP; SZ: granular cytoplasm and one large RB at the more rounded end. Zimmerman (1959) reported this species in minks in Germany and said the oocysts measured were L×W: 20.8–24×14.2–15.2; he also said that oocysts of *E. vison* "were only sporadically verified." Klopfer and Neumann (1970) said they found oocysts of *E. melis* (along with *E. vison* and *I.* (=*C.*) *laidlawi*) in 67/92 (73%) minks they examined in Israel, but how they reached this specific identification is unclear because it was not stated; they gave no measurements of oocysts or sporocysts. Anwar et al. (2000) and Newman et al. (2001) produced the most comprehensive work with *E. melis* in a European badger population in Wytham Woods, of the United Kingdom. In their initial epidemiological study, Anwar et al. (2000) first redescribed the structure of the sporulated oocyst and sporocysts and then looked closely at its prevalence and incidence in a stable population of badgers in Wytham Woods over a 13-month period. They found no evidence from their data that either the prevalence or the risk of infection with *E. melis* was different in males and females, either as cubs or adults. From this, they inferred that both exposure and susceptibility to infection are constant between the sexes. They also noted that the prevalence of *E. melis* decreased with age, which for such a ubiquitous parasite, suggested to them a change in the immune profile of the population from cub to adult, either through acquired immunity or through the death of innately susceptible individuals. Newman et al. (2001) followed up and expanded the

work of Anwar et al. (2000), collecting 1,502 fecal samples over a 3-year period in Wyndham Woods, to determine the consequences of infection with *E. melis* on growth and survival of this badger population by documenting and understanding whether prevalence and intensity of infection varied with sex, age, or season. *Eimeria melis* was the most prevalent parasite in the badger population studied by Newman et al. (2001), although oocysts of *Cystoisospora melis* also were present (see *Remarks* under *C. melis*, Chapter 14). They concluded there was no significant difference in intensity of infection between adult sexes, and the mean annual prevalence was only 8.5%. However, the mean annual prevalence of *E. melis* in cubs was 100% initially, and 66% across all years and seasons they studied. Intensity of infection (measured by oocysts/g feces) was also much greater in cubs than in adults; this led them to conclude that "cubs stand out as the population class most affected by *E. melis.*" This high infantile infection with *E. melis*, especially in male cubs, was associated with significantly retarded adult head–body length after 1 (1996) and 2 years (1997).

Badger life history may explain such high infection rates. Badger cubs are fossorial until 8 weeks of age and they do not emerge from their burrows until about 10-weeks-old; thus, during their first 10 weeks they defecate in subterranean latrines (sett chambers). Feces deposited in the setts contribute to a reservoir of high oocyst content that could sporulate and then transmit infection between annual cub cohorts (Newman et al., 2001). It is also possible that cubs could become infected via maternal transmission at parturition. Recrudescence of coccidia infections attributable to a compromised immune system during pregnancy has been recorded for infections with *Eimeria* species in rabbits (Hobbs et al., 1999). If our readers have an interest to follow up on this idea, alternative proposals for the high infection rate in cubs are given by Newman et al. (2001).

As a historical point of information, Pospesch was Pellérdy's name before he changed it (Levine and Ivens, 1981).

GENUS MUSTELA L., 1758 (17 SPECIES)

EIMERIA FURONIS HOARE, 1927

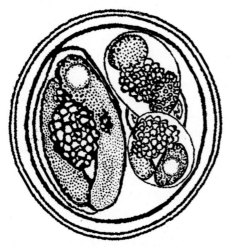

FIGURE 6.4 Original line drawing of the sporulated oocyst of *Eimeria furonis*. Modified from Fig. 33, Levine, N.D., Ivens, V., 1981. The Coccidian Parasites (Protozoa, Apicomplexa) of Carnivores, Illinois Biological Monograph No. 51. University of Illinois Press, Urbana, Illinois, USA, 249 p. The University of Illinois Press, Urbana, Illinois USA, has released the copyright.

Type host: *Mustela* (syn. *Putorius*) *putorius furo* (L., 1758), European Polecat (Domestic Ferret).

Type locality: Europe: United Kingdom: London.

Other hosts: *Neovison* (syn. *Mustela*) *vison* (Schreber, 1777), American Mink; *Mustela nigripes* (Audubon and Bachman, 1851), Black-Footed Ferret; *Mustela erminea* L., 1758, Ermine or Stoat.

Geographic distribution: Asia: Kazakhstan (former USSR); Europe: United Kingdom;

North America: USA: Michigan, Pennsylvania, Wyoming.

Description of sporulated oocyst: Oocyst shape: mostly spheroidal to slightly subspheroidal; number of walls, 2; wall characteristics: outer layer colorless, thin, whereas inner layer is thicker and yellowish; L×W: 12.8×12.0 (11–14×10–13); L/W ratio: 1.1; M, OR, PG: all absent. Distinctive features of oocyst: very small spheroidal form and lacking M, OR, and PG.

Description of sporocyst and sporozoites: Sporocyst shape: irregularly spindle-shaped, with one end blunter than the other, which is more rounded; L×W: 8–9×4; L/W ratio: ~2.2; SB: present, SSB, PSB: both absent; SR: present; SR characteristics: spheroidal aggregation of small granules; SZ: banana-shaped, with one end slightly more pointed than the other; one clear RB visible at the rounded end of SZ, and the N is "centrally situated." Distinctive features of sporocyst: spindle-shaped, with one end slightly flattened with a small SB, presence of a distinct SR, and absence of SB, SSB.

Prevalence: Hoare (1927) never gave the exact number of infected ferrets he found, stating only, "The total number of ferrets examined by me in the course of this work was about 50." Hoare (1927) found and described this species in/from a laboratory ferret. Nukerbaeva and Svanbaev (1973) reported *E. furonis* in 17/1,027 (<2%) *M. putorius* in Kazakhstan, and in a later survey (Nukerbaeva and Svanbaev, 1977), they reported this species in 2/7 (29%) ermines. Jolley et al. (1994) collected feces from *M. nigripes* in the field in 1982, 1984, and 1985, and said that their "small spherical to subspherical forms" were compatible with those of *E. furonis*; unfortunately, they neither gave the number of unique fecal samples collected nor did they indicate the number of those field samples that were infected with oocysts of this morphotype. They did, however, also collect feces from six captive black-footed ferrets, three of which were said to pass oocysts of *E. furonis*. Sledge et al. (2011) monitored the outbreaks of coccidiosis on three high-density, captive ferret populations. The first population, a ferret rescue group in the Detroit, Michigan area, USA, had 42 ferrets from <1- to >5-years-old. During June, 2005, >50% of the ferrets became affected/ infected with *E. furonis* and seven of them died. The second population, 63 ferrets on a private breeder farm/shelter in western Pennsylvania, USA, had 21 ferrets develop clinical signs of enteric disease and another 13 ferrets died (November–December, 2008), also, presumably, from *E. furonis* infection. The third population, a ferret shelter in eastern Pennsylvania, housed 62 ferrets; in October through mid-December, 2009, 20/63 (46%) developed severe diarrhea and four died, due to *E. furonis*. Pantchev et al. (2011) reported that 18/284 (6%) fecal samples from domestic ferrets examined by fecal flotation between 2002 and 2004 had detectable coccidian oocysts that were identified as *E. furonis*, *E. ictidea*, *I.* (=C.) *laidlawi*, and an unidentified *Isospora* species. Later, data from the same laboratory (IDEXX Veterinary Medical Lab, Ludwigsburg, Germany), from 2009 to 2010, showed that 21/253 (8%) fecal samples from domestic ferrets also had coccidian oocysts in their feces as demonstrated via flotation; these included nine with *E. furonis*, three with both *E. furonis* and *I.* (=C.) *laidlawi*, eight with only *I.* (=C.) *laidlawi*, and one with both *E. furonis* and *E. ictidea*.

Sporulation: Exogenous. Oocysts sporulated in 5–6 days at room temperature when placed in 0.5% chromic acid (Hoare, 1927) or in 5–6 days (Nukerbaeva and Svanbaev, 1973). Jolley et al. (1994) said that oocysts of this species (small spheroidal to subspheroidal forms) sporulated in "neither less than 48 nor more than 72 hours."

Prepatent and patent periods: Prepatent period was reported to be 5 days after experimental infection of a coccidium-free ferret, but the length of patency is unknown.

Site of infection: Epithelium of the small intestine, and the rectum, above the host cell nucleus (HCN) of each cell, mostly in the apices of the villi, but not in the crypts of Lieberkühn. Jolley et al. (1994) said that both merogony and gamogony stages were seen in the villar epithelial cells throughout the small intestine but were most prevalent in the jejunum, and that the endogenous stages of *E. furonis* were most commonly seen in the top one-third, but not in crypts or low basal regions of villi. Williams et al. (1996) described coccidian endogenous stages of what was "most likely *E. furonis*," in a ferret. In their case report on an infected 9-week-old ferret, they observed and measured meronts, merozoites, and oocysts in gall bladder and bile duct epithelial cells. Sledge et al. (2011), who examined histological sections of intestines from ferrets that had died during three different outbreaks in Michigan and Pennsylvania, USA, found numerous intracytoplasmic "coccidial stages" (meronts, macro-, and microgametocytes, oocysts) in superficial mucosal epithelial cells of the villus tips and occasional sloughed epithelial cells in the intestinal lumen.

Endogenous stages: Hoare (1935b) infected one ferret with a single dose of sporulated oocysts and killed it on day 6 PI, when oocysts were first found in its feces; nonetheless, a good number of developmental stages were present from meronts through gamonts through unsporulated oocysts, leading Hoare (1935b) to note that development did not proceed *pari passu* because multiple developmental stages were all well-represented; i.e., the various endogenous stages are indiscriminately mixed and do not exhibit an arrangement into age groups. The earliest endogenous stages visualized by Hoare (1935b) were spheroidal, 3–4 wide, with a relatively large nucleus containing a deeply-staining karyosome; he interpreted this to be either a trophozoite or an undivided young meront. Hoare (1935b) reported two merogonous stages. In the first (M_1), stumpy sausage-shaped merozoites (m_1), ~3–4 × 2, were budded off, leaving a cytoplasmic residuum; he illustrated ~14 m_1 in a single meront section (his Fig. 5, p. 113). In the M_2, the m_2s were longer and curved, ~6 × 1.3, with one end rounded, the other more pointed ("drawn out"), and a compact N near the rounded end. In the M_2, the m_2s appeared to lie within it rather than being budded off from it. Hoare (1935b) believed that the m_2s gave rise to gamonts. Macrogametocytes were described as spheroidal, ~8 wide, and contained darkly-staining globular inclusions; he reported the microgametocytes to be about the same size. Freshly developed oocysts within the tissues measured about 12.8 × 12.0. Jolley et al. (1994) said that the meronts of this species were small, with 16 or fewer merozoites, and that microgamonts and macrogametes/zygotes usually were seen in clusters, occurring most commonly in cells of the apical one-third of villi, as were the developing oocysts. Williams et al. (1996) measured meronts in biliary epithelial cells that were, L×W: 10.8–13 × 8.9–9.3; each meront had up to 16 merozoites, which measured 5.6–6.4 × 1.5–2.0 in longitudinally-cut tissue sections. Oocysts in tissue sections were ovoidal to spheroidal, 12.5 × 12.0 (Williams et al., 1996).

Cross-transmission: Hoare (1927) fed sporulated oocysts to a clean ferret and said he first saw oocysts appear in the feces 6 days PI. Later, Hoare (1935b) infected one ferret with clean oocysts of *E. furonis* and sacrificed the ferret on the day that oocysts first appeared in the feces, again day 6 PI. Nukerbaeva (1981a) used 5–7 × 10^3 oocysts of *E. furonis* from mink and infected two sables (*M. zibellina*), but they did not discharge oocysts. However, she did not state how long PI she continued to examine the animals for oocysts in their feces. Nukerbaeva (1981a) also used a mixture of 5–7 × 10^3 oocysts of *E. furonis* and *E. vison* from mink to infect another mink and said she found oocysts in the feces on days 4–7 PI.

Pathology: Hoare (1927) said that heavily infected ferrets had no obvious signs of disease; specifically, he said, "The infection did not appear to inconvenience the animals in any way, as no symptoms attributable to the infection were noted." This statement was a gross generalization since the ferrets he first examined were infected with one to three different coccidians (*I.* (=*C.*) *laidlawi*, *E. furonis*, *E. ictidea*). In his later work, with one ferret experimentally-infected only with *E. furonis*, he said the only effect was enlargement and an irregular arrangement of epithelial cells in the most heavily infected parts of the intestinal mucosa and denudation of some areas due to shedding of infected parts of the epithelium (Hoare, 1935a). Williams et al. (1996) studied the pathology of what was presumably *E. furonis* in the gall bladder and bile ducts and also measured clinical abnormalities in an infected ferret's blood. These included marked elevations of alkaline phosphatase (3,533 IT/L), total bilirubin (4.8 mg/dL), and moderately elevated alanine aminotransferase (853 IU/dL); in addition, the infected ferret's blood showed that it was "azotemic, hyperphosphatemic, hypoproteinemic, mildly hypoalbuminemic," and a complete blood count showed marked neutrophilic leukocytosis, a regenerative left shift, and macrocytic normochromic anemia. Gross examination showed the liver to be enlarged and pale, bile ducts were enlarged and firm, and the gall bladder was thickened up to eight times normal with moderate amounts of fibrous connective tissue and numerous lymphocytes, plasma cells, macrophages, and neutrophils. In the liver, interlobular bile ducts were duplicated and surrounded by abundant fibrous connective tissue. Meronts were present in ~20% of intact gall bladder and biliary epithelial cells, as well as in sloughed epithelial cells. Sledge et al. (2011) reported "severe enteric disease associated with *E. furonis* infection in ferrets." They evaluated and examined three unrelated, densely-populated ferret shelters and found that in each outbreak, there was high morbidity, an appreciable number of deaths, and ferrets of all ages were affected. Infected ferrets had acute onset of diarrhea, with feces usually containing digested blood, and other symptoms included anorexia, dehydration, weakness, lethargy, and weight loss. Clinical signs persisted in infected ferrets for 5–10 days prior to recovery or progressively worsened over a similar time frame leading to death. On necropsy they found marked atrophic enteritis associated with numerous intraepithelial and some extracellular coccidian endogenous stages. Sporulated oocysts recovered from the feces were identified as those of *E. furonis*, and a PCR assay on paraffin-embedded gut sections for the gene encoding the SSU rRNA yielded products with sequences identical to those described for *E. furonis*. Kaye et al. (2015) also described a case of biliary coccidiosis in an 18-month-old female, spayed pet ferret with severe anemia secondary to pure red cell aplasia; despite aggressive, supportive care, the ferret was euthanized and necropsy revealed intraepithelial coccidian parasite stages in the extrahepatic biliary tree. Histologically, the oocysts measured 13×12, meronts were 15×12, and contained up to 16 merozoites that were 5×2. Analysis of a fragment of the parasite's 18S rRNA gene using PCR amplification and DNA sequencing identified it as *E. furonis*, with 100% sequence identity.

Materials deposited: None.

Remarks: Hoare (1927) first became aware that coccidians were infecting laboratory ferrets when Dr. P.P. Laidlaw, working at the Wellcome Medical Research Council's Farm Laboratory, Mill Hill, London, encountered cases of coccidian infection among the experimental ferrets being used to investigate dog distemper. When Dr. Laidlaw made the material from ferrets available to Hoare, the latter found and described oocysts representing two eimerians (*E. ictidea*, *E. furonis*) and one isosporan (*I.* (=*C.*) *laidlawi*) (Hoare, 1927). He said that of the three coccidia he described, the two "*Eimeria* were most frequent and abundantly encountered, whereas those of the *Isospora* were found on a few occasions and in small numbers only." He mentioned that the percentage of coccidia-infected ferrets in the laboratory was much higher in those infected with distemper than in the healthy stock animals. Hoare (1927) also

examined a number of ferrets from London animal dealers, but said "no coccidia could be detected in them even after prolonged examinations." Hoare (1928) also reported this species in three "ferrets" with oocysts that were almost "globular," $11–14 \times 10–13$, without a M. Sporulated oocysts reported by Nukerbaeva and Svanbaev (1973) from minks in Kazakhstan were small ovoidal or spheroidal forms; spheroidal ones were 11 wide, whereas the short ovoidal ones were, $L \times W$: 13×11 ($12–14 \times 10–13$), L/W 1.2. Nukerbaeva and Svanbaev's (1973) oocysts had a two-layered wall, ~1 thick, and lacked OR, PG, M; its sporocysts were 6×4. In a later survey (Nukerbaeva and Svanbaev, 1977), they reported this species in 18/1,017 (<2%) minks and they found both spheroidal (11.2 wide) and ovoidal oocysts ($L \times W$: $12–14 \times 10–13$).

Williams et al. (1992) reported that this species had been identified in captive and free-ranging black-footed ferrets and occasionally may cause diarrhea and even death in kits during their stressful weaning process in captivity. This species is a natural parasite of the black-footed ferret (*M. nigripes*), and the coccidiosis, it causes is a problem primarily in ferret kits (Williams et al., 1992; Jolley et al., 1994; Williams and Thorne, 1996). Jolley et al. (1994) said the oocysts they saw had a pink, double-layered wall, and measured, $L \times W$ (n = 60): 12.6×11.9 ($11–15 \times 10–13$); L/W ratio: 1.1; M and PG: both absent, but a coarse, granular OR was visible. The sporocysts were described only as "elongate," with a SB and the SZ with RBs. Jolley et al. (1994) noted that mixed infections with *E. furonis* occurred, but it was much less prevalent than infection with *E. ictidea*, both in healthy ferrets and in those immunocompromised by canine distemper. Enteric coccidiosis due to infection with *E. furonis* typically has been reported to be subclinical rather than acute in ferrets, but the reports of Williams et al. (1992) and Sledge et al. (2011) indicate infection with *E. furonis* must be taken seriously because it can cause severe enteric disease (coccidiosis) with high morbidity and mortality in domestic ferrets. In the study of three ferret shelters by Sledge et al. (2011), it was interesting that few coccidial oocysts were observed in fecal samples pooled from diarrheic feces of their Group 1 ferrets, and the oocysts were never seen in fecal samples from their Group 2 and Group 3 ferrets. This is one of two *Eimeria* species now known to cause hepatic pathology in mustelids, but this is not unusual; several unidentified species with features of the Eimeriidae have been reported in the biliary epithelium of a dog (Lipscomb et al., 1989) and a cat (Neufeld and Brandt, 1974).

EIMERIA HIEPEI GRÄFNER, GRAUBMANN, AND DOBBRINER, 1967

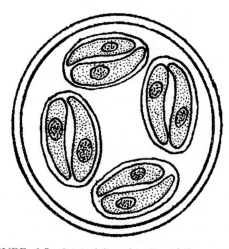

FIGURE 6.5 Original line drawing of the sporulated oocyst of *Eimeria hiepei*. *Modified from Fig. 44, Levine, N.D., Ivens, V., 1981. The Coccidian Parasites (Protozoa, Apicomplexa) of Carnivores, Illinois Biological Monograph No. 51. University of Illinois Press, Urbana, Illinois, USA, 249 p. The University of Illinois Press, Urbana, Illinois USA, has released the copyright.*

Type host: The type host is uncertain. No one is sure whether Gräfner et al. (1967) found this species in the European Mink, *Mustela lutreola* (L., 1758), or the American Mink, *Neovison vison* (Schreber, 1777) (Levine and Ivens, 1981;

Pellérdy, 1974a). Since this species was first described in East Germany, perhaps, we can assume it was from the European Mink.

Type locality: Europe: Germany (former East Germany).

Other hosts: *Neovison vison* (Schreber, 1777) (syns. *Mustela vison*, *Lutreola vison*), American Mink.

Geographic distribution: Europe: Germany; North America: USA: Wisconsin.

Description of sporulated oocyst: Oocyst shape: spheroidal to subspheroidal; number of walls, 2; wall characteristics: smooth, colorless; L × W (n = 50): 17 × 13; L/W ratio: 1.0–1.3; M, OR, PG: all absent. Distinctive features of oocyst: relatively small, nearly spheroidal body, and lacking M, OR, and PG.

Description of sporocyst and sporozoites: Sporocyst shape: ellipsoidal (line drawing); L × W: 6 × 4; L/W ratio: 1.5; SB, SSB, PSB, SR: all absent (line drawing); SZ: banana-shaped, with one end slightly pointed and the other end broadly rounded; no RB was visible, but a N was drawn in the lower third of the SZ. Distinctive features of sporocyst: thin, ellipsoidal wall, lacking SR, SB, SSB, and PSB.

Prevalence: Davis et al. (1953) confirmed a biliary coccidian in one adult female mink found dead on a fur farm near Madison, Wisconsin USA, which was almost certainly this species, but they did not describe the oocysts or name it.

Sporulation: Exogenous. Oocysts sporulated in 2 days at 24°C in 2.5% aqueous potassium dichromate ($K_2Cr_2O_7$) solution.

Prepatent and patent periods: Unknown.

Site of infection: Bile duct epithelial cells.

Endogenous stages: Gräfner et al. (1967) said there were two types of meronts, which they named Types A and B, in the bile duct epithelium. Type A meronts had 8 merozoites, whereas Type B meronts had 16 merozoites. Gräfner et al. (1967) suggested that Type A meronts formed first, but they could not verify that. When mature, Type A meronts were about 8 wide at their maximum, whereas Type B meronts were larger, ~12–15 wide. Merozoites in both types were described as banana-shaped and ~8×2 in size. Macrogametocytes were spheroidal to ovoidal, ~8–10 wide, whereas microgametocytes were spheroidal, ~8 wide.

Cross-transmission: None to date.

Pathology: Gräfner et al. (1967) said that the livers of infected mink contained yellowish, irregular nodules, or hollow structures that could be as large as a pea. Affected bile ducts were reported to contain detritus, leukocytes, eosinophils, meronts, gamonts, and unsporulated oocysts. Bile duct epithelial cells became swollen and proliferation of the bile duct mucosa was common. Earlier, Davis et al. (1953) said that the surface of the infected liver was pale, mottled, and had irregular, whitish, elevated areas from 0.25 to 1 cm wide. Microscopically, infected bile ducts were thickened by hyperplasia of the epithelium and were infiltrated by primarily plasma cells. The lumens of hyperplastic ducts were plugged with purulent exudate, necrotic debris, and numerous coccidian stages. Nodular areas were usually surrounded by well-defined fibrous capsules. Unfortunately, Davis et al. (1953) never identified the eimerian species which they say caused the pathology they reported. Since *E. hiepei* is the only eimerian known, to date, to exclusively infect cells of the liver and bile ducts with its endogenous stages in minks, we ascribe the pathology observed by Davis et al. (1953) to this form.

Materials deposited: None.

Remarks: The description of this species is modest by current day standards and certainly needs to be expanded on in much more detail. Additionally, we need to learn as much as we can about its biology and transmission because of its apparent pathogenicity to minks.

EIMERIA ICTIDEA HOARE, 1927

Synonym: *Eimeria melis* Zimmerman, 1959.

Type host: *Mustela* (syn. *Putorius*) *putorius furo* (L., 1758), European Polecat (Domestic Ferret).

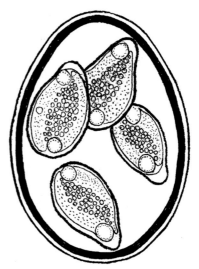

FIGURE 6.6   Original line drawing of the sporulated oocyst of *Eimeria ictidea*. *Modified from Fig. 56, Levine, N.D., Ivens, V., 1981. The Coccidian Parasites (Protozoa, Apicomplexa) of Carnivores, Illinois Biological Monograph No. 51. University of Illinois Press, Urbana, Illinois, USA, 249 p. The University of Illinois Press, Urbana, Illinois USA has released the copyright.*

Type locality: Europe: United Kingdom: London.

Other hosts: *Mustela eversmanii* Lesson, 1827, Steppe Polecat (?); *Mustela nigripes* (Audubon and Bachman, 1851), Black-footed Ferret; *Neovison vison* (Schreber, 1777) (syn. *Mustela vison* L., 1766), American Mink (Umurzakoff and Nukerbaeva, 1985).

Geographic distribution: Asia: Belarus (?), Kazakhstan (former USSR); Eastern Europe: Czech Republic; Europe: United Kingdom, Germany; North America: USA: Wyoming.

Description of sporulated oocyst: Oocyst shape: elongate-ovoidal to ellipsoidal; number of walls, 2; the outer is smooth, thin, colorless, and the inner is thicker and yellow; L×W: 23.6×17.5 (18–27×13–21); L/W ratio: 1.3; M: if present (?), small; OR: absent; PG: buds off the original sporoplasm but disappears before sporulation is completed. Distinctive features of oocyst: large ovoidal shape, and lacking both OR and PG; presence of a M is questionable, as Hoare (1927) said, "a small micropyle could sometimes be distinguished at one end," but he did not show one in his line drawing (Plate XXIV, Fig. 6, p. 321, Hoare, 1927).

Description of sporocyst and sporozoites: Sporocyst shape: irregularly ovoidal with one end broad and the other narrowed and slightly constricted; L×W: 11.5×6.5; L/W ratio: 1.8; SB: present, small, at the more constricted end; SSB, PSB: both absent; SR: present; SR characteristics: spheroidal aggregation of small and large granules usually clustered in the center of SP, between the SZ; SZ: banana-shaped, with one end slightly broader than the other; one RB at the more rounded end of SZ and the N is visible at midbody. Distinctive features of sporocyst: very thin wall, presence of a distinct SR, and absence of SB, SSB.

Prevalence: Not stated for ferrets in the original description by Hoare (1927), but Litvenkova (1969) said she found *E. ictidea* oocysts in 1/3 (33%) polecats in Belarus. Tinar (1985) examined 181 samples from two mink farms around Ankara, Turkey, for coccidia; of these, 150 were fecal pellets (presumably from different minks?), and the intestinal tracts from 31 animals. He found this species in 24/181 (13%) samples. Jolley et al. (1994) collected feces from *M. nigripes* in the field in 1982, 1984, and 1985, and said that the oocysts with "medium ovoidal forms" were compatible with those of *E. ictidea*; unfortunately, they neither gave the number of unique fecal samples collected nor did they indicate the number of those field samples that were infected with oocysts of this morphotype. They did, however, also collect feces from six captive black-footed ferrets, all of which they said passed oocysts of *E. ictidea*. Pantchev et al. (2011) reported 18/284 (6%) fecal samples from domestic ferrets examined by fecal flotation between 2002 and 2004 had detectable coccidian oocysts that were identified as *E. furonis*, *E. ictidea*, *I.* (=C.) *laidlawi*, and an unidentified *Isospora* species. Later, data from the same laboratory (IDEXX Veterinary Medical Lab, Ludwigsburg, Germany), from 2009 to 2010, showed that 21/253 (8%) fecal samples from domestic ferrets

also had coccidian oocysts in their feces via flotation; these included nine with *E. furonis*, three with both *E. furonis* and *I.* (=C.) *laidlawi*, eight with only *I.* (=C.) *laidlawi*, and one with both *E. furonis* and *E. ictidea*.

Sporulation: Exogenous. Oocysts sporulated in 3 days (Hoare, 1927) or in 40–44 hours at 20–25°C when in potassium "bichromate" solution (Svanbaev, 1956). Jolley et al. (1994) said that oocysts of this species (medium ovoidal form) sporulated in "no less than 48, nor more than 72 hours."

Prepatent and patent periods: Prepatent period is 7 days; length of patency is unknown.

Site of infection: Above the host cell nuclei in the epithelial cells of the villi, especially the tip, in the small intestine. Hoare (1935a,b) noted in one ferret infected only with *E. ictidea* that although the infection was extremely heavy, the distribution of endogenous stages in the mucous membrane was "patchy," in that the villi in some regions of the intestine were packed with stages, whereas in others they were entirely free from infection. Jolley et al. (1994) said that both merogony and gamogony stages were seen in the villar epithelial cells throughout the small intestine but were most prevalent in the jejunum. They said that gamogony occurred mainly in epithelial cells in the apical half of villi and "microgamonts with developing or fully formed microgametes were common near macrogametes/zygotes and oocysts in various stages of development."

Endogenous stages: Unlike the developmental stages of *E. furonis*, those of *E. ictidea* invade only epithelial cells in "free portions" of the villi, especially the tips, and these epithelial cells were never seen to harbor more than one parasite. As the parasite grows, always above the HCN, it gradually fills the entire space available within the host cell (Hoare, 1935b). Only one merogonous stage was seen by Hoare (1935b), "the final one with fully formed merozoites." This allowed him to conclude that all the SZ introduced with the single inoculum he used developed more or less simultaneously, and at the same rate such that the different endogenous stages are all grouped together. The merozoites he measured were elongate, 11×1, with one end rounded and the other slightly pointed, and had a compact N near the rounded end. After these merozoites penetrated other epithelial cells, they shortened, became rounded, and grew into gametocytes. Young macrogametocytes were, 9×7, with cytoplasm packed with granular material that is later transformed into dark-staining globules characteristic of a fully developed female gametocyte; this form elongates to $\sim 20 \times 7$, occupying the entire volume of the host cell. Hoare (1935b) said that microgametocytes and gametes differed from the corresponding stages of *E. furonis* only by having larger dimensions (which were not given). Freshly formed, unsporulated oocysts discharged in the feces measured, $\sim 23.6 \times 17.5$. Jolley et al. (1994) said they saw two morphological types of meronts in intestinal sections infected predominantly with *E. ictidea*; one commonly near the bases of the villi and rarely in the crypts and the second at or near the tips.

Cross-transmission: Hoare (1927) said "A large number of fully developed oocysts (in chromic acid) were washed and fed to a clean ferret," and that he detected unsporulated oocysts in the feces 7 days PI.

Pathology: Hoare (1927) said that heavily infected ferrets had no obvious signs of disease; specifically, "The infection did not appear to inconvenience the animals in any way, as no symptoms attributable to the infection were noted." The only effect was enlargement and an irregular arrangement of epithelial cells in the most heavily infected parts of the mucosa along with denudation of some areas due to shedding of infected parts of the epithelium. His statement, however, is a gross generalization since the ferrets he examined were infected with from one to three different coccidians that included *I.* (=*C.*) *laidlawi*, *E. furonis*, and *E. ictidea*. In his following papers (1935a,b), in which one ferret was experimentally infected only with oocysts of

E. ictidea, he noted that this parasite produced "a very marked tissue reaction of an unusual type," particularly when the extremity of a villus harbored a large number of late-stage meronts, gamonts, and unsporulated oocysts. There evidently is a tissue reaction that tends to isolate the infected (distal) portion of the villus from the noninfected (proximal) portion because an annular constriction begins to separate the two portions. This constriction involves both the epithelium and the villus core to a depth varying with the degree of its development. The constriction begins with a slight circular furrow in the epithelium and then increases in depth, penetrating more into the core until the villus assumes an irregular hour-glass shape with a narrow waist that separates the upper parasitized villus from the normal, uninfected lower epithelium of the villus. As the constriction deepens, the line between the infected extremity and the uninfected lower villus is supported only by the core of the villus. The upper infected portions show blood vessels of the lamina propria to be dilated and packed with erythrocytes with extravasation into surrounding tissue along with varying degrees of necrosis. Hoare (1935b) assumed that since the infected tip of the villus, with most of the epithelial cells occupied by parasites, ceased to perform its normal functions; this condition, in turn, served to stimulate the proliferative activity of epithelial cells at the base of the villi as the local destruction of epithelium would, with the result that new epithelial cells are pushed upward. However, reaching the obstruction prevents further advance of these new cells so the proliferating epithelium grows inward, forming a constriction of increasing depth around the core of the villus. This allows the healthy epithelium to become disconnected from the infected epithelium and forms a collar-like extension surrounding the tip of the villus. Pathological changes observed included dilatation of capillaries followed by congestion with erythrocytes, extravasation of these elements and, finally, focal necrosis of the infected villus tip. Hoare (1935b) also noted that none of these processes had the slightest effect on the coccidia, which continued their normal development. Jolley et al. (1994) said that free-ranging black-footed ferrets in Wyoming, USA, passed mainly oocysts of *E. ictidea*, but usually in small numbers, unless they became infected with canine distemper. Oocyst production in ferrets with distemper was always markedly higher, apparently because of "immunosuppression associated with the viral disease (Kauffman et al., 1982)."

Materials deposited: None.

Remarks: Hoare (1927) found and described oocysts representing two eimerians (*E. ictidea*, *E. furonis*) and one isosporan (*I.* (=C.) *laidlawi*) (see *Remarks* under *E. furonis*, above). He said that of the three coccidia he described, the two "*Eimeria* were most frequent and abundantly encountered, whereas those of the *Isospora* were found on a few occasions and in small numbers only." Hoare (1928) also reported this species in three "ferrets" with oocysts that were ellipsoidal, L×W: 18–27×13–21.

Ryšavý (1954) surveyed endemic and imported (zoo) vertebrates in the Czech Republic for coccidia and reported this species in the wild European polecat, *Mustela* (syn. *Putorius*) *putorius* and in its domesticated cousin, *Mustela* (syn. *Putorius*) *putorius furo* (domestic ferret). The oocysts he saw were, L×W: 21.9×16.9 (18–24.5×14–20); L/W ratio 1.3; with a very thin wall; M, PG, OR: all absent. Sporocysts were ellipsoidal, slightly pointed at one end (line drawing), L×W: 12.2×6.5; L/W ratio 1.9; SB; present (line drawing), but SSB, PSB: both absent; SR: present as a congregation of small granules in the center of SP; SZ: granular cytoplasm and one RB at the more rounded end. This species was found in polecats/ferrets in Moravia and around Prague. Svanbaev (1956) also examined polecats from Kazakhstan and said the SP and SZ he saw differed from those described by Hoare (1927). His ellipsoidal oocysts were L×W: 26×20 (25–28×20–21), L/W 1.3, with a bilayered wall, but

without M, OR, and PG. The short ellipsoidal SP were L×W: 8.7×8.5 (8–9×8–9), with an SR, and SZ were 6×4 (Svanbaev, 1956). Svanbaev (1956) likely was dealing with a different species. Zimmerman (1959) described two coccidian species, *E. vison* and *E. melis*, in mink in Germany, but Pellérdy (1965) concluded that *E. melis* oocysts seen by Zimmerman (1959) were actually oocysts of *E. ictidea*. Litvenkova (1969) did not describe the *E. ictidea* oocysts she found in one of three polecats in Belarus. Tinar (1985) measured oocysts from mink in Turkey, which were, L×W: 24.0×16.5 (23–28×15–19.5), L/W ratio: 1.5, with ovoidal sporocysts.

This species is a natural parasite of the black-footed ferret (*M. nigripes*) and the coccidiosis, diarrhea, and even death it causes is a problem primarily in ferret kits especially during their stressful weaning process during captivity (Williams et al., 1992; Jolley et al., 1994; Williams and Thorne, 1996). Jolley et al. (1994) said the oocysts they saw had a bilaminate wall and were, L×W (n=64): 23.2×15.5 (18–27×13–16), L/W ratio: 1.5; M and OR: both absent, but that a PG was formed. The sporocysts they described as elongate with a SB and a fine granular SR, but they gave no measurements, and the SZ had a prominent RB near their rounded end.

EIMERIA MUSTELAE IWANOFF-GOBZEM, 1934

Homonym: *Eimeria mustelae* (=*E. vison*) Kingscote, 1934a,b.

Type host: *Mustela nivalis* (L., 1766), Least Weasel.

Type locality: Asia: Kazakhstan (former USSR).

Other hosts: *Neovison vison* (Schreber, 1777) (syn. *Mustela vison* L., 1766), American Mink.

Geographic distribution: Asia: Kazakhstan, Turkmenistan (former USSR); Middle East: Turkey; Iceland; Europe: Austria (?); North America: USA: Illinois.

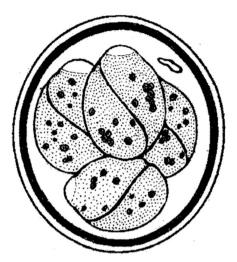

FIGURE 6.7 Original line drawing of the sporulated oocyst of *Eimeria mustelae*. *Modified from Fig. 4, Levine, N.D., 1948.* Eimeria *and* Isospora *in the mink (*Mustela vison*). Journal of Parasitology 34, 486–492, with permission from Allen Press, Inc., Lawrence, Kansas USA copyright holder.*

Description of sporulated oocyst: Oocyst shape: spheroidal or ellipsoidal; number of walls, 2; wall characteristics: outer is smooth, colorless, whereas inner is darker, almost appearing sculptured (original line drawing); L×W: 20 (18–26); L/W ratio: 1.0 for spheroidal forms and L×W: 22×19 (18–26×14–24); L/W 1.2 for ellipsoidal forms (Iwanoff-Gobzem, 1934, 1935); M, OR: both absent, but a PG is present. Distinctive features of oocyst: darker, inner oocyst wall and lacking M and OR, but having a distinct PG.

Description of sporocyst and sporozoites: Sporocyst shape: roughly ovoidal with a constriction at one end; L×W: 8×5; L/W ratio: 1.6; SB: present, as a large caplike structure; SSB, PSB: both absent; SR: present; SR characteristics: a few dispersed small granules; SZ: comma-shaped, broader at one end and pointed at the other, ~7×3; neither RB nor N were visible. Distinctive features of sporocyst: thin wall (line drawing), SR of only a few dispersed small granules, and presence of a large, cap-like SB.

Prevalence: Levine (1948) found this species in one mink from a fur farm in Illinois, USA. Frank

(1978) said she examined 40 *M. eversmanii* from "Illmitz in the European Soviet Union" (probably Austria), and found this species, but did not mention how many of the 40 were infected with it. Glebezdin (1978) examined three weasels in southwestern Turkmenistan and reported *E. mustelae* in two of them. Musaev and Veisov (1983) found it in 2/3 (66%) weasels in the Lenkoransk area in Azerbaijan. Tinar (1985) examined 181 samples from two mink farms around Ankara, Turkey, for coccidia; of these, 150 were fecal pellets (presumably from different individuals?), and the intestinal tracts from 31 animals. He reported this species in 11/181 (6%) samples. SkírNisson and Pálmadóttir (1993) reported oocysts of this species in 20/145 (14%) mink pups at 12/19 (63%) fur farms they surveyed in Iceland.

Sporulation: Exogenous. Oocysts sporulated in 3 days at room temperature in 2.5% aqueous potassium dichromate ($K_2Cr_2O_7$) solution.

Prepatent and patent periods: Unknown.

Site of infection: Unknown. Oocysts were recovered from feces and intestinal contents.

Endogenous stages: Unknown. However, Levine (1948) said he found a few oocysts in the duodenum, but most were in the ileum and large intestine.

Cross-transmission: None to date.

Pathology: Unknown.

Materials deposited: None.

Remarks: Kingscote (1934b) briefly described the sporulated oocysts of an *Eimeria* species he recovered in the summer of 1933, from the carcasses and feces of American mink, *N. vison*, which "had died from enteric coccidiosis" on ranches in Canada and the United States. He said that this eimerian was responsible for the disease of the mink, was an undescribed species, and for which he proposed to name, *Eimeria mustelae*. Unfortunately, he did not provide a line drawing or a photomicrograph of the sporulated oocyst, and without a type specimen to anchor the name it became a *species inquirenda*. While Kingscote was in the process of publishing a more complete description of his version of *E. mustelae*, the name became preoccupied when Iwanoff-Gobzem (1934), unaware of Kingscote's (1934b) name, used the same name to describe another eimerian from the weasel, *M. nivalis*, which was clearly different morphologically. As seemed to be par for the course at that time, Iwanoff-Gobzem (1934) described the oocysts she observed but published only a line drawing of two **un**sporulated oocysts (one spheroidal, one ellipsoidal) which, in our opinion, also rendered the form she named a *species inquirenda*. But Norman Levine (1948) came to the rescue when he published a more complete description of this mustelid eimerian and included a line drawing, which secured the name for Iwanoff-Gobzem (1934).

According to Levine (1948), oocysts in the mink were subspheroidal, L×W (n=50): 16×14 (13–18×12–15), L/W 1.1 (1.0–1.2), with a bilayered wall, lacking both M and OR, but a PG was present, and the oocysts he measured were somewhat smaller than those reported by Iwanoff-Gobzem (1934). Levine (1948) also never saw any spheroidal forms. Musaev and Veisov (1983) described spheroidal oocysts with a colorless, bilayered wall, ~2 thick. Their oocysts were, L×W: 23 (18–26) wide, L/W ratio, 1.0. Unfortunately, they measured only nine oocysts, only one of which was sporulated. Frank (1978) said she found this species in *M. nivalis* trapped near Lake Neusiedl, Austria, right on the border with Hungary but gave no morphological or prevalence data. In Turkey, Tinar (1985) measured oocysts from mink that were, L×W: 19.6×16.5 (16–23×15–19.5), L/W ratio: 1.2, with ovoidal sporocysts. The oocysts of this species reported by SkírNisson and Pálmadóttir (1993), in mink pups on fur farms in Iceland, were 14×13 (10–15×10–15). Glebezdin (1978) reported a survey on 2,350 wild mammals representing 25 species in southwestern Turkmenistan from 1974 to 1977; in *M. nivalis* he reported both spheroidal and ellipsoidal oocysts of *E. mustelae*; spheroidal forms were 20.8 (17–26) wide and ellipsoidal forms measured, L×W: 22.8×18.2(18–26×17–22);L/W ratio:1.1(1.0–1.2);

sporocysts were, L×W: 9.6×6.8 (8–11×6–8) L/W ratio: 1.4.

ISOSPORA ALTAICA SVANBAEV AND RACHMATULLINA, 1971

Type host: *Mustela altaica* Pallas, 1811, Mountain Weasel.

Remarks: This species name has been emended to *Cystoisospora altaica* N. Comb. (see Chapter 14, Sarcocystidae: Cystoisosporinae).

ISOSPORA GOUSSEVI MUSAEV AND VEISOV, 1983

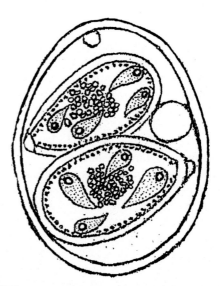

FIGURE 6.8   Original line drawing of the sporulated oocyst *of Isospora goussevi. From Fig. 3, Musaev, M.A., Veisov, A.M.M., 1983. New species of coccidia of the genera* Eimeria *and* Isospora *from weasel* (Mustela nivalis Lennans (sic), 1766). Izvestia Akademii Nauk Azerbaijdzhanskoi SSR, Seria Biologicheskich Nauk 5, 64–70. (in Russian). *Journal no longer exists, copyright not reassigned following collapse of the former USSR.*

Type host: *Mustela nivalis* (L., 1766), Least Weasel.

Type locality: Asia: Azerbaijan (former USSR).
Other hosts: None to date.

Geographic distribution: Asia: Azerbaijan.

Description of sporulated oocyst: Oocyst shape: ovoidal; number of walls, 1; wall characteristics: smooth, yellow, ~1.2 thick; L×W (n=14): 22.4×17.4 (22–25×16–19); L/W ratio: 1.4 (1.3–1.4); M: absent; OR: present as a spheroidal body, 4–5 wide; PG: present. Distinctive features of oocyst: presence of both PG and an OR.

Description of sporocyst and sporozoites: Sporocyst shape: ovoidal; L×W: 12×7 (10–13×6–8); L/W ratio: 1.7; SB: present as a nipple-like structure at one end of sporocyst; SSB: may also be present (line drawing); PSB: absent; SR: present; SR characteristics: small scattered granules in center of the SP (line drawing); SZ: elongate comma-shaped (line drawing), with a RB at the broadly rounded end. Distinctive features of sporocyst: small size, with both SB and SSB and a granular SR.

Prevalence: Musaev and Veisov (1983) measured 14 oocysts from a single weasel, but they did not say if this was the only one infected of the 14 weasels examined, or if there were others.

Sporulation: Exogenous. Oocysts sporulated in 96 hours in 2.5% aqueous $K_2Cr_2O_7$ at 25–30°C.

Prepatent and patent periods: Unknown.

Site of infection in definitive host: Unknown, although Musaev and Veisov (1983) said the oocysts they measured and described came from the contents of the large intestine.

Endogenous stages: Unknown.

Pathology: Unknown.

Materials deposited: None.

Etymology: This species was named after the Soviet protozoologist, Professor V.F. Goussev.

Remarks: There are other *Isospora*-like oocysts described from members of the genus *Mustela*, but all of them, to date, have sporocysts that lack a SB/SSB complex and this has led us to place such forms into the genus *Cystoisospora*, for reasons explained earlier. This species has not been reported since its original description, and it likely could be an isosporan from a bird the weasel had consumed, just passing through the intestine of this weasel.

ISOSPORA NIVALIS MUSAEV AND VEISOV, 1983

Type host: *Mustela nivalis* (L., 1766), Least Weasel.

Remarks: This species name has been emended to *Cystoisospora nivalis* N. Comb. (see Chapter 14, Sarcocystidae: Cystoisosporinae).

GENUS NEOVISON BARYSHNIKOV AND ABRAMOV, 1997 (2 SPECIES)

EIMERIA VISON (KINGSCOTE, 1934a,b) KINGSCOTE, 1935

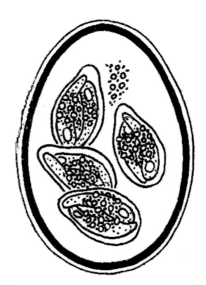

FIGURE 6.9 Original line drawing of the sporulated oocyst of *Eimeria vison*. *Modified from Fig. 12, Levine, N.D., Ivens, V., 1981. The Coccidian Parasites (Protozoa, Apicomplexa) of Carnivores, Illinois Biological Monograph No. 51. University of Illinois Press, Urbana, Illinois, USA, 249 p. The University of Illinois Press, Urbana, Illinois USA has released the copyright.*

Synonym: *Eimeria mustelae* Kingscote, 1934a,b; *Homonym*: *Eimeria mustelae* Iwanoff-Gobzem, 1934.

Type host: *Neovison vison* (Schreber, 1777) (syn. *Mustela vison* L., 1766), American Mink.

Type locality: North America: Canada: Ontario.

Other hosts: *Mustela* (syn. *Putorius*) *putorius furo* (L., 1758), European Polecat (Domestic Ferret).

Geographic distribution: Asia: Kazakhstan, Turkmenistan, Siberia (former USSR); Eastern Europe: Poland; Europe: Denmark, United Kingdom; Iceland; Middle East: Israel, Turkey; North America: Canada: Ontario; USA: Illinois, Wisconsin.

Description of sporulated oocyst: Oocyst shape: ovoidal; number of walls, 2; wall characteristics: ~0.75 thick, outer layer is thin, colorless, inner layer yellow–brown and thicker; L×W (n = 100): 20.3 × 14.6 (17–22 × 9–18); L/W ratio: 1.4; M, PG: both absent; OR: present as a small, granular body that is present immediately after sporulation is completed (Kingscote, 1934a,b). Distinctive features of oocyst: distinct ovoidal shape with a thick, dark inner wall, lacking M and PG, but with a granular OR.

Description of sporocyst and sporozoites: Sporocyst shape: pear-shaped; L×W: 10 × 5.5; L/W ratio: 1.8; SB, SSB, PSB: apparently all absent; SR: present; SR characteristics: spheroidal aggregation of small granules clustered in the center of SP; SZ: slightly curved, club-shaped, ~9.1 × 2.5, with one end slightly broader and the other tapered; a small RB is seen at the broader end, but a N was not visible. Distinctive features of sporocyst: pear shape, presence of a distinct SR, and absence of SB (?), SSB, PSB. We think it questionable that a SB was reported as not present, given the shape of the SP and that most SP of mammalian *Eimeria* species are known to possess a SB.

Prevalence: Kingscote (1934b) in his note in which he first named this form (as *E. mustelae*) said that "carcasses and feces of mink, which had died from enteric coccidiosis were obtained from the ranches in Canada and the United States," but he gave no numbers. In his follow-up paper (1934a) he mentioned that the "enzootic disease in an Ontario minkery… causes the death of many young animals and some adults," but again did not

mention prevalence. Levine (1948) said he found oocysts of this species in 1/2 (50%) mink, which had died suddenly in Illinois, USA; however, we believe he was dealing with a different species (see below). Zimmerman (1959) found *E. vison* in 21% of minks he examined in Poland. McTaggart (1960) found it in 3/200 (1.5%) minks from 42 farms in Britain. Klopfer and Neumann (1970) examined 92 mink fecal samples from nine farms in various parts of Israel and found 67/92 (73%) to be infected with oocysts of three coccidian species, which they identified as *E. vison*, *E. melis* (?), and *I.* (=*C.*) *laidlawi*; they were not precise in exactly how many infected minks shed oocysts of each of these three species stating, "In cases observed by us there was usually a mixed infestation of the two *Eimeria* species and of *Isospora*." Foreyt and Todd (1976) reported *E. vison* in mink on 18/29 (62%) mink ranches in Wisconsin, USA. Nukerbaeva and Svanbaev (1973, 1977) found it in 23/1,017 (2%) minks in Kazakhstan. Tinar (1985) examined 181 samples from two mink farms around Ankara, Turkey, for coccidia; of these, 150 were fecal pellets (presumably from different animals?), and the intestinal tracts from 31 animals. He found this species in 33/181 (18%) samples. SkírNisson and Pálmadóttir (1993) reported oocysts of this species in 9/145 (6%) mink pups at 4/19 (21%) fur farms they surveyed in Iceland. Hindsbo et al. (1995), in a long-term study (1986–93) in the middle of the island Zealander, Denmark, reported *E. vison* in mink kits, but not mink adults. Specifically, they examined 159 cages, each with one male and one female mink kits, and 139 adult minks; the mean prevalence of infection with *E. vison* (1987–93) in the kits was 6.4% (0%–22%). This allowed them to conclude there was a strong age-dependent resistance to this species in minks. The prevalence with *E. vison* in mink kits seen by Hindsbo et al. (1995) was lower than reported by Tinar (1985), and very much lower than the 83.5% infection rate reported by Jatusevich and Gerasimchik (1995).

Sporulation: Exogenous. Sporulation was almost completed on the 7th day when placed in 2.5% aqueous potassium dichromate ($K_2Cr_2O_7$)

solution at room temperature (Kingscote, 1934a,b), but Kingscote (1934a) said that sporozoites did not become perceptible (to him) until the 10th day after oocyst passage. However, in the same paper he said that the oocysts he recovered from experimental infections became infective on the seventh day PI. Levine (1948) said sporulation occurred in 3 days in $K_2Cr_2O_7$ solution at "room temperature," while McTaggart (1960) reported that oocysts took 5 days at "room temperature," Nukerbaeva and Svanbaev (1973) said sporulation was complete in 2–3 days, and Umurzakoff and Nukerbaeva (1985) reported sporulation to be 48–72 hours. This inconsistency presumably may be due to the differing "room temperatures."

Prepatent and patent periods: Prepatent period is 6 days and the patent period is 4 days according to Kingscote (1934a). In two different experiments, Nukerbaeva and Svanbaev (1974, 1977) infected minks with 100 and with 5,000 sporulated oocysts. Those receiving 5,000 oocysts started to discharge oocysts on day 6 PI, whereas those receiving 100 oocysts started patency on days 7 and 8 PI. Patency continued for about 15 days in both infections. Later, Umurzakoff and Nukerbaeva (1985) infected 12, 4.5–5-month-old minks with "various infective doses" of *E. vison* sporulated oocysts and said the prepatent period was 7 days and the patent period was 11 days.

Site of infection: Chiefly in the epithelial cells of the entire length of the small intestine according to Kingscote (1934a). Umurzakoff and Nukerbaeva (1985) said endogenous developmental stages were found both above and below the nucleus in epithelial cells of intestinal villi and that they localized in cells of the duodenum, jejunum, and ileum; they detected the highest number of stages in the central part of the small intestine.

Endogenous stages: Kingscote (1934a) studied and described endogenous development of this species in histological sections of the intestines of mink that had died during the course of the Ontario enzootic. Sporozoites became spheroidal shortly after cell invasion and began development in the supranuclear position, i.e., between the N and the cell's brush boarder. Early

development took place in the free extremity of the villus. As young meronts (M_1) increased in size, nuclear division produced 20–35 merozoites (m_1) that elongated and became spindle-shaped. Kingscote (1934a) did not know the exact number of merogonous stages but suggested that there were at least two types of meronts. As the number of merozoites increased via merogony, they penetrated further and further into the crypts of Lieberkühn, eventually invading and destroying the entire length of the epithelium of a villus, including the Goblet cells. After the final merogony, merozoites invaded cells in adjoining crypts to begin gamogony. These developing stages "increase rapidly in size and destroy the tissues that nourish them." The majority of gametocytes, according to Kingscote (1934a) became macrogametocysts; once fertilization occurred, developing zygotes and young oocysts increased in size, distended the crypts to several times their normal diameter and were gradually forced to the surface where they accumulated in white masses visible to the naked eye. Kingscote (1934a) estimated that each oocyst ingested resulted in the passage of app. 10,000 new oocysts. Unfortunately, Kingscote (1934a) did not measure any of the endogenous stages.

Umurzakoff and Nukerbaeva (1985), who experimentally-infected 20 5-month-old minks with $4-5 \times 10^5$ sporulated oocysts, found three merogonous stages preceding gamogony. Both young and mature M_1 were seen in duodenal epithelial cells 72 hours PI. They were spheroidal to ovoidal in shape, $L \times W$: 5.6–9.8 × 5.6; mature M_1 contained 8–12 m_1 that were 5 × 1.5, slightly curved, with one end more pointed than the other, and a mostly central N. The much larger M_2 measured, $L \times W$: 10–17 × 10–13, and were seen in the middle small intestine 140 hours PI; these contained 25–30 sausage-shaped, lightly curved m_2 that were 8.2 × 1.5, with a central N. Umurzakoff and Nukerbaeva (1985) then reported an unusual twist in this life cycle. They said that gamonts were seen in high numbers 168 hours PI. Young microgametocytes had a light cytoplasm and many small N that produced 90–100 elongated microgametes by multiple (mitotic?) divisions. These mature microgametocytes were asymmetrical-ovoidal in shape and, L×W: 11.2–19.6×8.4–14 in size. Macrogamonts had a very large N and wall-forming granules that increased in number as the macrogamont matured. Mature gamonts were reported to be ovoidal, L×W: 12.2–15.4×8.0–11.2. The twist to this cycle is that at 221 hours PI, after observing both micro- and macrogametes in abundance, Umurzakoff and Nukerbaeva (1985) saw a third generation of meronts that differed in size and in number of merozoites from the M_1 and M_2. These (presumably) M_3 were, L×W: 12–14×8.4–13.2, and contained 18–26 sickle-shaped m_3 that measured 5.5×0.5. Detecting these third-generation meronts and merozoites led the authors to conclude that merozoites produced from both M_2 and M_3 can "bring sexual stages into being." Developing unsporulated oocysts were seen both in epithelial cells and in the gut lumen beginning 172 hours PI and unsporulated oocysts were ovoidal, L×W: 19.5–26.7×15.2–16.4.

Cross-transmission: Kingscote (1934a,b) said he repeated fecal tests on a mink and two ferrets and found them to be free of coccidian oocysts. He then fed these three hosts "numbers of oocysts" (of *E. vison*) and "6 days later a mink and two ferrets commenced to pass oocysts, which disappeared entirely after 4 days" (Kingscote, 1934a). He also fed oocysts to two kittens, a rabbit, and a guinea pig, but these experimental recipients failed to become infected. Nukerbaeva and Svanbaev published two papers (1974, 1977) in which they added some confusion to the cross-transmission work they did with *Eimeria* and *Isospora* (=*Cystoisospora*) species from mink, foxes, cats, and dogs. Their 1977 cross-transmission paper was a duplicate of their 1974 paper, except for the tables that summarized their experiments. In their 1974 paper, the only Table they presented (page 37) said they infected a 5-month-old **mink** (Number 9) with oocysts of

E. vison from another mink and it began discharging oocysts on the sixth day PI. However, their 1977 paper (Table 12, page 79) introduced a typographical error that the oocysts of *E. vison* from a mink infected a 5-month-old **fox** (Number 9) that began discharging oocysts on the sixth day PI. Nukerbaeva and Svanbaev (1974, 1977) were not able to transmit this species from the mink to two 5-month-old foxes, *V. vulpes*, to two 5-month-old Arctic foxes, *V. lagopus*, or to a domestic dog, *C. lupus familiaris*. Nukerbaeva (1981a) used $5–7×10^3$ oocysts of *E. vison* from mink and infected two sables (*M. zibellina*), but they did not discharge oocysts. However, he did not state how long PI he continued to examine the animals for oocysts in their feces. Nukerbaeva (1981a) also used a mixture of $5–7×10^3$ oocysts of *E. furonis* and *E. vison* from mink to infect another mink and said he found oocysts in the feces on days 4–7 PI (presumably, respectively, for each eimerian, but this was not stated).

Pathology: During endogenous development there is rapid and extensive destruction of the intestinal epithelium. As the mucosa becomes progressively damaged, localized areas are devoid of their protective epithelial cells throughout the length of the small intestine. This destruction of epithelium results in exposure of underlying tissue, in which capillaries become congested, readily rupture, and numerous such hemorrhages result in bloody diarrhea. In long-standing infections, proliferation of fibrous connective tissue is conspicuous at the tips of the villi, which become swollen. Finally, this desquamation of the protective epithelium opens up numerous avenues for bacteria to enter the circulation to cause secondary infections, acute enteritis, or even systemic infections. In early stages of disease, minks do not leave their boxes and are hypersensitive to noise and movement. As the disease progresses, the stools become coated with mucous, streaked with blood, and ultimately, hemorrhagic diarrhea develops. At the same time, animals become increasingly weak, walk with an unsteady gait, the front paws turn inward, while the hindquarters often are swollen, and eventually become paralyzed. Their eyes protrude, and their coat becomes rough and lusterless, their temperature may reach 105°F, and their pulse becomes feeble and difficult to detect. In the terminal stage of disease they become susceptible to *Staphylococcus* infections that manifest as the formation of large boils at the site of any external injuries, usually around the head and neck (Kingscote, 1934a).

Materials deposited: None.

Remarks: Kingscote (1934b) published a short note naming a new coccidium, *Eimeria mustelae* from the American mink, *N. vison* (syn. *Mustela vison*); oocysts were described as noted above, but the description was somewhat incomplete and there was no line drawing or photomicrograph. Thus, without a type specimen to anchor the name, it became a *species inquirenda*. Kingscote (1934a) then published a more detailed description of *E. mustelae* along with a good line drawing, description of some endogenous stages, and photomicrographs of a sporulated oocyst, and infected tissue sections. He later realized that, however, while his second paper was in preparation or in press, the name *E. mustelae* became preoccupied because Iwanoff-Gobzem (1934) had used this name to describe a completely different species from *Mustela nivalis*, a weasel, from the USSR. Thus, Kingscote (1935) proposed *Eimeria vison* as a substitute for the homonym, and the detailed description, line drawing, and photomicrographs of tissue sections provided for *E. mustelae* by Kingscote (1934a,b) are actually for *E. vison*.

In commenting on the disease caused by *E. vison*, Kingscote (1934a) noted that many others had recognized a disease condition due to coccidiosis in mink in Germany, former Czechoslovakia, and other parts of Europe, and in Nebraska, Minnesota, and New York state in the United States, and he said that in 1933,

an enzootic disease in an Ontario mink farm caused the death of many young animals and some adults, leaving the survivors stunted; he later diagnosed the outbreak as due to coccidiosis caused by an *Eimeria* species for which he described the structure of the sporulated oocyst, part of the life cycle (endogenous stages), and some of the pathology (Kingscote, 1934a). He wrote that the disease occurred most frequently in the summer and early fall months, with most fatalities occurring from June through September, and he pointed out that unless the strictest sanitation is practiced, it soon spreads from pen to pen in mink ranches, and that kits and females seem to be the most susceptible. Fecal examinations showed that many animals can be carriers but show no obvious signs of sickness.

Levine (1948) also described oocysts from *N. vison* that had slightly larger dimensions than those given by Kingscote (1934a,b), but he felt they were sufficiently similar to it, to be the same species. Unfortunately, Levine (1948) was unaware of Kingscote's (1934a) paper, which we noted by its absence from his *References* section. We believe that Dr. Levine was observing oocysts of another *Eimeria* species, which we describe and name, below. According to McTaggart (1960), *E. vison* oocysts were ellipsoidal, sometimes ovoidal, or subspheroidal, with a bilayered wall, the outer is colorless and the inner is straw-colored; L×W (n=100): 22×15 (16.5–26×12–16.5); L/W ratio, 1.5 (1.2–1.9); M, OR: both absent. Nukerbaeva and Svanbaev (1973) said oocysts from mink in Kazakhstan were ovoidal to ellipsoidal with a bilayered wall, ~1.5 thick, and L×W: 20–22×14–15; their sporocysts were 7–10×6 with an SR, and SZs were 6×3. In a later survey (Nukerbaeva and Svanbaev, 1977) the *E. vision* oocysts they measured were, L×W: 24×15 (20–28×15–17). Foreyt and Todd (1976) collected 323 fecal samples on 29 mink ranches (22 counties) in Wisconsin, USA, from June to December, 1975. They found that 45/79 (57%) mink samples collected from ranches that fed dry pelleted rations contained coccidian oocysts, whereas 128/244 (52%) samples from ranches that fed a wet meat mixture contained oocysts. *Eimeria vison* was identified in minks on 18/29 (62%) of the ranches, but the number of animals with this species was not mentioned; only that "the coccidia of domestic mink in Wisconsin are prevalent and widespread." Tinar (1985) measured oocysts from mink in Turkey, which were, L×W: 23.2×16.4 (21–26×15–19.5), L/W ratio: 1.4, with spheroidal sporocysts. The oocysts of this species reported by SkírNisson and Pálmadóttir (1993), in mink pups on fur farms in Iceland, were L×W: 25×17 (22–31×15–19).

EIMERIA VISONLEVINEI (LEVINE, 1948) N. SP.

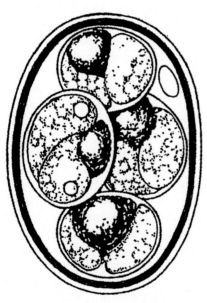

FIGURE 6.10 Line drawing of the sporulated oocyst *of Eimeria visonlevinei. Fig. 3, from Levine, N.D., 1948.* Eimeria *and* Isospora *in the mink (*Mustela vison*). Journal of Parasitology 34, 486–492, with permission from Allen Press, Inc., Lawrence, Kansas USA copyright holder.*

Synonym: *Eimeria vison* Levine, 1948.
Type host: *Neovison vison* (Schreber, 1777) (syn. *Mustela vison* L., 1766), American Mink.

Type locality: North America: USA: Illinois.
Other hosts: None to date.
Geographic distribution: North America: USA.
Description of sporulated oocyst: Oocyst shape: ellipsoidal; number of walls, 2; wall characteristics: outer is colorless, smooth, and inner is pale salmon pink, ~1.2 thick; L×W (n=100): 22.8×15.4 (20–26×13–17); L/W ratio: 1.5 (1.3–1.9); M, OR: both absent; PG: present as 1 to 4 or 5 refractile granules (however, Levine's line drawing showed only 1 ellipsoidal PG). Distinctive features of oocyst: distinct ellipsoidal shape, lacking M and OR, but 1 or more PG present.

Description of sporocyst and sporozoites: Sporocyst shape: ellipsoidal; L×W: 11×8 (ranges not given); L/W ratio: 1.4; SB, SSB, PSB: apparently all absent (line drawing) and not mentioned in the written description; SR: present; SR characteristics: large, coarsely granular, compact body in each SP (line drawing); SZ: broadly comma-shaped (line drawing), 9×3 in size, with a small RB at the broadly rounded end. Distinctive features of sporocyst: small size, lacking SB, SSB, PSB, but having a compact, granular SR.

Prevalence: Oocysts were recovered in 2/2 minks, which had died suddenly on a mink ranch in Illinois, USA (Levine, 1948).

Sporulation: Exogenous. Oocysts sporulated in 3 days in 2.5% aqueous $K_2Cr_2O_7$ at room temperature (Levine, 1948).

Prepatent and patent periods: Unknown.
Site of infection in definitive host: Unknown; however, Levine (1948) said, "a few oocysts were found in the duodenum, but they were more abundant in the ileum and large intestine."

Endogenous stages: Unknown.
Pathology: Unknown.
Materials deposited: None.
Etymology: For simplicity, we are combining Dr. Norman D. Levine's name to the specific epitaph he first used when, in our opinion, he misidentified the oocysts he found in Illinois mink as being those of *E. vison*.

Remarks: Levine (1948), apparently, was unaware of the detailed publication in which Kingscote (1934a) described the sporulated oocysts and some of the endogenous developmental stages of *E. vison* (as *E. mustelae*, before he had to change the name; see explanation under *E. vison*, above). The oocysts described by Levine (1948) differ significantly from those of *E. vison* (syn. *E. mustelae*), as described from mink by Kingscote (1934a). Their line drawings are quite distinctly different; *E. vison* oocysts are ovoidal, whereas oocysts described by Levine (1948) are distinctly ellipsoidal. Oocysts of *E. vison* as described by Kingscote (1934a) are, L × W: 20.3 × 14.6 (17–22 × 9–18), L/W ratio, 1.4 versus those described by Levine (1948), which are, L × W: 22.9 × 15.4 (20–25 × 15–16), L/W ratio, 1.5. Sporocysts of *E. vison* described by Kingscote (1934a) are pear-shaped, with one pointed end, L × W: 10 × 5.5, L/W ratio, 1.8 versus those described by Levine (1948), which are ellipsoidal, L × W: 11 × 8, L/W ratio, 1.4. Another big difference in the two descriptions is the sporulation times; Kingscote (1934a) said that sporulation continued from the 2nd to the 8th day and then, "on about the 10th day after the passage of the oocysts from the host, two sporozoites become perceptible within each sporocyst." Levine wrote, "sporulation was complete 3 days after the oocysts had been placed in a thin layer of 2.5% potassium dichromate in a Petri dish at room temperature." Lastly, Kingscote's (1934a) oocysts have a granular OR, but no PG, whereas Levine's oocysts have 1–5 PG, but no OR. For these reasons, we believe that Levine (1948) was looking at oocysts that were different than those first seen and described by Kingscote (1934a). Finally, Levine (1948) noted that the sporulated oocysts he found in the mink from Illinois, USA, were morphologically similar to those of *E. sibirica* from *M. zibellina*, sable; to those of *E. irara* from *Eira* (syn. *Galera*) *barbara*, tayra; and to those of *E. ictidea*, from *M. p. furo*, European polecat (domestic ferret).

He suggested that future experimental cross-infection studies might reduce them to synonymy. Clearly there is a need here for molecular studies to intervene.

ISOSPORA BIGEMINA (STILES, 1901) LÜHE, 1906

Synonyms: *Cytospermium villorum intestinalium canis* Rivolta, 1878, nomen nudum; *Coccidium rivolta* Grassi, 1879, *pro parte*; *Coccidium rivoltae* Leuckart, 1886, *pro parte*; *Coccidium bigeminum* Stiles, 1891, *pro parte*; *Coccidium bigeminum* var. *canis* Railliet and Lucet, 1891; *Diplospora bigemina* Martin, 1909; *Coccidium bigeminum* Wigdor, 1918, *pro parte*; *Isospora cati* Marotel, 1922, *pro parte*; *Lucetina bigemina* (Stiles, 1891) Henry and Leblois, 1926; *Isospora bigenina* Gousseff, 1933, lapsus; *Isospora bigemina* var. *bahiensis* de Moura Costa, 1956 (from Pellérdy, 1974a).

Type host: *Canis lupus familiaris* (syn. *C. familiaris*), L., 1758, Domestic Dog.

Other hosts: *Neovison vison* (Schreber, 1777) (syn. *Mustela vison* L., 1766), American Mink.

Remarks: This species has long been an enigma for parasitologists. Credit for the first naming, *Coccidium bigemina*, is given to Stiles (1891) for a parasite he saw developing in the lamina propria of a dog (Dubey and Fayer, 1976; Lindsay et al., 1997). In 1906, it was transferred to the genus *Isospora*, but the organism seen by Stiles (1891) is now known to clearly be a species of *Sarcocystis* (Lindsay et al., 1997). Wenyon (1926a) said there were two "races" of *I. bigemina*, differentiated by oocyst size, with the larger race developing in the lamina propria and excreted as sporulated oocysts or sporocysts (i.e., clearly a *Sarcocystis* species) and the smaller race developing in epithelial cells of the small intestine and excreted as unsporulated oocysts. This smaller "race" in dogs is now known to be *Hammondia heydorni*, which is obligatorily heteroxenous (Heydorn et al., 1975b; Lindsay et al., 1997). A small race of *I. bigemina* also is frequently reported from cats, but its oocysts are indistinguishable from those of *Toxoplasma gondii*, *Hammondia hammondi*, and some *Besnoitia* species.

ISOSPORA EVERSMANNI SVANBAEV, 1956

Type host: *Mustela eversmanii* Lesson, 1827, Steppe Polecat.

Remarks: This species name was emended to *Cystoisospora eversmanni* by Yi-Fan et al. (2012) (see Chapter 14, Sarcocystidae: Cystoisosporinae).

ISOSPORA LAIDLAWI HOARE, 1935a,b

Type host: *Mustela* (syn. *Putorius*) *putorius furo* (L., 1758), European Polecat (Domestic Ferret).

Remarks: This species name has been emended to *Cystoisospora laidlawi* Hoare, 1927, N. Comb. (see Chapter 14, Sarcocystidae: Cystoisosporinae).

ISOSPORA PAVLOVSKYI SVANBAEV, 1956

Type host: *Mustela eversmanii* Lesson, 1827, Steppe Polecat.

Remarks: This species name was emended to *Cystoisospora pavlovskyi* by Yi-Fan et al. (2012) (see Chapter 14, Sarcocystidae: Cystoisosporinae).

DISCUSSION AND SUMMARY

Other than the Canidae and Felidae, the members of the Mustelidae have been studied for internal parasites more than the other Carnivore families. Certainly, the value of the mink pelt trade and the desire to save the critically-endangered black-footed ferret are contributing

factors. Nonetheless, there still exists a tremendous ignorance about the apicomplexan coccidians that parasitize them. To our knowledge, the following 15 (of 22) Mustelidae genera and their 23 species do not have, and likely, have not been looked at for, intestinal eimeriid coccidia: *Aonyx* Lesson 1827 (2 species); *Enhydra* Flemming, 1822 (monotypic); *Hydrictis* Pocock, 1921 (monotypic); *Lontra* Gray, 1843 (4 species); *Lutrogale* Gray, 1865 (monotypic); *Pteronura* Gray, 1837 (monotypic); *Arctonyx* F.G. Cuvier, 1825 (monotypic); *Galictis* Bell, 1826 (2 species); *Gulo* Pallas, 1780 (monotypic); *Lycodon* Gervais, 1845 (monotypic); *Mellivora* Storr, 1780 (monotypic); *Melogale* I. Geoffroy Saint-Hilaire, 1831 (4 species); *Poecilogale* Thomas, 1883 (monotypic); *Taxidea* Waterhouse, 1839 (monotypic); *Vormela* Blasius, 1884 (monotypic). Species of seven mustelid genera have been studied in this regard, but only 9 of their combined 36 extant species have been looked at for coccidia, and from these 9 host species, 10 *Eimeria*, 12 *Cystoisospora*, 1 *Isospora*, and 1 *Hammondia* are known. In total, then, only 7/22 (32%) genera and 9/59 (15%) mustelid species have been studied, but most only once or on a very limited scale.

If we are to be able to understand whether closely related mustelids share and/or have similar or related eimerians, we need to understand which host species are most closely related to each other. Koepfli et al. (2008), using ~12,000 base pairs of mitochondrial and nuclear DNA from 22 gene segments, used multiple phylogenetic algorithms that resolved the Mustelidae into seven primary divisions of four major clades and three monotypic lineages.

The otters formed one clade, Lutrinae, which includes the seven genera listed above from Wilson and Reeder (2005). It is the sister clade to Mustelinae that includes the mink (*Neovison*) and true weasels (*Mustela*). These clades, in turn, are sister to a clade, Galictinae, which includes weasel-like species with aposematically-colored pelage (*Galictis*, *Ictonyx*, *Poecilogale*, *Vormela*). Ferret badgers (*Melogale*) form the fourth clade,

Helictidinae, a monotypic lineage that is sister to these three combined clades. The fifth major clade of Koepfli et al. (2008), Martinae, has two subclades, one with the hog-nosed and Eurasian badgers (*Arctonyx, Meles*), and the other containing the tayra (*Eira*), wolverine (*Gulo*), and martens (*Martes*). Finally, Koepfli et al. (2008) said that the earliest divergent species in their phylogenetic tree were the American badger (*Taxidea*) and then the honey badger (*Mellivora*), which form successive monotypic clades/lineages that are sister to all other mustelid genera. Their topology, however, is highly incongruent with a cladistic analysis based on morphology by Bryant et al. (1993).

Koepfli et al. (2008) used ancestral reconstruction of biogeographic areas to show that most of the modern diversification of the mustelids occurred in Eurasia, results consistent with two other observations, suggesting Eurasia was the center of mustelid diversification: (1) Eurasia contains the majority of extant species, with 34/59 (58%) known species either exclusively endemic to or having part of their distribution on, this continent; and (2) the earliest fossils of extant lineages, or those associated with the ancestors of extant lineages, are often found in Eurasia (Hunt, 1996). The mustelid fauna of Africa, North, and South America are composed of taxa from nearly all major clades/lineages, suggesting that *in situ* speciation has been a relatively minor component in the assembly of these faunas, and the combined molecular and fossil data suggest that different lineages of mustelids dispersed to Africa, North, and South America in successive waves (Koepfli et al., 2008). These kinds of modern studies give us a good idea of how the various mustelids are related and from whence and where they arrived. Now it behooves parasitologists to take to the field and gather the parasite data that will help them make sense of all the interesting host–parasite relationships waiting to be discovered.

Eimeriidae in the Caniformia Families Odobenidae, Otariidae, and Phocidae

EIMERIIDAE IN THE ODOBENIDAE ALLEN, 1880, OTARIIDAE GRAY, 1825, AND PHOCIDAE, GRAY, 1821

INTRODUCTION

Wilson and Reeder (2005) listed only the single genus *Odobenus*, with 1 species, *O. rosmarus*, the walrus, in the Odobenidae. There are 3 subspecies of walrus found throughout the Arctic regions, with Pacific walruses (*O. rosmarus divergens*) found in and around the Bering Sea, the Atlantic walrus (*O. rosmarus rosmarus*) found in the eastern and western Atlantic, and the Laptev walrus (*O. rosmarus laptevi*) found in the Laptev Sea. The Odobenidae and Otariidae share a common ancestor from which they diverged 19.5 (16.8–22.1) million years ago (MYA) (Hedges et al., 2006; Kumar and Hedges, 2011; Kumar et al., 2017). Walruses are distinct because of their size (males can exceed 1,200 kg, females up to 850 kg) and because both sexes have very large canine teeth (tusks) that can be up to 100 cm in males and 60 cm in females. Walruses are highly gregarious and can form herds of >2,000 individuals. One might expect

that aggregating in dense herds would facilitate fecal–oral transmission of directly-transmitted parasites and pathogens including coccidia and they would be common in walruses, but there have been no studies to test this perception.

There are 7 genera and 16 species in the Otariidae, the fur seals and sea lions, and, as noted above, they shared a common ancestor with the Odobenidae. *Callorhinus* is the most ancient genus in the family diverging from other otariids 9.6 (7.0–12.2) MYA. Approximately 6 (4.6–9.2) MYA, the remaining lineage split into two branches, one diverging 5.7 (3.4–7.9) MYA into *Zalophus* and *Eumetopias* and the second split 6.3 (3.9–8.6) MYA with one branch leading to the *Arctocephalus* and the second diverging 5.6 (2.9–8.3) MYA, giving rise to *Otaria* and the remaining branch splitting again 4.64 (2.87–6.42) MYA into the genera *Neophoca* and *Phocarctos* (Hedges et al., 2006; Kumar and Hedges, 2011; Kumar et al., 2017).

Species in the Otariidae are found on the coasts of the Pacific Ocean including North and South America, central and northern Asia, and on islands including the Galápagos archipelago. Otariids vary considerably in size ranging from 150–1,000 kg with males typically larger than females. Fur seals have a dense underfur that, at one time, made their pelts valuable and which

© 2018 Donald W. Duszynski published by Elsevier Inc. All rights reserved.

led to intense harvesting that drove many species close to extinction. Like many marine mammals, otariids are highly social and gather in large colonies during the breeding season where males oversee harems of females. Their high density in these colonies seems ideal for coccidia transmission.

There are 13 genera with 19 species of true or earless seals in the Phocidae, the ancestors of which diverged from a common ancestor with the Otariidae and Odobenidae, about 26 (23.1–28.9) MYA. This ancestral lineage split into two major clades 18.4 (15.0–21.8) MYA. One diverged 15.1 (12.3–17.9) MYA into the genus *Erignathus* and a branch that split 10 (6.2–13.9) MYA into the genera *Cystophora* and *Phoca*. The second major clade diverged several times to give rise to the genera *Monachus* (~13.5 MYA), *Mirounga* (~11.1 MYA), *Lobodon* (~7.6 MYA), *Ommatophoca* (~6.9 MYA), and finally *Leptonychotes* and *Hydrurga* (~4.74 MYA) (Hedges et al., 2006; Kumar and Hedges, 2011; Kumar et al., 2017). The Phocidae typically occur on coastlines above 30°N and 50°S latitude, and a few species are found on tropical coastlines and freshwater lakes and rivers. Seals vary in size from 90 kg ring seals to 3,600 kg elephant seals. Unlike otariids, seals lack external ears, and they are highly adapted to their aquatic environments; some species can dive to great depths for extended periods. The Weddell seal can dive to 600 m and stay underwater for up to 1 hour. Social structure and mating behaviors vary, but in general seals do not form large rookeries during the breeding season (Myers, 2000b). As mentioned for other gregarious marine mammals, one might expect eimeriid intestinal coccidia to be common in seals, but this is not necessarily true, as we see in this chapter. There are several reports of bona fide species of *Cystoisospora* (Chapter 14), *Sarcocystis* (Chapter 15), *Toxoplasma*, *Hammondia* or *Neospora* (Chapter 16), and *Cryptosporidium* (Chapter 17) reported in/from the marine mammals in these 3 families, but most reports of both the heteroxenous and homoxenous apicomplexans in marine mammals list them only as "sp." and the majority of these are given in Chapter 19. Below we cover only the monoxenous, intestinal Eimeriidae from these hosts.

SPECIES DESCRIPTIONS ODOBENIDAE

There are no eimeriid coccidians known from the only species of this carnivore family.

SPECIES DESCRIPTIONS OTARIIDAE

GENUS ARCTOCEPHALUS É. GEOFFROY SAINT-HILAIRE AND F.G. CUVIER, 1826 (8 SPECIES)

CYSTOISOSPORA ISRAELI KUTTIN AND KALLER, 1992

Type host: *Arctocephalus pusillus* (Schreber, 1775), Brown (South African) Fur Seal.

Remarks: Kuttin and Kaller (1992) described this species from the brown South African fur seal in Israel (See Chapter 14, Sarcocystidae: Cystoisosporinae).

GENUS OTARIA PÉRON, 1816 (MONOTYPIC)

Remarks: There is a single report (Iskander, 1984) of unsporulated oocysts in the feces and gametocytes in the intestinal epithelium scraped from the small intestine of a dead 5-year-old sea lion, *O. flavescens* (Shaw, 1800) (syn. *O. byronia* (de Blainville, 1820)), in the Giza Zoological Garden, Egypt. These unsporulated oocysts were identified by Iskander (1984) as *Isospora bigemina*, which we now know to be *Hammondia heydorni* (Lindsay et al., 1997) (see Chapter 16). However, the reliability of this identification is highly questionable because the oocysts were never allowed to sporulate and examined after sporocysts and sporozoites had formed. Thus, it is questionable how Iskander (1984) could have identified this coccidian to genus, let alone guess its species.

SPECIES DESCRIPTIONS
PHOCIDAE

GENUS *HALICHOERUS* NILSSON, 1820 (MONOTYPIC)

EIMERIA PHOCAE HSU, MELBY, AND ALTMAN, 1974a

Type host: *Phoca vitulina concolor* De Kay, 1842, Harbor Seal.

Other hosts: *Halichoerus grypus* (Fabricius, 1791) (?), Gray Seal.

Remarks: McClelland (1993) said that "fatal haemorrhagic enteritis associated with *Eimeria* sp. infection was… diagnosed in August 1992 in gray seals *H. grypus*," suggesting the infectious agent was *E. phocae*, but this statement is questionable. See *Remarks* under *E. phocae*, Genus *Phoca* (below).

GENUS *LEPTONYCHOTES* GILL, 1872 (MONOTYPIC)

EIMERIA ARCTOWSKI DRÓŻDŻ, 1987

See Dróżdż (1987, Fig. 4) for a modest photomicrograph of a sporulated (?) oocyst, which we are not able to reproduce here.

Type host: *Leptonychotes weddellii* (Lesson, 1826), Weddell Seal.

Type locality: Europe: South Shetlands, King George Island.

Other hosts: None to date.

Geographic distribution: Europe: South Shetlands.

Description of sporulated oocyst: Oocyst shape: ellipsoidal to "barrel-shaped;" number of walls, 2, ~2 thick; wall characteristics: covered with numerous small protuberances on entire surface; L × W: 46.0 × 28.1 (44–48 × 24–30); L/W ratio: 1.6; M: present as a funnel-shaped invagination of oocyst wall, ~5 wide; OR, PG: unknown and cannot be determined from the photomicrograph presented. Distinctive features of oocyst: thick rough wall covered with protuberances and a funnel-shaped M, ~5 wide.

Description of sporocyst and sporozoites: Sporocyst shape: not mentioned, but appear mostly subspheroidal in the photomicrograph; L × W: described only as 14–18 long; L/W ratio: unknown; SB: may be present, but we cannot tell for sure from the photomicrograph; SSB, PSB: both absent; SR: present; SR characteristics: large coarse granules (photomicrograph); SZ: no information given. Distinctive features of sporocyst: none.

Prevalence: Dróżdż (1987) said he found this "species" in 10/65 (15%) *L. weddellii* examined.

Sporulation: Exogenous, 7–10 days according to Dróżdż (1987), but he did not give details on the method used to make this determination.

Prepatent and patent periods: Unknown.

Site of infection: Unknown.

Endogenous stages: Unknown.

Cross-transmission: None to date.

Pathology: Unknown.

Materials deposited: None.

Remarks: By current standards, the description of this species is substandard and inadequate; however, Dróżdż (1987) published one photomicrograph of a (presumably) sporulated oocyst that allowed us to determine the structure of the sporocysts, which was not stated in his description. To our knowledge, this "species" has not been seen again since its original description, but… has anyone looked?

EIMERIA WEDDELLI DRÓŻDŻ, 1987

See Dróżdż (1987, Fig. 3) for a modest photomicrograph of a sporulated oocyst, which we are not able to reproduce here.

Type host: *Leptonychotes weddellii* (Lesson, 1826), Weddell Seal.

Type locality: Europe: South Shetlands, King George Island.

Other hosts: None to date.

Geographic distribution: Europe: South Shetlands.

Description of sporulated oocyst: Oocyst shape: ellipsoidal to slightly ovoidal; number of walls, 2, ~2 thick; wall characteristics: smooth, yellow-brown; L×W: 48.1×29.6 (45–52×28–30); L/W ratio: 1.6; M: present, ~3 wide; OR, PG: both absent, as best we can determine from the photomicrograph presented. Distinctive features of oocyst: large ellipsoidal with distinct M and lacking (?) OR and PG.

Description of sporocyst and sporozoites: Sporocyst shape: not mentioned, but appeared mostly spheroidal to subspheroidal in the photomicrograph; L×W: described only as 12–16 long; L/W ratio: unknown; SB: unknown if one is present, and we cannot determine if present or absent from the photomicrograph; SSB, PSB: both absent; SR: present; SR characteristics: large coarse granules or a few spheroidal globules (photomicrograph); SZ: no information given. Distinctive features of sporocyst: none.

Prevalence: Dróżdż (1987) said he found this "species" in 14/65 (21.5%) *L. weddellii* examined.

Sporulation: Exogenous, 9–10 days according to Dróżdż (1987), but he did not give details on the method used to make this determination.

Prepatent and patent periods: Unknown.

Site of infection: Unknown.

Endogenous stages: Unknown.

Cross-transmission: None to date.

Pathology: Unknown.

Materials deposited: None.

Remarks: By current standards, the description of this species is substandard and inadequate; however, Dróżdż (1987) published one photomicrograph of a (presumably) sporulated oocyst, which allowed us to determine some of the structures of the sporocysts that were not stated in his description. To our knowledge, this "species" has not been seen again since its original description. Dróżdż (1987) also "described" other unsporulated oocysts recovered in small numbers from *L. weddellii* feces that he referred to as "*Eimeria* species 2" and "*Eimeria* species 3." These unsporulated oocysts differed in external morphology from the others he found in Weddell seals, but because they were unsporulated, it was premature to place them into the genus *Eimeria*. These forms are relegated to *species inquirenda* (see Chapter 19).

GENUS *LOBODON* GRAY, 1844 (MONOTYPIC)

Remarks: Dróżdż (1987) described unsporulated oocysts recovered from crabeater seal (*L. carcinophagus*) feces that he referred to as "*Eimeria* species 1." However, because these oocysts never sporulated, it was premature to place them in the genus *Eimeria*. This form is relegated to *species inquirenda* (see Chapter 19).

GENUS *MIROUNGA* GRAY, 1827 (2 SPECIES)

ISOSPORA MIRUNGAE DRÓŻDŻ, 1987

Type host: *Mirounga leonina* (L., 1758), Southern Elephant Seal.

Remarks: This species name has been emended to *Cystoisospora mirungae* N. Comb. (see Chapter 14, Sarcocystidae: Cystoisosporinae).

GENUS PHOCA L., 1758
(2 SPECIES)

EIMERIA PHOCAE HSU, MELBY, AND ALTMAN, 1974a

Type host: *Phoca vitulina concolor* De Kay, 1842, Harbor Seal.

Type locality: North America: USA: Maine, Portland.

Other hosts: *Halichoerus grypus* (Fabricius, 1791) (?), Gray Seal.

Geographic distribution: North America: Canada: Nova Scotia, Sable Island; USA: Maine; Europe: Scotland: Shetland Islands.

Description of sporulated oocyst: Oocyst shape: ellipsoidal to slightly ovoidal; number of walls, 2, >3 in total thickness; wall characteristics: outer layer, ~¾ of total thickness, brownish-yellow, speckled, granular, rough with fine striations; inner is smooth, clear; L × W (n = 100): 43.9 × 26.6 (38–50 × 21–32); L/W ratio: 1.65; M: present, slightly sunken, ~4.4 wide; OR: 1–2 ovoidal or spheroidal masses present of many coarse granules; PG: 1 always present, prominent. Distinctive features of oocyst: large size, rough outer wall with distinct M, OR, and PGs all present.

Description of sporocyst and sporozoites: Sporocyst shape: elongate ovoidal to slightly ellipsoidal, slightly pointed at one end; L × W (n = 100): 16.3 × 8.9 (15–20 × 8–12); L/W ratio: 1.8 (1.4–2.1); SB: present as a prominent nipple-like structure at pointed end of sporocyst; SSB, PSB: both absent; SR: present; SR characteristics: large, spheroidal or ovoidal compact aggregation of coarse granules; SZ: banana-shaped, with one end broader than the other and they lie lengthwise in SP; each SZ has two clear RBs, one larger than the other; N: small, in middle of the SZ. Distinctive features of sporocyst: presence of SB, large SR with two RBs, and N visible in each SZ.

Prevalence: Hsu et al. (1974a) reported this species in 2/2 (100%) harbor seal pups they examined, one male and one female. The pups were estimated to be about 2-months-old when

(A)

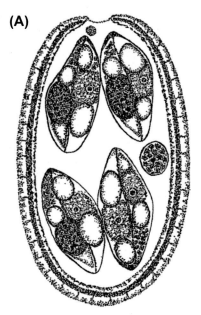

(B)

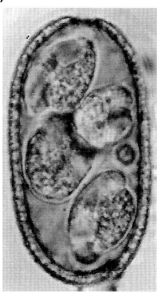

FIGURE 7.1   (A) Line drawing of the sporulated oocyst of *Eimeria phocae*. (B) Photomicrograph of *E. phocae*. (A) Fig. 1, *from Hsu, C.K., Melby, E.C., Altman, N.H., 1974a. Eimeria phocae n. sp. from the harbor seal* (Phoca vitulina concolor). *Journal of Parasitology 60 (3), 399–402, with permission of Allen Press, copyright holder.* (B) Fig. 3, from McClelland, G., 1993. *Eimeria phocae (Apicomplexa: Eimeriidae) in harbour seals* Phoca vitulina *from sable island, Canada. Diseases of Aquatic Organisms 17, 1–8, with permission of the editor and copyright holder.*

captured (Hsu et al., 1974b) and later examined. van Bolhuis et al. (2007) said that microscopic examination of intestinal tissues from 113 harbor seals that had died between 1999 and 2004 showed that only one was positive for *E. phocae*.

Sporulation: Exogenous. Oocysts sporulated in 48–52 hours when feces were placed into 2.5% potassium dichromate ($K_2Cr_2O_7$) solution at 26°C, and Hsu et al. (1974a) added that some oocysts sporulated in as few as 42 hours after leaving the host. McClelland (1993) studied sporulation in different media and at different temperatures. He found that the mean sporulation time of oocysts in 2.5% $K_2Cr_2O_7$ solution had a declining curvilinear relationship with temperature varying from 50 hours at 20°C to 1,300 hours (54 days) at 0.2°C. At 25°C, <10% of the oocysts sporulated, and no sporulation occurred at temperatures ≥30°C. Interestingly, McClelland (1993) also reported that oocysts in standing or aerated seawater were inhibited from sporulating, but after 30 days in seawater, >90% of the oocysts sporulated in ~50 hours after the water temperature was raised to 20°C.

Prepatent and patent periods: The prepatent period is thought to be 20–25 days, the time elapsed between a fatal case of coccidiosis in a captive harbor seal at Johns Hopkins University and the onset of symptoms in a second harbor seal held in the same facility (Hsu et al., 1974b). The patent period was reported to be 11 days (Hsu et al., 1974a), but McClelland (1993) reported that two seals with subclinical infections shed oocysts for 2 and 8 days, respectively, while a third infected seal shed oocysts for 4 days.

Site of infection: Lamina propria of villi in the colon and distal ileum.

Endogenous stages: Hsu et al. (1974a) did not observe any meronts in the two harbor seals they examined, but they did see, photograph, and measure gamonts in the lamina propria of the villi in the colon. Developing microgametocytes varied in shape and size, 90×65 (60–126 × 28–72); those developing microgametocytes were said to have invaginated cords with dividing nuclei. Ultimately, many microgametes were arranged in circular fashion in mature microgametocytes. Macrogametes in the lamina propria were, 36×25 (32–57×21–42), much smaller than developing microgametocytes. Several gamonts and oocysts were often present within the lamina propria of the same villus (Hsu et al., 1974a). McClelland (1993) reported that giant meronts occurred in colonies forming macroscopic nodules that extended from the submucosa to the intestinal lumen; these nodules (n=10) were 1.3×0.9 (0.9–1.5×0.75–1.1) mm in size and contained 800–1,200 individual meronts. Meronts were ovoidal to irregular in shape, and developing meronts were compartmentalized by invaginated cords of dividing nuclei, whereas more mature meronts contained merozoites. Mature meronts were 100×78 (80–128×64–85) and individual merozoites were 6–8×1–2, broader at one end, with a N slightly anterior to midbody. The fact that meronts occurred in large discrete colonies suggested to McClelland (1993) that they were second generation meronts, and that each colony may have arisen from single first-generation meronts. McClelland (1993) also found gamonts; his developing microgamonts (n=50) were 74×46 (52–120×29–60) and macrogamonts (n=50) were 32×26 (22–41×20–33). He also photographed oocysts, meronts, and gamonts and described symptoms and pathology.

Cross-transmission: None to date, but see *Remarks*, below.

Pathology: This species can be pathogenic, producing lethargy, anorexia, depression, loss of appetite, disinclination to move, diarrhea and/or dysentery, and death. Large numbers of endogenous stages and developing oocysts destroy epithelial cells causing extensive destruction of the lamina propria and the overlying mucosal tissues. Erythrocytes are found in the feces, and the most severe lesions occur in the colon and its lumen resulting in acute, diffuse hemorrhagic, necrotizing colitis. Numerous bacterial colonies were observed in these necrotic areas and in the crypts (Hsu et al., 1974a,b). Despite the ability of *E. phocae* to be pathogenic under some circumstances, seals in good physical condition can survive an infection (Lauckner, 1985). However, *E. phocae* is almost certainly implicated in disease and mortality of weak or undernourished juvenile harbor seals in the wild. For example, Munro and Synge (1991) described fatal hemorrhagic enteritis associated with a coccidial infection in two seal pups in a seal sanctuary in the Shetland Islands, Scotland, and noted that three other pups developed diarrhea and dysentery. Postmortem examination of the seal pups showed intestinal hemorrhage, large numbers of oocysts in the feces, marked destruction of the mucosa, and macrogametes in the lamina propria; they were almost certainly dealing with *E. phocae* infections, but they did not take time to measure oocysts or identify the species of *Eimeria*, even though they were aware of the papers of Hsu et al. (1974a,b) describing it.

McClelland (1993) also documented pathology caused by *E. phocae*. He reported 12 infections and reinfections with this species in 8 harbor seals, housed in tanks at Dalhousie University, between October, 1974, and April, 1975. Initial symptoms included vomiting, but he said most infections were mild or asymptomatic when small numbers of oocysts were being shed in the feces. However, lethargy, loss of appetite, and hemorrhagic diarrhea occurred when heavy oocyst output transpired. Actual "coccidiosis" in captive seals may be exacerbated by the stress of capture, confinement, change of diet, handling, poor sanitation, and overcrowding when *E. phocae* is present (Munro and Synge, 1991).

van Bolhuis et al. (2007) described fatal enterocolitis due to *E. phocae* infection in three juvenile harbor seals at a rehabilitation center in the Netherlands in 2003. The clinical signs they reported were lethargy, bloody feces, and intermittent convulsions and muscle tremors just before they died. They said the nervous signs

resembled those of nervous coccidiosis in calves. The main pathological finding was severe, diffuse, hemorrhagic enterocolitis with diffuse inflammatory changes in the lamina propria of the jejunal, ileal, cecal, and colonic mucosa, all of which were associated with the gamonts and oocysts of the endogenous development of *E. phocae*.

Materials deposited: None.

Remarks: This was the first species of *Eimeria* to be recorded from this family of carnivores, perhaps, because these animals spend most of their time in oceans making it difficult for parasitologists to collect feces for examination. The paper by Hsu et al. (1974a) should have alerted those who study diseases in marine mammals to be more vigilant and curious about potentially pathogenic organisms in their studies, but given the paucity of information available in this chapter, this certainly did not happen; it took another 13 years before other seals were examined for intestinal coccidia (see Dróżdż, 1987). The warning by Hsu (1974a,b) and McClelland (1993) should be especially relevant to those who work with seals and their relatives housed in laboratories and zoos.

Sporulated oocysts measured by McClelland (1993), from infected harbor seals collected at Sable Island, but housed in tanks at Dalhousie University, Halifax, were similar in most respects to those given by Hsu et al. (1974a). Sporulated oocysts were ellipsoidal with a yellowish-brown wall, ~3 thick, and a M that was ~4 wide; L × W (n = 100): 45.4 × 23.6 (42–47 × 22–25); L/W ratio: 1.9 (1.75–2.0); OR: 2, composed of coarse granules; PG: 1, prominent. Sporocysts were L × W (n = 100): 18.0 × 10.3 (15–21 × 9–12); L/W ratio: 1.7 (1.4–2.1); SP with a SB, but lacking SSB and PSB; SZ: with central N and two RBs.

McClelland (1993) created confusion regarding the specificity of *E. phocae* for harbor seals. When discussing Symptoms and Pathology (p. 3), he said he never detected oocysts in the feces of two gray seal (*Halichoerus grypus*) pups that shared facilities with seven harbor seals from February to June, 1975, including the period of April 3–15, when subclinical *E. phocae* infections were diagnosed in each of the harbor seals. However, in his Introduction (p. 1) he stated, "fatal haemorrhagic enteritis associated with *Eimeria* sp. infection was... diagnosed in August 1992 in gray seals *H. grypus* housed in the Life Sciences Centre, Dalhousie University, Halifax Nova Scotia (John Parsons, Biology Dept., Dalhousie University, pers. comm.)." Thus, it is not certain to us whether *E. phocae* can infect and cause disease in gray seals or not.

Finally, some authors have suggested frequent replacement of water in holding tanks of seawater to prevent *E. phocae* reinfections in captive seals (Hsu et al., 1974b; Lauckner, 1985; Munro and Synge, 1991). McClelland (1993), however, pointed out the fallacy of that logic when infections of harbor seals occurred repeatedly when they were held in outdoor tanks equipped with a flow-through system that delivered fresh, prefiltered seawater at a rate sufficient to replace its contents >10 times/day. He showed that oocysts sporulate in feces incubated under moist air but not when suspended in standing or aerated seawater and concluded that oocysts sporulate in seal haul-out areas where they become infected by ingesting or inhaling sporulated oocysts from soiled pelage during grooming or nursing. Captive seals also may ingest oocysts with food dragged across soiled haul-outs (McClelland, 1993).

GENUS *PUSA* SCOPOLI, 1771 (3 SPECIES)

Remarks: Kuiken et al. (2006) mentioned finding *Eimeria*-like oocysts in the cytoplasm of jejunal enterocytes in 1 of 18 *Pusa caspica* (Gmelin, 1788) (syn. *Phoca caspica*), Caspian seals, they necropsied. They did not try to identify or characterize them in any way. Thus, this form is relegated to *species inquirenda* (see Chapter 19).

DISCUSSION AND SUMMARY

Here we summarize what very little is known about eimeriid intestinal coccidians in 3 families of marine carnivorous mammals that include 21 genera comprising only 36 species. We know of no eimeriid coccidians described from 14 genera and 25 species: Odobenidae: *Odobenus* Brisson, 1762 (monotypic); Otariidae: *Arctocephalus* É. Geoffroy Saint-Hilaire and F. Cuvier, 1826 (8 species); *Callorhinus* J.E. Gray, 1859 (monotypic); *Eumetopias* Gill, 1866 (monotypic); *Neophoca* Gray, 1866 (monotypic); *Phocarctos* Peters, 1866 (monotypic); *Zalophus* Gill, 1866 (3 species); Phocidae: *Cystophora* Nilsson, 1820 (monotypic); *Erignathus* Gill, 1866 (monotypic); *Histriophoca* Gill, 1873 (monotypic); *Hydrurga* Gistel, 1848 (monotypic); *Monachus* Fleming, 1822 (3 species); *Ommatophoca* Gray, 1844 (monotypic); *Pagophilus* Gray, 1844 (monotypic). Thus, we know that 14/21 (67%) genera and 25/36 (69%) of the species in these families have not been studied sufficiently or never have been examined for eimeriid (or other) coccidia. Of the 11 host species in which oocysts have been reported, at least three reports are highly questionable because they are based on one host animal, few oocysts, and the oocysts reported were identified to genus without first being allowed to sporulate!

Only 5 intestinal coccidians (3 *Eimeria*, 2 *Cystoisospora*) have been named and described, three of these are not well-described, and all are reported from different species in the Phocidae. Based on our combined experience with numerous mammal families and genera across the Earth, it is difficult for us to imagine that all 36 species in the 3 families of marine carnivores do not harbor at least one eimeriid coccidian that is unique to each.

Only *E. phocae*, from harbor and gray (?) seals, has been reasonably well-studied. Sporulated oocysts have been measured and photographed, there is information on the endogenous developmental stages, and some of the pathology caused to the intestinal epithelium by these stages in infected seals has been well-documented. Beyond this, we know virtually nothing about the coccidia of marine carnivorous mammals except for the spotty reports of the heteroxenous species (Chapters 14–16) and *Cryptosporidium* (Chapter 17). Clearly there is much still to be learned about biodiversity and biology of coccidia in marine mammals. Given that many marine mammals spend a portion of the year in high-density breeding colonies, these provide ideal opportunities to collect fecal samples for examination. Because animals are concentrated, it seems this would also be a period when fecal–oral transmission of coccidia would be enhanced and coccidian prevalences would be at their highest.

Finally, as is true for many other carnivore species, a significant number of marine carnivores are of extreme concern to conservation biologists. The International Union for Conservation of Nature (IUCN) currently lists as vulnerable these 8 species: walrus (*Odobenus rosmarus*), northern fur seal (*Callorhinus ursinus*), and hooded seal (*Cystophora cristata*); near threatened: Steller sea lion (*Eumetopias jubatus*); and endangered: Galápagos fur seal (*Arctocephalus galapagoensis*), Australian sea lion (*Neophoca cinerea*), New Zealand sea lion (*Phocarctos hookeri*), and Galápagos sea lion (*Zalophus wollebaeki*). That is, at least 8/36 (22%) species in these families are on the IUCN lists. We need to study them before they, and their parasites, are gone forever.

Eimeriidae in the Caniformia Family Procyonidae

EIMERIIDAE IN THE PROCYONIDAE, GRAY, 1825

INTRODUCTION

The Procyonidae Gray, 1825, is a small New World family of carnivores comprising 6 genera and 14 species. Procyonids are most closely related to the Mustelidae and diverged from their most recent common ancestor approximately 29.3 (27.5–31.1) million years ago (MYA). Within the procyonids, the genus *Potos* (kinkajous) is the most ancient, diverging from the ancestors of other groups approximately 22.7 (19.9–25.5) MYA. The ancestral lineage split into two clades approximately 20.1 (16.2–24.1) MYA, one of which diverged 14.9 (8.7–21.1) MYA into the genera *Bassariscus* (ringtail, cacomistle) and *Procyon* (raccoon). The second clade diverged 14.9 (6.8–21.8) MYA, into the *Bassaricyon* (olingo) and a second lineage that diverged 9.2 (7.9–10.5) MYA, into the genera *Nasuella* (mountain coati) and *Nasua* (coati) (Hedges et al., 2006; Kumar and Hedges, 2011; Kumar et al., 2017).

In general, procyonids are omnivorous and are noted for their adaptability and problem-solving abilities. Many have banded tails and characteristic facial markings. Although at

one time thought to be closely related to bears (Ursidae) because of their bear-like body, omnivorous habits, and plantigrade locomotion (walking on the soles of their feet), recent molecular analyses have determined procyonids are more closely related to mustelids than bears (Nyakatura and Bininda-Emonds, 2012; Timetree.org, 2017). Species in the family inhabit a wide variety of habitats, and some are found living in close association with humans in urban and rural environments. One species, the raccoon (*P. lotor*), has been introduced widely, and it is now present in Austria, Azerbaijan, Belarus, Czech Republic, Denmark, France, Germany, Japan, Russia, Switzerland, and Uzbekistan (Wilson and Reeder, 2005). Sometimes procyonids, especially raccoons, are also kept as pets.

Procyonids are hosts for a variety of endo- and ectoparasites including ticks, mites, lice, protozoa (*Leishmania* spp., *Trypanosoma cruzi*), helminths (*Baylisascaris procyonis*, *Dirofilaria immitis*, *Trichinella pseudospiralis*), and they are reservoirs for viruses and bacteria of medical and veterinary concern such as canine distemper virus and rabies (Deem et al., 2000; Calvopina et al., 2004; Bern et al., 2011; Pozio, 2016). Concern is further amplified for several procyonid species, especially raccoons, because they are widely

© 2018 Donald W. Duszynski published by Elsevier Inc. All rights reserved.

distributed, increasing in number, and often live in close association with humans. For example, the nematode *B. procyonis* is extremely common in raccoons, and if a human becomes infected by ingesting viable eggs, it can result in *visceral larval migrans*, where larval worms migrate into brain tissue resulting in seizures and other neurologic symptoms. In North America, the prevalence in adult (70%) and juvenile (90%) raccoons is high (Sorvillo et al., 2002). Also of concern, the role of raccoons in the epidemiology of rabies has been well-documented. In 2015, 5,088 wildlife rabies cases were reported to the US Center for Disease Control from the 50 US states and Puerto Rico. Of these 1,619 (29.4%) were in raccoons (Birhane et al., 2017).

SPECIES DESCRIPTIONS

GENUS NASUA STORR, 1780 (2 SPECIES)

EIMERIA NASUAE CARINI AND GRECHI, 1938

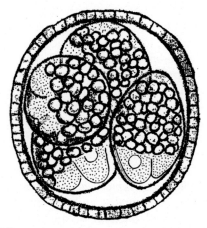

FIGURE 8.1 Original line drawing of the sporulated oocyst of *E. nasuae*. *Modified from Fig. 32 of Levine, N.D., Ivens, V., 1981. The Coccidian Parasites (Protozoa, Apicomplexa) of Carnivores, Illinois Biological Monograph No. 51. The University of Illinois Press, Urbana, Illinois, USA, 249 p. The University of Illinois Press, Urbana, Illinois, has released the copyright.*

Type host: *Nasua narica* (L., 1766) (syn. *Nasua nasica*), White-nosed Coati or Coatimundi.

Type locality: South America: Brazil.

Other hosts: None to date.

Geographic distribution: South America: Brazil.

Description of sporulated oocyst: Oocyst shape: spheroidal to subspheroidal (line drawing); number of walls, 2; wall characteristics: rough, with light radial striations that slightly protrude; L×W: 17–19×15–17 (means not given); L/W ratio: ~1.1; M, OR, PG: all absent. Distinctive features of oocyst: rough, thick, outer wall surface that appears striated and the lack of M, OR, and PG.

Description of sporocyst and sporozoites: Sporocyst shape: ovoidal; L×W: 10×8; L/W ratio: 1.25; SB: present; SSB and PSB: both absent; SR: present; SR characteristics: composed of large granules and spherules that occupy most of the space inside the SP (line drawing); SZ: sausage-shaped, longer than, and lying lengthwise within, the SP, so they are recurved back on themselves (line drawing); RB and N: not visible. Distinctive features of sporocyst: long SZ with SR that almost completely fills the SP and obscures the SZs.

Prevalence: Unknown.

Sporulation: Oocysts stored in 1% chromic acid at ambient temperature sporulated in 10–11 days.

Prepatent and patent periods: Unknown.

Site of infection: Unknown, oocysts recovered from intestinal content and feces.

Endogenous stages: Unknown.

Cross-transmission: Carini and Grechi (1938) tried to infect an older coati with (sporulated?) oocysts from the original host, but the infection failed. They attributed their failure to infect the older host to a previous immunity.

Pathology: Unknown.

Materials deposited: None.

Remarks: The description of this species is marginal by today's standards. It has not been reported since its original description, so its validity as a real species is questionable.

ISOSPORA ARCTOPITHECI RODHAIN, 1933

Synonym: *Isospora scorzai* Arcay-de-Peraza, 1967.

Type host: *Callithrix penicillata* (I. Geoffroy, 1812) (syn. *Hapale penicilatus*), Black Tufted-ear Marmoset.

Other hosts: Hendricks (1974, 1977) experimentally infected 5 carnivore genera/species demonstrating their suitability as definitive hosts including: *Canis familiaris* L., 1758, Domestic Dog (Canidae); *Eira barbara* (L., 1758), Tayra (Mustelidae); *Nasua nasua* (L., 1766), South American Coati, and *Potos flavus* (Schreber, 1774), Kinkajou (both Procyonidae); *Felis catus* L., 1758, Domestic Cat (Felidae).

Remarks: This species name has been emended to *Cystoisospora arctopitheci* N. Comb. (see Chapter 14, Sarcocystidae: Cystoisosporinae).

GENUS POTOS É. GEOFFROY SAINT-HILAIRE AND F.G. CUVIER, 1795 (MONOTYPIC)

EIMERIA POTI LAINSON, 1968

Type host: *Potos flavus* (Schreber, 1774), Kinkajou.

Type locality: Central America: Belize (former British Honduras), El Cayo District, Baking Pot.

Other hosts: None to date.

Geographic distribution: Central America: Belize.

Description of sporulated oocyst: Oocyst shape: ellipsoidal to cylindroidal; number of walls, 2; wall characteristics: colorless, smooth, ~0.8 in total thickness; L×W (n=5): 30×18 (26–31×17–20); L/W ratio: 1.7; M, OR, PG: all absent. Distinctive features of oocyst: elongate-ellipsoidal shape with M, OR, and PG all being absent.

Description of sporocyst and sporozoites: Sporocyst shape: ellipsoidal; L×W (n=5): 15×9 (14–15×8–9); L/W ratio: 1.7; SB: present, well-developed

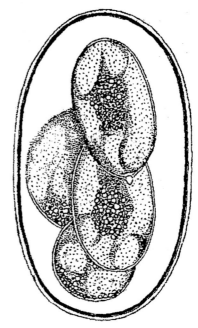

FIGURE 8.2 Original line drawing of the sporulated oocyst of *E. poti*. *Modified from Fig. 45 of Levine, N.D., Ivens, V., 1981. The Coccidian Parasites (Protozoa, Apicomplexa) of Carnivores, Illinois Biological Monograph No. 51. The University of Illinois Press, Urbana, Illinois, USA, 249 p. The University of Illinois Press, Urbana, Illinois, has released the copyright.*

as a small, nipple-, or plug-like structure (line drawing); SSB and PSB: both absent; SR: present; SR characteristics: composed of densely-packed globules in the center of the SP, between the SZ (line drawing); SZ: sausage-shaped, longer than, and lying lengthwise within, the SP so they are recurved back on themselves at their ends (line drawing); RB and N: not visible. Distinctive features of sporocyst: ellipsoidal shape with large L/W ratio, 1.7, SZs longer than SP, so they fold back on themselves at their ends.

Prevalence: Lainson (1968) found this species in the feces of 1/5 (20%) kinkajous examined.

Sporulation: Unknown.

Prepatent and patent periods: Unknown.

Site of infection: Unknown, oocysts recovered from feces.

Endogenous stages: Unknown.

Cross-transmission: None to date.

Pathology: Unknown.

Materials deposited: None.

Remarks: Unfortunately, Lainson (1968) was only able to observe and measure five sporulated oocysts, but they were sufficiently different from other species known at the time to justify his naming this form a new species.

ISOSPORA ARCTOPITHECI RODHAIN, 1933

Synonym: *Isospora scorzai* Arcay-de-Peraza, 1967.

Type host: *Callithrix penicillata* (I. Geoffroy, 1812) (syn. *Hapale penicilatus*), Black Tufted-ear Marmoset.

Other hosts: Hendricks (1974, 1977) experimentally infected 5 carnivore genera/species demonstrating their suitability as definitive hosts including: *Canis familiaris* L., 1758, Domestic Dog (Canidae); *Eira barbara* (L., 1758), Tayra (Mustelidae); *Nasua nasua* (L., 1766), South American Coati, and **Potos flavus** (Schreber, 1774), Kinkajou (both Procyonidae); *Felis catus* L., 1758, Domestic Cat (Felidae).

Remarks: This species name has been emended to *Cystoisospora arctopitheci* N. Comb. (see Chapter 14, Sarcocystidae: Cystoisosporinae).

GENUS PROCYON STORR, 1780 (3 SPECIES)

EIMERIA NUTTALLI YAKIMOFF AND MATIKASCHWILI, 1933

Type host: *Procyon lotor* (L., 1758), Raccoon.

Type locality: Asia: Russia, St. Petersburg (former Leningrad). See *Remarks* (below).

Other hosts: *Procyon pygmaeus* (Merriam, 1901), Pygmy Raccoon.

Geographic distribution: Europe: England (?); North America: Mexico: Quintana Roo; USA: Alabama, Florida, Georgia, Illinois, Iowa,

(A)

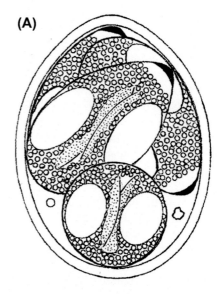

(B)

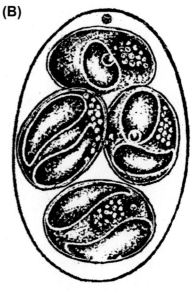

FIGURE 8.3   (A and B) Two original line drawings of sporulated oocysts of *Eimeria nuttalli*. *Modified from Figs. 28, 85, respectively, of Levine, N.D., Ivens, V., 1981. The Coccidian Parasites (Protozoa, Apicomplexa) of Carnivores, Illinois Biological Monograph No. 51. The University of Illinois Press, Urbana, Illinois, USA, 249 p. The University of Illinois Press, Urbana, Illinois, has released the copyright.*

Michigan, New York, Ohio. Inabnit et al. (1972) reported this species from 10/48 (21%) raccoons from Alabama, Georgia, and Michigan, but they did not provide details of where the 10 positive animals were collected.

Description of sporulated oocyst: Oocyst shape: ovoidal to ellipsoidal; number of walls, 1 (Inabnit et al., 1972; Adams et al., 1981) or two (Yakimoff and Matikaschwili, 1933); wall characteristics: external "layer" looks thicker and darker than the internal, 1.3–1.7 total thickness (Yakimoff and Matikaschwili, 1933), or smooth, colorless to yellowish-brown, and slightly thinner at one end, ~0.7 total thickness (Inabnit et al., 1972; Adams et al., 1981); L×W (n=50): 19.5×14 (17–23× 13–16); L/W ratio: 1.4 (Yakimoff and Matikaschwili, 1933), or L×W (n=100): 17.5×13.6 (12–21×11–15); L/W ratio: 1.3 (1.1–1.5) (Inabnit et al., 1972), or L×W (n=50): 18.4×14.2 (15–21× 12–17); L/W ratio: 1.3 (Adams et al., 1981); M and OR: both absent; PG: sometimes present (1–3 irregular, Inabnit et al., 1972). Distinctive features of oocyst: none noted.

Description of sporocyst and sporozoites: Sporocyst shape: slightly ovoidal; L×W: 7.5– 8.8×5.5–6.6 (means not given, Yakimoff and Matikaschwili, 1933) or L×W (n=100): 12.2×7.1 (9–13×5.5–11); L/W ratio: 1.7 (Inabnit et al., 1972), or L×W (n=50): 9×6.5 (8–11×5–7); L/W ratio: 1.4 (Adams et al., 1981); SB: not mentioned by Yakimoff and Matikaschwili (1933), but present as dark, dome-shaped body (Inabnit et al., 1972); SSB and PSB: both absent; SR: present; SR characteristics: composed of some residual granules/spherules clumped between SZ (Yakimoff and Matikaschwili, 1933; Adams et al., 1981), or many fine granules dispersed throughout SP sometimes obscuring SZ (line drawing, Inabnit et al., 1972); SZ: sausage-shaped, lying lengthwise in the SP; RB: one, a large clear globule at the more rounded end of SZ. Distinctive features of sporocyst: SZ sometimes becomes difficult to distinguish because of many disbursed SR granules, and in most cases, only the RB of the SZ can be observed (Inabnit et al., 1972).

Prevalence: Yakimoff and Matikaschwili (1933) wrote, "we examined eight American raccoons (*Procyon s. Notocyon lotor*) whose faeces, according to Darling, contained Coccidia of our species." From this, we presume that all eight animals examined had oocysts of this species. Found in 10/48 (21%) *P. lotor* from Michigan, Alabama, and Georgia (Inabnit et al., 1972); in 21/36 (58%) *P. lotor* from Illinois (Adams et al., 1981); in 6/61 (10%) *P. lotor* from Florida (Foster et al., 2004); in 10/28 (36%) *P. pygmaeus* from Cozumel Island, Mexico (McFadden et al., 2005); in 33/34 (97%) *P. lotor* from Collier County in 1973–74; in 1/1 from Indian River County in 1973; and in 7/10 (70%) from Monroe County, Florida in 1985 (Forrester, 1992).

Sporulation: Unknown.

Prepatent and patent periods: Unknown.

Site of infection: Unknown, oocysts recovered from intestinal content and feces.

Endogenous stages: Unknown.

Cross-transmission: None to date.

Pathology: Morgan and Waller (1940) conducted a postmortem examination of a sick raccoon collected at Garnavillo, Clayton County, Iowa, USA. The raccoon was submitted to the US Biological Survey unit in Ames, where it died 4 hours later. The next day the carcass was necropsied and the authors noticed a mild **catarrhal enteritis** and that the digestive tract was void of ingested materials. They reported a light coccidial infection with oocysts that were L×W: 20.2×14.3 and identified as *E. nuttalli*; however, they did not and could not confirm that the parasite was responsible for the enteritis seen and the lack of food in the gut.

Materials deposited: None.

Etymology: This species was named in honor of Professor G.H.G. Nuttall, the parasitologist (Yakimoff and Matikaschwili, 1933).

Remarks: The original description of this species is marginal by today's standards, and Yakimoff and Matikaschwili (1933) did not specify a locality where the raccoons they examined were collected. Inabnit et al. (1972) published a redescription of

E. nuttalli and listed the type locality as Leningrad, Russia, apparently assuming the eight raccoons examined by Yakimoff and Matikaschwili (1933) were collected there because the authors' address on the publication was Leningrad. Inabnit et al.'s (1972) redescription was based on oocysts recovered in 10/48 raccoons from Alabama, Georgia, and Michigan, USA. Comparing their description to that of Yakimoff and Matikaschwili (1933), they noted several differences including: their oocysts had 1–3 PG, the SP were larger, and a distinct SB was present. They also crushed oocysts to better observe SP features, a step Yakimoff and Matikaschwili (1933) did not take; thus, Inabnit et al. (1972) stated that the oocyst wall was single layered versus the implied notion that it was two layered ("double contoured") by Yakimoff and Matikaschwili (1933). Adams et al. (1981) said the oocysts they described differed from those of Inabnit et al. (1972) in oocyst wall color (none vs. yellowish-brown), and their sporocysts were smaller.

MacKinnon and Dibb (1938) recovered unsporulated oocysts from raccoons temporarily held in the Zoological Gardens at Regent's Park, London, England, that, based on dimensions, L×W: 18×15 (16.5–21×12–17), they suggested were likely *E. nuttalli*. Morgan and Waller's (1940) postmortem examination of the raccoon in Iowa, recovered oocysts that "closely resembled" *E. nuttalli*, being ovoidal, measuring, L×W (n=25): 20.2×14.3, and contained PGs. Dubey (1982a), in a study focused on *Baylisascaris procyonis* and *Eimeria procyonis* in raccoons collected in Ohio, USA, mentioned that *E. nuttalli* may have been present, but, because sporulated oocysts were not examined for 4 years, their morphology had deteriorated so that identification was not possible. McFadden et al. (2005) live-trapped critically-endangered pygmy raccoons, *P. pygmaeus*, on Cozumel Island, Quintana Roo, Mexico and found that 10/28 (36%) animals were infected. Rainwater et al. (2017) surveyed raccoons for parasites and diseases in Central Park, New York City, USA, and reported "coccidia" in 68/98

(69%) raccoons. They did not identify the species present in each sample but positively identified *E. nutalli* and *E. procyonis* in one sample.

EIMERIA PROCYONIS INABNIT, CHOBOTAR AND ERNST, 1972

Type host: *Procyon lotor* (L., 1758), Raccoon.
Type locality: North America: USA: southwestern Michigan. Inabnit et al. (1972) collected 43 raccoons from five counties in southwestern Michigan and fecal samples of three raccoons in Alabama and two from Georgia. They did not specify the state of the host(s) from which the oocysts of *E. procyonis* were isolated and described, but the odds dictate that it was from Michigan, so we designate it as the type locality.
Other hosts: None to date.
Geographic distribution: Asia: Japan; North America: USA: Alabama, Florida, Georgia, Michigan, New York, Ohio; South America: Brazil.
Description of sporulated oocyst: Oocyst shape: ellipsoidal to ovoidal; number of walls, 2 with LM (Inabnit et al., 1972; Adams et al., 1981) but 3 using TEM (see Fig. 10 in Duszynski et al., 1981); wall characteristics: outer layer rough with numerous radial striations, pitted and yellowish-brown, 1.5 thick, inner layer, 0.5 thick, and colorless to yellow (Inabnit et al., 1972), or outer layer slightly striated, tan, ~1.3 thick at sides and bottom, and 0.4–0.8 thick at top, inner layer brown, and 0.4 thick (Adams et al., 1981); L×W (n=100): 23.4×18.0 (16–29×13–24); L/W ratio: 1.2 (1.5–1.1) (Inabnit et al., 1972) or L×W (n=50): 25.1×20.2 (22–28×18–22); L/W ratio: 1.2 (Adams et al., 1981) or L×W (n=68): 19.6×14.6 (14–23×11–19); L/W ratio: 1.3 (Dubey, 1982a); M present as a smooth, thinner region at one end of the oocyst and ~5 wide (Inabnit et al., 1972) or not visible but probably present (Adams et al., 1981); OR: absent; PG: 1–3 present, irregularly-shaped. Distinctive features of oocyst: rough, thick, pitted outer wall that appears striated, with a M and 1–3 PG, and lacking an OR.

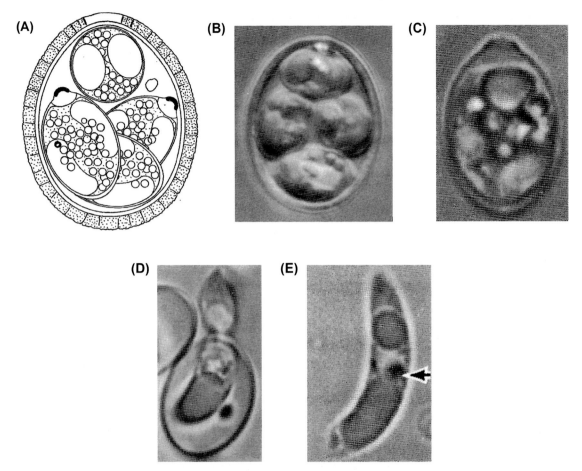

FIGURE 8.4 All images are of *Eimeria procyonis*. (A) Line drawing of a sporulated oocyst. (B) Photomicrograph of a sporulated oocyst. (C) Photomicrograph of an isolated sporocyst. (D) Photomicrograph of an SZ excysting from its SP. (E) Photomicrograph of an SZ; note two RB, on either side of the N. All photomicrographs originals. *(A) Modified Fig. 38, Levine, N.D., Ivens, V., 1981. The Coccidian Parasites (Protozoa, Apicomplexa) of Carnivores, Illinois Biological Monograph No. 51. University of Illinois Press, Urbana, Illinois, USA, p. 249. The University of Illinois Press has released the copyright.*

Description of sporocyst and sporozoites: Sporocyst shape: ovoidal; L×W (n=100): 12.1×9.3 (11.5–15×7–10); L/W ratio: 1.3 (Inabnit et al., 1972) or L×W (n=50): 13.1×8.6 (11–17×7–10); L/W ratio: 1.5 (Adams et al., 1981) or L×W (n=15): 8.9×6.8 (7–11×5–9); L/W ratio: 1.3 (Dubey, 1982a); SB: present at slightly pointed end of SP; SSB: present, as a homogenous flattened "plug" blocking narrow end of the sporocyst and wider than SB (line drawing);

PSB: absent; SR: present; SR characteristics: consisting of many large granules, each ~1 wide, forming an irregular mass often obscuring SZs; SZ: sausage-shaped (line drawing), often pushing against SSB causing it to vary in shape; Adams et al. (1981) observed a RB as a clear globule at the rounded end of SZ, but Duszynski et al. (1981) excysted SZ from their freed SP (see Fig. 8.4D) and described two RB, one large, ellipsoidal, filling posterior third of the SZ, and the second (sometimes absent), round, located in the anterior half of SZ, with N located between them; SZ free of their SP were L×W: 14.3×3.2 (13–16×3–4) (Duszynski et al., 1981). Distinctive features of sporocyst: distinct SB and SSB, SR of numerous large granules/globules, and SZ with a very large posterior RB.

Prevalence: This species was found in 32/48 (67%) *P. lotor* from Michigan, Alabama, and Georgia (Inabnit et al., 1972); in 9/36 (25%) *P. lotor* from Illinois (Adams et al., 1981); in 23/28 (82%) *P. lotor* from Ohio (Dubey, 1982a); in 51/61 (84%) *P. lotor* from Florida (Foster et al., 2004); in 19/34 (56%) *P. lotor* from Collier County, and 1/1 from Indian River County, Florida in 1973–74 (Forrester, 1992); and in 13/260 (5%) feral *P. lotor* from Hokkaido, Japan infected with *E. procyonis* and/or *Cystoisospora ohioensis* (Matoba et al., 2002).

Sporulation: Unknown.

Prepatent and patent periods: Unknown.

Site of infection: Meronts, gamonts, and unsporulated oocysts were found in epithelial cells at tips of the villi in small intestine (Dubey, 1982a).

Endogenous stages: Dubey (1982a) and Dubey et al. (2000a) found endogenous development in the villar epithelial cells of the small intestine (Fig. 8.5A). Uninucleate trophozoites (Fig. 8.5B), ~3×2, were located above the host cell nucleus. There were at least two kinds of meronts. Small mature meronts (Fig. 8.5C) first reported by Dubey (1982a) were L×W (n=19): 7×5.5 (5–9×4–7) and contained 4–10 (Dubey, 1982a) or 3–8 (Dubey et al., 2000a)

merozoites, without residual bodies. Small meronts were rare and found only at the tips of the villi in surface epithelial cells; they lacked residual bodies and their merozoites were L×W (n=6): 5×1.5 (Dubey, 1982a; Dubey et al., 2000a). Large mature meronts were seen in crypt glandular epithelial cells, measured up to 110 long, and often had central residual bodies surrounded by >50 merozoites (Fig. 8.5D and E), and their larger merozoites were sickle-shaped, with a nucleus toward their blunt ends. Some large meronts lacked central RBs (Fig. 8.5F). It appeared that not all merozoites developed simultaneously. Female gamonts with wall-forming bodies (Fig. 8.5B) measured L×W (n=37): 13.7×11.3 (10–18×8–14). Male gamonts (Fig. 8.5G) were L×W (n=17): 15.5×11.7 (12–21×9–12) and had a central residual body that was L×W (n=8): 8.1×5.5 (4–12×3–7). Male gametes were numerous and usually located near the periphery of gamonts. Unsporulated oocysts (Fig. 8.5H) were L×W (n=24): 15.5×11.8 (12–20×6–17), and the oocyst wall was rough, with the inner layer interrupted at the micropyle.

Cross-transmission: None to date.

Pathology: Dubey et al. (2000a) reported an outbreak of clinical coccidiosis in raccoons at the Wildlife Center in Lynnwood, Washington, USA. Following an outbreak of diarrhea with mortality, fecal samples from seven animals with diarrhea were pooled and sent to the Parasite Biology and Epidemiology Laboratory, Beltsville, Maryland, USA, for identification of

FIGURE 8.5 Photomicrographs of histologic sections from raccoons infected with *E. procyonis*. (A) Developing young meronts in glandular epithelium; note hyperinfection with parasite stages in most host cells. (B) Uninucleate trophozoites (*arrow heads*) and two macrogamonts with eosinophilic wall-forming bodies (*arrow*). (C) Small meront (*arrow*) with seven merozoites in surface epithelium. (D) Large meront with large central residual body containing degenerating materials. (E) Large meront with merozoites arranged in groups and a central mass containing merozoites. (F) Large meront without residual body; note elongated merozoites. (G) Microgamont (*small arrow*); also note, the small meront with four merozoites (*large arrow*). (H) Three unsporulated oocysts prior to their release into the intestinal lumen. *Fig. 2 and 3 from Dubey, J.P., 1982a. Baylisascaris procyonis and eimerian infections in raccoons. Journal of the American Veterinary Medical Association 181 (11), 1292–1294, with permission of the copyright holder, the JAVMA. Fig. 3A, D, F–I from Dubey, J.P., Garner, M.M., Rosenthal, B.M., DeGhetto, D., 2000a. Clinical coccidiosis in raccoons (Procyon lotor). Journal of Parasitology 86 (6), 1299–1303, with permission of Allen Press, Inc., Lawrence, Kansas, USA, copyright holder.*

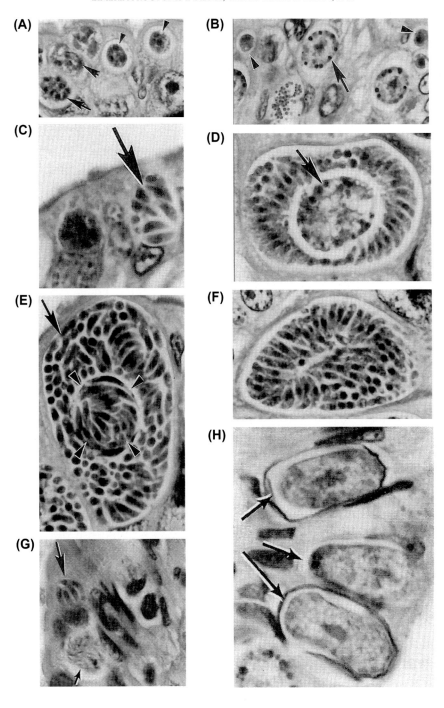

the coccidia. Five animals subsequently died, one was euthanized, and all were necropsied with tissues, including small intestine, prepared for histopathologic examination. Dubey et al. (2000a) examined the histological sections from the raccoons with clinical coccidiosis, and because *E. procyonis* is the most common eimerian in raccoons, they speculated that the pathology observed was due to it. Most stages observed in histological sections were large meronts occurring primarily in crypts of glandular epithelial cells, and some appeared to be in the submucosa.

At necropsy, all raccoons had reddened small intestines. One animal had a multifocally ulcerated small intestine with a jejunal **intussusception**, two animals had prolapsed rectums, and all raccoons had lesions associated with coccidian stages in the small intestine. Most sections had marked necrosis of the mucosa with superficial villous blunting and fusion, erosions or ulcers, crypt dilatation and necrosis, and superficial bacterial overgrowth, and the lamina propria was infiltrated with eosinophils, lymphocytes, and macrophages. Parasitized epithelial cells were necrotic, and there was hypertrophy of the cell nuclei, desquamation of epithelium, and coccidian stages in the lumen. One animal had pulmonary and hepatic congestion, one had suppurative inflammation and bacterial colonies in the mesenteric lymph nodes, and one animal had similar lymph nodes in the lungs. Dubey et al. (2000a) speculated that because only a few gamonts and no oocysts were observed in these histological sections, the meronts may be pathogenic and raccoons became sick before oocysts were formed. Alternatively, treatment with sulfadimethoxine may have affected the development of sexual stages. Numerous merozoites were observed in the intestinal lumen; this suggested to them that fecal smears, or smears of intestinal contents, should be examined for merozoites when diagnosing clinical coccidiosis in raccoons.

Materials deposited: USNPC 93689, photovoucher; 86352, phototype (Foster et al., 2004).

Remarks: The description of this species by Inabnit et al. (1972) was modest, at best, but it was consistent with the redescriptions of Adams et al. (1981) and differed slightly in oocyst and sporocyst dimensions and some qualitative characters. Inabnit et al. (1972) provided a line drawing but no photomicrograph and, unfortunately, they neither deposited the drawing or a photomicrograph in an accredited collection nor provided all of the quantitative and qualitative information needed (and expected) in a standardized species description. The oocysts observed by Dubey (1982a) were smaller than those of Inabnit et al. (1972) and of Adams et al. (1981), but because they possessed a rough outer wall and a micropyle, and were present in 23/28 raccoons, Dubey (1982a) and Dubey et al. (2000a) considered them to be *E. procyonis*.

Duszynski et al. (1981) observed sporozoite excystation by LM and used TEM to examine oocyst wall ultrastructure; they also provided photomicrographs of sporulated oocysts, sporocysts, sporozoites, and a cross section of the oocyst wall. After sporozoite excystation the sporocyst remained intact. The sporozoite excystation process was consistent with other Stieda body–possessing eimerian species described in the literature. The TEM micrographs showed the oocyst wall comprising three layers: an inner layer, 8–15 nm thick; a middle layer, 25–35 nm thick; and an outer layer of irregular thickness, 120–400 nm. The inner layer appeared discontinuous and consisted of electron-dense disc-shaped structures. The middle layer was electron lucent and consisted of a fine, granular matrix. Between the middle and outer layers there was a 12 nm-thick electron-lucent line. The outer layer comprised a granular electron-dense inner zone with knob-like protrusions and an outer region with electron-dense and electron-lucent material and irregularly-shaped membrane-bound vesicles. The oocyst wall structure was consistent with other coccidia having two to three prominent layers.

Foster et al. (2004) examined feces from live-trapped raccoons collected in Key Largo,

Florida, USA, for parasitic protozoa including coccidia and *Cryptosporidium* (see Chapter 17). They recovered *E. procyonis* from 51 raccoons examined but did not provide descriptions of the oocysts recovered. They did, however, submit a photovoucher and phototypes to the US National Parasite Collection because no previous photomicrographs had been deposited. They also noted that the prevalence of *E. procyonis* in raccoons from Key Largo was similar to prevalences reported by Inabnit et al. (1972) and Dubey et al. (2000a) but significantly greater than prevalences reported by Adams et al. (1981) and Forrester (1992). Matoba et al. (2002) found 4/260 (1.5%) feral raccoons from Hokkaido, Japan infected with eimerians. They observed one oocyst from a raccoon collected in Noporo Forest Park that resembled *E. procyonis* but were unable to confirm identification. They did provide a photomicrograph of the oocyst of *E.* cf. *procyonis* that measured $18–21 \times 22–23.5$, which is comparable to other reported oocyst dimensions for the species. Rainwater et al. (2017) surveyed raccoons for parasites and diseases in Central Park, New York City, USA, and reported coccidia in 68/98 (69%) raccoons. They did not identify the coccidian(s) present in each sample to species, but they did positively identify *E. nutalli* and *E. procyonis* in one sample.

ISOSPORA OHIOENSIS DUBEY, 1975c

Synonym: *Levinea ohioensis* (Dubey, 1975c) Dubey, 1977b.

Type host: *Canis lupus familiaris* (syn. *C. familiaris*), Domestic Dog.

Other hosts: *Procyon lotor* (L., 1758), Raccoon (?).

Remarks: Matoba et al. (2002) recovered oocysts resembling *I. ohioensis* from a raccoon collected in Noporo Forest Park, Hokkaido, Japan. Three oocysts were $L \times W$: 23.3×21.3. They noted that this could be a case of pseudoparasitism and

deferred specific identity until more detailed studies could be conducted. We concur with Matoba et al. (2002) that these oocysts represent spurious findings resulting from the raccoon having eaten an infected animal carcass or feces from infected dogs. It is well known that both sporulated and unsporulated oocysts of *Eimeria* and other apicomplexan genera and species can pass unchanged and unharmed through the intestinal tract of mammals that are not suitable hosts. This species name has already been emended to *Cystoisospora ohioensis* (Dubey, 1975c) Frenkel, 1977 (see Chapter 14, Sarcocystidae: Cystoisosporinae).

DISCUSSION AND SUMMARY

In spite of the fact there are only 6 genera and 14 species in this small carnivore family, there still exists a tremendous ignorance about the apicomplexan coccidians that parasitize them. To our knowledge, the following 3 genera and their 8 species, *Bassaricyon* J.A. Allen, 1876 (5 species), *Bassariscus* Coues, 1887 (2 species), and *Nasuella* Hollister, 1915 (monotypic) have likely never been examined for intestinal eimeriid coccidia.

Only 4 *Eimeria* species have been described from 3/14 (14%) species in this family, one from the raccoon, *P. lotor*, one from the pygmy raccoon, *P. pygmaeus*, one from the white-nosed coati, *N. narica*, and one from the kinkajou, *P. flavus*. Does this suggest that some coevolution and host specificity may be operating here? We really do not have the sample sizes and the data to know. The South American coati (*N. nasua*) and kinkajou (*P. flavus*), have also been experimentally infected with a single *Cystoisospora* species originally described from a marmoset. Can that experiment be repeated?

Thus, 11/14 (79%) of the species in this family have not been examined for coccidia. Of the named eimerian species, only *E. procyonis* has a type specimen deposited in an accredited museum. The lack of knowledge about eimerians from species in the family Procyonidae is concerning because the International Union for Conservation of Nature and Natural Resources (http://www.iucnredlist.org/) notes that populations of all species in the Procyonidae are decreasing except the raccoon, which is increasing, and the cacomistle (*Bassariscus sumichrasti*) and ringtail (*Bassariscus astutus*), have population trends that are unknown at this time. The IUCN lists the olinguito (*Bassaricyon neblina*) and western mountain coati (*Nasuella olivacea*) as near threatened, the eastern mountain coati (*Nasuella meridensis*) as endangered, and the pygmy raccoon (*Procyon pygmaeus*) as critically-endangered. As these host species decline in number and potentially become extinct, the opportunity to assess coccidian biodiversity in this group declines as well.

Perhaps because raccoons are abundant, widely distributed, and have colonized a number of new geographic regions, there has been more detailed work done on *E. procyonis* that occurs in this host relative to other wild carnivores and wildlife hosts. Detailed descriptions of oocysts and endogenous stages have been published for *E. procyonis* along with descriptions of oocyst ultrastructure and exogenous sporulation have been described as well. Here is a tractable carnivore host group in which every host species population could be surveyed with good sample sizes, and a lot of information gleaned on how many coccidia species actually exist in an entire family population. There must be a new graduate student in parasitology or mammalogy who could tackle this problem and answer a lot of basic questions, not the least of which would be to sequence some genes from all the coccidia fauna of procyonid hosts to test their relatedness. How interesting would that be?

Eimeriidae in the Caniformia Family Ursidae

EIMERIIDAE IN THE URSIDAE FISCHER DE WALDHEIM, 1817

INTRODUCTION

The Ursidae Fischer de Waldheim, 1817 is a family of carnivores comprising 5 genera and 8 species. All family members, generically referred to as "bears," are in the subfamily Caniformes and are most closely related to the Otariidae (eared seals), Odobenidae (walruses), and Phocidae (true seals), having diverged from a most recent common ancestor approximately 40 (37–43) million years ago (MYA) in Eurasia. Then, ~23.4 (17.8–28.9) MYA, the lineage split into two, with one branch leading to the monotypic genus *Ailuropoda* (giant panda, *A. melanoleuca*) and the second branch diverging 16.5 (10.4–22.6) MYA. This latter branch also resulted in two lineages: the first split off ~6.8 (4.4–9.2) MYA into the genera *Ursus* (4 species, black, brown, polar bears) and *Melursus* (sloth bear), whereas the second split off 6.49 (5.66–7.05) MYA into the monotypic genus *Tremarctos* (spectacled bear) (http://timetree.org/; Hedges et al., 2006; Kumar et al., 2017). At one time the inclusion of the giant panda in the family was in

debate, but molecular and karyotypic analyses confirmed that the giant panda is a true ursid (O'Brien et al., 1985; Pagès et al., 2008).

In general, bears are large animals with robust bodies. The Malayan sun bear (*Helarctos malayanus*) is the smallest species, ranging from 25 to 65 kg, and the polar bear (*U. maritimus*) is the largest weighing up to 800 kg. Extant species of bears are widely distributed, occurring in a variety of habitats ranging from arctic ice to tropical cloud forests in North America, Europe, Asia, and South America. There are no extant species in Africa, although fossil remains indicate that bears were present there at one time too. American black bears, in addition to occurring in temperate forests across the continent, are found in semidesert habitats in the southwestern United States and Mexico. A remnant population of brown bears is found in the Gobi Desert of southwestern Mongolia where they congregate at scattered, remote oases. Most bear species, with the exception of sows with cubs, lead solitary lives and are active primarily at dusk and dawn (**crepuscular**) or at night (**nocturnal**). Some temperate species undergo extended periods of lethargy or **torpor** during the winter, retreating to dens or caves where they rely on fat

© 2018 Donald W. Duszynski published by Elsevier Inc. All rights reserved.

reserves accumulated during the summer and fall for metabolic energy. Some physiologists do not consider this true "hibernation" because body temperature does not drop and the bear can be readily roused from lethargy, if startled. Others argue that this is hibernation because the bear's heart rate slows to almost half of its normal rate. Bear species that undergo torpor or hibernation often give birth during this period (Dewey and Myers, 2005). In general, bears are omnivorous and, depending on the species and season of year, a significant portion of their diet can consist of scavenged carcasses, vegetable matter (berries, roots, fruit), and arthropods, in addition to hunting live prey. Exceptions are the giant panda, with a diet that is 99% bamboo, and the polar bear that is almost exclusively carnivorous (Vaughn et al., 2011).

Compared with some other carnivore families, ursids have been examined for ecto- and endoparasites many times, but most of these surveys have concentrated on their intestinal and tissue helminths (e.g., Catalano et al., 2015; Bugmyrin et al., 2017). However, most parasites reported to infect Ursidae have limited veterinary or medical concern due to the restricted opportunity for transfer to domestic animals or humans because ursids live in remote areas and at low population densities. Two exceptions are the nematode, *Trichinella spiralis*, and the protist, *Toxoplasma gondii* (Chapter 16). There are numerous reports in the literature of human trichinellosis due to consumption of meat from brown, black, or polar bears in temperate, arctic, and subarctic regions (Dupouy-Camet et al., 2017), and the Center for Disease Control (2012) noted that, while reports of trichinellosis in the United States have declined over the last 40 years, the risk increased when eating undercooked wild bear meat.

Unfortunately, surveys for protists such as the coccidia (other than *T. gondii*) are rather limited in their scope and numbers. Here we report what little information seems to be known about these forms in members of the Ursidae.

SPECIES DESCRIPTIONS

GENUS *MELURSUS* MEYER, 1793 (MONOTYPIC)

ISOSPORA URSI AGRAWAL, AHLUWALIA, BHATIA, AND CHAUAN, 1981

Type host: *Melursus ursinus* (Shaw, 1791), Sloth Bear.

Other definitive hosts: None to date.

Remarks: This species name has been emended to *Cystoisospora ursi* N. Comb. (see Chapter 14, Sarcocystidae: Cystoisosporinae).

GENUS *URSUS* L., 1758 (4 SPECIES)

EIMERIA ALBERTENSIS HAIR AND MAHRT, 1970

Type host: *Ursus americanus* Pallas, 1780, American Black Bear.

Type locality: North America: Canada, Alberta, Cold Lake region (110°–111° W, 54.5 degrees N).

Other hosts: None to date.

Geographic distribution: North America: Canada: Alberta.

Description of sporulated oocyst: Oocyst shape: ellipsoidal; number of walls, 2; wall characteristics: smooth, brownish, thinner at the posterior end, outer wall is ~0.5 and becomes distinctly thicker at the anterior end to form a wider region lateral to the M, inner wall is ~1 thick, thinning at posterior end; L×W (n=50): 41.5×21.7 (36.5–44×19–22.5); L/W: 1.9; M: present, distinct, ~5.0 wide; M cap: absent; OR: usually present, compact mass of small granules that appear to be membrane-bounded (line drawing); PG: absent. Distinctive features of oocyst: distinct and wide M, usually possessing OR of compact granules but lacking a PG.

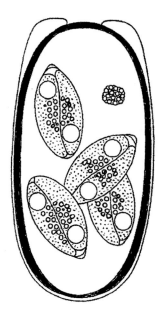

FIGURE 9.1 Original line drawing of the sporulated oocyst of *Eimeria albertensis. Modified from Fig. 36, Levine, N.D., Ivens, V. 1981. The Coccidian Parasites (Protozoa, Apicomplexa) of Carnivores, Illinois Biological Monograph No. 51. University of Illinois Press, Urbana, Illinois, USA. p. 248. The University of Illinois Press has released the copyright.*

Description of sporocyst and sporozoites: Sporocyst shape: ovoidal to elongate-ovoidal; L × W (n = 50): 14.7 × 7.7 (11–19 × 7–11); L/W ratio: 1.9; SB: present, small, translucent; SSB and PSB: both absent; SR: present; SR characteristics: centrally-located in SP as a group of small granules; SZ: vermiform, each with a prominent RB at the more rounded end. Distinctive features of sporocyst: SR of loose granules concentrated in center of SP and presence of a small, translucent SB.

Prevalence: Found in 4/52 (8%) black bears examined.

Sporulation: Exogenous. Hair and Mahrt (1970) said that feces collected from live-trapped bears were let to sporulate in a Petri dish containing 2.5% potassium dichromate ($K_2Cr_2O_7$) for 10 days at room temperature (22–24°C). However, they did not determine the percentage of successful sporulation during these 10 days.

Prepatent and patent periods: Unknown.

Site of infection: Unknown. Oocysts were collected from the feces.

Endogenous stages: Unknown.

Cross-transmission: None to date.

Pathology: Unknown.

Materials deposited: None to date.

Etymology: The specific epithet denotes the province of Alberta, Canada.

Remarks: The work by Hair and Mahrt (1970) was the first report of eimeriid coccidia from ursids in North America. In addition to *E. albertensis*, they also described *E. borealis* (see below) and 2 of the 52 (4%) fecal samples they examined from live-trapped bears were concurrently infected with both *Eimeria* spp. Prior to their work, only two coccidians had been described from bears: *E. ursi* from the brown bear, *U. arctos*, by Yakimoff and Matschoulsky (1935) and *Isospora* (syn. *Cystoisospora*) *fonsecai*, from the red bear, *Ursus arctos isabellius*, by Yakimoff and Matschoulsky (1940), both hosts from the former USSR. Sporulated oocysts of *E. albertensis* are morphologically quite distinct from those of *E. ursi* in size (36.5–44 × 19–22.5 vs. 13–15 × 10.5–13), shape (ellipsoidal vs. ovoidal), and the presence of a distinct M, which *E. ursi* lacks.

EIMERIA BOREALIS HAIR AND MAHRT, 1970

Type host: *Ursus americanus* Pallas, 1780, American Black Bear.

Type locality: North America: Canada, Alberta, Cold Lake region (110–111°W, 54.5°N).

Other hosts: None to date.

Geographic distribution: North America: Canada: Alberta.

Description of sporulated oocyst: Oocyst shape: ellipsoidal to slightly concave on one side; number of walls, 2; wall characteristics: smooth, colorless, thin, and slightly flattened at the anterior end that appears wrinkled: outer wall is

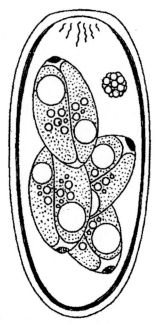

FIGURE 9.2   Original line drawing of the sporulated oocyst of *Eimeria borealis*. *Modified from Fig. 31, Levine, N.D., Ivens, V. 1981. The Coccidian Parasites (Protozoa, Apicomplexa) of Carnivores, Illinois Biological Monograph No. 51. University of Illinois Press, Urbana, Illinois, USA. p. 248. The University of Illinois Press, Urbana, Illinois, has released the copyright.*

~0.8 and inner wall is ~0.2 thick; L × W (n = 50): 30.2 × 14.8 (29–33 × 15–16); L/W 2.0; M: present, indistinct, ~3.0 wide; M cap: absent; OR: present as a compact mass of granules that appear to be membrane-bounded (line drawing); PG: absent. Distinctive features of oocyst: wrinkled appearance at the anterior end of the oocyst wall, possessing M and OR but lacking PG.

Description of sporocyst and sporozoites: Sporocyst shape: ovoidal; L × W (n = 50): 10.1 × 6.1 (7–11.5 × 4–7); L/W ratio: 1.7; SB: present, small, darkly-pigmented; SSB and PSB: both absent; SR: present; SR characteristics: disbursed granules in middle of SP; SZ: vermiform, each with a prominent, spheroidal RB at the more rounded end. Distinctive features of sporocyst: SR of disbursed granules in center of SP and presence of a darkly-pigmented SB.

Prevalence: Found in 3/52 (6%) of the black bears examined.

Sporulation: Exogenous. Hair and Mahrt (1970) said that feces collected from live-trapped bears were let to sporulate in a Petri dish containing 2.5% potassium dichromate ($K_2Cr_2O_7$) for 10 days at room temperature (22–24°C). However, they did not determine the degree of successful sporulation during these 10 days.

Prepatent and patent periods: Unknown.

Site of infection: Unknown. Oocysts were collected from the feces.

Endogenous stages: Unknown.

Cross-transmission: None to date.

Pathology: Unknown.

Materials deposited: None to date.

Etymology: The specific epithet denotes the boreal mixed wood forest that incorporates the Cold Lake region of Alberta.

Remarks: Sporulated oocysts of *E. borealis* are distinctly different from those of *E. albertensis* (above) in size, shape, and structure of the M. They also differ morphologically from those of *E. ursi* from the brown bear in the former USSR (Yakimoff and Matschoulsky, 1935) in that oocysts of the latter are spheroidal or ovoidal, much smaller (13–15 × 10.5–13) than those of *E. borealis*, and do not possess a M and OR. Two of the 52 (4%) fecal samples examined from live-trapped bears were concurrently infected with both *E. borealis* and *E. albertensis* (Hair and Mahrt, 1970).

EIMERIA URSI YAKIMOFF AND MATSCHOULSKY, 1935

Type host: *Ursus arctos* L., 1758, Brown Bear.

Type locality: Asia: Russia, Leningrad Oblast (now St. Petersburg), Leningrad Zoological Gardens.

Other hosts: None to date.

Geographic distribution: Asia: Russia, Leningrad Oblast.

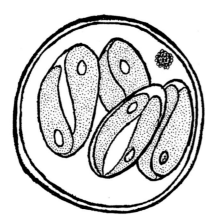

FIGURE 9.3 Original line drawing of the sporulated oocyst of *Eimeria ursi*. *Modified from Fig. 80, Levine, N.D., Ivens, V., 1981. The Coccidian Parasites (Protozoa, Apicomplexa) of Carnivores. Illinois Biological Monograph No. 51, The University of Illinois Press, Urbana, Illinois, USA. 249 p. The University of Illinois Press has released the copyright.*

Description of sporulated oocyst: Oocyst shape: spheroidal and ovoidal; number of walls, 1 (line drawings); wall characteristics: transparent, smooth, hyaline-like shell; L×W for ovoidal forms (n=21): 14.3×11.5 (13–15×11–13); L/W: 1.2 (Levine and Ivens, 1981) or 14.7×12.6 (Yakimoff and Matschoulsky, 1935); spheroidal forms ~13 wide (Levine and Ivens, 1981; Pellérdy, 1974a); M: present or absent (?); it is not evident in their line drawings; OR: absent; PG: present. Distinctive features of oocyst: relatively small size of oocysts, two forms of oocysts (spheroidal and ovoidal), both with very thin, smooth, hyaline-like outer wall, and absence of OR.

Description of sporocyst and sporozoites: Sporocyst shape: ellipsoidal (line drawing); L×W: 6.2×4.2 (ranges not given); L/W ratio: 1.5; SB: absent (line drawing); SSB and PSB: both absent (line drawing); SR: absent; SZ: elongate comma-shaped, lying head to tail (line drawing); RB: present at rounded end. Distinctive features of sporocyst: difficult to determine given how poorly they are described and drawn by Yakimoff and Matschoulsky (1935).

Prevalence: Found in 2/7 (29%) of the brown bears examined.

Sporulation: Exogenous. Oocysts were let to sporulate in 2% potassium dichromate ($K_2Cr_2O_7$) solution at 24°C. After 48 hours the sporoplasm divided into four sporoblasts, and after another 24 hours the sporoblasts transformed into sporocysts containing two sporozoites each.

Prepatent and patent periods: Unknown.

Site of infection: Unknown. Oocysts were collected from the feces.

Endogenous stages: Unknown.

Cross-transmission: Yakimoff and Matschoulsky (1935) infected one 2-month-old kitten per os with sporulated oocysts of *E. ursi*; the kitten did not discharge any oocysts for 34 days postinoculation.

Pathology: Unknown.

Materials deposited: None.

Remarks: This parasite was found in the feces of a bear housed in the Leningrad Zoological Gardens. The bear was imported from one of the northernmost parts of the former USSR, which may likely be the natural habitat for this eimerian. Rastegaïeff (1930) earlier had examined feces of one *U. arctos* from the Leningrad Zoo, but it was negative for coccidia. Yakimoff and Matschoulsky (1935) discussed that *E. ursi* may be a rodent eimerian because they noted the similarity of its sporulated oocysts to those of *Eimeria geomydis* reported by Skidmore (1929) from the plains pocket gopher (*Geomys bursarius* Shaw, 1800), which were similar in size and shape to those of *E. ursi* but differed because the latter possessed an SR and lacked a PG, both of which characterize *E. ursi*. Also, *G. bursarius* did not occur in the Leningrad Zoo. Yakimoff and Matschoulsky (1935) said they also saw, "another one, without M, measuring: the round oocystes from 18.95 by 31.95 in diameter and the oval oocystes from 23.16 to 33.68 by 21.05 to 29.47…this species is identical to *Isospora lacazei* Labbe."

ISOSPORA FONSECAI YAKIMOFF AND MATSCHOULSKY, 1940

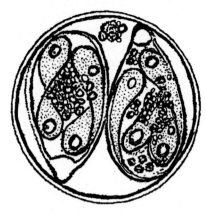

FIGURE 9.4 Original line drawing of the sporulated oocyst of *Isospora fonsecai*. *Modified from Fig. 21, Levine, N.D., Ivens, V., 1981. The Coccidian Parasites (Protozoa, Apicomplexa) of Carnivores, Illinois Biological Monograph No. 51. The University of Illinois Press, Urbana, Illinois, USA. 249 p. The University of Illinois Press, Urbana, Illinois, has released the copyright.*

Synonym: *Isospora lacazei* Labbé (1899) of Yakimoff and Matschoulsky (1935).

Type host: *Ursus arctos isabellinus* Horsfield, 1826 (syn. *Ursus pamirensis* Ognev, 1924), Brown or Red Bear.

Type locality: Asia: Republic of Uzbekistan (former USSR), Taschkent, Leningrad, and Kharkov Zoos.

Other hosts: None to date.

Geographic distribution: Asia: Russia, Uzbekistan (former USSR), Ukraine.

Description of sporulated oocyst: Oocyst shape: spheroidal, subspheroidal, to slightly ovoidal; number of walls, 2; wall characteristics: slightly pinkish, transparent, smooth, uniformly thick, ~1; in the Taschkent Zoo bear, L×W (n=10) of subspheroidal/ovoidal oocysts: 25.4×23.2 (22–32×20–30), L/W ratio: 1.1, and L×W (n=24) of spheroidal oocysts: 23.0 (18–26), L/W ratio: 1.0; in Kharkov Zoo bears, L×W of subspheroidal oocysts: 24.6×22.2 (22–28×20–26), L/W ratio: 1.1, and L×W of spheroidal oocysts: 23.2 (18.0–24.0),

L/W ratio: 1.0; and in Leningrad Zoo bears, L×W for subspheroidal/ovoidal oocysts: 26.4×24.0 (23–34×21–29), L/W ratio: 1.1, and L×W for spheroidal oocysts 24.6 (19–32); L/W ratio 1.0; M and OR: both absent; PG: present, usually one, sometimes two. Distinctive features of oocyst: variation in shape from spheroidal to subspheroidal to ovoidal with thin wall uniformly thick, ~1, lacking both M and OR but with one to two PG.

Description of sporocyst and sporozoites: Sporocyst shape: piriform or elongate ovoidal, distinctly pointed at one end (line drawing); L×W: 16×10 (14–18×8–12); L/W ratio: 1.6; SB: present on long, drawn-out neck of SP (line drawing); SSB: may or may not be present (line drawing), PSB: absent; SR: present; SR characteristics: large, dark granules scattered throughout SP (line drawing); SZ: elongate comma-shaped, lying head-to-tail (line drawing); RB: small, present at rounded end of SZ. Distinctive features of sporocyst: elongated, neck-like shape of anterior end of SP that supports the SB (line drawing by Yakimoff and Matschoulsky, 1940).

Prevalence: Prevalence in the Kharkov Zoo bear(s) not given. In the Leningrad Zoo, 2/7 (29%) brown bears were infected with oocysts of this species. In the Taschkent Zoo, the only brown bear examined was infected with oocysts of this species.

Sporulation: Exogenous, sporulation time and temperature not given. Oocysts were let to sporulate in 2% potassium dichromate ($K_2Cr_2O_7$) solution. The granular protoplasm was transformed into two hexagonal forms (pyramidal stages), and then the hexagonal forms were transformed into the sporocysts.

Prepatent and patent periods: Unknown.

Site of infection: Unknown. Oocysts were collected from the feces.

Endogenous stages: Unknown.

Cross-transmission: None to date.

Pathology: Unknown.

Materials deposited: None.

Remarks: This parasite was reported in bears from three different zoos (presumably all were

U. arctos) and the authors did not provide the origin of these animals, so its geographic distribution is uncertain. Yakimoff and Matschoulsky (1940) wondered whether it is really a bear parasite, or if it is a parasite of sparrows, because the bears often lick their paws contaminated by the soil where the sparrows defecate. However, because the oocysts of *I. fonsecai* were found in feces of brown bears at three different localities (Kharkov, Leningrad, and Taschkent Zoos), they concluded that it is indeed a parasite of bears.

DISCUSSION AND SUMMARY

There are no descriptions of eimeriid coccidia from the other 4 genera, all monotypic, in the Ursidae: *Ailuropoda* Milne-Edwards, 1870, *Helarctos* Horsfield, 1825, *Melursus* Meyer, 1793, and *Tremarctos* Gervais, 1855, although a Cystoisosporinae (*C. ursi*) is a parasite of *Melursus*.

Only 3 *Eimeria* species have been described from 2/8 (25%) species of Ursidae, two from black bears, *Ursus americanus*, in Canada, and one from the brown bear, *Ursus arctos*, in Russia. One species of *Isospora* has been described from brown bears (presumably) in zoos in Russia, Uzbekistan, and Ukraine, and 1 species of *Cystoisospora* is now known from a sloth bear in India. Thus, 5/8 (62.5%) species in the Ursidae

have not been examined for coccidia. Of the 4 described species in the Eimeriidae, none have a type specimen deposited in an accredited museum. As for many other carnivore families, genera, and species, this lack of knowledge is disconcerting. The IUCN lists 6/8 (75%) Ursidae as vulnerable and two (*U. americanus*, *U. arctos*) as species of least concern. Vulnerable species include the giant panda (*A. melanoleuca*, population trend increasing), sun bear (*H. malayanus*, decreasing), sloth bear (*M. ursinus*, decreasing), spectacled bear (*T. ornatus*, decreasing), polar bear (*U. maritimus*, unknown), and Asiatic black bear (*U. thibetanus*, decreasing). For the vulnerable host species, as populations decline and potentially become extinct, they will be accompanied by undescribed coccidian species that will likely be lost to science forever.

It is surprising that the 2 *Eimeria* species described from black bears have only been reported in Canada. Given the numerous published surveys for gastrointestinal parasites of black bears, it is curious that there are no reports of these or additional coccidian species from black bears south of Canada. To date no studies have proposed an explanation for this pattern, although it may be an artifact of limited sampling of other populations. As primarily solitary animals the prevalence of coccidia in bear populations is likely to be quite low.

10

Eimeriidae in the Feliformia Family Felidae

EIMERIIDAE IN THE FELIDAE FISCHER DE WALDHEIM, 1817

INTRODUCTION

The Felidae is a group of carnivores with two distinct lineages, the Felinae, consisting of 11 genera, 34 species, and the Pantherinae, with 3 genera and 6 species (Wozencraft, 2005). There is still, however, a great diversity of opinions as to how the various cat species should be classified, and classification schemes change dramatically as new species are discovered, better morphological measurements are made, and more and more genes are sequenced and compared for phylogenetic relatedness. For example, Romer (1968) divided the family into only 2 genera, *Felis* and *Acinonyx*; and 23 years later, Nowak (1991) said the Felidae consisted of 4 recent genera and 32 species. The most recent phylogenetic analyses support the taxonomy proposed by Wozencraft (2005). The Felidae are in the carnivore suborder Feliformia. They diverged from a common ancestor with the Viverridae, Hyaenidae, Herpestidae, and Eupleridae 40 (33–46) million years ago (MYA). The felids diverged 15.2 (12.3–18.1) MYA into two major (subfamily) lineages, Pantherinae and Felinae. The Pantherinae then

diverged 11.8 (8.3–16.3) MYA into the monotypic genus *Pardofelis* (marbled cat), and the second branch diverged 10.9 (6.5–15.3) MYA into the genera *Panthera* (lion, tiger, jaguar, and leopard) and *Neofelis* (clouded leopard and Sunda clouded leopard). The Felinae diverged 13 (8.5–16.4) MYA also into two branches. One branch split 11.5 (8.7–14.3) MYA giving rise to the genus *Puma* and a second lineage that underwent a fairly rapid radiation ~9–11 (5.1–13.5) MYA into the genera *Lynx* (lynx, bobcat), *Felis* (including domestic cat), *Prionailurus* (Iriomote, fishing, flat-headed, leopard, rusty-spotted cats), *Otocolobus* (monotypic, Pallas's cat), and *Leopardus* (margay, colocolo, kodkod, little spotted cat, ocelot, Geoffroy's cat, Andean mountain cat). The second branch in the Felinae diverged 13 (8.5–16.4) MYA into the genus *Acinonyx* (monotypic, cheetah) and a second lineage from which the genus *Catopuma* (bay cat, Asian golden cat) diverged 12.1 (9.4–15.6) MYA, the genus *Leptailurus* (monotypic, serval) diverged 8.1 (5.6–11.3) MYA, and finally split into the genera *Profelis* (monotypic, African golden cat) and *Caracal* (monotypic, caracal) 5.6 (1.9–11.3) MYA.

In the Felidae, the head, body length, weight, and color have significant variation. Head+body length vary from 337 to 2,800+ mm, tail length from 51 to 1,100 mm, weight from 5 to 306 kg, and

© 2018 Donald W. Duszynski published by Elsevier Inc. All rights reserved.

pelage can be gray to red to yellow-brown, there may be spots, rosettes, stripes, or none, and the tails are well-haired, but not bushy, and all cats have well-developed whiskers (Nowak, 1991). They have compact, muscular bodies. Their forefoot has five digits and the hind foot has four; and, in most species, the claws are retractile to prevent them from becoming blunted, and they are sharp and strongly curved to help them hold their prey.

SPECIES DESCRIPTIONS

SUBFAMILY FELINAE FISCHER DE WALDHEIM, 1817

GENUS ACINONYX BROOKES, 1828 (MONOTYPIC)

CYSTOISOSPORA RIVOLTA (GRASSI, 1879) FRENKEL, 1977

Type host: *Felis catus* L., 1758, Domestic Cat.
Remarks: Penzhorn et al. (1994) found oocysts in the feces of 2/16 (12.5%) cheetahs (*A. jubatus*) at the Hoedspruit Cheetah Breeding Centre, South Africa, which they identified as *I.* (syn. *C.*) *rivolta*, and zoo cheetahs in Egypt have been found infected with unidentified *Cryptosporidium* oocysts (Siam et al., 1994) (see Chapter 19). Nothing else is known about intestinal coccidians from cheetahs.

GENUS FELIS L., 1758 (7 SPECIES)

CYSTOISOSPORA FELIS (WENYON, 1923) FRENKEL, 1977

Synonyms: *Diplospora bigemina* Wasielewski, 1904, *pro parte*; *Isospora bigemina* Swellengrebel, 1914; *Isospora rivolta* Dobell and O'Connor, 1921; *Isospora cati* Marotel, 1921; *Lucetina felis* (Wenyon, 1923) Henry and Leblois, 1926; *Isospora felis* var. *servalis* MacKinnon and Dibb, 1938; *Levinea felis* (Wenyon, 1923) Dubey 1977a.

Type host: *Felis catus* L., 1758, Domestic Cat.
Remarks: Although *C. felis* was first discovered in the early 1900s, its name has undergone a number of changes over the last century. As emended by Frenkel (1977), it now properly belongs in the *Cystoisospora* (see Chapter 14).

CYSTOISOSPORA RIVOLTA (GRASSI, 1879) FRENKEL, 1977

Synonym: *Coccidium rivolta* Grassi, 1879; *Diplospora bigemina* Wasielewski, 1904 *pro parte*; *Isospora rivoltae* Dobell, 1919; *Isospora rivoltai* (Grassi, 1879) *auctores*; *Lucetina rivolta* (Grassi, 1879) Henry and Leblois, 1926; *Isospora novocati* Pellérdy, 1974b; *Levinea rivolta* (Grassi, 1879) Dubey, 1977a.

Type host: *Felis catus* L., 1758, Domestic Cat.
Remarks: Although the oocysts of this species were first discovered in the late 19th century, its name has undergone a number of changes over the last 120 years. As emended by Frenkel (1977), it now properly belongs in the *Cystoisospora* (see Chapter 14).

EIMERIA CATI YAKIMOFF, (1932) 1933

Type host: *Felis catus* L., 1758, Domestic Cat.
Type locality: Asia: Russia (former USSR), Leningrad.
Other hosts: *Felis chaus* Schreber, 1777, Jungle Cat.
Geographic distribution: Asia: India, Russia; Middle East: Iraq.
Description of sporulated oocyst: Oocyst shape: spheroidal, ovoidal, or ellipsoidal; number of walls, 1 (line drawing), but Levine and Ivens (1981) said there are 2 walls based on Gousseff (1933); wall characteristics: outer is smooth, colorless, and darker than inner layer; ellipsoidal oocysts were L×W (n=80): 20.8×17.1 (18–23×14–20); L/W ratio: 1.2, whereas spheroidal oocysts were 18 (16–22) wide; L/W ratio: 1.0; M, OR: both absent;

(A)   **(B)**

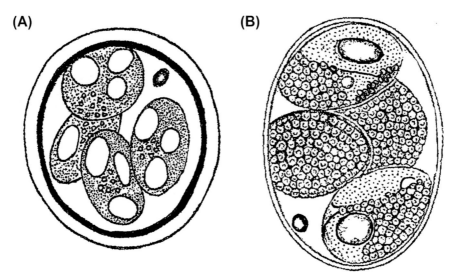

FIGURE 10.1   (A and B) Original line drawings of sporulated oocysts of *Eimeria cati*. *Modified from Figs. 76 and 78, Levine, N.D., Ivens, V., 1981. The Coccidian Parasites (Protozoa, Apicomplexa) of Carnivores, Illinois Biological Monograph No. 51. The University of Illinois Press, Urbana, Illinois, USA, 249 p. The University of Illinois Press, Urbana, Illinois USA, has released the copyright.*

PG: present. Distinctive features of oocyst: thin smooth wall(s), and the SPs almost completely fill the available space within the oocyst.

Description of sporocyst and sporozoites: Sporocyst shape: ovoidal; L × W: 11 × 6 (ranges not given); L/W ratio: 1.8; SB, SSB, PSB: all absent; SR: present; SR characteristics: a mass of many large globules that almost completely obscure the contents of the SP and, thus, hiding the SZ (Fig. 1, Yakimoff, 1933). Distinctive features of sporocyst: massive size of the SR.

Prevalence: Dubey and Pande (1963b) reported this species in 2/3 (67%) *F. chaus* they examined in India. Mirza (1970) reported it in 1/30 (3%) domestic cats in Iraq.

Sporulation: Exogenous. Dubey and Pande (1963b) said sporulation took 8 days to complete.

Prepatent and patent periods: Unknown.

Site of infection: Unknown. Oocysts were collected from the feces.

Endogenous stages: Unknown.

Cross-transmission: None to date.

Pathology: Unknown.

Materials deposited: None.

Remarks: Yakimoff (1932) named this species from the intestinal contents of a dead cat in Leningrad and gave preliminary measurements as listed above, but he did not provide a line drawing or photomicrograph with his new name, thus making it a *species inquirenda* or a *nomen nudum*. He redeemed himself a year later (Yakimoff, 1933) when he further described the oocysts from Leningrad and Azerbaijan and provided a line drawing. Gousseff (1933) found spheroidal, ovoidal, and ellipsoidal oocysts attributed to this species and described them as L × W: 18 × 16 (14–27 × 11–22); L/W ratio: 1.1, or spheroidal, 16 (12–16) wide; and SP were L × W: 7 × 4 (5–8 × 4–5); L/W 1.75; M, OR: both absent; PG: present. Dubey and Pande (1963b) said oocysts were subspheroidal to spheroidal, had an oocyst wall 1–2 thick, and composed of 2 layers, with the outer one thicker and the inner darker with a shining inner contour. Oocysts were L × W (n = 25): 21 × 19 (19–25 × 19–22); L/W ratio: 1.1; M, OR: both absent; PG: present as a single, ellipsoidal body (line drawing). The SP measured L × W (n = 20): 10–11 × 7, without a SB, but with a SR consisting of a few, scattered granules (Fig. 3, Dubey and Pande, 1963b). Mandal (1976) reported that subspheroidal to ellipsoidal oocysts of this species were L×W: 19–25×19–22; OR: absent; and ellipsoidal SP were L×W: 10–11×7, with a SR; Mandal (1976) clearly took his measurements directly from Dubey and Pande (1963b).

Although Dubey and Pande (1963b) reported what they called *E. cati* from *F. chaus* in India, the oocysts they described were quite different from those originally described from *F. catus* by Yakimoff (1933); the former authors described oocysts that were nearly spheroidal, with a thick wall of 2 distinct layers, and an SR that consisted of just a few scattered, small granules, whereas the latter author reported oocysts to be primarily ellipsoidal, with a thin, transparent wall, and a SR consisting of so many large globules that they almost completely obscured the SZ. Levine and Ivens (1981) thought this was "not an authentic parasite of cats." We tend to be in agreement with their appraisal and suggest that both sets of pseudoparasitic oocysts may be those of rodents passing through the digestive tract of the predators that ate them, especially, because no one has reported similar oocysts from either domestic or jungle cats as these independent sets of oocyst descriptions were first reported by Yakimoff (1933) and Dubey and Pande (1963b). And, as we note below, Dubey (1976) is now in agreement with this interpretation.

EIMERIA CHAUS RYŠAVÝ, 1954

Type host: *Felis chaus* Schreber, 1777, Jungle Cat.
Type locality: Europe: Czech Republic, Prague, Prague Zoo.
Other hosts: None to date.
Geographic distribution: Europe: Czech Republic.
Description of sporulated oocyst: Oocyst shape: broadly ovoidal to stoutly ellipsoidal (line drawing); number of walls, 1; wall characteristics: outer is thin, smooth, ~1.8 thick; L×W: 19.9×17.7

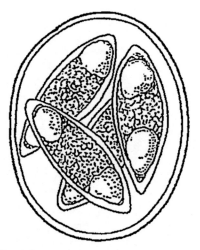

FIGURE 10.2 Line drawing of the sporulated oocyst of *Eimeria chaus*. Fig. 4g, from Ryšavý, B., 1954. *Příspěvek k poznání kokcidií našich i dovezených obratlovců (Contribution to the knowledge of our and imported vertebrates)*. Ceskoslovenska Parazitologie 1, 131–174, with permission of the Editor-in-Chief and copyright holder, Folia Parasitologica *(formerly* Ceskoslovenska Parazitologie*)*.

(18–24×14–22); L/W ratio: 1.1; M, OR, PG: all absent. Distinctive features of oocyst: smooth, 1-layered oocyst wall and absence of M, OR, and PG (line drawing).

Description of sporocyst and sporozoites: Sporocyst shape: spindle-shaped, elongate-ellipsoidal, slightly pointed at both ends (line drawing); L×W: (mean not given) 9–11×4–7; L/W ratio: unknown; SB: not mentioned in description but appears to be present at more pointed end of SP (line drawing); SSB, PSB: both absent; SR: present; SR characteristics: a group of granules in center of SP; SZ: not mentioned and not visible in line drawing. Distinctive features of sporocyst: elongate spindle-shape being slightly pointed at both ends.

Prevalence: Unknown.

Sporulation: Exogenous. Ryšavý (1954) said oocysts sporulated in 36–48 hours.

Prepatent and patent periods: Unknown.

Site of infection: Unknown. Ryšavý (1954) said the parasite was found in the small intestine.

Endogenous stages: Unknown.

Cross-transmission: None to date.

Pathology: Unknown.

Materials deposited: None.

Remarks: Levine and Ivens (1981) speculated that this may not be a genuine parasite of the jungle cat but might be a pseudoparasite. Ryšavý (1954) said the Prague Zoo was located near a swamp and that the cat had been imported from the Soviet Union. This species has not been seen since Ryšavý's (1954) original description, so Levine and Ivens (1981) may be correct.

EIMERIA FELINA
NIESCHULZ, 1924b

Type host: *Felis catus* L., 1758, Domestic Cat.

Type locality: Europe: The Netherlands.

Other hosts: *Felis chaus* Schreber, 1777, Jungle Cat; *Felis silvestris* Schreber, 1777, Wildcat; *Panthera leo* (L., 1758), Lion.

Geographic distribution: Asia: India; Russia; Europe: Belgium; The Netherlands; Spain.

Description of sporulated oocyst: Oocyst shape: long ellipsoidal to cylindroidal, with one end slightly flattened; number of walls, 2; wall characteristics: 0.8–1.5 thick, outer is smooth, thicker, and yellow-orange, whereas inner is darker with a shining inner contour; L × W: 24.0 × 14.5 (21–26 × 13–17); L/W ratio: 1.7 (Nieschulz, 1924b), or L × W (n = 100): 19 × 15 (15–19 × 11–17); L/W ratio: 1.3 (Dubey and Pande, 1963b); M, PG: both absent; OR: present, as a round mass of large granules (Fig. 1b, Nieschulz, 1924b) or as an "unorganized mass" (Fig. 12, Dubey and Pande, 1963b). Distinctive features of oocyst: elongate-cylindroidal form with a smooth outer wall, a darker inner wall, lacking M, PG but having a distinct OR.

Description of sporocyst and sporozoites: Sporocyst shape: broadly ovoidal; L × W (n = 25): 10 × 8 (8–10 × 6–8); L/W ratio: 1.3; SB: present,

(A)   **(B)**

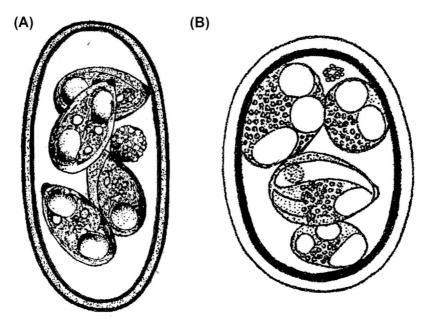

FIGURE 10.3   (A and B) Original line drawings of sporulated oocyst of *Eimeria felina*. *Modified from Figs. 61 and 64, Levine, N.D., Ivens, V., 1981. The Coccidian Parasites (Protozoa, Apicomplexa) of Carnivores, Illinois Biological Monograph No. 51. The University of Illinois Press, Urbana, Illinois, USA, 249 p. The University of Illinois Press, Urbana, Illinois USA, has released the copyright.*

prominent as a small cap at the narrower end of SP; SSB, PSB: both absent; SR: present, consisting of large granules sometimes in a single mass and sometimes scattered throughout SP (line drawing); SZ: comma-shaped, 8–9×2–3, with a large, spheroidal RB at their more rounded end. Distinctive features of sporocyst: distinct SB and a large RB at rounded end of SZ.

Prevalence: Dubey and Pande (1963b) found this species in 2/3 (67%) *F. chaus* they examined in India. Fameree and Cotteleer (1976) reported it from 5/252 (2%) cats in Belgium. Rodriguez and Carbonell (1998) looked at fecal samples from wild carnivores in central Spain and said that they found this species in 3/16 (19%) *F. silvestris* sampled.

Sporulation: Exogenous. Dubey and Pande (1963b) said sporulation was completed in 24 hours.

Prepatent and patent periods: Unknown.

Site of infection: Unknown. Oocysts were collected from the feces.

Endogenous stages: Unknown.

Cross-transmission: None to date.

Pathology: Unknown.

Materials deposited: None.

Remarks: Rastegaïeff (1929b, 1930) gave oocyst measurements as 20.7×16.2. Dubey and Pande (1963b) argued that oocysts of *E. felina* differed from other *Eimeria* species from cats only in the coloration of its oocyst wall and the character of its OR. Patnaik (1966) reported finding this species in a cat in Odisha, India. Levine and Ivens (1981) considered that this might be an authentic parasite of cats, but that it also could be a pseudoparasite. These reports appear to us to be rodent or avian *Eimeria* pseudoparasites.

EIMERIA HAMMONDI DUBEY AND PANDE, 1963b

Type host: Felis chaus Schreber, 1777, Jungle Cat.
Type locality: Asia: India.
Other hosts: None to date.
Geographic distribution: Asia: India.

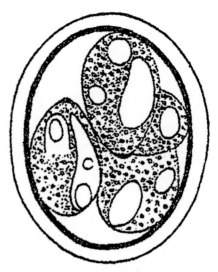

FIGURE 10.4 Line drawing of the sporulated oocyst of *Eimeria hammondi*. Fig. 5, modified from Dubey, J.P., Pande, B.P.P., 1963b. Observations on the coccidian oocysts from the Indian jungle cat (F. chaus). Indian Journal of Microbiology 3, 103–108, with permission of the Editor-in-Chief and copyright holder for IJM.

Description of sporulated oocyst: Oocyst shape: ellipsoidal; number of walls, 2, which were 1–2 thick; wall characteristics: outer is thicker and grayish, whereas the inner is darker with a shining inner contour; L×W (n=25): 24–29×19–22, means not given; L/W ratio: 1.1–1.3; M, OR, PG: all absent. Distinctive features of oocyst: small, ellipsoidal form with a lighter smooth outer wall and a darker inner wall and lacking M, OR, and PG.

Description of sporocyst and sporozoites: Sporocyst shape: broadly ovoidal; L×W (n=25): 12×8 (11–14×8–10); L/W ratio: 1.5; SB: present, described as vestigial, and visible only as a small thickening at the narrower end of SP; SSB, PSB: both absent; SR: present as granules distributed throughout the SP; SZ: comma-shaped, 8–10×2–3, with a centrally-placed N and 1 RB. Distinctive features of sporocyst: vestigial SB.

Prevalence: Dubey and Pande (1963b) found this species in 2/3 (67%) *F. chaus* they examined in India.

Sporulation: Exogenous. Dubey and Pande (1963b) said sporulation took 6 days to complete.

Prepatent and patent periods: Unknown.

Site of infection: Unknown. Oocysts were collected from the feces.

Endogenous stages: Unknown.

Cross-transmission: None to date.

Pathology: Unknown.

Materials deposited: None.

Etymology: This species was named in the honor of Dr. Datus M. Hammond, Professor of Zoology, Utah State University, Logan, Utah, USA.

Remarks: Dubey and Pande (1963b) said oocysts of *E. hammondi* differed from those of *E. canis* by having larger sporocysts and the presence of a SB. They differed from those of *E. felina* by lacking an OR, which oocysts of *E. felina* possess. They differed from those of *E. cati* because they have larger oocysts and lack a PG, which is present in *E. cati* sporulated oocysts. We are sad to suggest that this form, named after the great Dr. Datus Hammond, is invalid because we think the oocysts described by Dubey and Pande (1963b) represent those of a rodent coccidium the jungle cat had consumed before its feces were examined for oocysts.

EIMERIA MATHURAI DUBEY AND PANDE, 1963b

Type host: *Felis chaus* Schreber, 1777, Jungle Cat.

Type locality: Asia: India.

Other hosts: None to date.

Geographic distribution: Asia: India.

Description of sporulated oocyst: Oocyst shape: ellipsoidal to broadly spindle-shaped; number of walls, 2, which were 1–2 thick; wall characteristics: outer is smooth, thicker, and light yellow-green to pale yellow, whereas the inner is darker with a shining inner contour; L×W (n=25): 22×19 (20–28×16–20); L/W ratio: 1.2 (1.2–1.5); M, OR: both absent; PG: present, 1. Distinctive features of oocyst: ellipsoidal form with a smooth outer wall, a darker inner wall, lacking M, OR but having 1 distinct PG present.

Description of sporocyst and sporozoites: Sporocyst shape: broadly ovoidal; L×W (n=20): 11×8 (11–13×7–9); L/W ratio: 1.4; SB: present,

(A)   **(B)**

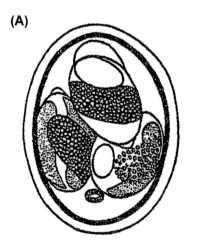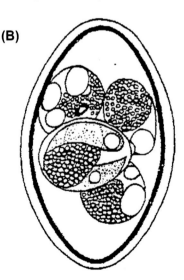

FIGURE 10.5   (A and B) Line drawings of two sporulated oocysts of *Eimeria mathurai*. *Figs. 8 and 9, modified from Dubey, J.P., Pande, B.P.P., 1963b. Observations on the coccidian oocysts from the Indian jungle cat* (Felis. chaus). *Indian Journal of Microbiology 3, 103–108, with permission of the Editor-in-Chief and copyright holder for IJM.*

prominent as a small cap at the narrower end of SP; SSB, PSB: both absent; SR: present as a large mass of many dark granules concentrated in the middle of the SP (line drawing); SZ: comma-shaped, 8–10×2–3, with a small, spheroidal RB at the rounded end. Distinctive features of sporocyst: distinct, cap-like SB.

Prevalence: Dubey and Pande (1963b) found this species in 2/3 (67%) *F. chaus* they examined in India.

Sporulation: Exogenous. Dubey and Pande (1963b) said sporulation took 6 days to complete.

Prepatent and patent periods: Unknown.

Site of infection: Unknown. Oocysts were collected from the feces.

Endogenous stages: Unknown.

Cross-transmission: None to date.

Pathology: Unknown.

Materials deposited: None.

Remarks: Dubey and Pande (1963b) argued the structure of these sporulated oocysts are distinct from those of *E. canis*, which has a M; from those of *E. felina* because they lack a PG; and from those of *E. chaus* because of oocyst shape and size and sporocyst structural differences. This species has not been recorded again since its original description, and there are no life cycles, cross-transmissions, or molecular data to suggest that these oocysts represent a real parasite of jungle cats. We think the oocysts described by Dubey and Pande (1963b) represent those of a rodent coccidium the jungle cat consumed prior to when its feces were examined for oocysts.

ISOSPORA ARCTOPITHECI RODHAIN, 1933

Synonym: *Isospora scorzai* Arcay-de-Peraza, 1967.

Type host: *Callithrix penicillata* (I. Geoffroy, 1812) (syn. *Hapale penicillatus*), Black Tufted-ear Marmoset.

Carnivore hosts: Hendricks (1974, 1977) said he found this species in 5 carnivore genera/species,

as definitive hosts, including the following: *Canis familiaris* L., 1758, Domestic Dog (Canidae); *Eira barbara* (L., 1758), Tayra (Mustelidae); *Nasua nasua* (L., 1766), South American Coati; and *Potos flavus* (Schreber, 1774), Kinkajou (both Procyonidae); *Felis catus* L., 1758, Domestic Cat (Felidae).

Remarks: This species name has been emended to *Cystoisospora arctopitheci* N. Comb. (see Chapter 14, Sarcocystidae: Cystoisosporinae). In addition to *C. arctopitheci*, there have been a variety of *Besnoitia, Cryptosporidium, Cystoisospora, Eimeria, Hammondia, Isospora, Sarcocystis,* and *Toxoplasma*-type oocysts found in the feces and *Hepatozoon* gamonts in blood of *Felis* spp. worldwide, but none of these have been identified to species, characterized sufficiently, or named (see Chapter 19).

GENUS *LEOPARDUS* GRAY, 1842 (9 SPECIES)

Remarks: *Cryptosporidium, Hepatozoon,* and *Isospora*-type organisms have been reported from time-to-time in the feces or blood of *Leopardus,* but none have been named or characterized to species (see Chapter 19).

GENUS *LYNX* KERR, 1752 (4 SPECIES)

CYSTOISOSPORA FELIS (WENYON, 1923) FRENKEL, 1977

Type host: *Felis catus* L., 1758, Domestic Cat.

Remarks: Triffitt (1927) reported *I.* (=*C.*) *felis* from a lynx that died in the Zoological Gardens of London, but she did not identify the host species, and Yakimoff et al. (1933b) reported *I.* (=*C.*) *felis* from Eurasian lynxes housed at the Leningrad Zoological Gardens (see Chapter 14). In addition, *Cryptosporidium, Eimeria, Hepatozoon, Isospora,* and *Sarcocystis*-type organisms have been reported from time-to-time in members of this genus, but none have been named or characterized to species (see Chapter 19).

GENUS *PRIONAILURUS* SEVERTZOV, 1858 (5 SPECIES)

ISOSPORA VIVERRINA AGRAWAL AND CHAUHAN, 1993

Type host: *Prionailurus* (syn. *Felis*) *viverrinus* (Bennett, 1833), Fishing Cat.

Remarks: Agrawal and Chauhan (1993) found numerous oocysts of an isosporan they described as a new species in the feces of a fishing cat from the Kanpur Zoo, India. This species name has been emended to *Cystoisospora viverrina* N. Comb. (see Chapter 14, Sarcocystidae: Cystoisosporinae).

GENUS *PUMA* JARDINE, 1834 (2 SPECIES)

Remarks: At least two *Sarcocystis*-type organisms have been reported from time-to-time in members of this genus, but none have been named or characterized to species (see Chapter 19).

SUBFAMILY PANTHERINAE POCOCK, 1917

GENUS *NEOFELIS* GRAY, 1867 (MONOTYPIC)

ISOSPORA LEOPARDI AGRAWAL, AHLUWALIA, BHATIA, AND CHAUHAN, 1981

Type host: *Neofelis nebulosa* (Griffith, 1821), Clouded Leopard.

Remarks: Agrawal et al. (1981) found oocysts of this form in the feces of one clouded leopard in the Lucknow Zoo, India. This species name has been emended to *Cystoisospora leopardi* N. Comb. (see Chapter 14, Sarcocystidae: Cystoisosporinae).

GENUS *PANTHERA* OKEN, 1816 (4 SPECIES)

CYSTOISOSPORA RIVOLTA (GRASSI, 1879) FRENKEL, 1977

Type host: *Felis catus* L., 1758, Domestic Cat.

Remarks: Yakimoff et al. (1933b) examined the fecal material of three lions, *P. leo*, and two tigers, *P. tigris*, in the Leningrad Zoological Gardens and found them all to be passing oocysts that, after sporulation, they identified as *I. rivolta*. This species name was emended to *C. rivolta* by Frenkel, 1977 (see Chapter 14, Sarcocystidae: Cystoisosporinae). There also have been a variety of "protozoa," "coccidia," *Cryptosporidium*, *Eimeria*, *Isospora*, and *Sarcocystis*-type oocysts found in the feces and *Hepatozoon* gamonts in blood, of *Panthera* spp. worldwide, but none of these have been identified to species, characterized sufficiently, or named (see Chapter 19).

EIMERIA ANEKALENSIS RAJASEKARIAH, HEGDE, GOWDA, RAHMAN, AND SUBBARAO, 1971

Type host: *Panthera pardus* (L., 1758), Leopard.
Type locality: Asia: India.
Other hosts: None to date.
Geographic distribution: Asia: India, Bangalore.
Description of sporulated oocyst: Oocyst shape: ovoidal, with one end slightly tapered; number of walls, 2 (line drawings); wall characteristics: outer is smooth and colorless; L×W: 26.5×19.8 (22–30×18–22); L/W ratio: 1.3; M: present; OR: absent; PG: present. Distinctive features of oocyst: presence of PG and a distinct M opening at the more pointed end of oocyst and lack of OR.

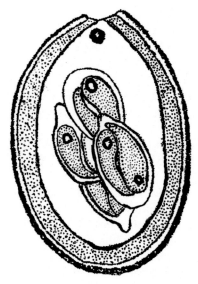

FIGURE 10.6 Original line drawing of the sporulated oocyst of *Eimeria anekalensis*. *Modified from Fig. 51, Levine, N.D., Ivens, V., 1981. The Coccidian Parasites (Protozoa, Apicomplexa) of Carnivores, Illinois Biological Monograph No. 51. The University of Illinois Press, Urbana, Illinois, USA, 249 p. The University of Illinois Press, Urbana, Illinois USA, has released the copyright.*

Description of sporocyst and sporozoites: Sporocyst shape: spindle-shaped; L×W: 12.3×7.4 (10–15×5–8); L/W ratio: 1.7; SB: present, as a clearly-defined nipple-like structure; SSB, PSB, SR: all absent; SZ: 9.7×3.9 (7–12×3–6); RB: small, present at rounded end of SZ. Distinctive features of sporocyst: distinct, nipple-like body at pointed end, lacking a SR.

Prevalence: Found in a "panther" cub that was kept at Dharmaram College, Bangalore.

Sporulation: Exogenous. Oocysts placed in 2.5% potassium dichromate ($K_2Cr_2O_7$) solution completed sporulation in 40–42 hours (Rajasekariah et al., 1971).

Prepatent and patent periods: Unknown.

Site of infection: Unknown. Oocysts were collected from the feces.

Endogenous stages: Unknown.

Cross-transmission: None to date.

Pathology: Unknown.

Materials deposited: None.

Etymology: The panther cub was caught in the hilly area of Anekal and this species is named after that location.

Remarks: Rajasekariah et al. (1971) found oocysts of this species in a panther cub kept at the Dharmaram College, Bangalore, India, but the description is sketchy and it has not been reported elsewhere since its original description. It remains to be determined if this form is a true parasite of *P. pardus*.

EIMERIA HARTMANNI
RASTEGAÏEFF, 1930

Type host: *Panthera tigris* (L., 1758), Tiger.

Type locality: Asia: Russia: Leningrad, Leningrad Zoo.

Other hosts: *Panthera pardus* (L., 1758), Leopard (?); Rajasekariah et al. (1971) reported

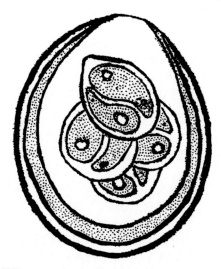

FIGURE 10.7 Original line drawing of the sporulated oocyst of *Eimeria hartmanni*. *Modified from Fig. 68, Levine, N.D., Ivens, V., 1981. The Coccidian Parasites (Protozoa, Apicomplexa) of Carnivores, Illinois Biological Monograph No. 51. The University of Illinois Press, Urbana, Illinois, USA, 249 p. The University of Illinois Press, Urbana, Illinois USA, has released the copyright.*

finding this species in a "panther" cub kept at Dharmaram College, Bangalore, India.

Geographic distribution: Asia: India, Russia.

Description of sporulated oocyst: Oocyst shape: elongate-ovoidal to slightly ellipsoidal; number of walls, 2 (line drawing); wall characteristics: outer is smooth, thinner, and darker than inner, whereas inner is thicker; L×W: 23×14 (only measurements given by Rastegaïeff, 1930) or 21.5×16.5 (20–22.5×14–19); L/W ratio: 1.3 (Rajasekariah et al., 1971); M: inconspicuous but present at markedly flattened end of oocyst; OR, PG: both absent. Distinctive features of oocyst: inconspicuous M that conspicuously flattens oocyst at one end.

Description of sporocyst and sporozoites: Sporocyst shape: spindle-shaped; L×W: 9.5–10×6–8 (means not given); L/W ratio: unknown; SB: present at slightly pointed end of SP; SSB, PSB, SR: all absent; SZ: no information presented. Distinctive features of sporocyst: small size with a small nipple-like SB at one end and lacking a SR.

Prevalence: Found in the only tiger (Rastegaïeff, 1930) and the only panther cub (Rajasekariah et al., 1971) examined, but on two continents.

Sporulation: Exogenous. Rajasekariah et al. (1971) said, "sporulation time was noted at 40–42 hours."

Prepatent and patent periods: Unknown.

Site of infection: Unknown. Oocysts were collected from the feces.

Endogenous stages: Unknown.

Cross-transmission: None to date.

Pathology: Unknown.

Materials deposited: None.

Etymology: Rastegaïeff (1930) named this species in honor of the famous German protozoologist, Mr. Hartmann.

Remarks: Rastegaïeff (1930), who first named this form, said, "As for the second coccidia, which has an egg-like form, the question is somewhat more difficult here. For some reason we did not succeed in cultivating this form and we cannot

say how much spores it gave. However, their egg-like shape, with strongly-flattened narrow end, differs greatly from the currently known 3 *Isospora*, as well as 2 *Eimeria*. We consider this coccid to be a new species. Leaving aside the question of the genus for the time being to further investigations." Nothing else was known about this "species" until Rajasekariah et al. (1971) said they found what likely was Rastegaïeff's (1930) coccidian in a panther cub in India and decided to "tentatively" complete the description. Levine and Ivens (1981) included this species in their book, still with a question about the genus identification, and said, "Rastegaïeff's form sounds suspiciously like a rabbit coccidium. Whether this is a true parasite of the tiger remains to be determined, as does whether it occurs in both the tiger and leopard." We agree, completely.

EIMERIA NOVOWENYONI RASTEGAÏEFF, 1930

Type host: *Panthera tigris* (L., 1758), Tiger.

Type locality: Asia: Russia: Leningrad, Leningrad Zoo.

Other hosts: *Panthera pardus* (L., 1758), Leopard (?); Rajasekariah et al. (1971) reported finding this species in a "panther" cub kept at Dharmaram College, Bangalore, India.

Geographic distribution: Asia: India; Russia.

Description of sporulated oocyst: Oocyst shape: spheroidal; number of walls, 2; wall characteristics: outer is thin, ~0.5 thick, whereas the inner is prominent, ~1.5 thick (see line drawing); L×W: 14–15 wide; L/W ratio: 1.0 (Rastegaïeff, 1929a, 1930) or L×W: 18–20 wide; L/W ratio: 1.0 (Rajasekariah et al., 1971); M, OR, PG: all absent. Distinctive features of oocyst: very small spheroidal shape with a thick inner wall.

Description of sporocyst and sporozoites: Sporocyst shape: ellipsoidal or slightly ovoidal (line drawing); L×W: 10×6; L/W ratio: 1.7; SB, SSB, PSB, SR: all absent, although it appears from the line drawing (Rastegaïeff, 1929a) that a

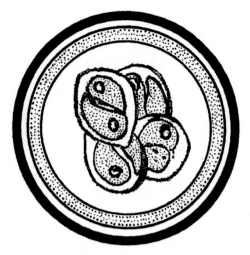

FIGURE 10.8 Original line drawing of the sporu-
lated oocyst of *Eimeria novowenyoni*. *Modified from Fig. 53,
Levine, N.D., Ivens, V., 1981. The Coccidian Parasites (Protozoa,
Apicomplexa) of Carnivores, Illinois Biological Monograph No. 51.
The University of Illinois Press, Urbana, Illinois, USA, 249 p. The
University of Illinois Press, Urbana, Illinois USA, has released the
copyright.*

small SB may, indeed, be present; SZ: granular at
their rounded end and clear at their pointed end
(Rajasekariah et al., 1971). Distinctive features
of sporocyst: very small size and lacking SB (?),
SSB, PSB, and SR.

Prevalence: Found in a "panther" cub that was
kept at Dharmaram College, Bangalore.

Sporulation: Exogenous. Rajasekariah et al.
(1971) said oocysts sporulated in 40–42 hours.

Prepatent and patent periods: Unknown.

Site of infection: Unknown. Oocysts were collected from the feces.

Endogenous stages: Unknown.

Cross-transmission: None to date.

Pathology: Unknown.

Materials deposited: None.

Remarks: This form is so poorly described
that it should be relegated to a *species inquirenda*.
Rastegaïeff (1929a, 1930), who named it from
a tiger, gave no structural information other
than the oocysts were small spheroids, and that
they had four SP after sporulation. We think it

is questionable whether this is a true parasite in
the first place, and we question whether it can
infect both tigers and leopards. This species has
not been seen since Rajasekariah et al. (1971) last
reported it. Levine and Ivens (1981) also question
its validity.

ISOSPORA BENGALENSI PATNAIK AND ACHARJYO, 1971

Type host: *Panthera tigris tigris* (L., 1758),
Bengal Tiger.

Remarks: Patnaik and Acharjyo (1971) found
oocysts of this form in the feces of a Bengal tiger
housed at the Nandankanan Zoological Park,
India. This species name has been emended to
Cystoisospora bengalensi N. Comb. (see Chapter
14, Sarcocystidae: Cystoisosporinae).

ISOSPORA FELINA PATNAIK AND ACHARJYO, 1971

Type host: *Panthera tigris tigris* (L., 1758),
Bengal Tiger.

Remarks: Patnaik and Acharjyo (1971) found
oocysts of this form in the feces of a Bengal tiger
housed at the Nandankanan Zoological Park,
India. This species name has been emended to
Cystoisospora felina N. Comb. (see Chapter 14,
Sarcocystidae: Cystoisosporinae).

ISOSPORA FELIS (WENYON, 1923) FRENKEL, 1977

Type host: *Felis catus* L., 1758, Domestic Cat.

Remarks: Yakimoff et al. (1933b) examined
fecal material of three lions, *P. leo*, and two
tigers, *P. tigris*, in the Leningrad Zoological
Gardens and found them all to be passing
oocysts that, after sporulation, they identified as
I. felis. This species name was emended to *C. felis*
by Frenkel, 1977 (see Chapter 14, Sarcocystidae:
Cystoisosporinae).

ISOSPORA LEONINA MANDAL AND RAY, 1960

Type host: *Panthera leo* (L., 1758), Lion.

Remarks: Mandal and Ray (1960) described "rhomboidal" oocysts of this form in the feces of one of two lion cubs housed in the Calcutta Zoological Garden, India. This species name has been emended to *Cystoisospora leonina* N. Comb. (see Chapter 14, Sarcocystidae: Cystoisosporinae).

ISOSPORA MOHINI AGRAWAL, AHLUWALIA, BHATIA, AND CHAUHAN, 1981

Type host: *Panthera leo* (L., 1758) (syn. *Leo leo* Frisch, 1775), Lion.

Remarks: Agrawal et al. (1981) found oocysts of this form in the feces of one lion cub in the Lucknow Zoo, India. This species name has been emended to *Cystoisospora mohini* N. Comb. (see Chapter 14, Sarcocystidae: Cystoisosporinae).

ISOSPORA PANTHERI AGRAWAL, AHLUWALIA, BHATIA, AND CHAUHAN, 1981

Type host: *Panthera leo* (L., 1758) (syn. *Leo leo* Frisch, 1775), Lion.

Remarks: Agrawal et al. (1981) found oocysts of this form in the feces of one lion in the Lucknow Zoo, India. This species name has been emended to *Cystoisospora pantheri* N. Comb. (see Chapter 14, Sarcocystidae: Cystoisosporinae).

ISOSPORA PARDUSI PATNAIK AND ACHARJYO, 1971

Type host: *Panthera pardus* (L., 1758), Leopard.

Remarks: Patnaik and Acharjyo (1971) found oocysts of this form in the feces of the only leopard cub sampled in the Nandankanan Zoological Park, India. This species name has been emended to *Cystoisospora pardusi* N. Comb. (see Chapter 14, Sarcocystidae: Cystoisosporinae).

DISCUSSION AND SUMMARY

We know of no eimeriid coccidia described from the 18 species in these 9 genera in the Felidae: *Acinonyx* Brookes, 1828 (monotypic); *Caracal* Gray, 1843 (monotypic); *Catopuma* Severtzov, 1858 (2 species); *Leopardus* Gray, 1842 (9 species); *Leptailurus* Severtzov, 1858 (monotypic); *Pardofelis* Severtzov, 1858 (monotypic); *Profelis* Severtzov, 1858 (monotypic); *Neofelis* Gray, 1867 (monotypic); and *Uncia* Gray, 1854 (monotypic).

As we can see from the entries above, there are a number of *Eimeria* species that have been found in felid feces. However, unless and until life cycle, cross-transmission, and/or molecular studies can confirm the validity of *Eimeria* species in felids, we concur with Dubey (1976), and many others, that these oocysts found in fecal samples all represent **spurious** findings resulting from the examination of cat feces that were sampled after the cats had eaten infected animal's carcasses or feces. Unsporulated oocysts of *Eimeria* species can pass unchanged and unharmed through the felid intestinal tract, and attempts to infect lab-reared cats with *Eimeria* species recovered in their feces have been unsuccessful (e.g., Streitel and Dubey, 1976). The only valid coccidia passing infective propagules in the feces, after undergoing some development in the cat intestine, are *Besnoitia*, *Cystoisospora*, *Hammondia*, *Sarcocystis*, and *Toxoplasma* species, and this leads us to an interesting observation. Members of the Felidae, and perhaps the Canidae, may be unique among mammal evolutionary lineages in that they have no coccidia in the apicomplexan family Eimeriidae (*Eimeria*, *Isospora* species) that parasitize them. Why not?

Eimeriidae in the Feliformia Family Herpestidae

EIMERIIDAE IN THE HERPESTIDAE BONAPARTE, 1845

INTRODUCTION

When biologists think about members of this family of small, carnivorous mammals, they think mostly of mongooses and meerkats, and some may even know the names: suricates, fossas, and kusimanse. These are mainly African, with an introduced genus widespread in Asia and southern Europe, and there are several small genera restricted to Madagascar. Most species are brown or gray, and a few are striped, but most are not. Their claws are not retractile and they tend to have small heads, pointed snouts, and short, rounded ears that are not as erect or pointed as their relatives, the **viverrids**. Many of these species have anal glands that secrete a foul-smelling substance, and the males have a **baculum**. Most are predators that feed on a wide range of animals such as small birds (including eggs) and mammals, reptiles (especially snakes), and a wide variety of crabs, insects, and other invertebrates (Myers, 2000a).

The place of origin (Africa or Eurasia) of the Herpestidae is unclear, but the family is inferred to have an Early Miocene origin, about 21–22 million years ago (MYA). Recent phylogenetic arrangements using DNA sequence data argue for an African origin even though the oldest known herpestid fossil was described from a European site (Roth, 1988). However, an African origin seems most parsimonious because it would imply a single migration event from Africa to Asia, probably through the Arabian microplate, allowing for the differentiation of the extant Asian *Herpestes* clade (Patou et al., 2009). Once they reached Asia, the divergent date for the Asian *Herpestes* (about 15 MYA) and the age of the most ancient fossil attributed to the Herpestidae from Europe (18 MYA) seem congruent with such a migration (Patou et al., 2009). The **monophyly** of this family is supported by morphological, **karyological**, and molecular characters; these combined data sets suggest the existence of two main **clades** or lineages, the social and the solitary mongooses (Patou et al., 2009).

The family consists of 14 genera and 33 species of small-bodied carnivores that are referred to as noted above: mongooses, kusimanse, meerkats, suricates, and fossas (Wozencraft, 2005). They are terrestrial animals, and primarily

© 2018 Donald W. Duszynski published by Elsevier Inc. All rights reserved.

diurnal, although a few mongoose species are nocturnal or **crepuscular**. Herpestids occupy a wide variety of habitats from deserts to tropical forests across their natural range in Africa and Asia. Several species are also found on islands (e.g., West Indies, Mauritius, Fiji, and others), where they were introduced in an attempt to control rodents and snakes, but now they are considered as invasive species on these islands. Only 1 genus, *Herpestes*, occurs in Asia and 1 species (*H. ichneumon*) is found in southern Europe where, likely, it was also introduced. Using both mitochondrial (cytochrome b and ND2) and nuclear (β-fibrinogen intron 7 and transthyretin intron 1) sequences from almost all known mongoose species, Patou et al. (2009) produced a well-resolved phylogeny of the Herpestidae and confirmed that the genus *Herpestes* is **paraphyletic**, with three distinct lineages. However, the morphological similarities of these lineages are so striking that the question emerges whether these species converged to this morphotype or retained some ancestral characteristics.

SPECIES DESCRIPTIONS

GENUS *HELOGALE* GRAY, 1862 (2 SPECIES)

ISOSPORA GARNHAMI BRAY, 1954

Type host: *Helogale parvula* (Sundevall, 1847), Common Dwarf Mongoose.

Other hosts: *Crossarchus obscurus* F.G. Cuvier, 1925, Common Kusimanse; *Herpestes edwardsi* (É. Geoffroy Saint-Hilaire, 1818) (syn. *Herpestes mungo* (Blanford, 1888)), Indian Gray Mongoose (Pellérdy, 1974a).

Remarks: This species name has been emended to *Cystoisospora garnhami* N. Comb. (see Chapter 14, Sarcocystidae: Cystoisosporinae).

ISOSPORA HOAREI BRAY, 1954

Type host: *Helogale parvula* (Sundevall, 1847) (syn. *Helogale undulatus* (Peters, 1852)), Common Dwarf Mongoose.

Other hosts: *Herpestes edwardsi* (É. Geoffroy Saint-Hilaire, 1818) (syn. *Herpestes mungo* (Blanford, 1888)), Indian Gray Mongoose (Pellérdy, 1974a).

Remarks: This species name has been emended to *Cystoisospora hoarei* N. Comb. (see Chapter 14, Sarcocystidae: Cystoisosporinae).

GENUS *HERPESTES* ILLIGER, 1811 (10 SPECIES)

EIMERIA JALPAIGURIENSIS BANDYOPADHYAY, 1982

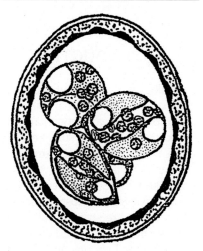

FIGURE 11.1 Original line drawing of the sporulated oocyst of *Eimeria jalpaiguriensis*. *Modified from Fig. 4, Bandyopadhyay, S.S., 1982. A new coccidium,* Eimeria jalpaiguriensis *n. sp. from a mongoose,* Herpestes edwardsi *(Geoffroy). Journal of the Bengal Natural History Society 1, 23–27.*

Type host: *Herpestes edwardsi* (É. Geoffroy Saint-Hilaire, 1818) (syn. *Herpestes mungo* (Blanford, 1888)), Indian Gray Mongoose.

Type locality: Asia: India, West Bengal, Jalpaiguri town.

Other hosts: None to date.

Geographic distribution: Asia: India.

Description of sporulated oocyst: Oocyst shape: ovoidal to subspheroidal; number of walls, 2; wall characteristics: outer wall is very thin, yellowish brown, inner wall is thick, ~1.5 thick, and marked with prominent convolutions; L×W: 21.6×19.0 (21–22.5×18–21); L/W ratio: 1.1; M, OR, PG: presumably all absent. Distinctive features of oocyst: thick, convoluted inner oocyst wall, and lacking M, OR, and PG.

Description of sporocyst and sporozoites: Sporocyst shape: ovoidal; L×W: 9.9×6.7 (9–11×6–7.5); L/W ratio: 1.5; SB: present as a small pointed structure at one end of sporocyst; SSB and PSB: both absent; SR: present; SR characteristics: 8–10 conspicuous globules disbursed between the SZ; SZ: described as long and broad, tapering toward one end, measuring 7.3×3.0 (6–9×2–3.5); RB: one, present as a clear globule at the broad end of SZ. Distinctive features of sporocyst: distinct small, pointed SB, and an SR as 8–10 clear globules.

Prevalence: Only 1/6 (17%) *H. edwardsi* examined by Bandyopadhyay (1982) had these oocysts in its feces when examined.

Sporulation: Oocysts sporulated in 72–96 hours in 2.5% potassium dichromate ($K_2Cr_2O_7$) solution when kept at room temperature (35–37°C).

Prepatent and patent periods: Unknown, oocysts were collected from the feces.

Site of infection: Unknown.

Endogenous stages: Unknown.

Cross-transmission: None to date.

Pathology: Unknown.

Materials deposited: None.

Remarks: Oocysts of this species resemble those of *E. newalai* in shape and in the shape and size of the sporocysts; they differ, however, in the structures of their oocyst walls, the SBs, and their SRs. Also oocysts of this species somewhat resemble those of *E. pandei* in size but differ in the structure of their oocyst walls and SRs.

EIMERIA NEWALAI DUBEY AND PANDE, 1963a

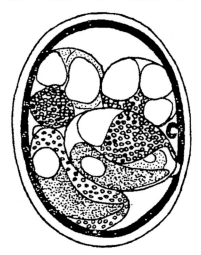

FIGURE 11.2 Original line drawing of the sporulated oocyst of *Eimeria newalai*. *Modified from Fig. 70, Levine, N.D., Ivens, V., 1981. The Coccidian Parasites (Protozoa, Apicomplexa) of Carnivores, Illinois Biological Monograph No. 51. University of Illinois Press, Urbana, Illinois, USA, 249 p. The University of Illinois Press, Urbana, Illinois, has released the copyright.*

Type host: *Herpestes edwardsi* (É. Geoffroy Saint-Hilaire, 1818) (syn. *Herpestes mungo* (Blanford, 1888)), Indian Gray Mongoose.

Type locality: Asia: India.

Other hosts: None to date.

Geographic distribution: Asia: India.

Description of sporulated oocyst: Oocyst shape: varied from ovoidal to ellipsoidal; number of walls, 2, ~0.8–1.5 in total thickness; wall characteristics: outer wall is yellow to orange, relatively thick, whereas inner wall is thin and darker; L×W: 19 (sic)×15 (15–19×11–17); L/W ratio: 1.3; M, OR, PG: presumably all absent. Distinctive features of oocyst: M, OR, and PG reported to be lacking, but a "small unorganized mass was constantly seen in all the oocysts examined," according to Dubey and Pande (1963a).

Description of sporocyst and sporozoites: Sporocyst shape: almost ovoidal; L×W: 10×8 (sic) (8–10×6–8); L/W ratio: 1.25; SB: present as a prominent nipple-like structure at pointed end of sporocyst; SSB and PSB: both absent; SR: present; SR characteristics: an irregular mass of large granules, or sometimes granules are disbursed in SP; SZ: comma- or sausage-shaped, with one end broad and the other end pointed, measuring 8–9 × 2–3; one RB present as a clear globule at the broad end of SZ. Distinctive features of sporocyst: SB at the distinctly pointed end.

Prevalence: Patnaik and Roy (sic) (1965) examined eight mongooses, seven were domesticated pets and one was a "captive wild-caught mongoose." Of these, 6/8 (75%) were passing unsporulated oocysts, but only 2/6 (33%) mongooses, the two youngest, passed oocysts of this species.

Sporulation: Pellérdy (1974a) said sporulation took 24 hours. Patnaik and Roy (1965) said sporulation took 3 days.

Prepatent and patent periods: Unknown, oocysts were collected from the feces.

Site of infection: Unknown.

Endogenous stages: Unknown.

Cross-transmission: None to date.

Pathology: Unknown.

Materials deposited: None.

Remarks: Patnaik and Roy (sic) (1965) said that they recovered oocysts of *E. newalai* in the feces of *H. edwardsi* and said that their oocysts were ellipsoidal, L × W: 17.0 × 14.4 (16–19 × 13–16); L/W ratio: 1.2 (1.1–1.25), with a colorless, uniformly-thick wall, and ovoidal sporocysts were L × W: 5.9 × 4.8, with a distinct SB, an SR, and comma-shaped SZ.

EIMERIA PANDEI (PATNAIK AND ROY (SIC), 1965) PATNAIK AND RAY, 1966

Synonym: *Eimeria pandeii* Patnaik and Roy (sic), 1965.

Type host: *Herpestes edwardsi* (É. Geoffroy Saint-Hilaire, 1818) (syn. *Herpestes mungo* (Blanford, 1888)), Indian Gray Mongoose.

Type locality: Asia: India: Uttar Pradesh, Mathura.

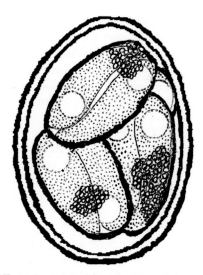

FIGURE 11.3 Original line drawing of the sporulated oocyst of *Eimeria pandei*. *Redrawn from Fig. 1h Patnaik, M.M., Roy, S.K.K., 1965. Coccidia of Indian mongoose* (Herpestes edwardsii). *Indian Journal of Animal Health 4 (1), 33–36, with permission of the Editor and copyright holder.*

Other hosts: None to date.

Geographic distribution: Asia: India.

Description of sporulated oocyst: Oocyst shape: ovoidal; number of walls, 2 (?), ~2 thick; wall characteristics: brownish-yellow, thinner at more pointed end; L × W (n = 20): 23.0 × 18.6 (22–24 × 17–19); L/W ratio: 1.2 (1.0–1.2+); M, OR, PG: all absent. Distinctive features of oocyst: oocyst thins at more pointed end, but M, OR, PG are all absent.

Description of sporocyst and sporozoites: Sporocyst shape: almost ellipsoidal or pyriform; L × W: 11 × 6; L/W ratio: 1.8; SB, SSB, PSB: all apparently absent; SR: present; SR characteristics: unknown; SZ: 9.5 long; RB, N: not mentioned. Distinctive features of sporocyst: none.

Prevalence: Patnaik and Roy (sic) (1965) examined eight mongooses, seven were domesticated pets and one was a "captive wild-caught mongoose." Six of seven (86%) hosts examined were shedding unsporulated oocysts representing 4 coccidian species. They said that four of six (67%) were older hosts and "preponderantly" harbored *I. hoarei* and *I. garnhami*, whereas the two younger animals shed oocysts of this species, in addition to those of *E. newalai* and *I. hoarei*.

Sporulation: Patnaik and Roy (sic) (1965) said that fecal material in 2.5% potassium dichromate ($K_2Cr_2O_7$) solution in Petri dishes at 32–35°C took 2 days to sporulate. Mandal (1976) reported that the sporulation time was 30–48 hours. Pellérdy (1974a) said sporulation takes 2 days, but he likely took this from Patnaik and Roy's (sic) (1965) paper.

Prepatent and patent periods: Unknown, oocysts were collected from the feces.

Site of infection: Mandal (1976) said this species was found in the intestine.

Endogenous stages: Unknown.

Cross-transmission: None to date.

Pathology: Unknown.

Materials deposited: None.

Etymology: This species was named in honor of Dr. B.P. Pande, Professor of Parasitology, Veterinary College, Mathura, India.

Remarks: Patnaik and Roy (sic) (1965) did not read their proofs very carefully because in their abstract, they named this species *I. pandeii* n. sp., and in the body of their published paper they originally named this form *E. pandeii*, which they said was a printing error; to comply with nomenclatural rules, they emended the name to *E. pandei* a year later (Patnaik and Ray, 1966); in addition, the second author's name was spelled Roy (1965) and Ray (1966), with the latter spelling being correct. Mandal (1976) reported ovoidal oocysts with a thick wall that measured 23 × 19 (23–24 × 17–19), but it looks like he took the measurements directly from the Patnaik and Roy (sic) (1965) paper.

ISOSPORA DASGUPTAI LEVINE, IVENS, AND HEALY, 1975

Synonyms: *Isospora rivolta* (Grassi, 1879) of Knowles and Das Gupta (1931); *Isospora garnhami* (small form) Bray, 1954 of Dubey and Pande (1963a) *pro parte*; *Isospora dasguptai* Levine, Ivens and Healy, 1975; [non] *Isospora rivolta* (Grassi, 1879) Wenyon, 1923; [non] *Isospora garnhami* Bray, 1954.

Type host: *Herpestes javanicus* (É. Geoffroy Saint-Hilaire, 1818) (syn. *Herpestes auropunctatus* (Hodgson, 1836)), Small Asian Mongoose.

Other hosts: *Herpestes edwardsi* (É. Geoffroy Saint-Hilaire, 1818) (syn. *Herpestes mungo* (Blanford, 1888)), Indian Gray Mongoose.

Remarks: This species name has been emended to *Cystoisospora dasguptai* N. Comb. (see Chapter 14, Sarcocystidae: Cystoisosporinae).

ISOSPORA HERPESTEI LEVINE, IVENS, AND HEALY, 1975

Type host: *Herpestes javanicus* (É. Geoffroy Saint-Hilaire, 1818) (syn. *Herpestes auropunctatus* (Hodgson, 1836)), Small Asian Mongoose.

Other hosts: *Herpestes edwardsi* (É. Geoffroy Saint-Hilaire, 1818) (syn. *Herpestes mungo* (Blanford, 1888)), Indian Gray Mongoose.

Remarks: This species name has been emended to *Cystoisospora herpestei* N. Comb. (see Chapter 14, Sarcocystidae: Cystoisosporinae).

ISOSPORA ICHNEUMONIS LEVINE, IVENS, AND HEALY, 1975

Synonym: *Isospora rivolta* (Grassi, 1879) of Balozet (1933).

Type host: *Herpestes ichneumon* (L., 1758), Egyptian Mongoose.

Remarks: This species name has been relegated to a *species inquirenda* (see Chapter 19).

ISOSPORA MUNGOI LEVINE, IVENS, AND HEALY, 1975

Synonyms: *Isospora garnhami* (large form) Bray, 1954 of Dubey and Pande (1963a).

Type hosts: *Herpestes edwardsi* (É. Geoffroy Saint-Hilaire, 1818) (syn. *Herpestes mungo* (Blanford, 1888)), Indian Gray Mongoose.

Remarks: This species name has been emended to *Cystoisospora mungoi* N. Comb. (see Chapter 14, Sarcocystidae: Cystoisosporinae).

ISOSPORA PELLERDYI (DUBEY AND PANDE, 1963a) DUBEY AND PANDE, 1964

Type host: *Herpestes edwardsi* (É. Geoffroy Saint-Hilaire, 1818) (syn. *Herpestes mungo* (Blanford, 1888)), Indian Gray Mongoose.

Remarks: This species name has been emended to *Cystoisospora pellerdyi* N. Comb. (see Chapter 14, Sarcocystidae: Cystoisosporinae).

GENUS SURICATA DESMAREST, 1804 (MONOTYPIC)

CYSTOISOSPORA TIMONI EL-GAYAR, HOLMAN, CRAIG, DEMAAR, WILSON, CHUNG, WOODS, NORRIS, AND UPTON, 2008

Type host: *Suricata suricatta* (Schreber, 1776), Meerkat, Suricate, Slender-tailed Meerkat.

Remarks: By the time El-Gayar et al. (2008) studied coccidians in meerkats, it was well-known that carnivores producing and passing isosporid-type oocysts that had sporocysts without SBs belonged in the *Cystoisospora* (not *Isospora*). We include this name here for completeness. The complete description is in Chapter 14 (Sarcocystidae: Cystoisosporinae).

DISCUSSION AND SUMMARY

We know of no **eimeriid** coccidia described from the 21 species in these 12 genera in the Herpestidae: *Atilax* F.G. Cuvier, 1826 (monotypic); *Bdeogale* Peters, 1850 (3 species); *Crossarchus*

F.G. Cuvier, 1825 (4 species); *Cynictis* Ogilby, 1833 (monotypic); *Dologale* Thomas, 1926 (monotypic); *Galerella* Gray, 1865 (4 species); *Ichneumia* I. Geoffroy Saint-Hilaire, 1837 (monotypic); *Liberiictis* Hayman, 1958 (monotypic); *Mungos* É. Geoffroy Saint-Hilaire and F.G. Cuvier, 1795 (2 species); *Paracynictis* Pocock, 1916 (monotypic); *Rhynchogale* Thomas, 1894 (monotypic); and *Suricata* Desmarest, 1804 (monotypic). Thus, only 2/14 (14%) genera and 5/33 (15%) species in this family have been examined for intestinal coccidia (*Crossarchus obscurus*, *Helogale parvula*, *Herpestes edwardsi* (syn. *Her. mungo*), *Her. javanicus* (syn. *Her. auropunctatus*), and *Her. ichneumon*.

Only 3 *Eimeria* species have been described/named from the members of this family, and we must remember/consider the possibility discussed with the Canidae (Chapter 4), that one or all three might be oocysts of the *Eimeria* species of prey items just passing through the intestine, and present in the feces of these herpestids, at the time fecal samples were collected. In each description we know the incidence of infection, but the sample sizes are tiny and we know nothing about the biology or life history of any of the three. Nothing is known about prepatent and patent periods, the sites of infection, endogenous developmental stages, or potential pathogenesis of these described species. And, there has been no cross-transmission work, and no type material has been deposited. The knowledge we have about the coccidians of Herpestidae is truly abysmal.

Six of the 7 *Isospora* species discovered from their herpestid hosts belong within the *Cystoisospora* because their sporocysts lack a SB, along with *Cystoisospora timoni*, which was discovered and named by El-Gayar et al. (2008) from the slender-tailed meerkat, *Suricata suricatta* (Schreber, 1776) from South Africa (see Chapter 14). *Isospora ichneumonis* has been relegated to a *species inquirenda*. It was given a name by Levine et al. (1975) for a form "described" by Balozet (1933) from *H. ichneumon* in Tunisia and thought to be *I. rivolta*. However, there was never a specimen, neither photomicrograph nor line drawing, to check the validity of Balozet's observation, so it can only be a *species inquirenda* or *nomen nudum*.

What an interesting group of animals this would be to work on from a parasitology point of view! There is a small number of very interesting animals in the Herpestidae, which makes it a tractable group in which virtually every species could be sampled throughout its range. Someone really needs to do this.

Eimeriidae in Feliformia Families–Eupleridae, Hyaenidae, Nandiniidae, and Viverridae

EIMERIIDAE IN THE EUPLERIDAE CHEN, 1850, HYAENIDAE GRAY, 1821, NANDINIIDAE POCOCK, 1929, AND VIVERRIDAE GRAY, 1821

INTRODUCTION

The Malagasy (Madagascar) carnivores are now placed into a single family, Eupleridae, with 7 genera and 8 species (Wozencraft, 2005) because they are believed to represent a single radiation; in the past decades, they were problematic with mammalian taxonomists since their discovery, and often placed as a separate subfamily within the Viverridae. Their species include fossas, fala-noucs, Malagasy civets, and Malagasy mongooses.

The Hyaenidae is thought to have evolved from a branch of the Viverridae; it has 3 recent genera and 4 species found in Africa and Asia and includes the aardwolf and hyenas. All 4 species have coarse guard hairs, a bushy tail, large heads, and forequarters, but rather weak hindquarters. They have blunt, nonretractile claws, and scent glands are present in their anal region, but males do not have a baculum. They all are mainly noc-turnal and generally inhabit not only grassland or bush country but also can be found in open forest. They walk on their digits giving the impression that they can trot tirelessly forever. Aardwolfs are primarily insectivores, whereas hyenas are scav-engers and predators of large game animals.

Wozencraft (2005) presents a substantive list of published papers arguing that *Nandinia bino-tata*, the African palm civet, should be placed in a monotypic family, Nandiniidae, based on the **plesiomorphic** condition of its auditory bullae and this has been confirmed by molecular data. This single species occurs from Guinea-Bissau to southern Sudan and south to Northern Angola and eastern Zimbabwe (Nowak, 1991). They are nocturnal and largely arboreal, living 30–50 m above the ground in various types of forest. Their diet consists of rodents, fruit, bird eggs, and large insects.

The Viverridae, a family with 15 genera and 35 species (Wozencraft, 2005), is one of the most problematic families of carnivores for taxono-mists, but evidence has accumulated that at least the Malagasy carnivores represent a single monophyletic origin and do not belong within the Viverridae, where they once were placed. The viverrids include binturongs and a diverse variety of civets, linsangs, and genets.

The Biology and Identification of the Coccidia (Apicomplexa) of Carnivores of the World
https://doi.org/10.1016/B978-0-12-811349-3.00012-8

121

© 2018 Donald W. Duszynski published by Elsevier Inc. All rights reserved.

SPECIES DESCRIPTIONS
EUPLERIDAE

There are no eimeriid coccidians known from any individual in the 7 genera and 8 species of this carnivore family.

SPECIES DESCRIPTIONS
HYAENIDAE

GENUS *HYAENA* BRISSON, 1762 (2 SPECIES)

ISOSPORA LEVINEI DUBEY, 1963a

Type host: *Hyaena brunnea* Brunnea, 1820 (syn. *Hyaena striata* A. Smith, 1826), Brown or Indian Hyena.
Remarks: This species name has been emended to *Cystoisospora levinei* N. Comb. (see Chapter 14, Sarcocystidae: Cystoisosporinae).

SPECIES DESCRIPTIONS
NANDINIIDAE

There are no eimeriid coccidians known from the only species of this carnivore family, *Nandinia binotata* (Gray, 1830), the African Palm Civet.

SPECIES DESCRIPTIONS
VIVERRIDAE

SUBFAMILY VIVERRINAE GRAY, 1821

GENUS *CIVETTICTIS* POCOCK, 1915 (MONOTYPIC)

ISOSPORA VIVERRAE ADLER, 1924

Type host: *Civettictis civetta* (Schreber, 1776) (syn. *Viverra civetta* Schreber, 1776), African Civet.

Remarks: This species name has been emended to *Cystoisospora viverrae* N. Comb., N. Sp. (see Chapter 14).

DISCUSSION AND SUMMARY

The Eupleridae is subdivided into 2 subfamilies. Subfamily Euplerinae Chenu, 1850, has 3 monotypic genera assigned to it (*Cryptoprocta* Bennett, 1833; *Eupleres* Doyère, 1835; *Fossa* Gray, 1865) and Subfamily Galidiinae Gray, 1865, has 4 genera including *Galidia* I. Geoffroy Saint-Hilaire, 1837 (monotypic); *Galidictis* I. Geoffroy Saint-Hilaire, 1839 (2 species); *Mungotictis* Pocock, 1915 (monotypic), and *Salanoia* Gray, 1865 (monotypic). There are virtually no other coccidian species reported from the individual members of this small felid family, the Eupleridae (see Chapters 14–17, and 19).

There are 2 other genera in the Hyaenidae, but we know of no valid, named eimeriid coccidia described from either of these 2 genera (*Crocuta* Kaup, 1828; *Proteles* I. Geoffroy Saint-Hilaire, 1824), both monotypic. There are, however, a variety of other coccidian species reported from a few individuals in the Hyaenidae that are identified in Chapters 14–17, and 19.

We suspect that no parasitologist has ever surveyed *N. binotata*, the African palm civet (Nandiniidae), for any kind of intestinal parasites. At least we are unable to find any such reference in the parasitological literature.

The Viverridae is a family consisting of about 35 species of carnivores called binturongs, civets, linsangs, and genets. These species are divided into 4 subfamilies. The Subfamily Paradoxurinae Gray, 1865, has 5 genera and 7 species: *Arctictis* Temminck, 1824 (monotypic); *Arctogalidia* Merriam, 1897 (monotypic); *Macrogalidia* Schwarz, 1910 (monotypic); *Paguma* Gray, 1831 (monotypic); *Paradoxurus* F.G. Cuvier, 1821 (3 species). The second group is the Subfamily Hemigalinae Gray, 1865, with 4 genera, all monotypic: *Chrotogale* Thomas, 1912; *Cynogale* Gray, 1837; *Diplogale* Thomas, 1912; and

Hemigalus Jourdan, 1837. The third group is the Subfamily Prionodontinae Pocock, 1933, with a single genus, *Prionodon* Horsfield, 1822 (2 species). The final grouping within the Viverridae is the Subfamily Viverrinae Gray, 1821, which includes the monotypic *Civettictis* (mentioned previously) and *Genetta* F.G. Couvier, 1816 (14 species), *Poiana* Gray, 1865 (2 species), *Viverra* L., 1758 (4 species), and *Viverricula* Hodgson, 1838 (monotypic). There is a variety of other coccidian species reported from a few individuals in the Viverridae, identified in Chapters 14–17, and 19, but not as many as we would suspect... or like to see. If there was ever a group of mammals that needed to be studied more intensively for their parasite fauna, these are them!

Adeleorina in the Carnivora

ADELEORINA LÉGER, 1911 IN THE CARNIVORA

INTRODUCTION

The Adeleorina is a poorly understood group of Apicomplexa parasites and is one of two groups within the Coccidia Leuckart, 1879, the other being the Eimeriorina Léger, 1911. Members of this group are united biologically by their use of **syzygy**, a characteristic method of gamete formation by which microgametes and macrogamonts are pressed together during their development (Adl et al., 2012). In the case of heteroxenous species, the conjugation of gamonts and subsequent sporogony most often occurs within an invertebrate *definitive* host and (mechanical) vector; the oocysts formed contain numerous sporocysts, and sporozoites are found in the hemocoel of the definitive host (Craig, 2001). When the vector is ingested, sporozoites are released, penetrate the gut of the vertebrate *intermediate* host, and enter the bloodstream to reach leukocytes and cells throughout the body to undergo merogony. Many of the species in this group have morphologically distinct meronts and merozoites during their asexual reproduction, which occurs in the vertebrate (intermediate) host.

The first-generation meronts (M_1) produce large merozoites (m_1) that are thought to initiate a second round of merogony in which the M_2 produces smaller m_2s, which then become the progenitors of gamonts (Barta, 2000). Merogony in the tissues ultimately gives rise to gamonts in white blood cells (WBCs) and tissue cysts; these tissue cysts may be a stage that can be transmitted by predation in carnivores, but this remains to be determined. Thus, the importance, if any, of predator–prey transmission among mammals is poorly understood (Craig, 1990, 2001).

The Adeleorina has 7 families of coccidia and includes those with both **homoxenous** and **heteroxenous** life cycles (Barta, 2000). One family, Hepatozoidae Wenyon, 1926b, has a single genus, *Hepatozoon* Wenyon, 1926b, with more than 300 species (Baneth et al., 2007; Ivanov and Tsachev, 2008); Barta (2000) suggested the genus is **paraphyletic**. Species in this genus infect various vertebrates including amphibia, reptiles, birds, and mammals, which are their *intermediate* hosts. The definitive hosts for these species are invertebrates that include mites, ticks, and various insects, and infection of the vertebrate host occurs when it ingests the infected invertebrate (i.e., not by its bite).

© 2018 Donald W. Duszynski published by Elsevier Inc. All rights reserved.

SPECIES DESCRIPTIONS

HEPATOZOON AMERICANUM VINCENT-JOHNSON, MACINTIRE, LINDSAY, LENZ, BANETH, SHKAP, AND BLAGBURN, 1997

Figures: For LM and/or TEM photomicrographs of cystic stages (Figs. 1–4), meronts (Figs. 6, 7), merozoites (Figs. 8, 9), gamonts (Figs. 13, 14), and zoites of *Hepatozoon americanum* see Figs. 1–15 in Vincent-Johnson et al. (1997).

Synonym: *Hepatozoon canis*.

Type intermediate host: *Canis lupus familiaris* (syn. *C. familiaris*), Domestic Dog.

Type locality: North America: USA: Alabama, Auburn.

Other intermediate hosts: *Canis latrans* Say, 1823, Coyote.

Type definitive host: Unknown for certain, but Vincent-Johnson et al. (1997) provided circumstantial evidence to suggest that *Amblyomma maculatum* Koch, 1844, Gulf coast tick, may be the definitive host because they observed *Hepatozoon* oocysts, sporocysts, and/or SZ in four *A. maculatum* adult ticks removed from one of their dogs that exhibited clinical signs of disease.

Geographic distribution: North America: USA: Southeastern states, including Alabama, Georgia, Louisiana, Mississippi, Oklahoma, and Texas.

Prevalence: Unknown, but Vincent-Johnson et al. (1997) described this species from 35/35 dogs exhibiting clinical signs that are typical for this species.

Cysts (intermediate host): Spheroidal to ovoidal, but highly variable in appearance, L×W (n=26): 186×150 (130–280×70–245); 1-several membranes with N surround a core, L×W (n=25): 77.8×65.0 (35–100×25–88); central mass of core, L×W (n=17): 46.5×41.1 (25–68×20–63) is surrounded by concentric rings of nonnucleated membranes. Core wall, ~3–5 thick, encloses the core and central mass, which has a large N.

Cysts are numerous, most often present in skeletal and cardiac muscle, pancreas, spleen, lymph nodes, liver, and lungs.

Meronts (intermediate host): Rare, present in a parasitophorous vacuole (PV), ~100×83; spheroidal to ovoidal, L×W (n=2): 188×162 (162–213×125–198); core, L×W (n=2): 85×79 (80–90×70–88), often surrounded by membranous layer with N; core wall, ~3–5 thick; central mass with 61–105 N, L×W (n=2): 58×52 (48–68×40–63). Merozoites, up to 117, randomly arranged, L×W (n=10): 7.5×2.7 (6–9×2–4). Meronts observed in skeletal muscle and lymph nodes.

Zoites (intermediate host): Subspheroidal to elongate, L×W (n=50): 6.3×5.0 (4–8×3–6), cytoplasm appears vacuolated. Present in granulomas within macrophage-like cells in the skeletal muscle.

Gamonts/gametocytes (intermediate host): Cylindroidal shape, found in cytoplasm of neutrophils and monocytes, L×W (n=20): 8.8×3.9 (8–10×3–5), seem to have a tail-like appendage not seen in leukocytes of *H. canis*. There is no thick fibril-like structure surrounding the PV as seen in *H. canis* gamonts.

Sporulated oocysts/sporocysts (definitive host): oocysts mostly spheroidal, L×W (n=24): 390×360 (310–480×260–460); L/W ratio (n=21): 1.1 (1.0–1.3); SP were spheroidal, L×W (n=58): 26.1×24.8 (20–30×20–29); L/W ratio (n=58): 1.05 (1.0–1.15).

Cross-transmission: None to date.

Pathology: Typically causes severe clinical signs of disease including fever, stiffness, gait abnormalities, lethargy, depression, mucopurulent ocular discharge, and weight loss (Barton et al., 1985; Macintire et al., 1997; Vincent-Johnson et al., 1997). In addition, dogs usually exhibit marked leukocytosis, with WBC counts from 20,000 to 200,000 cells/μL. Panciera et al. (2000) examined eight naturally-infected dogs and, also, experimentally-infected four dogs and two coyotes with *H. americanum*; they found that, in addition to skeletal and cardiac myositis, each of their experimentally-infected animals and seven of eight naturally-infected dogs had gross histopathologic osteo-proliferative lesions.

Materials deposited: In the US National Parasite Collection, Beltsville, Maryland. Cysts and pyogranulomas in H&E-stained sections of canine skeletal muscle with USNPC No. 87327. Gamonts present in canine leukocytes on modified Wright-Giemsa-stained blood smears as USNPC No. 87326.

Etymology: The specific name reflects the region of the world from which this parasite was described.

Remarks: This species was named by Vincent-Johnson et al. (1997) based on the clinical signs, histopathological findings, gamont size, gamont ultrastructure, serology results, and the inability to experimentally infect *Rhipicephalus sanguineus* (Latreille, 1806), the brown dog tick, which seems to be the natural definitive host for *H. canis* (below). This species differs from *H. canis* because definitive diagnosis is usually made by finding organisms in muscle biopsy. Johnson et al. (2008) collected cystozoites of *H. americanum* from experimentally-infected, lab-raised rodents and fed them to a *Hepatozoon*-free dog. They detected gamonts in blood smears 42 and 56 DPI, and PCR analysis of blood was positive for the 18S rRNA *Hepatozoon* gene on the days that gamonts were found. Meronts were detected histologically in skeletal muscle biopsy 90 DPI and sequencing confirmed that the parasite in the dog was *H. americanum*. Xenodiagnosis was conducted by replete feeding of *Ambylomma maculatum* larvae on the dog; 40 days after detachment, sporulated oocysts were recovered from recently molted nymphs.

HEPATOZOON CANIS (JAMES, 1905) WENYON, 1926b

Figures: For LM of a meront in the spleen of a dog from the Philippines, see Fig. 5, in Vincent-Johnson et al. (1997). For LM of developmental stages in the tick and SEM of oocysts and sporocyts in the tick, see Figs. 2–13, 14–17, respectively, in Baneth et al. (2007).

Type intermediate host: *Canis lupus familiaris* (syn. *C. familiaris*), Domestic Dog.

Type locality: Asia: India: Assam, Borjulie Tezpur.

Other intermediate hosts: *Acinonyx jubatus* (Schreber, 1775), Cheetah; *Canis latrans* Say, 1823, Coyote; *Canis mesomelas* Schreber, 1775, Black-backed Jackal; *Cerdocyon thous* (L., 1766), Crab-eating Fox; *Crocuta crocuta* (Erxleben, 1777), Spotted Hyena; *Felis catus* L., 1758, Domestic Cat; *Vulpes vulpes silacea* Miller, 1907, Red or Silver Fox; *Panthera leo* (L., 1758), Lion; *Panthera pardus* (L., 1758), Leopard, etc.

Type definitive host: *Rhipicephalus sanguineus* (Latreille, 1806), Brown Dog Tick.

Geographic distribution: Africa: Egypt, Nigeria; Asia: India, Japan; Eastern Europe: Bulgaria, Hungary; Europe: France, Italy, Portugal; Malaysia: Thailand; Middle East: Iran, Iraq, Israel, Turkey; Philippines; South America: Argentina, Brazil. Likely, worldwide.

Prevalence: Conceição-Silva et al. (1988) found 143/301 (48%) red foxes in Portugal to be infected with this species; however, they found only 50/1,752 (3%) domestic dogs from the same area to be infected. Baneth et al. (2001) found that 9/12 (75%) dogs inoculated with naturally-fed or percutaneously-injected ticks became infected and all showed seroconversion. O'Dwyer et al. (2001) examined blood smears of 250 dogs from rural areas of seven counties in Rio de Janeiro state, Brazil, for the prevalence of *H. canis*; these included 26 dogs from Seropédica, 82 from Itaguaí, 41 from Paracambi, 26 from Mangaratiba, 32 from Barra do Piraí, 32 from Piraí, and 11 from Miguel Pereira. Ticks found on dogs also were collected and identified. *Hepatozoon canis* was identified in 98/250 (39%) blood smears as were 4 tick species: *Amblyomma cajennense* on 59/250 (24%) dogs, *R. sanguineus* on 31/250 (12%) dogs, *A. aureolatum* on 7/250 (3%) dogs, and *A. ovale* on 5/250 (2%) dogs. O'Dwyer et al. (2001) pointed to a positive correlation between the presence of *A. cajennense* and *H. canis* infection. Baneth et al. (2007) found oocysts of *H. canis* in 17/20 (85%) hemolymph smears done 29 days postmolt from unfed adult ticks that had previously fed as nymphs on a naturally-infected dog. Cardoso et al. (2014) detected *H. canis* in 68/90 (76%) red foxes from eight districts in Portugal, using both molecular (PCR amplification of 18S rRNA gene fragments) and histopathological sections of multiple tissues (bone marrow, heart, hind leg muscle, jejunum, kidney, liver, lung, popliteal or axillary lymph nodes, spleen and/or tongue). Furtado et al. (2017) collected blood samples from domestic dogs from three regions of Brazil; 81/129 (63%) dogs were positive for *H. canis*, as determined by PCR nucleotide sequences of the 18S rRNA gene of *Hepatozoon*.

Cysts (*intermediate host*): Baneth and Shkap (2003) found small monozoic cysts in the spleen of two dogs naturally-infected and two experimentally-infected with *H. canis*. Cysts were ovoidal, L×W (n=8): 21.6×17.1 (17–25×14–21) in histopathologic sections and L×W (n=5): 23.6×18.7 (20–26×15–22) in cytologic preparations. Baneth et al. (2007) measured additional monozoic cysts in the spleen to be L×W (n=8): 21.0×17.1. These cysts contained a single curved zoite with a single N, but unlike meronts that develop within a host cell and compress the HCN, no relics of HCN were seen in these cysts, and they did not seem to be located within a host cell.

Meronts (*intermediate host*): With a characteristic wheel-spoke pattern typically seen in the spleen, lymph nodes, lungs, and liver of dogs (Vincent-Johnson et al., 1997). However, Conceição-Silva et al. (1988) found meronts to be numerous in the bone marrow, but scanty in the spleen and liver; they were ovoidal, L×W: 10.3–15.8×4.4–7.1; immature meronts, ~12 wide, with four N, also were found in the liver, as were mature meronts, ~16 wide, with 25–100+ merozoites. Merozoites released from the meront were pointed at both ends, ~5.8 long. Baneth et al. (2007) also reported merogony to occur mainly in the bone marrow and spleen and these meronts measured L×W (n=19): 30.6×28.9. The earliest finding of *H. canis* merogony in bone marrow was at 13 DPI (Baneth et al., 2007) and by 19 DPI an increasing number of meronts could be found in mononuclear host cells. Baneth et al. (2007) also reported seeing two types of meronts, one containing 2–4 macromerozoites and the other type with 20–30 micromerozoites; they proposed that the "micromerozoites are clearly the progenitors of gamonts, but the role of macromerozoites is less well understood."

Zoites (*intermediate host*): In histopathologic preparation zoites were L×W (n=8): 13.5×2.6 (10–19×2–4), with a N, 2.7 (2–3) wide, whereas zoites in cytological preparations measured L×W (n=5): 15.8×5.8 (12–18×4–8), with a N, 3.2 (2–4) wide. The cyst wall was ~1 thick (Baneth and Shkap, 2003).

Gamonts/gametocytes (*intermediate host*): cylindroidal shape, found in cytoplasm of neutrophils and monocytes, L×W (n=20): 11.0×4.3 (10–13×4–5) and a thick fibril-like structure surrounds the PV (Vincent-Johnson et al., 1997); L×W: 8–10×4–5, with a N, ~2–3 wide (Bentley, 1905); L×W: 9–11×4–6, with a "well-visible" N, in a 7-year-old male collie in Bulgaria (Ivanov and Kanakov, 2003). This stage was found in the blood neutrophils and spleen (Conceição-Silva et al., 1988). Baneth et al. (2007) measured micromerozoites in dog tissues to be L×W (n=13): 10.7×1.7; macromerozoites to be L×W (n=2): 15.0×6.7; and gamonts to be L×W (n=8): 9.7×5.4. **Parasitemia** (gamonts in WBC) varied significantly among infected dogs with some dogs exhibiting <1% parasitemia, whereas other similarly-infected dogs had parasitemias of 80% or higher (Baneth et al., 2007). Khoshnegah and Mlhri (2009), in Iran, gave examples of parasitemia approaching 100% of peripheral blood neutrophils in some dogs. Gamonts were first found in the peripheral blood at 28 DPI and a higher parasitemia was seen by 39 DPI.

Sporulated oocysts/sporocysts (definitive host): Gamonts within neutrophils of the vertebrate host needed about 24 hours to free themselves after ingestion by the tick; soon thereafter they aligned side-by-side in syzygy, their N enlarged, and their cells became crescent-shaped. At 48 hours in the tick, two types of cells were present: elongated cells with an eccentric N, presumed to be microgametes, and more rounded cells, also with an eccentric N, presumed to be macrogametes. At 4 days after the repletion of nymphs fed on a naturally-infected dog, zygotes or early oocysts, ~64×60, had formed with a dense, ovoidal N surrounded by a lighter staining zone; by 5 days after repletion, the oocysts were 86×86 wide and sporocyst formation had begun (Baneth et al., 2007). These stages were extracellular, not present within tick host cells. Baneth et al. (2007) found oocysts singly, in couples, or in clusters up to six, in unfed adult ticks, 13 days postmolt; these oocysts were L×W (n=2): 252.6×247.3 and their SP were L×W (n=2): 32.3×13.9. In unfed adult ticks at 35 days postmolt, oocysts were L×W (n=5): 309.8×255.8. Baneth et al. (2007) counted an average 7.5 (7–8) SZ in 14 SP. Vincent-Johnson et al. (1997) also measured *H. canis* oocysts and said they were mostly spheroidal, L×W (n=15): 214.8×192.9 (160–325×138–258); L/W ratio (n=15): 1.1 (1.0–1.3); and their SP were ellipsoidal, L×W (n=31): 35.6×25.7 (29–41×17–30); L/W ratio (n=31): 1.4 (1.1–1.8). In Japan, oocysts of *H. canis* were found in ticks, *Haemaphysalis longicornis* and *Hae. flava*, removed from dogs with hepatozoonosis (Murata et al., 1991).

Cross-transmission: None to date.

Pathology: *Hepatozoon canis* infections can range from being asymptomatic in dogs with low-level parasitemia to a severe, life-threatening illness with fever, lethargy, anemia, and emaciation in animals with very high parasitemia (Baneth et al., 2007). Sakuma et al. (2011) listed the characteristic hematological abnormalities in *H. canis* infections to include nonregenerative anemia, thrombocytopenia, neutrophilia, hyperproteinemia, hypoalbuminemia, polyclonal gammopathy, and increased concentrations of serum creatine kinase and alkaline phosphatase.

Materials deposited: None.

Remarks: Bentley (1905) examined the blood of English breed dogs in Assam, India; the dogs did not present any symptoms except slight anemia and a small temperature increase between 98 and 101°F. He noticed that many of the polymorphonuclear (PMN) leukocytes had nucleated, almost rectangular bodies ("vermicule-like body coiled on itself") in them that displaced the host cell nucleus. Bentley (1905) called the parasite "a leucocytozoan" and believed that he had found "the first haemogregarine reported as occurring in the blood of a mammalian host, and the first haemogregarine to be found as a parasite of the leukocytes." Bentley (1905) did not name his organism, but Christophers (1906) named the form seen by Bentley as *Leucocytozoon canis*. Miller (1908) described the genus *Hepatozoon* into which this canine parasite was eventually transferred by Wenyon (1926b). This species differed from a *H. americanum* infection because gamonts were common in peripheral blood smears. Conceição-Silva et al. (1988) reported that the gametocyte was the predominant stage of the cycle and was found in every organ except the bone marrow, where meronts were the most abundant stage. Baneth et al. (2001) experimentally transmitted *H. canis* to dogs with laboratory-reared ticks, *R. sanguineus* nymphs that fed on a naturally-infected dog or were percutaneously-injected with canine blood containing *H. canis*. Baneth et al. (2001) documented transstadial transmission of *H. canis* but could not demonstrate transovarial transmission. Later, Baneth et al. (2007) studied the chronological sequence of developmental stages in the life cycle of *H. canis*, both in *R. sanguineus* and in the domestic dog.

Forlano et al. (2005) studied transmission of *Hepatozoon* to dogs using 4 ixodid tick species: *Rhipicephalus sanguineus*, *Amblyomma aureolatum*, *A. ovale*, and *A. cajennense*. They collected engorged adult ticks of each species from dogs that were naturally-infested and positive for *Hepatozoon* and inoculated them orally into four negative dogs. Other ticks were dissected and examined for oocysts. Only the dog inoculated orally with the macerate of *A. ovale* became positive 63 DPI as seen by finding gametocytes in peripheral blood. Among all dissected ticks, Forlano et al. (2005) found only two oocysts; these were similar to those of *H. canis*, and both were recovered from a single *A. ovale* tick; they then inoculated SZ recovered from the oocysts intraperitoneally into a *Hepatozoon*-negative dog, and circulating gametocytes were detected 84 days later, thus demonstrating that *A. ovale* can be a vector of *H. canis* in Brazil.

Baneth et al. (2007) discussed the idea of *H. canis* transmission by cyst-bearing animals acting as transport hosts, when they are consumed, as an alternative cycle to the common route of infection of the vertebrate ingesting infected arthropod hosts containing oocysts. They noted that cysts with multiple layers of mucopolysaccharide material encircling a zoite were found in the muscles of dogs infected with *H. americanum*, but it is unknown whether these unique large cysts were homologous to the small cysts of *H. canis* or if they represented a different developmental stage. It is presently unknown whether transmission by predation occurs in these two *Hepatozoon* species by the ingestion of these cysts, but this mode seems likely. However, Baneth et al. (2013) firmly established that *H. canis* can, and does, infect *F. catus*, the domestic cat, when they established the validity of *H. felis* based on a phylogenetic analysis of 18S rRNA gene sequences. In that study they found two cats that were definitely infected by *H. canis*.

HEPATOZOON FELIS PATTON, 1908

Figures: For LM of meronts of *H. felis* within lung, myocardial, and striated muscles of cats, see Figs. 5–8, in Baneth et al. (2013).

Synonyms: *Haemogregarina felis domesticae* Patton, 1908; *Hepatozoon felis domesticae* (Patton, 1908) Wenyon, 1926b; *Leucocytozoon felis domestici* (Patton, 1908) Patton, 1908 in *Felis catus* L., 1758.

Type intermediate host: *Felis catus* L., 1758, Domestic Cat.

Type locality: Asia: India: Madras.

Other intermediate hosts: *Lycalopex gymnocercus* (G. Fischer, 1814), Pampas Fox (?); *Prionailurus bengalensis* (Kerr, 1792), Leopard Cat; *Prionailurus bengalensis euptilurus* (Elliot, 1871), Tsushima Leopard Cat; *Panthera onca* (L., 1758), Jaguar; *Prionailurus iriomotensis* Imaizumi, 1967 (syn. *P. bengalensis iriomotensis*), Iriomote Wild Cat.

Type definitive host: The arthropod host or hosts for this parasite is/are unknown. Sakuma et al. (2011) collected ectoparasites from a *H. felis*-infected male Iriomote cat in Japan and found large numbers of pubic lice (*Phthirus pubis*) and larvae and nymphs of the ticks *Amblyomma testudinarium* and *Haemaphysalis hystricis* on its caudal pinna, suggesting these should be looked at as possible definitive hosts.

Geographic distribution: Africa: Tanzania; Asia: India, Japan, Korea, Singapore; Europe: Spain; Middle East: Israel; South America: Argentina (?), Brazil.

Prevalence: Patton (1908) found gametocytes in the PMN leukocytes of 9/347 (~3%) cats in India, which he called *H. f. domestici*, but Wenyon (1926b) considered it impossible to differentiate the two and suggested both were *H. canis*. Laird (1959) found no examples of *Hepatozoon* infection in 39 blood smears of cats from Singapore, nor in 14 from Malaysia. Klopfer et al. (1973) necropsied 100 cats in Israel, 50 of which were dead cats submitted for rabies examination, and 50 of which were stray cats killed after being used in various lab experiments. They found 15/50 (30%) dead cats and 21/50 (42%) stray cats to be infected with a form they identified as *Hepatozoon* sp., but which we now believe to be *H. felis*. Kubo et al. (2006) examined 2 species of wild cats that live on Japanese islands, Iriomote wild cat on Iriomotejima Island (Okinawa Prefecture) and the Tsushima leopard cat on Tsushima Island (Nagasaki Prefecture); they found 17/30 (57%) Iriomote wild cats and 6/42 (14%) Tsushima leopard cats to be infected with a *Hepatozoon* species, which is almost certainly *H. felis*. Later, Kubo et al. (2010a) examined the hearts of five leopard cats (*P. bengalensis*) in Korea, both histologically and by phylogenetic analysis of the partial 18S rRNA gene sequence; they found 4/5 (80%) hearts to demonstrate meronts in tissue sections and to be PCR positive for *H. felis*-like gene sequences. Sakuma et al. (2011) found *H. felis* in 1/5 (20%) *P. iriomotensis* they captured three times in Japan, for ecological analysis; identity as *H. felis* was confirmed by PCR and amplified 18S rRNA gene fragment analysis. Baneth et al. (2013) PCR amplified *Hepatozoon* DNA from 55/152 (36%) blood samples of cats in Israel and from 19/19 (100%) additional cats determined to have the parasite by microscopy of histological sections. All of these cats were infected with *H. felis* except two, which were infected with *H. canis*. However, prevalence rates of infection vary dramatically from country-to-country. Studies using PCR in Spain have reported rates of 0.6%–4%–16% from different areas; a comparative study in Bangkok, Thailand, had rates of 32% in 300 cats, and a study from São Luis, Brazil, found the blood from only 1/200 (0.5%) cats to be infected with a *Hepatozoon* species that clustered with *H. felis* (de Bortoli et al., 2011; Baneth et al., 2013). Vilhena et al. (2013) assayed blood by real-time PCR from 320 domestic cats from regions in north and central Portugal for a number of vector-borne pathogens; they found 50/320 (16%) samples to be infected with *H. felis*. Furtado et al. (2017) collected blood samples from 30 jaguars from three regions of Brazil; all jaguars from the Pantanal (n = 22) and Cerrado (n = 4) and 3/4 (75%) from the Amazon were positive for *H. felis*. They also collected blood from domestic cats, and 7/22 (32%) of the cats also were

positive for *H. felis*, as determined by PCR nucleotide sequences of the 18S rRNA gene of *Hepatozoon*.

Cysts (intermediate host): Unknown. This stage has not yet been detected for *H. felis*.

Meronts (intermediate host): Prior to the report of Klopfer et al. (1973), the *Hepatozoon* species found in cats had only been described in neutrophil granulocytes; however, Klopfer et al. (1973) found meronts in the lumen of capillaries in the heart muscle that gave the impression of obstructing these markedly dilated capillaries. Two forms of meronts were observed: (1) meronts with nucleated formations resembling immature merozoites arranged in palisades and (2) meronts with its lumen either loosely or densely filled with merozoites. These meronts mostly were spheroidal, 22 (14–34) wide. Klopfer et al. (1973) also noted that more parasites localized in the wall of the left ventricle than in the right side. Kubo et al. (2006), who examined both Iriomote wild cats and Tsushima leopard cats in Japan, found the heart was the most common site of meront development, along with skeletal muscle in the tongue, masseter, thigh, and diaphragm; in fact, all of the infected cats had meronts in the heart, and in the Tsushima leopard cats no meronts were detected in any organs/tissues except the heart. Meronts were observed mostly between cardiac muscle cells, and all stages of development were identified: mononuclear zoites, immature meronts with peripherally arranged nuclei, mature meronts with immature merozoites around a central residuum, mature meronts filled with irregularly arranged merozoites, and ruptured meronts that were releasing merozoites. Meronts measured L × W (n = 21): 22.3 × 15.3 (16–29 × 11.5–20.5); L/W ratio: 1.5; merozoites were L × W (n = 8): 6.1 × 2.3 (5–7 × 2–2.5) (Kubo et al., 2006). Kubo et al. (2010a) examined histological tissue sections of the hearts of five leopard cats (*P. bengalensis*) in Korea; microscopically, they found meronts within parasitophorous vacuoles that were located between myocytes. The meronts were L × W (n = 3): 31 × 19 (25–39 × 15–24); L/W ratio: 1.6 and contained 28 (24–35) merozoites. Analysis of the 18S rRNA gene sequences of the *Hepatozoon* infecting these Korean leopards was 99.2%–99.8% identical to Brazilian and 97.0%–98.2% identical to Spanish isolates of *H. felis*. Baneth et al. (2013) measured meronts inside their capsule in skeletal muscle, myocardium, and lungs of domestic cats in Israel; they were L×W (n=13): 39.0×34.5; L/W ratio: 1.1; meront capsule width was 1.4; merozoites were L×W (n=14): 7.5×1.9; L/W ratio: 3.9; and merozoite N were L×W (n=14): 2.4×1.6; L/W ratio: 1.5. Meronts were round to ovoidal and their merozoites were dispersed within the meront without obvious pattern of arrangement.

Zoites (*intermediate host*): Unknown.

Gamonts/gametocytes (*intermediate host*): Very rare (see *Remarks*). However, Baneth et al. (2013) did measure gamonts located in the cytoplasm of neutrophils and monocytes, and sometimes compressing the HCN; they were L×W (n=13): 10.5×4.7; L/W ratio: 2.2; and the gamont N was L×W (n=12): 4×3.2. Gamonts were enveloped by a visible membrane.

Sporulated oocysts/sporocysts (*definitive host*): Unknown.

Cross-transmission: None to date.

Pathology: Klopfer et al. (1973) reported a mild perivascular infiltration of inflammatory cells surrounded some of the affected capillaries but noted that inflammatory reactions to meronts were scarce. Sakuma et al. (2011) captured a male Iriomote cat three times from January 2010 to January 2011 and noted that both parasitemia (gamonts in neutrophils) and serum creatine kinase levels increased during the year; even though neutrophils were infected with the capsule-like structure of the parasite gamont, both erythrocyte and leukocyte counts were normal, and the cat showed no outward signs of disease. Kubo et al. (2006) reported only a mild infiltration of mononuclear cells and/or mild fibrosis in the hearts of four Iriomote wild cats and one Tsushima leopard cat.

Materials deposited: None.

Etymology: The specific epitaph refers to the genus name of the type intermediate vertebrate host.

Remarks: Patton (1908) in India described this parasite in the peripheral blood, notably in the PMN leukocytes where, in his opinion, it presented morphological features that were identical to those of *H. canis* described a few years earlier (above). Because it occurred in the cat, Patton (1908) called it *Haemogregarina felis domesticae*. Laird (1959) observed that there were no further papers reporting infection with *Hepatozoon* in the half-century following Patton's original report. One reason might be that parasitemia in *H. felis* infections always seems to be exceptionally low. For example, Klopfer et al. (1973) never saw *Hepatozoon* gametocytes in the blood of 100 domestic cats studied in Israel, even though 36 animals had meronts in their myocardium. Baneth et al. (1998) could only detect gametocytes of *Hepatozoon* in 7/1,229 (0.5%) domestic cats at the ratio of about one gametocyte per 2,000 to 7,000 leukocytes. Kubo et al. (2006) never saw any peripheral leukocytes infected with gametocytes in their study of 72 island cats in Japan. And Sakuma et al. (2011) captured an Iriomote cat three times in 13 months: the first was January, 2010, and they detected no gamonts in leukocytes, the second time (December, 2010) parasitemia was 0.9%, and the third time it was 3.0% of neutrophils counted.

Although many authors had found and reported *Hepatozoon* organisms in various felids around the world, many were cautious and referred to *Hepatozoon*-like parasites without committing to a specific name, and others speculated they might have found *H. felis* Patton (1908). The recent development and use of PCR, with genus-specific primers for *Hepatozoon*-like organisms, allowed Baneth et al. (2013) to redescribe and establish *H. felis*, as a real species, based on the morphology of blood and tissue forms, and phylogenetic analysis of PCR sequenced fragments of the 18S rRNA gene. It is likely that *H. felis* is the predominant species infecting cats and wild felids worldwide and this distribution could be due to transmission by some ubiquitous vector such as a common flea, tick, or mite, and/or to alternative routes of transmission such as carnivorism and transplacental transmission. Baneth et al. (2013) also found a statistically significant association between outdoor access of cats and *H. felis* infection; they also found that two fetuses from *H. felis*-positive queens were positive by PCR of lung and amniotic fetal tissues suggesting possible transplacental transmission of this parasite as another strategy in its transmission.

Giannitti et al. (2012) examined one wild adult female Pampas gray fox in Rio Negro Province, Argentina; the animal showed severe incoordination and apparent blindness and was euthanized. The authors performed a complete necropsy and reported the fox was coinfected with canine distemper virus and a *Hepatozoon* that closely resembled *H. felis*, confirmed both by morphology and molecular evaluations. In fact, their sequenced 18S rRNA product was 99% identical to *H. felis* by BLAST analysis and it clustered with published *H. felis* sequences, but separately from *H. canis*, *H. americanum*, and other *Hepatozoon* species. This was the first time that *H. felis* was reported from a member of the Canidae, and the authors suggested the probable cause was immunosuppression due to the viral infection that exacerbated a preexisting *H. felis* infection that allowed increased merogony and the dissemination of *H. felis* into the host's tissues.

HEPATOZOON MUSTELIS NOVILLA, CARPENTER, AND KWAPIEN, 1980

Figures: For LM photomicrographs of liver (Fig. 6), lung (Fig. 10), hair follicles in the skin (Fig. 11), heart (Fig. 15) meronts, and aggregates with gametocytes or trophozoites (Fig. 14) of *Hepatozoon mustelis* see Novilla et al. (1980). They also have a TEM photomicrograph of a free merozoite (Fig. 13).

Type intermediate host: *Mustela eversmanni satunini* (Migulin, 1928), Siberian Polecat.

Type locality: Asia: Russia: Siberia.

Other intermediate hosts: Unknown.

Type definitive host: The arthropod host or hosts for this parasite is/are unknown. However, Novilla et al. (1980) suggested that a mosquito "is the likely cause" because of the many developing stages of this species found deep in the dermis and subcutaneous fat.

Geographic distribution: Asia: Russia: Siberia; North America: USA: Maryland, Patuxent Wildlife Research Center.

Prevalence: Forty-six Siberian polecats were shipped from the Voronezh State Preserve, Novosibirsk, Siberia, to the Patuxent Wildlife Research Center to serve as experimental prototypes of the endangered black-footed ferret (*Mustela nigripes*). A female in estrus was exposed to a male and a month later the dam delivered 11 kits; two were killed by cannibalism within 5–7 days, and 2 weeks after birth, the remaining kits developed dermal petechial and ecchymotic hemorrhages, anorexia, and were lethargic, dehydrated, and anemic, and seven kits died, whereas two kits survived and remained healthy, as did the dam and other members of the colony. All seven of the kits that died were infected with *Encephalitozoon cuniculi* (the likely cause of death) in multiple organs, and all seven kits that died had a concurrent infection with *H. mustelis*.

Cysts (intermediate host): Unknown. This stage has not yet been detected for *H. mustelis*.

Meronts (intermediate host): Microgranulomas and developing meronts in the seven infected kits were found in many areas of the skin (7/7), skeletal muscles (5/7), heart (7/7), liver (2/7), lungs (1/7), kidneys (4/7), and mesenteric lymph nodes (4/7) but not in the brain, intestine, or bone marrow. Virtually all sections of the skin, from head to the tail and toes, had meronts of *H. mustelis*. Thus, the skin, and particularly the hair follicles, appeared to be the predilection site of merogony because no developing stages were found in the spleen or bone marrow. Meronts were in aggregates of macrophages with little or no inflammatory reaction. Meronts varied in size, but the largest, under the skin, was 45×30

and contained about 40 merozoites. Individual merozoites averaged 9.6×3.3 and were seen within capillaries adjacent to granulomas.

Zoites (intermediate host): Trophozoites were seen within the cytoplasm of macrophages, but they were not measured nor were the macrophage cell types identified.

Gamonts/gametocytes (intermediate host): Not observed.

Sporulated oocysts/sporocysts (definitive host): Unknown.

Cross-transmission: None to date.

Pathology: Foci containing many mature meronts, some of which had ruptured, were characterized by focal infiltration with neutrophils, diffuse hemorrhages, and edema.

Materials deposited: None.

Etymology: The specific epitaph refers to the genus name of the type intermediate vertebrate host.

Remarks: In a symposium focused on the pathology encountered by zoo animals to certain parasitic infections, Novilla et al. (1980) named *H. mustelis* as a new species without providing mensural information other than what is summarized here, and no one has confirmed their observations or found it again since their original report. Their presentation focused mainly on nine, 17–20-days-old, *M. e. satunini*, born to a female from Siberia that had been shipped to Maryland, USA, for research purposes. The young polecats began squealing and became anorexic, lethargic, dehydrated, and anemic, and seven died. Necropsy of the pups revealed that they had a fatal systemic infection of *Encephalitozoon cuniculi* (the first reported from *M. eversmanni*) associated with meningoencephalitis, focal hepatitis, focal myocarditis, diffuse interstitial pneumonia, and focal nonsuppurative interstitial nephritis. Almost as an afternote, the authors mentioned a concurrent infection with a *Hepatozoon* sp. The fact that this was the first *Hepatozoon* sp. reported from this host suggested to them that the parasite was new, but they qualified their thoughts by saying, "The

species designation remains tentative until the vector is identified and the complete life cycle is elucidated." Once you give a species name, it becomes occupied. Period! To our knowledge, none of the authors followed this declaration with a formal naming of this species in a refereed publication, although their presentation is available in the published proceedings of the Symposium. We include their species designation here because a few authors, from time to time, refer to their paper as one "documenting" a *Hepatozoon* species in a mustelid.

HEPATOZOON PROCYONIS RICHARDS, 1961

Figures: For line drawings of gametocytes in raccoon heart section and blood cells, see Figs. 4, 5, in Richards (1961), and for LM of meronts within myofibers in raccoon tissue, see Fig. 3, in Clark et al. (1973).

Type intermediate host: *Procyon lotor* (L., 1758), Raccoon.

Type locality: North America: USA: Georgia.

Other intermediate hosts: *Nasua nasua* (L., 1766), South American Coati; *Procyon cancrivorus* (G. [Baron] Cuvier, 1898), Crab-eating Raccoon; *Procyon cancrivorus panamensis* (Goldman, 1913), Panamanian Crab-eating Raccoon.

Type definitive host: The arthropod host or hosts for this parasite is/are unknown.

Geographic distribution: Central America: Panamá: east of Panamá City on the Pacific side of the Isthmus; North America: USA: Georgia; South America: Brazil.

Prevalence: Richards (1961) found *H. procyonis* in heart tissues of 6/8 (75%) raccoons examined and saw gametocytes in 20/80 (25%) blood smears, but parasitized blood cells were found in only 3/6 (50%) raccoons with positive heart tissue sections. In raccoons trapped in pine hardwoods, 9/60 (15%) were infected with *H. procyonis*, whereas in a bottomland, hardwood swamp area, 11/20 (55%) raccoons were infected (Richards, 1961). Schneider (1968), in Panamá, reported *H. procyonis* from the only *P. c. panamensis* they purchased for the Gorgas Memorial Laboratory from an itinerant vendor. Clark et al. (1973) found that 57/65 (88%) adult raccoons, *P. lotor*, from 14 counties in Texas, USA, had developing gametocytes of *H. procyonis* in microgranulomas in their myocardium. Rodrigues et al. (2004, 2007) reported *H. procyonis* in 2/20 (10%) coatis trapped in an urban forest, and in the only *P. cancrivorus*, a captive female in the zoo of Campos dos Goytacazes.

Cysts (intermediate host): Unknown. This stage has not yet been detected for *H. procyonis*.

Meronts (intermediate host): Meronts and developing gametocytes were first seen in the heart tissue of raccoons, but none was found in the spleen (Richards, 1961). Meronts were ovoidal and measured L×W: 85×50, with the cyst wall inside a layer of host tissue. Richards (1961) estimated that mature meronts contained between 100 and 200 merozoites. Meronts were found only in the myocardium, but none in the liver, lungs, or spleen of *P. c. panamensis* by Schneider (1968), although he did not look at the bone marrow. The meronts he saw were cyst-like as indicated by a thin, limiting membrane, which was never thicker than 1.5, and usually thinner. Meronts were ovoidal to spheroidal, L×W (n=7): 40.3×27.1 (25–52×18–39); L/W ratio: 1.5. Mature meronts, or merocysts, were characterized by the presence of a large central body surrounded by individual merozoites. Mature merozoites had a compact N and measured (n=3): 8.7 (7.7–10) long; Schneider (1968) estimated there were >100 merozoites/meront. Meronts measured from *P. lotor* in Texas were smaller, L×W: 31.2×22.7, were found within myofibrils, and contained ~20 micromerozoites (Clark et al., 1973); these meronts were found mostly in cardiac and skeletal muscles (diaphragm, tongue), but in two instances meronts were found in splenic trabeculae.

Zoites (intermediate host): Unknown. This stage has not yet been detected for *H. procyonis*.

Gamonts/gametocytes (intermediate host): Gametocytes were first found in the monocytes of raccoons by Richards (1961). Each gametocyte was encased in a clear cyst (capsule), which had a narrow, recurved extension at one end. The capsule without the recurved tail was L×W: 10.9×5.4. Inside the capsule, the gametocyte was sausage-shaped and measured L×W: 9.5×4.3 with a N that was L×W: 7.0×3.8. In heart sections, gametocytes were numerous nearby developing meronts, often in clumps crowded between heart muscle fibers (Richards, 1961). Gametocytes were sparse in *P. c. panamensis* and found only in monocytes; none were ever seen in PMN leukocytes. Each gametocyte was usually in contact with the HCN or deeply embedded in it (Schneider, 1968); parasitized monocytes were not enlarged due to the presence of the gametocyte. Each gametocyte possessed a distinct capsule that was longer than the zoite inside it such that the unoccupied end bent back on itself or twisted to form a terminal flap (Schneider, 1968) or a recurved "tail" (Richards, 1961). The gametocytes themselves did not fold on themselves to form a "U" within their capsule but retained their cylindrical to ovoidal shape, not completely filling it. The gametocyte capsules, not including the free flap, measured L×W (n=20): 8.2×3.7 (7.5–8.7×3–4); L/W ratio: 2.2; the capsules plus the flap were L×W (n=9): 11.7×3.7 (10–12.5×3–4); L/W ratio: 3.2; and the zoite within the capsule was L×W (n=9): 5.5×2.5 (5–7×2–3); L/W ratio: 2.2 and had an oblong N, L×W (n=14): 3.5×2.3 (3–5×2–3); L/W ratio: 1.5 (Schneider, 1968). Clark et al. (1973) gave measurements of the gametocytes to be L×W: 7.5×3.9. The infected monocytes in *P. lotor* from Texas were enlarged (Clark et al., 1973) and neutrophils were not infected. Rodrigues et al. (2004, 2007) found gametocytes in two procyonids from Brazil, that they identified as *H. procyonis*, although the gametocytes they studied were found mainly in neutrophils (93%) and only rarely in monocytes (7%). Their gametocytes from *N. nasua* were L×W: 10.4×4.0; L/W ratio: 2.6; and the N was L×W: 4.2×2.0; L/W ratio: 2.1; and their gametocytes from *P. cancrivorus* measured L×W: 10.2×3.7; L/W ratio: 2.8; and the N was L×W: 4.0×2.0; L/W ratio: 2.0. The curved cytoplasmic projection, characteristic for this species, was seen in all gametocytes measured by Rodrigues et al. (2007).

Sporulated oocysts/sporocysts (definitive host): Unknown.

Cross-transmission: None to date.

Pathology: Infections are usually subclinical. Schneider (1968) saw only mild focal myocarditis, associated with pockets of infiltrating PMN leukocytes containing gametocytes in the heart of *P. c. panamensis* from Panamá. Clark et al. (1973) saw no clinical signs of disease or illness in infected, captive raccoons and no gross lesions referable to *Hepatozoon* infection were observed in infected tissues except for a focal accumulation of macrophages.

Materials deposited: Giemsa-stained blood film of mature gametocytes and sectioned heart tissue with meronts and developing gametocytes are deposited in the United States National Museum from raccoon number 6030 (Richards, 1961).

Etymology: The specific epitaph refers to the genus name of the type intermediate vertebrate host.

Remarks: Richards (1961) noticed that 8/11 (73%) of the raccoons he found to be positive for *H. procyonis* also were infected with *Trypanosoma cruzi*. The high rate of infection in raccoons in Texas, along with the length of their infections within the population (at least 2 years in captivity), suggested that the virulence of *H. procyonis* is low and that exposure, likely, is frequent. In addition, it seems that the parasitemia in blood cells is always quite low so studying blood smears is not the best way to diagnose an active infection. Clark et al. (1973) presented an interesting idea about transmission when they suggested that maturing meronts may become chemotactic because of the infiltration of mononuclear inflammatory cells into the adjacent

tissues. When the merozoites are released from their meronts, intense granulomatous inflammation occurs, and merozoites are phagocytized. They (1973) suggested that the fate of these phagocytized merozoites appeared to be important to the course of the infection because, presumably, at least some of the macrophages reenter the general circulation as monocytes with gametocytes.

Like the gametocytes of *H. ursi* (below), those of *H. procyonis* also have a beak-like structure. Both the shape and size of *H. procyonis* gametocytes are similar to those of *H. ursi* at 10.9×5.4 (Richards, 1961) and 10.4×4.0 (Rodrigues et al., 2007). However, *H. procyonis* meronts were principally found in the myocardium of raccoons and measured 40.3×27.1 versus the meronts of *H. ursi*, which were found only in the lungs of bears and measured 45.7×42.7.

HEPATOZOON URSI KUBO, UNI, AGATSUMA, NAGATAKI, PANCIERA, TSUBOTA, NAKAMURA, SAKAI, MASEGI, AND YANAI, 2008

Figures: For LM of zoites, meronts, lung nodules see Figs. 1–4, Uni et al. (2003) and Fig. 2, Kubo et al. (2008), and for TEM of various developmental stages see Fig. 5, Uni et al. (2003) and Fig. 5, Kubo et al. (2008).

Type intermediate host: *Ursus thibetanus japonicus* Schlegel, 1857, Japanese Black Bear.

Type locality: Asia: Japan, Gifu Prefecture.

Other intermediate hosts: None to date.

Type definitive host: The true definitive arthropod host or hosts for *H. ursi* is/are unknown. Uni et al. (2003) identified three ticks collected from their infected bears, *Ixodes ovatus*, *I. nipponensis*, and *Haemaphysalis flava*, but could not find oocysts in them. Kubo et al. (2008) collected 49 ticks from the skin of black bears they examined and identified 32 *Hae. japonica*, 3 *Hae. flava*, 10 *Dermacentor taiwanensis*, and 4 *Amblyomma testudinarium*. They (2008) found mature *Hepatozoon* oocysts in one *Hae. flava* and one *Hae. japonica*, both males. The oocyst in *Hae. flava* was L×W: 263.2×234.0; L/W ratio: 1.1; and the oocyst from *Hae. japonica* was L×W: 331.8×231.7; L/W ratio: 1.4. Oocysts had 40 and 50 sporocysts, respectively; these were subspheroidal, L×W (n=5): 31.2×27.0 (28–35×24–32); L/W ratio: 1.2. Each SP had 8–16 SZ and these measured L×W (n=4): 12.2×3.5 (10–14×3–4). However, oocyst morphology and size were similar to those of *Hepatozoon canis* found in *Hae. longicornis* and *Hae. flava*, collected from Japanese dogs, and Kubo et al. (2008) did not do the experimental transmission study or the genetic analysis of oocysts to separate them from *Hep. canis*. Thus, although Kubo et al. (2008) strongly suspected that these two *Haemaphysalis* tick species are the true definitive hosts for *Hepatozoon ursi*, they did not prove it.

Geographic distribution: Asia: Japan.

Prevalence: Uni et al. (2003) found this parasite, before it was named, in the lungs of 18/18 (100%) black bears in Fukui (9 bears), Shiga (5), and Gifu (4) Prefectures. Kubo et al. (2008) collected blood from the heart and the lungs from 35 Japanese black bears (22 males, 13 females) that had been killed in Gifu Prefecture and collected fresh blood from 9 additional bears (6 males, 3 females), also in Gifu; all 44 bears were positive for *Hepatozoon*.

Cysts (intermediate host): Tubercles formed of macrophages were found in all lobules of the lungs surrounded by squamous alveolar epithelial cells, and large alveolar epithelial cells enclosed zoites within the cytoplasm of the host cells, and these zoites had pushed the HCN to the margin of the cell. TEM of tubercles of macrophages showed large zoites within the macrophage. Nodules of merozoite/gametocyte-laden macrophages were observed in all 35 bear lungs examined by Kubo et al. (2008).

Meronts (intermediate host): Meronts and their merozoites were found in all lobules of the lungs of black bears but not in their liver, kidneys, heart, spleen, mesenteric lymph nodes, or skin. Meronts were subspheroidal to ovoidal, surrounded by a membrane, and mostly found between the alveoli, with a few in the pleura and in the connective

tissue (Uni et al., 2003). Meronts were characterized by peripherally arranged nuclei of the zoite and numerous internal merozoites. Mature meronts were L×W (n=10): 52.9×40.1; L/W ratio: 1.3 and were filled with many merozoites that were L×W (n=13): 4.9×2.0. Released merozoites were seen inside capillaries and between cells of the lung (Uni et al., 2003). In the descriptive study by Kubo et al. (2008), meronts were L×W (n=18): 45.7×42.7 (37–55×34–52); L/W ratio: 1.1, and each mature meront had ~80–130 merozoites and 0–5 residual bodies. Merozoites were L×W (n=8): 7.0×1.8 (6–8×1.5–2).

Zoites (intermediate host): Zoites were found within macrophages (Uni et al., 2003).

Gamonts/gametocytes (intermediate host): Gametocytes were found in leukocytes, probably neutrophils, in the peripheral blood. The parasitemia in the blood was 1.3–43 gametocytes/1,000 leukocytes. Kubo et al. (2008) studied 14 blood samples from bears and found *H. ursi* gametocytes in all of them but did not see any obvious hematological changes related to the presence of the parasite. Gametocytes were slightly curved, cigar-like, and had a beak-like protrusion at one end. Excluding their beak-like protrusion they were L×W (n=18): 10.9×3.3 (10.5–11.5×3–4).

Sporulated oocysts/sporocysts (definitive host): Kubo et al. (2008) found two oocysts, one in each of two ticks. The oocyst in *Hae. flava* was L×W: 263.2×234.0; L/W ratio: 1.1; and the oocyst from *Hae. japonica* was L×W: 331.8×231.7; L/W ratio: 1.4. Oocysts had 40 and 50 sporocysts, respectively; these were subspheroidal, L×W (n=5): 31.2×27.0 (28–35×24–32); L/W ratio: 1.2. Each SP had 8–16 SZ and these measured L×W (n=4): 12.2×3.5 (10–14×3–4). However, oocyst morphology and size were similar to those of *Hep. canis* found in *Hae. longicornis* and *Hae. flava*, collected from Japanese dogs, and Kubo et al. (2008) did not do the experimental transmission study, or the genetic analysis of oocysts, to separate them from *Hep. canis*. Thus, although Kubo et al. (2008) strongly suspected that these two *Haemaphysalis* tick species are the true definitive hosts for *Hep. ursi*, they did not prove it.

Cross-transmission: None to date.

Pathology: No inflammatory response was seen around *immature meronts* surrounded by a membrane. However, infiltration of inflammatory cells was found around degenerating tubercules and necrotic lesions in the lungs (Uni et al., 2003).

Materials deposited: The H&E-stained slide, with stained sections of *Hae. flava* containing *Hepatozoon* oocysts, is deposited in the National Museum of Nature and Science, Accession No. NSMT-Pr 240. The H&E-stained section of lung of bear N4 containing trophozoites and meronts and the Wright-Giemsa-stained blood smear of bear Sh2 with intraleukocytic gametocytes are deposited in the National Museum of Nature and Science, Tokyo, Japan, Accession No. NSMT-Pr 222a-b.

Etymology: The specific epitaph refers to the genus name of the type intermediate vertebrate host.

Remarks: The work by Uni et al. (2003) and Kubo et al. (2008) are the only two that document *Hepatozoon* infections in the family Ursidae. In Japanese black bears, only the lungs are infected by *H. ursi*. Wild martens (*Martes melampus*) in Japan also are infected by a *Hepatozoon* species that sometimes is found in the lungs, but the primary location for its meronts is the heart, peritoneal adipose tissue, and diaphragm.

The meronts of *Hep. ursi* are quite similar to those of *H. americanum* from dogs in both size and number of merozoites; however, *H. americanum* principally parasitizes skeletal muscles of American canids, whereas *Hep. ursi* parasitizes only the lungs of bears. The sizes of merozoites of the 2 species also are similar, but those of *H. ursi* are slightly smaller. The biggest defining difference between *Hep. ursi* and other *Hepatozoon* species is the shape and size of its gametocytes, especially the presence of its beak-like protrusion. Additionally, it always seems to be present in peripheral circulation of infected bears, whereas in some other *Hepatozoon* species, gametocytes in peripheral blood may be difficult to find.

DISCUSSION AND SUMMARY

Smith (1996) was the last person to summarize the number of *Hepatozoon* species known from vertebrates (amphisbaenians, anurans, birds, crocodilians, lizards, mammals, salamanders, snakes, tuatara, turtles) and, at that time, there were about 317 named species, of which 46 were from mammals and 3 were from carnivores (*H. canis*, *H. felis*, and *H. procyonis*). In the last two decades, dozens of new names have been added to these lists, with three from carnivores: *H. americanum* from North American canids, *H. mustelis* from the Siberian polecat, and *H. ursi* from the Japanese black bear were added to the known and named species from Carnivora. Baneth et al. (2013) redefined *H. felis* based on both morphology and sequence alignment and now estimates there are more than 340 species of *Hepatozoon* described to date.

As best we know, there are 6 valid species of *Hepatozoon*, described sufficiently and named, from carnivorous mammals in 6 families (Canidae, Felidae, Hyaenidae, Mustelidae, Procyonidae, and Ursidae), although "*Hepatozoon* spp." have been recorded from individual species in these and at least one other family, Viverridae (Schneider, 1968; Clark et al., 1973; Klopfer et al., 1973; Presidente and Karsta, 1975; Davis et al., 1978; Conceição-Silva et al., 1988; Mercer et al., 1988; Vincent-Johnson et al., 1997; Kubo et al., 2006; Kubo et al., 2010a; Furtado et al., 2017). In total, 7/15 (47%) carnivore families have one or more *Hepatozoon* species known from them.

When *Hepatozoon* zoites (gamonts) were first discovered in the WBCs of vertebrate hosts, it was considered sufficient to name a new parasite species each time a new host species was found to be infected because host specificity was considered to be an important taxonomic criterion for these coccidian species. Over the decades, as our knowledge increased, and especially with the advent of gene sequencing, we now know that certain *Hepatozoon* species are not host-specific and can infect a variety of reasonably unrelated host lineages (e.g., *H. canis*), and some *Hepatozoon* species found in many vertebrate groups have low host specificity for both definitive and intermediate hosts.

Although *H. felis* does not induce severe clinical symptoms in infected felids, such infectious diseases could threaten the existence of endangered species; thus it seems not only reasonable but also essential for conservation efforts to monitor infectious diseases in both threatened species and their domesticated cousins. Further studies are needed to find the definitive host for *H. felis*.

Sarcocystidae: Cystoisosporinae in the Carnivora

EIMERIORINA SARCOCYSTIDAE: CYSTOISOSPORINAE IN THE CARNIVORA

INTRODUCTION

Another major family within the Eimeriorina, Sarcocystidae Poche, 1913, has three sub-families, Cystoisosporinae Frenkel et al., 1987 (*Cystoisospora*), Sarcocystinae Poche, 1913 (*Sarcocystis, Frenkelia*), and Toxoplasmatinae Biocca, 1957 (*Besnoitia, Hammondia, Neospora, Toxoplasma*). Members of the Cystoisosporinae reported from carnivores are presented in this chapter. Members of the Sarcocystinae known from carnivores are detailed in Chapter 15, and the genera and species in the Toxoplasmatinae reported from carnivores are in Chapter 16.

Almost all of the coccidian species of carnivores covered in this chapter were initially described and named as species in the genus *Isospora* Schneider, 1881. This genus is characterized by having oocysts in the feces of the definitive host that are determined to contain two sporocysts, each with four sporozoites, but therein lies the problem. The members of this genus have been the source of intense scrutiny and controversy since the time it was named,

and especially after 1970, when we began to realize that *Besnoitia, Frenkelia* (?), *Hammondia, Neospora, Sarcocystis*, and *Toxoplasma* species all discharge *Isospora*-like oocysts containing two sporocysts, each with four sporozoites, and that their life cycles are not homoxenous as are those of *Eimeria, Cyclospora*, and *some Isospora* in the Eimeriidae.

Cystoisospora. Frenkel (1977, pp. 620, 625) erected the genus *Cystoisospora* to include those mammalian *Isospora* species with no Stieda body complex in their sporocysts, and with the ability to produce unique monozoic tissue cysts (MZTC) in intermediate or paratenic hosts, and these MZTC stages are a defining character in species of *Cystoisospora*. Frenkel (1977) made this decision because of earlier work he and Dubey (Frenkel and Dubey, 1972a) had done when they discovered the occurrence of tissue cyst stages of two intestinal coccidia of cats, *C. felis* and *C. rivolta*, in rodent paratenic hosts. Dubey and Frenkel (1972b) and then others a bit later (Dubey, 1975b, 1978a,b, Rommel and Zielasko, 1981) also demonstrated that extraintestinal (EIN) stages can occur in the tissues (mesenteric lymph nodes, liver, spleen, lungs, brain, musculature) of cats and dogs (definitive hosts) when fed sporulated oocysts of *C. felis* and *C. rivolta*, or *C. canis*, respectively. These

The Biology and Identification of the Coccidia (Apicomplexa) of Carnivores of the World
https://doi.org/10.1016/B978-0-12-811349-3.00014-1

© 2018 Donald W. Duszynski published by Elsevier Inc. All rights reserved.

expanded life cycles include MZTC typically found in mesenteric lymph nodes of intermediate/paratenic hosts (e.g., rodents). When either sporulated oocysts or infected intermediate hosts are ingested, the parasite undergoes merogony and gamogony in the intestinal epithelial cells of the carnivore definitive host and, ultimately, they discharge **un**sporulated oocysts with relatively thick walls (e.g., *C. felis*, *C. rivolta* of felids; *C. canis*, *C. ohioensis*, *C. vulpina* of canids). Thus, *Cystoisospora* species appear identical to *Isospora* species except for their ability to infect additional host species (Fayer and Dubey, 1987) and they all have sporocysts that lack any remnant of a Stieda body complex. Once molecular sequencing became an important tool, we began to learn that Frenkel (1977) was correct in separating heteroxenous isosporans into *Cystoisospora* species. Frenkel et al. (1987) then provided us with an important conceptual basis for thinking about all these "isosporans" by pointing out, "How we classify the heretofore unthought of cycles and stages is a scientific problem of taxonomy rather than of nomenclature." Their new taxonomic ideas on these seven genera (above) with heteroxenous life cycles reflects on the reproductive and transmission strategies of the parasites (as best we understand them), while maintaining the nomenclature. We believe that their (Frenkel et al., 1987) taxonomic concepts for the isosporid coccidia, in the interest of stability, uniqueness, and distinction is sound, and we refer to their concept in this and the next two chapters (except newer information on *Frenkelia*).

Carreno et al. (1998) and Franzen et al. (2000) using a phylogenetic analysis of the 18S rRNA gene were able to show that some *Cystoisospora* (formerly *Isospora*) species were more closely related to *Neospora*, *Sarcocystis*, and *Toxoplasma* species and belonged in the Sarcocystidae rather than the Eimeriidae. Barta et al. (2005) examined the morphology of the sporocysts along with the available molecular data and suggested assigning all *Isospora*-like species

that had sporocysts without Stieda bodies on/ in their sporocysts (from mammals) to the *Cystoisospora* and all such oocysts from birds, which had Stieda (and often sub-Stieda) bodies on their sporocysts, to the genus *Isospora*. Samarasinghe et al. (2008) further characterized the phylogenetic relationship of *Cystoisospora* to other related coccidian species by analyzing sequences of the rRNA internal transcribed spacer 1 (ITS-1); they also developed a PCR-RFLP assay, which should be of interest to some of our readers, to rapidly detect and differentiate *Cyclospora* species. Their study reinforced previous molecular work supporting that *Cystoisospora* species do not belong in the Eimeriidae and are best classified with the cyst-forming members of the Sarcocystidae. Thus, we have gone through the literature on *Isospora* species in carnivores with oocysts lacking a Stieda body on their sporocysts and have reassigned them to *Cystoisospora*. In the text we use "*I.* (=*C.*)" when referring to earlier work that used *Isospora* as the genus name of the species they studied but which we are now amending to *Cystoisospora*.

SPECIES DESCRIPTIONS

SUBORDER CANIFORMIA KRETZOI, 1938

CANIDAE FISCHER, 1817

GENUS CANIS L., 1758 (6 SPECIES)

CYSTOISOSPORA ARCTOPITHECI (RODHAIN, 1933) NOV. COMB.

Carnivore definitive host: Canis lupus familiaris L., 1758 (syn. *C. familiaris*), Domestic Dog.
Remarks: Hendricks (1974, 1977) said he found this species in five carnivore species, as

definitive hosts, including the domestic dog. For the complete species rendition, see *Eira* (Mustelidae), below.

CYSTOISOSPORA BURROWSI (TRAYSER AND TODD, 1978) ROMMEL AND ZIELASKO, 1981

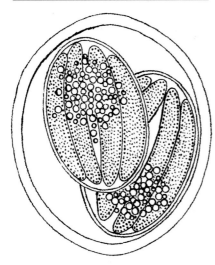

FIGURE 14.1 Original line drawing of the sporulated oocyst of *Cystoisospora burrowsi*. *Modified Fig. 16, Levine, N.D., Ivens, V. 1981. The Coccidian Parasites (Protozoa, Apicomplexa) of Carnivores. Illinois Biological Monograph No. 51, The University of Illinois Press, Urbana, Illinois USA. The University of Illinois Press has released the copyright.*

Synonym: *Isospora burrowsi* Trayser and Todd, 1978.

Type host: *Canis lupus familiaris* L., 1758 (syn. *C. familiaris*), Domestic Dog.

Type locality: North America: USA: North Carolina, Research Triangle Park (see footnote "a," p. 95, Trayser and Todd, 1978).

Other definitive hosts: None to date.

Known intermediate host: *Mus musculus* L., 1758, House Mouse (see Rommel and Zielasko, 1981).

Geographic distribution: Europe: Germany: Hannover/Hamburg; North America: USA: Illinois, North Carolina.

Description of sporulated oocyst: Oocyst shape: subspheroidal to slightly ellipsoidal; number of walls, 1; wall characteristics: smooth, yellow-green, ~1.0 thick; L×W: 20.3×17.3 (17–22×16–19); L/W ratio: 1.2 (1.0–1.4); M, OR, PG: all absent. Distinctive features of oocyst: smooth, transparent single-layered wall, and lack of M, OR, and PG.

Description of sporocyst and sporozoites: Sporocyst shape: subspheroidal to slightly ellipsoidal; L×W: 14.4×9.7 (12–16×8–11), L/W ratio: 1.5 (1.1–1.9); SB, SSB, PSB: all absent; SR: present; SR characteristics: an aggregation of large granules, 1.5–2.5 wide, usually located at one end of SP; SZ: sausage-shaped, with a blunt posterior end, and slightly tapering anterior end, 7×4 (6–8×4–5); RB: 1, present at broader end of SZ (not seen in line drawing). Distinctive features of sporocyst: very small size containing SZs that are exactly the same length as sporocyst (line drawing).

Prevalence: Unknown.

Sporulation: Exogenous. Sporulation was completed in 3 days at ~25°C.

Prepatent and patent periods: Prepatent period is 6 days, and patency lasts for 11 days (Trayser and Todd, 1978); or 6–9 days with patency lasting 4–12 days (Rommel and Zielasko, 1981). Rommel and Zielasko (1981) inoculated mice and rats with sporulated oocysts and "after infection through intermediate hosts," fed their tissues to dogs, and the prepatent period in beagles was 7–11 days with patency lasting 5–27 days.

Site of infection: Intestinal epithelial cells of the dog, in the posterior three-fifths of the small intestine, and in the cecum, both above and below the host cell nucleus (HCN). All stages were found in the tips of villar epithelial cells or in cells of the lamina propria (Trayser and Todd, 1978). Rommel and Zielasko (1981) also located endogenous stages in the lamina propria, at the tips of the villi, in the posterior two-thirds of the small intestine, as well as in the cecum and colon by 5 days postinfection (DPI).

Endogenous stages: Trayser (1973) and Trayser and Todd (1978) used a cloned culture from a single oocyst and passed it through dogs to get enough oocysts to study development in seven dogs, each of which was inoculated with 5×10^5 oocysts. Sporozoites entered epithelial cells on 1 DPI and developed into mature first-generation meronts (M_1) by 4 DPI; these measured L×W: 14.8×12.3 (11–18×9–18) in tissue sections and were tightly packed with first-generation merozoites (m_1) that measured 11.1×3.3 (8–14×3–3.5), with a mean of 5 m_1 in each M_1 section. Second-generation meronts (M_2) first were seen 5 DPI and became more numerous on 6 DPI; they were L×W: 25.8×18.3 (18–35×17–22) and contained loosely-arranged cylindroid m_2 with blunt ends and a subcentral N; these measured 16.2×4.9 (14–18×3–6). Mature microgamonts were seen 6 DPI and measured L×W (n=50): 19.8×14.1 (13–27×10–21) and contained many microgametes ~4–5×0.4. Macrogametes also were seen 6 DPI and were elongate-ovoidal to spheroidal; mature macrogametes were L×W (n=50): 17.1×11.5 (11–25×8–18), but eosinophilic wall-forming bodies were not seen.

Little is known about the MZTC stages of *C. burrowsi* from dogs in their intermediate host(s), unlike those stages in mice from *C. felis*, *C. rivolta*, *C. canis*, and *C. ohioensis*, which are all similar in their structure (Lindsay et al., 2014).

Cross-transmission: None to date.

Pathology: Uncertain. Penzhorn et al. (1992) reported acute diarrhea, often hemorrhagic, in young German shepherd dog litters in Pretoria, South Africa. They said they recovered oocysts of *I. canis* and *I. burrowsi/I. ohioensis* in fecal specimens of 26% of the bitches and 52% from their litters, but they could not find an association between shedding of oocysts by bitches and their litters nor was there an association between bouts of diarrhea and peaks of oocyst shedding.

Materials deposited: None.

Etymology: This species was named for Dr. Robert B. Burrows, Wellcome Research Laboratories, Burroughs Wellcome Co., Research Triangle Park, North Carolina, USA, who found the oocysts.

Remarks: Sporulated oocysts of this species are larger than those of *Hammondia heydorni* and smaller than those of *C. canis*, and the endogenous stages of *C. canis* and *C. burrowsi* differ significantly. Sporulated oocysts of *C. burrowsi* resemble oocysts of *C. ohioensis*, but differ by lacking a PG, and having smaller overall dimensions. Rommel and Zielasko (1981) isolated this strain of oocysts from dogs in Germany, did three passages in dogs, and said that oocysts from 8 experimentally-infected beagles measured L×W (n=380): 20.6×18.0 (17–24×15–22); L/W ratio: 1.1. They also emended the name to *Cystoisospora*.

CYSTOISOSPORA CANIS (NEMESÉRI, 1959) FRENKEL, 1977

Synonyms: *Diplospora bigemina* Wasielewsky, 1904 from a dog *pro parte*; *Isospora felis* (Wasielewsky, 1904) Wenyon, 1923 of *auctores* from the domestic dog; *Isospora bigemina* (Stiles, 1891) Lühe, 1906 of *auctores pro parte*; *Levinea canis* (Nemeséri, 1959) Dubey, 1977c; *Isospora canis* Nemeséri, 1959.

Type host: *Canis lupus familiaris* L., 1758 (syn. *C. familiaris*), Domestic Dog.

Type locality: North America: USA: Michigan, Detroit (by Hall and Wigdor, 1918).

Other definitive hosts: *Canis aureus* L., 1758, Golden Jackal; *Canis latrans* Say, 1823, Coyote; *Vulpes vulpes* (L., 1758) (syn. *Vulpes fulvus* (Desmarest, 1820)), Red or Silver-back Fox.

Known intermediate hosts: *Camelus dromedarius* L., 1758, One-humped Camel; *Felis catus* L., 1758, Domestic Cat (experimental as newborn kittens); *Mus musculus* L., 1758, House Mouse (experimental); *Ovis aries* L., 1758, Red Sheep.

Geographic distribution: Worldwide.

Description of sporulated oocyst: Oocyst shape: broadly ellipsoidal to slightly ovoidal; number of walls, 2; wall characteristics: outer is smooth, pale tan to light green; total thickness: 1.3–1.5,

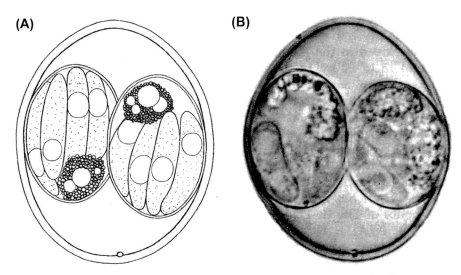

(A)   **(B)**

FIGURE 14.2   (A). Original line drawing of the sporulated oocyst of *Cystoisospora canis*, (B). Photomicrograph of a sporulated oocyst of *Cystoisospora canis*. *(A) Modified Fig. 1, Levine, N.D., Ivens, V. 1981. The Coccidian Parasites (Protozoa, Apicomplexa) of Carnivores. Illinois Biological Monograph No. 51, The University of Illinois Press, Urbana, Illinois USA. The University of Illinois Press has released the copyright. (B) From Dubey, J.P., 1976. A review of Sarcocystis of domestic animals and of other coccidia of cats and dogs. Journal of the American Veterinary Medical Association 169 (10), 1061–1078, with permission of the AVMA, copyright holder for the JAVMA.*

sometimes appears to be lined by a very thin membrane; L×W (n=50): 38×30 (34–42×27–33); L/W ratio: 1.3 (1.1–1.4); M, OR, PG: all absent. Distinctive features of oocyst: smooth, transparent two-layered wall, and lack of M, OR, and PG, all typical of *Cystoisospora* species; some oocysts may have a tiny "blob" adherent to the inside of the oocyst wall at the broad end.

Description of sporocyst and sporozoites: Sporocyst shape: ellipsoidal; L×W: 21×16 (18–24×15–18), L/W ratio: 1.3; SB, SSB, PSB: all absent; SR: present; SR characteristics: a prominent spheroidal body; SZ: sausage-shaped, with one subcentral, clear RB. Distinctive features of sporocyst: relatively large size, without SB, SSB and PSB, as is typical of SP of all *Cystoisospora* species.

Prevalence: Gassner (1940) found it in 19/320 (6%) dogs in Colorado, and Catcott (1946) found it in 4/113 (3.5%) dogs in Ohio, USA. Choquette and Gelinas (1950) found it in 23/155 (15%) dogs

in Montreal, Canada. Costa and Freitas (1959) examined 18 dogs in Belo Horizonet, Brazil and said 6/18 (33%) had oocysts of *I.* (=C.) *felis*; we now know, of course that the oocysts they saw almost certainly represented those of *I.* (=C.) *canis*. Nemeséri (1960) found it in 18/220 (8%) dogs in Hungary. Amaral et al. (1964) found it in 2/232 (1%) dogs in Brazil. Levine and Ivens (1965) found oocysts of *I.* (=C.) *canis* species in 22/139 (16%) dogs in Illinois, USA. Burrows (1968), in New Jersey, USA, found *I.* (=C.) *canis* in 139/835 (17%) dogs sampled over 12 years, beginning in 1956. Alcaino and Tagle (1970) found it in 30/1,505 (2%) dogs in Chile. Mirza (1970) found it in 5/54 (9%) dogs in Iraq. Lepp and Todd (1974) found it in only 6/308 (2%) dogs in Illinois, USA. Streitel and Dubey (1976) surveyed stray dogs in Ohio, USA, looking for stages of intestinal parasites; they found only 9/500 (2%) samples to have oocysts of *I.* (=C.) *canis*. Dubey et al. (1978a) reported *I.* (=C.) *canis*-like oocysts in 3/169 (2%) coyotes in Montana, USA. McKenna and Charleston (1980d) examined fecal samples from cats and dogs on the North Island of New Zealand and found 19/481 (4%) samples had oocysts they identified as *I. (=C.) canis*. Dubey (1982b) surveyed the feces for coccidians from a variety of wild carnivores from Montana, USA and reported *I. (=C.) canis*-like oocysts in the feces of 16/198 (8%) red foxes. Hoskins et al. (1982) examined fecal samples of dogs in Louisiana, USA from 1977 to 1980; they reported 2,800/4,058 (69%), mostly puppies <6-months-old, to shed oocysts of *I. (=C.) canis* and found no difference in infection rates between the sexes. Gothe and Reichler (1990) checked fecal samples of 100 randomly selected dog families in south Germany; they reported that the "excretion extent of the litters and their mothers was 16% and 8% for *I. canis*." Rodriguez and Carbonell (1998) looked at fecal samples from wild carnivores in central Spain and said they found *I. (=C.) canis* in 9/20 (45%) *V. vulpes*. Bugg et al. (1999) examined fecal samples collected from urban dogs at five sources (four pet shops, three refuges, six breeding kennels, eight veterinary clinics, two exercise areas) in the Perth metropolitan area, Western Australia, and *I. (=C.) canis* was detected in 29/421 (7%) samples, mostly from breeding kennels, puppies, and outdoor dogs. During a survey on endoparasites of dogs and cats in Freiburg, Germany, Barutzki and Schaper (2003) examined fecal samples of dogs by four different methods, and *I. (=C.) canis* was detected in 700/8,438 (8%) samples. Gompper et al. (2003) found oocysts of *I. (=C.) canis* in 1/23 (4%) *C. latrans* collected in Black Rock Forest near Cornwall, New York, USA; their identification was based on the size of oocysts in the feces, so it should be taken with caution. Cirak and Bauer (2004) examined fecal samples of dogs without diarrhea from three animal shelters in central Germany, to compare the effectivity of conventional coproscopical methods and a commercial coproantigen ELISA kit to detect *Cryptosporidium*; oocysts of *I. (=C.) canis*

were recorded in 5/270 (2%) dogs. Fontanarrosa et al. (2006) surveyed fecal samples of owned dogs in southern Buenos Aires, Argentina and detected oocysts of *I. (=C.) canis* in 66/2,193 (3%) samples, mostly in young dogs 0–6-months-old, and its prevalence decreased with increasing age. Rinaldi et al. (2006) examined canine fecal samples collected in Naples, Campania region, Italy, and oocysts of *I. (=C.) canis* were reported in 17/415 (4%) samples; however, because samples were collected from the ground, one may never know whether they all were really canine feces or not. Batchelor et al. (2007) examined fecal samples of pet dogs, most with diarrhea, in Lancashire, United Kingdom, from 2003 to 2005, and identified oocysts of *I. (=C.) canis* (size, morphology) in 232/4,526 (5%) samples, usually in dogs <6-months-old, with a higher prevalence of shedding in autumn. Palmer et al. (2008a) surveyed fecal samples of dogs from urban and rural areas across Australia, collected from 59 veterinary clinics (810 samples) and 26 refuges (590 samples), and *I. (=C.) canis* was detected in 15/1,400 (1%) dogs, mostly from refuges. From 1997 to 2007, Gates and Nolan (2009) surveyed dog fecal samples in Pennsylvania, USA, for the prevalence of endoparasites and identified *C. canis* in 80/6,555 (1%) samples, mostly dogs <1-year-old. Yamamoto et al. (2009) surveyed fecal samples of dogs in animal shelters, Saitama Prefecture, Japan and reported oocysts of *I. (=C.) canis* in only 5/906 (<1%) samples. Gingrich et al. (2010) studied fecal samples of domestic dogs from Santa Cruz (51 dogs), San Cristobal (17), and Isabela (29) islands of the Galápagos Archipelago and reported *I. (=C.) canis* oocysts in 4/80 (5%) samples from the Santa Cruz and Isabela islands. The dogs on the Galápagos Islands represent a unique population, because they are an introduced species. Mirzaei and Fooladi (2013) did a fecal survey of pet dogs in Kerman, Kerman Province, Iran and found *I. (=C.) canis* in 1/100 (1%) dogs. Neves et al. (2014) surveyed feces of asymptomatic pet dogs, and pet dogs with clinical signs from the Oporto urban area, northern Portugal; *C. canis* was detected in 14/175 (8%) asymptomatic dogs and in 26/193 (13%) dogs with clinical signs. Positive dogs from both groups were most often < 6-months-old. Takács et al. (2014) said they found *C. canis* oocysts in the feces of 3/20 (15%) wild golden jackals killed by hunters in Hungary; they failed to mention if they looked at sporulated oocysts or just measured unsporulated oocysts, so this record must be viewed with caution. Scorza and Lappin (2017) examined fecal samples of dogs on the Pine Ridge Indian Reservation, South Dakota, USA and reported *C. canis* oocysts in 2/84 (2%) dogs. Hermosilla et al. (2017) collected fecal samples of free-living European wolves (*C. lupus*) in mountainous areas of Gorski Kotar in Croatia; oocysts of *C. canis* were detected in 7/400 (2%) samples.

Sporulation: Exogenous. Lepp and Todd (1976) said sporulation took 48 hours at 20°C and 16 hours at 30 and 35°C. Oocysts sporulated after 48 hours at 27°C in Petri dishes in 2.5% aqueous potassium dichromate ($K_2Cr_2O_7$) solution (Hilali et al., 1992).

Prepatent and patent periods: The prepatent period is 9–11 DPI (Neméseri, 1960; Lepp and Todd, 1974; Dubey, 1975b; Lindsay et al., 1997) when dogs are fed oocysts. Dubey (1975b) reported the prepatent period was 8–9 DPI when dogs were fed infective mice, and Hilali et al. (1992) said the prepatent period was 3–6 DPI after dogs ate (presumably infected) camel meat and 5–8 DPI after eating (presumably infected) sheep meat. The patent period is long, about 4 weeks (Neméseri, 1960). Houk et al. (2013) experimented with a new strain of *C. canis* in a dog from Brazil when it was inoculated into beagle pups. The prepatent period was 9–10 DPI, and patency lasted 8–12 days.

Site of infection: In canids, development occurs mostly in the posterior one-third of the small intestine but can extend into the large intestine. Meronts are found mostly just beneath the epithelium, some are deeper in the lamina propria, but no meronts seem to occur in epithelial cells of the intestine. Macro- and microgamonts *do* occur in epithelial cells, subepithelial connective tissue of the small intestinal villi, and in the mucosa of the large intestine (Neméseri, 1969; Lepp and Todd, 1974). In intermediate/transport hosts, hypnozoites are in the mesenteric lymph nodes.

Endogenous stages: There are three merogonous stages in the definitive host gut. The first asexual division probably is by endodyogeny. The M_1 mature 5–7 DPI; they are ellipsoidal to spheroidal, L×W: 25×21 (16–38×11–23), with 14 (4–24) m_1 that are 10×4 (8–11×3–5) each with a central N and with one rounded end and the other pointed. The M_2 first appeared on 6 DPI and matured in ~24 hours. They are slightly ovoidal to spheroidal, L×W: 15×11 (12–18×8–13), with 3–12 banana-shaped m_2 that measured 12×4 (11–12×3–5), each with a central N that begins to divide, in some m_2, even before they leave the M_2. The M_3 mature on 7–8 DPI and were L×W: 24×17 (13–38×8–24), with ~26 (6–72) m_3 that seem not to be arranged in any particular order. The m_3 have a central N, with a prominent nucleolus, are rounded at one end, pointed at the other, and measured 11×2 (8–13×1.5–3). Earliest spheroidal gamonts were seen 7 DPI and were abundant 8–10 DPI. Microgamonts were L×W: 29×20 (20–38×14–26) and produced many microgametes, 5×1. Mature macrogamonts were ovoidal, L×W: 25×18 (22–29×14–23), with distinct eosinophilic granules. Oocysts appeared in tissue sections 8 DPI, and these measured L×W: 28–38×20–30.

Cross-transmission: da Rocha and Lopes (1971) tried to transmit sporulated oocysts of *I.* (=*C.*) *canis* to cats, but the infections failed. Loveless and Andersen (1975) infected three coyote pups with a mixed inoculum of 25,000 sporulated oocysts of *I.* (=*C.*) *canis* (60%) and *I.* (=*C.*) *rivolta* (40%) (now in the *C. ohioensis* complex) from the domestic dog; unsporulated oocysts of "*I. rivolta*" were found in the coyote pups' feces on 4 DPI and those of

I. (=*C.*) *canis* on 10 DPI. Oocysts of *I. canis* from the coyotes measured L × W: 36.8 × 30.7; L/W ratio: 1.2. Dubey (1975b) found that infections produced by *I.* (=*C.*) *canis* oocysts, or by tissues from *I.* (=*C.*) *canis*-infected mice, produced similar infections in dogs that discharged similar numbers of oocysts and had similar prepatent periods. Kittens and adult cats, including those immunosuppressed with drugs, did not shed oocysts after being inoculated orally with *I.* (=*C.*) *canis* sporulated oocysts (Neuméri, 1960; Rocha and Lopes, 1971; Dubey, 1975b; Levine and Ivens, 1981). However, both dogs and cats develop tissue infections with *I.* (=*C.*) *canis* after ingesting oocysts, as demonstrated using bioassay of their tissues (Dubey, 1975b; Lindsay et al., 2014). Sato (1976) infected dogs with oocysts of *I.* (=*C.*) *felis* and then challenged them with oocysts of *I.* (=*C.*) *canis*; no cross-infection occurred between canine and feline types. Sato (1976) also found that infection of dogs with sporulated oocysts of *I.* (=*C.*) *canis* produced complete immunity immediately after the patent period ended but that 21 days after patency ended, reinfection could be acquired, and the prepatent period of the challenge infection was shortened by 2–3 days, patency was shortened to about 7 days, and the number of oocysts discharged per g of feces decreased during patency. Hilali et al. (1992) fed nine dogs pooled heart and esophagus muscles from different numbers (15–30) of camels (*C. dromedarius*) and monitored their fecal output for 70 DPI. Four dogs began passing oocysts identified (after sporulation) as those of *I.* (=*C.*) *canis* on days 3, 3, 4, and 6 postinoculation (PI), and patency lasted 7, 3, 3, and 12 days, respectively. They also fed seven other dogs pooled heart and esophagus muscles from sheep (*O. aries*) and monitored their fecal output. Three of these dogs began passing oocysts of *I.* (=*C.*) *canis* 5, 6, and 8 DPI, with patent periods of 12, 13, and 13, respectively. Please note that all three dogs that shed *I.* (=*C.*) *canis* oocysts also passed oocysts of *I.* (=*C.*) *ohioensis* and one, in

addition, also passed sporocysts of one or more *Sarcocystis* species. This cross-transmission study was undertaken because Hilali et al. (1992) wanted to emphasize the public health importance of stray dogs that are in close association with humans and our food and companion animals.

Pathology: Neuméri (1960) said that 5,000 sporulated oocysts of the Hungarian strain produced no obvious signs of disease but that 50,000–80,000 oocysts caused dogs to be weak and lose their appetite 8–9 DPI, at which time they had dysentery-like diarrhea, with blood and mucus and a temperature of 39.5–40.3°C. Lepp and Todd (1974), on the other hand, saw no signs of pathology in dogs fed 200,000 sporulated oocysts in Illinois, USA. Levine and Ivens (1981) reported that there appears to be strain differences in the ability to produce pathology. Lindsay et al. (1997) reiterated the work of Lepp and Todd (1974) and said that disease was not produced in 6–8-week-old dogs inoculated with 1×10^5 or 1.5×10^5 sporulated oocysts and added that solid immunity follows primary infection, with no oocysts discharged by dogs after challenge. Houk et al. (2013) experimented with a new strain of *I.* (=*C.*) *canis* from a dog from São Paulo, Brazil; when six 6-week-old beagle pups, without a previous *Cystoisospora* infection (neither *I.* (=*C.*) *canis* nor *I.* (=*C.*) *ohioensis*), were inoculated with 5×10^4 sporulated oocysts of this strain, all six pups developed clinical disease and two required chemotherapy (sulfadimethoxine). The Houk et al. (2013) report confirmed that *C. canis* can be a primary pathogen for young dogs.

Materials deposited: None.

Remarks: Neuméri (1959, 1960) named this species twice, the first time in Hungarian, and the second time in German, and both times using the same six photomicrographs, four of oocysts and two of tissue sections. We presume that was the way things were expected to be done in those days. *Cystoisospora canis* has the largest oocysts of all the canine *Cystoisospora* species and, realistically, is the only one that can be reliably identified with LM. Levine and Ivens (1965) were among the first to summarize the species of isosporan coccidia found in dogs. They reiterated that *I.* (=C.) *canis* was first reported from a dog in Detroit, Michigan, USA by Hall and Wigdor (1918), who thought it was a large form of *I. bigemina*, whereas others found it in dogs from various places (e.g., England; US states of Maryland, Colorado, Ohio; Montreal, Canada; Australia) and referred to it as *I. felis* in dogs. Levine and Ivens (1965) also found one *Caryospora*-like oocyst with a single sporocyst and eight SZs in one dog infected with *I.* (=C.) *canis*; it measured L×W: 38×28, with its one sporocyst L×W: 23×22. They considered it to be an aberrant oocyst of *I.* (=C.) *canis*. Later, Matsui et al. (1989) showed that heat treatment can regularly transform sporocysts of *I.* (=C.) *canis* and other coccidians (*Eimeria*, *Isospora*, *Toxoplasma*) by transforming two sporocysts (*Isospora* sp.) into one and four sporocysts (*Eimeria* sp.) into two, each with eight sporozoites.

Roberts et al. (1972) and Speer et al. (1973) were the first investigators to use TEM to study the biology of *I.* (=C.) *canis*. Roberts et al. (1972) studied the fine structure of sporozoites and found they differed from those of *Eimeria* species in that they had crystalloid bodies in place of refractile bodies, one anterior and one posterior to the HCN. Speer et al. (1973) reported that the sporocyst wall was composed of two layers, with the inner layer 75% of the total thickness, and the outer layer was made up of four separate plates that separate along suture lines where the plates come together when exposed to trypsin and bile salts during excystation. Speer et al. (1973) said the release of *I.* (=C.) *canis* SZs is a process quite different than that seen in *Eimeria* species that have sporocysts with an SB (Speer et al., 1973). Markus (1983), using both LM and TEM, described three hypnozoites found in mouse mesenteric lymph nodes at 7 DPI with oocysts of *I.* (=C.) *canis*.

Fayer and Mahrt (1972) were the first to grow *I.* (=C.) *canis* sporozoites in cell culture (embryonic bovine kidney, embryonic bovine trachea, Madin–Darby canine kidney, embryonic canine intestine), where they discovered that daughter organisms were formed via endodyogeny, in a process similar to that seen in *Toxoplasma*, *Besnoitia*, and *Sarcocystis*. Mahrt (1973) reported both endodyogeny and merogony in Madin–Darby bovine kidney cell cultures. Mitchell et al. (2009) examined the development of *I.* (=C.) *canis* in two noncanine cell lines and the ultrastructure of the monozoic cysts that formed when grown on monolayers of bovine turbinate and African green monkey kidney cell lines. These cysts contained a single, centrally-located, crescent-shaped SZ surrounded by a thick cyst wall within a parasitophorous vacuole (PV), but no division or multinucleated stages were ever seen.

Schreck and Dürr (1970) reported that 1-day-old pups could be infected "if enough oocysts were used," and susceptibility to infection increased slowly with age until weaning, when there was a marked increase in susceptibility. Lepp and Todd (1974) said that 6-week-old dogs given ~100,000 oocysts were completely immune 2 months later and that 10-week-old dogs inoculated with 200,000 oocysts were completely immune 1 month after patency ended. Mandal (1976) reported finding *I.* (=C.) *canis* oocysts in domestic dogs in Calcutta, West Bengal, with oocysts that measured L×W: 38 (36–40)×32, L/W ratio: 1.2, and sporocysts that were L×W: 20×16, L/W ratio: 1.25, with a sporulation time of 15–20 hours (temperature not stated). Heine (1981) said he developed a simple trypsin digestion technique that helped him visualize "dormozoites" developing in the spleen, liver, mesentery, and some skeletal muscles, in mice that were experimentally inoculated with sporulated oocysts of *I.* (=C.) *burrowsi*, *I.* (=C.) *canis*, *I.* (=C.) *felis*, *I.* (=C.) *laidlawi*, *I.* (=C.) *ohioensis*, and *I.* (=C.) *rivolta*. However, he never showed any photographic evidence that he found these cryptic stages.

CYSTOISOSPORA DUTOITI (YAKIMOFF, MATIKASCHWILI, AND RASTEGAÏEFF, 1933a) NOV. COMB.

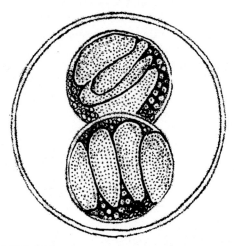

FIGURE 14.3 Original line drawing of the sporulated oocyst of *Cystoisospora dutoiti*. *Modified Fig. 81, Levine, N.D., Ivens, V., 1981. The Coccidian Parasites (Protozoa, Apicomplexa) of Carnivores. Illinois Biological Monograph No. 51, The University of Illinois Press, Urbana, Illinois USA. The University of Illinois Press has released the copyright.*

Synonym: *Eimeria dutoiti* Yakimoff, Matikaschwili, and Rastegaïeff, 1933a *lapsus calami*.

Type host: *Canis aureus* L., 1758, Golden Jackal.

Type locality: Asia: (former) USSR: Russia, Zoological Gardens of Leningrad (Transcaucasia).

Other definitive hosts: None to date.

Known intermediate host: None to date.

Geographic distribution: Asia: (former) USSR: Russia, Transcaucasia.

Description of sporulated oocyst: Oocyst shape: mostly spheroidal, but some are subspheroidal; number of walls, 1; wall characteristics: smooth, thin; L×W: subspheroidal forms 11.5×9.6 (10–13×9–11), L/W ratio: 1.1, and spheroidal forms 11 (9–13), L/W ratio: 1.0; M, OR, PG: all absent. Distinctive features of oocyst: small, spheroid, with a uniformly thin wall of single layer.

Description of sporocyst and sporozoites: Sporocyst shape: spheroidal; L×W: 6.6×6.6,

L/W ratio: 1.0; SB, SSB, PSB: all absent; SR: present; SR characteristics: an irregular mass of a few scattered granules at one end of sporocyst; SZ: pyriform and measured, 6–7×2, but neither N nor RB were visible. Distinctive features of sporocyst: small spheroidal shape without SB, SSB, PSB.

Prevalence: Yakimoff et al. (1933a) found oocysts of this form in the only jackal they examined from the Zoological Garden in Leningrad.

Sporulation: Exogenous. Yakimoff et al. (1933a) mentioned sporulating oocysts in 2.5% potassium "bichromate" solution but did not give a time for how long oocysts were incubated or at what temperature before they sporulated.

Prepatent and patent periods: Unknown.

Site of infection: Unknown.

Endogenous stages: Unknown.

Cross-transmission: None to date.

Pathology: Unknown.

Materials deposited: None.

Etymology: Yakimoff et al. (1933a) named this species in honor of the South African researcher and Director of the famous Transvaal Institute, Dr. P.J. DuToit.

Remarks: Yakimoff et al. (1933a) noted that the oocysts of this isosporan were very similar to those of *I.* (=C.) *theileri*, which he and Lewkowitsch (1932) had described the year before, also from a golden jackal, but believed these were better compared to the small form oocysts of *I. bigemina* (now known as *Hammondia heydorni*, see Chapter 16); they argued that their oocysts were more often round than any other shape and slightly bigger (12×10) than those of *H. heydorni* (11×10), which was stretching the truth just a little bit. Yakimoff et al. (1933a) mentioned their "interesting observation" that the jackal, closely related to the dog, possessed two different kinds of dog isosporans (*I. theileri*, *I. dutoiti*) than did the domestic dog (*I. canis*, *I. rivolta*) and that "the resolution of this question depends on further investigation." Pellérdy (1974a,b) said that the scanty data presented in the original description scarcely allowed the determination of this species as real, sound reasoning with which we can agree. However, we include it here only because it has been recognized by others since its description and in the hope someone will rediscover and redescribe it in the not too distant future. Glebezdin (1978) reported a survey on 2,350 wild mammals representing 25 species in southwestern Turkmenistan from 1974 to 1977; in *C. aureus* he found both spheroidal and ellipsoidal oocysts that he called *I. (C.) dutoiti*; his spheroidal oocysts were 10.6 (8–11) wide and the ellipsoidal oocysts measured L×W: 14.4×9.6 (11–17×8–11), L/W ratio: 1.4 (1.3–1.5) and had spheroidal sporocysts that were 10.4 (8–11) wide, L/W ratio: 1.0.

CYSTOISOSPORA NEORIVOLTA (DUBEY AND MAHRT, 1978), NOV. COMB.

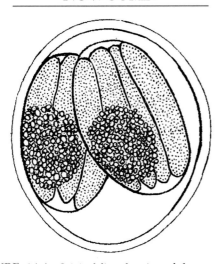

FIGURE 14.4 Original line drawing of the sporulated oocyst of *Cystoisospora neorivolta*. *Modified Fig. 14, Levine, N.D., Ivens, V., 1981. The Coccidian Parasites (Protozoa, Apicomplexa) of Carnivores. Illinois Biological Monograph No. 51, The University of Illinois Press, Urbana, Illinois USA. The University of Illinois Press has released the copyright.*

Synonyms: *Isospora rivolta* (Grassi, 1879) Wenyon, 1923 of Mahrt (1967); *Isospora neorivolta* Dubey and Mahrt, 1978.

Type host: *Canis lupus familiaris* L., 1758 (syn. *C. familiaris*), Domestic Dog.

Type locality: North America: USA: Illinois.

Other definitive host: *Canis latrans* Say, 1823, Coyote (?).

Known intermediate host: None to date.

Geographic distribution: North America: USA: Illinois.

Description of sporulated oocyst: Oocyst shape: ellipsoidal to slightly subspheroidal (line drawing); number of walls, 1; wall characteristics: smooth, colorless to pale yellow, total thickness ~0.8; L×W (in tissue sections): 12.6×11.4 (13–15×11–13), L/W ratio: 1.1; M, OR, PG: all absent (line drawing). Distinctive features of oocyst: no detailed description exists of the sporulated oocyst, only measurements of unsporulated oocysts in sections of dog intestine; thus, the only defining features are ellipsoidal shape, smooth outer wall, and lack of M, OR, and PG.

Description of sporocyst and sporozoites: Sporocyst shape: ellipsoidal (line drawing); L×W: unknown; L/W ratio: unknown; SB, SSB, PSB: all absent; SR: present; SR characteristics: a large, ellipsoidal compact granular mass (line drawing); SZ: sausage-shaped, almost as long as the SP, with one end broader and the other end slightly pointed; N, RB: no information given. Distinctive features of sporocyst: ellipsoidal shape without SB, SSB, or PSB and containing a large SR composed of compact granules.

Prevalence: Mahrt (1967) first found these oocysts in the feces of one dog submitted to the University of Illinois Small Animal Clinic; he then cloned it by feeding single oocysts to two coccidia-free beagle puppies. Thornton et al. (1974) did a survey of internal parasites of coyotes in southern Texas, USA and reported doing flotation on the feces of two of them and finding oocysts of *I. rivolta* in one of them. This was before Dubey and Mahrt's (1978) paper that revised the *I. rivolta* found in dogs to *I. (=C.) neorivolta*.

Sporulation: Exogenous. Mahrt (1968) studied sporulation at four different temperatures. At 20°C, 94% of the oocysts had sporulated and formed SZ by 48 hours. At 25°C, 97% of the oocysts had sporulated and formed SZ by 24 hours. At 30°C, 96% of the oocysts had sporulated and formed SZ by 16 hours. At 38°C, 93% of the oocysts had sporulated and formed SZ by 8 hours. Oocysts incubated at 50°C for 4 hours did not develop and failed to sporulate when reincubated at 30°C. At that time, Mahrt (1968) was working with *I. rivolta* from the dog, but this was before he and Dubey (Dubey and Mahrt, 1978) changed the name to *I.* (=*C.) neorivolta.*

Prepatent and patent periods: Mahrt (1967) said the prepatent period was 142–146 hours and the patent period lasted 19 (13–23) days.

Site of infection: All endogenous stages were found in the posterior one-half of the small intestine and rarely in the cecum and colon, with the largest number of all stages just anterior to the ileocecal valve. These stages occurred in the distal third of the villi, predominantly in subepithelial cells of the lamina propria, but a few stages also were seen in epithelial cells (Mahrt, 1967).

Endogenous stages: Mahrt (1967) was unable to determine the number of asexual stages, but based on oocyst production, he suggested there were at least two merogonous stages. Meronts he measured were L×W: 17–24 × 12–23 and contained 4–24 merozoites; meronts with mature merozoites were seen as early as 72 hours PI. These merozoites had slender curved bodies and measured 10.5–13.4 × 2.3–3.0. Mahrt (1967) also found mature gamonts at 6 DPI; mature microgametocytes were 13.4 × 8.7, with 50–70 microgametes that measured 5.8–6.4 × 0.6, and each had two posteriorly-directed flagella, 11–14 long. Mature macrogamonts were described to have a single large N, 4–5 wide, with a nucleolus ~1.7 wide, but Mahrt (1967) gave no measurements for them. Dubey and Mahrt (1978) studied endogenous development by feeding six 7-day-old dogs 5×10^5 oocysts and killing them 24, 48, 72, 96, 114, and 120 hours PI and preparing their intestinal tissues for histological study; they found at least four types of meronts. Type I meronts (M_1) were found 72 hours PI and measured L×W: 8.4 × 2.5 (6–10 × 2–3) and

had two (1–10) uninucleate merozoites (m_1); M_2 were found 96–120 hours PI, measured L×W: 9–18 × 7–18, means not given, and had 2–12 short, broad m_2, each with 1–3 N that were (n=4) 9 × 3.5 (8–12 × 3–5); M_3 were seen predominantly at 96 hours PI and measured L×W (n=26): 12.6 × 8.3 (7–25 × 4–16) and had 2–20 uninucleate m_3 that were (n=22), 10 × 2.5 (8–14 × 2–3); M_4 were seen mainly 120–144 hours PI, measured L×W: 9–18 × 7–18 (means not given), and had 4–30 short, thin m_4 that were 7.5 × 1.2 (7–8 × 1–1.5). Dubey and Mahrt (1978) found mature microgamonts were L×W: 14.2 × 10.1 (10–22 × 7–18), each with 30–50 microgametes arranged around a PAS-positive residual body. Macrogamonts were L×W: 12.6 × 10.8 (11–15 × 9–13).

Cross-transmission: Mahrt (1967) failed to infect three cats with the *I. rivolta* oocysts from dogs he worked with.

Pathology: According to Mahrt (1966) this species is only slightly pathogenic. Dubey and Mahrt (1978) noted only that microscopic lesions were limited to mild congestion and infiltration by neutrophils.

Materials deposited: None.

Remarks: Wenyon and Sheather (1925) were the first and perhaps the only workers to report on the endogenous stages of the dog *I. rivolta* (=*C. neorivolta*) from a dog with a natural infection, but they gave no drawings, descriptions, or measurements; they only mentioned to have seen meronts, micro-, and macrogametocytes. Mahrt (1967) described some of the endogenous stages in dogs using a cloned culture derived from a single oocyst and reported two asexual generations, with meronts containing mature merozoites as soon as 3 DPI. Dubey and Mahrt (1978) separated *I.* (=*C.) neorivolta* from *I.* (=*C.) ohioensis* because its endogenous stages develop predominantly in the lamina propria of the posterior half of the small intestine, whereas the endogenous stages of *I.* (=*C.) ohioensis* occur only in the epithelial cells of the villi throughout the small intestine. Additionally, although bi- and trinucleate merozoites were common in type II meronts, they were not observed in types I, III, or IV meronts (see Dubey and Mahrt, 1978), whereas multinucleated merozoites with up to 7–8 N are common in *I.* (=*C.*) *ohioensis* endogenous development. Dubey and Mahrt (1978) said that the 2–3 N found in their m_2s, within the same PV, suggested to them that two or more generations of merozoites may occur without leaving the host cell. Similar processes occur during the development of *I.* (=*C.*) *ohioensis* (Dubey, 1978b) and *I. canis* (Lepp and Todd, 1974) in dogs and in the development of *I.* (=*C.*) *felis* (Shah, 1971), *I.* (=*C.*) *rivolta* (Dubey and Frenkel, 1972b), and *Toxoplasma gondii* (Dubey and Frenkel, 1972a) in cats.

Unfortunately, the culture of oocysts that Mahrt (1967) used to initially describe the life cycle of *I.* (=*C.*) *neorivolta* was lost, so Dubey and Mahrt (1978) said they were unable to compare oocysts between *I.* (=*C.*) *neorivolta* and *I.* (=*C.*) *ohioensis*, when they named *I.* (=*C.*) *neorivolta*; they did, however, give oocyst size measurements for both, and for *I.* (=*C.*) *burrowsi* oocysts, but only as measured in sections of dog intestines infected with each species. Levine and Ivens (1981) said, "structural details and measurements of the oocysts of this species (*I.* (=*C.*) *neorivolta*) have

apparently not been published…(but) they are similar to those of *I. ohioensis*." In fact, detailed measurements of the sporulated oocysts of this species still have not been published in the public domain.

CYSTOISOSPORA OHIOENSIS (DUBEY, 1975c) FRENKEL, 1977

Synonyms: *Diplospora bigemina* Wasielewsky, 1904 from a dog *pro parte*; *Isospora rivolta* (Grassi, 1879) Wenyon, 1923 of *auctores* from the domestic dog; *Lucetina rivolta* (Grassi, 1879) Henry and Leblois, 1926 from the domestic dog; *Levinea ohioensis* (Dubey, 1975c) Dubey, 1977c (mostly from Levine and Ivens, 1981).

Type host: *Canis lupus familiaris* L., 1758 (syn. *C. familiaris*), Domestic Dog.

Type locality: North America: USA: Ohio, Columbus.

Other definitive hosts: *Canis latrans* Say, 1823, Coyote; *Canis lupus* L., 1758, Wolf; *Canis lupus dingo* Meyer, 1793, Dingo; *Nyctereutes procyonoides ussuriensis* Matschie, 1907, Raccoon

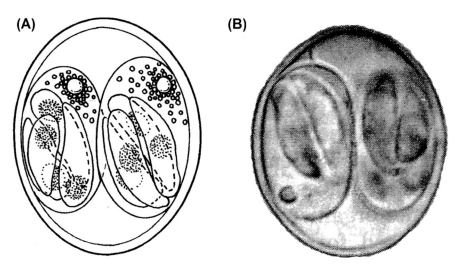

(A) **(B)**

FIGURE 14.5 (A). Line drawing of the sporulated oocyst of *Cystoisospora ohioensis*, (B). Photomicrograph of a sporulated oocyst of *C. ohioensis*. *(A) Fig. 1, from Dubey, J.P., 1975. Isospora ohioensis sp. n. proposed for* I. rivolta *of the dog. Journal of Parasitology 61 (3), 462–465, with permission of Allen Press, Inc., Lawrence, Kansas USA, copyright holder. (B) From Dubey, J.P., 1976. A review of* Sarcocystis *of domestic animals and of other coccidia of cats and dogs. Journal of the American Veterinary Medical Association 169 (10), 1061–1078, with permission of the AVMA, copyright holder for the JAVMA.*

Dog; *Vulpes vulpes* (L., 1758) (syn. *Vulpes fulvus* (Desmarest, 1820)), Red or Silver-back Fox (?).

Known intermediate hosts: *Felis catus* L., 1758, Domestic Cat; *Mus musculus* L., 1758, House Mouse; *Oryctolagus cuniculus* (L., 1758), European Rabbit (syn. *Lepus cuniculus*); *Ovis aries* L., 1758, Red Sheep.

Geographic distribution: Worldwide.

Description of sporulated oocyst: Oocyst shape: ellipsoidal to slightly ovoidal; number of walls, 2; wall characteristics: smooth, colorless to pale yellow, total thickness, ~0.8; L×W (n=50): 24×21 (21–27×19–23), L/W ratio: 1.2 (1.1–1.3); M, OR, PG: all absent. Distinctive features of oocyst: ellipsoidal/ovoidal shape with smooth, outer wall, and lack of M, OR, and PG.

Description of sporocyst and sporozoites: Sporocyst shape: ellipsoidal (line drawing); L×W (n=50): 17×12 (15–19×10–13), L/W ratio: 1.3 (1.2–1.4); SB, SSB, PSB: all absent; SR: present; SR characteristics: a large, compact granular mass lying at one end of SP or of a few scattered granules; SZ: banana-shaped, 10×3.5 (9–13×2.5–5), with one end broader and the other end slightly pointed; RB: usually one present at broader end. Distinctive features of sporocyst: generally ellipsoidal shape without SB, SSB, or PSB and containing a large SR composed of compact granules.

Prevalence: Nieschulz (1925, as per Levine and Ivens, 1981), found *I. (=C.) ohioensis* in 6/45 (13%) dogs in Utrecht, the Netherlands. It has been found in 4/113 (4%) dogs in Ohio, USA by Catcott (1946). Choquette and Gelinas (1950) recorded it in 34/155 (22%) dogs in Montreal, Canada. Costa and Freitas (1959) examined 18 dogs in Belo Horizonte, Brazil and said 1/18 (5.5%) had oocysts of *I. rivolta*; we now know, of course that the oocysts they saw almost certainly represented those of *I. (=C.) ohioensis*. Levine and Ivens (1965) found it in 24/139 (17%) dogs in Illinois, USA. Burrows (1968) found it in 43/835 (5%) dogs in New Jersey, USA. Alcaino and Tagle (1970) found it in 60/1,505 (4%) dogs in Chile, and Mirza (1970) found it in 7/54 (13%) dogs in Iraq. Mirzayans et al. (1972) recorded it from 5/115 (4%) dogs in Iran. Lepp and Todd

(1974) found it in 15/308 (5%) dogs, also in Illinois, USA. Streitel and Dubey (1976) found it in the feces 20/500 (4%) stray dogs, also in Ohio, USA. Arther and Post (1977) reported it in 2/82 (2%) coyotes in Colorado, USA. Dubey et al. (1978a) found *I. (=C.) ohioensis*-like oocysts in the feces of 5/169 (3%) adult coyotes in Montana, USA. Hoskins et al. (1982) examined dogs at the LSU Veterinary Teaching Hospital, Louisiana, USA from 1977 to 1980 and reported oocysts of *I. (=C.) ohioensis* in 1,177/4,058 (29%) samples in pups <6-months-old. Dubey (1982b) surveyed wild carnivores from Montana, USA and found its oocysts in the feces of 9/198 (4.5%) red foxes. McKenna and Charleston (1980d) examined fecal samples from dogs on the North Island of New Zealand and found 44/481 (9%) samples had oocysts they identified as *I. (=C.) ohioensis*. Bugg et al. (1999) examined fecal samples of urban dogs from four pet shops, three refuges, six breeding kennels, eight veterinary clinics, and two exercise areas in Perth, Western Australia and reported *I. (=C.) ohioensis* in 19/421 (4.5%) samples, mostly from breeding kennels and puppies from pet shops. During a survey of endoparasites, Barutzki and Schaper (2003) examined fecal samples of dogs in Freiburg, Germany, and *C. ohioensis* was identified in 1,434/8,438 (17%) samples. Gompper et al. (2003) said they found oocysts of *I. (=C.) ohioensis* in 6/23 (25%) *C. latrans* collected in the Black Rock Forest near Cornwall, New York, USA; their identification was based on the size of oocysts in the feces, so it should be taken with caution. Yamamoto et al. (2009) surveyed fecal samples of dogs in public animal shelters in the Saitama Prefecture, Japan and reported oocysts of *I. ohioensis* in 18/906 (2%) dogs. Hermosilla et al. (2017) surveyed fecal samples of wild European wolves (*C. lupus*) in mountainous areas of the Gorski Kotar region, Croatia and reported *I. (=C.) ohioensis* in 8/400 (2%) samples.

Sporulation: Exogenous. Sporulation was completed within 24 hours at 22–26°C (Dubey, 1975c), or oocysts sporulated after 36 hours at 27°C in Petri dishes, in 2.5% aqueous potassium dichromate ($K_2Cr_2O_7$) solution (Hilali et al., 1992), or sporulation took 4 days in 2.5% $K_2Cr_2O_7$ solution at 20–22°C (Arther and Post, 1977).

Prepatent and patent periods: Prepatent period is about 4.5 DPI with sporulated oocysts or 3.5 DPI after ingestion of infected mice (Dubey, 1978a). Hilali et al. (1992) said the prepatent period was 3, 5, and 5 DPI after three dogs ate (presumably infected) sheep meat, and patency in these dogs lasted 8, 5, and 12 days. Patency is 3–5 weeks in pups infected when they are 6–10-days-old and 1–2 weeks in pups infected when they are 4–384-days-old (Dubey, 1978a).

Site of infection: All endogenous stages in the dog definitive host were found in epithelial cells of the intestine.

Endogenous stages: Dubey (1978a) presented detailed photomicrographic evidence of the endogenous development in dogs using oocysts obtained from an infection with a single oocyst. He did not determine the number of merogonous stages, but said he saw two structurally-distinct meronts. Type I meronts were found in the jejunum and measured L × W: 9–19 × 2.5–4 (in tissue sections) and contained 2–8 merozoites, 11.1 × 3.1 (9–12 × 2.5–4). From 4 to 5 DPI merogony occurred throughout the small and large intestines, mostly in the ileum. "Type II meronts were about the same size as type I, but contained thinner merozoites." These meronts were L × W: 10.6 × 8.4 (6–12 × 5–12) and their merozoites were 7.0 × 1.5 (6–8 × 1–2). Gamonts were found in surface epithelial cells of the small intestine, cecum, and colon, but mostly in the ileum, 4–5 DPI. Macrogametes were L × W: 14.5 × 12.8 (sic) (13–17 × 11–12) in sections and L × W: 21.7 × 17.6 (21–26 × 17–25) in smears. Microgamonts were L × W: 15.3 × 11.4 (13–17 × 8–15) in sections and L × W: 27 × 19 (24–30 × 15–24) in smears and contained 20 to 50 microgametes.

Dubey (1978a) was unable to demonstrate MZTC or EIN stages of *I. (=C.) ohioensis* in sections of mesenteric lymph nodes, spleen, lung, liver, heart, skeletal muscle, and brain of dogs fed sporulated oocysts; however, bioassay in mice of mesenteric lymph nodes and spleen in dogs indicated that infective EIN or MZTC stages were present in these locations. Dubey and Mehlhorn (1978) studied the development of *I. (=C.) ohioensis* in mice after inoculating them with sporulated oocysts and examining their mesenteric lymph nodes using both LM and TEM. They learned that EIN organs of infected mice became infectious to dogs within 1 DPI and remained infectious up to at least 211 DPI with oocysts; and sporozoites of *I. (=C.) ohioensis* were found in lymphoreticular cells of mesenteric lymph nodes of mice from 1 to 374 DPI.

Cross-transmission: Heydorn (1973) found that the muscle, liver, lung, and brain tissue of mice that had been inoculated with oocysts of *I. (=C.) ohioensis* (=*I. bigemina* of the dog) caused specific pathogen free (SPF) dogs to shed oocysts in their feces from 5 to 27–33 DPI. In a series of experiments using both feline *I. (=C.) rivolta* and canine *I. (=C.) rivolta* (=*I. (=C.) ohioensis*), Dubey (1975c) showed that ingestion of feline *I. (=C.) rivolta* does not produce oocyst discharge in dogs, dogs can act as a transport host for feline *I. (=C.) rivolta* as do mice, hamsters, and rats, and cats can act as a transport host for canine *I. (=C.) rivolta* (=*I. (=C.) ohioensis*). Dubey (1975c) found that cats or mice infected with oocysts of this species from the dog did not produce oocysts but that the EIN organs of kittens or mice fed oocysts from dogs would cause dogs that ate these tissues to begin shedding oocysts; these results were verified by Dubey and Mehlhorn (1978). Loveless and Andersen (1975) transmitted this species from a dog to the coyote. Hilali et al. (1992) fed seven dogs pooled heart and esophagus muscle from 18 to 36 sheep (*Ovis aries*) and monitored their fecal output for 70 DPI. Three of these dogs passed oocysts of *I. (=C.) ohioensis* 3, 5, and 5 DPI, with patent periods of 8, 5, and 12 days, respectively. All three of the dogs that shed *I. (=C.) ohioensis* oocysts also passed oocysts and *I. (=C.) canis* and one, in addition, also passed sporocysts of one or more *Sarcocystis* species. Hilali et al. (1992) also inoculated two rabbits (presumably, *O. cuniculus*) with 20,000 sporulated oocysts of *I. ohioensis*; one was killed at 4 DPI and the other at 45 DPI. The one killed at 4 DPI was fed to two coccidia-free dogs, and the one killed at 45 DPI was fed to one coccidia-free dog. The dog fed the rabbit killed at 4 DPI passed *I. ohioensis* after a prepatent period of 8 days, whereas the dog fed the rabbit killed at 45 DPI shed no oocysts. The cross-transmission study undertaken by Hilali et al. (1992) was done to emphasize the public health importance of stray dogs that are in close association with humans and our food and companion animals.

Pathology: This species is usually nonpathogenic but sometimes can be mildly pathogenic. Dubey (1978b) found that 5/18 (28%) newborn pups fed either sporocysts or mouse tissues containing hypnozoites of *I. (=C.) ohioensis* developed diarrhea 3–4 DPI. Histologic lesions observed were necrotic with desquamation at the tips of the villi of the ileum and atrophy of the villi. Four 17-day-old dogs were fed homogenates of mesenteric lymph nodes and spleen from mice fed *I. (=C.) ohioensis* sporulated oocysts. Diarrhea was first observed at 3 DPI and microscopic lesions consisting of villous atrophy and necrosis of the intestinal epithelium were observed in the intestinal tissue sections of dogs examined 72 and 96 hours PI with mouse tissues. Pups >40-days-old acquired immunity within 1 week after ingesting sporulated oocysts, as evidenced by their failure to reshed oocysts on challenge. Dubey et al. (1978b) published a case report of a fatal coccidiosis event, "due to an *Isospora ohioensis*-like organism," in a 10-week-old female Chihuahua pup. The pup had diarrhea, dehydration, and weight loss before it died 7 days after the onset of its clinical signs. Lesions were limited to its intestinal tract beginning in the distal end of the small intestine and extending through the cecum and colon as histolytic lesions in the lamina propria; Dubey et al. (1978b) found numerous meronts and gamonts near these lesions. The parasite produced oocysts that were structurally similar to those of *I. (=C.) ohioensis*.

Materials deposited: None.

Remarks: The history of this name bears reiterating. Grassi (1879) first named it *Coccidium rivolta* describing oocysts from the cat. Wenyon (1923) reviewed the history of this organism and placed in into the genus *Isospora*. He also described it from the dog and considered the dog and cat species to be identical. Levine and Ivens (1965) first described oocysts of *I. (=C.) rivolta* from the feces of naturally-infected dogs, and Shah (1970a,b) described oocysts of *I. (=C.) rivolta* from the feces of naturally-infected cats. This further solidified the notion that *I. (=C.) rivolta* from cats and dogs were structurally identical and likely the same species, a view that was held until Dubey's (1975c) cross-transmission work supported their distinct life cycle differences and convinced him to name the dog form, *I. (=C.) ohioensis*. The oocysts of *I. (=C.) ohioensis* reported from coyotes by Arther and Post (1977) were L×W (n=50): 20.6×17.3 (17–23×15–21), L/W ratio: 1.2 (1.1–1.3), somewhat smaller than those described by Dubey (1975c), and sporocysts were ellipsoidal, L×W: 13×12. As noted earlier, Frenkel (1977) created the genus *Cystoisospora* for those dog and cat isosporans that had sporocysts without SBs and could be demonstrated to use other mammalian hosts to harbor their tissue stages and placed *I. (=C.) ohioensis* (and other species) into the genus *Cystoisospora*. Baek et al. (1993) confirmed finding oocysts of *I. (=C.) ohioensis* in dogs in Chonbuk Provence, Korea. Their oocysts took 96 hours to sporulate and measured L×W: 22.8×20.5 (21–24×19–22), L/W ratio: 1.1; lacking a M, OR, and PG. Sporocysts were L×W: 15.0×10.8 (13–17×10–12), L/W ratio: 1.4, lacking SB, SSB, PSB, but with a large SR consisting of a spheroidal hyaline body surrounded by several smaller granules. The prepatent period in the Korean dogs was 4 days.

GENUS NYCTEREUTES TEMMINCK, 1838 (MONOTYPIC)

CYSTOISOSPORA OHIOENSIS (DUBEY, 1975c) FRENKEL, 1977

Definitive host: *Nyctereutes procyonoides ussuriensis* Matschie, 1907, Raccoon Dog.

Remarks: Yakimoff and Matikaschwili (1933) identified *I. rivolta* (=*C. ohioensis*?) from 17/241 (7%) raccoon dogs in a fur farm in Voronezh, and from 81/135 (60%) in Novgorod, in the former USSR. Ovoidal/ellipsoidal oocysts were L×W: 21–30×18–25, and subspheroidal oocysts were L×W: 19–28×18–25; all lacked M, OR, and PG, and their sporocysts were L×W: 16.0×10.5 (14–18×9–13), L/W ratio: 1.5, and they lacked SB, SSB, and PSB, and all had a SR present. These oocysts may well have represented *C. ohioensis*, but because the original *I. rivolta* from dogs has now been divided into *I.* (=*C.*) *burrowsi*, *I.* (=*C.*) *neorivolta*, and *I.* (=*C.*) *ohioensis*, our conclusion is somewhat uncertain.

GENUS *VULPES* FRISCH, 1775
(12 SPECIES)

CYSTOISOSPORA BURIATICA (YAKIMOFF AND MATSCHOULSKY, 1940) NOV. COMB.

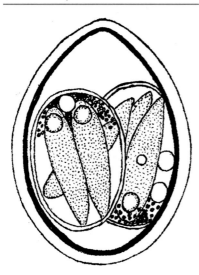

FIGURE 14.6 Original line drawing of the sporulated oocyst of *Cystoisospora buriatia*. *Modified Fig. 55, Levine, N.D., Ivens, V., 1981. The Coccidian Parasites (Protozoa, Apicomplexa) of Carnivores. Illinois Biological Monograph No. 51, The University of Illinois Press, Urbana, Illinois USA. The University of Illinois Press has released the copyright.*

Synonym: *Isospora buriatica* Yakimoff and Matschoulsky, 1940.

Type host: *Vulpes corsac* (L., 1768), Corsac Fox.

Type locality: Asia: Kazakhstan (former USSR).

Other definitive hosts: *Vulpes bengalensis* (Shaw, 1800), Bengal Fox; *Vulpes vulpes* (L., 1758) (syn. *Vulpes fulvus* (Desmarest, 1820)), Red or Silver-black Fox.

Known intermediate host: None to date.

Geographic distribution: Asia: Kazakhstan, Turkmenistan (former USSR); India.

Description of sporulated oocyst: Oocyst shape: ellipsoidal or ovoidal; number of walls, 2; wall characteristics: smooth, green or yellow-green (Svanbaev, 1956) or yellow with a dark shining inner contour (Dubey, 1963a), with total thickness 1.0–1.3; L×W (ellipsoidal forms): 25×19 (ranges unknown), L/W ratio: 1.3, and L×W (ovoidal forms): 32×25 (ranges unknown), L/W ratio: 1.3 (from Svanbaev, 1956), or 31×25 (29–33×22–25), L/W ratio 1.2–1.3; M, OR: both absent; PG: sometimes present (Svanbaev, 1956), or not (Dubey, 1963a). Distinctive features of oocyst: thick, smooth, two-layered, green or yellow wall, without M, OR, but with PG (occasionally).

Description of sporocyst and sporozoites: Sporocyst shape: elongate-ovoidal to ellipsoidal; L×W: mean unknown (15.5–17×10–13), L/W ratio: unknown (Svanbaev, 1956), or 19×12 (19–21×11–12), L/W ratio: 1.6; SB, SSB, PSB: all absent; SR: present; SR characteristics: an irregular mass of granules at one end of sporocyst; SZ: comma-shaped, with one end slightly more pointed than the other; SZs lie lengthwise in SP, and measured, 6–8×3–4 (Svanbaev, 1956), or 14–15×3–4, with a central N and a large RB at their more rounded end (Dubey, 1963a). Distinctive features of sporocyst: elongate-ovoidal to ellipsoidal shape, without SB, SSB, PSB, but possessing an SR.

Prevalence: Svanbaev (1956) found this form in the only corsac fox he examined. Dubey (1963a) found it in 4/4 (100%) *V. bengalensis* near Mathura, Uttar Pradesh, India, and Nukerbaeva and Svanbaev (1973) said they found this species in 149/1,199 (12%) *V. vulpes* in Kazakhstan.

Sporulation: Exogenous. Oocysts sporulated in 3–4 days when kept in 2% potassium dichromate solution ($K_2Cr_2O_7$) at 20–25°C (Svanbaev, 1956), or 2 days according to Dubey (1963a), or as early as 1–2 days (Nukerbaeva and Svanbaev, 1973).

Prepatent and patent periods: Unknown.

Site of infection: Unknown.

Endogenous stages: Unknown.

Cross-transmission: None to date.

Pathology: Unknown.

Materials deposited: None.

Remarks: Nukerbaeva and Svanbaev (1973) measured oocysts from *V. vulpes* in Kazakhstan and said they were ovoidal, L×W: 36×28 (31–45×25–31), L/W ratio: 1.3, with a two-layered wall that was 1.7–2.5 thick, and had ovoidal sporocysts, L×W: 20–22×11–14, and SZ: 10–13×4.6. Oocyst measurements by Svanbaev (1956), Dubey (1963a), and Nukerbaeva and Svanbaev (1973) are clearly different and may warrant separate species status (or not). Glebezdin (1978) reported a survey on 2,350 wild mammals representing 25 species in southwestern Turkmenistan from 1974 to 1977; in *V. corsac* he found ellipsoidal and ovoidal oocysts of *I.* (=*C.*) *buriatica* that were nearly identical to the original measurements provided by Yakimoff and Matschoulsky (1940).

CYSTOISOSPORA CANIVELOCIS ((WEIDMAN, 1915) WENYON, 1923) NOV. COMB.

Synonyms: *Isospora bigemina* var. *canivelocis* Weidman, 1915; *Isospora canivelocis* (Weidman, 1915) Wenyon, 1923; *Coccidium bigeminum* var. *canivelocis* Weidman, 1915; *Isospora bigeminum* var. *canivelocis* (Weidman, 1915) Mesnil, 1916; *Isospora canivecolis* (sic) (Weidman, 1915) Wenyon, 1923; *Isospora canivelocis* (Weidman, 1915) Wenyon, 1923 of *auctores*; *Lucetina canivelocis* (Weidman, 1915) Henry and Leblois, 1926.

Type host: *Vulpes velox* (Say, 1823), Swift Fox.

Type locality: Europe: Germany.

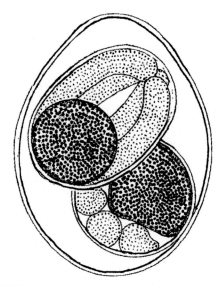

FIGURE 14.7   Original line drawing of the sporulated oocyst of *Cystoisospora canivelocis*. *Modified Fig. 27, Levine, N.D., Ivens, V., 1981. The Coccidian Parasites (Protozoa, Apicomplexa) of Carnivores. Illinois Biological Monograph No. 51, The University of Illinois Press, Urbana, Illinois USA. The University of Illinois Press has released the copyright.*

Other definitive hosts: *Vulpes vulpes* (L., 1758) (syn. *Vulpes vulgaris* Oken, 1816), Silver or Red Fox; *Vulpes* (syn. *Alopex*) *lagopus* (L., 1758), Arctic or Blue Fox (experimental).

Known intermediate host: None to date.

Geographic distribution: Asia: Russia: Kazakhstan, Turkmenistan (former USSR); Eastern Europe: Bulgaria; Estonia; Europe: Austria (?), Germany, Holland, Hungary, Iceland; North America: USA: Pennsylvania (Philadelphia Zoo).

Description of sporulated oocyst: Oocyst shape: subspheroidal to ellipsoidal; number of walls, 1; wall characteristics: smooth, yellow-orange to yellow-brown, with total thickness 1.2–1.6; L×W: ellipsoidal forms 33×28 (27–38×25–30), L/W ratio: 1.2 (Weidman, 1915), or 27×26 (24–32×20–32), L/W ratio: 1.0+ (Svanbaev, 1960), or 36×30 (33–39×27–32), L/W ratio 1.2 (Nieschulz and Bos, 1933), or 21–38×17–31 (means not given, Sprehn and Cramer, 1931), or 35×27 (30–39×23–30), L/W ratio: 1.3 (Golemansky and Ridzhakov, 1975);

M, OR, PG: all absent. Distinctive features of oocyst: oocysts variable in size, but all lack M, OR, and PG, and oocyst wall in older specimens sometimes collapses around sporocysts.

Description of sporocyst and sporozoites: Sporocyst shape: ellipsoidal; L×W: 14–16 wide, L/W ratio: unknown (Weidman, 1915), or 14–24×11–14, L/W ratio: unknown (Sprehn and Cramer, 1931), or 18×11 (16–20×9–12), L/W ratio: 1.6 (Svanbaev, 1960), or 11–17×9–11, L/W ratio: unknown (Golemansky and Ridzhakov, 1975); SB, SSB, PSB: all absent; SR: present; SR characteristics: an irregular mass of granules at one end of sporocyst; SZ: banana- or comma-shaped with one end more pointed than the other; SZs lie lengthwise in SP and measure 11 × 4 (10–12×3–4) (Svanbaev, 1960), or 12–15×3–4 (Golemansky and Ridzhakov, 1975). Distinctive features of sporocyst: a typical ellipsoidal shape without SB, SSB, PSB, and with a granular SR.

Prevalence: Svanbaev (1960) found this form in 6/18 (33%) foxes in the Alma Atinsk Oblast region, Kazakhstan. Golemansky and Ridzhakov (1975) found it in 22/146 (15%) red foxes in Bulgaria, and Nukerbaeva and Svanbaev (1973) said they found this species in 137/1,199 (11%) *V. vulpes* in Kazakhstan. Frank (1978) said she found this species in 3/5 (60%) red foxes she examined from "Illmitz in the European Soviet Union (probably Austria)." SkírNisson and Pálmadóttir (1993) reported oocysts of this species in 4/54 (7%) silver foxes on 2/7 (28.5%) fur farms and in 12/130 (9%) blue foxes on 3/7 (43%) fur farms they surveyed in Iceland.

Sporulation: Exogenous. Ridala (1936) said that after 72 hours, 75% of the oocysts sporulated when kept in moist surroundings at 18–24°C. Oocysts sporulated in 2–4 days when kept in 2% potassium dichromate solution ($K_2Cr_2O_7$) at 25°C (Svanbaev, 1960) or in 1 day (according to Weidman, 1915).

Prepatent and patent periods: The prepatent period was 5 days during experimental infections according to Nukerbaeva and Svanbaev (1977), both when oocysts were transmitted from *V. velox* to *V. lagopus* and from *V. lagopus* to *V. velox*; however, when oocysts were transmitted

from *V. velox* to *V. velox*, the prepatent period could be 5 or 6 days.

Site of infection: Unknown.

Endogenous stages: Unknown.

Cross-transmission: No one has attempted to cross-infect other animals with sporulated oocysts from the **type** host, swift fox, but Sprehn and Cramer (1931) using oocysts from the silver fox said they were unable to infect two domestic kittens, while Pellérdy (1955) could not infect a badger. Nieschulz and Bos (1933) could not transmit the larger oocysts of this form to a young dog. Nukerbaeva and Svanbaev published two identical papers (1974, 1977) with nearly identical tables. The only table in their 1974 paper (page 37) said they were able to transmit oocysts of *I.* (=*C.*) *laidlawi* and *E. vison* from mink to two other minks (Nos. 8, 9), whereas the table (No. 12, page 79) in their 1977 paper stated they were able to successfully transmit oocysts of *I.* (=*C.*) *laidlawi* and *E. vison* from mink to two foxes (Nos. 8, 9), *V. vulpes*, obviously a typographical error. In both tables, the prepatent period for *I.* (=*C.*) *laidlawi* was 8 days and for *E. vison* it was 6 DPI. Both papers (Nukerbaeva and Svanbaev, 1974, 1977) said they successfully infected four Arctic foxes, *V. lagopus* (Nos. 13–14, were 6-months-old; Nos. 15–16 were 40-days-old), with oocysts of *I.* (=*C.*) *canivelocis* they found in *V. vulpes*, and the prepatent period was always 5 DPI. Likewise, they collected *I.* (=*C.*) *canivelocis* oocysts from three *V. lagopus*, and successfully cross-transmitted it to three 5-month-old *V. vulpes* (Foxes 1–3), which all had prepatent periods of 5 days. They also took oocysts from two *V. vulpes* and infected two 5-month-old *V. vulpes*, which had prepatent periods of 5 and 6 days. Nukerbaeva and Svanbaev (1974, 1977) were unable to infect two 40-day-old cats, a dog, and two 5-month-old minks with oocysts derived from *V. vulpes*.

Pathology: Ridala (1936) described coccidiosis in two dead silver fox puppies. His observations documented that both pups had moderate colitis, moderate passive hyperaemia of the liver, fatty degeneration of the kidneys and cardiac muscle, and passive hyperaemia of the lungs. On necropsy of both pups, smear preparations showed abundant oocysts in mucous membrane of the small intestine, especially in the end part of the jejunum and ileum. Ridala (1936) measured sporulated oocysts to confirm they were *I.* (=*C.*) *canivelocis*. Oocysts were L × W (n = 150): 21–37 × 19–31 and sporocysts were L × W (n = 100): 17–21 × 13–16.

Materials deposited: None.

Remarks: The exact identity and defining characters of this species are problematic. Weidman (1915), who first described sporulated oocysts, said they were 27–38 in size. Sprehn and Cramer (1931) said they found this species in silver foxes in either Germany or Poland, but their population of oocysts had two size modes, small and large. The larger ones were slightly pointed at one end, whereas the smaller ones were broadly ovoidal and did not taper at the pole(s). They felt that this species from the fox identified as *I.* (=*C.*) *canivelocis* might, in fact, represent two species. Nieschulz and Bos (1933) also found what they identified as two size categories of this species in young silver foxes on a fur farm in the Netherlands; they kept the name *I.* (=*C.*) *canivelocis* for the larger form with oocysts 33–39 long and one pole clearly pointed, and renamed the smaller form, *Isospora vulpina*. Later, Bledsoe (1976a,b) said he found oocysts of *I.* (=*C.*) *vulpina* in silver foxes from Wisconsin, USA, but his oocysts were intermediate in size between the two size ranges given by Nieschulz and Bos (1933) for *I.* (=*C.*) *canivelocis* and *I.* (=*C.*) *vulpina*. Levine and Ivens (1981) suggested that because the only report of oocysts of *I.* (=*C.*) *canivelocis* from the swift fox is that of Weidman (1915), more swift foxes need to be examined for coccidia to help clarify what are the morphometrics of the oocysts within them. The oocysts measured by Nukerbaeva and Svanbaev (1973) in silver foxes were ovoidal, L × W: 29 × 26 (28–31 × 25–28), L/W ratio: 1.1 and had a two-layered yellow-orange wall, 1.5 thick, and their sporocysts were 14–20 × 10–13. Frank (1978) said she found this species in *V. vulpes* trapped near

Lake Neusiedl, Austria, right on the border with Hungary but gave no morphological or prevalence data. Pellérdy (1974a) said that the type host for this species was *V. vulpes*, but he was mistaken as noted by Levine and Ivens (1981). Oocysts identified as *I.* (=*C.*) *canivelocis* were reported by SkírNisson and Pálmadóttir (1993), in mink pups on fur farms in Iceland, to be 36 × 29 (31–41 × 25–34). Glebezdin (1978) reported a survey on 2,350 wild mammals representing 25 species in southwestern Turkmenistan from 1974 to 1977; in *V. vulpes* he found ellipsoidal oocysts of *I.* (=*C.*) *canivelocis* that measured, L × W: 32.6 × 27.4 (28–36 × 25–31), L/W ratio: 1.1 (1.1–1.2) and sporocysts were L × W: 18.7 × 12.9 (14–22 × 11–14), L/W ratio: 1.4. Upton (pers. comm., 1999) said the oocyst of this species was morphologically identical with *I.* (=*C.*) *canis*, even being tapered at one end, but no one to that time (or to the present) had done the appropriate cross-transmission studies to confirm or dispute this identity crisis.

CYSTOISOSPORA PAVLODARICA (NUKERBAEVA AND SVANBAEV, 1973) NOV. COMB.

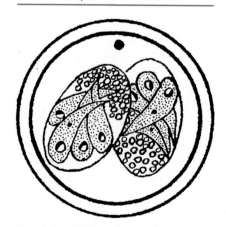

FIGURE 14.8 Original line drawing of the sporulated oocyst of *Cystoisospora pavlodarica*. A rendition of Fig. 1, Nukerbaeva, K.K., Svanbaev, S.K., 1973. Koktsidii pushnykh zverei v Kazakhstane. (Coccidia of fur-bearing mammlas in Kazakhstan). Vestnik Sel'skokhoziaistvennoi Nauki Kazakhstana 12, 50–54. (In Russian).

Synonym: *Isospora pavlodarica* Nukerbaeva and Svanbaev, 1973.

Type host: *Vulpes vulpes* (L., 1758) (syn. *Vulpes fulvus* (Desmarest, 1820)), Red or Silver Fox.

Type locality: Asia: Kazakhstan (former USSR).

Other definitive host: *Vulpes* (syn. *Alopex*) *lagopus* (L., 1758), Blue or Arctic Fox.

Known intermediate host: None to date.

Geographic distribution: Asia: Kazakhstan (former USSR).

Description of sporulated oocyst: Oocyst shape: short-ovoidal to spheroidal; number of walls, 2; wall characteristics: ~1.4 thick; L×W: short-ovoidal forms 22–25×20–22, L/W ratio: unknown (means not given), and spheroidal forms 20–22, L/W ratio: 1.0; M, OR; both absent; PG: present, small, but only found in "some oocysts." Distinctive features of oocyst: smooth, single-layered wall (line drawing), and one small PG, but lacking M and OR.

Description of sporocyst and sporozoites: Sporocyst shape: ovoidal; L×W: 13×7, L/W ratio: 1.9; SB, SSB, PSB: all absent; SR: present; SR characteristics: multiple granules scattered at one end of SP; SZ: elongate comma-shaped (line drawing), with one small, clear RB at rounded end. Distinctive features of sporocyst: typical short-ellipsoidal shape without SB, SSB, PSB and with a SR of granules.

Prevalence: Nukerbaeva and Svanbaev (1973) found it in 19/1,199 (1.6%) *V. vulpes* in Kazakhstan.

Sporulation: Exogenous. Nukerbaeva and Svanbaev (1973) said sporulation occurred in 3–4 days.

Prepatent and patent periods: Unknown.

Site of infection: Unknown, but Nukerbaeva and Svanbaev (1973) said it occurred in the intestine.

Endogenous stages: Unknown.

Cross-transmission: None to date.

Pathology: Unknown.

Materials deposited: None.

Remarks: Nukerbaeva and Svanbaev (1973) said, "the oocysts differ from those known before by smaller size, shape of spores, and presence of polar granule. That is why we named this species as new." To view a photomicrograph of a sporulated oocyst, see Nukerbaeva (1981b, Fig. 21).

CYSTOISOSPORA TRIFFITTI (NUKERBAEVA AND SVANBAEV, 1973) NOV. COMB.

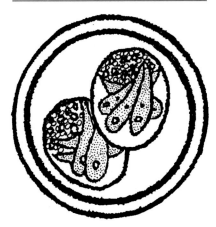

FIGURE 14.9 Original line drawing of the sporulated oocyst of *Cystoisospora triffitti*. A rendition of Fig. 2, Nukerbaeva, K.K., Svanbaev, S.K., 1973. *Koktsidii pushnykh zverei v Kazakhstane*. (Coccidia of fur-bearing mammlas in Kazakhstan). *Vestnik Sel'skokhoziaistvennoi Nauki Kazakhstana* 12 50–54. (In Russian).

Synonym: *Isospora triffitti* Nukerbaeva and Svanbaev, 1973.

Type host: *Vulpes* (syn. *Alopex*) *lagopus* (L., 1758), Blue or Arctic Fox.

Type locality: Asia: Kazakhstan (former USSR).

Other definitive host: *Vulpes vulpes* (L., 1758) (syn. *Vulpes fulvus* (Desmarest, 1820)), Red or Silver Fox.

Known intermediate host: None to date.

Geographic distribution: Asia (former USSR): Georgia, Kazakhstan.

Description of sporulated oocyst: Oocyst shape: broadly ovoidal to spheroidal; number of walls, 2; wall characteristics: smooth, light gray, ~1 thick; L×W: broadly ovoidal forms 11–13×10–11, L/W ratio: unknown (means not given), and sphe-roidal forms, 11–13, L/W ratio: 1.0; M, OR, PG: all absent. Distinctive features of oocyst: small, mostly spheroidal form with a smooth wall, ~1 thick, and lacking M, OR, and PG.

Description of sporocyst and sporozoites: Sporocyst shape: ovoidal to slightly ellipsoi-dal; L×W: 6×4, L/W ratio: 1.5; SB, SSB, PSB: all absent; SR: present; SR characteristics: granules scattered at one end of SP; SZ: elongate comma-shaped (line drawing), with one clear RB at rounded end. Distinctive features of sporocyst: typical short-ellipsoidal shape without SB, SSB, PSB, and with a SR of granules.

Prevalence: Nukerbaeva and Svanbaev (1973) found it in 17/1,199 (1%) *V. lagopus* in Kazakhstan.

Sporulation: Probably exogenous; time is unknown.

Prepatent and patent periods: Unknown.

Site of infection: Unknown, but Nukerbaeva and Svanbaev (1973) said it occurred in the intestine.

Endogenous stages: Unknown.

Cross-transmission: None to date.

Pathology: Unknown.

Materials deposited: None.

Remarks: Based on their morphological simi-larity of the sporulated oocysts, Triffitt (1927) said these oocysts belonged to *I. bigemina*, which was described by Stiles (1892) in cats. However, Nukerbaeva and Svanbaev (1973) said their exper-iments "in cross-transmission demonstrated that the coccidia of cats and fox are highly specific."

CYSTOISOSPORA VULPINA (NIESCHULZ AND BOS, 1933) FRENKEL, 1977

Synonyms: *Isospora vulpina* Nieschulz and Bos, 1933; *Isospora aprutina* Mantovani, 1965, emend. Pellérdy, 1974a; *Isospora vulpina* var. *aprutina* (Nieschulz and Bos, 1933) Mantovani, 1965; *Isospora vulpina* var. *vulpina* (Nieschulz and Bos, 1933) Mantovani, 1965.

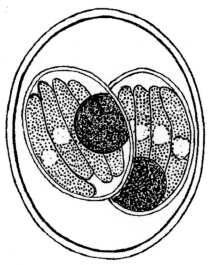

FIGURE 14.10 Original line drawing of the sporulated oocyst of *Cystoisospora vulpina*. *Modified Fig. 25, Levine, N.D., Ivens, V., 1981. The Coccidian Parasites (Protozoa, Apicomplexa) of Carnivores. Illinois Biological Monograph No. 51,* The University of Illinois Press, *Urbana, Illinois USA. The University of Illinois Press has released the copyright.*

Type host: *Vulpes vulpes* (L., 1758) (syn. *Vulpes fulvus* (Desmarest, 1820)), Red or Silver Fox.

Type locality: Europe.

Other definitive hosts: *Vulpes bengalensis* (Shaw, 1800), Bengal Fox; *Vulpes* (syn. *Alopex*) *lagopus* (L., 1758), Blue or Arctic Fox; *Canis lupus famil-iaris* L., 1758 (syn. *C. familiaris*), Domestic Dog (experimental).

Known intermediate host: *Mus musculus* L., 1758, House Mouse.

Geographic distribution: Europe: Bulgaria, Holland, Iceland, Italy; North America: USA: Washington, Wisconsin; Asia (former USSR): Georgia, Kazakhstan.

Description of sporulated oocyst: Oocyst shape: broadly ellipsoidal; number of walls, 1; wall characteristics: smooth, yellow, ~1.3 thick; L×W: ellipsoidal forms 24.9×21.4 (21–32×19–27), L/W ratio: 1.2 (Nieschulz and Bos, 1933), or 27×23 (21–34×19–28), L/W ratio: 1.2 (Dunlap, 1956), or 24.5×21 (22–28×18–22), L/W ratio: 1.2 (Mantovani, 1965), or 25.2×19.6 (22–28×17–22),

L/W ratio: 1.3 (Nukerbaeva and Svanbaev, 1973), or 25 × 20 (20–31 × 16–24), L/W ratio: 1.25 (Golemansky and Ridzhakov, 1975), or 30 × 24 (25–38 × 21–32), L/W ratio 1.25 (Bledsoe, 1976a, b); M, OR, PG: all absent. Distinctive features of oocyst: oocyst without M, OR, PG, and the smooth wall sometimes collapses around the sporocysts after sporulation.

Description of sporocyst and sporozoites: Sporocyst shape: slightly ovoidal to ellipsoidal; L × W: 15 × 11 (13–18 × 9–13), L/W ratio: 1.4 (Nieschulz and Bos, 1933), or 18.5 × 13 (17–20 × 12–14), L/W ratio: 1.4 (Mantovani, 1965), or 12.6 (sic) × 11.2 (14–17 × 11–14), L/W ratio: 1.1 (Nukerbaeva and Svanbaev, 1973), or 16–19 × 10–13 (mean not given) (Golemansky and Ridzhakov, 1975), or 18 × 13 (15–23 × 11–16), L/W ratio: 1.4 (Bledsoe, 1976a,b); SB, SSB, PSB: all absent; SR: present; SR characteristics: a large, compact, spheroidal mass of granules that appears membrane-bounded; SZ: elongate sausage-shaped, lie lengthwise in SP, and measured 10–12 × 2–3 (Golemansky and Ridzhakov, 1975); neither N nor RB were visible. Distinctive features of sporocyst: elongate-ovoidal to ellipsoidal shape without SB, SSB, PSB.

Prevalence: Golemansky and Ridzhakov (1975) found this species in 26/146 (18%) *V. vulpes* in Bulgaria. Bledsoe (1976a, b) found and identified only this species in *V. vulpes* in Wisconsin, USA, Mikeladze (1978) reported it in foxes in Georgia (former USSR), and Nukerbaeva and Svanbaev (1973) found it in 62/1,199 (5.2%) *V. vulpes* in Kazakhstan. In Iceland, SkírNisson and Pálmadóttir (1993) found oocysts they identified as this species in 8/54 (15%) *V. vulpes* pups on 4/7 (57%) fur farms they surveyed; they also found it in 25/130 (19%) *V. lagopus* pups on 8/15 (53%) fur farms sampled; all pups sampled were between 8- and 10-weeks-old.

Sporulation: Exogenous. Oocysts sporulated in 2 days at 25°C in 2.5% potassium dichromate ($K_2Cr_2O_7$) solution (Bledsoe, 1976a,b) or in 2–3 days (Nukerbaeva and Svanbaev, 1973).

Prepatent and patent periods: Dunlap (1956) said the prepatent period in the silver fox was 6 days,

and Bledsoe (1976a,b) said it was 6–7 days in a dog. Dunlap (1956) said the patent period lasted 5 days in the silver fox, and Bledsoe (1976a,b) said it was 7 days in the dog. Nukerbaeva and Svanbaev (1974, 1977) said it had a prepatent period of 6 days.

Site of infection: Unknown.

Endogenous stages: Unknown.

Cross-transmission: Neither Nieschulz and Bos (1933) nor Mantovani (1965) were able to transmit this species to young dogs. Bledsoe (1976a,b) was able to transmit oocysts from the silver fox to beagle puppies both directly via sporulated oocysts and by feeding the pups mice that had been fed sporulated oocysts 5–6 months previously. Pups that ingested infected mice began passing oocysts on 5 DPI. Bledsoe (1976a,b) also was able to transfer the infection from dog to dog via sporulated oocysts. It seems clear from the photomicrographs that the oocysts he studied were not *I. canis*. Nukerbaeva and Svanbaev (1974, 1977) in a series of cross-infection experiments, using oocysts they identified as *I.* (=*C.*) *vulpina* harvested from *V. vulpes*, said they infected four Arctic foxes, *V. lagopus* (Nos. 13–14, 6-months-old; Nos. 15–16, 40-days-old), and all had a prepatent period of 6 days; likewise, when they took oocysts from three *V. lagopus* and inoculated them into three *V. vulpes*, all red foxes became infected and the prepatent period also was 6 days. They also took oocysts from one *V. vulpes* and infected another 5-month-old *V. vulpes*, which had a prepatent period of 6 days. Finally, they were unable to infect two 40-day-old cats with oocysts produced by *V. vulpes*.

Pathology: Unknown.

Materials deposited: None.

Remarks: Mantovani (1965) thought that the oocysts and sporocysts he measured were different from those measured by Nieschulz and Bos (1933), but we agree with Levine and Ivens (1981) that these differences do not seem significant enough to name theirs a different species. In addition, Pellérdy (1974a) said that Mantovani (1965) first named the species he found in a fox *I. vulpina* var. *vulpina* to distinguish it from

I. vulpina var. *aprutina*, which he described from *V. vulpes*, but that after corresponding with him (Pellérdy) several times, he (Mantovani) canceled his two varieties. Nukerbaeva and Svanbaev (1973) measured oocysts from silver foxes in Kazakhstan, which were subspheroidal, L×W: 25.2×19.6 (22–28×17–22), L/W ratio: 1.3, had a two-layered oocyst wall that was 1.3 thick, but may have had a small (?) residuum; their sporocysts were spheroidal, 11–13 wide, or ovoidal, 14–17×11–14. Based on the oocyst measurements given by the various authors cited above, it seems probable that more than one species of coccidia are being confused, and some of the coccidia, including the original description, may be referring, at least in part, to *I. (=C.) ohioensis*, *I. (=C.) neorivolta*, or *I. (=C.) burrowsi*. The *I. (=C.) vulpina* of Bledsoe (1976a, b) may represent a synonym of *I. (=C.) vulpis* Galli-Valerio, 1931, but the original description of the latter species is so poor that it is difficult to tell. The oocysts measured by SkírNisson and Pálmadóttir (1993) and identified as *I. vulpina* were L×W: 27×23 (22–30×18–28) and L/W ratio: 1.2. Glebezdin (1978) reported a survey on 2,350 wild mammals representing 25 species in southwestern Turkmenistan from 1974 to 1977; in *V. vulpes* he found ellipsoidal oocysts of *I. (=C.) vulpina* that measured L×W: 26.2×23.6 (22–31×20–25) and L/W ratio: 1.1, and sporocysts were L×W: 16.7×10.5 (14–20×8–11), L/W ratio: 1.6.

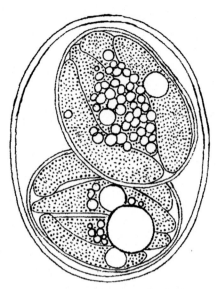

FIGURE 14.11 Original line drawing of the sporulated oocyst of *Cystoisospora sengeri*. Modified Fig. 47, Levine, N.D., Ivens, V., 1981. The Coccidian Parasites (Protozoa, Apicomplexa) of Carnivores. Illinois Biological Monograph No. 51, The University of Illinois Press, Urbana, Illinois USA. The University of Illinois Press has released the copyright.

MEPHITIDAE BONAPARTE, 1845

GENUS *SPILOGALE* GRAY, 1865 (4 SPECIES)

CYSTOISOSPORA SENGERI (LEVINE AND IVENS, 1964) NOV. COMB.

Synonym: *Isospora sengeri* Levine and Ivens, 1964.

Type host: *Spilogale putorius ambarvalis* (Bangs, 1898), Eastern Spotted Skunk.

Type locality: North America: USA: Florida, Clewiston.

Other definitive hosts: None to date.

Known intermediate host: None to date.

Geographic distribution: North America: USA: Arkansas, Florida.

Description of sporulated oocyst: Oocyst shape: ellipsoidal, sometimes slightly squared at one end; number of walls, 1; wall characteristics: smooth, colorless to pale yellow, very thin with total thickness 0.6–0.8; L×W (n=50): 20×15 (16–23×12–18), L/W ratio: 1.3 (1.1–1.5); M, OR, PG: all absent. Distinctive features of oocyst: smooth, transparent single-layered wall, M, OR, PG all absent, and the thin oocyst wall can be depressed between sporocysts.

Description of sporocyst and sporozoites: Sporocyst shape: slightly ellipsoidal, sometimes with one side slightly flattened; L×W (n=50): 12×10 (10–14×8–12), L/W ratio: 1.2 (1.1–1.4); SB, SSB, PSB: all absent; SR: present; SR characteristics: composed of one or more globules or as a loose group of granules, or both; SZ: elongate sausage-shaped with one end slightly more pointed than the other; SZ lie lengthwise in SP, each with a clear, subcentral N, but RBs were not visible. Distinctive features of sporocyst: ellipsoidal shape without SB, SSB, PSB, and with SR.

Prevalence: Levine and Ivens (1964) found this form in the only skunk they examined. Lesmeister et al. (2008) found oocysts, which they identified as this species, in the feces of 9/29 (31%) *S. putorius*, including 5/13 (38%) females and 4/16 (25%) males, in western Arkansas, USA, but their oocysts were not measured or photographed.

Sporulation: Unknown. The fecal sample examined by Levine and Ivens (1964) was taken from a wild spotted skunk in Florida, USA, and then sent to Rodney Mead at Montana State University, Missoula, and Mr. Mead then sent the sample to Levine and Ivens at the University of Illinois, Champaign, Illinois, USA. Lesmeister et al. (2008) did not mention how they sporulated their oocysts.

Prepatent and patent periods: Unknown.

Site of infection: Unknown.

Endogenous stages: Unknown.

Cross-transmission: None to date.

Pathology: Unknown.

Materials deposited: None.

Remarks: The oocysts seen, reported, and measured by Levine and Ivens (1964) actually may represent a *Sarcocystis* species because they said, "In some instances the oocyst wall was stretched tightly around the sporocysts, while in a few, it was depressed between the sporocysts." These are characteristics typical of *Sarcocystis* oocysts. Our view is that *I*. (=*C*.) *sengeri* may represent a species of *Sarcocystis*, but in the *Remarks* of their original description, Levine and Ivens (1964) argued, "free sporocysts of *I. sengeri* were never seen, and the oocyst wall was relatively thick and sturdy." Thus, for the moment at least, we place it as a *Cystoisospora* species.

CYSTOISOSPORA SPILOGALES (LEVINE AND IVENS, 1964) NOV. COMB.

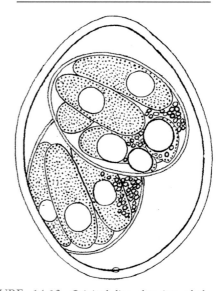

FIGURE 14.12 Original line drawing of the sporulated oocyst of *Cystoisospora spilogales*. *Modified Fig. 74, Levine, N.D., Ivens, V., 1981. The Coccidian Parasites (Protozoa, Apicomplexa) of Carnivores. Illinois Biological Monograph No. 51, The University of Illinois Press, Urbana, Illinois USA. The University of Illinois Press has released the copyright.*

Synonym: *Isospora spilogales* Levine and Ivens, 1964.

Type host: *Spilogale putorius ambarvalis* (Bangs, 1898), Eastern Spotted Skunk.

Type locality: North America: USA: Florida, Clewiston.

Other definitive hosts: None to date.

Known intermediate host: None to date.

Geographic distribution: North America: USA: Arkansas, Florida.

Description of sporulated oocyst: Oocyst shape: ovoidal, ellipsoidal, or sometimes asymmetrical; number of walls, 1; wall characteristics: smooth, colorless to pale gray or yellow, with total thickness 1.0–1.2; L×W (n=50): 34×26 (29–38×22–28), L/W ratio: 1.4 (1.2–1.5); M, OR: both absent; PG: reported as absent, but Levine and Ivens (1964) said that a "tiny bleb of material adheres to the inside of the broad end of the oocyst wall," which we interpret may be a PG or a small OR. Distinctive features of oocyst: smooth, transparent single-layered wall without M, but it has a "tiny bleb" of material on the inside of the oocyst wall, seen in both unsporulated and sporulated oocysts.

Description of sporocyst and sporozoites: Sporocyst shape: ellipsoidal; L×W (n=75): 19×14 (17–22×13–16), L/W ratio: 1.4 (1.1–1.5); SB, SSB, PSB: all absent; SR: present; SR characteristics: consisted of one or more large globules, and some residual granules; SZ: sausage-shaped, with a clear, subcentral N, but RBs were not visible. Distinctive features of sporocyst: ellipsoidal shape without SB, SSB, PSB, but with a SR.

Prevalence: Levine and Ivens (1964) found this form in the only skunk they examined. Lesmeister et al. (2008) found oocysts, which they identified as this species in the feces of 9/29 (31%) *S. putorius*, including 4/13 (31%) females and 5/16 (31%) males, in western Arkansas, USA, but they did not measure or photograph oocysts.

Sporulation: Unknown. The fecal sample examined by Levine and Ivens (1964) was taken from a wild spotted skunk in Florida, USA, and then sent to Rodney Mead at Montana State University, Missoula, and Mr. Mead then sent the sample to Levine and Ivens at the University of Illinois, Champaign, Illinois, USA. Lesmeister et al. (2008) did not mention how they sporulated their oocysts.

Prepatent and patent periods: Unknown.
Site of infection: Unknown.
Endogenous stages: Unknown.
Cross-transmission: None to date.
Pathology: Unknown.
Materials deposited: None.

Remarks: The oocysts seen, reported, and measured by Levine and Ivens (1964) may be a valid *Cystoisospora* species, but no one has found it again since the original description.

MUSTELIDAE FISCHER, 1817

SUBFAMILY LUTRINAE BONAPARTE, 1838

GENUS *LUTRA* BRISSON, 1762 (3 SPECIES)

CYSTOISOSPORA LUTRAE (TORRES, MODRÝ, FERNÁNDEZ, ŠLAPETA, AND KOUDELA, 2000) NOV. COMB.

Synonym: *Isospora lutrae* Torres, Modrý, Fernández, Šlapeta and Koudela, 2000.

Type host: *Lutra lutra* (L., 1758), European Otter.

Type locality: Europe: Spain: Brozas, province of Cáceres (40°6′ N, 6°8′ W).

Other definitive hosts: None to date.

Known intermediate host: None to date.

Geographic distribution: Europe: Spain.

Description of sporulated oocyst: Oocyst shape: slightly subspheroidal to spheroidal; number of walls, 2, about 1 thick; wall characteristics: outer layer smooth, colorless; L×W: 32.1×29.6 (27.5–33×28–31), L/W ratio: 1.0 (1.0–1.1); M, OR, PG: all absent. Distinctive features of oocyst: mostly spheroidal shape with a smooth, transparent outer wall, and without M, OR, PG.

Description of sporocyst and sporozoites: Sporocyst shape: ellipsoidal; L×W: 18.2×14.4 (17–19×14–16), L/W ratio: 1.3 (1.2–1.4); SB, SSB, PSB: all absent; SR: present; SR characteristics: spheroidal granules scattered among the SZ; SZ: spindle-shaped, 12.4×2.5 with both anterior and posterior RBs. Distinctive features of sporocyst: highly scattered granules of SR, and spindle-shaped SZ, each with two RB and SP lack SB, SSB, PSB.

Prevalence: Only 1/10 (10%) otters examined were found to be naturally-infected.

Sporulation: Mostly exogenous; unsporulated oocysts, oocysts in early stages of sporulation,

(A) **(B)**

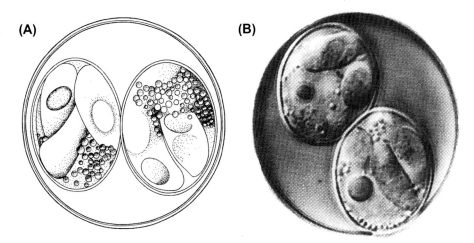

FIGURE 14.13 (A). Line drawing of the sporulated oocyst of *Cystoisospora lutrae*. (B). Photomicrograph of a sporulated oocyst of *C. lutrae*. *(A) and (B) Reprinted by permission from Springer Nature and copyright Clearinghouse, publisher of Systematic Parasitology 47 (1), 59–63, Torres, Modrý, Fernández, Šlapeta, Koudela. 2000.* Isospora lutrae *n. sp. (Apicomplexa: Eimeriidae), a new coccidium from the European otter* Lutra lutra *(L.) (Carnivora: Mustelidae) from Spain.*

and a few sporulated oocysts were observed in fresh fecal samples from otters. Oocysts sporulated within 12 hours at 22°C in 2.5% aqueous potassium dichromate ($K_2Cr_2O_7$).

Prepatent and patent periods: Unknown.

Site of infection: Unknown; oocysts recovered from feces.

Endogenous stages: Unknown.

Cross-transmission: None to date.

Pathology: Unknown.

Materials deposited: Phototypes of sporulated oocysts are in the Institute of Parasitology, Academy of Sciences of the Czech Republic, České Budějovice (Coll. No. R-126/99).

Remarks: Torres et al. (2000) described and named *I.* (=*C.*) *lutrae* from the European otter, in Spain. Interestingly, in late 2000, von Cord Gottschalk (2000), apparently unaware of the paper by Torres et al. (2000), published another new species description of an *Isospora*-like oocyst, which he also named *I.* (=*C.*) *lutrae*, from *L. lutra* in Germany. Based on the morphology of their sporulated oocysts these two "species" are clearly different. However, based on independent phylogenetic analyses discussed in earlier chapters (e.g., Carreno and Barta, 1999; Franzen et al., 2000; Barta et al., 2005; Samarasinghe et al., 2008), we believe it is prudent to emend the names of *Isospora*-like oocysts, having sporocysts without Stieda bodies, into the genus *Cystoisospora* (Sarcocystidae), as we do here.

There are now about 13 *Isospora*-like "species" described and named from hosts in the Mustelidae (Galli-Valerio, 1932; Hoare, 1927; Levine and Ivens, 1964; Musaev and Veisov, 1983; Nukerbaeva, 1981a,b; Pellérdy, 1974a; Prasad, 1961b; Svanbaev and Rachmatullina, 1971; Svanbaev, 1956) and all of these names are emended here and placed into the *Cystoisospora*.

CYSTOISOSPORA GOTTSCHALKI NOV. COMB., N. SP.

Synonym: *Isospora lutrae* von Cord Gottschalk, 2000.

Type host: *Lutra lutra* (L., 1758), European Otter.

Type locality: Europe: Germany: Ostprignitz, Zippelsförde, Conservation Station of Brandenburg.

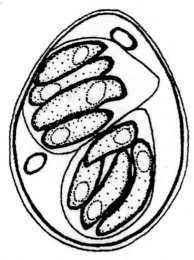

FIGURE 14.14   Line drawing of the sporulated oocyst of *Cystoisospora gottschalki. From von Cord Gottschalk, H., 2000. Eine neue mustelidenkokzidie aus* Lutra lutra *(L.). (A new mustelid coccidia from* Lutra lutra *L.). Der Zoologische Garten 70 (6), 361–368. (In German, English summary). with kind permission of the Copyright Coordinator, Global Rights Department, Elsevier, for* der Zoologische Garten.

Other definitive hosts: None to date.

Known intermediate host: None to date.

Geographic distribution: Europe: Germany.

Description of sporulated oocyst: Oocyst shape: ovoidal, subspheroidal, or spheroidal (although the line drawing shows a distinct ovoidal form); number of walls, 2 (line drawing); wall thickness, 1.5 (1.4–1.8) thick at the apex, 1.8 thick at the midsection, and 2.1 (1.8–3.2) thick at the basal part of the oocyst; wall characteristics: outer layer is smooth, colorless; L×W (n = 106): 32.9 × 26.3 (25–38 × 21–31), L/W ratio: 1.25; M, OR: both absent; PG: present as one or two ellipsoidal bodies. Distinctive features of oocyst: distinctly ovoidal shape with a wall that varies in thickness from the apex to the base of the oocyst, and the presence of two PGs.

Description of sporocyst and sporozoites: Sporocyst shape: ovoidal (line drawing); L×W (n = 106): 18.2 × 14.4 (15–22 × 12–16), L/W ratio: 1.3; SB, SSB, PSB: all absent; SR: present; SR characteristics: a small, compact, spheroidal

mass of granules, but may be absent; SZ: sausage-shaped (line drawing) with one RB at more rounded end. Distinctive features of sporocyst: ovoidal shape with a SR that is present shortly after sporulation is completed but may disappear with time.

Prevalence: "Frosted" feces from 1/1 (100%) "wounded" *L. lutra* was examined and found to be naturally-infected with two oocyst morphotypes representing one isosporan-type oocyst described here and an eimerian oocyst that was not described because it never fully sporulated.

Sporulation: Exogenous; von Cord Gottschalk (2000) said that sporulation begins in about 5 hours and is completed in a few days, presumably after being discharged by the host in its feces (?), but no further details were given (e.g., temperature, incubation solution, etc.).

Prepatent and patent periods: Unknown.

Site of infection: Unknown; oocysts recovered from feces.

Endogenous stages: Unknown.

Cross-transmission: None to date.

Pathology: Unknown. However, von Cord Gottschalk (2000) reported the wounded otter "died from pneumonia and secondary coccidiosis in Brandenburg, Germany."

Materials deposited: None.

Remarks: In early 2000, Torres et al. described and named *I.* (=*C.*) *lutrae* from the European otter, in Spain. Near the end of 2000, von Cord Gottschalk (2000), apparently unaware of the paper by Torres et al. (2000), published a new species description of an *Isospora*-like oocyst, which he also named *I.* (=*C.*) *lutrae*, from *L. lutra* in Germany. Based on the morphology of their sporulated oocysts these two "species" are clearly different so we decided to name this form after the original author. In Chapter 5, we discussed the appropriate placement of *Isospora*-like oocysts, having sporocysts without Stieda bodies, into the Sarcocystidae supported by several phylogenetic analyses, repeated independently, with the same results (Carreno and

Barta, 1999; Franzen et al., 2000; Barta et al., 2005; Samarasinghe et al., 2008) to support our conclusion to transfer and emend *I*. (=*C*.) *lutrae* named by von Cord Gottschalk (2000) to *Cystoisospora gottschalki* after the author who first described it.

SUBFAMILY MUSTELINAE FISCHER, 1817

GENUS *EIRA* C.E.H. SMITH, 1842 (MONOTYPIC)

CYSTOISOSPORA ARCTOPITHECI (RODHAIN, 1933) NOV. COMB.

Synonyms: *Isospora scorzai* Arcay-de-Peraza, 1967; *Isospora arctopitheci* Rodhain, 1933.

Type host: *Callithrix penicillata* (I. Geoffroy, 1812) (syn. *Hapale penicilatus*), Black Tufted-ear Marmoset.

Type locality: Unknown (see *Remarks* in Duszynski, 2016, p. 21).

Other definitive hosts: This is one of the most studied coccidians of nonhuman primates (Lindsay et al., 1997). Hendricks (1974, 1977)

said he found this species in six other nonhuman primate genera and species and also reported it in five carnivore genera/species, as definitive hosts, including: *Canis lupus familiaris* (syn. *C. familiaris*), Domestic Dog (Canidae); *Eira barbara* (L., 1758), Tayra (Mustelidae); *Nasua nasua* (L., 1766), South American Coati, and *Potos flavus* (Schreber, 1774), Kinkajou (both Procyonidae); *Felis catus* L., 1758, Domestic Cat (Felidae).

Known intermediate host: None to date.

Geographic distribution: Cosmopolitan.

Description of sporulated oocyst: Oocyst shape: slightly subspheroidal; number of walls, 2, about 1 thick; wall characteristics: outer layer is smooth, colorless; inner is light yellow-brown; L×W: 27.7×24.3 (23–33×20–27), L/W ratio: 1.1 (1.05–1.3); M, OR, PG: all absent. Distinctive features of oocyst: subspheroidal shape, smooth outer wall that is easily deformed in handling, especially in concentrated sugar solution used for flotation, and without M, OR, and PG.

Description of sporocyst and sporozoites: Sporocyst shape: ellipsoidal; L×W: 17.6×12.5 (13–20×10–16), L/W ratio: 1.4 (1.2–1.6); SB, SSB, PSB: all absent; SR: present; SR characteristics: a compact mass of large globules; SZ: sausage- or

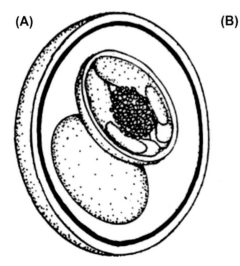 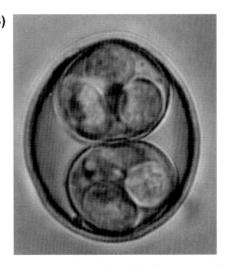

FIGURE 14.15 (A) Line drawing of the sporulated oocyst of *Cystoisospora arctopitheci*. (B). Photomicrograph of a sporulated oocyst of *C. arctopitheci*. Both figures originals.

banana-shaped with one end rounded and containing a distinct RB. Distinctive features of sporocyst: voluminous SR, ~10.2×6.9, composed of spheroidal, coarse granules in the middle of the SP.

Prevalence: 1/1 (100%) in the type host and from 50% to 100% in other naturally-infected hosts. As per Hendricks (1977), the following carnivore species were found to be susceptible to experimental infection via oocysts recovered from the feces of an infected marmoset, *S. geoffroyi*: 2/2 (100%) *C. familiaris*, 1/1 (100%) *E. barbara*, 3/4 (75%) *F. catus*, 2/2 (100%) *N. nasua*, and 2/2 (100%) *P. flavus*.

Sporulation: Exogenous. Oocysts sporulated in 2 days at room temperature (? °C) in 1% chromic acid in Belgium; 4 days in 2.5% aqueous potassium dichromate ($K_2Cr_2O_7$) at 24°C in Panamá.

Prepatent and patent periods: Prepatent period 5–6 days and the patent period is 3–55 days in experimentally-infected primates (Hendricks, 1977).

Site of infection: Epithelial cells of the small intestinal villi, principally the jejunum; no parasites were found in any EIN tissue (Olcott et al., 1982).

Endogenous stages: Hendricks and Walton (1974) said they transmitted this species from *C. capucinus* to *S. geoffroyi* and Olcott et al. (1982) described the endogenous stages in *S. geoffroyi*. They found developmental stages 1–7 DPI and said that asexual development was principally by several cycles of endodyogeny that resulted in ~16 merozoites within one PV. Gamogony occurred 5–7 DPI. Oocysts were present only as early as the 7 DPI, when sloughing of the epithelium began to occur.

Cross-transmission: Hendricks (1974) reported that he successfully transmitted this species, via oocysts, and achieved patent infections in six genera of New World primates and five genera of carnivores (see *Prevalence*, above).

Pathology: Intestinal pathology leading to death was recorded in 4/13 (31%) marmosets (Olcott et al., 1982) that had been experimentally-infected with *C. arctopitheci*, but there is no report to date about any pathology caused in infected carnivores.

Materials deposited: A photoneotype of a sporulated oocyst is in the US National Parasite Collection as USNPC No. 87407.

Remarks: The unusually large and diverse range of reported definitive hosts for *I. (=C.) arctopitheci* seems atypical and suggests to us that further experimental studies are needed to verify or reject these initial findings.

GENUS ICTONYX KAUP, 1835 (2 SPECIES)

CYSTOISOSPORA AFRICANA (PRASAD, 1961b) NOV. COMB.

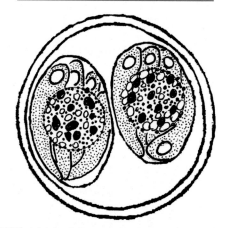

FIGURE 14.16   Original line drawing of the sporulated oocyst of *Cystoisospora africana*. *Modified Fig. 22, Levine, N.D., Ivens, V., 1981. The Coccidian Parasites (Protozoa, Apicomplexa) of Carnivores. Illinois Biological Monograph No. 51, The University of Illinois Press, Urbana, Illinois USA. The University of Illinois Press has released the copyright.*

Synonym: *Isospora africana* Prasad, 1961b.
Type host: *Ictonyx (Poecilictis) libyca* (Hemprich and Ehrenberg, 1833), Saharan Striped Polecat.
Type locality: Africa: Egypt.
Other definitive hosts: None to date.
Known intermediate host: None to date.

Geographic distribution: Africa: Egypt.

Description of sporulated oocyst: Oocyst shape: spheroidal; number of walls, 2; wall characteristics: smooth, pale yellow, membranous, uniform in total thickness; L×W: 26 (25.5–27), L/W ratio: 1.0; M, OR, PG: all absent. Distinctive features of oocyst: perfect spheroidal shape with smooth, two-layered wall and without M, OR, and PG.

Description of sporocyst and sporozoites: Sporocyst shape: ovoidal; L×W: 15–16.5×10–12 (mean not given); L/W ratio: ~1.4 (extrapolated from ranges); SB, SSB, PSB: all absent; SR: present; SR characteristics: described only as "prominent;" SZ: 13.5×3.0, club-shaped, with a prominent RB at the slightly rounded end. Distinctive features of sporocyst: without SB, SSB, PSB.

Prevalence: Prasad (1961b) found this form in 1/3 (33%) fecal samples from the type host.

Sporulation: The process of sporulation was completed in 36 hours at 23°C.

Prepatent and patent periods: Unknown.

Site of infection: Unknown.

Endogenous stages: Unknown.

Cross-transmission: Prasad (1961b) attempted to infect one kitten with a mixture of sporulated oocysts that contained three morphotypes of isosporan-like oocysts that he isolated from *I. libyca*. Fecal samples from that cat were examined "for a fortnight" (2 weeks), but no oocysts that conformed to this form (species?) were ever detected.

Pathology: Although Prasad (1961b) said the infection in the only positive polecat "was fairly heavy," no signs of distress were observed in that animal.

Materials deposited: None.

Remarks: The fecal samples examined by Prasad (1961b) were collected from the type host trapped in Africa (Egypt) and brought to the London School of Hygiene and Tropical Medicine by Dr. Harry Hoogstraal. They were kept in 2.5% aqueous potassium dichromate ($K_2Cr_2O_7$) to allow for sporulation. The sporulated oocyst of this species differed from those of *I*. (=C.) *hoogstraali*, also from *I. libyca* (Prasad,

1961b), by lacking a visible M and a PG. Oocyst of this form resemble those of *C*. (*I*.) *vulpina* described from the fox (Nieschulz and Bos, 1933), but oocysts of the latter are broadly ellipsoidal, 21–32×19–24, whereas oocysts of this species are strictly spheroidal measuring 25.5 wide.

CYSTOISOSPORA HOOGSTRAALI (PRASAD, 1961b) NOV. COMB.

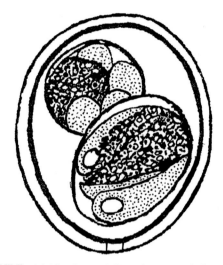

FIGURE 14.17 Original line drawing of the sporulated oocyst of *Cystoisospora hoogstraali*. Modified Fig. 42, Levine, N.D., Ivens, V., 1981. The Coccidian Parasites (Protozoa, Apicomplexa) of Carnivores. Illinois Biological Monograph No. 51, The University of Illinois Press, Urbana, Illinois USA. The University of Illinois Press has released the copyright.

Synonym: *Isospora hoogstraali* Prasad, 1961b.

Type host: *Ictonyx* (*Poecilictis*) *libyca alexandrae*, Saharan Striped Polecat.

Type locality: Africa: Egypt.

Other definitive hosts: None to date.

Known intermediate host: None to date.

Geographic distribution: Africa: Egypt.

Description of sporulated oocyst: Oocyst shape: mostly ellipsoidal; number of walls, 2; wall characteristics: outer is smooth, colorless, whereas inner is thinner, with a button-like M; L×W: 38×33 (37–41×32–34), L/W ratio: 1.2; M; present as a button-like structure between the two layers of the oocyst wall; OR; absent; PG: present in some oocysts. Distinctive features of oocyst: ellipsoidal shape and a smooth, transparent two-layered wall with a button-like M between the layers (shown as 2 parallel lines in his drawing).

Description of sporocyst and sporozoites: Sporocyst shape: ovoidal; L×W: 19–21 × 13–15, L/W ratio: 1.4; SB, SSB, PSB: all absent; SR: present; SR characteristics: a compact mass composed of small granules that occupies about one-half of the sporocyst (line drawing); SZ: club-shaped, 18–19 × 4.5–6, with one large, clear RB at the rounded end. Distinctive features of sporocyst: relatively large size, without SB, SSB, PSB, but with a large, compact SR, and club-shaped SZ.

Prevalence: Prasad (1961b) found this species in 1/3 (33%) fecal samples from the type host. This was the same host in which he also found *I. (=C.) africana*.

Sporulation: The process of sporulation was completed in 24 hours at 23°C.

Prepatent and patent periods: Unknown.

Site of infection: Unknown.

Endogenous stages: Unknown.

Cross-transmission: Prasad (1961b) attempted to infect one kitten with a mixture of sporulated oocysts that contained three morphotypes of isosporan-like oocysts that he isolated from *I. libyca*. Fecal samples from that cat were examined "for a fortnight" (2 weeks), and he claimed that oocysts of this morphotype were observed on the 9th and 10th days PI but not subsequently and that "this experiment was repeated after a fortnight on the same kitten with similar results."

Pathology: Although Prasad (1961b) said the infection in the only positive polecat "was fairly heavy," no signs of distress were observed in that animal.

Materials deposited: None.

Remarks: Prasad (1961b) said that the sporulated oocysts of *I. (=C.) hoogstraali* differed from those of *I. (=C.) laidlawi* recovered from *Mustela*

putorius L., 1758 (Hoare, 1927), the European polecat, in shape and size, and by possessing a visible M and PG, and from those of *I. (=C.) africana* and *I. (=C.) zorillae*, both also from *I. (P.) libyca alexandrae*, the Saharan striped polecat, by the same features.

CYSTOISOSPORA ZORILLAE (PRASAD, 1961b, EMEND. PELLÉRDY, 1963) NOV. COMB.

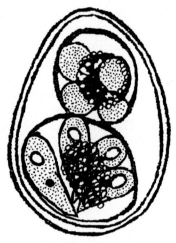

FIGURE 14.18 Original line drawing of the sporulated oocyst of *Cystoisospora zorillae*. *Modified Fig. 40, Levine, N.D., Ivens, V., 1981. The Coccidian Parasites (Protozoa, Apicomplexa) of Carnivores. Illinois Biological Monograph No. 51, The University of Illinois Press, Urbana, Illinois USA. The University of Illinois Press has released the copyright.*

Synonyms: *Isospora bigemina* var. *zorillae* Prasad, 1961b; *Isospora zorillae* (Prasad, 1961b) emend. Pellérdy, 1963.

Type host: *Ictonyx (Poecilictis) libyca alexandrae*, Saharan Striped Polecat.

Type locality: Africa: Egypt.

Other definitive hosts: None to date.

Known intermediate host: None to date.

Geographic distribution: Africa: Egypt.

Description of sporulated oocyst: Oocyst shape: mostly ovoidal; number of walls, 1; wall characteristics: very thin; L×W (n=50): 12×10

(10–14 × 8–12), L/W ratio: 1.2; M, OR, PG: all absent. Distinctive features of oocyst: very small size with a single, smooth, transparent outer wall.

Description of sporocyst and sporozoites: Sporocyst shape: ovoidal; L × W: 6–8 × 5, L/W ratio: 1.4; SB, SSB, PSB: all absent; SR: present; SR characteristics: a prominent, compact, ovoidal mass composed of small granules (line drawing); SZ: sickle-shaped, with one end broadly rounded and the other ending in a blunt point, ~6 × 3, with clear RB at the more rounded end. Distinctive features of sporocyst: very small size, without SB, SSB, PSB, but with a large, compact SR, and sickle-shaped SZ.

Prevalence: Prasad (1961b) found this species in 1/3 (33%) fecal samples from the type host. This was the same host in which he also found *I.* (=C.) *africana* and *I.* (=C.) *hoogstraali*.

Sporulation: The process of sporulation was completed in >2 days at 23°C.

Prepatent and patent periods: Unknown.

Site of infection: Unknown.

Endogenous stages: Unknown.

Cross-transmission: Prasad (1961b) attempted to infect one kitten with a mixture of sporulated oocysts that contained three morphotypes of isosporan-like oocysts that he isolated from *I. libyca*. Fecal samples from that cat were examined "for a fortnight" (2 weeks), but no oocysts that conformed to this form (species?) were ever detected.

Pathology: Although Prasad (1961b) said the infection in the only positive polecat "was fairly heavy," no signs of distress were observed in that animal.

Materials deposited: None.

Remarks: The measurements of sporulated oocysts of this species agree with those of the small form/race of what was formerly *I. bigemina*, but because Prasad (1961b) was unable to transmit sporulated oocysts of this form to one kitten, he decided to call it a variety of *I. bigemina*, a designation with which we disagree. It is now known that the small race of *I. bigemina* in

dogs is *Hammondia heydorni* (see Lindsay et al., 1997). However, some colleagues think this may be a *Sarcocystis* species (Upton, unpublished).

GENUS MARTES PINEL, 1792 (8 SPECIES)

CYSTOISOSPORA MARTESSII (NUKERBAEVA, 1981a) NOV. COMB.

To view a photomicrograph of a sporulated oocyst, see Fig. 1d in Nukerbaeva (1981a).

Synonym: *Isospora martessii* Nukerbaeva, 1981a.

Type host: *Martes zibellina* (L., 1758), Sable.

Type locality: Asia: Siberia (former USSR).

Other definitive hosts: None to date.

Known intermediate host: None to date.

Geographic distribution: Asia: Siberia (former USSR).

Description of sporulated oocyst: Oocyst shape: spheroidal to short-ovoidal to distinctly ovoidal; number of walls, 2; wall characteristics: smooth outer surface, ~1.5 thick; L × W (ovoidal forms): 25.2–28.0 × 16.8–22.4, (short-ovoidal forms): 19.6 × 16.8, (spheroidal forms): 16.8; L/W ratio: 1.0–1.2; M, OR, PG (?): all absent. Distinctive features of oocyst: variation in shape from spheroidal to short-ovoidal to distinctly ovoidal.

Description of sporocyst and sporozoites: Sporocyst shape: ovoidal; L × W: 11.2–16.8 × 8.4–11.2 (means not given); L/W ratio: unknown; SB, SSB, PSB: presumably all absent, although not specifically stated; SR: present; SR characteristics: composed of coarse granules; SZ: described only as "elongated;" neither RB nor N were mentioned. Distinctive features of sporocyst: without SB, SSB, PSB, but with a SR of coarse granules.

Prevalence: Nukerbaeva (1981a) found 24/320 (7.5%) sables in the Altai region of Siberia infected with from one to three coccidian species but neglected to mention which of the 24 sables was infected with which species. She did say, however, "infection was higher in summer (15.1%) compared to spring (4.7%)."

Sporulation: Presumably exogenous; Nukerbaeva (1981a) said sporulation time was 48–72 hours after she placed oocysts in 2% potassium dichromate ($K_2Cr_2O_7$) solution.

Prepatent and patent periods: Unknown.

Site of infection in definitive host: Nukerbaeva (1981a) said it was located in the "gut."

Endogenous stages: Unknown.

Cross-transmission: Nukerbaeva (1981a) used a mixture of $5–7 \times 10^3$ oocysts of *I. (=C.) martessii* from a sable and was able to infect another sable in which oocysts were discharged 7 DPI. She also infected two minks (presumably, *Neovison vison*, but this was not stated) with oocysts of *I. (=C.) martessii*, but they did not discharge oocysts. However, she did not state how long PI she continued to examine the animals for oocysts in their feces.

Pathology: Unknown.

Materials deposited: None.

Remarks: The description of this "species" provided by Nukerbaeva (1981a) was marginal, indeed, even when the most lenient descriptive criteria are applied. The only reason we include it here is that she provided a photomicrograph, which we are unable to reproduce here because of its poor quality, but which we think represents what we consider a "typical" cystoisosporoid-type oocyst from a carnivore. This species has not been seen since its original publication (Nukerbaeva, 1981a).

GENUS *MELES* BRISSON, 1762 (3 SPECIES)

CYSTOISOSPORA MELIS (PELLÉRDY, 1955) NOV. COMB.

Synonyms: *Lucetina* sp. Kotlán and Pospesch, 1933; *Isospora melis* (Kotlán and Pospesch, 1933) Pellérdy, 1955 of Pellérdy (1965).

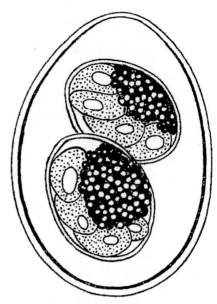

FIGURE 14.19 Original line drawing of the sporulated oocyst of *Cystoisospora melis*. Modified Fig. 72, Levine, N.D., Ivens, V., 1981. The Coccidian Parasites (Protozoa, Apicomplexa) of Carnivores. Illinois Biological Monograph No. 51, The University of Illinois Press, Urbana, Illinois USA. The University of Illinois Press has released the copyright.

Type host: *Meles meles* (L., 1758) (syn. *Meles taxus* Boddaert, 1785), European Badger.

Type locality: Eastern Europe: Hungary, Budapest Zoological Gardens.

Other definitive hosts: None to date.

Known intermediate host: None to date.

Geographic distribution: Eastern Europe: Hungary.

Description of sporulated oocyst: Oocyst shape: mostly ovoidal, but some are asymmetrical; number of walls, 2; wall characteristics: smooth, ~1.8 thick; L×W (n=12): 26–34×20–27, means not given, L/W ratio: unknown (Kotlán and Pospesch, 1933), or 27–31×18–24, means not given, L/W ratio: unknown (Pellérdy, 1955), or L×W (n=50): 32.8×26.9 (26–38×24–30), L/W ratio: 1.2 (1.1–1.6) (Anwar et al., 2000); M, OR, PG: all absent. Distinctive features of oocyst: typical ovoidal shape for *Cystoisospora* species and lacking M, OR, and PG.

Description of sporocyst and sporozoites: Sporocyst shape: fusiform or ellipsoidal; L×W: 14–16×12 (means not given), L/W ratio: unknown (Kotlán and Pospesch, 1933), or 21.5×14.0 (19–24×12–17), L/W ratio: 1.6 (1.3–1.9) (Anwar et al., 2000); SB, SSB, PSB: all absent; SR: present; SR characteristics: a prominent mass composed of many granules (line drawing); SZ: 14.2×4.0 (10–20×3–5) with one tapering end and one rounded end with a RB. Distinctive features of sporocyst: without SB, SSB, PSB, and with an SR, a "typical" *Cystoisospora* sporocyst.

Prevalence: Present in 3/4 (75%) badgers examined by Kotlán and Pospesch (1933); these included three badgers that had died at the Zoological Gardens, Budapest (two of which were infected with this species) and one wild-caught badger. Anwar et al. (2000) examined badgers from Wytham Woods, Oxfordshire, United Kingdom and found 91/259 (35%) to be infected with this species and 51/91 (56%) also were concurrently infected with *Eimeria melis*. Anwar et al. (2000) said there was no significant interaction between age and sex for either *C. melis* or *E. melis* infection; that is, there was no detectable difference in the prevalence rate between males and females as adults and cubs.

Sporulation: Exogenous, 2–3 days in 2% potassium dichromate ($K_2Cr_2O_7$) solution (Kotlán and Pospesch, 1933; Pellérdy, 1955, 1965), or 72 hours at $25\pm2°C$ when placed in Petri dishes containing a thin layer of 2.5% $K_2Cr_2O_7$ solution (Anwar et al., 2000).

Prepatent and patent periods: Prepatent period is 5 days (Kotlán and Pospesch, 1933) or 7–8 days (Pellérdy, 1965).

Site of infection in definitive host: Unknown.

Endogenous stages: Unknown.

Cross-transmission: Kotlán and Pospesch (1933) could not transmit this species to the domestic cat. Kotlán and Pospesch (1933) and Pellérdy (1965) said that their lack of ability to infect cats provided evidence that *I.* (=*C.*) *melis* is neither *I.* (=*C.*) *felis* nor *I.* (=*C.*) *rivolta* from the cat, and that it is different from *I.* (=*C.*) *canivelocis*

"from the fox because all attempts to transmit oocysts derived from the cat and the fox to the badger, or from the badger to the cat and the fox have definitely failed."

Pathology: Unknown.

Materials deposited: None.

Remarks: Pellérdy (1959) agreed with Bray (1954) that from the descriptions available, the oocysts of *I.* (=*C.*) *garnhami* cannot be differentiated from those of *I.* (=*C.*) *melis*, but he concluded, "the coccidium in the badger should be referred to as *I. melis* (Kotlán and Pospesch, 1933) Pellérdy, 1955, and the coccidium in the mongoose as *I. garnhami* Bray, 1954," based on cross-infection work cited earlier in his paper (also see *Remarks* under *C. garnhami*, below). Glebezdin (1978) surveyed 2,350 wild mammals representing 25 species in southwestern Turkmenistan, from 1974 to 1977; in *M. meles* he found oocysts of *I.* (=*C.*) *melis* that measured L×W: 31.3×21.8 (29–34×20–25), L/W ratio: 1.4 (1.3–1.5), and sporocysts were L×W: 15.4×12.2 (14.5–17×11–14), L/W ratio: 1.3. In their epidemiological study of coccidia in European badgers of the United Kingdom, Anwar et al. (2000) said there was no evidence that either the prevalence or the risk of infection with *I.* (=*C.*) *melis* was different in males and females, either as cubs or adults. From this they inferred that both exposure and susceptibility to infection are constant between the sexes. In addition, the intensity of infection with *I.* (=*C.*) *melis* (measured as oocysts/g feces) did not vary by age, sex, or interaction with *E. melis* when both co-occurred. As we noted earlier, there is evidence that some of the *Cystoisospora* are facultatively heteroxenous. Although badgers are mustelid carnivores, their dietary habits show them to be generalist or opportunist feeders. According to Kruuk (1978), in Wytham and through much of the United Kingdom they feed predominantly on earthworms (*Lumbricus terrestris*), supplemented by other invertebrates, with rodents only rarely eaten. Because 35% of the badgers studied in Wytham harbored *I.* (=*C.*) *melis*, it seemed unlikely by Anwar et al. (2000)

that their source of infection was vertebrate prey and/or that earthworms are transmitting the parasite to badgers.

GENUS *MUSTELA* L., 1758 (17 SPECIES)

CYSTOISOSPORA ALTAICA (SVANBAEV AND RACHMATULLINA, 1971) NOV. COMB.

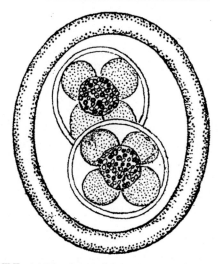

FIGURE 14.20 Original line drawing of the sporulated oocyst of *Cystoisospora altaica*. A rendition of Figure 'a,' *Svanbaev, S.K., Rachmatullina, N.K., 1971. The question on coccidia from fur-bearing animals in Kazachstan. Akademia Nauk Kazakhskoi SSR, Trudy Instituta Zoologii 31, 165–170. (In Russian).*

Synonym: *Isospora altaica* Svanbaev and Rachmatullina, 1971.

Type host: *Mustela altaica* Pallas, 1811, Mountain Weasel.

Type locality: Asia: Kazakhstan (former USSR), Almaty (former Alma-Ata) Region.

Other definitive hosts: None to date.

Known intermediate host: None to date.

Geographic distribution: Asia: Kazakhstan (former USSR).

Description of sporulated oocyst: Oocyst shape: spheroidal to ovoidal; number of walls, 2; wall characteristics: smooth outer surface, ~3–4 in total thickness; L × W (ovoidal forms): 33.3 × 27.7 (28–34 × 25–28), L/W ratio: 1.2 (1.1–1.2), whereas spheroidal forms were 27.7 wide, L/W ratio: 1.0; M, OR, PG: all absent. Distinctive features of oocyst: thick outer wall, lacking M, OR, PG.

Description of sporocyst and sporozoites: Sporocyst shape: spheroidal to slightly ovoidal; L × W: 11–17 × 14–17 (means not given), L/W ratio: unknown; spheroidal forms were 11.1 wide; L/W ratio 1.0; SB, SSB, PSB: all absent; SR: present; SR characteristics: a prominent, spheroidal mass composed of small granules that appeared to be membrane-bounded (line drawing); SZ: described as spheroidal, ~5.6 wide; neither RB nor N were visible in the SZ. Distinctive features of sporocyst: without SB, SSB, PSB, but with a spheroidal SR that may be membrane-bounded.

Prevalence: Svanbaev and Rachmatullina (1971) found this species in 2/56 (3%) of the type host.

Sporulation: Presumably exogenous.

Prepatent and patent periods: Unknown.

Site of infection in definitive host: Unknown, although Svanbaev and Rachmatullina (1971) said it was located in the gut.

Endogenous stages: Unknown.

Cross-transmission: None to date.

Pathology: Unknown.

Materials deposited: None.

Remarks: Svanbaev and Rachmatullina (1971) said the sporulated oocysts of this species were morphologically most similar to those of *I.* (=*C.*) *pavlovskyi*, which Svanbaev had described in 1956, from the steppe polecat (*M. eversmanii*) in Kazakhstan, and which Yi-Fan et al. (2012) also found in polecats in China. Oocysts of *C. altaica* are smaller than those of *C. pavlovskyi* (33 × 28 vs. 38.5 × 30), have a much thicker wall (3–4 vs. 1.6–1.8) and their sporocysts also are much smaller (11–17 × 14–17 vs. 19 × 16). These differences allowed Svanbaev and Rachmatullina (1971) to conclude with confidence that the two forms were separate species.

CYSTOISOSPORA EVERSMANNI (SVANBAEV, 1956) EMEND. YI-FAN, LE, YIN, JIANG-HUI, AND DUSZYNSKI, 2012

Synonym: *Isospora eversmanni* Svanbaev, 1956.

Type host: *Mustela eversmanii* Lesson, 1827, Steppe Polecat.

Type locality: Asia: Kazakhstan (former USSR).

Other definitive host: *Mustela putorius* L., 1758, European Polecat (syn. *Mustela vison* de Sélys Longchamps, 1839).

Known intermediate host: None to date.

Geographic distribution: Asia: China, Kazakhstan (former USSR); Europe: Austria (?).

Description of sporulated oocyst: Oocyst shape: spheroidal to slightly ellipsoidal; number of walls, 2; wall characteristics: ~1–1.4 thick; L×W: 20.3 (range not given), L/W ratio: 1.0 (Svanbaev, 1956), or L×W: 16.8–22.4, L/W ratio: 1.0 (Nukerbaeva and Svanbaev, 1973), or L×W (n=50): 18.5×14.8 (16–20×12–16), L/W ratio: 1.3 (1.1–1.6) (Yi-Fan et al., 2012); M, OR, PG: all absent. Distinctive features of oocyst: none, a typical *Cystoisospora* oocyst.

Description of sporocyst and sporozoites: Sporocyst shape: subspheroidal to slightly ellipsoidal; L×W: 11.5×9.8 (10–13.5×9–11), L/W ratio: 1.2 (1.1–1.5); SB, SSB, PSB: all absent; SR: present; SR characteristics: a prominent, compact, ovoidal mass composed of small granules occupying ~1/3 of SP; SZ: sausage-shaped, with both ends broadly rounded, ~5.2×3.3; neither RB nor N were visible in the SZ. Distinctive features of sporocyst: small size, without SB, SSB, PSB, but with a large, compact SR, and sausage-shaped SZ.

Prevalence: Nukerbaeva and Svanbaev (1973, 1977) found this species in 2/1,017 (0.2%) minks

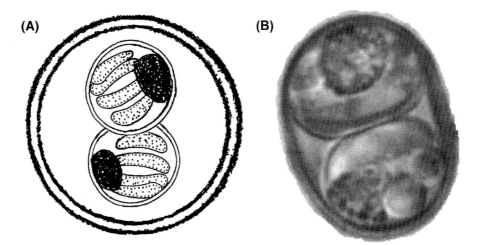

FIGURE 14.21   (A). Original line drawing of the sporulated oocyst of *Cystoisospora eversmanni*, (B). Original photomicrograph of a sporulated oocyst of *C. eversmanni*. *(A) Modified Fig. 82, Levine, N.D., Ivens, V., 1981. The Coccidian Parasites (Protozoa, Apicomplexa) of Carnivores. Illinois Biological Monograph No. 51, The University of Illinois Press, Urbana, Illinois USA. The University of Illinois Press has released the copyright. (B) From Yi-Fan, C., Le, Y., Yin, D., Jiang-Hui, B., Duszynski, D.W., 2012. Emendation of 2* Isospora *species (Apicomplexa: Eimeriidae) infecting the steppe polecat,* Mustela eversmanii *Lesson, 1827, in China, to the genus* Cystoisospora *(Apicomplexa: Sarcocystidae). Comparative Parasitology 79, 147–152, with permission from the authors and the Editor and copyright holder of* Comparative Parasitology.

in Kazakhstan, Frank (1978) said she found it in 5 *M. eversmanii* from "Illmitz in the European Soviet Union (probably Austria)," and Yi-Fan et al. (2012) found it in of 3/6 (50%) polecats in China.

Sporulation: Exogenous. Oocysts sporulated in 43–45 hours at 20–25°C in 2.5% aqueous $K_2Cr_2O_7$ (Svanbaev, 1956).

Prepatent and patent periods: Unknown.

Site of infection in definitive host: Unknown.

Endogenous stages: Unknown.

Cross-transmission: None to date.

Pathology: Unknown.

Materials deposited: Phototypes in the USNPC in Beltsville, Maryland, USA: USNPC No. 104109; symbiotype host specimen (see Frey et al., 1992) of *M. eversmanii* in the Qinghai–Tibet Plateau Biological Specimen Museum (QPBSM No. 6905; collected by Y. F. Cao, L. Yang, and G. S. Wu, 18 August 2010).

Remarks: Svanbaev (1956) originally described oocysts of *I. eversmanni* from a polecat in Kazakhstan (former USSR), but they were poorly characterized in his description and little additional structural data were provided when he and Nukerbaeva later reported these oocysts from *M. putoris* (Nukerbaeva and Svanbaev, 1973, 1977). Nukerbaeva and Svanbaev (1973) said that the SP were pear-shaped or ovoidal, 11.2×8.4, with seed-shaped SZ and that neither OR nor SR were present. Frank (1978) said she found this species in *M. eversmanii* trapped near Lake Neusiedl, Austria, on the border with Hungary, but gave no morphological or prevalence data. Oocysts of this species were not seen again until Yi-Fan et al. (2012) more completely described the structural features of both the oocyst and its sporocysts from *M. eversmanii* in Qinghai Province, China. Most of the measurements of oocysts and sporocysts, above, are from the work of Yi-Fan et al. (2012). Oocysts from Svanbaev's (1956) original description were reported as spheroidal, ~20 wide, with a wall ~1 thick, and Nukerbaeva and Svanbaev (1973) said spheroidal oocysts were 17–22 wide

with a two-layered wall, ~1.4 thick, and sporocysts, 11×8. Yi-Fan et al. (2012) recommended that all of the coccidia with non-Stieda body isosporan-like oocysts with thick walls that have been described from carnivores should be reexamined and their names should be emended into the genus *Cystoisospora*, as we are doing in this book.

CYSTOISOSPORA LAIDLAWI (HOARE, 1927) NOV. COMB.

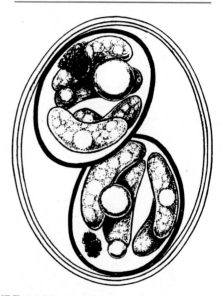

FIGURE 14.22 Line drawing of the sporulated oocyst of *Cystoisospora laidlawi*. *Figure 5, from Levine, N.D., 1948. Eimeria and Isospora of the mink* (Mustela vison). *Journal of Parasitology 34 (6), 486–492, with permission of Allen Press, Inc., Lawrence, Kansas USA, copyright holder.*

Synonym: *Isospora laidlawi* Hoare, 1927.

Type host: *Mustela* (syn. *Putorius*) *putorius furo* (L., 1758), European Polecat (Domestic Ferret).

Type locality: Europe: England: London.

Other definitive hosts: *Neovison vison* (Schreber, 1777), American mink; *Vulpes vulpes* (L., 1758) (syn. *Vulpes fulvus* (Desmarest, 1820)), Red or Silver Fox.

Known intermediate host: None to date.

Geographic distribution: Eurasia: Turkey; Europe: England, Iceland; Asia: Kazakhstan (former USSR); North America: Illinois, Wisconsin.

Description of sporulated oocyst: Oocyst shape: mostly ovoidal; number of walls, 2; wall characteristics: a thick, yellowish inner layer, and a thin colorless outer layer; L×W: 34×28 (31–37×25–31), L/W ratio: 1.2; M, OR, PG: all absent. Distinctive features of oocyst: none, this oocyst has a "typical" *Cystoisospora*-like oocyst.

Description of sporocyst and sporozoites: Sporocyst shape: ellipsoidal; L×W: 20.8×14.4 (ranges not given), L/W ratio: 1.4; SB, SSB, PSB: all absent; SR: present; SR characteristics: a bulky mass of coarse granules that sometimes occupies >50% of the SP volume (line drawing); SZ: sausage-shaped, with one end broadly rounded and the other ending in a slight point, with clear RB at the more pointed end, and the N is centrally-located. Distinctive features of sporocyst: typical *Cystoisospora*-like SP, without SB, SSB, PSB, but with a large, compact SR.

Prevalence: Hoare (1927) found this species in 2/3 (67%) fecal samples from the type host. McTaggart (1960) found this species in 5/200 (2.5%) minks, from 42 farms in Britain. Klopfer and Neuman (1970) examined 92 mink fecal samples from nine farms in various parts of Israel and found 67/92 (73%) to be infected with oocysts of three coccidia species, which they identified as *E. vison*, *E. melis* (?), and *I.* (=*C.*) *laidlawi*; they were not precise in how many infected minks shed oocysts of each of these three species stating, "In cases observed by us there was usually a mixed infestation of the two *Eimeria* species and of *Isospora*." Foreyt and Todd (1976) collected 323 fecal samples on 29 mink ranches (22 counties) in Wisconsin, USA, from June to December, 1975. They found that 45/79 (57%) mink samples collected from ranches that fed dry pelleted rations contained coccidian oocysts, whereas 128/244 (52%) samples from ranches that fed a wet meat mixture contained oocysts. This species, which they called *I. laidlawi*, was identified in mink on 26/29 (90%) of the ranches,

but the number of animals with this species was not mentioned; only that "the coccidia of domestic mink in Wisconsin are prevalent and widespread." Nukerbaeva and Svanbaev (1973, 1977) found it in 20/1,017 (2%) minks in Kazakhstan. In a separate study reported for the first time in their 1977 paper, Nukerbaeva and Svanbaev looked at 408 minks in Alakulsk (Taldi-Kurgansk region), Imantavsk (Koktschetavsk region), and Zyrianovsk (Vostochno-Kazakhstansk region) during July and August, 1971, and reported *I.* (=*C.*) *laidlawi* to be the most prevalent coccidian with an overall prevalence of 4%. Tinar (1985) examined mixed samples from two mink farms near Ankara, Turkey for coccidia; of these, 150 were fecal pellets (presumably from different animals?) and the intestinal tracts from 31 animals. He found this species in 36/181 (20%) samples. SkírNisson and Pálmadóttir (1993) reported oocysts of this species in 28/145 (19%) mink pups at 13/19 (68%) fur farms in Iceland. Hindsbo et al. (1995) studied mink kits and adults from 1986 to 1993, on the island Zealander, Denmark, and reported *I.* (=*C.*) *laidlawi* in both. Specifically, they examined 139 cages, each with an adult mink; the mean prevalence of infection with *I.* (=*C.*) *laidlawi* in the adults was 24% and infection was significantly lower in adults than in kits. This allowed them to conclude there was a strong age-dependent resistance to this species in mink.

Sporulation: The process of sporulation was completed in 4 days at room temperature while in 0.5% chromic acid (Hoare, 1927), or in 3 days at room temperature (McTaggart, 1960), or in 2 days (Nukerbaeva and Svanbaev, 1973).

Prepatent and patent periods: Nukerbaeva and Svanbaev (1977) said they infected one 5-month-old mink with oocysts from another mink and the prepatent periods was 8 DPI. Nukerbaeva (1981b) later said that oocysts were discharged in the feces on 7 DPI.

Site of infection: According to McTaggart (1960) infections were confined to the posterior three-fifths of the intestine.

Endogenous stages: Unknown.

Cross-transmission: Nukerbaeva and Svanbaev (1974, 1977) added some confusion to the cross-transmission work they did with *Eimeria* and *Isospora* (=*Cystoisospora*) species from minks, foxes, cats, and dogs. Their 1977 cross-transmission paper was a duplicate of their 1974 paper, except for the tables that summarized their experiments. In their 1974 paper, their table (page 37) said they infected a 5-month-old mink (No. 8) with oocysts of *I.* (=*C.*) *laidlawi* from a mink and it discharged oocysts on the 8th DPI. However, in their 1977 paper, Table 12 (page 79) added a typographical error that the oocysts of *I.* (=*C.*) *laidlawi* from a mink infected a 5-month-old fox, *V. vulpes*, which began discharging oocysts on the 8th DPI. This was clearly incorrect. Nukerbaeva and Svanbaev (1974, 1977) were unable to transmit this species from mink to two 5-month-old red foxes, *V. vulpes* (foxes 6, 7), or to two 5-month-old Arctic foxes, *V. lagopus* (foxes 19, 20), or to one domestic dog, *C. lupus familiaris*. Nukerbaeva (1981a) used $5-7 \times 10^3$ oocysts of *I.* (=*C.*) *laidlawi* from mink (presumably, *N. vison*, but this was not stated) and fed them to two sables, *M. zibellina*, but did not produce an infection. However, it was not stated how many DPI she continued to examine the animals for oocysts in their feces. She also infected one mink with oocysts of *I.* (=*C.*) *laidlawi* from another mink and found oocysts discharged in the feces on 7 DPI.

Pathology: During their dissection of minks, Bell and Trelkeld (1948) said they found severe enteritis that they attributed to *I.* (=*C.*) *laidlawi*. Head (1959) examined 896 mink carcasses in Edinburgh, England, from 1949 to 1959, and found that coccidiosis caused the death of only one animal. McTaggart (1960) examined 200 minks from the same sample as did Head (1959), looking specifically for coccidia; he found this species in 5/200 (2.5%) minks from 42 farms in Britain. A few of the five infected animals had "very many" oocysts in the intestinal tract, and he said they were associated with "macroscopic lesions in the intestine." Nonetheless, the implication is that this species is not pathogenic in mink, even under conditions of severe husbandry that can occur on fur farms.

Materials deposited: None.

Remarks: The sporulated oocysts of this species somewhat resemble those described as *I. canivelocis* (*Coccidium bigeminum* var. *canivelocis*) by Weidman (1915) from the American fox, *V. velox*, in which oocysts were L×W: 25–40×25–30. However, in the fox parasite, the SR is tiny, and the SZs have an irregular arrangement within the sporocyst. Levine (1948) described similar oocysts from the mink as ellipsoidal, L×W (n=5): 34.0×26.5 (32–36×26–27), L/W ratio: 1.3, with a two-layered wall, the outer colorless and the inner yellow, and without M, OR, and PG; Levine's (1948) ellipsoidal sporocysts lacked SB, SSB, PSB, but had a small SR and SZ were sausage-shaped. McTaggart (1960) described oocysts from mink as mostly ovoidal, sometimes ellipsoidal, and occasionally subspheroidal, L×W (n=100): 35×29 (30–38.5×25–34), L/W ratio: 1.2 (1.0–1.5), with a two-layered wall, outer being colorless and inner being slightly yellow, and without M, OR, and PG; these sporocysts were L×W: 23×17 (19–27.5×14–20), L/W ratio: 1.35, with a SR. McTaggart (1960) mentioned that on one occasion an oocyst was observed that contained only one large sporocyst with four SZ and measured L×W: 35.2×27.7, with a sporocyst L×W: 28.6×19.8, and SZ were 19.8×5.5, with a SR 16.5 wide. Nukerbaeva and Svanbaev (1973) measured oocysts from mink in Kazakhstan that were ovoidal, L×W: 33.8×28.0 (31–37×25–31), L/W ratio: 1.2, with a two-layered wall, without M, PG, or OR; sporocysts were spheroidal, 14–15 wide with a SR, but without SB, SSB, and PSB. Tinar (1985) measured oocysts from mink in Turkey, which had a two-layered wall and were L×W: 34.2×27.5 (32.5–36×26–29), L/W ratio: 1.2, with ovoidal sporocysts. The oocysts of this species reported by SkírNisson and Pálmadóttir (1993), in mink pups on fur farms in Iceland, were L×W: 34×26 (30–36×23–30). Hindsbo et al.'s (1995) study from 1986 to 1993 showed this species was present in all years, in both kits and adults, but the prevalence in kits (37/151, 24.5%) was statistically significantly higher than it was in adults (4/125, 3%). Jatusevich and Gerasimchik (1995) reported a 57% coccidia infection in 3-month-old kits, but less than 12% infection in adult mink. These studies allowed Hindsbo et al. (1991, 1995) to conclude there was a strong age-dependent resistance to this species in mink.

CYSTOISOSPORA NIVALIS (MUSAEV AND VEISOV, 1983) NOV. COMB.

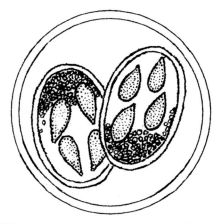

FIGURE 14.23 Original line drawing of the sporulated oocyst of *Cystoisospora nivalis. A rendition from Musaev, M.A., Veisov, A.M. 1983. New species of coccidia of the genera* Eimeria *and* Isospora *from weasel* (Mustela nivalis Lennans *(sic), 1766). Izvestia Akademii Nauk Azerbaijdzhanskoi SSR, Seria Biologicheskich Nauk 5, 64–70. (In Russian). Journal no longer exists, copyright not reassigned after the collapse of the former USSR.

Synonym: *Isospora nivalis Musaev and Veisov, 1983.*

Type host: *Mustela nivalis* (L., 1766), Least Weasel.

Type locality: Asia: Azerbaijan (former USSR).

Other definitive hosts: None to date.

Known intermediate host: None to date.

Geographic distribution: Asia: Azerbaijan (former USSR).

Description of sporulated oocyst: Oocyst shape: ovoidal to spheroidal; number of walls, 1; wall characteristics: smooth, colorless, slightly yellow, 1.4 thick; L×W (n=13): 20.6×18.4 (20–23×18–21), L/W ratio: 1.1; M, OR, PG: all absent. Distinctive features of oocyst: small spheroidal shape with a thick single-layered wall and lacking M, OR, and PG.

Description of sporocyst and sporozoites: Sporocyst shape: ellipsoidal or ovoidal; L×W: 12.5×8.0 (12–13×7–9), L/W ratio: 1.6; SB, SSB, PSB: all absent; SR: present; SR characteristics: a collection of granules forming a cluster at one end of the SP; SZ: described as lemon- or pear-shaped. Distinctive features of sporocyst: a typical *Cystoisospora*-like sporocyst, ellipsoidal, without SB, SSB, PSB, but with a SR composed of a clump of granules at one end of the SP.

Prevalence: Not stated.

Sporulation: Exogenous. Oocysts sporulated in 72 hours in 2.5% aqueous $K_2Cr_2O_7$ at 25–30°C.

Prepatent and patent periods: Unknown.

Site of infection in definitive host: Unknown, although Musaev and Veisov (1983) said that the oocysts they measured were collected from contents in the large intestine.

Endogenous stages: Unknown.

Pathology: Unknown.

Materials deposited: None.

Remarks: Musaev and Veisov (1983) said that the weasel harboring oocysts of this species was collected on summer pasture in the Batabag Shahbusk region of the Nakhitschevansk in Azerbaijan. This species has not been reported since its original description.

CYSTOISOSPORA PAVLOVSKYI (SVANBAEV, 1956) EMEND. YI-FAN, LE, YIN, JIANG-HUI, AND DUSZYNSKI, 2012

Synonym: *Isospora pavlovskyi Svanbaev, 1956.*

Type host: *Mustela eversmanii* Lesson, 1827, Steppe Polecat.

Type locality: Asia: Kazakhstan (former USSR).

Other definitive hosts: None to date.

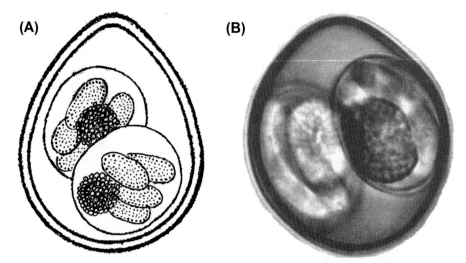

FIGURE 14.24 (A). Original line drawing of the sporulated oocyst of *Cystoisospora pavlovskyi*, (B). Original photomicrograph of a sporulated oocyst of *C. pavlovskyi*. (A) *Modified Fig. 87, Levine, N.D., Ivens, V., 1981. The Coccidian Parasites (Protozoa, Apicomplexa) of Carnivores. Illinois Biological Monograph No. 51,* The University of Illinois Press, Urbana, Illinois USA. *The University of Illinois Press has released the copyright.* (B) *From from Yi-Fan, C., Le, Y., Yin, D., Jiang-Hui, B., Duszynski, D.W., 2012. Emendation of 2* Isospora *species (Apicomplexa: Eimeriidae) infecting the steppe polecat,* Mustela eversmanii Lesson, 1827, *in China, to the genus* Cystoisospora *(Apicomplexa: Sarcocystidae). Comparative Parasitology 79, 147–152, with permission from the authors and the Editor and copyright holder of* Comparative Parasitology.

Known intermediate host: None to date.

Geographic distribution: Asia: China, Kazakhstan (former USSR).

Description of sporulated oocyst: Oocyst shape: ovoidal; number of walls, 2; wall characteristics: smooth, colorless, ~1.6–1.8 total thickness; L×W: 38.5×30.0 (37–40×29–31), L/W ratio: 1.3 (Svanbaev, 1956), or L×W (n=50): 32.2×27.3 (29–36×26.5–28.5), L/W ratio: 1.2 (1.1–1.4) (Yi-Fan et al., 2012); M, PG: both absent, but an OR may (Svanbaev, 1956) or may not (Yi-Fan et al., 2012) be present. Distinctive features of oocyst: distinct ovoidal shape with a thick, smooth, transparent outer wall, but without M, PG and possibly without an OR.

Description of sporocyst and sporozoites: Sporocyst shape: ellipsoidal or ovoidal; L×W: 18.9×16.0 (19×15.5–17), L/W ratio: 1.2 (Svanbaev, 1956), or L×W (n=50): 19.5×14.4 (18–21×12–15), L/W ratio: 1.4 (1.2–1.5) (Yi-Fan et al., 2012); SB, SSB, PSB: all absent; SR: present; SR characteristics: a prominent, spheroidal to ellipsoidal mass composed of small granules that takes up about one-half the volume of the SP; SZ: elongate sausage-shaped, with broadly rounded ends, ~7×5 (6–7×5–6). Distinctive features of sporocyst: large size, without SB, SSB, PSB, but with a large, compact, spheroidal to ovoidal SR.

Prevalence: 2/6 (33%) steppe polecats in China were infected.

Sporulation: Exogenous. Oocysts sporulated in 38–45 hours in 2.5% aqueous $K_2Cr_2O_7$ at 20–25°C (Svanbaev, 1956).

Prepatent and patent periods: Unknown.

Site of infection in definitive host: Unknown.

Endogenous stages: Unknown.

Pathology: Unknown.

Materials deposited: Phototypes in the USNPC in Beltsville, Maryland, USA: USNPC No. 104110; symbiotype host specimen (see Frey et al., 1992) of *M. eversmanii* in the Qinghai–Tibet Plateau Biological Specimen Museum (QPBSM No. 6905; collected by Y. F. Cao, L. Yang, and G.S. Wu, 18 August 2010).

Remarks: Svanbaev (1956) originally described oocysts of *I. pavlovskyi* from the polecat in Kazakhstan (former USSR), but they were poorly characterized in that description. Oocysts of this species were not seen again until Yi-Fan et al. (2012) more completely described the structural features of both the oocyst and its sporocysts from *M. eversmanii* in Qinghai province, China. The measurements of oocysts and sporocysts, above, are from the work of both authors. Svanbaev (1956) said that an OR arises during sporulation, but his original line drawing does not show an OR to be present. The sporulated oocysts of this species somewhat resemble those of *C.* (=*I.*) *laidlawi* Hoare, 1927 but differ in the shape and size of their sporocysts and the much larger SR in the latter. Yi-Fan et al. (2012) redescribed sporulated oocysts and did not see/report an OR; they also recommended that all of the coccidia with non-Stieda body, isosporan-like oocysts with thick walls that have been described from carnivores should be reexamined, and their names should be emended into the genus *Cystoisospora*, as we are doing in this book.

GENUS NEOVISON BARYSHNIKOV AND ABRAMOV, 1997 (2 SPECIES)

CYSTOISOSPORA LAIDLAWI (HOARE, 1927) NOV. COMB.

Other definitive host: *Neovison vison* (Schreber, 1777), American mink.

Remarks: McTaggart (1960) in Britain, Klopfer and Neuman (1970) in Israel, Foreyt and Todd (1976) in Wisconsin, USA, Nukerbaeva and Svanbaev (1973, 1977) in Kazakhstan, Tinar (1985) in Turkey, SkírNisson and Pálmadóttir (1993) in Iceland, and Hindsbo et al. (1995), in Denmark, all reported finding this species in mink. See the full species description, above, under the type definitive host.

OTARIIDAE GRAY, 1825

GENUS ARCTOCEPHALUS É. GEOFFROY SAINT-HILAIRE AND F.G. CUVIER, 1826 (8 SPECIES)

CYSTOISOSPORA ISRAELI KUTTIN AND KALLER, 1992

See Kuttin and Kaller (1992, Fig. 2) for two photomicrographs of sporulated (?) oocysts of *Cystoisospora israeli*, which we are not able to reproduce here.

Type host: *Arctocephalus pusillus* (Schreber, 1775), Brown (South African) Fur Seal.

Type locality: Asia (Near East): Israel.

Other definitive hosts: None to date.

Known intermediate host: None to date.

Geographic distribution: Asia (Near East): Israel.

Description of sporulated oocyst: Oocyst shape: ellipsoidal or slightly ovoidal (photomicrograph); number of walls, 2; wall characteristics: smooth; L×W: 28.5×21 (27–30×20–22), L/W ratio: 1.4; M, OR, PG: all absent. Distinctive features of oocyst: ovoidal shape, with one end slightly pointed (photomicrographs), smooth oocyst outer wall, lacking M, OR, PG.

Description of sporocyst and sporozoites: Sporocyst shape: spheroidal; L×W: 11–15 wide, L/W ratio: 1; SB, SSB, PSB: all absent; SR: present; SR characteristics: numerous coarse granules spread throughout SP such that SZ are barely visible (photomicrographs, Fig. 2); SZ: no description presented. Distinctive features of sporocyst: without SB, SSB, PSB, but with a massive SR of coarse granules that obscure the SZ.

Prevalence: Kuttin and Kaller (1992) found oocysts of this species in the stool of one 7-year-old female fur seal that had been kept in captivity in Israel for 5 years, while being housed with other fur seals.

Sporulation: Presumably exogenous, but unknown.

Prepatent and patent periods: Unknown.

Site of infection in definitive host: Unknown. Oocysts were collected from the feces.

Endogenous stages: Unknown.

Pathology: The infected fur seal had diarrhea with very dark, fluid, mucoid feces and had lost weight from 57.7 to 47.8 kg when symptoms were discovered.

Materials deposited: None.

Remarks: By current standards, the description of this species is modest; however, Kuttin and Kaller (1992) published four photomicrographs, two (their Fig. 1) of unsporulated oocysts and two (their Fig. 2) of presumably sporulated oocysts, although their sporocysts may not have been completely developed, or the SR is composed of so many coarse granules that they completely fill the SP and obscure the SZ. The fur seal in question was treated *per os* twice daily for 2 days with tablets of Resprim Forte® (Teva Pharmaceutical Industries, Israel) containing 800 mg sulfamethoxazole and 160 mg trimethoprim. This treatment was repeated after 10 days. After treatment stopped, the diarrhea stopped, the fur seal gained weight, and no oocysts could be found in the feces. To our knowledge, this species has not been seen again since its original description, but we have no knowledge that there have been additional surveys to look for coccidia in these, and most other marine carnivores.

PHOCIDAE GRAY, 1821

GENUS *MIROUNGA* GRAY, 1827 (2 SPECIES)

CYSTOISOSPORA MIRUNGAE (DRÓŻDŻ, 1987) NOV. COMB.

See Dróżdż (1987, Fig. 1) for a photomicrograph of sporulated oocysts of *Cystoisospora mirungae*, which we are not able to reproduce here.

Synonym: Isospora mirungae Dróżdż, 1987.

Type host: *Mirounga leonina* (L., 1758), Southern Elephant Seal.

Type locality: Europe: South Shetlands, King George Island.

Other definitive hosts: None to date.

Known intermediate host: None to date.

Geographic distribution: Europe: South Shetlands.

Description of sporulated oocyst: Oocyst shape: ellipsoidal or slightly ovoidal; number of walls, 2; wall characteristics: transparent, grey, thin, smooth; L × W: 20.2 × 12.2 (18–22 × 12–14), L/W ratio: 1.65; M, OR, PG: all absent. Distinctive features of oocyst: ellipsoidal shape, thin oocyst wall, lacking M, OR, PG.

Description of sporocyst and sporozoites: Sporocyst shape: spheroidal; L × W: 8–10 wide, L/W ratio: 1; SB, SSB, PSB: all absent; SR: present; SR characteristics: granules spread among the SZ (his photomicrograph, Fig. 1); SZ: no description given. Distinctive features of sporocyst: without SB, SSB, PSB, but with a SR.

Prevalence: Dróżdż (1987) found oocysts of this species in 4/8 (50%) 3-month-old elephant seals, born on King George Island.

Sporulation: Presumably exogenous, but unknown.

Prepatent and patent periods: Unknown.

Site of infection in definitive host: Unknown. Oocysts were collected from the feces.

Endogenous stages: Unknown.

Pathology: Unknown.

Materials deposited: None.

Remarks: By current standards, the description of this species is substandard and inadequate; however, Dróżdż (1987) published one photomicrograph of two (presumably) sporulated oocysts, which allowed us to determine the structure of the sporocysts, which was not stated in his description. To our knowledge, this "species" has not been seen again since its original description, but... has anyone looked?

PROCYONIDAE GRAY, 1825

GENUS NASUA STORR, 1780 (2 SPECIES)

CYSTOISOSPORA ARCTOPITHECI (RODHAIN, 1933) NOV. COMB.

Carnivore definitive host: Nasua nasua (L., 1766), South American Coati.

Remarks: Hendricks (1974, 1977) said he found this species in five carnivore species, as definitive hosts, including the South American coati. For the complete species rendition, see *Eira* (Mustelidae), above.

GENUS PROCYON STORR, 1780 (3 SPECIES)

CYSTOISOSPORA CHOBOTARI (LEVINE AND IVENS, 1981) NOV. COMB.

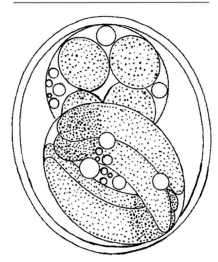

FIGURE 14.25 Original line drawing of the sporulated oocyst of *Cystoisospora chobotari*. *Modified Fig. 37, Levine, N.D., Ivens, V., 1981. The Coccidian Parasites (Protozoa, Apicomplexa) of Carnivores. Illinois Biological Monograph No. 51, The University of Illinois Press, Urbana, Illinois USA. The University of Illinois Press has released the copyright.*

Synonyms: Isospora sp. Inabnit, Chobotar and Ernst, 1972; *Isospora chobotari* Levine and Ivens, 1981.

Type host: Procyon lotor (L., 1758), Raccoon.

Type locality: North America: USA: Michigan.

Other definitive hosts: None to date.

Known intermediate host: None to date.

Geographic distribution: North America: USA.

Description of sporulated oocyst: Oocyst shape: ellipsoidal to subspheroidal; number of walls, 1; wall characteristics: smooth, brown, ~1 thick; L × W (n = 100): 16.8 × 13.7 (16–18.5 × 12.5–15.5), L/W ratio: 1.2; M, OR, PG: all absent. Distinctive features of oocyst: a "typical" *Cystoisospora* oocyst, lacking M, OR, PG.

Description of sporocyst and sporozoites: Sporocyst shape: spheroidal; L × W (n = 100): 11.2 × 9.1 (9.5–11.5 × 8–10), L/W ratio: 1.2; SB, SSB, PSB: all absent; SR: present; SR characteristics: 1–4 randomly scattered, variably sized globules spread among the SZ (line drawing); SZ: one end blunt, the other end pointed, without visible RB or N. Distinctive features of sporocyst: without SB, SSB, PSB, but with a SR.

Prevalence: Inabnit et al. (1972) recovered these isosporan oocysts from 1/43 (2%) raccoons collected in Michigan.

Sporulation: Presumably exogenous, but unknown.

Prepatent and patent periods: Unknown.

Site of infection in definitive host: Unknown. Oocysts were collected from the feces.

Endogenous stages: Unknown.

Pathology: Unknown.

Materials deposited: None.

Etymology: The species epitaph was given by Levine and Ivens (1981) in honor of Dr. Bill Chobotar, Professor, Andrews University, Berrien Springs, Michigan, USA.

Remarks: Inabnit et al. (1972) preferred to delay assigning a name to this form until experimental studies on host specificity were completed. However, such studies were not forthcoming, and Levine and Ivens (1981) decided to name their *Isospora* sp. in honor of Dr. Chobotar.

GENUS *POTOS* É. GEOFFROY-SAINT-HILAIRE AND F.G. CUVIER, 1795 (MONOTYPIC)

CYSTOISOSPORA ARCTOPITHECI (RODHAIN, 1933) NOV. COMB.

Carnivore definitive host: *Potos flavus* (Schreber, 1774), Kinkajou.

Remarks: Hendricks (1974, 1977) said he found this species in five carnivore species, as definitive hosts, including the kinkajou. For the complete species rendition, see *Eira* (Mustelidae), above.

URSIDAE FISCHER DE WALDHEIM, 1817

GENUS *MELURSUS* MEYER, 1793 (MONOTYPIC)

CYSTOISOSPORA URSI (AGRAWAL, AHLUWALIA, BHATIA, AND CHAUAN, 1981) NOV. COMB.

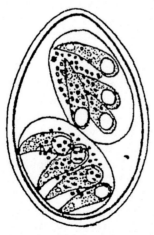

FIGURE 14.26   Line drawing of the sporulated oocyst of *Cystoisospora ursi. Fig. 4, from Agrawal, R.D., Ahluwalia, S.S., Bhatia, B.B., Chauhan, P.P.S., 1981. Note on mammalian coccidia at Lucknow zoo.* Indian Journal of Animal Science 51 (1–6), *125–128, with permission of the Editor and the copyright holder for IJAS.*

Synonym: *Isospora ursi* Agrawal, Ahluwalia, Bhatia, and Chauan, 1981.

Type host: *Melursus ursinus* (Shaw, 1791), Sloth Bear.

Type locality: Asia: India, Uttar Pradesh, Lucknow, Lucknow Zoo (Prince of Wales Zoological Gardens).

Other definitive hosts: None to date.

Known intermediate host: None to date.

Geographic distribution: Asia: India (however, this parasite was found in a zoo animal).

Description of sporulated oocyst: Oocyst shape: strongly ovoidal; number of walls, 2; wall characteristics: 1.5 thick, outer yellow-green, inner dark brown; L×W: 37.4×24.5 (35–43×20–30), L/W ratio: 1.5 (1.4–1.7); M, OR, PG: all absent. Distinctive features of oocyst: relatively big, distinctly egg-shaped oocyst with dark brown inner wall, and lacking M, OR, PG.

Description of sporocyst and sporozoites: Sporocyst shape: broadly ellipsoidal; L×W: 18.7×13.0 (16–22×10–16), L/W ratio: 1.4; SB, SSB, PSB: all absent; SR: present; SR characteristics: clumps of dark granules or sometimes granules are spread among the SZ; SZ: "elongated," laying nearly parallel, with the broader end carrying a refractile globule and the other tapering; L×W: 12.9×3.6 (12–14×3–4); RB: present; N: not seen. Distinctive features of sporocyst: without SB, SSB, PSB, but with a SR.

Prevalence: Unknown, but probably only one sloth bear was examined.

Sporulation: Presumably exogenous.

Prepatent and patent periods: Unknown.

Site of infection in definitive host: Unknown. Oocysts were collected from the feces.

Endogenous stages: Unknown.

Cross-transmission: None to date.

Pathology: Unknown.

Materials deposited: None.

Remarks: Oocysts of this form were found in the feces of a sloth bear kept at the Lucknow Zoo in India, so its true geographic distribution is unknown. To our knowledge, there are no other coccidian species yet described from *M. ursinus*.

SUBORDER FELIFORMIA KRETZOI, 1945

FELIDAE FISCHER DE WALDHEIM, 1817

SUBFAMILY FELINAE FISCHER DE WALDHEIM, 1817

GENUS ACINONYX BROOKES, 1828 (MONOTYPIC)

CYSTOISOSPORA RIVOLTA (GRASSI, 1879) FRENKEL, 1977

Type host: *Felis catus* L., 1758, Domestic Cat.

Remarks: Penzhorn et al. (1994) found oocysts in the feces of 2/16 (12.5%) cheetahs (*A. jubatus*) at the Hoedspruit Cheetah Breeding Centre, South Africa, that they identified as *I*. (=*C*.) *rivolta*. Spheroidal to slightly ellipsoidal oocysts they measured were L×W (n=20): 24.1×22.8 (21–27.5×20–27.5), L×W ratio: 1.05; M, OR, PG: all absent; and broadly ellipsoidal sporocysts were L×W (n=20): 14.0×12.7 (11–16×10–15) (their Table 1), L×W ratio: 1.1; SB, SSB, PSB: all absent; SR: present as an irregular-shaped compact mass of many large granules (their Fig. 1). A complete description of *C. rivolta* appears below under the type host, *F. catus*.

GENUS *FELIS* L., 1758 (7 SPECIES)

CYSTOISOSPORA ARCTOPITHECI (RODHAIN, 1933) NOV. COMB.

Carnivore definitive host: *Felis catus* L., 1758, Domestic Cat.

Remarks: Hendricks (1974, 1977) said he found this species in five carnivore species, as definitive hosts, including the domestic cat.

For the complete species rendition, see *Eira* (Mustelidae), above.

CYSTOISOSPORA FELIS (WENYON, 1923) FRENKEL, 1977

Synonyms: *Diplospora bigemina* Wasielewski, 1904, *pro parte*; *Isospora bigemina* Swellengrebel, 1914; *Isospora rivolta* Dobell and O'Connor, 1921; *Isospora cati* Marotel, 1921; *Lucetina felis* (Wenyon, 1923) Henry and Leblois, 1926; *Isospora felis* var. *servalis* Mackinnon and Dibb, 1938; *Levinea felis* (Wenyon, 1923) Dubey, 1977c.

Type host: *Felis catus* L., 1758, Domestic Cat.

Type locality: Europe: Germany.

Other definitive hosts: *Felis chaus* Schreber, 1777, Jungle Cat (cited in Moudgil, 2015); *Felis silvestris* Schreber, 1777, European Wildcat (as cited in Prasad, 1961b, and others); *Leopardus pardalis* (L., 1758), Ocelot (syn. *Felis pardalis* as cited in Lainson, 1968, and others); *Leptailurus serval* (Schreber, 1776), Serval (syn. *Felis serval* as cited in Mackinnon and Dibb, 1938, and others); *Lynx lynx* (L., 1758), Lynx (Triffitt, 1927, cited in Yakimoff et al., 1933b); *Lynx pardinus* (Temminck, 1827), Iberian Lynx (in Rodriguez and Carbonell, 1998); *Panthera leo* (L., 1758), Lion (syn. *Leo leo* as cited in Yakimoff et al., 1933b, and others; syn. *Felis leo* as cited in Yakimoff and Matschulsky, 1940, and others); *Panthera onca* (L., 1758), Jaguar (syn. *Leo onca* as cited in Barreto and de Almeida, 1937); *Panthera tigris* (L., 1758), Tiger (syn. *Leo tigris* as cited in Yakimoff et al., 1933b, Prasad, 1961b, and others); Hybrid (*Panthera tigris tigris*, Bengal Tiger × *Panthera leo persica*, African Lion) (see Chaudhuri and Choudhury, 1982).

Known intermediate hosts: *Bos taurus* L., 1758, Aurochs (Fayer and Frenkel, 1979); *Canis lupus familiaris* L., 1758 (syn. *C. familiaris*), Domestic Dog (Dubey, 1975b); *Felis catus* L., 1758, Domestic Cat (Dubey and Frenkel, 1972b); *Gallus gallus domesticus* (L., 1758), Domestic Chicken; *Mesocricetus auratus* (Waterhouse, 1839), Golden Hamster

(A)   **(B)**

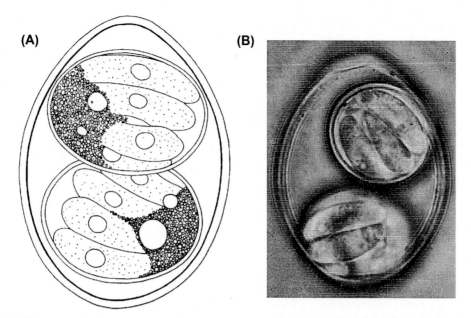

FIGURE 14.27   (A). Original line drawing of the sporulated oocyst of *Cystoisospora felis*, (B). Photomicrograph of a sporulated oocyst of *C. felis*. *(A) Modified Fig. 69, Levine, N.D., Ivens, V., 1981. The Coccidian Parasites (Protozoa, Apicomplexa) of Carnivores. Illinois Biological Monograph No. 51, The University of Illinois Press, Urbana, Illinois USA. The University of Illinois Press has released the copyright. (B) Fig. 21, from Shah, H.L., 1970b. Sporogony of the oocysts of* Isospora felis *Wenyon, 1923 from the cat. Journal of Protozoology 17 (4), 609–614, with permission from John Wiley and Sons, copyright holder and publisher, Journal of Eukaryotic Microbiology (formerly the Journal of Protozoology).*

(Frenkel and Dubey, 1972a); *Mus musculus* L., 1758, House Mouse (Frenkel and Dubey, 1972a; Christie et al., 1976; Dubey and Streitel, 1976b); *Rattus norvegicus* (Berkenhout, 1769), Brown or Norway Rat (Frenkel and Dubey, 1972a).

Geographic distribution: Asia: India, Japan, Russia; Australia: New South Wales; Europe: Belgium, Germany, Portugal, Spain, the Netherlands; Middle East: Iraq; North America: Mexico: Mexico City; USA: Illinois, Iowa, Missouri, New Jersey, Ohio; South America: Brazil, Chile; probably the most common parasite of cats, worldwide.

Description of sporulated oocyst: Oocyst shape: ovoidal; number of walls, 1; wall characteristics: smooth, colorless, ~1.3 thick, apparently lined by a thin membrane; L × W: 45 × 33 (39–48 × 26–37), L/W ratio: 1.4 (Wenyon, 1923),

or L × W: 42.5 × 32 (32–53 × 26–43), L/W ratio: 1.3 (Levine and Ivens, 1981), or L × W (n = 40): 42 × 31 (38–51 × 27–39), L/W ratio: 1.35 (Shah, 1971); M, OR, PG: all absent. Distinctive features of oocyst: large size, distinct ovoidal shape with a thin, smooth, transparent outer wall, but without M, PG, and OR.

Description of sporocyst and sporozoites: Sporocyst shape: ellipsoidal; L × W: 23 × 18 (20–26 × 17–22), L/W ratio: 1.3 (Shah, 1971; Levine and Ivens, 1981); SB, SSB, PSB: all absent; SR: present; SR characteristics: a prominent, spheroidal to ellipsoidal mass composed of granules that takes up about one-half the volume of the SP; SZ: elongate sausage-shaped, with one end slightly narrowed, 10–15 long. Distinctive features of sporocyst: large size, without SB, SSB, PSB, but with a large, compact, spheroidal to ovoidal SR; in other words, a typical *Cystoisospora*-type sporocyst.

Prevalence: Tomimura (1957) selected and examined the feces of young cats from Osaka Prefecture, Japan, from 1951 to 1952, and reported that 27/200 (13.5%) were suffering from coccidiosis; 19/200 (9.5%) were infected with *I.* (=*C.*) *felis* and 5/200 (2.5%) with both *I.* (=*C.*) *felis* and *I.* (=*C.*) *rivolta*. Alwar and Lalitha (1958) surveyed cats in Madras, India and found 7/50 (14%) cats with oocysts of *I.* (=*C.*) *felis*. Patnaik (1966) reported finding this species in a cat in Orissa, Odisha, India. Burrows (1968) in New Jersey, USA found *I.* (=*C.*) *felis* in 62/237 (26%) cats sampled over 12 years beginning in 1956. Burrows and Hunt (1970) also in central New Jersey found *I.* (=*C.*) *felis* in 203/757 (27%) stray cats sampled from Monmouth and Burlington counties. Shah (1970a) found *I.* (=*C.*) *felis* in 17/130 (13%) cats in Illinois, USA. Niak (1972) detected it in 2/18 (11%) cats in Liverpool, Great Britain; their oocysts measured L×W: 27.5–32.0×20–27. Torres et al. (1972) examined cats from Valdivia City, Chile and found 13/100 (13%) to be passing oocysts of *I.* (=*C.*) *felis*. Dubey (1973) found oocysts of this species in 88/510 (17%) domiciled cats in Kansas City, USA. Nery-Guimaraes and Lage (1973) studied the prevalence and life cycle of both *I.* (=*C.*) *felis* and *I.* (=*C.*) *rivolta* in domestic cats; they reported 30/125 (24%) cats had *I.* (=*C.*) *felis* and noted that its endogenous stages were usually found between the HCN and the brush boarder of infected epithelial cells and that the size and numbers of merozoites and microgametocytes were larger than those of *I.* (=*C.*) *rivolta*. Iseki et al. (1974) did a fecal survey of cats in Osaka, Japan and found oocysts they identified as *I.* (=*C.*) *felis* in 10/100 (10%) cats, and Ito et al. (1974) found oocysts in 39/446 (9%) cats in the Saitama area in Tokyo, Japan. Christie et al. (1976) surveyed feces from cats, all >3-months-old, from a humane shelter in Ohio, USA and found 62/1,000 (6%) to have oocysts of *I.* (=*C.*) *felis*. These oocysts were orally inoculated into mice after sporulation

and proved to be infectious for mice, "as indicated by the serial passage of this species from cats to mice to cats." Wilkinson (1977) studied a "cat colony" that was established by a large pet-food manufacturing company in Brisbane, Queensland, Australia, to test various formulations of cat food. He found 49/58 (84.5%) of the cats examined to be infected with *I.* (=*C.*) *felis*; treatment with a 20% solution of sulfadimethoxine at a dose of 50 mg/kg body weight in their food for 14 days, successfully eradicated the infections. Boch and Walter (1979) reported four species of coccidia in cats in Germany, including *I.* (=*C.*) *felis* in 20/694 (3%) cats they surveyed. McKenna and Charleston (1980a), working on the North Island, New Zealand, examined fecal samples from domestic cats and identified oocysts of *I.* (*C.*) *felis* in 89/508 (17.5%) samples. Coman et al. (1981) examined fecal samples of feral, mostly adult, cats from Victoria and New South Wales, Australia and detected oocysts of *I.* (=*C.*) *felis* in 12/300 (4%) samples. Nichol et al. (1981a) examined fecal samples of feral cats from London and Sheffield urban areas, England and found oocysts of *I.* (=*C.*) *felis* in 3/69 (4%) samples. Nichol et al. (1981b) surveyed domestic cats from London, England and detected *I.* (=*C.*) *felis* oocysts in 18/947 (2%) samples, all in cats <3-years-old. Chaudhuri and Choudhury (1982) reported finding oocysts of *I.* (=*C.*) *felis* in a fresh fecal sample from a white tiger (*P. t. tigris*) in the Calcutta Zoological Garden, India. The oocysts they found were ovoidal and measured L×W (n=50): 46×31 (41–49.5×29–34), L/W ratio: 1.5; M, OR, PG: all absent, and sporocysts were ellipsoidal, L×W (n=50): 21×16 (20.5–24×16–19), L/W ratio: 1.3; SB, SSB, PSB: all absent; SR: composed of lots of granules; SP were sausage-shaped and measured (n=10) 12.7×3.9 (12–15×3–4), each with a large RB at its more rounded end. Chaudhuri and Choudhury (1982) said that sporulation was complete in 64–72 hours at room temperature; they also said the "affected tiger lost appetite and strength," and its "feces turned liquid, almost watery, and were of extremely foul odor." Chhabra et al. (1984) examined fecal samples of domestic cats from North India (Delhi, Rishikesh, Lucknow) and saw oocysts of *I.* (=*C.*) *felis* in 20/118 (17%) scats. Ogassawara et al. (1986) examined fecal samples of domestic cats from different areas of São Paulo, Brazil and found oocysts of *I.* (=*C.*) *felis* in 19/215 (9%) cats, mostly <6-months-old. Uga et al. (1989) examined rectal contents of 507 cats in Hyogo Prefecture, Japan and reported *I.* (=*C.*) *felis* oocysts, but the number of positive samples was not stated. Meloni et al. (1993) examined fecal samples of cats from eight Aboriginal communities in the west Kimberley region, Western Australia and detected oocysts of *I.* (=*C.*) *felis* in 5/33 (15%) samples. Rodriguez and Carbonell (1998) looked at fecal samples from wild carnivores in central Spain and found *I.* (=*C.*) *felis* in 5/16 (31%) *F. silvestris* and in 2/9 (22%) *Lynx pardinus*. Barutzki and Schaper (2003) examined fecal samples of cats in Freiburg, Germany and reported *I.* (=*C.*) *felis* in 485/3,167 (15%) samples. McGlade et al. (2003) examined multiple fecal samples from 125 domestic cats from five pet shops, four breeding establishments, three refuge facilities, privately owned, and boarding cats in Perth, Western Australia and reported oocysts of *I. felis* in 19/418 (4.5%) samples, being most prevalent in pet shop kittens. Cirak and Bauer (2004) examined fecal samples of non-diarrhetic cats in Germany and found oocysts of *I.* (=*C.*) *felis* in 7/100 (7%) cats. Palmer et al. (2008a) surveyed fecal samples of cats across Australia, which were collected from 59 veterinary clinics (572 samples) and 26 refuges (491 samples), and *I.* (=*C.*) *felis* was found in 59/1,063 (6%) cats, mostly from refuges. Tzannes et al. (2008) examined cat fecal samples from mainland Great Britain, Northern Ireland, the Isle of Man, and the Channel Islands. Three populations of cats were surveyed: (1) 1,355 domestic cats displaying signs of gastrointestinal disease; (2) 48 domestic cats with signs of gastrointestinal disease; (3) 45 pet cats with no gastrointestinal signs of illness, and oocysts of *I.* (=*C.*) *felis*

were detected only in domestic cats displaying disease, where 46/1,355 (3%) cats were positive. Arbabi and Hooshyar (2009) examined fecal samples of stray cats in the Kashan region, Iran and reported oocysts of *I.* (=*C.*) *felis* in 6/113 (5%) samples. Gates and Nolan (2009) surveyed fecal samples of cats at the University of Pennsylvania, USA and oocysts of *I.* (=*C.*) *felis* were detected in 43/1,566 (3%) samples, mostly in cats <3-years-old. Yamamoto et al. (2009) surveyed feces of cats in animal shelters in Saitama Prefecture, Japan and found *I.* (=*C.*) *felis* in 48/1,079 (4.5%) cats.

Sporulation: Exogenous. Tomimura (1957) said that sporulation of *I.* (=*C.*) *felis* oocysts occurred in ~14 hours when placed in 1% aqueous chromic acid at 28°C. Shah (1969, 1970b) said sporulation was completed in 2 days or less when in 2.5% potassium dichromate ($K_2Cr_2O_7$) solution: 40 hours at 20°C, 24 hours at 25°C, 12 hours at 30°C, and 8 hours at 38°C. No sporulation occurred, and the oocysts died when exposed to 45–50°C.

Prepatent and patent periods: The prepatent period was reported to be 7 days (Tomimura, 1957; Chessum, 1972; Dubey, 1976), 7–8 days (Lickfeld, 1959; Shah, 1971), 7–11 days (Dubey and Frenkel, 1972a; Lindsay et al., 1997), 8–10 days (Frenkel and Dubey, 1972a), 7–10 days (Dubey and Streitel, 1976b), and 5–13 days (Powell and McCarley, 1975). Dubey and Frenkel (1972b) said the prepatent period in kittens consuming oocysts of *I.* (=*C.*) *felis* was 7–11 DPI but converted to 4–8 DPI after consuming EIN tissues of kittens infected with *I.* (=*C.*) *felis*. Christie et al. (1976) said the prepatent period in cats, after mouse passage, was 6–7 DPI for *I* (=*C.*) *felis*. Tomimura (1957) said the patent period was 16–20 days, Shah (1971) said patency lasted 10–11 days, with peak oocyst production on the sixth day, Chessum (1972) said it was 16 days, and Powell and McCarley (1975) said the patent period lasted 7–20 days.

Site of infection in definitive host: Endogenous stages occur in epithelial cells of the distal parts of the villi in the ileum and sometimes in the duodenum and jejunum of the small intestine. Shah (1971) never found endogenous stages at the base of the villi, in goblet cells, in the crypts of Lieberkühn, or in the cecum, colon, or other organs. Lindsay et al. (1997), however, said it developed in enterocytes in the small intestine and occasionally in the cecum.

Endogenous stages: Shah (1969, 1971) used a strain of *I. felis* he derived from a single oocyst to study the life cycle of *I.* (=C.) *felis* and mostly confirmed an earlier life cycle study by Lickfeld (1959). There are three generations of meronts. First-generation meronts (M_1) were seen in small numbers 120 hours PI, in greatest numbers at 96 hours PI, and were present up to 120 hours PI. Mature M_1 were $L \times W$ (n=8): 23×16 ($11-30 \times 10-23$) and contained 16–17 banana-shaped merozoites (m_1) that measured $L \times W$ (n=10): 13×4 ($11-15 \times 3-5$). The m_1s entered new epithelial cells and gave rise to M_2 first seen 96 hours PI, and by 120 hours PI contained 2–10 m_2. Mature M_2 were $L \times W$ (n=8): 20×15 ($12-30 \times 10-22$), and m_2s measured $L \times W$ (n=10): 13×4 ($10-15 \times 3-5$). Shah (1971) said that at 120 hours PI the m_2 were uninucleate, but by 144 hours PI they turned into large multinucleate forms, some of which changed to ovoidal forms from their more typical banana-shape, without leaving the PV in which they developed. These gave rise to spindle-shaped M_3 enclosed within the same PV, and mature M_3 (cysts) were $L \times W$ (n=11): 22×17 ($14-36 \times 13-22$), with banana-shaped m_3s that measured $L \times W$ (n=12): 7×2 ($6-8 \times 1-2$); these m_3 were most plentiful 168 hours PI but persisted as long as 216 hours PI, with 36–70 m_3 per M_3. The m_3s, which Lickfeld (1959) called micromerozoites because of their size, began the sexual cycle. Mature macrogametes measured $L \times W$ (n=10): 18×10 ($16-22 \times 8-13$). Mature microgametocytes were observed between 192 and 216 hours PI and measured $L \times W$ (n=10): 46×26 ($24-72 \times 18-32$); each contained 36 to >70 microgametes, and the latter measured 6×0.8 ($5-7 \times 0.8$) and each had two flagella (Shah, 1969,

1971). Dubey and Frenkel (1972b) fed tissues of kittens infected with *I.* (=C.) *felis* for 5–104 days to newborn kittens, some of which eventually shed oocysts in their feces as follows: 3/5 fed liver and spleen mixture; 4/4 fed mesenteric lymph nodes; 1/5 fed brain, muscle mixtures, and 1/5 fed lung mixture. Frenkel and Dubey (1972a) and Powell and McCarley (1975) found tissue multiplication "sarcocysts" in mouse muscle that were up to 150 wide and often extended the full length of the muscle fiber. Bradyzoites in these cysts were sausage-shaped and measured $L \times W$ (n=20): 12.5×4.5 ($10-15 \times 3-5$). There seems to be no evidence that tissue or intestinal stages of *I.* (=C.) *felis* are transmitted transplacentally from mother cats to their kittens (Dubey, 1977a). Pelster (1973) was the first to study and describe the fine structure of the macrogametes of *I.* (=C.) *felis* and to diagrammatically explain it. Ferguson et al. (1980c) did an ultrastructural study of the development of later generations of merozoites of *I.* (=C.) *felis*, 6 DPI in the cat gut, and documented the process of endodyogeny similar to that described for endozoites of *T. gondii* and provided morphological evidence for the close relationship of *I.* (=C.) *felis* to members of the Sarcocystidae, in support of Frenkel's (1977) classification. This ultrastructural evidence of endodyogeny during *I.* (=C.) *felis* endogenous development was supported again by Daly and Markus (1981).

Cross-transmission: Böhm (1923) was one of the first to initiate cross-transmission work with dog and cat coccidia. He fed some oocysts (presumably *C. canis*?), which were previously infective to one dog, to a kitten, and a human volunteer and monitored their feces for 1 month; he never saw oocysts. He then fed oocysts of *I.* (=C.) *felis* to a 2-month-old fox terrier puppy on three consecutive days and monitored its feces for 67 DPI but never found oocysts to be discharged. Based on this work, he concluded that the large oocysts in cats (*C. felis*) and dogs (*C. canis*) are not mutually cross-infective and, therefore, are distinct species. However, in a note that gives the appearance of trying to discredit Böhm's (1923) work, Andrews (1926b) suggested, "Böhm's negative results may be due either to his method of examination of feces or the fact that he may have used animals that had been previously infected and were, therefore, immune." However, the evidence and argument Andrews (1926a, b) provided were so muddled that they only served to confuse this issue for the next half century. To wit, Andrews (1926b) infected eight dogs with different batches of oocysts from cats that contained either I. (=C.) felis or I. (=C.) rivolta or both ("…oocysts of feline origin of one or both of the two larger species of Isospora."). He reported that two dogs, "showed infection parasitologically, though the attacks were mild, and of the remaining four, three showed clinical evidence (diarrhea) of infection, though no oocysts were found in their feces," and, "the fecal examinations of the last two…were both positive clinically and parasitologically." Andrews (1926b) also infected one cat with oocysts from a dog and said the cat "showed a typical, though somewhat belated, case of coccidiosis clinically and parasitologically." From these limited cross-infections, Andrews (1926b) concluded that he had "conclusive parasitological evidence" that dog and cat isosporans were interchangeable!

Kotlán and Pospesch (1933) were not able to produce a patent infection in a young badger, M. meles, with I. (=C.) felis oocysts. Shah (1970a) inoculated 1×10^5 sporulated oocysts of I. (=C.) felis into four 1.5-month-old, coccidia-free puppies, but patent infections did not occur. da Rocha and Lopes (1971) tried to transmit I. (=C.) felis to dogs, but the infections failed. Nery-Guimaraes and Lage (1973) studied the prevalence and life cycle of both I. (=C.) felis and I. (=C.) rivolta in domestic cats; they tried twice to administer sporulated oocysts of I. (=C.) felis per os to seven puppies, but the dogs "did not produce Isospora infections." Sato (1976) infected cats with oocysts of I. (=C.) canis and then challenged them with oocysts of C. felis; no cross-infection occurred between canine and feline types. We now know

that patent infections do not occur in dogs fed I. (=C.) felis oocysts (Neméséri, 1959, 1960; Shah, 1969, 1970a; Dubey et al., 1970; da Rocha and Lopes, 1971; Nery-Guimaraes and Lage, 1973; Dubey, 1975b; Guterbock and Levine, 1977; others). Frenkel and Dubey (1972a) were the first to demonstrate that mice, rats, and hamsters, infected with sporulated oocysts of I. (=C.) felis, and then fed to kittens 10–67 DPI, resulted in coccidial infections to those kittens. This was the first time that this coccidium, hitherto considered a single-host parasite, demonstrated transmission by carnivorism and doing so indicated new epidemiological implications. Nukerbaeva and Svanbaev (1974, 1977) collected oocysts of I. (=C.) felis from domestic cats and tried to transmit this species to two 5-month-old foxes (V. vulpes), two 40-day-old Arctic foxes (V. lagopus), and two 1-year-old minks (N. vison), but none of these animals became infected. They were successful in transmitting it to a control cat, which shed oocysts in its feces on the 7th DPI. Powell and McCarley (1975) found sarcocysts, which they thought were similar to those of S. muris, in mice from the Iowa State University Mouse Genetics Laboratory. Muscle tissues of these mice were fed to cats and 5/8 (63%) developed intestinal infections and discharged oocysts of I. (=C.) felis. Sporulated oocysts of I. (=C.) felis were then fed to mice and at the 100th DPI the mice had developed sarcocysts that were visible macroscopically. Three other cats were fed muscle tissue from experimentally-infected mice and all three developed I. (=C.) felis infections. Their work demonstrated that this "isosporan" life cycle in cats can use the mouse as an intermediate host in which cyst-like structures that resemble sarcocysts of Sarcocystis species develop; however, dogs fed infected/infective mice do not shed oocysts (Guterbock and Levine, 1977). Dubey and Frenkel (1972b) fed I. (=C.) felis sporocysts to kittens and killed them at intervals so they could feed suspensions of their EIN tissues to clean, < 1-day-old, kittens. They found that the lungs were positive for I. (=C.) felis infective stages for 10 DPI, the brain and skeletal muscles for 12 DPI, the liver and spleen were positive for *I.* (=*C.*) *felis* up to 45 DPI, and mesenteric lymph nodes were infective up to 104 DPI. The prepatent period in these kittens ranged from 4 to 8 DPI versus 7–11 DPI after ingesting sporulated oocysts. Frenkel and Dubey (1972a) fed *I.* (=*C.*) *felis* oocysts to mice and found tissue stages in the lungs, livers, spleens, and mesenteric lymph nodes for up to 67 DPI; when these mice were fed to newborn kittens, the prepatent period in the kittens was 5–6 DPI versus 8–10 DPI in kittens fed sporulated oocysts. Frenkel and Dubey (1972a) found that the same tissues in Norway rats and golden hamsters also could develop infective tissue stages after being fed *I.* (=*C.*) *felis* oocysts. Mehlhorni and Markus (1976), using TEM, described the ultrastructure of these tissue stages in the mesenteric lymph nodes of mice fed sporulated oocysts of *I.* (=*C.*) *felis*. Sato (1976) found that infection of cats with sporulated oocysts of *I.* (=*C.*) *felis* produced complete immunity immediately after the patent period ended, but that 21 days after patency ended, reinfection could be acquired, but that the prepatent period of the challenge infection was shortened by 2–3 days, patency was shortened to about 7 days, and the number of oocysts discharged per g of feces decreased during patency. Dubey and Streitel (1976b) compared feeding sporulated oocysts to cats by feeding them *C. felis* MZTC-infected tissue stages of mice fed similar numbers of oocysts. They found that the prepatent period of *I.* (=*C.*) *felis* was slightly shorter and that the number of oocysts excreted by cats was similar regardless of inoculum. de Oliveira et al. (2007) demonstrated that orally-infective stages of *I.* (=*C.*) *felis* can form in gerbils (*Meriones unguiculatus*), guinea pigs (*Cavia porcellus*), rabbits (*Oryctolagus cuniculus*), and chickens (*Gallus gallus domesticus*) producing oocysts when fed to cats.

Pathology: The pathogenicity of *I.* (=*C.*) *felis* is controversial. This species seems to be slightly pathogenic under "normal" infection circumstances. Andrews (1926a) said he observed enteritis, emaciation, weakness, depression, dysentery, and sometimes death in kittens experimentally-infected with *I.* (=*C.*) *felis*, but Hitchcock (1955), in hindsight, thought these signs of pathology were due to feline distemper because none of the 18 kittens he fed 100,000 sporulated oocysts showed signs of any disease. Tomimura (1957), in contrast, reported watery diarrhea, anorexia, a small rise in temperature, failure to digest food, depression, weakness, anemia, emaciation, and weight loss in experimentally-infected cats, with heavy infections being fatal, but Tomimura (1957) neglected to state how many oocysts he gave or how many kittens (or cats?) were used in his experiments. Tomimura (1957) also said that erythrocyte numbers decreased and leukocyte numbers increased 3 DPI, especially lymphocytes and eosinophils. Lainson (1968) reported on a pet ocelot (*L. pardalis*) of a family in the El Cayo District of Belize, which became very sick when 3-months-old, showing symptoms of abdominal pain, emaciation, and passing watery, loose stools; upon examination, oocysts of *I.* (=*C.*) *felis* were found in the stools, along with smaller oocysts that did not sporulate. However, there was no proof offered of a cause and effect relationship. Shah (1969) also saw no clinical signs of disease in 1.5–2-month-old kittens fed up to 150,000 sporulated oocysts. Powell and McCarely (1975) found that 1/5 (20%) cats with a patent infection of *I.* (=*C.*) *felis* for 20 days was emaciated, lethargic, and had hemorrhagic diarrhea. This cat was treated with sulfadimethoxine and stopped shedding oocysts 4 days later. The other four infected cats showed no clinical signs of infection with the exception of some mild diarrhea. In mice with heavy infections, the muscles were nearly replaced by the sarcocysts, and the mice were weak and moved with difficulty (Powell and McCarely, 1977). Chaudhuri and Choudhury (1982) said that a hybrid "tigon" infected with *I. felis* suffered inappetence and feebleness and had liquid feces and hemorrhagic diarrhea. Hutchison et al. (1981) used scanning electron microscopy to study the small intestine of four SPF cats inoculated with 1×10^5 sporulated *I.* (=*C.*) *felis* oocysts at 168 hours (two cats) and 200 hours PI (two cats). The greatest degree of disruption was observed in the ileum due to the high parasite density there; infected villi tended to be shorter and less closely packed than those in uninfected cats, and numerous swollen enterocytes were seen, including ruptured enterocytes during parasite escape from them. Hutchison et al. (1981) commented that *I.* (=*C.*) *felis* produced "similar, but more severe mucosal alterations in the cat small intestine than that brought about by *T. gondii* during its development." Dubey (1993) said that for many years, both *I.* (=*C.*) *felis* and *I.* (=*C.*) *rivolta* were thought to be serious pathogens of cats, causing abdominal pain, diarrhea, vomiting, and neurologic and respiratory signs attributed to infections with either or both species. However, most often, intestinal bacterial and viral infections were excluded from etiological consideration when investigators found isosporan oocysts in the feces of sick cats. Dubey (1993) pointed out that under monospecific infections clinical disease has not been produced in cats raised under coccidia-free conditions; however, he cautioned: (1) clinical coccidiosis can be found in young cats, especially when concurrent with malnutrition, weaning stress, and concurrent viral and/or bacterial infections; (2) certain strains of both *I.* (=*C.*) *felis* and *I.* (=*C.*) *rivolta* might be more virulent than others; and (3) reactivation of latent coccidial infections might occur during immunosuppression.

Materials deposited: None.

Remarks: Wenyon (1923) provided a literature review of the coccidia of cats and dogs, up to that time, and our readers are encouraged to study the details of that review. Apparently, our knowledge on dog and cat coccidia began when Finch (1854) recorded changes in the intestinal epithelium of cats during food absorption. For decades thereafter, most investigators assumed that cats and dogs harbored only one coccidium, usually described under the name *Isospora bigemina* (Stiles, 1891). Dobell (1919, p. 177) began to dispel the myth when he stated there is no really conclusive evidence to prove that the *Isospora* from the cat was the same as that of the dog or that both were varieties of one species. Finally, Reichenow (1921) first asserted that the form in the dog was (probably) distinct from the one in the cat.

The early history of the life cycle studies of the endogenous development of *I.* (=*C.*) *felis* can be traced to Hitchcock (1954), Lickfeld (1959), and Shah (1969, 1971). The accounts of the first two authors differed so much that Mahrt (1967) suggested they probably were studying different species. Unfortunately, neither used a cloned species to begin their infections, as did Shah (1969, 1970a,b), so they may have had different species or a mixed infection of two species. The results that Hitchcock (1954) reported differed at almost every developmental stage from that of Shah, whereas the results reported by Lickfeld (1959) had strong similarities to that of Shah, but were not as complete; both authors, for example, completely missed the second-generation of merogony. Thus, the structural and developmental information presented here relies mostly on the data of Shah (1969, 1971).

Ryšavý (1954) measured oocysts identified as *C.* (=*I.*) *felis* that were L × W: 41 × 33 (37–47 × 28.5–35), L/W ratio: 1.2, with sporocysts 16–18 × 12–14; he said he found these oocysts in the red fox, *V. vulpes*, the Eurasian lynx, *L. lynx*, the Jungle cat, *F.* (=*Chaus*) *chaus*, and in the domestic cat, *F. catus* (=*F. ocreata domestica*), all animals in and around Prague, Czech Republic. Bearup (1954) reported *I.* (=*C.*) *felis* in cats and dogs in Sydney, Australia. These oocysts were ovoidal and measured L × W: 42.5 × 33.5 (37.5–47.5 × 30–40), L/W ratio: 1.3. Patnaik (1966) reported finding this species in a cat in Orissa, Odisha, India. Fayer and Thompson (1974) were among the first to report the development of *I.* (=C.) *felis* in cultured cells using monolayers of human embryonic intestine, esophageal epithelium, amnion, lung, and epitheloid carcinoma of the cervix (HeLa) cells, as well as cells from embryonic bovine trachea, canine kidney, and chick kidney. They noted that pairs of daughter organisms developed by endodyogeny and probably merogony. Tejero and Arcay-de-Peraza (1982) reported that macrophages from the peritoneal exudate of rats were invaded *in vitro* by sporozoites and merozoites of *C. felis* and Gutiérrez and Arcay (1987) reported they could grow up to three generations of meronts, and the development of the gametogonic phase as far as the differentiation into zygotes, in chorioallantoic membranes of the chick embryo.

Powell and McCarley (1975) said that oocysts (n=20) measured 37.5×29.5 (31–42×25–33), L/W ratio, 1.3. Powell and McCarley (1975) also said that an isolate of *I.* (=C.) *felis* used in their lab produced sarcocysts in mice, but Ruiz and Frenkel (1976) considered a more likely explanation when they said the mice used by Powell and McCarley (1975) were likely infected with both sarcocysts of *S. muris* and the monozoic cysts of *I.* (=C.) *felis*. Mehlhorn and Markus (1976) studied the stages of *I.* (=C.) *felis* in the mesenteric lymph nodes of mice 25 DPI with sporulated oocysts; these stages occurred singly within PVs in host cell cytoplasm and were sporozoite-like, having a large crystalloid body, ~5.5 long, posterior to their N. Mehlhorn and Markus (1976) called these parasites *"waiting stages,"* with a biological function similar to that of the tissue cyst stages of other isosporan coccidia (e.g., *Toxoplasma, Sarcocystis,* etc.). Smith and Frenkel (1978) noted that lab mice housed in the same room as cats that shed sporulated sporocysts of *S. muris,* occasionally developed muscle sarcocysts "spontaneously." They said that cat feces never came in contact with mouse cages, but

they did see German cockroaches (*Blatella germanica*) in the same room from time-to-time. To assess the role of *B. germanica,* and the American cockroach (*Periplaneta americana*) in transmission, cockroaches were exposed to cat feces that contained oocysts of *I.* (=C.) *felis* and *Toxoplasma gondii.* They found that oocysts of *I.* (=C.) *felis* were transmitted to mice only by *B. germanica,* and only for 2 days. Fayer and Frenkel (1979) fed a mixture of from $100×10^3$ to $570×10^3$ sporulated oocysts of *I.* (=C.) *felis* and *I.* (=C.) *rivolta,* from a Costa Rican cat, to two calves in each of two experiments. Weight gains for all calves were normal and no gross lesions were observed. Calves were killed 26 to 115 DPI, and calf organs were pooled, ground, and fed to two coccidia-free cats in each experiment. All cats fed organs from the inoculated calves shed unsporulated *I.* (=C.) *felis* oocysts from 4 to 10 days later and unsporulated *I.* (=C.) *rivolta* oocysts from 2 to 11 days later. McKenna and Charleston (1980b) and others have shown that infections of *I.* (= C.) *felis* in mice produced monozoic cysts in the lungs, liver, lymph nodes and spleen, but not sarcocysts in the muscles. Ferguson et al. (1980a) studied the ultrastructure of macrogametogenesis and the structure of the macrogamete of *I.* (= C.) *felis* within epithelial cells of the small intestine of infected cats at 8 and 9 DPI; they also documented the ultrastructure of microgametogenesis and the structure of microgametes of *I.* (= C.) *felis* within the PV inside epithelial cells of the small intestine of a cat at 8 DPI (Ferguson et al., 1980b). Chaudhuri and Choudhury (1982) reported finding oocysts of *I.* (=C.) *felis* in the feces of a "tigon," a hybrid cross between a Bengal tiger (*P. tigris tigris*) and an African lion (*P. leo persica*) from a zoo in Calcutta, India. The ovoidal oocysts they measured were L×W (n=35): 46×31 (41–49×29–34), L/W ratio: 1.5; M, OR, PG: all absent; ellipsoidal sporocysts were L×W (n=35): 21.1×16.3 (20–24×15–19), L/W ratio: 1.3; SB, SSB, PSB: all absent; SR: present; SR characteristics: as a mass of granules comprising about one-fourth of the space within SP; sausage-shaped SZ were (n = 8): 12.7 × 3.9 (12–15 × 3–4), each with a RB at the broader end. McKenna and Charleston (1982) studied the activation and excystation of I. (=C.) felis sporozoites and found activation under a wide range of in vitro conditions. The presence of bile appeared to be essential for this process to occur, but the presence of trypsin did not.

Singla et al. (2009) published a case report of a stray female kitten that suffered from acute diarrhea, dehydration, weakness, and severe anemia. The cat died before any treatment was attempted. Fecal flotation revealed the presence of oocysts of I. (=C.) felis. Necrotic enteritis and endogenous stages of I. (=C.) felis (mainly oocysts) in the intestine were observed in histopathological sections. However, which part of the intestine affected was not given. The information where this case occurred (city, country) is also not given (perhaps India?). Necropsy revealed the concurrent infection with several adult tapeworms, Taenia taeniaeformis. Moudgil (2015), in his masters' thesis, said he recovered oocysts of I. (=C.) felis in the feces of both jungle cats and Asian lions; oocysts from the jungle cat were L × W: 44.7 × 28.2 (38–52 × 23.5–33), L/W ratio: 1.6, whereas those from the Asian lion measured L × W: 41.8 × 27.3 (38–52 × 23.5–33), L/W ratio: 1.5.

Cats that recover from an intestinal infection with I. (=C.) felis are resistant to reinfection, and there is no evidence of cross-immunity between I. (=C.) felis, I. (=C.) rivolta, and T. gondii. Lindsay et al. (1997) pointed out that I. (=C.) felis and T. gondii seem to have evolved an unusual relationship in cats. Those that have previously recovered from a T. gondii infection will re-excrete T. gondii oocysts if they receive a primary challenge with I. (=C.) felis oocysts. Cats that have a primary I. (=C.) felis infection followed by a primary T. gondii develop strong immunity to T. gondii and will not re-excrete T. gondii oocysts when challenged with I. (=C.) felis oocysts. The mechanism or significance of this relationship is unknown.

CYSTOISOSPORA FRENKELI ARCAY, 1981

For a photomicrograph, which we are unable to reproduce, of a sporulated oocyst of Cystoisospora frenkeli, see Fig. 1 in Arcay (1981).

Synonym: Isospora frenkelia Arcan-de-Peraza, 1976.

Type host: Felis catus L., 1758, Domestic Cat.

Type locality: South America: Venezuela, Caracas, Catia area.

Other definitive hosts: None to date.

Known intermediate hosts: Mus musculus L., 1758, House Mouse; Rattus norvegicus (Berkenhout, 1769), Brown or Norway Rat.

Geographic distribution: South America: Venezuela.

Description of sporulated oocyst: Oocyst shape: ellipsoidal; number of walls, 2; wall characteristics: smooth, colorless; L × W: 27.5 × 22.2 (ranges not given), L/W ratio: 1.2; M, PG, OR: all absent. Distinctive features of oocyst: not many; "typical" slightly ellipsoidal shape and lacking M, PG, and OR.

Description of sporocyst and sporozoites: Sporocyst shape: subspheroidal; L × W: 14.5 × 13.6 (ranges not given), L/W ratio: 1.1; SB, SSB, PSB: all absent; SR: not mentioned but apparently present (Fig. 1, Arcay, 1981); SR characteristics: aggregated or scattered granules (Fig. 1, Arcay, 1981); SZ: not mentioned. Distinctive features of sporocyst: none, a typical cystoisosporan SP, without SB, SSB, PSB, and with a SR composed of various numbers of granules that either are aggregated or scattered in the SP.

Prevalence: Found in the only cat they studied from the Catia area in Caracas.

Sporulation: Exogenous. Arcay (1981) said sporulation occurred in 5 days when oocysts and cat feces were placed in 2% potassium dichromate ($K_2Cr_2O_7$) and kept at room temperature.

Prepatent and patent periods: Arcay (1981) reported that the prepatent period could be from 7 to 26 days but that the patent period was very short, only 2–3 days.

Site of infection in definitive host: Large intestine (Arcay, 1981).

Endogenous stages: Arcay (1981) had difficulty studying this parasite in the cat because of its very low reproductive potential that resulted in "the scarce presence of some phases of the parasite endogenous cycle." In cats, she could only find a few first-generation meronts within PVs and mostly found macrogametocytes, also within PVs, later during the infection. Because of the low reproductive capacity of the endogenous stages in cats, Arcay (1981) decided to study development in the chicken embryo chorioallantoic membrane (MCA). Arcay-de-Peraza (1976; Arcay, 1981) collected sporozoites from oocysts from a cat and seeded them onto the MCA of chicken embryos and "studied the development of the parasite in its schizogonic and gametogonic phases until the formation of zygotes." She then compared the stages they found on the MCA to similar, albeit limited, structures found in histological slides of experimentally-infected cat intestines. About 6 hours after SZ were inoculated onto the MCA, first-generation meronts (M_1) were mature, measured 4.7×4.3, contained a large N, and had 8, 16, or 32 m_1 that were 2.6×1.4. Parasites on the MCA grew both in epithelial cells of the allantois and in the chorion and conjunctiva between these embryonic layers. After 4 days, well-defined M_2 and M_3 were reported, especially in the conjunctiva; M_2 were 14.6×8.0, and their m_2 were 2×1.8, whereas M_3 were 14×9 and had more elongated m_3 that were 2.1×1.6. Microgametocytes were ellipsoidal, 10.5×6.5, with numerous comma-shaped microgametes. Globular meronts, 10–14.6 wide, were frequently seen within blood vessels of the MCA, within the endothelium of the blood vessel. Developmental stages were most abundant in the conjunctiva of the MCA at 5 DPI and in the chorion after 6 DPI. By 9–12 DPI, parasite endogenous development began to decline (Arcay, 1981).

Cross-transmission: Arcay (1981) said that *C. frenkeli* is capable of forming cystic stages in the lymphoid organs of rats and mice, as well as in the pulmonary parenchyma and in the bronchial epithelium of the rat. In experimental oral infections of immunosuppressed white lab mice (Arcay-de-Peraza, 1976; Arcay, 1981), she observed, "stages of development of *Isospora* in the intestinal epithelium, having found differentiation of gametes and zygotes." She also said, "schizont-like structures with very fine and small zoites have been found in the intestinal villi crypts of the mouse, as well as in the axillary and inguinal lymph nodes, and in the spleen." Kittens fed with visceral macerate and lymphatic nodules of experimentally-infected rodents produced unsporulated oocysts with a prepatent period of 6 DPI. In mice and rats, she reported tissue stages in lymph nodes and pulmonary parenchyma, whereas in the bronchial epithelium of rats she observed some structures she said were "of the gamogony cycle of the parasite."

Pathology: In cats, the only pathology noted by Arcay (1981) was that macrogametocytes within the mucosal glands caused disorganization and lysis of the invaded cells; this resulted in the increase in goblet cells. In mice-administered sporulated oocysts and immunosuppressants *per os*, adenopathies of the cervical and inguinal lymph nodes were observed by Arcay (1981), and cyst forms containing groups of zoites appeared in lymph nodes 1–6 months PI. In gray mice babies fed viscera of experimentally-infected white mice, similar structures also were observed in cervical and abdominal lymph nodes, as well as phases of gametogony; Arcay (1981) further reported both merogony and gametogony were found in the intestinal epithelium of these mice. In rats, Arcay (1981) said that cervical and abdominal adenopathies were present in addition to pseudocysts and "evolutionary forms of the endogenous cycles" in the small intestine. In the lungs of rats, gametogony was observed in the bronchial epithelium as well as areas of diffuse congestion and leukocytic infiltrates, and within pulmonary blood vessels there was an abundance of polymorpho-nuclear leukocytes and eosinophils, and in the rats' thymus there were broken pseudocysts that showed the release of their zoites.

Materials deposited: None.

Etymology: Arcay-de-Peraza (1976) said she coined this name "in honor of the distinguished Dr. J.K. Frenkel."

Remarks: Arcay-de-Peraza (1976) committed the cardinal sin of naming a new species when she coined the name *"Isospora frenkelia"* in an abstract, submitted for presentation before the fourth Latin America Congress of Parasitology, 7–11 December, 1976, in San Jose, Costa Rica. She presented little data in her abstract and, of course, no type specimen can be put forward in an abstract and, thus, the name became a *nomen nudum*. It was not until 5 years later that she resurrected the name in a refereed publication (Arcay, 1981), with photomicrographs of one sporulated (?) oocyst (poor) and of tissue sections of several asexual and sexual endogenous stages. Arcay-de-Peraza (1976) studied the development of this new form in chicken embryos on the MCA because "we do not know its cystic development in an intermediate host that allows it to be defi-nitely located as an organism belonging to the *Toxoplasma*." Later, Dr. Arcay finally published her full description of *C. frenkeli* (Arcay, 1981) and noted that this cystoisosporan has very low reproductive capacity in its endogenous cycle in cats. Both in the single cat sent to her laboratory and in healthy, experimentally-infected kittens, she could find only very small numbers of first-generation meronts, no second or third genera-tion meronts, no microgametocytes, only a few macrogametocytes of diverse stages of develop-ment and only a small number of unsporulated oocysts in the feces, including in cats immuno-suppressed with cortisone acetate. In addition, only 3/14 (21%) 2-month-old kittens infected *per os* with oocysts of *C. frenkeli* became infected, and these shed only small numbers of unsporu-lated oocysts. This forced her to study develop-mental stages in chick embryos as she and her

colleagues had done earlier with *I. felis* (unpub-lished abstract). Having found cystic stages in the lymphoid organs and in the lungs of both rats and mice, she felt justified in placing this organism in the *Cystoisospora*. She concluded her new species description with this state-ment, "…we have observed that *C. frenkeli* sp. n. not only develops tissue cysts in the lymphoid organs of rats and mice, but also develops schi-zogony and gametogony stages of enteric char-acteristics in the bronchial epithelium of rats and in the intestinal epithelium of experimen-tally infected mice."

CYSTOISOSPORA (?) NEOTOMAFELIS (GALAVÍZ-SILVA, MERCADO-HERNÁNDEZ, RAMÍREZ-BON, ARRENDONDO-CANTÚ, AND LAZCANO-VILLARREAL, 1991) NOV. COMB.

View a photomicrograph of a sporulated oocyst in Galavíz-Silva et al. (1991, Fig. 17), which we are not able to reproduce here.

Synonym: *Sarcocystis neotomafelis* Galavíz-Silva, Mercado-Hernández, Ramírez-Bon, Arrendondo-Cantú, and Lazcano-Villarreal, 1991.

Definitive host (experimental): *Felis catus* L., 1758, Domestic Cat.

Type locality: North America: Mexico, Nuevo Leon, Municipality of Doctor Coss (95° 52′ 05″ N, 99° 02′ 01″ W).

Other definitive hosts: Unknown.

Known intermediate host: *Neotoma micropus* Baird, 1855, Southern Plains Woodrat.

Geographic distribution: North America: Mexico.

Description of immature oocyst: Oocyst shape: subspheroidal; number of walls, 2; wall charac-teristics: two layers of uniform thickness; L×W (n=60): 44.4–45.1×36.7–40.7 (means not given), L/W ratio: unknown; M, OR, PG: apparently all absent (photomicrograph). Distinctive features of oocyst: relatively big, with two-layered outer wall that maintains its integrity during passage through the cat intestinal tract, and lacking M, OR, PG.

Description of sporocyst and sporozoites: Sporocyst shape: subspheroidal to slightly ellipsoidal; L×W: 24.3–29.9, L/W ratio: ~1.0; SB, SSB, PSB: all absent; SR: present; SR characteristics: irregular clumps of dark granules spread among the SZ (photomicrograph); SZ: fusiform; RB, N: not mentioned. Distinctive features of sporocyst: without SB, SSB, PSB, but with a SR.

Prevalence: Tissue cysts were found in muscle fibers in the facial subcutaneous tissues or in the muscles of the legs, genital, and perianal muscles of 37/129 (29%) wild-caught *N. micropus* that included 21/70 (30%) females and 16/59 (27%) males.

Sporulation: Exogenous. Oocysts were passed unsporulated in the feces of experimentally-infected kittens and sporulation of oocysts from the feces took 4–7 days of incubation in 2.5% potassium dichromate ($K_2Cr_2O_7$) solution.

Prepatent and patent periods: The prepatent period varied from 5 to 16 days and the patent period varied from 6 to 21 days in 17 experimentally-infected kittens.

Site of infection, definitive host: Galavíz-Silva et al. (1991) said that sexual stages were found throughout the length of the small intestine, with the heaviest concentration in the jejunum. Microgamonts, macrogametes, and immature oocysts infected cells of the intestinal lamina propria immediately below the epithelium crypts of Lieberkühn, tunica propria, and intestinal villi.

Site of infection, intermediate host: Cysts were in the muscle fibers of woodrats, *N. micropus*.

Endogenous stages, definitive host: Macrogametes, microgamonts, and immature oocysts were observed principally in the jejunum. Subspheroidal macrogametes were L×W (n=35): 5.9×4.8 and were in a PV that measured 8.5 wide. Microgamonts were also in a PV that was 7.5 wide, containing the spheroidal

microgametes that measured L×W (n=9): 6.8×1.9.

Endogenous stages, intermediate host: Macroscopic cysts were visible within muscle fibers in the subcutaneous tissue of facial, digastric muscle, legs, anus, prepuce and meaty panicle. Tissues most frequently infected were masseter muscles, the forward region of infraorbital foramen between medial masseter tendons, the prepuce, panniculus, proximal region of the legs, and the perianal muscles. These cysts ("sarcocysts?") were macroscopic, and when removed from the tissue measured 0.5–2.0 mm wide; bradyzoites in the inner periphery of the cysts were crescent-shaped, 7.7–12.2 × 1.5–3.1.

Cross-transmission: Cysts in woodrat muscles were inoculated *per os* into 17 newborn kittens, 5 pups, and 5 crotalids. Infection developed only in all 17 newborn kittens (Galavíz-Silva et al., 1991)

Pathology: Unknown.

Materials deposited: None.

Remarks: Based on morphological observations made by both LM and TEM, and repeated transmission experiments, Galavíz-Silva et al. (1991) described a parasite they called, *S. neotomafelis*, involving the woodrat, *N. micropus*, as an intermediate host and the domestic cat as the definitive host. However, when cats were fed tissues from woodrats, they shed oocysts with a distinct, two-layered wall, and these oocysts took 4–7 days to sporulate once outside the cat. However, one of *the* defining characteristics of the genus *Sarcocystis* is that, as far as we know, complete sporulation of the oocyst occurs within the intestinal cells of the definitive host resulting in the shedding of sporulated sporocysts in the feces after they have ingested sarcocyst-infected tissues from the intermediate host. No one seems to have noticed this before. Odening (1998) listed this species as one of the 189 in his *Sarcocystis* species names list, and Dubey et al. (2015a) provided structural and biological information on *S. neotomafelis* (Tables 21.2, 23.1) and considered this a valid species of *Sarcocystis* (Tables 24.1, 24.4). We think that Galavíz-Silva et al. (1991) either may have been dealing with two distinct parasite genera or they misinterpreted the muscle cysts in woodrats to be sarcocysts of a *Sarcocystis* species. Clearly, the woodrats they examined seem to have harbored tissue cysts that resemble sarcocysts, and when they fed woodrat tissue to cats (and dogs and rattlesnakes), they never saw free sporocysts in the feces; either they missed them or none of these were the appropriate definitive hosts for these particular sarcocysts. However, the authors did not look into these woodrats for microscopic (monozoic) dormozoites in the mesenteric lymph nodes, and perhaps it was stages like these that produced the large unsporulated oocysts eventually recovered by Galavíz-Silva et al. (1991). The other possibility is that *C. neotomafelis* forms large muscle cysts in woodrats just as *C. felis* infects muscle cysts in mice and forms large, macroscopic cysts in them.

CYSTOISOSPORA RIVOLTA (GRASSI, 1879) FRENKEL, 1977

Synonyms: *Coccidium rivolta* Grassi, 1879; *Coccidium rivoltae* Leuckart, 1896 *pro parte*; *Coccidium bigeminum* Stiles, 1891 *pro parte*; *Diplospora bigemina* Wasielewski, 1904 *pro parte*; *Isospora rivoltae* Dobell, 1919; *Isospora rivoltai* (Grassi, 1879) *auctores*; *Lucetina rivolta* (Grassi, 1879) Henry and Leblois, 1926; *Isospora novocati* Pellérdy, 1974a,b; *Levinea rivolta* (Grassi, 1879) Dubey, 1977c.

Type host: *Felis catus* L., 1758, Domestic Cat.

Type locality: Europe: Italy.

Other definitive hosts: *Canis lupus dingo* Meyer, 1793, Dingo (?); *Canis lupus familiaris* L., 1758, Domestic Dog (?); *Felis chaus* Schreber, 1777, Jungle Cat; *Felis silvestris* Schreber, 1977, Wild Cat; *Leopardus pardalis* (L., 1758), Ocelot; *Lynx lynx* (L., 1758), Lynx; *Panthera leo* (L., 1758), Lion (syn. *Leo leo* as cited in Yakimoff et al., 1933b); *Panthera onca* (L., 1758), Jaguar (syn. *Leo onca* as cited in Barreto and de Almeida, 1937); *Panthera*

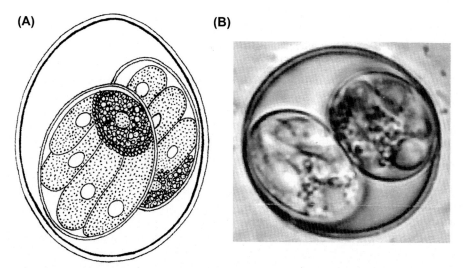

(A)   **(B)**

FIGURE 14.28   (A). Original line drawing of the sporulated oocyst of *Cystoisospora rivolta*, (B). Photomicrograph of a sporulated oocyst of *C. rivolta*. *(A) Modified Fig. 65, Levine, N.D., Ivens, V., 1981. The Coccidian Parasites (Protozoa, Apicomplexa) of Carnivores. Illinois Biological Monograph No. 51, The University of Illinois Press, Urbana, Illinois USA. The University of Illinois Press has released the copyright. (B) Figure 1, Penzhorn, B.L., Booth, L.M., Meltzer, D.G.A., 1994.* Isospora rivolta *recovered from cheetahs. Journal of the South African Veterinary Association 65 (1), 2, with permission from the Editor, and copyright holder for JSAVA.*

pardus (L., 1758), Leopard; *Panthera tigris* (L., 1758), Tiger (syn. *Leo tigris* as cited in Yakimoff et al., 1933b, Prasad, 1961b).

Known intermediate host: *Bos taurus* L., 1758, Aurochs; *Cavia porcellus* (L., 1758), Guinea Pig; *Cricetus cricetus* (L., 1758), Golden Hamster; *Felis catus* L., 1758, Domestic Cat; *Gallus gallus domesticus* (L., 1758), Domestic Chicken; *Meriones unguiculatus* (Milne-Edwards, 1867), Mongolian Gerbil; *Mus musculus* L., 1758, House Mouse; *Oryctolagus cuniculus* (L., 1758), European Rabbit; *Rattus norvegicus* (Berkenhout, 1769), Brown or Norway Rat.

Geographic distribution: Asia: India; Australia: New South Wales, Sydney; Europe: Spain.

Description of sporulated oocyst: Oocyst shape: ovoidal to subspheroidal; number of walls, 2; wall characteristics: smooth, colorless, and the outer layer is easily removed by treatment with sodium hypochlorite; L×W (n=100): 25.4×23.4 (23–29×20–26), L/W ratio: 1.1; M, PG, OR: all absent. Distinctive features of oocyst: not many; "typical" subspheroidal shape and lacking M, PG, and OR.

Description of sporocyst and sporozoites: Sporocyst shape: ellipsoidal; L×W (n=100): 17.2×15.0 (13–21×10–15), L/W ratio: 1.1; SB, SSB, PSB: all absent; SR: present; SR characteristics: either aggregated or scattered granules; SZ (live): elongate banana-shaped, 12.4×2.8 (10–14×2.5–3). Distinctive features of sporocyst: small to medium size, without SB, SSB, PSB, and with a SR composed of only a few granules, either aggregated or scattered in the SP.

Prevalence: Alwar and Lalitha (1958) surveyed cats in Madras, India and found 2/50 (4%) cats examined to have oocysts of *I. (=C.) rivolta*. Mimioğlu et al. (1960) said they found oocysts of *I. (=C.) rivolta* in 1/39 (2%) domestic dogs they examined in Ankara, Turkey (probably *I. canis*). Burrows and Hunt (1970), in central New Jersey, USA, found *I. (=C.) rivolta* in 11/757 (<2%) stray cats sampled from Monmouth and Burlington counties. Torres et al. (1972) examined cats from Valdivia City, Chile for parasites and found 7/100 (7%) to be passing oocysts of *I. (=C.) rivolta*. Dubey (1973) found oocysts of *I. (=C.) rivolta* in 48/510 (9%) domiciled cats in Kansas City, USA. Nery-Guimaraes and Lage (1973) studied the prevalence and life cycle of both *I. (=C.) rivolta* and *I. (=C.) felis* in domestic cats; they reported 18/125 (14%) cats had *I. (=C.) rivolta* and noted that its endogenous stages were usually found between the HCN and the basal membrane of infected epithelial cells and that the size and numbers of merozoites and microgametocytes were smaller than those of *I. (=C.) felis*. Iseki et al. (1974) did a fecal survey on cats in Osaka, Japan and found oocysts they identified as *I. (=C.) rivolta* in 5/100 (5%), whereas Ito et al. (1974) found oocysts in only 2/446 (<0.05%) cats in the Saitama area in Tokyo. Christie et al. (1976) surveyed feces from cats, all >3-months-old, from a humane shelter in Ohio, USA, looking for stages of intestinal parasites. They found 32/1,000 (3%) samples to have oocysts of *I. (=C.) rivolta*. These oocysts were orally inoculated into mice after sporulation and proved to be infective for mice, "as indicated by the serial passage of this species from cats to mice to cats." The prepatent period in cats, after mouse passage, was 5–6 days for *I. (=C.) rivolta*. Guterbock and Levine (1977) did a fecal survey of cats in east central Illinois, USA and found 52/217 (24%) cats to be passing oocysts of *I. (=C.) rivolta*. Boch and Walter (1979) reported four species of coccidia in cats in Germany, including *I. (=C.) rivolta* in 35/694 (5%) cats they surveyed. McKenna and Charleston (1980a), working on the North Island, New Zealand, examined fecal samples from domestic cats and identified oocysts of *I. (=C.) rivolta* in 10/508 (2%) samples. Coman et al. (1981) examined fecal samples of feral, mostly adult, cats from three different habitat types: (1) national parks and wildlife reserves; (2) remote mountainous areas; (3) miscellaneous sites (rubbish heaps, picnic reserves, camping grounds) in southeastern Australia (Victoria, Western New South Wales). Oocysts of *I. (=C.) rivolta* were detected in 9/300 (3%) samples. Specific antibodies to feline panleukopenia virus (79%), feline calicivirus (77%), and feline herpes virus (11%) were concurrently detected in these examined cats. Nichol et al. (1981b) surveyed the prevalence of intestinal parasites in domestic cats in the London area, England and found *I.* (=*C.*) *rivolta* in 8/947 (<1%) samples in cats less than 5-years-old. Chhabra et al. (1984) examined fecal samples of domestic cats from North India (Delhi, Rishikesh, Lucknow), and oocysts identified as *I.* (=*C.*) *rivolta* were detected in 13/118 (11%) samples. Ogassawara et al. (1986) examined fecal samples of domestic cats from different areas of the city of São Paulo, Brazil; they reported finding oocysts of *I.* (=*C.*) *rivolta* in 8/215 (4%) fecal samples, mostly in animals either <6-months-old or those that were 10–24-months-old. Meloni et al. (1993) examined fecal samples of cats from eight Aboriginal communities in the west Kimberley region, Western Australia, and *I.* (=*C.*) *rivolta* was detected in 3/33 (9%) samples. Rodriguez and Carbonell (1998) looked at fecal samples from wild carnivores in central Spain and said they found oocysts of *I.* (=*C.*) *rivolta* in 7/16 (44%) *F. silvestris*, 1/9 (11%) *Lynx pardinus*, and 3/20 (15%) *V. vulpes* sampled. During a survey on endoparasites of dogs and cats in Germany, Barutzki and Schaper (2003) examined fecal samples of cats in Freiburg, Germany; oocysts of *I.* (=*C.*) *rivolta* were detected in 253/3,167 (8%) samples. McGlade et al. (2003) examined fecal samples of 125 domestic cats from five pet shops, four breeding establishments, three privately-owned refuge facilities, and boarding cats in metropolitan Perth, Western Australia, and oocysts of *I.* (=*C.*) *rivolta* were detected in 6/418 (<2%) samples, being most prevalent in pet shop kittens, whereas it was not detected in cats from private owners. Cirak and Bauer (2004) examined fecal samples of cats from three animal shelters in central Germany, and all cats were without diarrhea. Oocysts of *I.* (=*C.*) *rivolta* were recorded in 10/100 (10%) cats. Palmer et al. (2008a) surveyed fecal samples of cats from both urban and rural areas across Australia, which were collected from 59 veterinary clinics (572 samples) and 26 refuges (491 samples); they reported *I.* (=*C.*) *rivolta* oocysts in 29/1,063 (3%) cats, mostly from the refuges. Arbabi and Hooshyar (2009) examined fresh fecal samples of stray cats trapped and necropsied in

urban and rural areas of the Kashan region, central Iran; they detected oocysts of *I.* (=*C.*) *rivolta* in 6/113 (5%) samples. Yamamoto et al. (2009) surveyed fecal samples of cats in public animal shelters in the Saitama Prefecture, Japan, and their examinations revealed the presence of *I.* (=*C.*) *rivolta* in 24/1,079 (2%) cats.

Sporulation: Exogenous. Bearup (1954) said sporulation was completed in 4 days. Mandal (1976) said sporulation was completed in 2–3 days. Dubey (1979b) said sporulation was completed within 24 hours at 24°C (22–26°C), 12 hours at 30°C, and 8 hours at 37°C.

Prepatent and patent periods: Dubey and Frenkel (1972b) said the prepatent period in kittens consuming sporulated oocysts was 5–7 days, and it was the same for kittens consuming EIN tissues of cats infected with *I.* (=*C.*) *rivolta*. Dubey (1979b) reported that the patent period was 4–7 days and patent periods ranged from 2 to several weeks for cats ingesting sporulated oocysts.

Site of infection in definitive host: Asexual and sexual developmental stages occurred throughout the small intestine, in epithelial cells of the villi, and in the glands of Lieberkühn. Most of these stages were found below the HCN and pushed the HCN toward the lamina propria giving the false impression of a subepithelial location.

Endogenous stages: Frenkel and Dubey (1972a) found tissue multiplication stages in the skeletal muscle of mice fed sporulated oocysts. Dubey and Frenkel (1972b) fed tissues of kittens infected with *I.* (=*C.*) *rivolta* for 5–21 days to newborn kittens, some of which eventually shed oocysts in their feces as follows: 3/5 fed liver and spleen mixture; 1/5 fed mesenteric lymph nodes; and 0/5 fed brain, muscle, and lung mixtures. Pelster (1973) was the first to study and describe the fine structure of the macrogametes of *I.* (=*C.*) *rivolta* and to diagrammatically explain it. Brösigke et al. (1982) were the first, we think, to demonstrate "sleeping" stages (dormozoites) in the tissue of mice after they were infected with sporulated oocysts of *I.* (=*C.*) *rivolta*. They noted that in some cases a cyst-like sheath developed around these zoites from the 7 DPI onward; these dormozoites measured $12–15 \times 3$. Spleen, liver, and mesenteric lymph nodes ("mesenterium") showed the highest levels of infection, and they reported the dormozoites were found in all organs except the brain during heavy infections. They also reported that there was no transmission of dormozoites through the placenta to the fetus but that oral transmission from mouse to mouse was possible from the time of infection until 7 DPI.

Dubey (1993) studied endogenous developmental stages in cats fed sporulated oocysts, in newborn cats fed mice that were infected with intra- and extracellular zoites in their mesenteric lymph nodes and spleens, and in mice fed sporocysts. In mice fed $10^5–10^6$ sporocysts, sporozoites most frequently invaded their mesenteric lymph nodes and remained there for at least 23 months; they also invaded the spleen, liver, and skeletal muscles, but these zoites could not be passed from mouse to mouse. Dubey (1993) regularly found both intra- and extracellular single parasites in mouse lymph nodes, and they increased in size with time; on 1 DPI, zoites were $L \times W$: 6.8×4.9 $(6–8 \times 4–6)$ and on 31 DPI, zoites were 13.4×6.9 $(11–17 \times 6–9)$. Some zoites also developed a covering sheath (or cyst wall), and at 31 DPI those with the sheath measured $L \times W$: 23.1×10.2 $(18–30 \times 8–13)$. After 7 DPI, the majority of zoites were sheathed. In cats fed $10^5–10^6$ sporocysts, Dubey (1993) was not able to determine exactly the number of merogonous stages with any certainty but said there were at least three structurally different meronts. Type I meronts measured $L \times W$: 8.5×5.1 $(6–13 \times 3–6)$, with 2–8 merozoites that were $7.8–2.2$ $(7–10 \times 2–3)$; he could not determine if these divided by binary division or endodyogeny. Type II meronts "were a collection of 1–5 multinucleated merozoite-shaped meronts" in a PV that measured $L \times W$: 12.6×9.8 $(9–18 \times 9–13)$, with uninucleate, binucleate, and multinucleate zoites that contained up to eight nuclei; these merozoites probably divided several times without leaving the PV. Type III meronts measured $L \times W$: 13.9×11.1 $(7–24 \times 4–21)$ and contained 2–30 slender merozoites, $5–6 \times 1–1.5$. Dubey (1993) designated these meronts as

types instead of generations (as with *Eimeria* species) because at least type I divided by division into 2, probably by endodyogeny, a process similar to that seen in *T. gondii* and *I.* (=*C.*) *ohioensis* (Dubey and Frenkel, 1972a; Dubey, 1978a). Mature microgamonts were $L \times W$: 11.3×8.0 $(9–15 \times 6–9)$ in tissue sections and 21.5×14 in smears and contained up to 70 microgametes. Macrogamonts measured $L \times W$: 13.3×9.0 $(11–18 \times 5–13)$ in tissue sections and 18×16 in smears. Both oocyst-induced and mouse-induced cycles in newborn kittens were identical.

Matsui et al. (1993b) infected four mice with 2.3×10^5 sporulated oocysts of *I.* (=*C.*) *rivolta*, sacrificed them 7 DPI, and detected ensheathed zoites in mouse mesenteric lymph nodes. Infected mouse mesenteric lymph nodes and spleens were then fed to donor cats that were killed on 3 DPI, when Matsui et al. (1993b) found numerous merozoites in the cats' intestinal mucosa and a few more "zoites" in the cats' mesenteric lymph nodes. The intestinal mucosa and internal organs (liver, mesenteric lymph nodes, spleen) from these cats were then fed to two (first recipient) cats. These first recipient cats were killed on 9 DPI and their EIN organs were fed to two second recipient cats, both of which started shedding oocysts in their feces on 7 or 9 days after feeding. Matsui et al. (1993b) concluded that merozoites and zoites may invade EIN organs of first recipient cats. In a parallel study, perhaps even using some of the same laboratory mice and cats, Matsui et al. (1993a) found that both the merozoites and ensheathed zoites of *I.* (=*C.*) *rivolta* in cats are infectious for mice, and grow into ensheathed zoites, and when these mice are fed to cats, the cats shed oocysts from 5 to 6 DPI.

Cross-transmission: Dubey et al. (1970) failed to infect healthy dogs with oocysts of *I.* (=*C.*) *rivolta* from cats, as did Pellérdy (1974b). Frenkel and Dubey (1972a) were the first to demonstrate that mice, rats, and hamsters infected with sporulated oocysts of *I.* (=*C.*) *rivolta* and then fed to kittens 10–67 DPI, resulted in coccidial infections to those kittens. This was the first time that this coccidian, hitherto considered a single-host parasite, demonstrated transmission by carnivorism, and doing so indicated new epidemiological implications. Nery-Guimaraes and Lage (1973) studied the prevalence and life cycle of both *I. (=C.) felis* and *I. (=C.) rivolta* in domestic cats; they tried twice to administer sporulated oocysts of *I. (=C.) rivolta per os* to seven puppies, but the dogs "did not produce *Isospora* infections." Nukerbaeva and Svanbaev (1974, 1977) collected oocysts from domestic cats and tried to transmit this species to two 5-month-old foxes (*V. vulpes*), two 40-day-old Arctic foxes (*V. lagopus*), and two 1-year-old minks (*N. vison*), but none of these animals became infected. They were successful in transmitting it to a control cat, which shed oocysts in its feces on the 8th DPI. Dubey and Streitel (1976b) compared feeding sporulated oocysts to cats by feeding them *I. (=C.) rivolta* MZTC-infected tissue stages of mice fed similar numbers of oocysts. They found that the prepatent period of *I. (=C.) rivolta* was the same and that the number of oocysts excreted by cats was similar regardless of inoculum. Dubey (1979b) showed that sporulated oocysts of *I. (=C.) rivolta* will excyst in mice, and the liberated SZ most frequently infect their mesenteric lymph nodes and their MZTC increase in size for the first 31 days and remain viable (infective) for up to 23 months. MZTC of *I. (=C.) rivolta* also are found in the spleen, liver, and skeletal muscle of mice, but these MZTC are not transmissible from mouse to mouse either orally or by intraperitoneal inoculation of infected tissue. de Oliveira et al. (2007) demonstrated that orally-infective stages of *I. (=C.) rivolta* can form in gerbils (*M. unguiculatus*), guinea pigs (*C. porcellus*), rabbits (*O. cuniculus*), and chickens (*G. g. domesticus*) producing oocysts when fed to cats.

Pathology: *Cystoisospora rivolta* is pathogenic for newborn but not for weaned cats. Newborn cats fed 10^5 sporocysts or mice infected with intra- and extracellular zoites usually develop diarrhea 3–4 DPI; microscopically, desquamation of the tips of their villi and cryptitis occurs in the ileum and cecum in association with developmental stages (meronts, gamonts) of the parasite (Dubey, 1979b).

Materials deposited: None.

Remarks: Ryšavý (1954) measured oocysts identified as *I. (=C.) rivolta* that were 25 × 19 (20–28.5 × 16–20), L/W ratio: 1.3, with sporocysts 12–14; he said he found these oocysts in the red fox, *V. vulpes*, the Eurasian lynx, *L. lynx*, the jungle cat, *F.* (syn. *Chaus*) *chaus*, and in the domestic dog, *C. lupus familiaris*, all animals in and around Prague, Czech Republic; in all likelihood, of course, the oocysts identified from the canids were one or more species in the *I. (=C.) ohioensis* complex. Bearup (1954) reported *I. (=C.) rivolta* in cats and dogs and in a dingo in Sydney, Australia. These oocysts were spheroidal to ovoidal and measured L × W: 25.5 × 23.0 (23–28 × 20.5–27.5), L/W ratio: 1.1; sporocysts averaged L × W: 16.5 × 12.5, with sausage-shaped SZ, 10 × 3. Dubey and Pande (1963b) examined three jungle cats, *F. chaus*, in India (exact location not given), and recovered or isolated oocysts of *I. (=C.) rivolta*. The number of *I. (=C.) rivolta*-positive jungle cats was not stated. The authors only said that two jungle cats harbored "coccidian oocysts;" however, they also recorded the presence of four *Eimeria* spp. and "cryptosporidial oocysts." Patnaik (1966) reported finding this species in a cat in Orissa, Odisha, India. Fayer (1972a) was the first to grow feline *I. (=C.) rivolta* in mammalian cell cultures including feline kidney, embryonic bovine kidney, and Madin–Darby canine kidney cell cultures. Pellérdy (1974b) proposed the name *I. novocati* for *I. (=C.) rivolta* from the cat because he believed that *I. (=C.) rivolta* was initially discovered and described from the dog by Grassi (1879). However, Wenyon (1923) did an historical review of the literature on the coccidia of cats and dogs and concluded that *I. (=C.) rivolta* was first discovered in the cat and later in the dog. Dubey (1975c) agreed with Wenyon's (1923) assessment and, after having read Wenyon's (1923) paper, so do we. Based on these historical facts, Pellérdy's (1974b) name must be considered a *nomen nudum*.

Mandal (1976) said that ovoidal oocysts were 10–25×15–22, lacked an OR, and sporocysts measured 16×10 and had a SR. Dubey (1977a) infected eight 12–24-month-old SPF female cats *per os* with cysts in the brains of mice infected with *T. gondii* (0 DPI), and then with 10^4 sporulated oocysts of *I.* (=*C.*) *rivolta* and *I.* (=*C.*) *felis* (39 DPI), and, finally, with cysts of the CR-4 strain of *Hammondia hammondi*. He then caged four males, and all eight females became pregnant and delivered 48 healthy kittens. One kitten became infected with *T. gondii*, but Dubey (1977a) thought it was because of fecal contamination; he was unable to demonstrate that any of these organisms were transmitted transplacentally by the queens to the remaining 47 newborn kittens. Smith and Frenkel (1978) noted that lab mice housed in the same room as cats that shed sporulated sporocysts of *S. muris*, occasionally developed muscle sarcocysts "spontaneously." They said that cat feces never came in contact with mouse cages, but they did see German cockroaches (*Blatella germanica*) in the same room from time-to-time. To assess the role of *B. germanica* and the American cockroach (*Periplaneta americana*) in transmission, cockroaches were exposed to cat feces that contained oocysts of *I. rivolta* and *T. gondii*. They found that oocysts of *I.* (=*C.*) *rivolta* were transmitted to mice by both cockroach species for at least 10 days. Fayer and Frenkel (1979) fed a mixture of from 100×10^3 to 570×10^3 sporulated oocysts of *I.* (=*C.*) *felis* and *I.* (=*C.*) *rivolta*, from a Costa Rican cat, to two calves in each of two experiments. Weight gains for all calves were normal and no gross lesions were observed. Calves were killed 26 to 115 DPI and calf organs were pooled, ground, and fed to two coccidia-free cats in each experiment. All cats fed organs from the inoculated calves shed unsporulated *I.* (=*C.*) *felis* oocysts from 4 to 10 days later and unsporulated *I.* (=*C.*) *rivolta* oocysts from 2 to 11 days later. Fayer and Frenkel (1979) also fed sporulated oocysts of *I.* (=*C.*) *rivolta* to calves to look for clinical signs of infection for 26–115 DPI, but no gross lesions, microscopic lesions, or parasites were found

in any of the experimentally-infected calves. However, although *I.* (=*C.*) *rivolta* was not pathogenic in calves, oocysts were shed by cats that ingested organs from calves infected with a mixture of *I.* (=*C.*) *felis* and *C. rivolta* oocysts. McKenna and Charleston (1982) studied the activation and excystation of *I.* (=*C.*) *rivolta* sporozoites and found activation under a wide range of *in vitro* conditions. The presence of bile appeared to be essential for this process to occur, but the presence of trypsin did not.

Matsui et al. (1993c) heated fresh, unsporulated oocysts of *I.* (=*C.*) *rivolta* at 50°C for 5 min and then immersed them in cold 2% potassium dichromate ($K_2Cr_2O_7$) solution and incubated them at 25°C to observe sporulation. After 39 hours, 43% of the oocysts had developed the morphology of *Caryospora*-type oocysts; that is, with one SP containing eight SZ rather than the typical *Isospora*-type oocyst with two SP, each with four SZ. They then inoculated mice and cats with only *Caryospora*-type sporulated oocysts. Four coccidia-free cats given these *Caryospora*-type oocysts started shedding oocysts 6–7 DPI, similar to those cats given the normal *I. rivolta* oocysts and in similar numbers. When mesenteric lymph nodes and spleens of four mice given *Caryospora*-type oocysts were fed to four other cats, the cats shed oocysts starting 6–9 DPI. Freshly passed oocysts from cats fed mouse tissues or *Caryospora*-type oocysts were incubated in 2% $K_2Cr_2O_7$ at 25°C and all of them developed into *Isospora*-type oocysts after sporulation. In an earlier study, Matsui et al. (1989) reported that some isosporan oocysts developed into *Tyzzeria*- or *Caryospora*-type oocysts and some eimerian oocysts developed into *Isospora*-type oocysts after sporulation following heat treatment at 50°C for 5 min. All of these transformed sporulated oocysts contained eight sporozoites with the number of sporocysts varying from zero to two. The underlying mechanisms for this transformation are not understood. Moudgil (2015), in his masters' thesis, said he recovered oocysts of *I.* (=*C.*) *rivolta* in the feces of a leopard; these oocysts measured 25.4×21.5 (23.5–28×19–23.5), L/W ratio: 1.2.

GENUS *LEOPARDUS* GRAY, 1842 (9 SPECIES)

CYSTOISOSPORA FELIS (WENYON, 1923) FRENKEL, 1977

Type host: *Felis catus* L., 1758, Domestic Cat.

Other definitive host: *Leopardus pardalis* (L., 1758), Ocelot.

Remarks: Lainson (1968) reported a pet ocelot of a family in the El Cayo District, Belize, that became very sick when 3-months-old, showing symptoms of abdominal pain, emaciation, and passing watery, loose stools; on examination oocysts of *I.* (=*C.*) *felis* were found in the stools. For full species description of *C. felis*, see above.

GENUS *LEPTAILURUS* SEVERTZOV, 1858 (MONOTYPIC)

CYSTOISOSPORA FELIS (WENYON, 1923) FRENKEL, 1977

Type host: *Felis catus* L., 1758, Domestic Cat.

Other definitive host: *Leptailurus serval* (Schreber, 1776), Serval.

Remarks: Mackinnon and Dibb (1938) said they found oocysts of *I.* (=*C.*) *felis* in 1/2 (50%) of the servals they examined (see full species description of *C. felis*, above).

CYSTOISOSPORA RIVOLTA (GRASSI, 1879) FRENKEL, 1977

Type host: *Felis catus* L., 1758, Domestic Cat.

Other definitive host: *Leptailurus serval* (Schreber, 1776), Serval.

Remarks: Ryšavý (1954) measured oocysts identified as *I.* (=*C.*) *rivolta* that were 25×19 (20–28.5 × 16–20), L/W ratio: 1.3, with sporocysts 12–14; he said he found these oocysts in the Eurasian lynx, *L. lynx*.

GENUS *LYNX* KERR, 1752 (4 SPECIES)

CYSTOISOSPORA FELIS (WENYON, 1923) FRENKEL, 1977

Type host: *Felis catus* L., 1758, Domestic Cat.

Other definitive host: *Lynx lynx* (L., 1758), Eurasian Lynx.

Remarks: Yakimoff et al. (1933b) examined fecal material of three *L. lynx*, at the Leningrad Zoological Gardens (1), and a menagerie at Gandscha (2), and found them all to be passing oocysts that they identified as *I.* (=*C.*) *felis*, when they sporulated. These oocysts from the Gandscha lynxes were L×W (n=100): 45.5×35.0 (39.5–50 × 31–40), L/W ratio: 1.3; M, OR, PG: all absent; ovoidal sporocysts were L×W (n=100): 23–25 × 18–22 (means not given). The oocysts from the lynx in Leningrad were L×W (n=50): 36×29 (30–42 × 24.5–33), L/W ratio: 1.2; M, OR, PG: all absent; sporocysts were L×W (n=50): 21–22 × 17–18 (ranges not given); they provided four line drawings, but no other information was given.

GENUS *PRIONAILURUS* SEVERTZOV, 1858 (5 SPECIES)

CYSTOISOSPORA VIVERRINA (AGRAWAL AND CHAUHAN, 1993) NOV. COMB.

Synonym: *Isospora viverrina* Agrawal and Chauhan, 1993.

Type host: *Prionailurus* (syn. *Felis*) *viverrinus* (Bennett, 1833), Fishing Cat.

Type locality: Asia: India: Uttar Pradesh, Kanpur Zoo.

Other definitive hosts: None to date.

Known intermediate host: None to date.

Geographic distribution: Asia: India.

Description of sporulated oocyst: Oocyst shape: ellipsoidal, with one end slightly narrower; number of walls, 2; wall characteristics: smooth, ~1.3

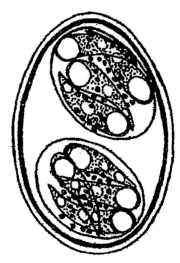

FIGURE 14.29   Line drawing of the sporulated oocyst of *Cystoisospora viverrina*. *Fig. 1, Agrawal, R.D., Chauhan, P.P.S., 1993. On a new coccidium* Isospora viverrina *from fishing cat (Felis viverrina). Indian Journal of Animal Sciences 63, 628–629, with permission of the Editor and the copyright holder for IJAS.*

thick; outer is yellow, whereas inner is yellow-brown; L×W (n=15): 31.9×26.6 (31–33×25–27), L/W ratio: 1.2; M, OR, PG: all absent. Distinctive features of oocyst: none, a "typical" cystoisosporan-type oocyst from a felid, without M, OR, or PG.

Description of sporocyst and sporozoites: Sporocyst shape: ovoidal; L×W (n=15): 19.9×14.6 (10–21×13–16), L/W ratio: 1.4; SB, SSB, PSB: all absent; SR: present; SR characteristics: coarsely-granular scattered particles throughout the SP; SZ: banana-shaped, 12.6×4.0 (12–13×3–5) with broadly rounded ends that contain one prominent, spheroidal RB, whereas smaller spheroidal RB was seen at the pointed end, with a central N. Distinctive features of sporocyst: without SB, SSB, PSB, but with a large, scattered SR of numerous small granules and RBs at each end of the SZ, with a central N.

Prevalence: Found in the only fishing cat examined in the Kanpur Zoo, India.

Sporulation: Exogenous. Sporulation took 4 days when strained feces were left in 2.5% potassium dichromate ($K_2Cr_2O_7$) solution, presumably at room temperature.

Prepatent and patent periods: Unknown.
Site of infection in definitive host: Unknown.
Endogenous stages: Unknown.
Cross-transmission: None to date.
Pathology: Unknown.
Materials deposited: None.

Remarks: Agrawal and Chauhan (1993) found numerous oocysts of an isosporan they described as a new species in the feces of a fishing cat from the Kanpur Zoo, India. They provided only line drawings of the sporulated oocyst, a sporocyst, and a SZ. They compared the dimensions of this form only to those of *I. bigemina* (large form) from domestic dogs, cats, foxes, and a polecat, to *I.* (=*C.*) *rivolta* from domestic dogs and cats and the dingo, and to *I.* (=*C.*) *felis* from the domestic cat, with all their descriptive information coming from Pellérdy (1974a). To our knowledge, this species has never been found again in any felids.

SUBFAMILY PANTHERINAE POCOCK, 1917

GENUS *NEOFELIS* GRAY, 1867 (MONOTYPIC)

CYSTOISOSPORA LEOPARDI (AGRAWAL, AHLUWALIA, BHATIA, AND CHAUHAN, 1981) NOV. COMB.

Synonym: *Isospora leopardi* Agrawal, Ahluwalia, Bhatia, and Chauhan, 1981.

Type host: *Neofelis nebulosa* (Griffith, 1821), Clouded Leopard.

Type locality: Asia: India: Uttar Pradesh, Lucknow Zoo.

Other definitive hosts: None to date.

Known intermediate host: None to date.

Geographic distribution: Asia: India.

Description of sporulated oocyst: Oocyst shape: ovoidal; number of walls, 2; wall characteristics: smooth; outer is yellowish, whereas inner is dark brown, ~1.5 thick; L×W: 41.0×25.2 (39–45×23–27), L/W ratio: 1.6 (1.5–1.7); M, OR, PG: all absent. Distinctive features of oocyst: distinctly

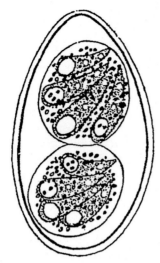

FIGURE 14.30 Line drawing of the sporulated oocyst of *Cystoisospora leopardi*. Fig. 3, Agrawal, R.D., Ahluwalia, S.S., Bhatia, B.B., Chauhan, P.P.S., 1981. Note on mammalian coccidia at Lucknow Zoo. *Indian Journal of Animal Sciences* 51 (1–6), 125, 128, with permission of the Editor and the copyright holder for IJAS.

ovoidal shape, a smooth, two-layered wall, but without M, PG, and OR.

Description of sporocyst and sporozoites: Sporocyst shape: ovoidal; L×W: 18.0×17.3 (16–20×16–19), L/W ratio: 1.0; SB, SSB, PSB: all absent; SR: present; SR characteristics: scattered small granules throughout the SP; SZ: banana-shaped, 13×4.3 (11.5–16×4–5) with broadly rounded ends that contain one prominent, spheroidal RB. Distinctive features of sporocyst: without SB, SSB, PSB, but with a large, scattered SR of numerous small granules.

Prevalence: Unknown; presumably collected from only one clouded leopard in the Lucknow Zoo, India.

Sporulation: Exogenous.

Prepatent and patent periods: Unknown.

Site of infection in definitive host: Unknown.

Endogenous stages: Unknown.

Cross-transmission: None to date.

Pathology: Unknown.

Materials deposited: None.

Remarks: Agrawal et al. (1981) said the oocysts of this species differed from the three species

described from the closely related lion (*P. leo*), was the only species reported from the clouded leopard, and on the basis of the distinctly ovoidal shape, their large size, and scattered granules of its SR. This species description is modest by any standard and we include it here only because the authors included a line drawing. To our knowledge, this species has not been found since its original description.

GENUS PANTHERA (L., 1758) (4 SPECIES)

CYSTOISOSPORA BENGALENSI (PATNAIK AND ACHARJYO, 1971) NOV. COMB.

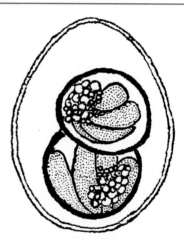

FIGURE 14.31 Original line drawing of the sporulated oocyst of *Cystoisospora bengalensi*. Modified from Fig. 4, Patnaik, M.M., Acharjyo, L.N., 1971. Notes on the coccidian parasites of wild mammals in captivity at Nandankanan. *Orissa Veterinary Journal* 6 (3/4), 133–135.

Synonym: *Isospora bengalensi* Patnaik and Acharjyo, 1971.

Type host: *Panthera tigris tigris* (L., 1758), Bengal Tiger.

Type locality: Asia: India, Odisha, Bhubaneswar, Nandankanan Zoological Park.

Other definitive hosts: None to date.

Known intermediate host: None to date.

Geographic distribution: Asia: India.

Description of sporulated oocyst: Oocyst shape: ovoidal to broadly ovoidal; number of walls, 1 (line drawing); wall characteristics: smooth, thin; L × W: 40 × 30 (ranges not given), L/W ratio: 1.3; M, OR, PG: all absent. Distinctive features of oocyst: large size with ovoidal shape, a smooth, single-layered wall, but without M, PG, and OR.

Description of sporocyst and sporozoites: Sporocyst shape: ovoidal; L × W: 11.0 × 9.5 (ranges not given), L/W ratio: 1.2; SB, SSB, PSB: all absent (line drawing); SR: present; SR characteristics: a prominent, spheroidal mass composed of small granules that takes up about two-thirds the volume of the SP; SZ: banana-shaped, 8.8 × 2.8; no information given on RB or N. Distinctive features of sporocyst: without SB, SSB, PSB but with a large, compact, spheroidal SR.

Prevalence: Apparently found in the only Bengal tiger sampled in Nandankanan Zoological Park by Patnaik and Acharjyo (1971).

Sporulation: Exogenous. Oocysts required 72 hours to sporulate when maintained in 2.5% potassium dichromate ($K_2Cr_2O_7$) solution at room temperature.

Prepatent and patent periods: Unknown.

Site of infection in definitive host: Unknown.

Endogenous stages: Unknown.

Cross-transmission: None to date.

Pathology: Unknown.

Materials deposited: None.

Remarks: This species was unknown to Levine and Ivens (1981). The original description by Patnaik and Acharjyo (1971) is marginal and we would relegate to a *species inquirenda* except for the fact that the authors included a line drawing. Patnaik and Acharjyo (1977) later published a "short communication" pointing out that Mandal and Chakravarty (1964) had published a description of *Isospora*-type oocysts from a crow in India (*Corvus splendens* Vieillot, 1817) and named a new species for them as *I. bengalensis*. The sporocysts of the Mandal and Chakravarty (1964) species are distinct in that they possess a SB. Nonetheless, even though the specific epitaphs are spelled slightly differently, Patnaik and Acharjyo (1977) thought it

necessary to change the name of the isosporan they had found in the Bengal tiger (*I. bengalensi*) to *Isospora nandankanani* because, "some are apt to consider the name of the feline species as an homonym of the form from avian host." Although this was a reasonable thought, the action was unnecessary in spite of the similar spellings. In addition, they apparently misspelled the epitaph because in the reprints they sent to colleagues, they inked-in "*nandankanansis*" as the correct spelling of their proposed name change; that name becomes a *nomen nudum*. To our knowledge, this "species" has not been found or reported since its original description.

CYSTOISOSPORA FELINA (PATNAIK AND ACHARJYO, 1971) NOV. COMB.

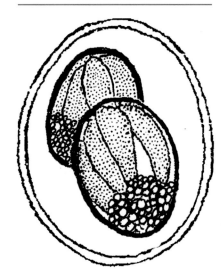

FIGURE 14.32 Original line drawing of the sporulated oocyst of *Cystoisospora feline. Modified from Figure 3, Patnaik, M.M., Acharjyo, L.N., 1971. Notes on the coccidian parasites of wild mammals in captivity at Nandankanan. Orissa Veterinary Journal 6 (3/4), 133–135.*

Synonym: *Isospora felina* Patnaik and Acharjyo, 1971.

Type host: *Panthera tigris tigris* (L., 1758), Bengal Tiger.

Type locality: Asia: India, Odisha, Bhubaneswar, Nandankanan Zoological Park.

Other definitive hosts: None to date.

Known intermediate host: None to date.

Geographic distribution: Asia: India.

Description of sporulated oocyst: Oocyst shape: ellipsoidal; number of walls, 1 (line drawing); wall characteristics: smooth, thin; L × W: 25 × 20 (ranges not given), L/W ratio: 1.25; M, OR, PG: all absent (line drawing). Distinctive features of oocyst: small size with ellipsoidal shape, a smooth, single-layered wall, but without M, PG, and OR.

Description of sporocyst and sporozoites: Sporocyst shape: ovoidal; L × W: 21 × 15 (ranges not given), L/W ratio: 1.4; SB, SSB, PSB: all absent (line drawing); SR: present; SR characteristics: a prominent, spheroidal mass composed of small granules that takes up about one-third the volume of the SP; SZ: banana-shaped, 10 × 3 (ranges not given). Distinctive features of sporocyst: without SB, SSB, PSB, but with a large, compact, spheroidal SR.

Prevalence: Apparently found in the only Bengal tiger sampled in Nandankanan Zoological Park, India by Patnaik and Acharjyo (1971).

Sporulation: Exogenous. Oocysts required 48 hours to sporulate when maintained in 2.5% potassium dichromate ($K_2Cr_2O_7$) solution at room temperature.

Prepatent and patent periods: Unknown.

Site of infection in definitive host: Unknown.

Endogenous stages: Unknown.

Cross-transmission: None to date.

Pathology: Unknown.

Materials deposited: None.

Remarks: This species was unknown to Levine and Ivens (1981). The original description is marginal by every measure and we would relegate to a *species inquirenda* except for the fact that the authors included a line drawing. This "species" has not been found or reported since its original description.

CYSTOISOSPORA FELIS (WENYON, 1923) FRENKEL, 1977

Type host: *Felis catus* L., 1758, Domestic Cat.

Other definitive hosts: *Panthera leo* (L., 1758), Lion; *Panthera tigris* (L., 1758), Tiger.

Remarks: Yakimoff et al. (1933b) examined fecal material of three lions, *P. leo*, and two tigers, *P. tigris*, in the Leningrad Zoological Gardens and found them all to be passing oocysts that they identified as *I.* (=*C.*) *felis*, when they sporulated. These oocysts from the lions were L × W (n = 75): 44.5 × 33.6 (38–50 × 29–36), L/W ratio: 1.3; M, OR, PG: all absent; ovoidal sporocysts were L × W (n = 75): 29.7 × 18.0 (ranges not given), L/W ratio: 1.7. The oocysts from the tigers were L × W (n = 30): 39.5 × 30.5 (34–45 × 22–35), L/W ratio: 1.3; M, OR, PG: all absent; sporocysts were L × W (n = 30): 20–22 × 16.5 (ranges not given). Line drawings were given for both, but no other information was provided.

CYSTOISOSPORA LEONINA (MANDAL AND RAY, 1960) NOV. COMB.

FIGURE. A modest photomicrograph of a sporulated oocyst of *C. leonina* is in Mandal and Ray (1960), *Bulletin of the Calcutta School of Tropical Medicine* 8, p. 107, but we were unable to reproduce it here.

Synonym: *Isospora leonina* Mandal and Ray, 1960.

Type host: *Panthera leo* (L., 1758), Lion.

Type locality: Asia: India: Calcutta, Zoological Garden.

Other definitive hosts: None to date.

Known intermediate host: None to date.

Geographic distribution: Asia: India.

Description of sporulated oocyst: Oocyst shape: ovoidal; number of walls, 2; wall characteristics: outer is orange, ~1.5 thick, and the inner is colorless, ~1 thick; L × W: 31.8 × 28.2 (30–32 × 28–31),

L/W ratio: 1.1; M, OR: both absent; Mandal and Ray (1960) did not mention if a PG is present or absent, but Patnaik and Acharjyo (1970) said that a small PG, "adjacent to the greater side" was sometimes present in sporulated oocysts (whatever that means). Distinctive features of oocyst: two-layered thick wall, ~2.5 total thickness, without M, OR, but with a small PG.

Description of sporocyst and sporozoites: Sporocyst shape: ovoidal; L×W: means not given (16–20×13.5–15), L/W ratio: unknown; SB, SSB, PSB: all absent; SR: present; SR characteristics: a coarsely-granular mass that assumes the form of a solid mass, 4.5 wide, about 2 days after sporulation; SZ: sausage-shaped, 9.5 long (Mandal, 1976) or 12×3 (Patnaik and Acharjyo, 1970), but no information was given on visibility of RB or N. Distinctive features of sporocyst: without SB, SSB, PSB, but with a large, compact SR.

Prevalence: Mandal and Ray (1960) apparently found oocysts of this species in 1/2 (50%) lion cubs that were showing diarrhea.

Sporulation: Exogenous. Mandal and Ray (1960) said that unsporulated oocysts kept in 2.5% potassium dichromate ($K_2Cr_2O_7$) solution completed their sporulation in 24–48 hours at 33°C. Patnaik and Acharjyo (1970) said sporulation was completed in 5 days but did not mention the temperature at which they were incubated.

Prepatent and patent periods: Unknown.

Site of infection in definitive host: Unknown.

Endogenous stages: Unknown.

Cross-transmission: Mandal and Ray (1960) tried to infect "a clean 20-days-old pup with numerous mature oocysts of *Isospora leonina*." They examined the dog's feces for 15 DPI, but never found it to pass oocysts.

Pathology: Unknown.

Materials deposited: None.

Remarks: Mandal and Ray (1960) described the oocyst shape as "rhomboidal," but their photomicrograph of a sporulated oocyst shows it to be clearly ovoidal, with one end slightly pointed. Patnaik and Acharjyo (1970) reported this species from an African lion and said the oocysts were 32×29 (30–33×28–30), L/W ratio: 1.1, with a thin wall and without a M; they also provided a primitive line drawing of a sporocyst, and they seemed convinced that this species is distinct from other *Isospora*-type species recorded from felids. Levine and Ivens (1981) questioned whether or not this was a true parasite of the lion. This question remains to be answered.

CYSTOISOSPORA MOHINI (AGRAWAL, AHLUWALIA, BHATIA, AND CHAUHAN, 1981) NOV. COMB.

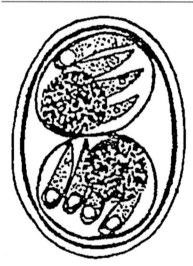

FIGURE 14.33 Line drawing of the sporulated oocyst of *Cystoisospora mohini*. Fig. 2, Agrawal, R.D., Ahluwalia, S.S., Bhatia, B.B., Chauhan, P.P.S,. 1981. Note on mammalian coccidia at Lucknow zoo. *Indian Journal of Animal Sciences* 51 (1–6), 125–128, with permission of the Editor and the copyright holder for IJAS.

Synonym: *Isospora mohini* Agrawal, Ahluwalia, Bhatia, and Chauhan, 1981.

Type host: *Panthera leo* (L., 1758) (syn. *Leo leo* Frisch, 1775), Lion.

Type locality: Asia: India: Uttar Pradesh, Lucknow Zoo.

Other definitive hosts: None to date.

Known intermediate host: None to date.

Geographic distribution: Asia: India.

Description of sporulated oocyst: Oocyst shape: ovoidal to broadly ellipsoidal; number of walls, 2; wall characteristics: smooth; outer is yellow-green, whereas inner is dark brown, total thickness ~1.5; L×W: 23.0×17.3 (19–27×14–20), L/W ratio: 1.3 (1.2–1.4); M, OR, PG: all absent. Distinctive features of oocyst: small size with ovoidal shape, a smooth, two-layered wall, but without M, PG, and OR.

Description of sporocyst and sporozoites: Sporocyst shape: ovoidal; L×W: 13.0×7.9 (11.5–19×7–10), L/W ratio: 1.6; SB, SSB, PSB: all absent; SR: present; SR characteristics: a prominent, spheroidal mass composed of small granules that take up about one-third the volume of the SP; SZ: banana-shaped, 9.4×2.2 (8–11×2–3) with broadly rounded ends that contain one prominent, spheroidal RB. Distinctive features of sporocyst: without SB, SSB, PSB, but with a large, compact, spheroidal SR.

Prevalence: Unknown; presumably collected from only one lion in the Lucknow Zoo, India.

Sporulation: Exogenous.

Prepatent and patent periods: Unknown.

Site of infection in definitive host: Unknown.

Endogenous stages: Unknown.

Cross-transmission: None to date.

Pathology: Unknown.

Materials deposited: None.

Remarks: Agrawal et al. (1981) said this species differed from isosporans at their time on the basis of its shape, the smaller size range of oocysts (18.7–27.4×14.4–20.2), and its sporocysts and small elongate SZ. This species description is modest, and we include it here only because the authors included a line drawing. To our knowledge, this species has not been found since its original description.

CYSTOISOSPORA PANTHERI (AGRAWAL, AHLUWALIA, BHATIA, AND CHAUHAN, 1981) NOV. COMB.

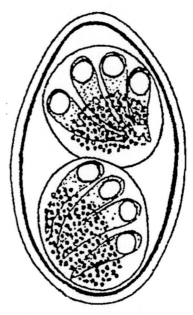

FIGURE 14.34 Line drawing of the sporulated oocyst of *Cystoisospora pantheri*. *Fig. 1, Agrawal, R.D., Ahluwalia, S.S., Bhatia, B.B., Chauhan, P.P.S,. 1981. Note on mammalian coccidia at Lucknow zoo. Indian Journal of Animal Sciences 51 (1–6), 125–128, with permission of the Editor and the copyright holder for IJAS.*

Synonym: *Isospora pantheri* Agrawal, Ahluwalia, Bhatia, and Chauhan, 1981.

Type host: *Panthera leo* (L., 1758) (syn. *Leo leo* Frisch, 1775), Lion.

Type locality: Asia: India: Uttar Pradesh, Lucknow Zoo.

Other definitive hosts: None to date.

Known intermediate host: None to date.

Geographic distribution: Asia: India.

Description of sporulated oocyst: Oocyst shape: ellipsoidal; number of walls, 2; wall characteristics: smooth, ~1.5 thick; outer is light yellow, and inner is dark brown; L×W: 36.7×22.3 (33–40×20–26), L/W ratio: 1.6 (1.5–1.9); M, OR, PG: all absent. Distinctive features of oocyst: ellipsoidal shape, slightly pointed at one end, with a smooth, two-layered wall, but without M, PG, and OR.

Description of sporocyst and sporozoites: Sporocyst shape: ovoidal; L×W: 17.3×14.4 (14–20×11.5–15.5), L/W ratio: 1.2; SB, SSB, PSB: all absent; SR: present; SR characteristics: a prominent, spheroidal to ellipsoidal mass composed of small granules that takes up about one-half the volume of the SP; SZ: banana-shaped, 12.2×3.6 (11.5–14×3–4), with broadly rounded ends that contain one prominent, spheroidal RB. Distinctive features of sporocyst: large size, without SB, SSB, PSB, but with a large, compact, spheroidal to ovoidal SR.

Prevalence: Unknown; presumably collected from only one lion in the Lucknow Zoo, India.

Sporulation: Exogenous.

Prepatent and patent periods: Unknown.

Site of infection in definitive host: Unknown.

Endogenous stages: Unknown.

Cross-transmission: None to date.

Pathology: Unknown.

Materials deposited: None.

Remarks: Agrawal et al. (1981) said this species differed from *I. leonina* (Mandal and Ray, 1960) and *Isospora* sp. (Pande et al., 1970) because *I.* (=C.) *pantheri* has larger, ellipsoidal oocysts, lacks a PG that is present in *I. leonina*, and its SZs may be slightly larger, and those of *I. pantheri* differ from the latter in oocyst shape, being larger, 33–40×20–26 *vs.* 23–33×20–28, with a larger L/W ratio, 1.5–1.9 *vs.* 1.1–1.4, and the sporocyst shapes were different. This species description is modest by every standard, and we include it here only because the authors included a line drawing. To our knowledge, this species has not been found since its original description.

CYSTOISOSPORA PARDUSI (PATNAIK AND ACHARJYO, 1971) NOV. COMB.

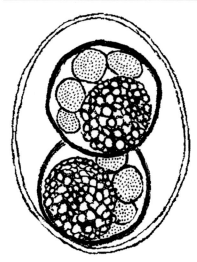

FIGURE 14.35 Original line drawing of the sporulated oocyst of *Cystoisospora pardusi. Modified from Fig. 2, Patnaik, M.M., Acharjyo, L.N., 1971. Notes on the coccidian parasites of wild mammals in captivity at Nandankanan. Orissa Veterinary Journal 6 (3/4), 133–135.*

Synonym: *Isospora pardusi* Patnaik and Acharjyo, 1971.

Type host: *Panthera pardus* (L., 1758), Leopard.

Type locality: Asia: India, Odisha, Bhubaneswar, Nandankanan Zoological Park.

Other definitive hosts: None to date.

Known intermediate host: None to date.

Geographic distribution: Asia: India.

Description of sporulated oocyst: Oocyst shape: ovoidal; number of walls, 1 (line drawing); wall characteristics: smooth, thin; L×W: 45×33 (40–49×30–36), L/W ratio: 1.4; M, OR, PG: all absent (line drawing). Distinctive features of oocyst: large size with ovoidal shape, a smooth, single-layered wall, but without M, PG, or OR.

Description of sporocyst and sporozoites: Sporocyst shape: spheroidal (line drawing); L×W: 22.5×18 (ranges not given), L/W ratio: 1.25; SB, SSB, PSB: all absent; SR: present; SR characteristics: a prominent, spheroidal mass, 18×12, composed of small granules that takes up about three-fourths the volume of the SP; SZ: "elongate," 15×4.5. Distinctive features of sporocyst: without SB, SSB, PSB, but with a large, compact, spheroidal SR.

Prevalence: Apparently found in the only leopard cub sampled in Nandankanan Zoological Park, India by Patnaik and Acharjyo (1971).

Sporulation: Exogenous. Oocysts required 72 hours to sporulate when maintained in 2.5% potassium dichromate ($K_2Cr_2O_7$) solution at room temperature.

Prepatent and patent periods: Unknown.
Site of infection in definitive host: Unknown.
Endogenous stages: Unknown.
Cross-transmission: None to date.
Pathology: Unknown.
Materials deposited: None.

Remarks: This species was unknown to Levine and Ivens (1981). The original description is marginal by every measure, and we would relegate to a *species inquirenda* except for the fact that the authors included a line drawing. This "species" has not been found or reported since its original description.

CYSTOISOSPORA RIVOLTA (GRASSI, 1879) FRENKEL, 1977

Type host: *Felis catus* L., 1758, Domestic Cat.
Other definitive hosts: *Panthera pardus* (L., 1758), Leopard; *Panthera tigris* (L., 1758), Tiger.

Remarks: Yakimoff et al. (1933b) examined fecal material of two tigers, *P. tigris*, and one leopard, *P. pardus*, in the Leningrad Zoological Gardens and found them all to be passing oocysts that they identified as *I.* (=*C.*) *rivolta*, when they sporulated. The oocysts from the tigers were $L \times W$ (n=50): 22.1×16.5 ($18-25 \times 13-20$), L/W ratio: 1.3; M, OR, PG: all absent; sporocysts were $L \times W$ (n=50): $14-18 \times 11-13$ (means not given). The oocysts from the leopard were $L \times W$ (n=20): 23.0×17.5 ($20-25.5 \times 15-21$), L/W

ratio: 1.3; M, OR, PG: all absent; sporocysts were $L \times W$ (n=20): $13-15 \times 11-12$ (means not given). Yakimoff et al. (1933b) included three line drawings, but no other information was provided.

FAMILY HERPESTIDAE BONAPARTE, 1845

GENUS CROSSARCHUS F.G. CUVIER, 1825 (4 SPECIES)

CYSTOISOSPORA GARNHAMI (BRAY, 1954) NOV. COMB.

Type host: *Helogale parvula* (Sundevall, 1847) (syn. *Helogale undulatus* (Peters, 1852)), Common Dwarf Mongoose.
Other definitive host: *Crossarchus obscurus* F.G. Cuvier, 1925, Common Kusimanse.

Remarks: Bray (1959) mentioned the postmortem examination of a specimen of *C. obscurus* that had been made by Professor H. Vogel, Liberian Institute of the American Foundation for Tropical Medicine, and the oocysts were transferred to Bray for identification. Bray (1959) reported that sporogony was completed in 3 days, revealing isosporan oocysts, which he identified as those of *I.* (=*C.*) *garnhami* (see below for full species description).

GENUS HELOGALE GRAY, 1862 (2 SPECIES)

CYSTOISOSPORA GARNHAMI (BRAY, 1954) NOV. COMB.

Synonym: *Isospora garnhami* Bray, 1954.
Type host: *Helogale parvula* (Sundevall, 1847) (syn. *Helogale undulatus* (Peters, 1852)), Common Dwarf Mongoose.
Type locality: Africa: Kenya, Kitui District.
Other definitive hosts: *Crossarchus obscurus* F.G. Cuvier, 1925, Common Kusimanse; *Herpestes*

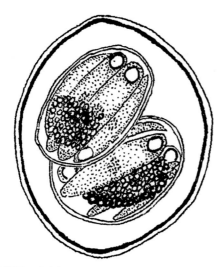

FIGURE 14.36 Original line drawing of the sporulated oocyst of *Cystoisospora garnhami*. *Modified from Fig. 62, Levine, N.D., Ivens, V., 1981. The Coccidian Parasites (Protozoa, Apicomplexa) of Carnivores. Illinois Biological Monograph No. 51, The University of Illinois Press, Urbana, Illinois USA. The University of Illinois Press has released the copyright.*

edwardsi (É. Geoffroy Saint-Hilaire, 1818) (syn. *Herpestes mungo* (Blanford, 1888)), Indian Gray Mongoose (Pellérdy, 1974a).

Known intermediate host: None to date.

Geographic distribution: Africa: Kenya, Liberia; Asia: India.

Description of sporulated oocyst: Oocyst shape: short-ellipsoidal; number of walls, 2; wall characteristics: a thin, fragile outer layer, and a thick, tough and elastic inner layer; L × W: 28.6 × 24.5 (26–32 × 22–28), L/W ratio: 1.2; M, OR, PG: all absent. Distinctive features of oocyst: two-layered wall, inner is thin and fragile, whereas outer is thicker, tough, and elastic, without M, OR, and PG.

Description of sporocyst and sporozoites: Sporocyst shape: spheroidal to ellipsoidal; L × W: 13.8 × 11.5 (12–15 × 11–12), L/W ratio: 1.2; SB, SSB, PSB: all absent; SR: present; SR characteristics: an irregular mass of coarse granules; SZ: sausage-shaped with one end slightly more pointed than the other, lie lengthwise in SP, and

measure 13.7 × 2.3, with a central N and a hyaline spheroidal RB at their more rounded end. Distinctive features of sporocyst: typical ellipsoidal shape, without SB, SSB, PSB and with a SR composed of coarse granules.

Prevalence: Bray (1954) found 10/10 *H. undulatus rufula* (syn. *Helogale parvula*) infected with oocysts of this form. The feces of all 10 animals were collected in Kenya by Professor P.C.C. Garnham and sent to Bray in the London School of Hygiene and Tropical Medicine. Dubey and Pande (1963a,b) recorded this species in 4/4 mongooses, *H. edwardsi* (syn. *H. mungo*) in India.

Sporulation: Exogenous. Bray (1954) said that about 30% of the oocysts of this form started sporulation in freshly passed feces and about 2% were completely sporulated. The remainder of the oocysts took 3 days to complete sporogony at 22°C when placed in 4% sodium dichromate solution ($Na_2Cr_2O_7$), and in 0.25% chromic acid. Dubey and Pande (1963a) said oocysts sporulated in 24 hours.

Prepatent and patent periods: Unknown.

Site of infection: Bray (1954) found the majority of oocysts of this form mostly in the large intestine and rectum.

Endogenous stages: Bray (1954) saw only three meronts in one small patch of the ileum; he did not measure them but said they contained from 12 to 24 merozoites. All stages of gamogony occurred in the lower small intestine and in the large intestine where young gametocytes were found in epithelial cells of the villi, usually in the distal end of each enterocyte. Microgametocytes had "apparently aimless patterning of nuclei" and were found mostly at the distal end of enterocytes. Mature microgametocytes were ellipsoidal, 23 × 22 in fixed tissues, with a large ellipsoidal residual body and the microgametes arranged haphazardly around it. One microgametocyte he saw contained 403 microgametes. Macrogametocytes had a tendency to develop toward the base of the enterocytes, forcing the HCN to one side or to the distal end of the cell. Mature macrogametocytes were 24 × 22 in fixed tissue.

Cross-transmission: Bray (1954) was unable to infect a coccidia-free ferret (*Mustela putorius furo*) or a newly-weaned kitten with sporulated oocysts of this form (but see *Remarks*, below).

Pathology: Bray (1954) could see no macroscopic changes in the alimentary tract of a mongoose infected with this species even though it still passed numerous oocysts nor did he notice any visible signs of distress in infected animals. Dubey and Pande (1963a) said the intestinal lining of infected mongooses "did not reveal any macroscopic lesions."

Materials deposited: None.

Remarks: The 10 mongooses examined by Bray (1954) all were infected with oocysts of two distinct morphotypes; the larger ones are described here, and the smaller forms he described and named *I.* (=*C.*) *hoarei* (see below). He argued that these oocysts from the mongoose were quite distinct from those of *I.* (=*C.*) *felis*, which are much larger, and those of *I. bigemina*, now known to be a form of *Sarcocystis*. He also noted that these oocysts are similar to those of *I.* (=*C.*) *rivolta* from cats and said, "their lack of infectivity for the kitten supports" their differentiation. Finally, Bray (1954, 1959) said that sporulated oocysts of *I.* (=*C.*) *garnhami* were indistinguishable from those first described as an unnamed *Lucetina* (=*Isospora*) species (Kotlán and Pospesch, 1933), from the badger (*M. meles*), but later named by Pellérdy (1955) as *I. melis*. In his cross-infection experiments with a ferret and a cat, he infected both with a combination of both oocyst forms. He observed that the ferret remained free of coccidial infection for 2 months PI, but the kitten began to discharge large, ovoidal oocysts 46 × 36 (40–48 × 35–40) 7 days after feeding; he concluded these larger oocysts were those of *I.* (=*C.*) *felis* and, thus, he said the kitten was refractory to infection by the two species he used in the inoculum. However, he did not mention how the kitten became infected spontaneously with oocysts of *I.* (=*C.*) *felis*. He also observed two aberrant oocysts of this form, one contained a single sporocyst with

eight sporozoites (like a *Caryospora* oocyst), and the second had three immature sporocysts. In his later paper, Bray (1959) reported receiving a local mongoose, *Cross. obscurus*, from a colleague, Professor H. Vogel, Liberian Institute of the American Foundation for Tropical Medicine (Harbel), which also had isosporan oocysts in its fecal material. Oocysts completed sporulation in 3 days and measured 26.6 × 19.7 (22–30 × 18–22), L/W ratio: 1.35; "all other measurements and in general morphology these oocysts were indistinguishable from those of *I. garnhami*." Bray (1959) had no doubt in his mind that this coccidium from *Cross. obscurus* from Liberia was also *I.* (=*C.*) *garnhami*. He also was adamant that the *Isospora* sp. of *Meles* "is morphologically identical with *I. garnhami*." This led him to postulate that because "the host specificities among *Isospora* of carnivores are uncertain," and "until carefully controlled cross-infection experiments can be done, the *Isospora* species in *Meles* should be referred to as *Isospora garnhami* (Kotlán and Pospesch, 1933) Bray, 1954 (Bray, 1959)." Pellérdy (1959) agreed with Bray (1954) that from the descriptions available, the oocysts of *I.* (=*C.*) *garnhami* cannot be differentiated from those of *I.* (=*C.*) *melis*, but concluded that "the coccidium in the badger should be referred to as *Isospora melis* (Kotlán and Pospesch, 1933) Pellérdy, 1955, and the coccidium in the mongoose as *Isospora garnhami* Bray, 1954," based on cross-infection work cited earlier in his paper. We believe that until genes in these various cystoisosporans from these disparate host species can be sequenced, it would be most prudent to keep the current terminology.

Dubey and Pande (1963a) recovered two kinds of oocysts from *H. edwardsi* (syn. *H. mungo*) and regarded both as *I.* (=*C.*) *garnhami*. Larger oocysts (n = 50) were ellipsoidal and were L × W: 27–34 × 23–27, with a two-layered wall, ~1–2 thick, consisting of a yellow-green outer, and a thinner, darker inner layer; sporocysts were L × W: 19–21 × 12–14, with a SR. Their (1963) smaller oocysts were spheroidal to ellipsoidal, L×W: 19–22×16–19, with sporocysts, L×W: 14–17×8–11. They concluded that both size forms belonged to this single species. Patnaik and Roy (1965) also found ovoidal to ellipsoidal oocysts in *H. edwardsi*, which they also regarded as *I.* (=*C.*) *garnhami*; their oocysts were ellipsoidal to ovoidal with a yellowish, two-layered wall and measured L×W (n=25): 23×42 (sic) (23–26×18–23), and had a L/W ratio: 1.1 (1.1–1.3); sporocysts were L×W:14×10 (12.5–14.5×6–12.5), L/W: 1.4; a large, granular SR was present. They said these oocysts sporulated in 1–2 days. The reports of finding *I.* (=*C.*) *garnhami* in *Herpestes* should be considered with caution.

Singh (1962, unpublished dissertation) believed *I.* (=*C.*) *rivolta* described from this host conformed to the description of *I.* (=*C.*) *garnhami* in every respect.

CYSTOISOSPORA HOAREI (BRAY, 1954) NOV. COMB.

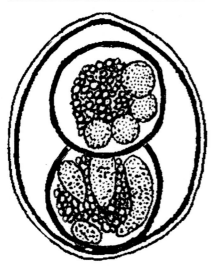

FIGURE 14.37 Original line drawing of the sporulated oocyst of *Cystoisospora hoarei*. *Modified Fig. 48, Levine, N.D., Ivens, V., 1981. The Coccidian Parasites (Protozoa, Apicomplexa) of Carnivores. Illinois Biological Monograph No. 51, The University of Illinois Press, Urbana, Illinois USA. The University of Illinois Press has released the copyright.*

Synonym: *Isospora hoarei* Bray, 1954.

Type host: *Helogale parvula* (Sundevall, 1847) (syn. *Helogale undulatus* (Peters, 1852)), Common Dwarf Mongoose.

Type locality: Africa: Kenya, Kitui District.

Other definitive host: *Herpestes edwardsi* (É. Geoffroy Saint-Hilaire, 1818) (syn. *Herpestes mungo* (Blanford, 1888)), Indian Gray Mongoose (Pellérdy, 1974a).

Known intermediate host: None to date.

Geographic distribution: Africa: Kenya; Asia: India.

Description of sporulated oocyst: Oocyst shape: ellipsoidal; number of walls, 2; wall characteristics: outer is colorless, and inner is darker and more fragile; L×W: 17.3×14.8 (16–19×13–17), L/W ratio: 1.2; M, OR, PG: all absent. Distinctive features of oocyst: two-layered wall, very thin and fragile, without M, OR, and PG.

Description of sporocyst and sporozoites: Sporocyst shape: spheroidal; L×W: 9×9 (9–10×8–9), L/W ratio: 1.0; SB, SSB, PSB: all absent; SR: present; SR characteristics: a large, mostly spheroidal mass of coarse granules in center of SP; SZ: sausage-shaped, slightly tapering at one end, 7.2×1.8, without a RB at either end. Distinctive features of sporocyst: typical ellipsoidal shape, without SB, SSB, PSB, and with a SR composed of coarse granules.

Prevalence: Bray (1954) found 10/10 *H. undulatus rufula* (syn. *Helogale parvula*) infected with this form.

Sporulation: Exogenous. Oocysts took 4 days to complete sporogony at 22°C when placed in 4% sodium dichromate solution ($Na_2Cr_2O_7$) or in 0.25% chromic acid solution.

Prepatent and patent periods: Unknown.

Site of infection: Majority of oocysts of this form were found in the duodenum and jejunum.

Endogenous stages: Bray (1954) was not able to find any meronts in his preserved tissues, but he did report mature macrogametes, 16×14, and mature microgamonts, 17×16. In one microgamont he counted 117 microgametes.

Cross-transmission: Bray (1954) was unable to infect a coccidia-free ferret (*Mustela putorius furo*) or a newly-weaned kitten with sporulated oocysts of this form (but see *Remarks*, above for *C. (=I.) garnhami*).

Pathology: Bray (1954) could see no macroscopic changes in the alimentary tract of a mongoose infected with this form even though it still was passing numerous oocysts nor did he notice any visible signs of distress in infected animals.

Materials deposited: None.

Remarks: Bray's (1954) observations on, and description of, endogenous development for this species should be regarded with caution because he was observing a mixed infection with *I. (=C.) garnhami*, so his interpretations of which stages fit which species is questionable. Patnaik and Roy (1965) said they found oocysts of this species in *H. edwardsi* and measured them; their oocysts were spheroidal or subspheroidal, occasionally ellipsoidal, with a yellowish outer wall and were: L×W (n=25): 19.0×17.6 (sic) (19–21×16 (?)), L/W ratio: ~1.1; M, OR: both absent, but a tiny PG may have been present (line drawing); ellipsoidal sporocysts were L×W (n=25): 10–12×8–10; SZ were banana- or sausage-shaped, and sporulation for these oocysts took 2–3 days.

GENUS *HERPESTES* ILLIGER, 1811

CYSTOISOSPORA DASGUPTAI (LEVINE, IVENS, AND HEALY, 1975) NOV. COMB.

Synonyms: *Isospora rivolta* (Grassi, 1879) of Knowles and Das Gupta (1931); *Isospora garnhami* (small form) Bray, 1954 of Dubey and Pande (1963a); *Isospora dasguptai* Levine, Ivens, and Healy, 1975; [non] *Isospora rivolta* (Grassi, 1879) Wenyon, 1923; [non] *Isospora garnhami* Bray, 1954.

Type host: *Herpestes javanicus* (É. Geoffroy Saint-Hilaire, 1818) (syn. *Herpestes auropunctatus* (Hodgson, 1836)), Small Asian Mongoose.

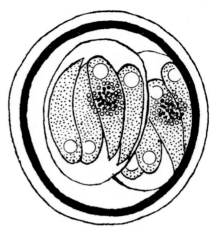

FIGURE 14.38 Original line drawing of the sporulated oocyst of *Cystoisospora dasguptai*. Modified Fig. 63, Levine, N.D., Ivens, V., 1981. *The Coccidian Parasites (Protozoa, Apicomplexa) of Carnivores. Illinois Biological Monograph No. 51*, The University of Illinois Press, Urbana, Illinois USA. *The University of Illinois Press has released the copyright.*

Type locality: Asia: India, Calcutta (?).

Other definitive host: *Herpestes edwardsi* (É. Geoffroy Saint-Hilaire, 1818) (syn. *Herpestes mungo* (Blanford, 1888)), Indian Gray Mongoose.

Known intermediate host: None to date.

Geographic distribution: Asia: India.

Description of sporulated oocyst: Oocyst shape: ellipsoidal to ovoidal; number of walls, 2; wall characteristics: not mentioned; L×W: 20.6×17.2 (19–22×16–19), L/W ratio: 1.2; M, OR, PG: all absent. Distinctive features of oocyst: only that the M, OR, and PG are all absent.

Description of sporocyst and sporozoites: Sporocyst shape: ellipsoidal; L×W: mean not given, 14–17×8–11, L/W ratio: unknown; SB, SSB, PSB: all absent; SR: present, but no details are given; SZ: sausage-shaped, slightly tapering at one end, and may have a clear globule at the broader end, but no other details are known. Distinctive features of sporocyst: typical ellipsoidal shape, without SB, SSB, PSB and with a SR composed of some granules.

Prevalence: Unknown.

Sporulation: Exogenous. Knowles and Das Gupta (1931) said oocysts were passed unsporulated and Dubey and Pande (1963a) said sporulation was completed in 1 day.

Prepatent and patent periods: Unknown.

Site of infection: Unknown.

Endogenous stages: Unknown.

Cross-transmission: Unknown.

Pathology: Unknown.

Materials deposited: None.

Remarks: These were the first *Isospora*-like oocysts reported from mongooses when Knowles and Das Gupta (1931) reported it in the small Asian mongoose (*H. javanicus* (syn. *H. auropunctatus*)) in India and called it *I.* (=*C.*) *rivolta*. They said the oocyst dimensions "fit in" with those of *I.* (=*C.*) *rivolta* reported from cats and dogs; however, Levine et al. (1975) pointed out that the Knowles and Das Gupta (1931) description, and their tiny, nondescript line drawing, did not resemble the descriptions of *I.* (=*C.*) *rivolta* from the dog (Levine and Ivens, 1965) or from the cat (Shah, 1969, 1970a,b). Three decades later, Dubey and Pande (1963a) also reported it in the Indian gray mongoose (*H. edwardsi*), and they called it the small form of *I.* (=*C.*) *garnhami*. Levine et al. (1975) based their description (given above) on the drawing and text of Knowles and Das Gupta (1931) and Dubey and Pande (1963a). They (Levine et al., 1975) further argued that the oocysts of this form are smaller than those of *I.* (=*C.*) *garnhami* from the African mongoose, *H. undulata rufula*, and differed from it in host genus, oocyst and sporocyst shape, and in having a thick oocyst outer wall.

CYSTOISOSPORA HERPESTEI (LEVINE, IVENS, AND HEALY, 1975) NOV. COMB.

Synonym: *Isospora herpestei* Levine, Ivens, and Healy, 1975.

Type host: *Herpestes javanicus* (É. Geoffroy Saint-Hilaire, 1818) (syn. *Herpestes auropunctatus* (Hodgson, 1836)), Small Asian Mongoose.

Type locality: Asia: India (see *Prevalence*, below).

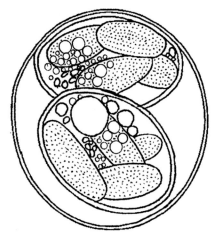

FIGURE 14.39 Original line drawing of the sporulated oocyst of *Cystoisospora herpestei*. Modified Fig. 46, *Levine, N.D., Ivens, V., 1981. The Coccidian Parasites (Protozoa, Apicomplexa) of Carnivores. Illinois Biological Monograph No. 51, The University of Illinois Press, Urbana, Illinois USA. The University of Illinois Press has released the copyright.*

Other definitive host: *Herpestes edwardsi* (É. Geoffroy Saint-Hilaire, 1818) (syn. *Herpestes mungo* (Blanford, 1888)), Indian Gray Mongoose.

Known intermediate host: None to date.

Geographic distribution: North America: USA: Georgia; Asia: India; Virgin Islands (?).

Description of sporulated oocyst: Oocyst shape: ellipsoidal to subspheroidal; number of walls, 1; wall characteristics: thin (<0.4 thick), smooth, colorless, delicate, and collapses easily; L×W (n=50): 19.9×15.4 (18–24×13–18), L/W ratio: 1.3; M, OR, PG: all absent. Distinctive features of oocyst: extremely thin oocyst wall that collapses easily.

Description of sporocyst and sporozoites: Sporocyst shape: ellipsoidal, with a sporocyst wall that looks slightly thicker than the oocyst wall; L×W (n=50): 12.9×9.3 (11–15×8–11), L/W ratio: 1.4; SB, SSB, PSB: all absent; SR: present as a few scattered small and large granules; SZ: sausage-shaped, with both ends of equal diameter; RB and N were not visible. Distinctive features of sporocyst: typical ellipsoidal shape, without SB, SSB, PSB, with SZ that have both ends of equal diameter, and a SR of only a few scattered granules of various sizes.

Prevalence: This species was found in a specimen of *H. edwardsi* examined by Levine et al. (1975); they said that "mongooses" were imported from India, to the Virgin Islands, and then to Georgia, USA, but they did not say how many mongooses were examined or were infected.

Sporulation: Exogenous. Oocysts were placed in 2% potassium dichromate ($K_2Cr_2O_7$) for 5 days at room temperature to facilitate sporulation and afterward placed into 10% formalin solution. Levine et al. (1975) said that oocysts sporulated in both solutions.

Prepatent and patent periods: Unknown.

Site of infection: Unknown.

Endogenous stages: Unknown.

Cross-transmission: None to date.

Pathology: Levine et al. (1975) believed this coccidium to be pathogenic because some of the mongooses passing it had diarrhea.

Materials deposited: None.

Remarks: The oocysts of this form differ from those of all other species with isosporan-type oocysts reported from mongooses. These oocysts are similar in size and shape to those of *I.* (=*C.*) *dasguptai*, but differ in having a thin, single-layered wall, sporocyst walls thicker than its oocyst wall, and having SZs that did not narrow at one end. They differed from those of *I.* (=*C.*) *garnhami* and *I.* (=*C.*) *hoarei* in host genus.

CYSTOISOSPORA MUNGOI (LEVINE, IVENS, AND HEALY, 1975) NOV. COMB.

Synonyms: *Isospora garnhami* (large form) Bray, 1954 of Dubey and Pande (1963a); [non] *Isospora garnhami* Bray, 1954; *Isospora mungoi* Levine, Ivens, and Healy, 1975.

Type host: *Herpestes edwardsi* (É. Geoffroy Saint-Hilaire, 1818) (syn. *Herpestes mungo* (Blanford, 1888)), Indian Gray Mongoose.

Type locality: Asia: India.

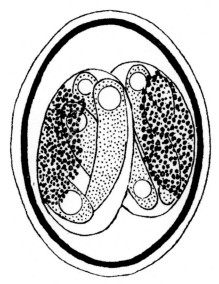

FIGURE 14.40 Original line drawing of the sporulated oocyst of *Cystoisospora mungoi*. Modified Fig. 60, Levine, N.D., Ivens, V., 1981. The Coccidian Parasites (Protozoa, Apicomplexa) of Carnivores. Illinois Biological Monograph No. 51, The University of Illinois Press, Urbana, Illinois USA. The University of Illinois Press has released the copyright.

Other definitive hosts: None to date.

Known intermediate host: None to date.

Geographic distribution: Asia: India.

Description of sporulated oocyst: Oocyst shape: ellipsoidal with rounded ends; number of walls, 2; wall characteristics: outer is thicker, yellow-green, whereas inner is darker; 1–2 in total thickness; L×W: 34×27 (sic) (27–34×23–27), L/W ratio: 1.3; M, OR, PG: all absent. Distinctive features of oocyst: a two-layered wall, lacking M, OR, and PG, and the oocyst shape varies after sporulation with the position of the sporocysts.

Description of sporocyst and sporozoites: Sporocyst shape: ellipsoidal; L×W: 21×14 (sic) (19–21×12–14), L/W ratio: 1.5; SB, SSB, PSB: all absent; SR: present, but no details were given; SZ: sausage-shaped, slightly tapering at one end, with one clear RB at more rounded end. Distinctive features of sporocyst: typical ellipsoidal shape, without SB, SSB, PSB and with a SR composed of some granules.

Prevalence: Unknown.

Sporulation: Exogenous. Dubey and Pande (1963a) said sporulation was complete in 1 day.

Prepatent and patent periods: Unknown.

Site of infection: Unknown.

Endogenous stages: Unknown.

Cross-transmission: None to date.

Pathology: Unknown.

Materials deposited: None.

Remarks: This species, as named by Levine et al. (1975), is Dubey and Pande's (1963a) large form of *I*. (=C.) *garnhami*, however, it differs from *I*. (=C.) *garnhami* in host genus and continent, and by having a thick (vs. a thin) oocyst wall and in having larger sporocysts. These seemed reasons enough for Levine et al. (1975) to coin a new species name for this form.

CYSTOISOSPORA PELLERDYI (DUBEY AND PANDE, 1964) NOV. COMB.

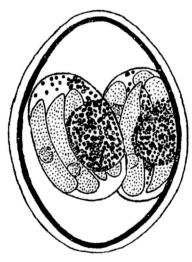

FIGURE 14.41 Original line drawing of the sporulated oocyst of *Cystoisospora pellerdyi*. *Modified Fig. 73, Levine, N.D., Ivens, V., 1981. The Coccidian Parasites (Protozoa, Apicomplexa) of Carnivores. Illinois Biological Monograph No. 51, The University of Illinois Press, Urbana, Illinois USA. The University of Illinois Press has released the copyright.*

Synonyms: *Isospora knowlesi* Dubey and Pande, 1963a,b; *Isospora pellerdyi* (Dubey and Pande, 1963a) Dubey and Pande, 1964; [non] *Isospora knowlesi* Ray and Das Gupta, 1937.

Type host: *Herpestes edwardsi* (É. Geoffroy Saint-Hilaire, 1818) (syn. *Herpestes mungo* (Blanford, 1888)), Indian Gray Mongoose.

Type locality: Asia: India.

Other definitive hosts: None to date.

Known intermediate host: None to date.

Geographic distribution: Asia: India.

Description of sporulated oocyst: Oocyst shape: ovoidal; number of walls, 2, 1–2 in total thickness; wall characteristics: outer is thicker, yellow to orange, and inner is darker; L×W (n=50): 28×23 (27–30×20–25), L/W ratio: 1.2; M, OR, PG: all absent. Distinctive features of oocyst: nothing distinctive but lacking M, OR, and PG.

Description of sporocyst and sporozoites: Sporocyst shape: ellipsoidal; L×W (n=25): 15×11 (sic) (17–19×12–24), L/W ratio: 1.4 (?); SB, SSB, PSB: all absent; SR: present; SR characteristics: a large, ellipsoidal mass of coarse granules in center of SP (line drawing); SZ: sausage-shaped, tapering toward a point at one end, 13–15×2–3; no mention of a RB, but line drawing shows the presence of a N in the middle third of SZ. Distinctive features of sporocyst: typical ellipsoidal shape, without SB, SSB, PSB, and with a SR composed of coarse granules.

Prevalence: Unknown.

Sporulation: Exogenous. Oocysts took only 1–2 days to sporulate.

Prepatent and patent periods: Unknown.

Site of infection: Unknown.

Endogenous stages: Unknown.

Cross-transmission: None to date.

Pathology: Unknown.

Materials deposited: None.

Remarks: Dubey and Pande (1963a) first named this form *Isospora knowlesi*, but because this name was preoccupied (for an isosporan parasite of a lizard), they emended it to *I. pellerdyi* in 1964; the latter is a senior synonym to *I. dubeyi*, created by Patnaik and Roy (1965) (Pellérdy, 1974a).

GENUS *SURICATA* DESMAREST, 1804 (MONOTYPIC)

CYSTOISOSPORA TIMONI EL-GAYAR, HOLMAN, CRAIG, DEMAAR, WILSON, CHUNG, WOODS, NORRIS, AND UPTON, 2008

Type host: *Suricata suricatta* (Scheber, 1776), Meerkat, Suricate, Slender-tailed Meerkat.

Type locality: Africa: South Africa (see *Remarks*, below).

Other definitive hosts: None to date.

Known intermediate host: None to date.

Geographic distribution: Africa: South Africa; North America: USA: Kansas, Texas.

Description of sporulated oocyst: Oocyst shape: spheroidal to subspheroidal; number of walls, 2, ~1.5 thick; wall characteristics: outer is smooth and both layers are of equal thickness; L × W (n = 45): 25.9 × 24.8 (22.5–30 × 20–27), L/W ratio: 1.1 (1.0–1.2); M, OR, PG: all absent. Distinctive features of oocyst: nothing distinctive about its nearly spheroidal shape; lacking M, OR, and PG.

Description of sporocyst and sporozoites: Sporocyst shape: ellipsoidal; L × W (n = 45): 15.3 × 12.8 (12.5–17.5 × 10–14), L/W ratio: 1.2 (1.0–1.3); SB, SSB, PSB: all absent; SR: present; SR characteristics: a large cluster of hundreds of small homogeneous granules; SZ: sausage-shaped, rounded at both ends; N: visible, slightly posterior to midpoint of SZ; no mention of a RB, but one appears to be present at each rounded end of SZ (line drawing). Distinctive features of sporocyst: typical ellipsoidal shape, without SB, SSB, and PSB, SR composed of a large cluster of homogeneous granules, and El-Gayar et al. (2008) mentioned the presence of a crystalloid body that is "difficult to discern," posterior to the N.

Prevalence: Unknown. Composite fecal samples collected during quarantine at the Zoo in Kansas, USA, contained numerous oocysts, whereas follow-up fecal samples collected 10 weeks later from individual meerkats showed only 2/10 (20%) passing oocysts.

Sporulation: Exogenous. Oocysts were shed unsporulated but became fully sporulated within 24 hours when placed into 2.5% aqueous potassium dichromate ($K_2Cr_2O_7$) at room temperature, ~23°C (El-Gayar et al., 2008).

(A) 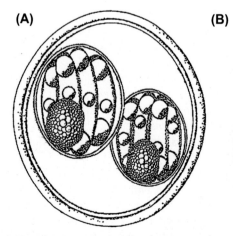   **(B)**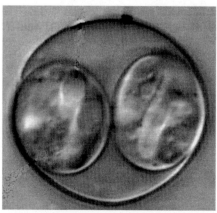

FIGURE 14.42   (A). Line drawing of the sporulated oocyst of *Cystoisospora timoni*. (B). Photomicrograph of the sporulated oocyst of *C. timoni*. *(A) and (B) From El-Gayar, A.K., Holman, P.J., Craig, T.M., Demaar, T.W., Wilson, S.C., Chung, P., Woods, K.M., Norris, C., Upton, S.J., 2008. A new species of coccidia (Apicomplexa: Sarcocystidae) from the slender-tailed meerkat Suricata suricatta (Schreber, 1776) from South Africa. Acta Protozoologica 47 (1), 69–76, with permission of the Editor, and the copyright holder for Acta Protozoologica.*

Prepatent and patent periods: Unknown.

Site of infection: Unknown.

Endogenous stages: Unknown.

Cross-transmission: None to date.

Pathology: Manharth (2004) reported a 2002 survey of North American institutions holding meerkat populations and said 3/33 (9%) reported coccidiosis as a health concern. El-Gayar et al. (2008) said that up to the time of their report, a history of coccidiosis in meerkats, including mortalities, had been documented for more than a decade at the Gladys Porter Zoo in Brownsville, Texas, USA.

Materials deposited: Phototypes (USNM No. 100,231) were deposited in the US National Parasite Museum, now the National Museum of Natural History, Department of Invertebrate Zoology, Smithsonian Museum Support Center, Suitland, Maryland, USA.

Etymology: The trivial name is derived from the Greek philosopher Timon of Philius (320–230 BC), who promoted skepticism through satire.

Remarks: El-Gayar et al. (2008) found this species in two different populations of meerkats. One population of 10 animals was in quarantine at the time, having been recently imported from South Africa and were destined to be housed at the Sedgwick County Zoo, Wichita, Kansas, USA. The second population of meerkats, in which oocysts were discovered, had been housed at the Gladys Porter Zoo, Brownsville, Texas, USA, for 14 years before their feces were examined for oocysts. Thus, because imported animals (South Africa) and resident meerkats (Texas) were both found to harbor this species, El-Gayar et al. (2008) concluded that this parasite must have originated in South Africa, which is why we list it as the type locality.

Cystoisospora timoni oocysts are morphologically distinct from other cystoisosporans in related hosts. Their spheroidal/subspheroidal oocysts differed from those of *C. dasguptai* from the small Asian mongoose (*H. javanicus*) in India, which are smaller and ovoidal/ellipsoidal. Sporulated oocysts of *C. garnhami* from the dwarf mongoose (*H. parvula*), in Kenya, are

more ellipsoidal and have a thin, fragile outer layer and a thick, tough, elastic inner layer not present in those of *C. timoni*. Oocysts of *C. herpestei* from the small Indian mongoose (*H. javanicus*) in India, and those from *C. hoarei* from the dwarf mongoose (*H. parvula*) in Kenya, both tend to be smaller than those of *C. timoni*, whereas those of *C. mungoi* from the Indian gray mongoose (*H. edwardsi*) in India tend to be larger. *Cystoisospora pellerdyi* sporulated oocysts also from the Indian gray mongoose are ovoidal with a yellow outer layer that is thicker and a darker inner layer. Finally, oocysts of *C. viverrae* from the civet cat (*Civettictis civetta*), in Sierra Leone and South Africa, are smaller in size than those of *C. timoni*.

HYAENIDAE GRAY, 1821

GENUS *HYAENA* BRISSON, 1762 (2 SPECIES)

CYSTOISOSPORA LEVINEI (DUBEY, 1963a) NOV. COMB.

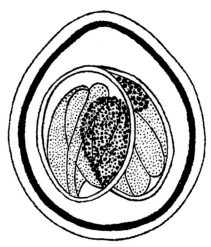

FIGURE 14.43 Original line drawing of the sporulated oocyst of *Cystoisospora levinei*. *Modified Fig. 77, Levine, N.D., Ivens, V., 1981. The Coccidian Parasites (Protozoa, Apicomplexa) of Carnivores. Illinois Biological Monograph No. 51, The University of Illinois Press, Urbana, Illinois USA. The University of Illinois Press has released the copyright.*

Synonym: *Isospora levinei* Dubey, 1963a.

Type host: *Hyaena hyaena* (L., 1758) (syn. *Hyaena striata* Zimmerman, 1777), Striped Hyaena.

Type locality: Asia: India, Mathura.

Other definitive hosts: None to date.

Known intermediate host: None to date.

Geographic distribution: Asia: India.

Description of sporulated oocyst: Oocyst shape: ovoidal; number of walls, 2, 1–2 thick; wall characteristics: outer is smooth, thicker, yellow-green and inner is darker with a shining contour; L×W (n=50): 27×25 (23–29×22–26), L/W ratio: 1.1 (1.0–1.2); M, OR, PG: all absent. Distinctive features of oocyst: nothing distinctive about its typical ovoidal shape; lacking M, OR, and PG.

Description of sporocyst and sporozoites: Sporocyst shape: ellipsoidal; L×W (n=20): 18×14 (16–18×11–14), L/W ratio: 1.3; SB, SSB, PSB: all absent; SR: present; SR characteristics: a few refractile bodies embedded in many dark granular bodies; SZ: sausage-shaped, rounded at both ends; N: visible, slightly posterior to mid-point of SZ, which were rounded at one end and pointed at the other, but no mention was made of seeing a RB or N; SZ measured, 10–14×3–4. Distinctive features of sporocyst: typical ellipsoidal shape, without SB, SSB, and PSB, SR composed of many granules.

Prevalence: Unknown. Dubey (1963a) found these oocysts in one hyaena.

Sporulation: Exogenous. Oocysts completed sporulation within 24 hours (Dubey, 1963a).

Prepatent and patent periods: Unknown.

Site of infection: Unknown.

Endogenous stages: Unknown.

Cross-transmission: None to date.

Pathology: Unknown.

Materials deposited: None.

Etymology: The trivial name was given in honor of Dr. Norman D. Levine, Professor of Parasitology, College of Veterinary Medicine, University of Illinois, Urbana, Illinois, USA.

Remarks: During an investigation of wild carnivores, one specimen of *H. hyaena* was necropsied by Dubey (1963a) in the Department of Parasitology, in the College of Veterinary Sciences and Animal Husbandry, Mathura, India. Dubey (1963a) studied both sporulated and unsporulated oocysts. Because this was the first record, ever, of an isosporan in *Hyaena*, Dubey (1963a) was confident and comfortable naming it as new and did so in honor of Dr. Levine.

VIVERRIDAE GRAY, 1821

SUBFAMILY VIVERRINAE GRAY, 1821

GENUS *CIVETTICTIS* POCOCK, 1915 (MONOTYPIC)

CYSTOISOSPORA VIVERRAE (ADLER, 1924) NOV. COMB.

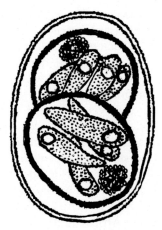

FIGURE 14.44 Original line drawing of the sporulated oocyst of *Cystoisospora viverrae*. *Modified Fig. 75, Levine, N.D., Ivens, V., 1981. The Coccidian Parasites (Protozoa, Apicomplexa) of Carnivores. Illinois Biological Monograph No. 51, The University of Illinois Press, Urbana, Illinois USA. The University of Illinois Press has released the copyright.*

Synonym: *Isospora viverrae* Adler, 1924.

Type host: *Civettictis civetta* (Schreber, 1776) (syn. *Viverra civetta* Schreber, 1776), African Civet.

Type locality: Africa: Sierra Leone, Freetown.

Other definitive hosts: None to date.

Known intermediate host: None to date.

Geographic distribution: Africa: Sierra Leone.

Description of sporulated oocyst: Oocyst shape: ellipsoidal; number of walls, 1; wall characteristics: thin, smooth (line drawing); L×W: 23×19 (19–28×15–25), L/W ratio: 1.2; M, OR, PG: all absent. Distinctive features of oocyst: small size with a thin wall, without M, OR, and PG.

Description of sporocyst and sporozoites: Sporocyst shape: ellipsoidal; L×W: 12.5–15.2×8–11, mean not given, L/W ratio: unknown; SB, SSB, PSB: all absent; SR: present; SR characteristics: a mass of several coarse granules at one end of SP (line drawing); SZ: sickle-shaped, broader at one end, slightly tapering at the other, 9–11×3, with a RB at the more rounded end. Distinctive features of sporocyst: typical spheroidal to subspheroidal shape, without SB, SSB, PSB and with a SR composed of coarse granules.

Prevalence: Adler (1924) found this species in 3/3 heavily-infected civet cats.

Sporulation: Exogenous. Oocysts took 3 days to complete sporulation (Adler, 1924).

Prepatent and patent periods: Unknown.

Site of infection: All endogenous stages were found in epithelial cells of the lower half of the small intestine; very few cells were infected in the basal parts of each villus, but enterocytes in the distal parts of each villus were heavily-infected.

Endogenous stages: Adler (1924) did not clearly state that he saw multiple merogonous generations although he did say merozoites varied in size from 4–10×1–2; he attributed this variation to the number of merozoites per meront. The largest meronts were about 10–18 wide with 4–13 merozoites of variable size, and each merozoite "may or may not contain a residual body." Adler (1924) felt that "normal" meronts contained eight merozoites, whereas abnormal meronts contained either more or less than eight, with the size of the merozoites dependent on the number within each meront. His interpretation led Levine and Ivens (1981) to speculate there may be up to three generations of meronts. Adler (1924) reported that there were about 30 times more macrogametes as microgamonts. Mature microgamonts were 16–25 wide and contained ~200 biflagellate microgametes, each about 10 long, and grouped around two residual bodies. Macrogametes were deeply staining and attained almost the same size as the oocysts. Fertilization was reported to take place inside the host cell and Adler (1924) said he saw as many as 9 or 10 microgametes inside a single macrogamete. After fertilization, the first division of the sporoplasm took place inside the parasitized enterocyte or in the lumen of the gut.

Cross-transmission: Adler (1924) was unable to infect two cats, three kittens, and two young dogs with this species.

Pathology: Adler (1924) attributed the death of two young civets to infection by this species. He said they passed blood, mucus, and large numbers of oocysts in their feces and that the subepithelial tissue was markedly hyperemic with enterocytes in the distal parts of the villi heavily-infected whereas few cells in the basal parts of the villi were infected. In some sections of the infected intestine the distal villar epithelium was destroyed (Adler, 1924).

Materials deposited: None.

Remarks: Adler (1924) said the definitive host was *Viverra civetta*, but species in the genus *Viverra* occur only in eastern Asia (India, Burma, Cambodia, Vietnam, Thailand, etc.), not in Africa, so the appropriate host designation is *C. civetta* (Wilson and Reeder, 2005). Oocysts of this species are approximately the same size as those of *C.* (=*I.*) *rivolta* but differ by having oocysts passed containing two sporoblasts, whereas in the latter, oocysts are passed unsegmented. Also, *C.* (=*I.*) *rivolta* is capable of infecting both dogs and cats, but this species does not infect cats or dogs.

DISCUSSION AND SUMMARY

The Caniformia branch of the Carnivora consists of 9 families composed of 72 genera with 165 species (Wilson and Reeder, 2005). There is at least one named *Cystoisospora* species in 7/9 (78%) families, but none are reported yet in the monotypic families Odobenidae (walrus) and Ailuridae (red panda). In the Canidae, only 3/13 (23%) genera and 9/35 (26%) species have been documented to host 10 named *Cystoisospora* species, as definitive hosts, with 5 *Cystoisospora* species in *Canis* and *Vulpes* each, and 1 species (*C. ohioensis*) shared with *Nyctereutes*. In the Mephitidae, only 1/4 (25%) genera and 1/12 (8%) species have been studied, but 2 *Cystoisospora* species are now known from *S. putorius*, the Eastern spotted skunk. In the Mustelidae, 7/22 (32%) genera and 11/59 (19%) species have been studied and found to play host to 13 different named *Cystoisospora* species. In the Otariidae, only 1/7 (14%) genera and 1/16 (6%) species have been examined, and a single, unique species was found. In the Phocidae, 1/13 (8%) genera and 1/19 (5%) species have 1 *Cystoisospora* species that is unique to it. In the Procyonidae, 3/6 (50%) genera and 3/15 (20%) species harbor the only *Cystoisospora* species known from that group. And in the Ursidae, 1/5 (20%) genera and 1/8 (12.5%) species have been examined for and documented to harbor one *Cystoisospora* species, also unique to *Melursus*. In total, we have knowledge that about 29 distinct species of *Cystoisospora* are known to be present in 7/9 (78%) families, 17/72 (24%) genera with 27/165 (16%) species in the Caniformia branch of the Carnivora.

The Feliformia branch of the Carnivora consists of 6 families composed of 54 genera with 121 species (Wilson and Reeder, 2005), but its members have not been as well studied for Sarcocystidae species as have those in the Caniformia. There are no named *Cystoisospora* species in 41 genera and 100 species from this felid lineage. In the Felidae, 8/14 (57%) genera including 14/40 (35%) of their species have been found to harbor 12 named *Cystoisospora* species that mostly are unique to the family. In the Herpestidae 3/14 (21%) genera and 5/33 (15%) species have 7 *Cystoisospora* species described

from them; *Hel. parvula* has 2 species, whereas *Her. edwardsi* has reportedly been found to host 6 different *Cystoisospora* species. The Hyaenidae is a small family with only 3 genera and 4 species; *C. levinei* was recorded in 1/3 (33%) genera and in 1/4 (25%) species. The Viverridae is a much larger lineage, but its members have not been examined to any extent for *Cystoisospora*; only 1/15 (7%) genera and only 1/35 (3%) species in the family have been examined and it was found to play host to a *Cystoisospora* species unique to it. Thus, 21 *Cystoisospora* species are known to be present in 4/6 (67%) families, 13/54 (24%) genera, and in 21/121 (17%) species in the Feliformia branch of the Carnivora.

To summarize for all Carnivora, with the exceptions of domestic and laboratory dogs and cats, only a handful of wild and zoo carnivore specimens and species have had their feces examined for *Cystoisospora* coccidians in 11/15 (73%) families, which include only 30/126 (24%) genera and 48/286 (17%) species. From these few studies to date, 50 named *Cystoisospora* species have been described, or about one per each carnivore species that has been examined. We believe it likely that all Carnivora species can serve as definitive hosts for at least one *Cystoisospora* species unique to it. If our assumption is reasonable, then there may be another 250 *Cystoisospora* species yet to be discovered just from carnivores.

Of the 50 known *Cystoisospora* species descriptions, how many of these are truly meaningful? The data are very difficult to interpret because there is so little of it. We know the intermediate host for only 8 species. We have some prevalence data on 39 of these species, but in most cases, they derive from the original and only survey and are based on trivial numbers of individual hosts sampled. We know the site of infection in the definitive host and perhaps a little about some the endogenous developmental stages for about 17 species. Cross-transmission, via oocysts or via infected intermediate hosts, has been done with 20 *Cystoisospora* species, but mostly to only one other host species, and in small numbers. At least 11 of the known *Cystoisospora* species are thought to be mildly pathogenic in their definitive host, but we know little or nothing about the pathogenic nature of the other 39 *Cystoisospora* species. The prepatent and patent periods are known for about 12 species, and sporulation time is generally known to be >24 hours in two-thirds of the 50 species, but it is ≤24 hours in 10 of them. Perhaps these later forms are really *Sarcocystis* species? It certainly would be nice to have molecular data on these forms to answer that question so we can better understand the biology and evolutionary tendencies of these forms. Only 21 of the 50 described and named species also have been found at a later time by someone other than the individual(s) who described them; were the oocysts found in the other 29 merely spurious forms of prey items just passing through the gut of the carnivore that ate them? Sadly, only five *Cystoisospora* species have any type of voucher specimens deposited in accredited museums to anchor their names. We could go on, but this is depressing enough. Clearly, there is an enormous amount of basic work to be done, and basic biology to be learned, just on the *Cystoisospora* species that live in Carnivora species.

Sarcocystidae: Sarcocystinae in the Carnivora

INTRODUCTION

Sarcocystinae Poche, 1913 is the second subfamily within the Sarcocystidae Poche, 1913 and contains two genera (*Sarcocystis*, *Frenkelia*). The third subfamily is Toxoplasmatinae Biocca, 1957 (*Besnoitia*, *Hammondia*, *Neospora*, *Toxoplasma*) and those organisms that infect carnivores will be reported in Chapter 16.

Sarcocystis **Lankester, 1882**. The history of the initial discovery of a *Sarcocystis* species and the later discovery of an obligatory two-host life cycle has been reviewed many times (Frenkel, 1974; Dubey, 1976; Levine, 1986; Dubey et al., 1989b; Duszynski and Couch, 2013; Dubey et al., 2015a; others) and need not be repeated here. Although the first sarcocysts in skeletal muscles were reported by Miescher in 1843 as "milky white threads" in a house mouse in Switzerland, the first sarcocysts found in **carnivore** muscles were discovered by Huet (1882), who found them in skeletal muscle of a sea lion that died in the Jardin des Plantes de Paris, France; the sarcocysts were 300–400 long and 20–30 wide. Lankester (1882) introduced the genus name for these Miescher's tubules to reflect what he saw, muscle (Gk. *sarco*, flesh. muscle) and cyst (Gk. *cyst*, bladder, bag), thus, *Sarcocystis*. Blanchard (1885) restudied Huet's material and named the organism *Miescheria hueti* and Labbé (1899) transferred this parasite to the genus *Sarcocystis*. The real beginning of our understanding of the life cycle of these (typically) muscle parasites did not occur until the seminal studies by Fayer (1970, 1972b) who was the first to observe transformation of bradyzoites from muscle cysts in grackles (*Quiscalus quiscula*) into gametocytes and oocysts in cell culture, and this was soon followed by Rommel et al. (1972) who described the shedding of sporulated sporocysts from cats after they ingested sarcocyst-infected mutton (a.k.a. *Sarcocystis tenella*).

Smith and Frenkel (1978) found sarcocysts in skeletal muscles of 4/15 (27%) lab mice housed in the same room as cats that had shed sporulated sporocysts of *Sarcocystis muris*. They noted that cat feces never came in proximity with mouse cages, but they did see German cockroaches (*Blatella germanica*) in the same room from time to time. To assess the role of *B. germanica* and the American

© 2018 Donald W. Duszynski published by Elsevier Inc. All rights reserved.

cockroach (*Periplaneta americana*) in transmission, cockroaches were exposed to cat feces that contained oocysts/sporocysts of *S. muris*, *Isospora felis*, and *Toxoplasma gondii*. They found that *S. muris* sporocysts, which remained infectious in cat feces for at least 20 days, were transmitted to mice by *P. americana* for at least 20 days, and by *B. germanica* for five days postexposure to infected cat feces. Later, Smith and Frenkel (1978) searched their lab records and noted that sporocysts of *S. muris* remained infectious for at least 119 days at 21°C in 2% aqueous sulfuric acid (H$_2$SO$_4$).

Levine and Tadros (1980) listed 93 species of named *Sarcocystis* from all vertebrate hosts. Levine and Ivens (1981), used part of that list, but covered only the coccidian parasites of carnivores in which they listed about 38 named *Sarcocystis* species, some of which were tentative. Levine (1986) updated the list along with Tadros and, in just the 6 years between publications, the named *Sarcocystis* species was 122, a 24% increase. Odening (1998) revised the species name-systematics of *Sarcocystis* a dozen years later and listed 189 *Sarcocystis* species names, another 35% increase (although he considered some of the names to be *species inquirendae*). Dubey et al. (2015a) published an extensive treatise on *Sarcocystis* species in humans and other animals, and we refer to it extensively here; they listed 195 names as valid (their Table 24.1), 49 *Sarcocystis* species names as invalid (Table 24.2), and 83 names (*Sarcocystis* sp.) that have never received a binomial. We encourage interested readers in all disciplines to use these references should they be interested in maximizing *Sarcocystis* species data for any particular host species group. The data on *Sarcocystis* species in this chapter are presented differently from our species presentations in other chapters, with our focus principally on *Sarcocystis* species found only in Carnivora species.

It is our intent to be as inclusive as we can be of every *Sarcocystis* species (binomial) named to date in every carnivore, whether as a definitive host, an intermediate host, or both. In the interest of space, however, we give a complete rendition only of the *Sarcocystis* species discovered and named since 1986, when Levine's last list was published. Thus, for the 46/122 (38%) *Sarcocystis* species in carnivores covered by Levine (1986), we list their names, hosts, distributions, and a few pertinent remarks, principally referencing work that followed the notations given in Levine (1986). For *Sarcocystis* species discovered and named after 1986, and for those few species that Levine (1986), Odening (1998), or Dubey et al. (2015a) neglected to list, we will attempt to present all of their known life cycle details as we do the descriptions for eimeriid species in Chapters 3–13.

***Frenkelia* Biocca, 1968.** Compartmentalized, thin-walled cysts found in the brains of a variety of rodents (*Myodes* (syn. *Clethrionomys*) and *Microtus* species) were originally named *Toxoplasma microti* Findlay and Middleton, 1934. Frenkel (1953, 1956) found similar organisms in *Microtus modestus* from Montana, USA, and separated them from *Toxoplasma* because he could not transmit it by passage into mice, so he tentatively designated them as "M-organism," (for *Microtus*). The name was changed to *Frenkelia* by Biocca (1968) who designated the type species as *Frenkelia microti* (syn. *T. microti*). In those early days, the developmental stages in rodents and their ultrastructure were studied, but the definitive host and complete life cycle(s) were unknown (Frenkel, 1974). Rommel and Krampitz (1975) described the first life cycle when they fed infected bank voles (*My. glareolus* (syn. *C. glareolus*)) to buzzards (*Buteo buteo*) and later recovered sporocysts in the feces that were identical to sporocysts describied by others as *Isospora buteonis* from hawks and owls. *Frenkelia* cysts were thin-walled and only known to occur in the brains of small mammals (Rodentia). As our knowledge accumulated, all of the few *Frenkelia* species known used rodents as intermediate hosts, where they lived in the central nervous system (usually the brain), and carnivorous birds were always the definitive hosts that shed infective sporocysts in their feces. Species of *Frenkelia* were differentiated from those of *Sarcocystis* by the morphology and location of cysts in rodents, and *Frenkelia* species were differentiated by host specificity. However, as more and more *Sarcocystis* life cycles and developmental stages became known, the differences between the two genera have blurred. Odening (1998) said, "The continued maintenance of the genus *Frenkelia* Biocca, 1968 (with two species) separate from *Sarcocystis* is no longer tenable, because there are neither morphological nor developmental features which can be used for distinguishing the two genera." The minor features used initially to distinguish the two genera are now known in several *Sarcocystis* species that have small mammals as intermediate hosts and birds of prey as definitive hosts, and all seem to have the transmission electron microscopy (TEM) type 1 sarcocyst wall structure. Finally, we know of no *Frenkelia* species ever recorded from carnivorous mammals and, with the development of molecular tools during the last three decades, a number of investigators indicated that the genus *Frenkelia* is a synonym of *Sarcocystis* (see Dubey et al., 2015a for a list of references). Thus, only *Sarcocystis* species in carnivores are summarized, below.

SPECIES DESCRIPTIONS

SUBORDER CANIFORMIA KRETZOI, 1938

AILURIDAE GRAY, 1843

GENUS *AILURUS* F.G. CUVIER, 1825 (MONOTYPIC)

SARCOCYSTIS NEURONA DUBEY, DAVIS, SPEER, BOWMAN, DE LAHUNTA, GRANSTROM, TOPPER, HAMIR, CUMMINGS, AND SUTER, 1991b

Definitive hosts: *Didelphis albiventris* Lund, 1840, White-eared Opossum; *Didelphis marsupialis* L., 1758, Common Opossum; *Didelphis virginiana* Kerr, 1792, Virginia Opossum.

Intermediate host: *Ailurus fulgens* F.G. Cuvier, 1825, Red Panda.

Remarks: Zoll et al. (2015) used TEM, immunohistochemistry (IHC), polymerase chain reaction (PCR), and nucleic acid sequencing to determine that one or more *Sarcocystis* species infected two neonatal male red pandas. Using PCR and nucleic acid sequencing of partial 18S rRNA, and the first internal transcribed spacer (ITS-1), region, they confirmed a *Sarcocystis* species that shared 99% sequence homology to *Sarcocystis neurona*. Theirs was the first report of sarcocystosis in red pandas (even though the identity of the species was not conclusively determined). *Sarcocystis neurona* is an economically important pathogen and it likely is closely related to *Toxoplasma gondii* and *Neospora caninum*. For more complete information on *S. neurona*, see Genus *Procyon* below for the natural intermediate host, *P. lotor*. Zoll et al. (2015) also believed another *Sarcocystis* species may have been present in these pandas (see Chapter 19).

CANIDAE FISCHER, 1817

GENUS CANIS L., 1758 (6 SPECIES)

SARCOCYSTIS ALCESLATRANS DUBEY, 1980b

Synonym: *Sarcocystis* sp. Type A of Colwell and Mahrt (1981).

Definitive hosts: *Canis latrans* Say, 1823, Coyote; *Canis lupus familiaris* (syn. *C. dingo*) L., 1758, Domestic Dog.

Intermediate host: *Alces alces* (L., 1758), Eurasian Elk, Moose.

Geographic distribution: North America: USA: Montana; Canada: Alberta.

Remarks: Dubey (1980b) looked at moose, bison (*Bison bison* (L., 1758)), and pronghorn antelope (*Antilocapra americana* (Ord, 1815)) in Montana and found sarcocysts in muscles of all three species. Muscle tissue with sarcocysts from the moose was fed to laboratory-reared coyotes and domestic dogs. Twelve days post-inoculation (DPI), both *C. latrans* and *C. l. familiaris* shed sporocysts in their feces. Sporocysts were, L × W: 14.5 × 8.8 (14–17 × 8.5–10.5); L/W ratio: 1.6. Two morphologically distinct sarcocysts (thin-walled, thick-walled) were found in the moose muscles and Dubey (1980b) provided this name for the thin-walled sarcocysts. It was not established whether the bison and the pronghorn shared the same *Sarcocystis* species with the moose. Colwell and Mahrt (1981) reported two distinct sarcocysts from the musculature of *A. alces* from Alberta, Canada, which they compared by electron microscopy. Their fusiform type A cysts differed from the spherical type B cysts in the appearance and thickness of the primary cyst wall, organization of cyst interior, and the presence of a secondary cyst wall around type B. Odening (1998) was convinced that his type A sarcocysts were identical to those of *S. alceslatrans*. Dubey and Blagburn (1983) tried to infect one 7-month-old raccoon with 1 kg of meat over 7 days, from a moose infected with sarcocysts of *S. alceslatrans* and that had been shot near Bozeman, MT, but the raccoon remained uninfected for at least 5 weeks post-inoculation (PI). Levine (1986) included this species in his summary of valid *Sarcocystis* species names, and Dubey et al. (2015a) listed it in their alphabetical list of valid (Table 24.1) and named *Sarcocystis* species (Table 24.4).

SARCOCYSTIS ARIETICANIS HEYDORN, 1985

Definitive host: *Canis lupus familiaris* (syn. *C. familiaris*) L., 1758, Domestic Dog.

Intermediate host: *Ovis aries* L., 1758, Red Sheep.

Geographic distribution: Asia: India; Japan; Australia: Northwest Territory; Western Australia; Europe: Germany; Slovakia; Middle East: Iran; Saudi Arabia; Turkey; North America: USA: Texas. Most likely, worldwide in distribution.

Remarks: Since Heydorn (1985) first discovered this parasite in sheep in Europe, it has been found in that host on most continents, and sarcocysts are not infective to domestic cats (see references in Dubey et al., 2015a). This species was listed in Levine's (1986) review of valid *Sarcocystis* species through 1985. Heydorn and Melhorn (1987), using TEM, examined the ultrastructure of developmental stages, including two generations of meronts, merozoites, and gamogony. Dubey et al. (1988b) found sarcocysts of this species in the muscles of 18/512 (3.5%) adult ewes from the northwestern United States and Texas. Odening et al. (1995) identified this species by light microscopy (LM) and electron microscopy in muscle samples from six wild and two captive European mouflons (*O. aries musimon*) in Germany, purportedly the first time *S. arieticanis* was recorded from wild sheep. Odening (1998) also listed this as a valid species and considered it a sibling species to *S. hircicanis*, separated from it based on intermediate host specificity. Giannetto et al. (2005) used Dubey et al.'s (1989b) classification of 24 sarcocyst types to identify sarcocysts of this species (as type 7) in 38/50 (76%) diaphragm samples from sheep in Sicily, Italy. Dubey et al. (2015a) reviewed what is known about the structure of sarcocysts in sheep muscles, life cycle information known to date, and pathogenicity of *S. arieticanis* for sheep (less than *S. tenella*).

SARCOCYSTIS AUCHENIAE BRUMPT, 1913

Synonyms: *Sarcocystis lama-canis* Gorman, Alcaino, Muñoz and Cunazza, 1984; *Sarcocystis tilopodi* Quiroga, Lombardero & Zorrilla, 1969; *Sarcocystis guanicoe-canis* Gorman, Alcaino, Muñoz and Cunazza, 1984.

Definitive host: *Canis lupus familiaris* (syn. *C. familiaris*) L., 1758, Domestic Dog.

Intermediate host: *Lama glama* (L., 1758) (syn. *Lama guanicoe* (Müller, 1776)) Guanaco, Llama, Alpaca.

Geographic distribution: Most likely, worldwide in distribution (see Dubey et al., 2015a).

Remarks: A sarcocyst observed in a llama (*Lama glama*) was named *Sarcocystis aucheniae*, but no other detail was provided (Brumpt, 1913). Quiroga et al. (1969), in Argentina, found sarcocysts in *Lama guanicoe* and named the species *S. tilopodi*, based on its finding in a different species of *Lama*. Gorman et al. (1984), in Chile, found macroscopic and microscopic sarcocysts in *L. guanicoe* and transmitted the infection to four dogs, but four cats that were fed the same infected meat did not excrete sporocysts. They (1984) suggested that the parasite in *L. glama* be named *S. lama-canis* and the parasite in *L. guanicoe* should be called *S. guanicoe-canis* (Quiroga et al., 1969). However, both *Lama* species names are synonymous and considered to be the same species. In Germany, both microscopic and macroscopic sarcocysts were found in *L. glama* (Schneider et al., 1984). One dog and one cat were fed isolated macroscopic sarcocysts; only the dog excreted oocysts. Additionally, another cat fed infected meat also did not excrete sporocysts. These experiments confirmed the findings of Gorman et al. (1984) that sarcocysts from llamas are transmissible to dogs but not cats; sporocysts from dogs were: L × W: 15 × 10 (13–16 × 9–11), L/W ratio: 1.5, the prepatent period was 11 days, and the patent period was 21 days. The sarcocysts of this species are surrounded by a folded primary cyst wall that formed cauliflower-like protrusions into the muscle fiber in which it grows. The protrusions have numerous microfilaments and the cyst wall forms numerous tiny vesicles.

Although the idea that two species of *Sarcocystis* (*S. aucheniae* and "*S. lamacenis*," possibly *S. lamacanis*) infect alpacas has been suggested by some (Leguía, G., 1991; Mason and Orr, 1993), critical examination of the literature led Odening (1998) and Dubey et al. (2015a) to conclude that there is only one valid name, *S. aucheniae*, to represent the form with macroscopic sarcocysts. Odening (1998) also suggested that the separation of species only with reference to the hosts is not appropriate, especially in llamas, because both alpacas and llamas are domesticated forms of the guanaco and, therefore, represent only one species, *L. glama*. Dubey et al. (2015a) suggested that a new name can be proposed for the species with microscopic sarcocysts when its structure and definitive host(s) are described. Some authors have called the form with microscopic sarcocysts *S. lamacanis* (Gabor et al., 2010), whereas others have called it *S. lamacensis* (Rooney et al., 2014). Levine (1986) said that *S. lama-canis* named by Gorman et al. (1984) was a junior synonym of *S. aucheniae*. Because there is no morphological description of the microsarcocyst of the llama, the closest description is an illustration in a histologic section of heart of a llama (Fig. 1, Dubey et al., 1989b); thus, the names *S. guanicoe-canis*, *S. lama-canis*, *S. lamacensis* should be considered either *nomen dubia* or *species inquirendae* at this time. Carletti et al. (2013) recently sequenced the complete 18S rRNA gene from llamas and concluded that the large sarcocyst form of *S. aucheniae* in South America is the same as that described in alpacas in Australia and, likely, Europe as well, having been transported with the hosts from South America.

SARCOCYSTIS BAIBACINACANIS UMBETALIEV, 1979

Synonym: *Sarcocystis baibacina* Umbetaliev, 1979 (see Odening, 1998, and Dubey et al., 2015a).

Definitive hosts: *Canis lupus* L., 1758, Wolf; *Canis lupus familiaris* (syn. *C. familiaris*) L., 1758, Domestic Dog; *Vulpes vulpes* (L., 1758), Red or Silver Fox.

Intermediate hosts: *Marmota baibacina* Kastschenko, 1899, Gray Marmot; *Marmota bobak* (Müller, 1776), Bobak Marmot; *Marmota caudata* (Geoffroy, 1844), Long-tailed Marmot.

Geographic distribution: Asia: Kazakhstan, former USSR.

Remarks: Sporocysts are up to 17 long. Levine (1986), Odening (1998), and Dubey et al. (2015a) considered this as a valid species because both the definitive and intermediate host species were known. However, Dubey et al. (2015a) did not list this species name in their "Table 14.2: *Sarcocystis* species sporocysts in feces of dogs." There is no other information about this "species," and the original manuscript was not available to us (*nos non videbo illum*).

SARCOCYSTIS BERTRAMI DOFLEIN, 1901

Synonyms: *Isospora rivolta* sporocysts of Gassner (1940) and Levine and Ivens (1965) *pro-parte*; *Isospora bigemina* large form of Mehlhorn et al. (1975b) and Heydorn et al. (1975a) *pro parte*; *Endorimospora bertrami* (Dolfein, 1901) Tadros and Laarman, 1976; *Sarcocystis asinus* Gadaev, 1978; *Sarcocystis equicanis* Rommel and Geisel, 1975; *Hoareosporidium pellerdyi* Pande, Bhatia, and Chauhan, 1972; and *Sarcocystis fayeri* Dubey, Streitel, Stromberg, and Toussant, 1977 (?) (from Levine, 1986).

Definitive host: *Canis lupus familiaris* (syn. *C. familiaris*) L., 1758, Domestic Dog.

Intermediate hosts: *Equus asinus* L., 1758, Ass; *Equus caballus* L., 1758, Horse; *Equus burchellii antiquorum* C.H. Smith, 1841, Burchell's Zebra; *Equus kiang holdereri* Matschie, 1911, Kiang.

Geographic distribution: Africa: Egypt; Europe: Austria; Germany; Great Britain; according to Odening (1998) this species likely is found worldwide.

Remarks: This name was first proposed by Doflein (1901) for sarcocysts in a horse that he found in the esophagus and leg muscles, but no other information was given. Because there are no archived specimens, it is impossible to determine the validity of the species. Rommel and Geisel (1975) thought the form they saw in the horse was a new species, but Levine and Ivens (1981) considered it a synonym and they summarized what limited information was (and still is) known about the location of endogenous stages, oocyst/sporocyst structure, sporulation, and pathogenicity of *S. bertrami*. They (1981) also added an important discussion, *vis-à-vis* the different named forms described from horses, *S. bertrami*, *S. equicanis*, and *S. fayeri* (see their *Remarks*, pp. 39–41) that have been used and described by others (Doflein, 1901; Rommel and Geisel, 1975; Göbel, 1976; Dubey et al., 1977a,b; Levine, 1977). Levine (1986) included this species in his summary of 122 valid *Sarcocystis* species names. Odening (1998) included this species in his summary of 189 valid *Sarcocystis* species names and said that he considered it similar to *S. fayeri* because they both have type 11 sarcocysts (Dubey et al., 1989a). Dubey et al. (2015a) added that sarcocysts in horse muscle cells attain their maximum length, ~15 mm, when the horse is 4 years old.

SARCOCYSTIS CAMELI (MASON, 1910) BABUDIERI, 1932

Synonyms: *Sarcocystis camelicanis*; *Sarcocystis camelocanis*; *Sarcocystis miescheri*; *Sarcocystis* sp. of Ghaffar et al. (1979).

Definitive host: *Canis lupus familiaris* (syn. *C. familiaris*) L., 1758, Domestic Dog.

Intermediate hosts: *Camelus dromedarius* L., 1758, One-humped Camel; *Camelus bactrianus* L., 1758, Bactrian Camel.

Geographic distribution: Africa: Egypt, Ethiopia, Morocco, Somalia, Sudan; Asia: India, Mongolia, former USSR; Middle East: Afghanistan, Iran, Iraq, Jordan; Saudi Arabia.

Remarks: The prevalence of *Sarcocystis* sarcocysts in camels is high. Mason (1910) was the first to see sarcocysts in striated and heart muscle of camels; he reported two types of sarcocysts: those with a thicker, striated wall, ~1–2 thick, and those with a thinner wall,

<1 thick. Initially, he believed they were different stages of the same species and named it *S. cameli*. Brumpt (1913) placed all sarcosporidia then known into the genus *Sarcocystis*, listed this species as *S. cameli* Mason, 1910, and said only that is was found in camel muscles in Egypt, and it was more common in older animals. Hilali and Mohamed (1980) examined meat samples from camel carcasses in a slaughter house in Cairo City, and found 41/112 (37%) to have microscopic sarcocysts of *S. cameli* in their muscles. The cysts varied in size from L × W: 33–389 × 22–33 and had a striated cyst wall that was 1.2 thick. Hilali and Mohamed (1980) infected each of three dogs and three cats with ~250 g of infected meat; after a prepatent period of 10, 11, and 14 days, each dog began to shed sporocysts in its feces, and the patent period in the dogs lasted for periods of 69, 71, and 73 days. No cats discharged sporocysts for a period of 69 days. The sporocysts discharged by the dogs measured L × W: 12 × 9, on average. Levine (1986) listed this species as one of the 122 names he considered to be valid species of *Sarcocystis* at that time. Dubey et al. (1989b) later attributed this name only to the thick, striated-wall form, whereas the thin-walled form was named *S. ippeni* by Odening (1997). Hilali et al. (1992) fed nine dogs pooled heart and esophagus muscle from different numbers (15–30) of camels (*C. dromedarius*) and monitored their fecal output, via salt flotation, for 70 DPI. Five dogs began passing sporocysts of *S. cameli* on 10 or 11 DPI and patency lasted for 8–26 days, respectively. Odening (1998) listed this species as one of the 189 valid species of *Sarcocystis* in his thorough review of the genus. Motamedi et al. (2011) were the first to employ molecular methods to develop a restriction map for this species. Dubey et al. (2015a) said that this species is found in striated muscles of the tongue, esophagus, and heart. Dubey et al. (2017a) found five macroscopic sarcocysts from the muscles of two adult *C. dromedarius* in Iraq and studied their ultrastructure; they concluded that it was the first confirmation of macroscopic sarcocysts from the one-humped camel as *S. cameli*.

SARCOCYSTIS CANINUM DUBEY, SYKES, SHELTON, SHARP, VERMA, CALERO-BERNAL, VIVIANO, SUNDAR, KHAN, AND GRIGG, 2015c

For light and electron micrographs of tissue cysts and zoites of this species see Figs. 3–7 in Dubey et al. (2014).

Definitive type host: Unknown.

Type locality: North America.

Other definitive hosts: Unknown.

Intermediate type host: *Canis lupus familiaris* (syn. *C. familiaris*) L., 1758, Domestic Dog.

Other intermediate hosts: Unknown.

Geographic distribution: North America: Canada, USA.

Description of sporulated oocyst: Unknown.

Description of sporocyst and sporozoites: Unknown.

Prevalence: Dubey et al. (2015c) detected sarcocysts of this species in muscle biopsies of all four dogs they examined. Two of the four infected dogs had sarcocysts only of this form, whereas the other two infected dogs had sarcocysts of both *S. caninum* and *S. svanai* (see below). The four infected dogs were from geographically separate areas, ruling out a common meal as their source of infection, and the intensity of sarcocysts in the muscles of all four dogs was similar, suggesting that these were not **spurious** infections.

Sporulation: Unknown, but likely endogenous with sporulated, infective sporocysts shed in the feces of the definitive host.

Prepatent and patent periods: Unknown.

Site of infection, definitive host: Unknown.

Site of infection, intermediate host: Striated muscles.

Endogenous stages, definitive host: Unknown.

Endogenous stages, intermediate host: Sarcocysts of this species were L × W: 1.2 mm × 75 μm. By LM the sporocyst wall was thin, smooth, and without striations, but by TEM the sarcocyst wall was a "type 9" (Dubey et al., 1989b), 1–2 thick, and contained villar protrusions that lacked microtubules. Bradyzoites (n = 13) were L × W: 6–7.5 × 2–3 under the LM, whereas they measured (n = 6) 7.5–9 long under TEM. The granular substance layer of the sarcocyst wall continued into the interior of the sarcocyst as septa that separated individuals and groups of metrocytes and bradyzoites. Metrocytes were ovoidal, with few organelles, whereas bradyzoites had a double-layered pellicle with electron-dense thickening at the conoidal end and organelles that included 1–3 rhoptries with electron-dense centers, numerous micronemes often arranged in rows, a large mitochondrion, numerous amylopectin granules, but they were absent or rare near the micronemes, a micropore, and a terminal or subterminal nucleus.

Cross-transmission: None to date.

Pathology: Unknown.

Materials deposited: Specimens deposited in the US National Parasite Collection (USNPC), Division of Invertebrate Zoology and National Museum of Natural History, Smithsonian Institution, Washington, DC (under US National Museum [USNM]). H&E-stained histological sections from Dog B (Colorado), syntype specimens of *S. caninum*, USNM No. 1251650; voucher specimens of H&E-stained sections from Dog C (Montana), USNM No. 1251651; H&E-stained sections from Dog D (British Columbia, Canada), USNM No. 1251652; H&E-stained sections from Dog A (British Columbia, Canada), USNM No. 1251649. DNA sequences are deposited in GenBank, Accession Nos. KM362427 (Dog D), KM362428 (Dog B).

Remarks: We know the domestic dog can act as the definitive host for numerous *Sarcocystis* species, but the reports of sarcocysts in the muscles of domestic dogs (and cats, and wild felids and wild canids) are relatively rare and, as a result, nothing is known about their life cycles. Dubey et al. (2014) summarized this literature noting that muscle sarcocysts were found in one dog from India (Sahasrabudhe and Shah, 1966), one dog from Georgia, USA (Hill et al., 1988), one dog from Alabama, USA (Blagburn et al., 1989), and one dog from Kenya (Bwangamoi et al., 1993), none of which were associated with clinical disease.

Clinical myositis associated with numerous sarcocysts has only been reported in a dog from Canada (Chapman et al., 2005), and two dogs from Colorado, USA (Sykes et al., 2011). In addition, there are two named species that involve dogs and have unusual life cycles, *S. canis* and *S. neurona*. The former species has been reported in several hosts, including dogs, but only meronts and merozoites are known (see below). The latter species, *S. neurona*, has an unusual life cycle with dogs and other species acting as intermediate (or aberrant) hosts, whereas the opossum, *Didelphis virginiana*, is the definitive host (see Duszynski, 2016, pp. 118–120).

Dubey et al. (2014) had the opportunity to examine preserved, infected muscle tissues from dogs in British Columbia, Canada (2), Colorado (1), and Montana (1) that had been identified and preserved by others (Chapman et al., 2005; Sykes et al., 2011). Examining this material with LM, TEM, and PCR, they were able to distinguish *S. caninum* from others and identify and name it as new because it has a structurally distinct sarcocyst wall and by its phylogenetic resolution using the 18S rRNA and rpoB genetic markers. They pointed out that the structure of the sarcocyst wall is considered a useful tool for distinguishing *Sarcocystis* species within a given host and that Dubey et al. (1989b) and Dubey and Odening (2001) characterized 37 "types" of sarcocyst walls based on their ultrastructure. The sarcocyst wall of *S. caninum* is unique with respect to its villar protrusions because they do not have tubules that extend into the ground substance. Phylogenetic analysis of gene sequences showed that *S. caninum* was similar but not identical to *S. canis* and *S. arctosi*, parasites found in polar bears (*Ursus maritimus*) and brown bears (*U. arctos*), respectively. However, the 18S rRNA region sequence of *S. caninum* showed 100% identity to that of *S. arctica*, which is known to infect Arctic foxes (*Vulpes lagopus*). The rpoB sequence for *S. caninum* was most similar to *S. canis*, but its sarcocysts are unknown. Genetic evidence indicates that *S. caninum* is different molecularly from *S. canis* at both the 18S rRNA and the rpoB loci; the DNA sequences from *S. caninum* and *S. svanai* were similarly resolved from each other at the 18S rRNA locus. Dubey et al. (2015b) suggested that this observation supported infection by two different but related species of *Sarcocystis*, rather than coinfection by two different strains of *S. caninum* that each possessed a different, maternally inherited apicoplast organellar genome that was polymorphic at rpoB. Gjerde and Josefsen (2015) argued that the ITS-1 region sequences of *S. arctica* (KF601306, KF601311), which they produced, were nearly identical with two sequences (JX993923, JX993924) of the *Sarcocystis* species from two Colorado dogs (Sykes et al., 2011), which Dubey et al. (2015b) claimed to be a separate species (*S. caninum*) because they disregarded the high identity between these ITS-1 sequences.

SARCOCYSTIS CANIS DUBEY AND SPEER, 1991

For light and electron micrographs of tissue cysts and zoites of this species see Figs. 1–13 in Dubey and Speer (1991).

Definitive type host: Unknown.

Type locality: North America: USA: Illinois, Ottawa.

Other definitive hosts: Unknown.

Intermediate type host: *Canis lupus familiaris* (syn. *C. familiaris*) L., 1758, Domestic Dog.

Other intermediate hosts: *Monachus schauinslandi* Matschie, 1905, Hawaiian Monk Seal; *Eumetopias jubatus* (Schreber, 1776), Steller Sea Lion; *Zalophus californianus* (Lesson, 1828), California Sea Lion.

Geographic distribution: North America: USA: Alaska, Illinois, Maryland; Central America: Costa Rica; Western Pacific: USA: Hawaii.

Description of sporulated oocyst: Unknown.

Description of sporocyst and sporozoites: Unknown.

Prevalence: A *Sarcocystis*-like parasite was associated with hepatitis (Dubey et al., 1991a), encephalitis (Dubey and Slife, 1990), and dermatitis (Dubey et al., 1991c), each in one Rottweiler dog. These reports led Dubey and Speer (1991) to study three additional infected Rottweiler dogs (two from Illinois, one from Maryland) and to name *S. canis* after studying merogony in their tissue stages. Berrocal and López (2003) diagnosed the first case of pulmonary *S. canis* in a 10-week-old Rottweiler in Guanacaste, Costa Rica. Yantis et al. (2003) found *S. canis* in one Hawaiian monk seal that died in captivity at the Kewalo Basin Facility in Honolulu, Hawaii, and Welsh et al. (2014) also reported *S. canis* associated with hepatitis in a Steller sea lion from Alaska; in the latter, intrahepatocellular meronts were found among areas of necrosis and inflammation. The report by Welsh et al. (2014) was the first from a sea lion. Gingrich et al. (2010) surveyed fecal samples of nondiarrhetic domestic dogs from Santa Cruz (51 dogs), San Cristobal (17 dogs), and Isabela (29 dogs) islands of the Galápagos Archipelago. The dogs often roamed throughout the towns and were not routinely administered anthelmintics, and their veterinary care was limited. Fecal samples were examined by salt and sucrose centrifugation/flotation methods, and *S. canis* was detected in 3/97 (3%) samples from Santa Cruz and Isabela islands. The dogs on the Galápagos Islands represent a unique population and are classified as an introduced species.

Sporulation: Unknown, but likely endogenous with sporulated, infective sporocysts shed in the feces of the definitive host.

Prepatent and patent periods: Unknown.

Site of infection, definitive host: Unknown.

Site of infection, intermediate host: Cytoplasm of neural cells, hepatocytes, leukocytes, and dermal and other cells in dogs.

Endogenous stages, definitive host: Unknown.

Endogenous stages, intermediate host: Meronts divided only by endopolygeny. Mature meronts, L × W: 5–25 × 4–20, were with 6–40 merozoites, which were 4–6 × 1.0 in tissue sections and 5–7 × 1.0 in smears. Both meronts and merozoites reacted with *Sarcocystis cruzi* antiserum but not *T. gondii*, *N. caninum*, or *Caryospora bigenetica* antisera. All parasite stages were located free within host cell cytoplasm without a parasitophorous vacuole (PV). Intracellular merozoites (n = 5) measured via TEM were L × W: 4.5 × 1.7 (4.3–4.8 × 1.5–1.8) and lacked rhoptries.

Cross-transmission: None to date.

Pathology: Berrocal and López (2003) examined one of eight littermate puppies. All the puppies were born healthy and vaccinated for canine parvovirus at 4 weeks of age. One of their puppies received its parvovirus booster 10 weeks later, but on the following day it developed diarrhea, became weak, and started vomiting. Three of the pup's littermates also developed clinical signs that included salivation, convulsions, and other neurological signs. The owner decided not to have a postmortem examination of the other three pups. The puppy examined by Berrocal and López (2003) was eventually diagnosed with canine distemper, but numerous meronts and merozoites were scattered throughout the alveolar walls. Canine distemper predisposes dogs to secondary infections so Berrocal and López (2003) were unable to determine the extent to which *S. canis* endogenous stages contributed to the demise of the puppy. Yantis et al. (2003) found that the monk seal they examined from Hawaii was icteric and the liver was friable, and its lesions included random hepatic

necrosis and cholestasis. They determined that the parasite divided by endopolygeny, merozoites sometimes formed rosettes around a central residual body, and ultrastructurally merozoites lacked rhoptries. Theirs was the first report of *S. canis* in *M. schauinslandi*, an endangered pinniped in US waters. Welsh et al. (2014) reported pathology from a Steller's sea lion found floating in Muir Inlet at Glacier Bay National Park, Alaska. Its liver did not show gross evidence of hepatitis and was not icteric; histologically, however, the liver was congested and had multifocal areas of necrosis with hemorrhage, fibrin thrombi, pyknotic debris, and rare neutrophils. Scattered necrotic hepatocytes contained *S. canis* merozoites and meronts.

Materials deposited: Syntypes from the skin of their No. 2 dog are deposited in the USNM Helminthological Collection, USDA, No. 81893; paratypes of liver from Dog No. 1 are deposited as USNM Helminthological Collection No. 81894.

Etymology: Specific epitaph is the generic name of the type host.

Remarks: Dubey and Speer (1991) justified naming this species since its meronts closely resembled those of *Sarcocystis* because they lacked rhoptries, divided by endopolygeny, were located directly within the host cell cytoplasm without a PV, and stained with anti-*Sarcocystis* serum. They stated that this was the only species known to form meronts in dog tissues. The meronts of this form were somewhat unique because they had a residual body, whereas meronts of "conventional" *Sarcocystis* species lack a residual body at least at the LM level. This species also differed from the *Sarcocystis* species associated with encephalomyelitis in horses and raccoons because the latter forms were confined to the central nervous system (Dubey and Speer, 1991). Dubey and Speer (1991) elaborated in their discussion on the structural, biological, and immunological differences between *S. canis* and *T. gondii*, *N. caninum*, and *Caryospora* species. Increasing reports of *Sarcocystis* species in marine mammals raises the question about the significance of sarcocystosis in pinniped populations (seals) as a whole, especially those species experiencing significant population declines such as Hawaiian monk seals and Steller sea lions. Odening (1998) listed this species as one of the 189 species of *Sarcocystis* in his thorough review of the genus, but he said it should be a *species inquirenda* at the time because no sarcocyst stage was known then. Dubey et al. (2015a) listed this as a valid species of *Sarcocystis* (their Tables 23.1, 24.1, and 24.4).

SARCOCYSTIS CAPRACANIS FISCHER, 1979

Synonym: *Sarcocystis capracanis* El-Rafaii, Abdel-Baki, and Selim, 1980, *lapsus calami*.

Definitive hosts: *Canis latrans* Say, 1823, Coyote; *Canis lupus familiaris* (syn. *C. familiaris*) L., 1758, Domestic Dog; *Cerdocyon thous* (L., 1766), Crab-eating Dog; *Vulpes* (syn. *Alopex*) *corsac* (L., 1768), Corsac Fox; *Vulpes vulpes* (L., 1758), Red or Silver Fox.

Intermediate host: *Capra hircus* L., 1758, Goat.

Geographic distribution: Africa: Egypt; Asia: India; Japan; Europe: Germany; Middle East: Iraq; Jordan; South America: Brazil; South Pacific: Philippines. Probably worldwide.

Remarks: Fischer (1979) worked out the life cycle of this species in Germany and found sarcocysts containing metrocytes in the brain, heart, and striated muscles of experimentally-infected goats on 43 DPI. The sarcocysts were L × W: 130–800 × 50–70 and had thick, striated walls, ~2.8 thick. Aryeetey et al. (1980) fed dogs raw goat meat containing *Sarcocystis* sarcocysts and the sporocysts they shed were inoculated orally into 11 dwarf goats (*C. aegagrus hircus*). Goats were killed on 12, 20, 21, 23, 30, 31, 43, 56, 65, 92, and 118 DPI and mature meronts were found in the cytoplasm of endothelial cells of the veins in the liver, spleen, kidney, and brain. Although degenerated meronts were present in the brain,

host cells around the parasitized cells showed no reactions. Following asexual development, sarcocyst maturation took place in about a month so that on the 65th DPI numerous infectious, banana-shaped merozoites (~15 long) along with some metrocytes (~12 long) were present in the sarcocysts, and they could be seen reproducing by endodyogeny. The sarcocysts of *S. capracanis* had broad protrusions and occurred in all experimentally-infected goats. El-Refaii et al. (1980), Heydorn and Haralambidis (1982), Pereira and Lopes (1982), and Barham et al. (2005) confirmed its transmission to various canids. Levine and Ivens (1981) received unpublished data from a colleague in India, Dr. D.K. Pethkar, who found two types of microscopic sarcocysts in Indian goats. One type had a radially-striated wall, 2–4 thick, and the other had a smooth, thin wall with hair-like processes. Pethkar was able to transmit his sarcocysts (both morphotypes?) to domestic dogs. Levine and Ivens (1981) reasoned that Pethkar's sarcocysts with thick, striated walls may be the same species as *S. capracanis*. They (1981) also stated *S. capracanis* is apparently not *S. moulei* Neveu-Lemaire, 1912, from the domestic goat because that latter form has very large sarcocysts. Pereira and Lopes (1982) confirmed that *C. thous* can act as a definitive host for *S. capracanis*. Heydorn and Haralambidis (1982) fed sporocysts to goats and found first-generation meronts and merozoites in multiple organs (heart, liver, spleen, lungs, brain, mesenteric lymph nodes) 10–15 DPI, mainly in the endothelial cells of arteries; second generation meronts were found in all the same tissues 20–23 DPI. Dubey (1983a) used five littermates of 6-week-old *V. vulpes*, three species of *Sarcocystis* that previously had been isolated from and identified in their intermediate hosts (cattle, sheep, goats) in Montana, USA, and oocysts and tissue cysts of *T. gondii* to conduct a series of cross-transmission experiments. One fox (No. 2) was fed two mice infected with tissue cysts of *T. gondii*; 21 DPI with *T. gondii*, this fox was fed sarcocyst-infected goat meat and shed

S. capracanis-like sporocysts 10 DPI; sporocysts measured L × W (n = 20): 13–14 × 8–10. One goat was fed 1×10^7 of these sporocysts and suddenly became comatose and was in acute respiratory failure on 13 DPI, when it was euthanized; first-generation meronts were found in sections of the arteries of the small intestine and kidneys. A second goat fed 1×10^6 sporocysts died of acute sarcocystosis 19 DPI, and numerous second generation meronts were found in the kidneys and other tissues. A third goat fed 1×10^4 sporocysts was mildly anemic, but otherwise normal and numerous cross-striated sarcocysts were found in its muscles at necropsy, 70 DPI. Dubey and Blagburn (1983) tried to infect one 6-month-old male raccoon with sarcocysts of *S. capracanis* from five experimentally infected goats that had been inoculated with 10,000 sporocysts of *S. capracanis* from a dog, 96 DPI, but the raccoon remained uninfected for at least 5 weeks PI. Cawthorn et al. (1986) studied the *in vitro* excystation of sporozoites from their sporocysts in three *Sarcocystis* species, including *S. capracanis*, and found they could get improved rates of excystation by pretreating sporocysts with an aqueous sodium hypochlorite (NaOCl) solution followed by incubation in excysting fluid.

Odening (1998) included this species as one of 189 valid *Sarcocystis* species names in his very thorough summary paper, but added that *S. capracanis* was not morphologically discernable from *S. tenella*, which he called a sibling species, but that it did differ from *S. tenella* "by intermediate host specificity and molecular genetic features" (as per Tenter et al., 1992). Barham et al. (2005) surveyed 826 goats slaughtered in the winter season in northern Iraq, and found three morphologically distinct types of sarcocysts, macrocysts (both fat and thin), and microcysts; macrocysts were reported to occur in 281/826 (34%) goats and microcysts in 801/826 (97%). Macrocysts were not identified, but microcysts, which were found in the esophagus, striated, and cardiac muscles, were identified as

S. capracanis; these microcysts were elongated, spindle- or spiral-shaped, L × W: 529 × 62 (446–645 × 42–78), with a cyst wall of 3.2 (2.1–4.0) that was striated, with minute finger-like villar protrusions, corresponding to those seen by Heydorn and Haralambidis (1982). Barham et al. (2005) fed goat meat containing numerous sarcocysts (microcysts) to four cats and four dogs; cats did not shed sporocysts, but they did not mention how long they continued to monitor cat feces PI. Dogs did become infected and gamogony occurred in their small intestine, and 7–8 days after eating sarcocyst-infected muscle, sporocysts appear in dog feces that were L × W: 14.9 × 9.5 (12–15 × 9–10), L/W ratio: 1.6. Barham et al. (2005) said the prepatent period in dogs was 12–14 days, and the patent period can be several weeks, up to 64–66 days.

This species does not seem to be pathogenic for dogs, except for 1–2 days of inappetence and mild watery diarrhea (Barham et al., 2005), but in goats that ingest large numbers of sporocysts it causes fever and anemia, and some goats die 20–65 DPI. Levine and Ivens (1981) summarized most of the details of the biology and life cycle. Levine (1986) listed *S. capracanis* as a valid species of *Sarcocystis* found in carnivores as did Odening (1998). Dubey et al. (2015a), in their review of this species included information on structure and life cycle, pathogenicity, protective immunity, and clinical disease in naturally infected goats.

SARCOCYSTIS CAPREOLICANIS ERBER, BOCH, AND BARTH, 1978

Synonyms: "Cyst wall type 6" of Entzeroth, 1982a,b; *Sarcycystis capreoli* in Levine (1988), Dubey et al. (1989b) and Navarrete et al. (1990); *Sarcocystis capreoli* Levchenko, 1963 (?).

Definitive hosts: Canis lupus familiaris (syn. *C. familiaris*) L., 1758, Domestic Dog; *Vulpes velox* (Say, 1823), Swift Fox: *Vulpes vulpes* (L., 1758), Red or Silver Fox.

Intermediate host: *Capreolus capreolus* (L., 1758), European Roe Deer.

Geographic distribution: Europe: wherever roe deer are found.

Remarks: Neither Pellérdy (1974a), nor Levine and Ivens (1981), nor Levine (1986) referred to a published paper by Levchenko (1963), but Levine (1986) suggested that *S. capreolicanis* is a synonym of *S. capreoli*. Erber et al. (1978) were the first to describe sarcocysts with hair-like protrusions in roe deer and, after having transmitted it via sporocysts shed by dogs to at least one roe deer and finding identical sarcocysts in a deer necropsied 122 DPI, they called this species *S. capreolicanis*. Erber et al. (1978) also fed muscles from *Sarcocystis*-infected roe deer to 16 domestic cats, 2 wildcats (*Felis silvestris*), 2 jungle cats (*Felis chaus*), and 2 bobcats (*Lynx rufus*) but none shed sporocysts of *Sarcocystis*. Erber et al. (1978) also fed roe deer muscles to a cat, dog, and fox, but only the dog and fox shed *Sarcocystis* sporocysts. Odening (1998) included this species as one of the 189 valid *Sarcocystis* species names in his very thorough summary paper, but added that *S. capreolicanis* was similar to *S. rangi* and to *Sarcocystis* species type IIB of Atkinson et al. (1993) from *O. virginianus* in North America. Odening (1998) also added that it was "very probably" also to be found in *Cervus elaphus* (cf. Wesemeier and Sedlaczek, 1995b), *Dama dama*, and zoo-born *Cervus unicolor* (Odening, 1997; Odening et al., 1999) in Europe. Gjerde (2012) characterized the morphology of *S. capreolicanis* sarcocysts with LM and SEM, defined the molecular characteristics of the 18S rRNA gene, and did a phylogenetic analysis of *S. capreolicanis* (and *S. silva*) in *C. capreolus* in Norway. In the phylogenetic analysis, *S. capreolicanis* was placed together with other species with hair-like surface protrusions, which indicated to Gjerde (2012) that they are sibling species with a common ancestor. His phylogeny also placed *S. capreolicanis* among other species known to be transmitted

by canines, corroborating the results of Erber et al. (1978). Dubey et al. (2015a) identified *S. capreolicanis* in *C. capreolus* and said the dog and red fox were valid definitive hosts that shed sporocysts, L × W: 12–18 × 9–11. We are unable to find any papers attributable to Levchenko in our combined comprehensive review of the literature. Thus we think that *S. capreolicanis* as described by Erber et al. (1978) is the appropriate name for one of the *Sarcocystis* species commonly found in roe deer muscles.

SARCOCYSTIS CERVICANIS HERNANDEZ, NAVARRETE, AND MARTINEZ, 1981

Definitive host: *Canis lupus familiaris* (syn. *C. familiaris*) L., 1758, Domestic Dog.

Intermediate host: *Cervus elaphus* L., 1758 (syn. *Cervus canadensis* Erxleben, 1777), Red Deer, Elk, Wapiti.

Geographic distribution: Probably worldwide.

Remarks: Levine (1986) said that the relationship of this species to *S. wapiti* is unknown. Odening (1998) included this species as one of the 189 valid *Sarcocystis* species names in his summary paper but added that *S. cervicanis* was probably a synonym of *S. grueneri*, together with *S. alceslatrans* and *S. wapiti* (see Odening, 1997; Odening et al., 1999). Dubey et al. (2015a) listed this species as one of 10 valid *Sarcocystis* species for this intermediate host and its three subspecies; the other nine are: *S. hjorti* Dahlgren and Gjerde, 2010a; *S. ovalis* Dahlgren and Gjerde, 2008; *S. elongata* (Gjerde, 2013) Gjerde 2014c; *S. truncata* (Gjerde, 2013) Gjerde 2014c; *S. hardangeri* Gjerde, 1984b,c (also found in reindeer); *S. tarandi* Gjerde, 1984a,e (also found in reindeer); *S. cervicanis* Hernandez-Rodriguez, Navarrete and Martinez-Gomez, 1981; *S. wapiti* Speer and Dubey, 1982; and *S. sybillensis* Dubey, Jolley, and Thorne, 1983.

SARCOCYSTIS CRUZI (HASSELMANN, 1923) WENYON, 1926b

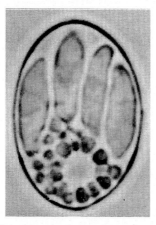

FIGURE 15.1 Photomicrograph of a sporocyst (Fig. 2) of *Sarcocystis cruzi. From Fayer, R., Leek, R.G., 1973. Excystation of* Sarcocystis fusiformis *sporocysts from dogs. Proceedings of the Helminthological Society of Washington 40 (2), 294–296, with permission of the senior author and the Editor. Comparative Parasitology, copyright of the Helminthological Society of Washington, with permission.*

Synonyms: *Miescheria cruzi* Hasselmann, 1923 *pro parte*; *Coccidium bigeminum* Stiles, 1891, *pro parte*; *Coccidium bigemina* var. *canis* Railliet and Lucet, 1891, *pro parte*; *Sarcocystis fusiformis* Railliet, 1897 of Babudieri (1932) and *auctores*, *pro parte*; [non] *Sarcocystis fusiformis* (Railliet, 1897) Bernard and Bauche, 1912; *Sarcocystis iturbei* Vogelsang, 1938; *Sarcocystis marcovi* Vershinin, 1975, *pro parte*; *Sarcocystis bovicanis* Heydorn, Gestrich, Mehlorn, and Rommel, 1975b; *Isospora rivolta* sporocysts of Gassner (1940), Levine and Ivens (1965), and *auctores*, *pro parte*; *Isospora bigemina* large form of Mehlhorn, Senaud, Heydorn, and Gestrich (1975a) *pro parte*; *Lucetina bigemina* (Stiles, 1891) Henry and Leblosi, 1926, *pro parte*; *Cryptosporidium vulpis* Wetzel, 1938; *"Cryptosporidium"* of Bearup (1954) *pro parte*; *Sarcocystis* sp. of Golemansky and Ridzhakov (1975); *Endorinospora hirsuta* (Moulé, 1888) Tadros and Laarman, 1976.

Definitive hosts: *Canis lupus* L., 1758, Wolf; *Canis l. familiaris* (syn. *C. familiaris*) L., 1758, Domestic Dog; *Canis latrans* Say, 1823, Coyote; *Cerdocyon thous* (L., 1758), Crab-eating Dog; *Nyctereutes procyonoides* (Gray, 1834), Raccoon Dog; *Vulpes vulpes* (L., 1758), Red or Silver Fox; *Procyon lotor* (L., 1758), Raccoon (Fayer et al., 1976; Levine, 1986).

Intermediate hosts: *Bison bison* (L., 1758), American Bison; *Bison bonasus* (L., 1758), European Bison; *Bos frontalis* Lambert, 1804, Gaur; *Bos javanicus* d'Alton, 1823, Banteng; *Bos taurus* L., 1758, Aurochs; *Bubalus bubalis* (L., 1758), Water Buffalo.

Geographic distribution: Africa: Egypt; Nigeria; Uganda; Asia: China; India; Japan; Malaysia; Philippines; South Korea; Thailand; Vietnam; Australia; Middle East: Iran; Turkey; Europe: Belgium; Czech Republic; England; Germany; Italy; Lithuania; New Zealand; North America; many states; South America: Argentina; Brazil; Uruguay. Clearly its distribution is worldwide.

Remarks: The history of this species name is especially convoluted and there are two contradictory arguments regarding it. One that has been most widely accepted as valid, and in line with the International Code of Zoological Nomenclature, is that proposed by Levine (1988) and Dubey et al. (1989b), which maintains that the correct (valid) name is *S. cruzi* and the name *S. bovicanis* is a junior synonym.

Wetzel (1938) found mature sporocysts in the feces of 1/2 (50%) red fox puppies received at his institute in Germany; he named the species *Cryptosporidium vulpis*. It is likely that these sporocysts were either those of *S. cruzi* or of *S. miescheriana*. Fayer and Leek (1973), after several unsuccessful attempts, were finally able to demonstrate that sporocysts first had to be exposed to a 1:1 mixture of CO_2 and air before sporozoites would excyst from their sporocyst *in vitro*. At the time, they worked with sporocysts from dogs but called it *S. fusiformis*. Later that year, Fayer (1973) was the first to report transmission of *Sarcocystis* from a dog, via sporocysts, to a bovine host (also using the name *S. fusiformis*); he inoculated five calves with suspensions of 250,000–1 million sporocysts from dogs and four became acutely ill. Infected calves had anorexia, cachexia, weight loss, anemia, and accelerated heart rates. Fayer (1973) examined 18 different tissues from infected calves histologically and found meronts in all tissues from 4/5 (80%), with the greatest numbers within endothelial cells of blood vessels of the kidneys. By all measures, *S. cruzi* is the most pathogenic *Sarcocystis* species in cattle. Acute disease occurs in calves experimentally infected with sporocysts from canine feces. Clinical signs are anorexia, pyrexia, anemia, cachexia, and weight loss; infected calves become moribund and often die between 30 and 35 DPI with 10^5 to 10^6 sporocysts (Dubey, 1976).

Fayer (1974) inoculated coccidia-free dogs with sporocysts of *S. cruzi* (called *S. fusiformis* at the time), but all dogs failed to pass sporocysts within 18 and 32 DPI, whereas three groups of dogs fed raw bovine heart, with sarcocysts, passed sporocysts 13–22 days later. After these dogs stopped passing sporocysts they were fed infected bovine heart a second time and began passing sporocysts 9 and 11 days later. Other dogs fed with raw bovine heart were killed 1–8, 10, 11, and 13 DPI and sections of their small intestines demonstrated macrogamonts, oocyst wall formation, and sporogony in the lamina propria of the villi, being most abundant in the distal jejunum and proximal ileum. Microgamonts were not seen or identified. Mehlhorn et al. (1975b) described the sarcocysts of this species (syn. *S. fusiformis*), by both LM and TEM, in the muscles of calves experimentally infected with sporocysts of what was then called the large form of *Isospora bigemina* from dogs. Fayer (1977a) inoculated 21 dogs with either experimentally-infected or naturally-infected beef and found the prepatent period ranged from 9 to 33 days with seven dogs shedding their first sporocysts on 12 DPI. These dogs were still shedding sporocysts for the length of his experiments, 40 and 60 days. Fayer and Leek (1979) found merozoites of this species in blood smears of calves exhibiting signs of acute sarcocystosis after oral infection with sporocysts from dogs. They took whole blood containing merozoites from calves and transfused it into two uninfected calves, and large numbers of intramuscular sarcocysts were found in both transfused recipients, indicating that *S. cruzi* (syn. *S. bovicanis*) had been transmitted between intermediate hosts of the same species by blood transfusion.

Levine and Ivens (1981) summarized the location of gamonts, gametes, and oocysts/sporocysts in the lamina propria of the villi of the small intestine and included information on oocyst/sporocyst structure, sporulation times, merogony in the intermediate host(s), prepatent and patent periods, various cross-transmission studies, and what we knew then about the pathogenic nature and immunology in both definitive and intermediate hosts. Levine and Ivens (1981) also did a lengthy review in their *Remarks* section (pp. 29–31) on the historical confusion that various authors have had in correctly naming this species (and see *Synonyms*, above). For example, Fayer and Johnson (1974) were able to take sporocysts from dogs and produce sarcocysts in calves that were fed these sporocysts. They also traced the development of the parasite and found meronts in adrenal glands, cecum, cerebellum, cerebrum, diaphragm, esophagus, eye, auricle and ventricle of the heart, ileum, jejunum, kidney, liver, lung, mesenteric lymph nodes, pancreas, spleen, skeletal muscle, testicle, thyroid, tongue, and urinary bladder; but they called the parasite *S. fusiformis*. Fayer et al. (1976) did a large-scale study in Maryland, USA, feeding sarcocyst-infected bovine tissues to a variety of carnivores (cats, dogs, skunks, ferrets) and omnivores (primates, rodents, lagomorphs) but once again called the parasite *S. fusiformis*. Farmer et al. (1978) surveyed feces from 123 working sheepdogs in Gwynedd, from 33 greyhounds from the London area, and from 41 red foxes killed on Anglesey or in the Bangor area of England. They found sporocysts of *Sarcocystis* spp. in 35/123 (28%) sheepdogs, 8/33 (24%)

greyhounds, and 7/41 (17%) red foxes (their Table 1, p. 79). Based only on sporocyst dimensions, they said that *S. cruzi* sporocysts were identified in 13/47 (sic) (28%) samples examined (Farmer et al., 1978, Table 2, p. 79).

This species undergoes at least three sequential generations of asexual development in its intermediate host. First-generation meronts develop inside endothelial cells of small arteries throughout the body, about 15–16 DPI (Fayer, 1977b). Second-generation meronts also develop in endothelial cells of capillaries throughout the body, 26–33 DPI (Fayer and Johnson, 1973); and, later, intramuscular sarcocysts develop in diaphragm, esophagus, skeletal muscles, and tongue of the cow as early as 33–54 DPI (Fayer and Johnson, 1974; Fayer, 1979). Interestingly, merozoites from second-generation meronts were observed in the peripheral blood on 27 DPI by Gestrich et al. (1975) and that observation was followed up by Fayer (1979, using the name *S. bovicanis*) who infected a 2-month-old male calf with ~350,000 sporocysts of *S. bovicanis* and then took blood smears on 27, 28, 29 DPI. The calf died on 29 DPI of acute sarcocystosis. Fayer (1979) found merozoites free in the blood and within large and small leukocytes (mostly lymphocytes); on 27 DPI only a few merozoites were observed, but on 28 and 29 DPI, 19–50 merozoites were observed per blood smear and these merozoites were multiplying via endodyogeny. Fayer's (1979) work showed that merozoites can multiply in the blood stream to increase their reproductive potential; however, Fayer (1979) added that this additional asexual stage may be significant from the standpoint of immunity and pathology related to metabolites or other parasite products from multiplication as well as debris from the parent organism would be released directly into the blood stream and within lymphocytes.

Dubey (1983a,b) used five littermates of 6-week-old *V. vulpes*, three species of *Sarcocystis* that previously had been isolated from and identified in their intermediate hosts (cattle,

sheep, goats) in Montana, USA, and oocysts and tissue cysts of *T. gondii* to conduct a series of cross-transmission experiments. Two foxes (Nos. 3, 4) were each fed 350 sporulated oocysts of the GT-1 strain of *T. gondii*. Thirty-three DPI with *T. gondii*, fox No. 3 was fed meat from a calf that had been experimentally infected with 5×10^5 sporocysts of the B1 isolate of *S. cruzi* 84 days prior to necropsy; 42 DPI with *T. gondii*, fox No. 4 was fed meat from a calf that had been experimentally infected with 5×10^5 sporocysts of the B1 isolate of *S. cruzi* 93 days prior to necropsy. Foxes Nos. 3 and 4 shed *S. cruzi*-like sporocysts 9 DPI; the sporocysts measured L × W (n = 20): 14–16 × 9–10.5. One calf fed these sporocysts was febrile (40–41°C) on 15, 25, 26, 27, 28 DPI; on 27 DPI it had watery diarrhea, appeared dull, and was euthanized the next day because of weakness and inappetence. At necropsy, petechial hemorrhages were seen throughout muscles and viscera and these were particularly severe in the heart. Single and dividing merozoites were found in mononuclear cells of the blood at 21 and 28 DPI and second-generations meronts were found in kidneys and several other tissues. Cawthorn et al. (1986) studied the *in vitro* excystation of sporozoites from their sporocysts in three *Sarcocystis* species, including *S. cruzi*, and found they could get improved rates of excystation by pretreating sporocysts with an aqueous sodium hypochlorite (NaOCl) solution followed by incubation in excysting fluid. Dubey and Blagburn (1983) tried to infect one 9-month-old raccoon with sarcocysts of *S. cruzi* from an infected calf that had been inoculated with 287,000 sporocysts of *S. cruzi* 86 DPI, but the raccoon remained uninfected for at least 5 weeks PI. Levine (1986) listed *S. cruzi* as a valid species of *Sarcocystis* found in carnivores. Böttner et al. (1987) surveyed muscle samples microscopically of 500 beef cattle slaughtered in New Zealand and found 100% to be infected; of these, 98% were infected with the thin-walled cysts of *S. cruzi*. Gajadhar and Marquardt (1992) studied beef carcasses from an abattoir in Colorado, USA, which were both condemned for eosinophilic myositis and those that were unaffected. In their work, Gajadhar and Marquardt (1992) examined sarcocysts by LM and TEM and showed that sarcocysts, affected by cellular response in condemned carcasses, as well as those found unaffected by cellular responses, were consistent with those of *S. cruzi*, and their transmission experiments confirmed that dogs, but not cats, were the definitive hosts. Odening (1998) included this species as one of the 189 valid *Sarcocystis* species names in his very thorough summary paper and said that *S. cruzi* was similar to both *S. poephagicanis* from the yak and to *S. levinei* from the water buffalo (see Xiao et al., 1993). Dubey et al. (2015a) did a thorough literature review and gave detailed information and references on the structure of the life cycle, pathogenicity, including gross and microscopic lesions, abortion and neonatal mortality, natural outbreaks, protective immunity, and molecular and genetic diversity of *S. cruzi*.

Fischer and Odening (1998) isolated sarcocysts of *S. cruzi* from a zoo-born dwarf zebu (*B. taurus*) and a zoo-born bison (*B. bison*) and compared sequenced PCR products of their 18S rRNA genes; sequences of both isolates from these different host species always showed a very high, nearly complete identity to each other both within all or only the conserved overlapping nucleotides, verifying they were the same species. Li et al. (2002) used a PCR-based analysis of the 18S rRNA gene to examine *S. cruzi*-like sarcocysts from water buffalo in Yunnan, China; 15 water buffalo isolates were compared with 10 *S. cruzi* isolates from cattle. Restriction fragment length polymorphism (RFLP) patterns for both sets of isolates were found to be identical with all the 12 restriction enzymes used. They also found that variation between samples from Kunming and Gengma (both in Yunnan) was undetectable at these loci, which led them to conclude that *S. cruzi* was able to use the water buffalo as an intermediate host, and it is not restricted

to cattle. Over the last decade, much relevant work using both morphological studies at all levels (LM, TEM, SEM), and PCR amplification of several loci (18S rRNA, 28S rRNA, ITS-1, cox1) of *Sarcocystis* sarcocysts in various wild and domesticated Artiodactyla species, has been done in Norway and a few other countries, by Gjerde et al. (Gjerde, 2012; 2013, 2014a,b,c; Gjerde and Josefsen, 2015; Gjerde, 2016a,b; Gjerde et al., 2017). Regarding *S. cruzi*, Gjerde (2016b) excised 200 individual sarcocysts from 12 beef cattle samples from five countries (Argentina, Brazil, Germany, New Zealand, Uruguay) and genomic DNA was extracted from 147 of these sarcocysts. Using PCR amplification and sequencing of the partial cox1 gene and three regions of nuclear ribosomal DNA (complete 18S rRNA, complete ITS-1 region, and partial 28S rRNA gene) he compared results with previous molecular identifications to evaluate the regions for species delimitations and phylogenetic inferences. Based on his molecular characterizations and sarcocyst morphology, 22 microscopic sarcocysts (1 × 0.1), with hair-like protrusions, were assigned to *S. cruzi*; these sarcocysts of *S. cruzi* came from beef samples from Argentina and Uruguay.

SARCOCYSTIS ERDMANAE ODENING, 1997

Definitive host: *Canis lupus familiaris* (syn. *C. familiaris*) L., 1758, Domestic Dog.

Remarks: For more complete information on *Sarcocystis erdmanae* see Genus *Mephitis*, below.

SARCOCYSTIS FAYERI DUBEY, STREITEL, STROMBERG, AND TOUSSANT, 1977b

Definitive host: *Canis lupus familiaris* (syn. *C. familiaris*) L., 1758, Domestic Dog.

Intermediate hosts: *Equus burchellii burschelii* Schinz, 1845, Burchell's Zebra; *Equus burchellii chapmanni* Layard, 1866, Burchell's Zebra; *Equus caballus* L., 1758, Horse; *Equus hemionus* Pallas, 1775 (syn. *Equus onager* Boddaert, 1785), Onager; *Equus zebra* L., 1758, (syn. *Equus hartmannae* Matschie, 1898), Mountain Zebra.

Geographic distribution: Europe: Germany; Middle East: Turkey; North America: USA: Indiana, Ohio, Wisconsin. Probably worldwide in distribution.

Remarks: Levine and Ivens (1981) included this species and pointed out how little is known about it, since its discovery in Ohio, USA. Levine (1986) said that this species may turn out to be a synonym of *S. bertrami*, and Odening (1998) agreed this species was quite similar to *S. bertrami*. Sarcocysts are found primarily in the skeletal muscles but rarely in the heart of infected horses. Odening (1998) said that *S. fayeri* probably also was found in the European hare, *Lepus europaeus* Pallas, 1778, as per Odening et al. (1994c, 1996b). Dubey et al. (2015a) provided some life cycle information on the endogenous development in horses. This species seems to be only mildly pathogenic in ponies and adults. Dubey et al. (2015a) briefly discussed the prevalence of natural infections and clinical disease and then summarized what little other information was available on *Sarcocystis* spp. in horses (their Table 11.1).

SARCOCYSTIS FEROVIS DUBEY, 1983b

Photomicrograph of a sporulated oocyst (Fig. 4), one LM section of infected coyote gut (Fig. 3), and two TEM photomicrographs of sarcocysts of *Sarcocystis ferovis* (Figs. 1 and 2) are found in Dubey (1983b).

Definitive host: *Canis latrans* Say, 1823, Coyote.

Intermediate host: *Ovis canadensis* Shaw 1804, Bighorn Sheep.

Geographic distribution: North America: USA: Montana, near Gardner.

Remarks: Dubey (1983b) necropsied a 6-year-old ram that was shot in Montana, USA. He found no macroscopic sarcocysts in the tongue, heart, esophagus, diaphragm, or other muscles. However, under LM, microscopic sarcocysts were found in squash preparations of muscles from the legs, abdomen, diaphragm, heart, eye, tongue, and esophagus. Sarcocysts in the tissues measured L × W (n = 31): 173 × 57 (30–780 × 30–100); L/W ratio: 3.0, were septate, had a smooth, thin wall (0.6 thick), and contained numerous bradyzoites that were L × W (n = 10): 10–14 × 3–3.5. Portions of these tissues were ground and stored at 4°C, and the next day were fed over a period of three days to one lab-raised, female, 8-month-old coyote. On 9 DPI, the coyote began shedding oocysts and sporocysts in its feces. It was killed on 12 DPI and unsporulated and sporulated oocysts were found just below the epithelium and occasionally the lamina propria of infected villi was infiltrated with neutrophils. Sporulated oocysts measured L × W (n = 14): 19.6 × 14.0 (17.5–21 × 14–15), L/W ratio: 1.4; individual sporocysts were L × W (n = 52): 13.6 × 9.7 (13–15 × 9–11), L/W ratio: 1.4; and living SZ were L × W (n = 10): 7.0–8.5 × 2. Dubey (1983b) infected two goats (*C. hircus*), five sheep (*O. aureus*), and an ox (*B. taurus*) with from 1 to 25 million sporocysts retrieved from the infected coyote; they were necropsied from 17 to 70 DPI, but none showed any signs of infection. Levine (1986) listed this name as a valid *Sarcocystis* species. Odening (1998) also listed this form as one of the 189 *Sarcocystis* species in his review. Dubey et al. (2015a) do not list it in their Table 14.2: "*Sarcocystis* species sporocysts in feces of dogs," but they do list it, with the coyote as the definitive host, in their Table 18.2 "*Sarcocystis* species in other wild ruminants and large animals."

SARCOCYSTIS GRUENERI YAKIMOFF AND SOKOLOFF, 1934

Definitive host: *Canis lupus familiaris* (syn. *C. familiaris*) L., 1758, Domestic Dog (?)

Remarks: For more complete information on *S. grueneri*, see Genus *Vulpes*, below.

SARCOCYSTIS HEMIONILATRANTIS HUDKINS AND KISTNER, 1977

Definitive hosts: *Canis latrans* Say, 1823, Coyote; *Canis lupus familiaris* (syn. *C. familiaris*) L., 1758, Domestic Dog.

Intermediate hosts: *Capreolus capreolus* L., 1758, European Roe Deer; *Odocoileus hemionus* (Rafinesque, 1817), Mule Deer.

Geographic distribution: North America: USA: Montana, Oregon.

Remarks: Fifteen coyote pups, ~2–3 weeks old, were captured from dens in eastern Oregon, USA, and raised in medium isolation facilities. They were fed freshly ground skeletal muscle from a mule deer infected with sarcocysts, and all of them shed sporocysts in their feces, intermittently, from 12 to 36 DPI. Sporocysts were L × W (n = 80): 14.4 × 9.3 (14–16 × 9–11); L/W ratio: 1.5 (Hudkins and Kistner, 1977). They then fed 11 mule deer fawns with sporocysts from coyotes that ranged in dosage levels from 1×10^6, 2.5×10^5, and 5×10^4, and all became infected and clinically ill. Nine of the 11 died between 27 and 63 DPI with sporocysts. Clinical signs included anorexia, weight loss, pyrexia, and weakness. Hudkins and Kistner (1977) were unable to infect a calf, *B. taurus*, or two lambs, *O. aries*, with sporocysts from the coyote. Speer et al. (1980) determined the prepatent (9–13 days) and patent periods (31–35 days) in coyotes that had ingested infected mule deer musculature and described the endogenous sexual development of *S. hemionilatrantis* in the lamina propria of the coyote small intestine. They (1980) found sporulated and unsporulated oocysts that were L × W: 21.3 × 17.5, L/W ratio: 1.2; and sporocysts measured L × W: 16.2 × 9.9, L/W ratio: 1.6. Dubey and Blagburn (1983) tried to infect one 7-month-old raccoon with 1 kg of meat, over 7 days, from a mule deer infected with sarcocysts of *S. hemionilatrantis* that had been shot near Bozeman, MT, but the raccoon remained uninfected for at least 5 weeks PI. Entzeroth (1983) did a TEM study of merogony preceding cyst formation of what likely were early stages of *S. hemionilatrantis* in roe deer (*C. capreolus*) in Germany; he inoculated 2×10^4–10^5

sporocysts, recovered from dogs, into roe deer fawns, and killed them at 33, 45, and 49 DPI, when all three became seriously ill. Transforming merozoites and meronts were found in myofibroblasts, satellite cells, and endothelial cells of the deer muscle tissues on 25 and 49 DPI. Dubey and Speer (1985) found three distinct types of sarcocysts in 130/153 (85%) samples of mule deer (*O. hemionus*) muscle around Bozeman, Montana, USA, and described the ultrastructure of their sarcocyst walls, one of which was *S. hemionilatrantis*, but they did not mention how many of their infected deer were infected with each species. Levine (1986), Odening (1998), and Dubey et al. (2015a) all listed this as a valid *Sarcocystis* species, and other information on various developmental stages in the life cycle are available from them. Levine (1986) pointed out that the relationship of this species to *S. gracilis* Rátz, 1908, in *C. elaphus*, to *S. grueneri* Yakimoff and Sokoloff, 1934 in *C. elaphus*, to *S. cervi* Destombes, 1957, in Vietnam deer, and to other unnamed and poorly described *Sarcocystis* species from other deer and elk remains to be determined. Odening (1998) thought this species was similar to *S. odocoileocanis*. Again, given the pathogenic nature of *S. hemionilatrantis* in deer, there is still a lot of important work to be accomplished in these hosts.

SARCOCYSTIS HIRCICANIS HEYDORN AND UNTERHOLZNER, 1983

Definitive host: *Canis lupus familiaris* (syn. *C. familiaris*) L., 1758, Domestic Dog.

Intermediate host: *Odocoileus hemionus* (Rafinesque, 1817), Mule Deer.

Geographic distribution: Asia: India; Japan; Europe: Germany (?); Middle East: Jordan. Probably worldwide in distribution.

Remarks: Levine (1986) included *S. hircicanis* in his list of 122 valid *Sarcocystis* species known to that time. Odening (1998) also listed this form as one of the 189 *Sarcocystis* species in his review, said that the domestic goat was the intermediate host, and indicated that *S. arieticanis* might be a sibling species differing only in intermediate host specificity. Dubey et al. (2015a) added only information on the gross structure of the sarcocysts in deer and pointed out that very little else is known about this species.

SARCOCYSTIS HORVATHI RÁTZ, 1908

Synonyms: *Sarcocystis gallinarum* Krause and Goranoff, 1933; *Sarcocystis* v. Rátz, 1908 of Kalyakin and Zasukhin (1975) *lapsus calimi*; *Sarcocystis horwati* Rátz, 1908 of Kalyakin and Zasukhin (1975) *lapsus calimi*.

Definitive hosts: *Canis lupus familiaris* (syn. *C. familiaris*) L., 1758, Domestic Dog (Munday et al., 1977) (?); *Felis catus* L., 1758, Domestic Cat (Golubkov, 1979) (?).

Intermediate host: *Gallus gallus* (L., 1758), Red Jungle Fowl or Chicken.

Geographic distribution: Australia; Asia: Azerbaijan, Russia; Europe: Bulgaria, Czech Republic, Germany, Hungary; North America: USA: Mississippi; Oceana: Papua New Guinea.

Remarks: There is considerable confusion about the species of *Sarcocystis* that infect chickens. Rátz (1908, 1909), in Hungary, first described sarcocysts in chicken muscle that were up to 1 mm long, with a wall that was 1.8–2.7 thick, and named it *S. horvathi*. Later, Krause and Goranoff (1933), in Bulgaria, proposed the name *S. gallinarum*, for chicken sarcocysts they described as up to 10 mm long, with banana-shaped bradyzoites that were 7–13 × 2–4.5, but Levine and Tadros (1980) synonymized *S. gallinarum* with *S. horvathi*. Mehlhorn et al. (1976) described the ultrastructure of muscle sarcocysts in chickens from Australia and Papua New Guinea, but they did not describe bradyzoites. Munday et al. (1977) published a case report about a *Sarcocystis* species causing severe myositis in three fowls in Papua New Guinea and two from Tasmania, Australia; in all, they saw sarcocysts in histological sections of 35/78 (45%) free-ranging fowls

(chickens) in New Guinea. The sarcocysts they described were up to 2 mm long and 45 µm in diameter, with a 2.5–3.0 µm thick wall that was striated. The pathology seen in 3/78 (4%) Papua New Guinea birds included muscular weakness that resulted in a "duck-sitting" posture and histologically showed nutritional myopathy (white muscle disease). They said the myositis was focal rather than diffuse and accompanied by scattered areas of myonecrosis associated with macrophages, lymphocytes, and a few heterophils and giant cells. One 6-week-old, coccidia-free dog was fed sarcocyst-infected flesh from a chicken, and on 7 DPI discharged small numbers of sporocysts that were L × W: 11.5 × 8.0 (10–13 × 7–8.5), L/W ratio: 1.4; the pup was killed 10 DPI and oocysts in its jejunal scrapings (L × W: 15 × 11) were "dosed" into three 1-day-old chicks. The chicks were examined 90 DPI, but no sarcocysts were detected in sections of muscles "despite an intensive search." Their cross-transmission work *suggested* a dog was the intermediate host.

Golubkov (1979), in Russia, added confusion when working with sarcocysts of *S. horvathi* in naturally-infected chickens and *S. rileyi* in ducks; he infected dogs and cats with muscle sarcocysts (presumably of both species) and got sporocyst production in the feces of both carnivores, but he neglected to say which *Sarcocystis* species they were positive for or even whether or not the dogs and cats he used had ever been fed any kind of meat before the experiments. Then Wenzel et al. (1982), in Germany, found sarcocysts in 45/241 (19%) free-range chickens. They reported two types of sarcocysts based on the shape of the bradyzoites. Sarcocysts with banana-shaped bradyzoites, L × W: 9–12.5 × 2.5–3.0, were considered to be *S. horvathi*, but a dog, cat, polecat, marten, and goshawk fed infected chicken muscle did not excrete sporocysts (Dubey et al., 2015a). The second type of sarcocyst (Wenzel et al., 1982) contained lancet-shaped bradyzoites that were L × W: 12–15 × 2.5–3.0, and Odening (1997) named the species with lancet-shaped bradyzoites to be *S. wenzeli* (see below). Pecka (1988, 1990), in the Czech Republic, reported sarcocysts of *S. horvathi*, with banana-shaped cystozoites 10–12 × 3.5 in 2/30 (7%) hens and with lancet-shaped cystozoites 12–14 × 4 in one bird. Levine and Ivens (1981) summarized this species mostly from the work of Munday et al. (1977) and Golubkov (1979). Levine (1986) listed this as a valid *Sarcocystis* species and included the dog and the cat as definitive hosts with the domestic chicken as an intermediate host; Odening (1998), however, listed it as a valid species but not the cat as a definitive host. Dubey et al. (2005) did not find *Sarcocystis* sporocysts in the feces of cats that were fed breast muscle from over 2,000 chickens from grocery stores in the United States nor did Dubey (2010) find sarcocysts in hearts from more than 1,000 free-range chickens from different countries (although muscles were not examined microscopically). In Azerbaijan, Memmedov (2010) found sarcocysts he considered to be *S. horvathi* in pectoral and esophageal muscles of chicken hens. Dubey et al. (2015a) summarized the *Sarcocystis* of chickens by identifying *S. horvathi* as one of the two valid species infecting domestic chickens, but noting the uncertainty of whether dogs, or cats, or both, or neither of them are the definitive hosts. Dubey et al. (2015a) cited all the known contributing authors and their work on sarcocyst and bradyzoite size and structures, the limited cross-transmission work that has been done to date, and prevalences in various countries with such surveys, and they mentioned this species in their Tables 1.4, 24.1, and 24.4.

SARCOCYSTIS LEVINEI DISSANAIKE AND KAN, 1978

Excellent photomicrographs of a sporulated oocyst (Fig. 8) and sporocyst (Fig. 9), two LM sections of sarcocysts (Figs. 1 and 2), and five TEM photomicrographs of sarcocysts *S. levinei* (Figs. 3–7) are found in Dissanaike and Kan (1978).

Synonym: "Large form of *Isospora bigemina*" of Wenyon and Sheather (1925) and Wenyon (1926a) in dogs from Sri Lanka.

Definitive host: *Canis lupus familiaris* (syn. *C. familiaris*) L., 1758, Domestic Dog.

Intermediate host: *Bubalus bubalis* (L., 1758), Water Buffalo.

Geographic distribution: Africa: Egypt; Asia: China; India; Malaysia; Philippines; Vietnam; Middle East: Iran; Turkey; South America: Brazil.

Remarks: Levine and Ivens (1981) confirmed that gamonts, gametes, zygotes, oocysts, and sporocysts are in the lamina propria of the dog small intestine and sarcocysts in the striated muscles of buffalo. They also summarized what was known about sarcocysts in buffalo muscle cells, and Levine (1986) listed this as a valid species of *Sarcocystis*. Huong et al. (1997b) redescribed *S. levinei* because the original description was a mixture of this species and of *S. buffalonis*. In tissue sections, *S. levinei* sarcocysts are microscopic, up to 640 long and 95 wide; ultrastructurally, they have a thin wall (<1 thick) with a minute undulating surface and smooth, hair-like villar protrusions arising at irregular intervals from the cyst wall. Dogs, but not cats, fed water buffalo hearts infected with sarcocysts of this form shed sporocysts that were L × W: 14.0–16.5 × 9.5–10.5 on 14–16 DPI. Odening (1998) in his compilation of *Sarcocystis* names, listed this as a valid species. He also pointed out that *S. levinei* is similar to *S. cruzi*, and was formerly mixed with *S. buffalonis*. Dubey et al. (2015a) listed *S. levinei* as one of four species being pathogenic for buffalo and summarized some of the morphological and geographical data in their Figs. 10.1 A, B and Table 10.2. Natural infections with *Sarcocystis* species in water buffalo are quite frequent.

SARCOCYSTIS MICROS WANG, WEI, WANG, LI, ZHANG, DONG, AND XIAO, 1988

Definitive type host: *Canis lupus familiaris* (syn. *C. familiaris*) L., 1758, Domestic Dog.

Type locality: Asia: China, Qinghai Province.

Other definitive hosts: Unknown.

Intermediate type host: *Ovis ammon* (L., 1758), Argali.

Other intermediate host: *Ovis aries* L., 1758, Red Sheep.

Geographic distribution: Asia: China.

Description of sporulated oocyst: Oocyst shape: ovoidal to nearly rectangular, with one thin membrane (wall) stretched over the two SP; L × W: 18.5 × 13.3 (18–19 × 13–13.5); L/W ratio: 1.4; M, OR, PG: all absent. Distinctive features of oocyst: typical thin-walled *Sarcocystis*-type, which usually breaks down releasing sporocysts into the intestinal lumen.

Description of sporocyst and sporozoites: Sporocyst shape: ellipsoidal; L × W: 14 × 9 (14 × 6–9); L/W ratio: 1.5; SB, SSB, PSB: all absent; SR: present; SR characteristics: a compact mass of granules, 4.5 (4–5) wide; SZ: banana-shaped, L × W: 9.5 × 2.3 (9–10 × 2–2.5), each with one RB. Distinctive features of sporocyst: none; a "typical" *Sarcocystis*-type SP, lacking SB, SSB, PSB and with a distinct, granular SR.

Prevalence: Wang et al. (1988) found sarcocysts of this species in 2/21 (10%) sheep from "certain sheep farms."

Sporulation: Endogenous with sporulated, infective sporocysts shed in the feces of the definitive host.

Prepatent and patent periods: Dogs began to shed sporulated oocysts and free sporocysts 13–14 DPI with infected sheep heart muscle.

Site of infection, definitive host: Unknown.

Site of infection, intermediate host: Sarcocysts seemed to localize in the myocardium, mostly under the endocardium and fewer in myocardium fibers.

Endogenous stages, definitive host: Unknown.

Endogenous stages, intermediate host: Under LM, sarcocysts were pupa-shaped, wedge-shaped, or ovoidal with L × W (n = 50): 210 × 76 (160–310 × 50–80); L/W ratio: 2.8, with obvious surface striations. Sarcocyst walls were ~1.3 thick and closely attached to the muscle fiber but with no secondary cyst wall. Sarcocysts were full of bradyzoites, with undistinguishable septa that separate peripheral and central zones of the sarcocyst. Bradyzoites were ~8.5 × 3.0, with a terminal, round N located at its blunt, more-rounded end. Wang et al. (1988) saw rhoptries "coming out of the conoid" and described micronemes as short and rod-shaped, about 0.15 long and 0.04 wide. These were seen clustered in the anterior part of the bradyzoites and arranged both vertically and horizontally.

Sarcocysts also were examined with the TEM. Under TEM, the cyst wall was 1.1–1.4 thick, consisting of a microvilli layer and a granular layer. Microvilli were T-shaped, 0.6–0.7 wide in their middle, and 1.3 wide at their tip. Microvilli were "neatly arranged" on the granular layer. The granular layer was 0.5–0.8 thick and septa were extended inward separating the cyst into several chambers. The membrane of bradyzoites was only ~0.01 thick and had micropores.

Cross-transmission: Six (likely domestic) cats and six dogs, all checked to be free from having sporocysts in their feces, were divided into two groups with four dogs/cats serving as experimental hosts and two dogs/cats as controls. All animals were housed individually. The four cats and dogs in the experimental-infection groups were fed heart tissue from one of the two infected sheep; the authors estimated that each animal received about 15,000 sarcocysts (Wang et al., 1988). Only dogs shed oocysts and sporocysts in their feces, whereas the four infected cats and the two control dogs and two control cats never shed oocysts or sporocysts.

Pathology: Unknown.

Materials deposited: None.

Remarks: Wang et al. (1988) compared the LM and TEM mensural characters of the sarcocysts they found in sheep heart to the sarcocysts in the other four sheep *Sarcocystis* species known at that time: *S. gigantea*, *S. medusiformis*, *S. ovicanis*, and *S. arieticanis*. By comparing the shape and size of the sarcocysts, the intermediate hosts, the prepatent periods, and the size of the sarcocysts produced, they concluded they were dealing with a new species and named it. Odening (1998) in his compilation of *Sarcocystis* names listed this as a valid species and noted that the sarcocyst was "presumably" a TEM type 27 (cf. Dubey et al., 1989b). Dubey et al. (2015a) did not mention this species.

SARCOCYSTIS MIESCHERIANA (KÜHN, 1865) LABBÉ, 1899

Synonyms: *Coccidium bigeminum* Stiles, 1891, *pro parte*; *Coccidia bigeminum* var. *canis* Railliet and Lucet, 1892; *Cryptosporidium vulpis* Wetzel 1938 *pro parte*; *Isospora bigemina* large form of Mehlhorn et al. (1975b) and Heydorn et al. (1975a) *pro parte*; *Endorimospora miescheriana* (Kühn) Tadros and Laarman, 1976; *Lucetina bigemina* (Stiles, 1891) Henry and Leblois, 1926 *pro parte*; *Miescheri utriculosa* Harz, 1887 *pro parte*; *Sarcocystis miescheriana* (1843) of Panasyuk, Mintyugov, Pyatov, Zyablov, and Golovin (1971) *lapsus calami*; *Sarcocystis miescheri* Lancaster, 1882; *Sarcocystis bigemina* (Stiles, 1891) Levine, 1977; *Sarcocystis suicanis* Erber, 1977; *Synchrytium miescherianum* Kühn, 1865.

Definitive hosts: *Canis aureus* L., 1758, Golden Jackal; *Canis lupus* L., 1758, Wolf; *Canis lupus familiaris* (syn. *C. familiaris*) L., 1758, Domestic Dog; *Procyon lotor* (L., 1758), Raccoon (Levine, 1986); *Vulpes vulpes* (L., 1758), Red or Silver Fox.

Intermediate host: *Sus scrofa* L., 1758, Wild Boar.

Geographic distribution: Africa: Egypt; Asia: China; India; Japan; Philippines; Europe: Lithuania; Switzerland; Middle East: Iran; North America: USA: Iowa and 28 other states (Dubey et al., 2015a).

Remarks: This is the type species for the genus *Sarcocystis*. Brumpt (1913) placed all sarcosporidia then known into the genus *Sarcocystis* and listed this species as *S. miescheriana* Kühn, 1885. He said it was a very frequent parasite in pig muscle. Wetzel (1938) found mature sporocysts in the feces of 1/2 (50%) red fox puppies received at his institute in Germany; he named the species *Cryptosporidium vulpis*. It is likely that these sporocysts were either those of *S. cruzi* or *S. miescheriana*. Boch et al. (1978) said they found this species (syn. *S. suicanis*) in 59/122 (48%) infected slaughter pigs in southern Germany. Levine and Ivens (1981) summarized all that was known at that time on endogenous stages and sporulation in the definitive host, prevalence, oocyst and sporocyst structures and sizes, the prepatent period, pathogenicity in intermediate hosts, what little cross-transmission had been done, and a lengthy discourse on who had confused it with *S. cruzi*, *S. tenella* and *S. bertrami*, also from the dog. Levine (1986) listed this species as one of the 122 names he considered as valid species of *Sarcocystis* at that time using the authorities given above, as did Odening (1998). Sarcocysts in wild and domestic pigs are L × W: 1,500 × 200 and found in the skeletal and cardiac muscles; the wall is 3–6 thick and appears radially striated. Endogenous development in the pig includes at least two generations of merogony, and mature sarcocysts can be found as early as 27 days after ingestion of sporocysts. Subclinical effects on pigs can be as simple as modest weight loss, but when large numbers of sporocysts are ingested, pigs become moribund with a variety of symptoms that can lead to death. Dubey et al.'s (2015a) thorough review of the literature mentions *S. miescheriana* 56 times (not including literature cited titles) and provides the reader with information on the pathogenicity and protective immunity in detail and includes Table 6.1, of the developmental stages of this species that are known in pigs, and Tables 6.2 and 6.3 summarizing numerous surveys where *S. miescheriana* has been documented in both domestic and wild boars.

SARCOCYSTIS MIHOENSIS SAITO, SHIBATA, KUBO, AND ITAGAKI, 1997

A photomicrograph of an isolated sporocyst (Fig. 8) of *S. mihoensis*, along with LM (Figs. 1 and 2), SEM (Figs. 3 and 4), and TEM micrographs (Figs. 5–7) of sarcocysts are found in Saito et al. (1997).

Definitive type host: *Canis lupus familiaris* (syn. *C. familiaris*) L., 1758, Domestic Dog.

Type locality: Asia: Japan, Honshu, Ibaraki Prefecture, Miho Village.

Other definitive hosts: Unknown.

Intermediate type host: *Ovis aries* L., 1758, Red Sheep.

Other intermediate hosts: Unknown.

Geographic distribution: Asia: Japan.

Description of sporulated oocyst: Not mentioned by Saito et al., (1997).

Description of sporocyst and sporozoites: Sporocyst shape: ellipsoidal (their Fig. 8); L × W (n = 50): 15–16 × 8–9; L/W ratio: unknown, means not given; SB, SSB, PSB: all absent; SR: present; SR characteristics: a compact, subspheroidal mass of large granules; SZ: not mentioned. Distinctive features of sporocyst: none; a "typical" *Sarcocystis*-type SP, lacking SB, SSB, PSB and with a distinct, granular SR.

Prevalence: This species was found in 2/16 (12.5%) sheep from a farm in Ibaraki Prefecture, Japan.

Sporulation: Endogenous with sporulated, infective sporocysts shed in the feces of the definitive host.

Prepatent and patent periods: Prepatent period in two female 6-month-old mongrel dogs was 11 days, and the patent period lasted for 46–49 days.

Site of infection, definitive host: Unknown but presumably the intestinal epithelium.

Site of infection, intermediate host: Sarcocysts were found in the diaphragm (greatest numbers), masseter, and muscles in the neck, dorsal regions, brachium, and thigh of infected sheep.

Endogenous stages, definitive host: Unknown but likely intestinal mucosa.

Endogenous stages, intermediate host: Fresh sarcocysts were 1,300–2,100 long by 200–300 wide, with a thick wall, 10–12 wide, and a palisade-like structure. Clear compartments were seen within the sarcocyst and histological examination showed that villar protrusions of the wall were radially-arranged. Bradyzoites were numerous but were not measured, and a few metrocytes

were seen situated along the cyst wall (Figs. 1 and 2, Saito et al., 1997). SEM showed that villar protrusions were finger-like, L × W: 8–10 × 2–2.5 and attenuated gradually from the base to about two-third of the length. TEM showed microtubules in the villar protrusions.

Cross-transmission: Both dogs inoculated with sarcocysts in sheep muscle passed sporulated sporocysts, but two female cats, 6- and 12-months-old, respectively, did not pass sporocysts.

Pathology: Unknown.

Materials deposited: None.

Remarks: There seem to be only four other *Sarcocystis* species reported from sheep. *Sarcocystis tenella*, *S. arieticanis*, and now *S. mihoensis* use dogs as definitive hosts, whereas *S. gigantea* and *S. medusiformis* use the cat as the definitive host. The species with sheep-canid life cycles seem to have much smaller sarcocysts than the sheep-felid species. Also, sporocysts are slightly larger in the sheep-canid species than those in the sheep-felid species, but the differences are not significant. Odening (1998), in his compilation of *Sarcocystis* names, listed this as a valid species and noted that the sarcocyst was a TEM type 24 (cf. Dubey et al., 1989b). Dubey et al. (2015a) pointed out the rarity of this species. Nothing more seems to be known about *S. mihoensis*.

SARCOCYSTIS ODOCOILEOCANIS CRUM, FAYER, AND PRESTWOOD, 1981

Synonym: *Sarcocystis* sp. of Entzeroth et al. (1982a,b).

Definitive hosts: *Canis latrans* Say, 1823, Coyote; *Canis lupus familiaris* (syn. *C. familiaris*) L., 1758, Domestic Dog; *Urocyon cinereoargenteus* (Schreber, 1775), Gray Fox; *Vulpes vulpes* (L., 1758), Red or Silver Fox.

Intermediate hosts: *Odocoileus virginianus* (Zimmermann, 1780), White-tailed Deer; *Bos taurus* L., 1758, Aurochs; *Ovis aries* L., 1758, Red Sheep; *Cervus nippon* Temminck, 1838, Sika Deer.

Geographic distribution: North America: USA: Alabama, Florida, Michigan, Montana, South Carolina, Texas, Virginia, Wisconsin; Canada: Alberta, Ontario.

Remarks: Crum et al. (1981) obtained venison meat from 24 white-tailed deer from South Carolina, Florida, Virginia, and West Virginia; diaphragm, esophagus, heart, loin, thigh muscle, and tongue were transported to their lab at the University of Georgia, Athens. Infected tissues were determined by finding sarcocysts in esophagus, heart, and tongue. Infected meat from each state was pooled, ground in a food mill, and fed daily for 2–4 days to different potential definitive hosts that included: 10 dogs, 2 cats, and 1 raccoon (South Carolina); 1 dog, 2 opossums, and 2 raccoons (Florida); 1 cat, 1 opossum, and 2 raccoons (West Virginia); and 2 cats, 2 dogs, 1 opossum, and 2 raccoons (Virginia). All 13 dogs fed sarcocyst-infected venison from Florida, South Carolina, and Virginia passed sporocysts in their feces. These sporocysts were L × W (n = 195): 15.2 × 10.7 (13–16 × 9–12), L/W ratio: 1.4, prepatency varied from 8 to 16 DPI (mean = 11.6), and the patent period lasted ~38 days. These sporocysts were fed to white-tailed deer (3), calves (2), a sheep, and lambs (4), which developed sarcocysts in their tissues, principally cardiac and striated muscles. Sarcocysts in skeletal muscle of deer 104 DPI with sporocysts measured L × W: 264 × 40 (150–536 × 30–51); unfortunately, Crum et al. (1981) did not discuss the structure of the sarcocyst wall, although it appears to be relatively thick and striated in their photomicrographs (their Figs. 3 and 4A–C). From these data they were able to name this species, *S. odocoileocanis* (see also, Chapter 19, *Sarcocystis* sp. of Entzeroth et al., 1982b). Levine (1986) listed this as one of his 122 valid species of *Sarcocystis*. Lindsay et al. (1988) looked at the prevalence of *S. odocoileocanis* in white-tailed deer in Alabama, USA, as well as the prevalence of sarcocysts in the tissues they examined. They found sarcocysts in 30/34 (88%) white-tailed deer and recorded that hearts were infected less often, 13/34 (38%)

than were tongues, 30/34 (88%). They also fed infected tongues to a gray fox that excreted sporocysts 8 DPI, and four days later it was killed to harvest sporocysts that were used to experimentally infect two mixed breed goats with 50,000 or 500,000 sporocysts. Goats were euthanized at 122 DPI, but neither of the goats developed clinical signs of infection, nor could tissue sarcocysts be found. Odening (1998), in his compilation of *Sarcocystis* names, also listed this as a valid species; he noted that the sarcocyst was a TEM type 17 (cf. Dubey et al., 1989b) and that this species was similar to *S. hemionilatrantis*. Dubey et al.'s (2015a) thorough review of the literature summarizes morphological and biological features of this species in their Tables 1.2, 1.3, 14.2, 18.1, 24.1, and 24.4, and in their Figs. 1.10E and 1.49A.

SARCOCYSTIS PECKAI ODENING, 1997

Synonyms: *Sarcocystis* sp. of Wenzel et al. (1982); *Sarcocystis* sp. of Pecka (1988).

Definitive type host: *Canis lupus familiaris* (syn. *C. familiaris*) L., 1758, Domestic Dog.

Type locality: Europe: Germany.

Other definitive hosts: *Felis catus* L., 1758, Domestic Cat (?).

Intermediate type host: *Phasianus colchicus* L., 1758, Common Pheasant, Ring-necked Pheasant.

Other intermediate hosts: *Gallus gallus* (L., 1758), Red Jungle Fowl (?).

Geographic distribution: Europe: former Czechoslovakia, Germany.

Description of sporulated oocyst: Not available.

Description of sporocyst and sporozoites: Sporocyst shape: not mentioned but likely ovoidal with blunt ends; L × W: 13–15 × 9–11; L/W ratio: unknown, means not given; SB, SSB, PSB: all (apparently) absent; SR: not mentioned; SR characteristics: not mentioned; SZ: not mentioned. Distinctive features of sporocyst: none; a "typical" *Sarcocystis*-type SP, lacking SB, SSB, PSB and with a distinct, granular SR.

Prevalence: Wenzel et al. (1982) found two different types of sarcocysts in the muscles of 3/36 (8%) pheasants in Germany; the first type, according to them (1982), corresponded to *S. horvathi* Rátz, 1909, whereas the second type, found only in the breast musculature, likely belonged to this species, although they did not name it. Pecka (1988), in the former Czechoslovakia, found two types of sarcocysts in the musculature of pheasants that he said were similar to those reported by Wenzel et al. (1982). In all, 46/90 (51%) *P. colchicus* from two localities apparently had sarcocysts of both types; 21/63 (33%) pheasants in the pheasantry of Jindřichův Hradec, and 25/27 (93%) pheasants in the pheasantry of Třeboň. Pecka (1988) also reported that 3/30 (10%) *G. gallus* hens in Bohemia had sarcocysts of the same two types in breast and femoral muscles.

Sporulation: Unknown, but likely endogenous with sporulated, infective sporocysts shed in the feces of the definitive host.

Prepatent and patent periods: Pecka (1988) said that dogs fed muscles from an infected pheasant began passing sporocysts on 6–8 DPI, and the patent period lasted until 50 DPI (i.e., ~42–44 days long).

Site of infection, definitive host: Pecka (1988) reported oocysts were found in enterocytes in the whole length of the small intestine of the dog that was killed at 10 DPI.

Site of infection, intermediate host: Pecka (1988) found sarcocysts in breast and femoral striated muscles.

Endogenous stages, definitive host: Unknown.

Endogenous stages, intermediate host: Meronts, L × W: 7.1–7.8 × 5.2–6.0, were found in capillaries in the heart musculature of pheasants after they were fed oocysts/sporocysts. Sarcocysts in striated muscles were nearly 2,000 long and 80 wide. The sarcocyst wall was 3.2 thick and formed thin, finger-like protrusions that were L × W: 1.8–2.3 × 0.8–0.9, and all of these measurements corresponded to the unnamed *Sarcocystis* species of Wenzel et al. (1982).

Cross-transmission: Pecka (1988) fed seven pheasants "with oocysts obtained from dogs" and found meronts on 8 DPI and sarcocysts morphologically homologous with the cystic stage from naturally-infected pheasants in the muscles of birds 5 weeks PI. Dogs were then fed sarcocysts in muscles from the experimentally-infected birds and they passed oocysts from 6–8 DPI.

Pathology: Unknown.

Materials deposited: None.

Remarks: Wenzel et al. (1982), in Germany, gave the first well-documented finding of *Sarcocystis* species in pheasants when they reported two distinct types of sarcocysts. The first type of sarcocysts had banana-shaped (type I) cystozoites and were identified as *S. horvathi*, and the second, type II cystozoites were lancet-shaped, which they did not name. Pecka (1988), in the former Czechoslovakia, found the same two sarcocyst types in pheasant breast and femoral muscles, took some measurements, and fed dogs sarcocyst-infected muscles, and they produced sporocysts. These oocysts/sporocysts were then fed to (presumably) uninfected pheasants and sarcocysts were found in their muscles in 5 weeks. One of the uncertainties of this paper is that Pecka (1988) admits to finding two distinct types of sarcocysts in pheasants, that all infected pheasants had both types of sarcocysts and when dogs were infected with sarcocyst-infected muscles they passed oocysts/sporocysts. However, it was never quite clear that Pecka (1988) actually separated the two sarcocyst types in his feeding experiments, so the question of which sarcocyst actually produced the oocysts/sporocysts in dogs remains, *S. horvathi* or the species with lancet-shaped cystozoites? In spite of this uncertainty, Odening (1997) decided to name this second form *S. peckai*. Odening (1998), in his compilation of 189 *Sarcocystis* names, listed this as a valid species and said it was similar to *S. wenzeli*, but he separated it from that species by intermediate host specificity "and some metrical differences." On the other hand, Dubey et al. (2015a) only mentioned this species twice; in Table 17.2 they listed the bradyzoites to be lancet-shaped, and measured 14–16 × 2–3 and the pheasant as an intermediate host, but in their Table 24.2 they listed *S. peckai* as an invalid species.

SARCOCYSTIS POEPHAGICANIS WEI, CHANG, DONG, WANG, AND XIA, 1985

Definitive type host: *Canis lupus familiaris* (syn. *C. familiaris*) L., 1758, Domestic Dog.

Type locality: Asia: China.

Other definitive hosts: Unknown.

Intermediate type host: *Bos grunniens* L., 1766 (syn. *Poephagus grunniens* Gray, 1843), Yak.

Other intermediate hosts: Unknown.

Geographic distribution: Asia: China.

Description of sporulated oocyst: Not available from Wei et al. (1985).

Description of sporocyst and sporozoites: Sporocyst shape: ovoidal with blunt ends; L × W: 14.6 × 10.6 (10.5–18.5 × 7–14); L/W ratio: 1.4; SB, SSB, PSB: all absent; SR: present; SR characteristics: not mentioned; SZ: not mentioned. Distinctive features of sporocyst: none; a "typical" *Sarcocystis*-type SP, lacking SB, SSB, PSB, and with a distinct, granular SR.

Prevalence: Unknown, not available from Wei et al. (1985).

Sporulation: Unknown but likely endogenous with sporulated, infective sporocysts shed in the feces of the definitive host.

Prepatent and patent periods: Prepatent period in puppies is 7–9 days, and the patent period lasted for 13–26 days.

Site of infection, definitive host: Unknown.

Site of infection, intermediate host: Striated muscles.

Endogenous stages, definitive host: Unknown.

Endogenous stages, intermediate host: Sarcocysts were macroscopic, ovoidal, ~0.3 mm long with a thin wall and a secondary cyst wall; SEM showed that the sarcocyst wall has a generally smooth, honeycomb-like appearance (Wei et al., 1985; Dubey et al., 2015a, Table 18.2). Bradyzoites were not measured.

Cross-transmission: Wei et al. (1990) tried to infect 10 oocyst-free domestic kittens, *F. catus*, with 4,000 individual sarcocysts dissected from yaks, but the cats never passed oocysts in their feces. Wei et al. (1990) also experimentally infected white rats, mice, guinea pigs, domestic rabbits, and chicks with sarcocysts from yaks, but no sporocysts were ever detected in fecal examinations. Finally, Wei et al. (1990) then infected all of the above animals with sporocysts (from their dogs), but no sarcocysts were detected in the muscles of all animals in necropsy 90 DPI with the sporocysts.

Pathology: Unknown.

Materials deposited: None.

Remarks: Levine (1986) did not include this species in his list of 122 valid *Sarcocystis* species. Odening (1998), in his compilation of 189 *Sarcocystis* names, listed this as a valid species; he said it was similar to *S. cruzi* and to *S. levinei* (*sensu* Huong et al., 1997b) and added that its sarcocysts were "TEM type 6/7 (originally type 7, Dubey et al., 1989b)." Dubey et al. (2015a) cited it as a valid species from the dog, and mentioned it five times (Tables 1.4, 14.2, 18.2, 24.1, and 24.4). Wei et al. (1990) fed 4,000 individual sarcocysts dissected from yaks to 20 oocyst-free puppies and found sporocysts in their feces. We had Wei et al.'s (1990) paper translated by colleagues in China, and the measurements of sporocysts in dog feces are given above; however, Dubey et al. (2015a) listed oocyst size for this species to be L × W: 15.4–27.8 × 14.2–25.2 (their Table 14.2) and then listed dog oocysts of this species to be L × W: 14.6 × 10.6 (their Table 18.2), which actually is the size of the sporocysts reported by Wei et al. (1990). Stojecki et al. (2012) listed 32 valid species of *Sarcocystis* from selected domesticated intermediate hosts (mostly mammals, two birds), selecting from Tenter (1995), with modifications of Elsheikha and Mansfield

(2007) and Olias et al. (2009); definitive hosts were listed when they were known. They considered *S. poephagicanis* a valid species and listed the dog as the definitive host.

SARCOCYSTIS SVANAI DUBEY, SYKES, SHELTON, SHARP, VERMA, CALERO-BERNAL, VIVIANO, SUNDAR, KAHN, AND GRIGG, 2015c

For light and electron micrographs of tissue cysts and zoites of this species see Figs. 8–10 in Dubey et al. (2014).

Definitive type host: Unknown.

Type locality: North America (Canada: British Columbia; USA: Colorado, Montana; see Dubey et al., 2015c).

Other definitive hosts: Unknown.

Intermediate type host: *Canis lupus familiaris* (syn. *C. familiaris*) L., 1758, Domestic Dog.

Other intermediate hosts: *Lycalopex gymnocercus* (G. Fischer, 1814), Pampas Fox.

Geographic distribution: North America: Canada, USA.

Description of sporulated oocyst: Unknown.

Description of sporocyst and sporozoites: Unknown.

Prevalence: Dubey et al. (2014) detected sarcocysts of this species in muscle biopsies of 2/4 (50%) dogs they examined. Both infected dogs also were infected with sarcocysts of *S. caninum*. One infected dog was from Montana, whereas the other was from Colorado. This geographic separation should rule out a common meal as their source of infection, and the intensity of sarcocysts in the muscles of both dogs was similar, suggesting that these were not spurious infections. Scioscia et al. (2017) were able to identify *S. svanai* sarcocysts in 22/36 (61%) *L. gymnocercus* samples examined by microscopic and molecular methods, with the tongue and masseter muscles most frequently infected.

Sporulation: Unknown, but likely endogenous with sporulated, infective sporocysts shed in the feces of the definitive host.

Prepatent and patent periods: Unknown.

Site of infection, definitive host: Unknown.

Site of infection, intermediate host: Striated muscles of digital flexor, biceps, triceps.

Endogenous stages, definitive host: Unknown.

Endogenous stages, intermediate host: Only three sarcocysts of this species were found by TEM; the sarcocyst wall was thin, ~0.5, and its parasitophorous vacuolar membrane (Pvm) undulated with tiny blebs (invaginations), without villar protrusions. Bradyzoites with numerous micronemes were toward the upper one-fourth of the conoidal end. Up to four rhoptries per section were with electron-dense contents. Numerous amylopectin granules were toward the upper three-fourths of the bradyzoite.

Cross-transmission: None to date.

Pathology: Unknown.

Materials deposited: Specimens deposited in the USNPC, Division of Invertebrate Zoology and National Museum of Natural History, Smithsonian Institution, Washington, DC (under USNM). H&E-stained histological sections from Dog B (Colorado), syntype specimens of *S. caninum*, USNM No. 1251650; voucher specimens of H&E-stained sections from Dog C (Montana), USNM No. 1251651. DNA sequences are deposited in GenBank, Accession No. KM362428 (Dog B).

Etymology: Named after the host dog in Sanskrit, *svanai*.

Remarks: Dubey et al. (2014) had the opportunity to examine preserved, infected muscle tissues from dogs in British Columbia, Canada (2), Colorado (1), and Montana (1) that had been identified and preserved by others (Sykes et al., 2011; Chapman et al., 2005). Examining this material with LM, TEM, and PCR, they were able to distinguish *S. svanai* sarcocysts from others and identify and name it as new. The structure of *S. svanai* and *S. caninum* sarcocysts can be distinguished from those of *S. neurona* because the villar protrusions in *S. neurona* sarcocysts have tubules that extend into the ground substance, whereas villar tubules are absent in both *S. svanai* and *S. caninum*. The sarcocyst wall of *S. svanai* is structurally similar to that of *S. arctosi* sarcocysts from the brown bear (*Ursus arctos*) from Alaska, USA but very distinct from *S. caninum* (above), and all of their bradyzoites are structurally distinct. This species has a unique phylogenetic resolution using the 18S rRNA and rpoB genetic markers. Phylogenetic analysis of the two rpoB sequence types were unique from all published sequences available in GenBank, with the closest relationship of the *S. svanai* rpoB sequence being to *S. carpestris*, the first named *Sarcocystis* in the badger (Cawthorn et al., 1983). Scioscia et al. (2017) were able to use PCR products from pooled muscles to show the highest identity by BLAST (99%) with *S. svanai* sequence (KM362428) from a North American dog. They also examined sarcocysts by TEM and found the wall to be thin, <1, with minute undulations and tiny evaginations and without evident villar protrusions. They referred to this as a "type 1" sarcocyst wall. Because *S. svanai* naturally infects *L. gymnocercus* in such high prevalence, Scioscia et al. (2017) suggested that the Pampas fox was a natural intermediate host, even though the definitive host of *S. svanai* remains unknown.

SARCOCYSTIS SYBILLENSIS DUBEY, JOLLEY, AND THORNE, 1983

Photomicrograph of two sporulated oocysts (Fig. 11), a sporocyst (Fig. 12), five LM sections of sarcocysts (Figs. 1–5), and five TEM photomicrographs of sarcocysts of *S. sybillensis* (Figs. 6–10) are found in Dubey et al. (1983).

Synonym: *Sarcocystis cervi* von Hessling, 1854 of Drost (1977) (?).

Definitive host: *Canis lupus familiaris* (syn. *C. familiaris*) L., 1758, Domestic Dog.

Intermediate host: *Cervus elaphus* L., 1758 (syn. *Cervus canadensis* Erxleben, 1777), Red Deer, Elk, Wapiti.

Geographic distribution: North America: USA: Wyoming.

Remarks: Dubey et al. (1983) fed four elk with sporocysts from a 2-month-old dog, which had been fed heart and skeletal muscles of a naturally-infected elk that was part of a herd maintained at the Sybille Wildlife Research Unit, Wyoming Fish and Game Department. The elk were clinically normal throughout their experiment, while two structurally different sarcocysts developed in their muscles. There were a few thin-walled sarcocysts they identified as *S. wapiti* and numerous thick-walled sarcocysts to which they gave a new name, *S. sybillensis*. Elk were killed 88–90 DPI, and their sarcocysts fixed and examined by LM and TEM. Most sarcocysts seen were immature with a thin wall (<1 thick) that had filamentous protrusions. Sarcocysts from skeletal muscle, sectioned longitudinally were L × W (n = 10): 506.2 × 28.7 (373–637 × 22–45), the metrocytes measured were L × W (n = 11): 8.8 × 5.4 (7–10.5 × 4–7), and the bradyzoites were L × W (n = 12): 10.6 × 3.3 (9.5–12 × 2.5–4). The one dog fed infected meat shed oocysts and sporocysts 14 DPI; oocysts were L × W (n = 10): 21.4 × 15.9 (20–23 × 15–17), L/W ratio: 1.3, whereas individual sporocysts measured L × W (n = 50): 15.5 × 10.7 (15–17 × 10.5–12), L/W ratio: 1.4, and their SZ were L × W (n = 15): 10.5 × 2.8 (9–12.5 × 2.5–3.5). Levine (1986) listed this species as one of the 122 names he considered to be a valid species of *Sarcocystis* at that time. Odening (1998), in his compilation of 189 *Sarcocystis* names, listed this as a valid species and added that it had a TEM type 12 sarcocyst wall (of Dubey et al., 1989b). Dubey et al.'s (2015a) thorough review of the literature summarized morphological and biological features of this species in their Tables 1.2, 1.3, 14.2, 18.1, 24.1, and 24.4 and in their Figs. 1.10L and 1.47A.

SARCOCYSTIS TARANDIVULPES GJERDE, 1984d

Definitive host: *Canis lupus familiaris* (syn. *C. familiaris*) L., 1758, Domestic Dog.

Remarks: For more complete information on *S. tarandivulpes*, see Genus *Vulpes*, below.

SARCOCYSTIS TENELLA (RAILLIET, 1886a,b) MOULÉ, 1886

Synonyms: *Miescheria tenella* Railliet, 1886a,b of *auctores*, *pro parte*; *Coccidium bigemina* Stiles, 1891 *pro parte*; *Coccidium bigeminum* var. *canis* Railliet and Lucet, 1891 *pro parte*; *Cryptosporidium* sp. Bearup, 1954, in dingo (?); *Endorimorpora ovicanis* (Heydorn, Gestrich, Mehlhorn, and Rommel, 1975b) Tadros and Laarman, 1976; *Hoareosporidium pellerdyi* Pande, Bhatia, and Chauhan, 1972 (?); *Isospora rivolta* free sporocysts of Gassner (1940) and *auctores*; *Isospora bigemina* large form of Mehlhorn et al. (1975b) and Heydorn et al. (1975a) *pro parte*; *Lucetina bigemina* (Stiles, 1891) Henry and Leblois, 1926 *pro parte*; *Sarcocystis ovicanis* Heydorn, Gestrich, Mehlhorn, and Rommel, 1975b.

Definitive hosts: *Canis latrans* Say, 1823, Coyote; *Canis lupus* L., 1758, Wolf; *Canis lupus familiaris* (syn. *C. familiaris* Meyer, 1793) L., 1758, Domestic Dog; *Vulpes vulpes* (L., 1758), Red or Silver Fox.

Intermediate hosts: *Ovis ammon* (L., 1758), Argali; *Ovis aries* L., 1758, Red Sheep.

Geographic distribution: Africa: Nigeria; Republic of Senegal; Asia: India; Japan; Australia: Northwest Territories; Western Australia; Europe: Austria; Czech Republic; England (?); Germany; Romania; Slovakia; Middle East: Iran; Jordan; Turkey; North America: USA: Maryland, Montana, Texas; South America: Brazil. Probably worldwide in its distribution.

Remarks: Ashford (1977) traced the history of the naming of this species as follows. The muscle stages were first named by Railliet (1886a,b), who differentiated the small sarcocysts from the large sarcocysts, naming the former *Miescheria tenella* and the latter *Balbiania gigantea*. Subsequently, the two species/forms were united under the name *S. tenella* by authors who considered their sarcocysts to represent different ages of the same parasite, which is obviously a mistake (Ashford, 1977). The small sarcocysts are now assigned to this species, *S. tenella*, and known to be transmitted by dogs to sheep, whereas the large sarcocysts are now known as *S. gigantea* and known to be transmitted to sheep by cats. Stiles (1891, 1892) described paired sporocysts in the intestine of dogs, which he called *Coccidium bigemina* (=*Isospora bigemina*); those sporocysts closely resemble others found by Munday et al. in dogs (Munday and Corbould, 1973; Munday and Rickard, 1974; Munday et al., 1975) and by Ashford (1977) in foxes, so *I. bigemina* (of Stiles) may well be a synonym of *S. tenella*. Brumpt (1913) placed all sarcosporidia then known into the genus *Sarcocystis* and listed this species as *S. tenella* Railliet, 1886a. He said the parasite lives in the muscles of sheep in a cyst, L × W: ~500 × 50–100. Mehlhorn and Scholtyseck (1973) were the first to study the fine structure of the sarcocyst stage of *S. tenella* in the esophageal musculature of sheep. Seneviratna et al. (1975) surveyed sheep from an abattoir in Detroit, Michigan, USA, and identified sarcocysts in 578/789 (73%) adults and in 12/108 (11%) lambs; this led Dubey (1976) to state that *Sarcocystis* infections in sheep occur worldwide, and it is generally accepted that *S. tenella* is nonpathogenic in sheep. Ashford (1977) found macroscopic sarcocysts in the esophagi of naturally-infected sheep but did not examine the tissues histologically to determine if microscopic sarcocysts also were present. He fed these sheep esophagi to five live foxes trapped and collected near Liverpool and said he successfully infected them eight times with sheep esophagi. Leek et al. (1977) orally inoculated eight Dorset lambs with sporocysts of this species (which they called *S. ovicanis*). Two lambs got 1×10^5 or 2×10^5 sporocysts and became clinically ill but recovered and were killed 67 and 88 DPI, when numerous intramuscular cysts were found in their skeletal and cardiac muscles. Three lambs received 1×10^5 sporocysts and three lambs received 1×10^6 sporocysts. The first three (1×10^5) became acutely ill with anemia, inappetence, weight loss, fever, and reduced serum protein, and all died 27–29 DPI. The three that received 1×10^6 sporocysts all died 24 or 25 DPI, and it was found that hemorrhage involving the striated muscle and visceral organs was the most obvious lesion. The hearts were severely affected, and meronts were found in vascular endothelial cells of all inoculated lambs. Dogs fed sarcocysts from these lambs produced sporocysts 11 to 37 DPI, cats fed similar stages produced no sporocysts, and dogs fed tissues containing only early meronts, but no sarcocysts, produced no sporocysts. Farmer et al. (1978) surveyed feces from 123 working sheepdogs in Gwynedd, from 33 greyhounds from the London area, and from 41 red foxes killed on Anglesey or in the Bangor area of England. They found sporocysts of *Sarcocystis* spp. in 45/123 (36.5%) sheepdogs, 8/33 (24%) greyhounds, and 7/41 (17%) red foxes (Table 1, p. 79, Farmer et al., 1978). Based only on sporocyst dimensions, they said that *S. tenella* (syn. *S. ovicanis*) sporocysts were identified in 30/47 (64%) sheepdog, in 6/8 (75%) greyhound, and in all five red fox samples they examined (Table 3, p. 79, Farmer et al., 1978). Fayer and Leek (1979) found merozoites of this species in blood smears of lambs exhibiting signs of acute sarcocystosis after oral infection with sporocysts from dogs. They took whole blood containing merozoites from lambs and transfused it into two uninfected lambs, and large numbers of intramuscular sarcocysts were found in both transfused recipients, indicating that *S. tenella* (syn. *S. ovicanis*) had been transmitted between intermediate hosts of the same species by blood transfusion. Levine and Ivens (1981) covered information on prevalences, oocyst/sporocyst structure and sizes, gamogony and sporulation in the definitive host, merogony and sarcocyst development in the intermediate host, prepatent and patent periods in the definitive host, pathogenicity in both definitive (mild) and intermediate (high) hosts, cross-transmission known to that time, and *in vitro* cultivation. Dubey (1983a) used five littermates of 6-week-old *V. vulpes*, three species of *Sarcocystis* that previously had been isolated from and identified in their intermediate hosts (cattle, sheep, goats) in Montana, USA, and oocysts and tissue cysts of *T. gondii* to conduct a series of cross-transmission experiments. One fox (No. 5) was fed sarcocyst-infected sheep meat and shed *S. tenella*-like sporocysts 8 DPI; these sporocysts measured L × W (n = 16): 12.5–14 × 7.5–9. Two lambs were fed 5×10^5 of these sporocysts, and they became anemic on 25 DPI; one died 26 DPI and the other was euthanized 27 DPI. A third lamb fed 1×10^4 sporocysts remained asymptomatic and was killed 60 DPI. Numerous second-generation meronts were found in the tissues of lambs necropsied 26 and 27 DPI, and numerous cross-striated sarcocysts and nonsuppurative myositis were found in the lamb necropsied 60 DPI. Dubey and Blagburn (1983) tried to infect one 10-month-old female raccoon with sarcocysts of *S. tenella* from an infected lamb that had been inoculated with 50,000 sporocysts of *S. tenella* 79 DPI, but the raccoon remained uninfected for at least 5 weeks PI. Cawthorn et al. (1986) studied the *in vitro* excystation of sporozoites from their sporocysts in three *Sarcocystis* species, including *S. tenella* and found they could get improved rates of excystation by pretreating sporocysts with an aqueous sodium hypochlorite (NaOCl) solution followed by incubation in excysting fluid. Heydorn and Karaer (1986) used a pure isolate of *S. tenella* (syn. *S. ovicanis*) sporocysts from dogs to study its presarcocyst development in sheep; sporocysts from these dogs measured L × W: 13–15 × 9–10. One young lamb was inoculated with five million sporocysts and three other lambs were inoculated with 30 million sporocysts each. Two of the latter hosts were killed on 14 DPI, during the first rise in body temperature, and the other two lambs were killed 24 DPI, during the second period of fever when one died, and the other was moribund. Lambs killed on 14 DPI had both mature and premature first-generation meronts in endothelial or subendothelial cells of small arteries and arterioles, and a few meronts were seen in endothelial cells of capillaries. The most affected organs were mesenteric lymph nodes, kidneys, spleen, and cardiac and skeletal musculature. On 24 DPI many second-generation meronts were found predominantly in endothelial cells of capillaries and also in some arteries and arterioles in all the same organs. In the livers of both lambs examined on 24 DPI, most meronts were in endothelial cells of branches of the portal veins, but the most heavily infected organs on 24 DPI were the kidneys and mesenteric lymph nodes (Heydorn and Karaer, 1986). Dubey et al. (1988b) found sarcocysts of this species in the muscles of 430/512 (84%) adult ewes from the northwestern United States and Texas. Odening et al. (1995) identified this species by LM and TEM in muscle samples from six wild and two captive European mouflons (*O. aries musimon*) in Germany, purportedly the first time *S. tenella* was recorded from wild sheep.

Levine (1986) listed this species as one of the 122 names he considered as valid species of *Sarcocystis* at that time. Dubey et al. (1989b) recorded a case of fatal perinatal sarcocystosis in a lamb, which they attributed to *S. tenella*. Odening (1998), in his compilation of 189 *Sarcocystis* names, listed this as a valid species and added that it had a TEM type 14 sarcocyst wall (of Dubey et al., 1989b); he also added that *S. tenella* was "similar to *S. capracanis* (sibling species), but separated from that species by intermediate host specificity and molecular genetic characters (Tenter et al., 1992)." Dubey et al.'s (2015a) thorough review of the literature provides the reader with information on the structure of sarcocysts in sheep muscles, the life cycle and timing of parasite development (merogony) within sheep, pathogenic symptoms, clinical disease, and consequences of infection for sheep, including the effects on parturition and reproduction. They (2015a)

also included a small section on immunity in sheep and the consequences of prophylactically administered anticoccidial drugs.

SARCOCYSTIS TILOPODI QUIROGA, LOMBARDERO, AND ZORILLA, 1969

Synonym: *Sarcocystis guanicoe-canis* Gorman, Alcaino, Muñoz, and Cunazza, 1984.

Definitive host: *Canis lupus familiaris* (syn. *C. familiaris*) L., 1758, Domestic Dog (see Gorman et al., 1984).

Intermediate host: *Lama glama* (L., 1758) (syn. *Lama guanicoe* (Müller, 1776)), Guanaco, Llama.

Geographic distribution: Probably worldwide (see Dubey et al., 2015a).

Remarks: Levine (1986) listed this as a valid *Sarcocystis* species name with the dog as a definitive host and a llama as an intermediate host, but Dubey et al. (2015a) considered this name to be a synonym of *S. aucheniae* Brumpt, 1913.

SARCOCYSTIS TROPICALIS (MUKHERJEE AND KRASSNER, 1965) LEVINE AND TADROS, 1980

Synonym: *Isospora tropicalis* Mukherjee and Krassner, 1965.

Definitive host: *Canis aureus* L., 1758, Golden Jackal.

Intermediate host: Unknown.

Geographic distribution: Asia: India.

Remarks: This may be a valid species of *Sarcocystis* in carnivores, but we know virtually nothing about it. Mukherjee and Krassner (1965) described it as a species of *Isospora*, but that was at a time when we knew little about the life cycle of *Sarcocystis*; they (1965) did not find oocysts in the feces, although oocysts with very thin walls stretching over the sporocysts were found in the intestinal contents. Free sporocysts in the feces were L × W: 15–16 × 10–12, and banana-shaped

SZ were L × W: 8–10 × 3–4. Mukherjee and Krassner (1965) fed sporocysts to a (presumably) clean Indian fox, *Vulpes bengalensis*, which died 12 DPI. There were no sporocysts in its feces the first 7 DPI, but they said there were many sporocysts in the gut contents when they necropsied the fox on the 12th DPI. Pellérdy (1974a) thought it unlikely that the sporocysts found in the fox intestine on day 12 were produced by the sporocysts that were inoculated, and Levine and Ivens (1981) agreed. Then, Levine (1986) listed this form as a valid *Sarcocystis* species, but Odening (1998), in his compilation of 189 *Sarcocystis* names, listed this as a *species inquirenda*, and Dubey et al. (2015a) mentioned it only once, listing it as an invalid *Sarcocystis* species (their Table 24.2).

SARCOCYSTIS WAPITI SPEER AND DUBEY, 1982

Photomicrographs of a sporulated oocyst (Fig. 1), a sporocyst (Fig. 2), an LM section through a sarcocyst (Fig. 3), and five TEM photomicrographs of sarcocysts of *S. wapiti* (Figs. 4–8), are found in Speer and Dubey (1982).

Synonym: *Sarcocystis cervi* von Hessling, 1954 of Drost (1977), in part (?) (from Levine, 1986).

Definitive hosts: *Canis latrans* Say, 1823, Coyote; *Canis lupus familiaris* (syn. *C. familiaris*) L., 1758, Domestic Dog.

Intermediate host: *Cervus elaphus* L., 1758 (syn. *Cervus canadensis* Erxleben, 1777), Red Deer, Elk, Wapiti.

Geographic distribution: Probably worldwide.

Remarks: Margolin and Jolley (1979), Dubey (1980a), Fayer et al. (1982), and perhaps others, demonstrated that sarcocysts found in the muscles of elk are infectious for coyotes, which will produce oocysts/sporocysts in their feces after ingesting infected muscle. Speer and Dubey (1982) named this species from North American elk and provided detailed measurements and photomicrographs (both LM and TEM) on morphology of tissue sarcocysts, oocysts, and sporocysts, along with good photomicrographs of the latter two structures. Levine (1986) said that this name may be a synonym of *S. cervicanis*. Sarcocysts in the various muscles of elk were both micro- and macroscopic, had a thin primary cyst wall with septa, and were L × W: 652 × 322. These sarcocysts contained many bradyzoites (16.1 × 2.4) but only a few metrocytes (11.2 × 4.6). Both dogs and coyotes fed elk muscle infected with sarcocysts began shedding oocysts/sporocysts in their feces on 10 DPI, but a cat also infected with *S. wapiti* sarcocysts never passed oocysts and/or sporocysts. Sporulated oocysts were L × W: 20.3 × 15.6, L/W ratio: 1.3, and its sporocysts were L × W: 15.9 × 10.6, L/W ratio: 1.5. Oocysts were found in the lamina propria of the distal one-third of the villi of the coyote small intestine. Dubey and Blagburn (1983) tried to infect a 7-month-old raccoon with 1 kg of meat (over 7 days) from an elk infected with sarcocysts of *S. wapiti* that had been shot near Bozeman, MT, but the raccoon remained uninfected for at least 5 weeks PI. Odening (1998), in his compilation of 189 *Sarcocystis* names, listed this as a valid species and added that it had a TEM type 2/8 sarcocyst wall (originally type 2, Dubey et al., 1989b). Odening (1998) also said *S. wapiti* was "probably a synonym of *S. grueneri*, including *S. alceslatrans* and *S. cervicanis*." Dubey et al. (2015a) listed this species in four of their tables (Tables 1.3, 18.1, 24.1, and 24.4) and considered it a valid species.

SARCOCYSTIS WENZELI ODENING, 1997

Synonyms: *Sarcocystis gallinarum* Krause and Goranoff, 1933; *Sarcocystis* sp. of Wenzel et al., (1982).

Definitive type host: *Canis lupus familiaris* (syn. *C. familiaris*) L., 1758, Domestic Dog.

Type locality: Europe: Germany.

Other definitive host: *Felis catus* L., 1758, Domestic Cat (?).

Intermediate type host: *Gallus gallus domesticus* (L., 1758), Domestic Chicken.

Other intermediate hosts: Unknown.

Geographic distribution: Asia: China; Europe: Czech Republic; Oceana: Papua New Guinea.

Description of sporulated oocyst: Unknown.

Description of sporocyst and sporozoites: Sporocyst shape: ellipsoidal; L × W: 13.0 × 8.6; L/W ratio: 1.5; SB, SSB, PSB: all absent; SR: present; SR characteristics: granules in SP; SZ: not described. Distinctive features of sporocyst: none; a "typical" *Sarcocystis*-type SP, lacking SB, SSB, PSB and with a distinct, granular SR.

Prevalence: Wenzel et al. (1982) found sarcocysts in 45/241 (19%) free-range chickens but not in any of 207 battery-raised chickens in Germany; in China, Mao and Zuo (1994) found sarcocysts in most of the carcass muscles of 6/284 (2%) free-range chickens in Kunming, but no sarcocysts were found in heart muscles; Chen et al. (2012) also found it in 17/191 (9%) free-range chickens from Yunnan, China.

Sporulation: Not stated, but likely endogenous with sporulated, infective sporocysts shed in the feces of the definitive host.

Prepatent and patent periods: Unknown.

Site of infection, definitive host: Unknown.

Site of infection, intermediate host: Striated muscles.

Endogenous stages, definitive host: Unknown.

Endogenous stages, intermediate host: Unknown.

Cross-transmission: None to date.

Pathology: Unknown.

Materials deposited: None.

Remarks: Wenzel et al. (1982) reported two types of sarcocysts that were based on the shape of bradyzoites. Sarcocysts with banana-shaped bradyzoites were considered to be *S. horvathi* of Rátz (1909) (see above), whereas sarcocysts containing lancet-shaped bradyzoites, 12–18 × 2.5–3.0, were considered to be another species. Both dogs and cats fed sarcocysts shed sporocysts that were L × W: 11.6 × 9.2, L/W ratio: 1.3 (Wenzel et al., 1982); they then fed 1,000–10,000 sporocysts (either dog or cat origin) to 90 chickens and killed chickens at intervals for histological study. No stages were found in chickens killed 1–15 DPI, but meronts/young sarcocysts were detected at 16 DPI (which seems very early when compared with other species). At 40 DPI sarcocysts were immature, and at 71 DPI they were said to be mature. Both dogs and cats fed chickens 88 DPI excreted sporocysts, but it was not clear which type of sarcocysts were used (Wenzel et al., 1982; Dubey et al., 2015a).

Odening (1997) named the sarcocysts with lancet-shaped bradyzoites (of Wenzel et al., 1982) to be *S. wenzeli*. Sarcocysts reported by Mao and Zuo (1994) that contained lancet-shaped bradyzoites, L × W: 14.3 × 2.9, also became *S. wenzeli*; the cyst wall was said to be identical to those sarcocysts seen in Australia and Papua New Guinea by Mehlhorn et al. (1976). Mao and Zuo (1994) reported that 4/6 (66%) 2-month-old dogs, and 5/8 (62.5%) cats excreted sporocysts after consuming naturally-infected muscles of chickens; sporocysts were L × W: 13.0 × 8.6, L/W ratio: 1.5. Sporocysts (500,000; source not stated) were fed to five 2-week-old chickens that were killed 20, 33, 63, 116, and 128 DPI. Sarcocysts were not observed at 20 DPI, immature sarcocysts were reported at 33 DPI, and mature sarcocysts were found 63, 116, and 128 DPI (Mao and Zuo, 1994). Chen et al. (2012) said that their sarcocysts were thread-like, L × W: 1,093 × 65 (334–3,169 × 41–117), had septa, and had dense, short finger-like protrusions that appeared radially striated. Their sarcocyst wall was 2.4 (1.4–3.5) thick, and bradyzoites were lancet-shaped, L × W: 14.6 × 2.5 (12–18 × 2–3). Ultrastructurally, the sarcocyst wall had stubby villar protrusions that corresponded to the "type 9" class from Dubey et al. (1989b). Chen et al. (2012) thus confirmed the previous work of Mao and Zuo (1994) finding *S. wenzeli* in chickens of the Kunmiing region of China. This species was not mentioned by Levine (1986) in his review of valid taxonomic names of *Sarcocystis* species. Odening (1998), in his compilation of 189

Sarcocystis names, listed this as a valid species and added that it had a TEM type 9 sarcocyst wall (of Dubey et al., 1989b). Dubey et al. (2015a) summarized the *Sarcocystis* of chickens by identifying *S. wenzeli* as one of the two valid species infecting domestic chickens but noted the uncertainty of whether dogs, or cats, or both, or neither of them are the definitive hosts for this species. They cited all the known contributing authors on chicken *Sarcocystis* species and their work on sarcocyst and bradyzoite sizes and structures, the limited cross-transmission work that has been done, prevalences in various countries with surveys, and they mentioned this species in their Tables 1.4, 24.1, and 24.4 (Dubey et al., 2015a).

SARCOCYSTIS SPECIES

Finally, there are another 45+ accounts of *Sarcocystis* being identified only to genus, either from oocysts/sporocysts in fecal materials or from sarcocysts in the muscles of various *Canis* species including domestic dogs, wolves, coyotes, and even the black-backed jackals, from which no named species has yet been documented (see Chapter 19). We know there are hundreds more such reports in the literature worldwide, but our sampling is presented to demonstrate how widespread such superficial identifications have been (and continue to be) and how much work is yet to be accomplished.

GENUS CERDOCYON C.E.H. SMITH, 1839 (MONOTYPIC)

SARCOCYSTIS CAPRACANIS FISCHER, 1979

Definitive host: *Cerdocyon thous* (L., 1766), Crab-eating Dog.
Remarks: For more complete information on *S. capracanis*, see Genus *Canis*, above.

SARCOCYSTIS CRUZI (HASSELMANN, 1923) WENYON, 1926a

Definitive host: *Cerdocyon thous* (L., 1758), Crab-eating Dog.
Remarks: For more complete information on *S. cruzi*, see Genus *Canis*, above.

SARCOCYSTIS SPECIES

To our knowledge, there is only one report of *Sarcocystis* fecal stages from *Cerdocyon brachyurus*, the maned wolf, in Brazil (see Chapter 19).

GENUS CUON HODGSON, 1838 (MONOTYPIC)

SARCOCYSTIS SPECIES

There is one report of a *Sarcocystis* life cycle involving the dhole, *Cuon alpinus*, in India, but an appropriate application of a binomial name was not done (see Chapter 19).

GENUS LYCALOPEX BURMEISTER, 1854 (6 SPECIES)

SARCOCYSTIS SVANAI DUBEY, SYKES, SHELTON, SHARP, VERMA, CALERO-BERNAL, VIVIANO, SUNDAR, KAHN, AND GRIGG, 2015b

Intermediate host: *Lycalopex gymnocercus* (G. Fischer, 1814), Pampas Fox.
Remarks: For more complete information on *S. svanai*, see Genus *Canis*, above.

GENUS *LYCAON* BROOKES, 1827 (MONOTYPIC)

SARCOCYSTIS SPECIES

There are at least three reports of *Sarcocystis* intestinal stages found in *Lycaon pictus*, the African wild dog, in Zambia and South Africa (see Chapter 19).

GENUS *NYCTEREUTES* TEMMINCK, 1838 (MONOTYPIC)

SARCOCYSTIS CRUZI (HASSELMANN, 1923) WENYON, 1926a

Definitive host: *Nyctereutes procyonoides* (Gray, 1834), Raccoon Dog.
Remarks: For more complete information on *S. cruzi*, see Genus *Canis*, above.

SARCOCYSTIS GRUENERI YAKIMOFF AND SOKOLOFF, 1934

Definitive host: *Nyctereutes procyonoides* (Gray, 1834), Raccoon Dog.
Remarks: For more complete information on *S. grueneri*, see Genus *Vulpes*, below.

SARCOCYSTIS RILEYI (STILES, 1893) LABBÉ, 1899

Definitive host: *Nyctereutes procyonoides* (Gray, 1834), Raccoon Dog.
Remarks: For more complete information on *S. rileyi*, see Genus *Mephitis*, below.

SARCOCYSTIS TARANDIVULPES GJERDE, 1984c

Definitive host: *Nyctereutes procyonoides* (Gray, 1834), Raccoon Dog.

Remarks: For more complete information on *S. tarandivulpes*, see Genus *Vulpes*, below.

SARCOCYSTIS SPECIES

There are at least three reports of *Sarcocystis* sarcocysts found in the muscles of *N. procyonoides* in Russia and Japan, but no identifications to species were made (see Chapter 19).

GENUS *UROCYON* BAIRD, 1857 (2 SPECIES)

SARCOCYSTIS ODOCOILEOCANIS CRUM, FAYER, AND PRESTWOOD, 1981

Definitive host: *Urocyon cinereoargenteus* (Schreber, 1775), Gray Fox.
Remarks: For more complete information on *S. odocoileocanis*, see Genus *Canis*, above.

GENUS *VULPES* FRISCH, 1775 (12 SPECIES)

SARCOCYSTIS ALBIFRONSI KUTKIENĖ, PRAKAS, AND SRUOGA, 2012

For LM (Fig. 1A) and TEM photomicrographs (Figs. 1B–D) of sarcocysts and their surface structures, and a sporulated sporocyst (Fig. 1E) see Kutkienė et al. (2006), and for the phylogenetic tree for bird *Sarcocystis* species based on gene sequence of ITS-1 region see Kutkienė et al. (2012, Fig. 1).
Synonym: *Sarcocystis* sp. (cyst type III) of Kutkienė, Sruoga, and Butkauskas, 2009.
Definitive type host: *Vulpes* (syn. *Alopex*) *lagopus* (L., 1758), Arctic or Blue Fox.
Type locality: Eastern Europe: Lithuania: Šilutė district, near the Baltic Sea.
Other definitive hosts: None to date.

Intermediate type host: *Anser albifrons* (Scopoli, 1769), Greater White-fronted Goose.

Other intermediate hosts: None to date.

Geographic distribution: Eastern Europe: Lithuania.

Description of sporulated oocyst: Unknown.

Description of sporocyst and sporozoites: Sporocyst shape: ellipsoidal; L × W (n = 37): 12 × 8 (10–13 × 7–9); L/W ratio: 1.5; SB, SSB, PSB: all absent; SR: present; SR characteristics: small granules scattered in SP (Fig. 1E, Kutkienė et al., 2006); SZ: not described, but more or less comma-shaped (photomicrographs). Distinctive features of sporocyst: none; a "typical" *Sarcocystis*-type SP, lacking SB, SSB, PSB and with a distinct, granular SR.

Prevalence: All three *A. albifrons* shot on the coast of the Baltic Sea near Curonian Bay were infected with sarcocysts. All three fox cubs fed infected leg muscle became infected.

Sporulation: Endogenous with sporulated, infective sporocysts shed in the feces of the definitive host.

Prepatent and patent periods: Prepatent period was 13 DPI (cub 2) or 14 DPI (cub 3).

Site of infection, definitive host: Unknown, but likely in the intestinal mucosa.

Site of infection, intermediate host: Sarcocysts were found in the muscles of the leg, breast, and neck.

Endogenous stages, definitive host: Not reported, but certainly in the epithelial cells of the small intestine as interpreted from the pathology caused in cub 1.

Endogenous stages, intermediate host: Microcysts were ribbon-shaped up to 4 mm long and 750 μm wide. The cyst wall had teat- or finger-like protrusions, ~2.4 high, with gaps between them. Within these protrusions were numerous fibrillar elements that extended from the villi tips into the ground substance of the cyst. Small invaginations of the primary cyst wall and spots of electron-dense material appeared circular in cross sections. Sarcocysts were divided into large chambers by septa that contained almost straight cystozoites that measured L × W (n = 36): 11.4 × 1.7 (10–13.5 × 1.5–2.5). Kutkienė et al.

(2006) said these sarcocysts had type-9 tissue cyst walls after Dubey et al. (1989b).

Cross-transmission: None to other potential carnivores.

Pathology: All three fox cubs developed severe diarrhea on days 2–3 after ingesting raw goose leg muscle infected with sarcocysts. Cubs 1 and 2 were fed 18–20 g of raw muscle when they were 25-days-old and cub 3 was fed ~100 g of infected leg muscle when it was 30-days-old. Cub 1 died 3 DPI and its intestine showed severe inflammation. Cubs suffered diarrhea for 3–4 DPI.

Materials deposited: TEM material and histological preparations are deposited at the Laboratory of Molecular Ecology of the Institute of Ecology, Nature Research Centre, Vilnius, Lithuania. Gene sequences are deposited in GenBank with accession Nos. EU502868 (18S rDNA), EF079885 (28S rDNA), JF520780 (ITS-1 region).

Etymology: The Latin name of the white-fronted goose is used for a species name.

Remarks: Early studies by Kutkienė et al. (e.g., Kutkienė and Sruoga, 2004) alerted them that infection of white-fronted geese with *Sarcocystis* species in their area was high; for example, 89/144 (62%) geese examined had muscle sarcocysts with two types of cysts, which they called type I and type III. Kutkienė et al. (2006) isolated type III sarcocysts from the legs, breasts, and neck muscles of three hunter-killed *A. albifrons*; they fixed the sarcocysts for LM and TEM and offered a brief description of the sarcocyst wall. They also fed infected leg muscles to three *V. lagopus* cubs that had been isolated from their mother at 19-days-old and maintained separately in metallic cages in a clean room until they were infected. However, although they had both structural and life cycle information, they neglected at that time to name their species. Kutkienė et al. (2012) stated, "data on the ultrastructure of the cyst wall are not enough to describe new species and answer the question about host specificity of the species," but that molecular studies, particularly sequencing DNA of the ITS-1 region, can help solve this problem. Thus, they did a phylogenetic analysis of 12 bird *Sarcocystis* species and included *S. neurona* (horses) and *S. cruzi* (cattle) as outgroups in the phylogenetic tree. Using that molecular data, in combination with their earlier life cycle and morphological data, they named two new *Sarcocystis* species, *S. albifronsi* (above) from *Anser albifrons*, and *S. anasi* from the mallard duck (*Anas platyrhynchos* L., 1758), for which the definitive host is still unknown (and, thus, is not included in this chapter). Dubey et al. (2015a) listed *S. albifronsi* as a valid species (their Table 24.1).

SARCOCYSTIS ALCES DAHLGREN AND GJERDE, 2008

For light (Fig. 1) and scanning electron micrographs (Fig. 2) of sarcocysts and their surface structures and phylogenetic placement on an inferred Bayesian tree based on 18S rRNA (Fig. 6) see Dahlgren and Gjerde (2008). For LM photomicrographs of sporulated oocysts and sporocysts (Figs. 3C and D) see Dahlgren and Gjerde (2010b).

Definitive type host: *Vulpes vulpes* (L., 1758), Red or Silver Fox (selected as their type host because red foxes are common in Norwegian forests and known to commonly feed on carcasses of moose that have died).

Type locality: Europe: Norway: Oslo, Akershus, Oppland, and Østfold Counties in Southeastern Norway.

Other definitive hosts: *Vulpes* (syn. *Alopex*) *lagopus* (L., 1758), Arctic or Blue Fox.

Intermediate type host: *Alces alces* (L., 1758), Eurasian Elk or Moose.

Other intermediate hosts: Unknown.

Geographic distribution: Europe: Norway.

Description of sporulated oocyst: Oocyst shape: ellipsoidal, with 1 thin wall; L × W: 17.5 × 12.5 (15–20 × 10–15); L/W ratio: 1.4; M, OR, PG: all absent. Distinctive features of oocyst: typical thin-walled *Sarcocystis*-type, which usually

breaks down releasing sporocysts into the intestinal lumen.

Description of sporocyst and sporozoites: Sporocyst shape: ellipsoidal; L × W: 14–15 × 10; L/W ratio: unknown; SB, SSB, PSB: all absent; SR: present; SR characteristics: spheroidal mass of small granules (Figs. 3C and D in Dahlgren and Gjerde, 2010b); SZ: not described, but more or less banana-shaped (photomicrographs). Distinctive features of sporocyst: none; a "typical" *Sarcocystis*-type SP, lacking SB, SSB, PSB and with a distinct, granular SR.

Prevalence: In the moose intermediate host, these sarcocysts were the predominant cyst type in the diaphragm and esophagus, found in 24/34 (69%) moose (Dahlgren and Gjerde, 2008). Dahlgren and Gjerde (2008, 2010b) said that *S. alces* is the most prevalent *Sarcocystis* species in Norwegian moose. Mucosal scrapings showed that all 12 foxes became infected with one of the two *Sarcocystis* species (*S. alces*, *S. hjorti*) in moose muscle, but molecular findings in fecal and mucosal-scraping samples only confirmed that 2/6 (33%) *V. vulpes* and 2/6 *V. lagopus* had oocysts/sporocysts of *S. alces* (Table 2, Dahlgren and Gjerde, 2010b).

Sporulation: Endogenous with sporulated, infective sporocysts shed in the feces of the definitive host.

Prepatent and patent periods: Prepatent period is ~14 days, while the length of patency was not given.

Site of infection, definitive host: Oocysts and sporocysts were found in the intestinal mucosa of both fox species.

Site of infection, intermediate host: The esophagus was the most heavily infected muscle, but sarcocysts also were commonly found in the diaphragm, whereas the number of sarcocysts was small in moose hearts. Esophageal sarcocysts were generally larger (longer and thicker) compared with those in the diaphragm.

Endogenous stages, definitive host: Unknown. Only unsporulated and sporulated oocysts were seen in the intestinal scrapings from *V. vulpes* and *V. lagopus* (Dahlgren and Gjerde, 2010b).

Endogenous stages, intermediate host: In skeletal muscle, sarcocysts were spindle-shaped, L × W: 3–5.5 × 0.3–0.4 mm. In cardiac muscle, sarcocysts were sac-like, 0.5–0.6 × 0.2–0.3 mm. By LM, the cyst wall was smooth, with no discernible protrusions, but ultrasound treatment showed very short surface protrusions in some cysts, with a regular pattern of small dots, aligned in rows, across the cyst surface. All cysts in cardiac muscle were small and sac-like. By SEM, the cyst surface was divided into numerous polygonal to rounded convex areas by intersecting shallow grooves, corresponding to the internal compartments of the cysts, delimited by septa. The entire surface of the cysts was provided with short platform-like protrusions, which were regularly distributed in parallel rows running lengthwise on the cysts. Individual cysts had protrusions that were fairly uniform in size and shape, but their outline in different cysts varied between regular squares, rectangles, hexagons, or more polygonal or rounded objects. Square protrusions were ~0.8×0.8, and the distance between them, within each longitudinal row, was ~1.2; rectangular areas between four adjacent protrusions were ~1.2 × 1.0. Areas between the protrusions were pitted due to numerous small invaginations of the surface membrane, whereas the flat, distal surface of each protrusion was smooth. Height of the protrusions was <0.2 (Dahlgren and Gjerde, 2008).

Cross-transmission: None to date.

Pathology: Dahlgren and Gjerde (2010b) reported that 7/12 (58%) foxes in their two experiments had reduced feed intake, soft feces and/or vomited between 6 and 10 DPI and one fox had diarrhea and vomited on the 13th DPI, but they did not mention which of the two fox species fed infected moose meat experienced these symptoms. Later in their paper, they suggested that these symptoms "were most likely associated with the *Hammondia* infection" also documented in these hosts because *Hammondia*

heydorni infection in dogs have been associated with diarrhea (Abel et al., 2006).

Materials deposited: The complete 18S rRNA gene sequence has been deposited in GenBank with accession no. EU282018. Sarcocysts excised from muscular tissues from moose, and photographs from LM and SEM examinations of the sarcocyst wall are on deposit at the Natural History Museum, Oslo, Norway, collection no. NHMO-Prot00001.

Etymology: Because the species seems to be prevalent in moose, Dahlgren and Gjerde (2008) assigned the Latin name for moose as its specific epitaph.

Remarks: When Dahlgren and Gjerde (2008) first proposed the name for this species, their description was based on sarcocysts excised from muscular tissues of moose, LM and SEM photomicrographs of the sarcocyst wall, and phylogenetic separation from other *Sarcocystis* species on an inferred Bayesian tree based on 18S rRNA. Dahlgren and Gjerde (2009) studied several *Sarcocystis* species in Norwegian roe deer (*C. capreolous*) by morphological (SEM) identification and determined their phylogenetic relationships by DNA amplification and sequencing of the 18S rRNA gene. They showed that sarcocysts of *S. gracilis* were similar to those of *S. alces* in moose (Dahlgren and Gjerde, 2008), which also lack deep invaginations of the cyst surface, but that other distinct features still separated sarcocysts of *S. gracilis* from those of *S. alces*. The protrusions on *S. gracilis* sarcocysts are more rounded, higher, narrower, and more densely packed on the surface than the protrusions on *S. alces* cysts. The shorter protrusions on cysts of *S. alces* are nearly invisible by LM (except after ultrasound treatment), resulting in a smooth surface, as opposed to the crenated margin of *S. gracilis* sarcocysts. Dahlgren and Gjerde (2010b) later fed muscle sarcocysts from moose to six silver foxes (*V. vulpes*) and six blue foxes (*V. lagopus*). The foxes were euthanized 7–28 DPI and intestinal scrapings and fecal samples were screened microscopically for *Sarcocystis*

oocysts/sporocysts, which were later identified to species, by species-specific primers,
and sequence analysis of the 18S rRNA gene.
Molecular identification showed that the oocysts/
sporocysts belonged to two species, *S. alces* and
S. hjorti, even though sarcocysts in moose muscle
were only identified as *S. hjorti* prior to infections of foxes. Dahlgren and Gjerde (2010b) concluded that their study proved both fox species
are definitive hosts for both *Sarcocystis* species,
as had been inferred from phylogenetic position
of these forms earlier (2008). Dubey et al. (2015a)
listed this as a valid species (their Table 24.1).

SARCOCYSTIS ALECTORIVULPES PAK, SKLYAROVA, AND PAK, 1989

Definitive host: *Vulpes* (syn. *Alopex*) *corsac* (L.,
1758), Corsac Fox.
Type locality: Asia: Kazakhstan.
Other definitive host: *Vulpes vulpes* (L., 1758),
Red or Silver Fox.
Intermediate type host: *Alectoris chukar* (Gray,
1830), Chukar Partridge.
Other intermediate hosts: Unknown.
Geographic distribution: Asia: Kazakhstan.
Description of sporulated oocyst: Unknown.
Description of sporocyst and sporozoites:
Unknown.
Prevalence: Unknown.
Sporulation: Unknown, but likely endogenous
with sporulated, infective sporocysts shed in the
feces of the definitive host.
Prepatent and patent periods: Unknown.
Site of infection, definitive host: Unknown, but
likely in the intestinal mucosa.
Site of infection, intermediate host: Unknown.
Endogenous stages, definitive host: Unknown.
Endogenous stages, intermediate host: Unknown.
Cross-transmission: Unknown.
Pathology: Unknown.
Materials deposited: None.
Remarks: We were unable to obtain a copy of
this publication, so the information presented

herein is from Odening (1998). Dubey et al.
(2015a) mentioned this species three times, but
only in Tables 17.2, 24.1, and 24.4, did not discuss it, but considered it a valid species.

SARCOCYSTIS ARCTICA GJERDE AND SCHULZE, 2014

For light micrographs of tissue cysts (Figs. 1
and 2) and phylogenetic analyses (Figs. 3 and
4) using genomic DNA sequences at 4 loci, see
Gjerde and Schulze (2014).
Definitive type host: Unknown.
Type locality: Europe: Norway, Finnmark
County, Vadsø municipality.
Other definitive hosts: None to date.
Intermediate type host: *Vulpes* (syn. *Alopex*)
lagopus (L., 1758), Arctic or Blue Fox.
Other intermediate hosts: Unknown.
Geographic distribution: Europe: Norway,
Finnmark, and Trøndelag Counties.
Description of sporulated oocyst: Unknown.
Description of sporocyst and sporozoites:
Unknown.
Prevalence: Gjerde and Schulze (2014) found
this species in 2/2 arctic foxes in Norway and
the sarcocysts in fox 1, collected in 2011 from
Finnmark County, were much more numer-
ous than those in fox 2, collected in 2013 from
Trøndelag County.
Sporulation: Unknown, but likely endogenous
with sporulated, infective sporocysts shed in the
feces of the definitive host.
Prepatent and patent periods: Unknown.
Site of infection, definitive host: Unknown, but
likely in the intestinal mucosa.
Site of infection, intermediate host: Muscle cells
of the myocardium, diaphragm, masseter, and
musculus extensor digitalis communis.
Endogenous stages, definitive host: Unknown.
Endogenous stages, intermediate host: Sarcocysts
in fox 1 were spindle-shaped to thread-like, 1–12 ×
0.1–0.25 mm in the extensor muscle, and 1–6 ×
0.1–0.2 mm in the diaphragm, and the larger cysts

could be seen grossly. All isolated sarcocysts had the same surface structure with short knob-like or dome-shaped protrusions that gave sarcocysts a serrated outline. Protrusions were ~1.0–1.5 mm wide at their base and 0.5–1.0 μm high. Sarcocysts were subdivided by septa into many compartments, each with numerous cystozoites (but these were not measured). Sarcocysts from the muscles of fox 1 and two sarcocysts derived from the tongue muscle of fox 2 were successfully PCR amplified and sequenced at one or more loci, including 18S rRNA, ITS-1, 28S rRNA, and *cox1*, and all isolates could be assigned to the same *Sarcocystis* species, which Gjerde and Schulze (2014) named as new. They (2014) also said that in pairwise BLAST sequences, *S. arctica* was 99.9% identical with GenBank sequence JN256676 (*Sarcocystis* sp. MTI) from a Rottweiler dog from Montana, USA, but only 99.0% identical with sequence JN256677 (*Sarcocystis* sp. CO1) from a golden retriever dog in Colorado, USA (Sykes et al., 2011). This allowed them to conclude that, based on the 18S rRNA sequence, the two US dogs likely host two separate *Sarcocystis* species, of which one is consistent with their *S. arctica*, whereas based on the ITS-1 sequences, identical to those of *S. arctica*, both US dogs seem to harbor their *S. arctica*. Supporting that idea, TEM of the sarcocysts from those dogs had short villar protrusions consistent with the protrusions seen by LM (Fig. 3, Sykes et al., 2011) by them (Gjerde and Schulze, 2014).

Cross-transmission: Unknown.

Pathology: Apparently no pathology was seen because Gjerde and Schulze (2014) found no associated tissue reaction in H&E-stained muscle sections, other than a slight compression of the neighboring muscle fibers.

Materials deposited: Nucleotide sequences of *S. arctica* are deposited in GenBank, under accession nos. KF601301-KF601327. Two partial *cox1* sequences obtained from the arctic fox in this study were originally deposited in GenBank (KF601326, KF601327) under the species name *S. arctica*, but Gjerde and Josefsen (2015) later assigned these sequences to *S. lutrae* for reasons explained below. Histological sections of sarcocysts and DNA samples are deposited in the Department of Food Safety and Infection Biology, the Norwegian University of Life Sciences, Oslo, Norway.

Etymology: The specific epitaph is derived from the common name of the intermediate host, the arctic fox.

Remarks: Most often, carnivores act as definitive hosts for *Sarcocystis* species, with herbivores as intermediate hosts, and some omnivores acting in both capacities (although not usually for the same *Sarcocystis* species). However, as we see here, and in Chapter 19, many carnivores, including canids (*Canis, Nyctereutes, Vulpes*), skunks (*Mephitis*), mustelids (*Martes, Meles, Millivora, Mustela, Neovison*), otarids (*Callorhinus*), phocids (*Erignathus, Phoca, Pusa*), procyonids (*Procyon*), ursids (*Ursus*), felids (*Felis, Puma, Panthera*), and herpestids (*Helogale, Mungos*) have been found to harbor muscular sarcocysts. In addition, the pathogenic species *S. neurona* may form extraintestinal sarcocysts in many carnivores, as well as horses, but these sarcocysts are usually confined to the central nervous system. There are only a few instances where authors tried to characterize muscle sarcocysts by molecular methods, mainly using short fragments of the 18S rRNA gene or the ITS-1 locus, but no specific identifications were made and these species had a fairly high sequence identity at the 18S rRNA gene with various *Sarcocystis* species using birds as intermediate hosts (Gillis et al., 2003; Dubey et al., 2010a; Larkin et al., 2011; Sykes et al., 2011). Gjerde and Schulze (2014) said that this species from arctic foxes in Norway differed from all other named *Sarcocystis* species deposited in GenBank but that "it might be identical to an unnamed *Sarcocystis* species from dogs in the United States."

Finally, because *S. albifronsi* can use the arctic fox as a definitive host (Kutkienė et al., 2012), Gjerde and Schulze (2014) suggested this may indicate that their species, *S. arctica*, may have a similar life cycle, where foxes are only aberrant or incidental intermediate hosts of a species that normally cycles among birds or at least uses birds as its preferred intermediate host. However, because they found *S. arctica* in two widely separated foxes in different years, and because it may even be the same species found in two unrelated dogs in the United States, it seemed more likely to them that *S. arctica* primarily uses canids as intermediate hosts and mammals or avian carnivores or scavengers as definitive hosts. The arctic fox itself, through cannibalism, might also be a suitable definitive host, but this was not tested. Dubey et al. (2015a) mentioned this species four times (their Tables 19.1, 23.2, 24.1, and 24.4) and did not discuss it but considered it a valid species.

SARCOCYSTIS CAPRACANIS FISCHER, 1979

Definitive hosts: *Vulpes* (syn. *Alopex*) *corsac* (L., 1768), Corsac Fox; *Vulpes vulpes* (L., 1758), Red or Silver Fox.

Remarks: For more complete information on *S. capracanis*, see Genus *Canis*, above.

SARCOCYSTIS CAPREOLICANIS ERBER, BOCH, AND BARTH, 1978

Definitive hosts: *Vulpes velox* (Say, 1823), Swift Fox; *Vulpes vulpes* (L., 1758), Red or Silver Fox.

Remarks: For more complete information on *S. capreolicanis*, see Genus *Canis*, above.

SARCOCYSTIS CITELLIVULPES PAK, PERMINOVA, AND ESHTOKINA, 1979

Definitive hosts: *Mustela eversmanii* Lesson, 1827, Steppe Polecat; *Vulpes* (syn. *Alopex*) *corsac* (L., 1758), Corsac Fox; *Vulpes vulpes* (L., 1758), Red or Silver Fox.

Intermediate host: *Spermophilus* (syn. *Citellus*) *fulvus* (Lichtenstein, 1823), Yellow Ground Squirrel.

Geographic distribution: Asia: Kazakhstan (former USSR).

Remarks: Levine and Ivens (1981) said the sporocysts were L × W: 10–13 × 7–10, and sarcocysts were found in muscles of *S. fulvus*. They also said that sarcocysts in the muscles of the ground squirrel are 30–9,000 × 20–600 in size, the prepatent period in the red and corsac foxes was 7–8 days, and the patent period lasted 7–14 days in these hosts. Levine (1986) listed this species as a valid, named *Sarcocystis* species, gave no other information, and did not list the original reference. Odening (1998) included this species as one of the 189 valid *Sarcocystis* species names in his summary paper and said it was quite similar to *Sarcocystis putorii*. We were not able to secure a copy of this paper, but we listed the complete reference in our literature cited. Dubey et al. (2015a) said the sarcocysts were up to 8 mm long, with a thick (1.4–3.5), striated wall, but they then listed *Sarcocystis citellivulpes* (Table 24.2) as an invalid species of *Sarcocystis*.

SARCOCYSTIS CORSACI PAK, 1979

Definitive host: *Vulpes* (syn. *Alopex*) *corsac* (L., 1758), Corsac Fox.

Intermediate host: *Vulpes* (syn. *Alopex*) *corsac* (L., 1758), Corsac Fox.

Geographic distribution: Asia: Kazakhstan (former USSR).

Remarks: Odening (1998) included this species as one of the 189 valid *Sarcocystis* species names in his summary paper on named species of *Sarcocystis* and listed the corsac fox as both definitive and intermediate hosts. We were not able to secure a copy of this paper but listed the complete reference in our literature cited. Odening (1998) recommended finding Pak et al., 1984, in Anon (1984). Dubey et al. (2015a) said the sarcocysts were up to 8.2 mm long and had a sarcocyst wall of two layers, with the total wall thickness

2.1–2.8 and containing bradyzoites that measured 7.0–8.4 × 1.4–2.8 (their Table 19.1); they also listed it as a valid species (Tables 24.1 and 24.4).

SARCOCYSTIS CRUZI (HASSELMANN, 1923) WENYON, 1926a

Definitive host: *Vulpes vulpes* (L., 1758), Red or Silver Fox.

Remarks: For more complete information on *S. cruzi*, see Genus *Canis*, above.

SARCOCYSTIS GRACILIS RÁTZ, 1909

For light and electron micrographs of tissue cysts and zoites of this species see Figs. 6–9 in Odening et al. (1994a).

Synonyms: *Sarcocystis* sp. type 1 of Erber et al., 1978; "Thin-walled cysts, type Rh2" of Bergmann and Kinder, 1976; "Cyst wall type 5" of Entzeroth, 1982a; *Sarcocystis sibirica* Matschoulsky, 1947b, in Dubey et al. (1989b), Sugár et al. (1990) and Navarrete et al. (1990).

Definitive type host: *Vulpes vulpes* (L., 1758), Red or Silver Fox.

Type locality: Europe: Germany.

Other definitive hosts: *Vulpes* (syn. *Alopex*) *lagopus* (L., 1758), Arctic or Blue Fox.

Intermediate type host: *Capreolus capreolus* (L., 1758), European Roe Deer.

Other intermediate hosts: *Capreolus pygargus* (Pallas, 1771), Siberian Roe Deer; *Bos taurus* L., 1758, Aurochs.

Geographic distribution: Europe: Germany, Poland, throughout the range of *C. capreolus*.

Description of sporulated oocyst: Oocyst shape: irregular, with one thin wall; L × W: 20 × 15; L/W ratio: 1.3; M, OR, PG: all absent. Distinctive features of oocyst: typical thin-walled *Sarcocystis*-type, which usually breaks down releasing sporocysts into the intestinal lumen.

Description of sporocyst and sporozoites: Sporocyst shape: subellipsoidal; L × W

(n = 100): 15 × 10 (12–18 × 9–11); L/W ratio: 1.5; SB, SSB, PSB: all absent; SR: present; SR characteristics: unknown; SZ: not described. Distinctive features of sporocyst: none; a "typical" *Sarcocystis*-type SP, lacking SB, SSB, PSB, and with a distinct, granular SR.

Prevalence: Erber et al. (1978) found sarcocysts they thought represented three distinct species in 392/421 (93%) roe deer from Germany, but they did not state specifically how many of the infected deer had only this species. Sedlaczek and Wesemeier (1995) found this species in 58/66 (88%) roe deer they examined between 1992 and 1994 from locations in Germany (n = 35) and Poland (n = 31) and 17/58 (29%) infected roe deer harbored only *S. gracilis*, whereas the remaining 41 infected deer were infected by two or three species.

Sporulation: Endogenous with sporulated, infective sporocysts shed in the feces of the definitive host.

Prepatent and patent periods: Erber et al. (1978) said, "the prepatent period needs 10–14 days, the patent period lasts 50 days at least." Gjerde (2012) listed the prepatent period as 9 days.

Site of infection, definitive host: Intestinal mucosa.

Site of infection, intermediate host: Muscle cells of the tongue, esophagus, heart, diaphragm, and skeleton (thigh, loin, thorax, ribs).

Endogenous stages, definitive host: Unknown.

Endogenous stages, intermediate host: Sarcocysts in the esophagus measured L × W (n = 11): 916 × 144 (440–1,431 × 73–257), those in the heart were L × W (n = 28): 282 × 78 (110–551 × 51–121), and those in the skeletal musculature were L × W (n = 62): 1,904 × 150 (110–2,937 × 59–330). Bradyzoites (n = 5) were 12.5–15.6 × 3.1–3.9 (Sedlaczek and Wesemeier, 1995).

By LM, the sarcocyst wall appeared smooth but showed a cogged wheel or stamp-like periphery that was distinctly visible at the "apical" part of the cyst with short, stubby-like villar protrusions at the tip of the cyst. TEM showed a cyst wall with stubby-like protrusions that appeared in irregular intervals of 0.4–2.2. These protrusions had different shapes and sizes and their core was more or less compact than the granular layer of the wall. The cyst wall formed bubble-like elevations between the protrusions.

Cross-transmission: None to date.

Pathology: Unknown.

Materials deposited: None.

Remarks: Sarcocysts in *C. capreolus* were described for the first time in Germany by Theodor von Hessling (1854), and his form was later named *S. gracilis* by Rátz (1909), in Hungary. Brumpt (1913) placed all sarcosporidia then known into the genus *Sarcocystis* and listed this species as *S. gracilis* Von Rátz, 1910, and said that it was found only in the muscles of deer. Bergmann and Kinder (1976) and Entzeroth (1982a) reported on the TEM of *S. gracilis* sarcocysts, but the authors did not classify the sarcocysts to a particular species. It was first recognized as a distinct species when Erber et al. (1978) assigned this name to one of three sarcocyst types (type 1), which they described by LM from roe deer in Germany because it matched the original description of *S. gracilis*. Levine and Ivens (1981) did not include this species in their monograph because it was not known then that a carnivore was the definitive host. Levine (1986) did list this species as one of the 122 names he considered as valid species of *Sarcocystis* at that time but said the relationship between this species to *S. capreoli* and *S. sibirica* is unknown. Entzeroth (1985) studied and detailed the sarcocyst wall of this species in *C. capreolus* muscles using LM, SEM, and TEM. Sedlaczek and Wesemeier (1995) complemented the species description by TEM and LM photomicrographs but reiterated that *S. gracilis* is morphologically similar to a *Sarcocystis* sp. described by Odening et al. (1994a) from the European badger, *M. meles*, and they said it was possible that *S. sibirica* Matschoulsky, 1947b is a synonym of *S. gracilis*. Odening (1998) listed this species as one of the 189 names in his summary list of *Sarcocystis* species names and said *S. gracilis* probably infects *M. meles* as an accidental intermediate host. Kutkienė (2001) examined

muscle preparations from 24 roe deer hunted in Lithuania using only LM but was able to distinguish *S. gracilis* sarcocysts from those of *S. capreolicanis*, *Sarcocystis* cf. *hofmanni*, and *Sarcocystis* sp. Dahlgren and Gjerde (2009) examined sarcocysts of several *Sarcocystis* species in Norwegian roe deer (*C. capreolus*) using PCR amplification, and sequencing of the 18S rRNA gene and SEM. Their conclusions were that when comparing SEM findings of *S. gracilis* with SEM descriptions reported by others, the previous papers seemed to contain discrepancies between which species the micrographs allegedly represented and the species they actually depicted. They said that Entzeroth (1985) described *S. gracilis* cysts by LM, SEM, and TEM and that his SEM micrographs (Figs. 4 and 5) are indeed of *S. gracilis*, whereas (in their opinion) his LM (Fig. 2) and TEM micrographs (Fig. 3) were a different species, very similar to the *Sarcocystis* sp. with type 3 cysts described by Erber et al. (1978) or *S.* cf. *hofmanni* sarcocysts described by Sedlaczek and Wesmeier (1995). Continuing their historical reconstruction, Dahlgren and Gjerde (2009) said that Stolte et al. (1996a) presented LM and SEM pictures (Plate VI) of cysts that they assumed were of *S.* cf. *hofmanni*, but their SEM micrographs (Plate VIc) showed a cyst surface consistent with that of *S. gracilis* and with their own description of this species by LM, SEM, and TEM in a subsequent paper (Stolte et al., 1998). Aside from this confusion as to which species is shown, the above-mentioned papers present cysts of *S. gracilis* with a similar surface structure to the sarcocysts reported by Dahlgren and Gjerde (2009). By LM, sarcocysts of *S. gracilis* were indistinguishable from those of *S. tarandivulpes* in reindeer (Gjerde, 1985a), but SEM micrographs by Dahlgren and Gjerde (2009) and previous TEM studies showed that elaborate arrangement of deep invaginations on the sarcocyst surface between rows of protrusions, which are found on sarcocysts of *S. tarandivulpes* (Gjerde, 1985a), are not present on *S. gracilis* sarcocysts. Gjerde (2012) completed the life cycle by feeding *S. gracilis*-infected roe deer muscle to two *Vulpes* spp., described sporulated oocysts of *S. gracilis* in the intestinal mucosa of its definitive hosts, and found *Sarcocystis* sporocysts in their feces 9 days later. Dubey et al.'s (2015a) review of the literature mentioned *S. gracilis* 12 times and summarized morphological, geographical, and other data (in their Tables 1.3, 14.2, 18.1, 19.1, 23.1, 24.1, 24.3, and 24.4).

SARCOCYSTIS GRUENERI YAKIMOFF AND SOKOLOFF, 1934

Definitive hosts: *Canis lupus familiaris* (syn. *C. familiaris*) L., 1758, Domestic Dog (?); *Nyctereutes procyonoides* (Gray, 1834), Raccoon Dog (see *Remarks*, below); *Vulpes* (syn. *Alopex*) *lagopus* (L., 1758), Arctic or Blue Fox (?); *Vulpes vulpes* (L., 1758), Red or Silver Fox (?).

Intermediate hosts: *Capreolus capreolus* (L., 1758), European Roe Deer; *Cervus elaphus* L., 1758, Red Deer; *Cervus nippon* Temminck, 1838, Sika Deer; *Rangifer tarandus* (L., 1758), Reindeer; *Dama dama* (L., 1758), Fallow Deer.

Geographic distribution: Europe: Norway.

Remarks: The naming of this species is a bit convoluted, but the history is nicely compiled by Gjerde and Bratberg (1984) and Gjerde (1984a). To wit, Yakimoff and Sokoloff (1934) coined this species name for "Sarkozysten" they described in reindeer and maral (*Cervus canadensis asiaticus*), but they used the term not to describe muscle cysts but rather individual organisms (their "spores") within the sarcocysts, and the organisms as a group became synonymous with "Sarcosporidia." Yakimoff and Sokoloff (1934) did not describe the muscle cysts in the reindeer, they only reported the findings of Bergman (1913), Hadwen (1922), and Grüner (1927), and the pictures presented were those of Grüner (1927) according to the careful reading of the original papers by Gjerde and Bratberg (1984). Yakimoff and Sokoloff (1934) did make some smears from a piece of reindeer cardiac muscle and from blood in the heart of the maral. In these smears they found structures (organisms?) they thought were spores of *Sarcocystis*, but the actual identity of these spores is anyone's guess, and the point is that they never observed any sarcocysts. Later, Yakimoff and Gousseff (1936) gave a description of both sarcocysts and their cystozoites obtained from cardiac and skeletal muscles of reindeer and identified them as *S. grüneri*. Gjerde and Bratberg (1984) examined skeletal and cardiac muscle of reindeer from northern Norway by LM and found three different types of sarcocysts in the skeletal muscles: thick-walled macroscopic cysts with a fibrillar layer (type I), thick-walled microscopic cysts (type 2), and thin-walled microscopic cysts (type 3), whereas in the cardiac muscles they found only type 3 sarcocysts. As already mentioned, Gjerde and Bratberg (1984) felt the original description of *S. grueneri* was sadly inadequate, which led them to do cross-infection studies. Different groups of domestic dogs and silver and blue foxes were fed sarcocyst-infected skeletal muscle, cardiac muscle, microisolated macrocysts, or combinations of these infectious materials. All canid species shed sporocysts after a prepatent period of 11–17 days, and the authors believed there were enough similarities in the sporocysts to conclude that "*Sarcocystis* sp. with type 3-cysts in all likelihood is identical with *Sarcocystis grueneri*." Using the description by Yakimoff and Gousseff (1936) and the descriptive and cross-transmission work of Gjerde and Bratberg (1984), it should have been reasonable to conclude that the name *S. grueneri* can safely be assigned to the species in reindeer with thin-walled, type 3 sarcocysts found in cardiac and skeletal muscles. However, later in the same year, Gjerde (1984a) cast some doubt on their previous cross-transmission work (Gjerde and Bratberg, 1984) by stating, "while any of the 3 other species could have caused the shedding of *Sarcocystis* sporocysts by foxes and dogs given skeletal muscle in their experiments. It is also possible that some of the thin-walled cysts in skeletal muscle really were cysts of *S. grueneri* according to the new definition, even though such a mixed infection has not been detected in the present (Gjerde, 1984a) investigation." That is to say, that Gjerde (1984a) wanted to redefine the definition of *S. grueneri* by limiting it to thin-walled sarcocysts in cardiac muscle, while considering the thin-walled sarcocysts in skeletal muscle to be a different, "for the time being, not renamed" species. Gjerde (1984d) gave cardiac muscle from two reindeer, which had been slaughtered at an abattoir in northern Norway, to one raccoon dog. The muscle was infected with sarcocysts of *S. grueneri*, and 10 DPI, the raccoon dog began shedding sporocysts that measured L × W (n = 180): 13.9 × 10.1 (12–16 × 9–11), L/W ratio, 1.4, and the patent period lasted at least 16 days. Levine and Ivens (1981) did not mention this species. Gjerde (1985b) documented the ultrastructure of the sarcocysts of *S. grueneri* from cardiac muscle of reindeer. Levine (1986) listed this as a valid name of a *Sarcocystis* species with the reindeer as the intermediate host and several canids as definitive hosts. Sarcocysts in reindeer muscle are sack-like with rounded ends and measured L × W: 580 × 140 and bradyzoites measured L × W: 13.9–16.5 × 2.4–4.8. When dogs were fed muscles infected with sarcocysts they shed sporocysts that measured L × W: 12–16 × 9–11. Wesemeier and Sedlaczek (1995a,b) found sarcocysts in both the fallow and the red deer that they thought looked like *S. grueneri*. Odening (1998) listed this species in his comprehensive inventory of 189 *Sarcocystis* species and suggested that *S. alceslatrans*, *S. cervicanis*, and *S. wapiti* were probably synonyms of this species. Dubey et al. (2015a) listed this species in their Tables 14.2, 18.1, 24.1, 24.3, and 24.4, which cover most of the information known about *S. grueneri*.

SARCOCYSTIS HJORTI DAHLGREN AND GJERDE, 2010a

Light and scanning electron micrographs of sarcocysts (Figs. 1 and 2) of this species are in Dahlgren and Gjerde (2010a). For LM photomicrographs of sporulated oocysts and sporocysts (Figs. 3C, D), see Dahlgren and Gjerde (2010b).

Definitive type host: *Vulpes vulpes* (L., 1758), Red or Silver Fox (selected as their type host because red foxes are common in Norwegian forests and known to commonly feed on carcasses of deer that have died).

Type locality: Europe: Norway, Hordaland, and Rogaland Counties.

Other definitive host: *Vulpes* (syn. *Alopex*) *lagopus* (L., 1758), Arctic or Blue Fox.

Intermediate type host: *Cervus elaphus* L., 1758, Red Deer.

Other intermediate host: *Alces alces* (L., 1758), Eurasian Elk or Moose.

Geographic distribution: Europe: Norway.

Description of sporulated oocyst: Oocyst shape: ellipsoidal, with one thin wall; L × W: 17.5 × 12.5 (15–20 × 10–15); L/W ratio: 1.4; M, OR, PG: all absent. Distinctive features of oocyst: typical thin-walled *Sarcocystis*-type, which usually breaks down releasing sporocysts into the intestinal lumen (note that Dahlgren and Gjerde, 2010b, did not distinguish between the oocysts of *S. hjorti* vs. those of *S. alces* when they recorded these measurements).

Description of sporocyst and sporozoites: Sporocyst shape: ellipsoidal; L × W: 14–15 × 10; L/W ratio: unknown; SB, SSB, PSB: all absent; SR: present; SR characteristics: spheroidal mass of small granules (Figs. 3C, D in Dahlgren and Gjerde, 2010b); SZ: not described, but more or less banana-shaped (photomicrographs). Distinctive features of sporocyst: none; a "typical" *Sarcocystis*-type SP, lacking SB, SSB, PSB, and with a distinct, granular SR (note that Dahlgren and Gjerde, 2010b, did not distinguish between the sporocysts of *S. hjorti* vs. those of *S. alces* when they recorded these measurements).

Prevalence: Dahlgren and Gjerde (2010a) reported sarcocysts of this species in the diaphragm and/or esophagus muscle of 35/37 (95%) red deer they examined and only 6/37 (16%) had these sarcocysts in cardiac muscle, as best they could tell. Mucosal scrapings showed that all 12 foxes became infected with one of the two *Sarcocystis* species (*S. alces* and *S. hjorti*) in moose muscle, but molecular findings in fecal and mucosal-scraping samples only confirmed that 2/6 (33%) *V. vulpes* and 3/6 (50%) *V. lagopus* had oocysts/sporocysts of *S. hjorti* (Table 2, Dahlgren and Gjerde, 2010b).

Sporulation: Sporulated, infective sporocysts shed in the feces of the definitive host.

Prepatent and patent periods: Prepatent period is ~14 days; the patent period is not known.

Site of infection, definitive host: Oocysts and sporocysts were found in the intestinal mucosa of both fox species.

Site of infection, intermediate host: Sarcocysts of this species were found mostly in the diaphragm and esophagus and to a lesser degree in the heart muscle of infected deer.

Endogenous stages, definitive host: Unknown. Only unsporulated and sporulated oocysts were seen in the intestinal scrapings from *V. vulpes* and *V. lagopus* (Dahlgren and Gjerde, 2010b).

Endogenous stages, intermediate host: Using LM, sarcocysts in the esophagus and diaphragm were slender, spindle-shaped, L × W: ~1.0–3.1 × 0.08–0.2 mm; they had thin, flexible, hair-like protrusions, ~10–12 µm long. Much smaller cysts found in the heart were sack-like, L × W: 0.25–0.35 × 0.1 mm. Under SEM, the sarcocyst surface had numerous flexible, slender, hair-like protrusions, at least, L × W: 10 × 0.4 at the base, and narrowing toward their tips. Protrusions were regularly distributed in rows across the sarcocyst surface with a fairly uniform distance between their bases.

Cross-transmission: None to date.

Pathology: Dahlgren and Gjerde (2010b) reported that 7/12 (58%) foxes in their two experiments had reduced feed intake, soft feces, and/or vomited between 6 and 10 DPI and one fox had diarrhea and vomited on the 13th DPI, but they did not mention (1) which of the two fox species fed infected moose meat experienced these symptoms nor (2) which of the two parasite species, *S. alces* or *S. hjorti*, might be responsible for these symptoms. Later in their paper, they suggested that these symptoms "were most likely associated with the *Hammondia* infection also documented in these hosts because *H. heydorni* infection in dogs have been associated with diarrhoea" (Abel et al., 2006).

Materials deposited: Sarcocysts excised from muscular tissues from red deer and photomicrographs from LM and SEM of the sarcocyst wall are deposited at the National History Museum, Oslo, Norway, collection no. NHMO-Prot 00006. The complete 18S rRNA gene sequence is deposited in GenBank with accession no. GQ250990. This rRNA sequence of *S. hjorti* is identical with that of the unnamed *Sarcocystis* species, type E, from the moose that is deposited in GenBank with accession no. EU282017 (Dahlgren and Gjerde, 2008).

Etymology: The species name is derived from the Scandinavian common word for red deer and also partly comprising the Norwegian word for species of the family Cervidae.

Remarks: When Dahlgren and Gjerde (2010a) first proposed the name *S. hjorti*, their description was based on sarcocysts excised from muscular tissues of red deer, *C. elaphus*, LM and SEM photomicrographs of the sarcocyst wall, and phylogenetic separation from other *Sarcocystis* species on an inferred Bayesian tree, based on 18S rRNA gene sequences. They initially thought that these small sarocysts were similar to those of *S. cervicanis* in the red deer (Hernández-Rodriguez et al., 1981), and *S. wapiti* (Speer and Dubey, 1982), and *S. grueneri* in reindeer (Gjerde, 1986); however, molecular analyses demonstrated that they were dealing with a different species that they named *S. hjorti*. Sarcocysts with similar hair-like protrusions as those seen in *S. hjorti* were earlier reported in red deer and elk; Wesemeier and Sedlaczek (1995a), in Germany, reported such cysts in both free-ranging red deer and in a red deer and an elk that had been born and raised in a zoo, and they (Wesemeier and Sedlaczek, 1995a) called this species *S.* cf.

capreolicanis because it resembled that species described earlier in roe deer (Erber et al., 1978). Kutkienė (2003) also referred a "hairy" cyst she found in red deer in Lithuania, to S. cf. *capreolicanis*. Neither of the previous authors (1995a, 2003) mentioned the work by Dubey et al. (1983), who described a species they named *S. sybillensis* from elk in the United States. Most important, in the paper by Dubey et al. (1983), sarcocysts of *S. sybillensis* were described to have a thick wall, up to 8 wide, noting this feature as a major morphological difference from thin-walled sarcocysts of *S. wapiti*, which also occurred in the elk they examined. But Dahlgren and Gjerde (2010b) went on to argue that in standard histological sections under LM, sarcocysts with hair-like protrusions appear thin walled (like those of *S. hjorti*), a mistake that they contend has been repeated in different papers describing sarcocysts including those for *S. cruzi* (cattle, Mehlhorn et al., 1975b; Dubey et al., 1982), *S. arieticanis* (sheep, Heydorn, 1985), and *S. hircicanis* (goats, Heydorn and Unterholzner, 1983). In addition, sarcocysts with hair-like protrusions were said to be indistinguishable in histological sections from sarcocysts with delicate ribbon-like protrusions such as *S. cervicanis* (red deer), *S. wapiti* (elk), and *S. grueneri* (reindeer) because all would appear thin walled. Subsequent more thorough studies (Gjerde and Bratberg, 1984; Gjerde, 1986) showed that these thin-walled sarcocysts represented two species, *S. grueneri*, with ribbon-like protrusions, and *S. rangi*, with hair-like protrusions. This led Dahlgren and Gjerde (2010b) to contend that the thick-walled cyst described by Dubey et al. (1983, their Fig. 5) is not consistent with a species with hair-like protrusions, but rather with a cyst with finger-like protrusions like those of *S. tarandi* of reindeer and red deer.

Dahlgren and Gjerde (2010b) also suggested that Saito et al. (1995) made a similar interpretation when the latter authors said *Sarcocystis* species in Japanese sika deer resembled *S. sybillensis* of elk because, in histological sections, the sarcocysts from sika deer have a thick wall with hairy protrusions (Fig. 2, Saito et al., 1995), but

reevaluating their data, Dahlgren and Gjerde (2010b) said the species seen by Saito et al. (1995) was indistinguishable from *S. tarandi* in reindeer and red deer and, as a result, they considered *S. sybillensis* in elk (Dubey et al., 1983) to represent *at least* two different species, one with finger-like protrusions, and one with hair-like protrusions. Because of these conflicting interpretations of sarcocyst structure at the LM and SEM levels, Dahlgren and Gjerde (2010b) chose the name *S. hjorti* for species with hair-like protrusions in red deer and moose in Norway and suggested that *S. sybillensis* "be considered a nomen dubium until it has been restricted to only one species with clearly defined sarcocyst morphology and molecular characteristics."

Dahlgren and Gjerde (2010b) later fed muscle sarcocysts from moose to six silver foxes (*V. vulpes*) and six blue foxes (*V. lagopus*). The foxes were euthanized 7–28 DPI, and intestinal scrapings and fecal samples were screened microscopically for *Sarcocystis* oocysts/sporocysts, which were later identified to species, by species-specific primers and sequence analysis of the 18S rRNA gene. Molecular identification showed that the oocysts/sporocysts belonged to two species, *S. alces* and *S. hjorti*, even though sarcocysts in moose muscle were only identified as *S. hjorti* prior to infections of foxes. Dahlgren and Gjerde (2010b) concluded that their study proved both fox species are definitive hosts for both *Sarcocystis* species as had been inferred from phylogenetic position of these forms earlier (2008). This was the first study in which molecular methods verified the results of transmission experiments used to determine the definitive host(s) of cervid *Sarcocystis* species, and they noted an important distinction; the life cycle of some species in cervids has been determined by feeding potential definitive hosts muscles infected with *Sarcocystis* sarcocysts, followed by screening their feces or intestinal mucosa to find oocysts/sporocysts, and then assuming that the sporocysts belong to the single species identified as sarcocysts (rightly or wrongly) in the intermediate host, which may not be the case. Dubey et al. (2015a) mentioned this species four times (Tables 18.1, 23.1, 24.1, and 24.4) and did not discuss it but considered it a valid species.

SARCOCYSTIS LUTRAE GJERDE AND JOSEFSEN, 2015

Intermediate host: *Vulpes* (syn. *Alopex*) *lagopus* (L., 1758), Arctic or Blue Fox.

Remarks: For more complete information on *S. lutrae*, see Genus *Lutra*, below.

SARCOCYSTIS MIESCHERIANA (KÜHN, 1865) LABBÉ, 1899

Definitive host: *Vulpes vulpes* (L., 1758), Red or Silver Fox.

Remarks: For more complete information on *S. miescheriana*, see Genus *Canis*, above.

SARCOCYSTIS ODOCOILEOCANIS CRUM, FAYER, AND PRESTWOOD, 1981

Definitive host: *Vulpes vulpes* (L., 1758), Red or Silver Fox.

Remarks: For more complete information on *S. odocoileocanis*, see Genus *Canis*, above.

SARCOCYSTIS RANGI GJERDE, 1984b

Definitive hosts: *Vulpes* (syn. *Alopex*) *lagopus* (L., 1758), Arctic or Blue Fox; *Vulpes vulpes* (L., 1758), Red or Silver Fox.

Intermediate host: *Rangifer tarandus* (L., 1758), Reindeer.

Geographic distribution: Europe: Norway, Setesdal Vesthei.

Remarks: Gjerde (1985a) reported the first experimental transmission of *S. rangi*, from a reindeer shot in southern Norway, to a fox. Esophagus and the diaphragm were obtained

from the wild reindeer and sarcocysts therein were microisolated from these tissues and classified by Gjerde (1985a) according to their size, shape, and cyst wall structure. Gjerde (1985a) identified the sarcocysts of two species, *S. tarandivulpes* and *S. rangi*. Those of *S. tarandivulpes* were spindle-shaped, L × W: 470–1,000 × 55–220, and had minute knob-like cyst surface protrusions. The sarcocysts of *S. rangi* were slender, L × W: 4,000–10,000 × 75–125, and had fine hair-like surface protrusions. Gjerde (1985a) took *S. rangi* sarcocysts along with small amounts of surrounding tissue and fed them to a blue fox. Sporocysts of *Sarcocystis* were first detected in fox feces on the 11th DPI and the fox was still passing sporocysts when the experiment was terminated 9 days later. These sporocysts measured L × W (n = 55): 14.6 × 10.2 (13–15.5 × 9.5–11), L/W ratio, 1.4. This allowed Gjerde (1985a) to conclude, "that the fox is a suitable definitive host for *S. rangi*." Later the same year Gjerde (1985b) described the ultrastructure of the cysts of *S. rangi* from skeletal muscle of *R. t. tarandus*. Levine (1986) listed this form as one of his 122 valid species. Odening (1998), in his compilation of 189 *Sarcocystis* names, listed this as a valid species and added that it had a TEM type 6/7 sarcocyst wall (originally type 7, Dubey et al., 1989b). He also said *S. rangi* was similar to *S. capreolicanis* and to *Sarcocystis* sp. type II B of Atkinson et al. (1993) from *O. virginianus*. Dubey et al. (2015a) verified that this is a valid *Sarcocystis* species (their Tables 24.1 and 24.4) in cervids, with cigar-shaped sarcocysts, 2,106 × 400, long hair-like villar protrusions up to 12.6 × 0.3–0.6, and bradyzoites that measured 12.4–16.5 × 2.4–4.6 (Table 18.1) and that this is one of the few species that has had molecular markers studied (18S rDNA).

SARCOCYSTIS RILEYI (STILES, 1893) LABBÉ, 1899

Definitive host: *Vulpes vulpes* (L., 1758) Red or Silver Fox.

Remarks: For more complete information on *S. rileyi*, see Genus *Mephitis*, below.

SARCOCYSTIS TARANDIVULPES GJERDE, 1984c

Definitive hosts: *Canis lupus familiaris* (syn. *C. familiaris*) L., 1758, Domestic Dog (?); *Nyctereutes procyonoides* (Gray, 1834), Raccoon Dog; *Vulpes* (syn. *Alopex*) *lagopus* (L., 1758), Arctic or Blue Fox; *Vulpes vulpes* (L., 1758), Red or Silver Fox (?).

Intermediate host: *Rangifer tarandus* (L., 1758), Reindeer.

Geographic distribution: Europe: Norway, Hardangervidda.

Remarks: Gjerde (1984c) obtained skeletal muscle from five wild reindeer and skeletal muscle and a heart from a sixth animal in southern Norway and examined them by LM for sarcocysts. All skeletal muscles were infected with sarcocysts that Gjerde (1984c) initially identified as "*Sarcocystis* sp.;" he also found different sarcocysts that he identified as *S. hardangeri* in skeletal muscles of 2/6 (33%) reindeer, and the single heart he examined, apparently, had only sarcocysts of *S. grueneri*. Gjerde (1984c, Experiment 1) fed four *V. lagopus* only skeletal muscle that he purported to contain only sarcocysts of *S.* sp., and he fed two *V. lagopus* (Experiment 2) skeletal muscle containing sarcocysts of both *S.* sp. and *S. hardangeri*. The four foxes in the first experiment began shedding *Sarcocystis* sporocysts on 10, 11, 12 DPI, and the two foxes in the second experiment shed sporocysts on 10 and 12 DPI. Foxes in both groups continued to shed sporocysts until the experiments ended (25, 23 DPI, respectively), demonstrating a patent period of at least 14–16 days. Sporocysts shed by all six foxes were nearly identical in size.

Having said that, Gjerde's (1984c) reasoning became a bit circular, and he reached a conclusion to rename his "*Sarcocystis* sp." with its new moniker, *S. tarandivulpes*. Gjerde (1984c) reiterated that Gjerde and Bratberg (1984) described two morphotypes of thick walled and one of thin-walled sarcocysts from reindeer, with only the thin-walled cysts in cardiac muscle, "which they assumed belonged to the same species as the thin-walled cysts in skeletal muscle." Gjerde and Bratberg (1984) went on to name the thin-walled cysts in both cardiac and skeletal muscle as *S. grueneri*. But then Gjerde (1984d) added, "when fresh preparations of micro-isolated cysts were examined, the thin-walled cysts could be further differentiated as cysts of 2 different species parasitizing cardiac and skeletal muscle, respectively (Gjerde, 1984a)." *Sarcocystis grueneri* was considered the species having sarcocysts without cyst wall protrusions in cardiac muscle, whereas his "*Sarcocystis* sp." designated the species having sarcocysts with very short, knob-like protrusions in skeletal muscle (Gjerde, 1984d). This led him to conclude, "*Sarcocystis* sp. must have been the main or single contributor to the sporocyst shedding observed in experiment 1, establishing the fox as definitive host for this species. The sporocysts shed by the foxes in experiment 2 in the present investigation, and those passed by silver foxes, blue foxes, and dogs given skeletal muscle of domestic reindeer (by Gjerde and Bratberg, 1984), must therefore also have been, wholly or in part, sporocysts of *Sarcocystis* sp." He therefore proposed *Sarcocystis tarandivulpes* as the replacement name for *Sarcocystis* sp. based on the above reasoning. He did conclude, however, "Much research is needed to further elucidate the life cycle of *S. tarandivulpes* and *S. grueneri*, and to determine the difference between the 2 species in cyst ultrastructure and type of muscle tissue invaded." Amen! Gjerde (1984d) gave skeletal muscle infected with four *Sarcocystis* species to a raccoon dog, and the raccoon dog began shedding sporocysts on 10 DPI and continued to do so for at least 16 more days. These sporocysts measured L × W (n = 180): 14.0 × 10.1 (12–16 × 9–11), L/W ratio, 1.4. Gjerde (1985c) described the ultrastructure of the sarcocysts of *S. tarandivulpes* from skeletal muscles of reindeer. Levine (1986) listed this form as one of his 122 valid species. Odening (1998), in his compilation of 189 *Sarcocystis* names, listed this as a valid species and added that it had a TEM type 25 sarcocyst wall (originally type 17, Dubey et al., 1989b). Dubey et al. (2015a) listed this species in their Tables 18.1, 24.1, and 24.4.

SARCOCYSTIS TENELLA (RAILLIET, 1886a,b) MOULÉ, 1886

Definitive host: *Vulpes vulpes* (L., 1758), Red or Silver Fox.

Remarks: For more complete information on *S. tenella*, see Genus *Canis*, above.

SARCOCYSTIS WETZELI (SUGÁR, 1980) N. COMB.

Synonym: *Isospora wetzeli* Sugár, 1980.

Definitive host: *Vulpes vulpes* (L., 1758), Red or Silver Fox.

Type locality: Eastern Europe: Bulgaria.

Other definitive host: None to date.

Intermediate type host: Unknown.

Other intermediate hosts: Unknown.

Geographic distribution: Eastern Europe: Bulgaria.

Description of sporulated oocyst: Oocyst shape: a typical sarcocystid oocyst wall of variable shape, as a membrane-like structure enclosing both SPs; number of walls, 1; wall characteristics: colorless, thin; L × W: 15–19 × 13–16; L/W ratio: unknown; M, OR, PG: all absent. Distinctive features of oocyst: none, the one-layered wall is so thin and attached to the sporocysts as to be almost invisible.

Description of sporocyst and sporozoites: Sporocyst shape: ellipsoidal; L × W: 13–16 × 6.5–10; L/W ratio: unknown; SB, SSB, PSB: all absent; SR: present; SR characteristics: a large mass of aggregated granules packing one end of SP; SZ: sausage-shaped, L × W: 9–10 × 3–4. Distinctive features of sporocyst: none; a "typical" *Sarcocystis*-type SP, lacking SB, SSB, PSB and with a distinct, granular SR.

Prevalence: Sugár (1980) reported finding oocysts and sporocysts in 2/48 (4%) red foxes in Bulgaria.

Sporulation: Endogenous sporulation; Sugár (1980) said he saw both oocysts and sporocysts in both the small and large intestines.

Prepatent and patent periods: Unknown.

Site of infection, definitive host: Sugár (1980) said that sporulated oocysts were seen in the last third section of the small intestine, and sporocysts were found from there and throughout the large intestine.

Site of infection, intermediate host: Unknown.

Endogenous stages, definitive host: Unknown.

Endogenous stages, intermediate host: Unknown.

Cross-transmission: None to date.

Pathology: Not stated.

Materials deposited: None.

Remarks: Sugár (1980) reported these sporulated oocysts and free sporocysts in the small and large intestines and feces of two foxes at a time when we were just beginning to learn about the complex life cycle of *Isospora/Cryptosporidium/Sarcocystis* species. That is, when ruptured *Sarcocystis* oocysts would release their sporocysts, and when these naked sporocysts were found in the feces, various investigators would name them as new *Cryptosporidium* species. In fact, at the end of his paper he quoted from Pellérdy (1974a) saying, "Evidently Pellérdy was right in his conclusion that 'It is not improbable that this *Cryptosporidium* of the fox corresponds in fact with the sporocysts of some *Isospora* species.'" Levine and Ivens (1981) did not see this publication before they published their treatise on coccidian parasites of carnivores. Levine (1986) did not mention this form. Odening (1998) included *S. wenzeli*, which he named (Odening, 1997), a parasite of galliform birds and dogs and cats, but made no mention of *S. wetzeli*; likewise, Dubey et al. (2015a) also did not make mention of the paper by Sugar nor of this species.

SARCOCYSTIS SPECIES

We included 11 additional accounts of *Sarcocystis* being identified only to genus, either from oocysts/sporocysts in fecal materials or from sarcocysts in the muscles of various *Vulpes* species (see Chapter 19). Certainly there are dozens, likely hundreds, more such reports in the literature worldwide; our sampling is presented to demonstrate how widespread such superficial identifications have been (and continue to be) and how much work is yet to be accomplished.

MEPHITIDAE BONAPARTE, 1845

GENUS *MEPHITIS* É. GEOFFROY SAINT-HILAIRE AND F.G. CUVIER, 1795 (2 SPECIES)

SARCOCYSTIS ERDMANAE ODENING, 1997

Synonym: *Sarcocystis* sp. of Erdman (1978).

Definitive type host: *Canis lupus familiaris* (syn. *C. familiaris*) L., 1758, Domestic Dog.

Intermediate type host: *Mephitis mephitis* (Schreber, 1776), Striped Skunk.

Geographic distribution: North America: USA: Iowa.

Remarks: Ms. Erdman (1978) was a freshman veterinary student at Iowa State University, Ames, Iowa, USA, when she published a one-page paper in which she described finding microscopic sarcocysts up to 300 long, in heart, diaphragm, esophagus, and iliopsoas muscles in each of three *M. mephitis* collected in Green County. She fed all four types of muscle to each of four 8–12-week-old puppies; 10 days later, two of the pups began passing sporocysts that averaged L × W: 12 × 10. No other

information (e.g., photomicrographs of the sarcocysts, oocysts, and/or sporocysts in dog feces) was given. Odening (1997) decided to name Erdman's parasite, *S. erdmanae*, but with the lack of any other descriptive information, it is our opinion it would have been best to keep this form as a *species inquirenda*. Odening (1998) reconfirmed his opinion that *S. erdmanae* was a good species when he included it among the 189 *Sarcocystis* species names he listed but gave no additional information or data. Dubey et al. (2015a) reprinted Erdman's original, but minimal, mensural data (their Table 19.1), and listed Odening's (1997) name as a valid species of *Sarcocystis* (their Tables 24.1 and 24.4). We believe this is a mistake.

SARCOCYSTIS MEPHITISI DUBEY, HAMIR, AND TOPPER, 2002c

For light and electron micrographs of tissue cysts and zoites of this species see Figs. 1–4 in Dubey et al. (2002c).

Definitive type host: Unknown.

Type locality: North America: USA: Oregon, Corvallis area.

Other definitive hosts: Unknown.

Intermediate type host: *Mephitis mephitis* (Schreber, 1776), Striped Skunk.

Other intermediate hosts: Unknown.

Geographic distribution: North America: USA: Oregon, but Dubey et al. (2002b) suggested this species may exist in the remainder of the United States, wherever *M. mephitis* are found.

Description of sporulated oocyst: Unknown.

Description of sporocyst and sporozoites: Unknown.

Prevalence: Dubey et al. (2002c) found sarcocysts of this species in 4/5 (80%) *M. mephitis* they examined from Oregon.

Sporulation: Unknown.

Prepatent and patent periods: Unknown.

Site of infection, definitive host: Unknown.

Site of infection, intermediate host: Sarcocysts were found in tongue, heart, masseter, diaphragm, and esophagus muscles in the four infected skunks examined.

Endogenous stages, definitive host: Unknown.

Endogenous stages, intermediate host: Dubey et al. (2002c) found two types of sarcocysts in skunk muscles, thick-walled cysts (type A), and thin-walled cysts (type B). They proposed the name *S. mephitisi* for the type A sarcocysts. These sarcocysts measured L × W (n = 10): 400 × 120, with a wall that was up to 6 thick. Ultrastructurally, the sarcocyst wall had evenly spaced villar protrusions up to 5 × 1; these were constricted at their base, expanded in the middle, and with blunt tips. The protrusions had numerous microtubules and septa were prominent. Bradyzoites were 11 × 3.2 and contained organelles normally found in *Sarcocystis* bradyzoites; numerous micronemes were scattered in the anterior one-third of the bradyzoite. Electron-dense granules were absent in villar microtubules of this species.

Cross-transmission: None to date.

Pathology: Unknown.

Materials deposited: Sections in muscles of skunks are deposited in the USNPC, No. 91628.

Etymology: This species is named after the genus and species of the host.

Remarks: Dubey et al. (2002c) argued that, among all the available taxonomic criteria, the structure of villar protrusions (Vp) on the sarcocyst wall is the most reliable and that the data accumulated over the years now allows the Vp structures on sarcocysts to be divided into 36 different types. Based on their reasoning that the Vp structure on the sarcocyst wall of this form was distinctly different from all 36 types of sarcocyst walls reported previously (Dubey et al., 1989b; Dubey and Odening, 2001) and that they were justified in naming this form as a new species, Dubey et al. (2015a) listed this species four times (their Tables 1.2, 19.1, 24.1 and 24.4).

SARCOCYSTIS RILEYI (STILES, 1893) LABBÉ, 1899

Synonyms: *Balbiania riley* Stiles, 1893; *Sarcocystis rileyi* (Stiles, 1893) Minchin, 1903; *Sarcocystis anatina* Krause and Goranoff, 1933.

Definitive hosts: *Mephitis mephitis* (Schreber, 1776), Striped Skunk; *Didelphis virginiana* Kerr, 1792, Virginia Opossum (?); *Nyctereutes procyonoides* (Gray, 1834), Raccoon Dog; *Vulpes vulpes* (L., 1758) Red or Silver Fox.

Intermediate hosts: *Anas acuta* L., 1758 (syn. *Dafila acuta*), American or Northern Pintail; *Anas americana* Gmelin, 1789 (syn. *Mareca americana*), American Wigeon; *Anas carolinensis* Gmelin, 1789, Green-winged Teal; *Anas clypeata* L., 1758 (syn. *Spatula clypeata*), Northern Shoveler; *Anas crecca* Gmelin, 1789, Green-winged Teal; *Anas discors* (L., 1766) (syn. *Querquedula discors*), Blue-winged Teal; *Anas fulvigula* Ridgway, 1874, Mottled Duck; *Anas platyrhynchos* L., 1758, Domestic Duck, Wild Mallard; *Anas rubripes* (Brewster, 1910), American Black Duck; *Aix sponsa* (L., 1758), Wood Duck; *Anas strepera* L., 1758, Gadwall; *Aythya affinis* (Eyton, 1838), Lesser Scaup; *Aythya americana* (Eyton, 1838), Redhead; *Aythya marila* (L., 1761), Greater Scaup; *Aythya valisineria* (Wilson, 1814), Canvasback; *Bucephala albeola* (L., 1758) (syn. *Anas albeda* L., 1758), Bufflehead; *Melanitta deglandi* (Bonaparte, 1850), White-winged Scooter.

Geographic distribution: Central America: Panamá; Europe: England, Finland, Lithuania, Norway, Sweden; North America: USA: Louisiana; Mexico. Probably found worldwide, wherever wild ducks are found.

Remarks: Wicht (1981) and Cawthorn and Rainnie (1981) published back-to-back papers in the *Journal of Wildlife Diseases* showing that the striped skunk can act as the definitive host for *S. rileyi* of ducks. Levine and Ivens (1981) briefly summarized the work of Golubkov (1979), mentioned above under *S. horvathi* (from chickens), where he infected dogs and cats with both *S. rileyi* and *S. horvathi*, but did not make it clear whether both *Sarcocystis* species produced infections in dogs *and* cats. Levine and Ivens (1981) concluded by saying, "It would certainly be unusual if both the dog and cat were definitive hosts of the same species," although we now know that some animals can act both as intermediate and definitive host for some *Sarcocystis* species (Dubey et al., 2002c). Later, Levine (1986) listed *S. rileyi* as one of his 122 valid species but made no mention of Golubkov's (1979) work and listed the skunk and the opossum as definitive hosts. Odening (1998), in his compilation of 189 *Sarcocystis* names, listed this as a valid species and added that it had a TEM type 23 sporocyst wall. Dubey et al. (2015a) discussed the confusion caused by Golubkova's (1979) paper and listed several relevant survey papers (Cornwell, 1963; Chabreck, 1965; Dubey et al., 2003a; Kutkienė et al., 2011) as well as what we now know about genetic diversity and some molecular characteristics of *S. rileyi* (Dubey et al., 2010c; Gjerde, 2014a; Prakas et al., 2014). Prakas et al. (2015) found sporocysts of *Sarcocystis* in the feces of 4/23 (17%) and in the mucosal scrapings of 4/20 (20%) red foxes and in small intestinal mucosal scrapings of 7/13 (54%) raccoon dogs hunted in Lithuania. Sporocysts from red foxes measured L × W (n = 16): 12.9 × 8.1, L/W ratio: 1.6, whereas those from raccoon dogs were L × W (n = 54): 12.1 × 8.1, L/W ratio: 1.5. Using species-specific PCR and subsequent sequencing, the ITS-1 region partial sequences of oocyst/sporocyst from small intestine mucosal scrapings from six raccoon dogs and three red foxes, both were identified to belong to *S. rileyi*. This is good evidence, but controlled cross-transmission experiments are needed for ultimate confirmation.

GENUS *SPILOGALE* GRAY, 1865 (4 SPECIES)

SARCOCYSTIS SPECIES

There is at least one report of *Sarcocystis* sporocysts found in the feces of *Spilogale putorius* in Arkansas, USA, but no identification to species was made (see Chapter 19).

MUSTELIDAE FISCHER, 1817

SUBFAMILY LUTRINAE BONAPARTE, 1838

GENUS *ENHYDRA* FLEMMING, 1822 (MONOTYPIC)

SARCOCYSTIS NEURONA DUBEY, DAVIS, SPEER, BOWMAN, DE LAHUNTA, GRANSTROM, TOPPER, HAMIR, CUMMINGS, AND SUTER, 1991b

Definitive hosts: *Didelphis virginiana* Kerr, 1792, Virginia Opossum; *Didelphis albiventris* Lund, 1840, White-eared Opossum; *Didelphis marsupialis* L., 1758, Common Opossum.

Intermediate host: *Enhydra lutris* (L., 1758), Sea Otter.

Geographic distribution: North America: Canada, USA.

Remarks: Rosonke et al. (1999) first reported *S. neurona* in histologic sections of brain of a captive sea otter housed in a public aquarium in Oregon, USA. Lindsay et al. (2000a, 2001a) and Miller et al. (2001a) isolated *S. neurona* in cell cultures inoculated with neural tissue of two encephalitic free-ranging sea otters from California, USA. Dubey et al. (2001c) found sarcocysts from two naturally infected sea otters that they characterized biologically, ultrastructurally, and genetically as *S. neurona*. Thomas et al. (2007) examined California and Washington state sea otters from 1985 to 2004 and found 39/344 (11%) had histopathological evidence of significant protozoal meningoencephalitis. Using morphology and immunohistochemical labeling they identified the aetiological agents of infection to be *S. neurona* (n = 22), *T. gondii* (n = 5), or dual infection with both organisms (n = 12), and active *S. neurona* was present in all dual infections. In *S. neurona* meningoencephalitis, multifocal to diffuse gliosis was widespread in gray matter, and consistently present in the molecular layer of the cerebellum. The disease was diagnosed more frequently in the then (2007) expanding population of Washington sea otters (10/31, 32%) than in the declining California population (29/313, 9%). Those sea otters that had displayed neurological signs prior to death had active *S. neurona* encephalitis supporting Thomas et al.'s (2007) conclusion that *S. neurona* is the most significant protozoan pathogen in sea otter central nervous systems. Miller et al. (2009) published a case report on three *E. l. nereis* that were diagnosed with putative meningoencephalitis in 2004. Histologically, they found meronts, free merozoites, and tissue cysts in the brain of all three otters. Immature tissue cysts from the brain of one otter were examined by TEM and the structural features found were compatible with prior descriptions of *S. neurona* tissue cysts. DNA amplification using panspecific 18S rDNA primers and additional sequencing at the ITS-1 locus confirmed that all three otters were infected with *S. neurona*; no other *Sarcocystis* species were detected in the brains or in the skeletal muscles of these three animals by IHC or PCR. Barbosa et al. (2015) sampled 227 marine mammals,

most with clinical or pathological evidence of potential disease and, using a nested PCR assay, tested them for the presence of coccidian parasites. They found an overall prevalence of infection for *S. neurona* in 136/227 (60%) animals, including 4/6 (67%) northern sea otters. This parasite is an important cause of protozoal encephalitis among marine mammals in the northeastern Pacific Ocean, and their work identified a unique, new molecular signature (Ag type XIII MS type hh) to help identify *S. neurona* isolates responsible for fatal infections in marine mammals. All but one individual with single genotype XIII infections, and all with coinfections (with *T. gondii*) that included type XIII had marked to severe protozoal encephalitis, and all died of protozoal disease, demonstrating that this genotype is highly pathogenic and an important cause of mortality in marine mammals. Barbosa et al. (2015) pointed out that in recent decades, small mammals such as the Virginia opossum have been observed to shift their geographic ranges northward, both due to global warming of surface temperatures and the likely increased availability of food sources from human population expansions. They warned that as the range of the opossum expands, new *S. neurona* genotypes, such as type XIII, may emerge to cause infection in susceptible host species not previously exposed to these pathogens such as marine mammals. So, we have been warned! For more complete information on *S. neurona*, see Genus *Procyon*, below for the natural intermediate host, *P. lotor*.

SARCOCYSTIS SPECIES

There is at least one report of mature sarcocysts of *Sarcocystis* being found in the skeletal muscles and tongue of *E. lutris* in Washington, USA, but these were not *S. neurona* and no identification to species was made (see Chapter 19).

GENUS *LUTRA* BRISSON, 1762 (3 SPECIES)

SARCOCYSTIS LUTRAE GJERDE AND JOSEFSEN, 2015

Definitive type host: Unknown.

Type locality: Europe: Norway.

Intermediate type host: *Lutra lutra* (L., 1758), European Otter.

Other intermediate host: *Vulpes* (syn. *Alopex*) *lagopus* (L., 1758), Arctic or Blue Fox.

Geographic distribution: Europe: Norway: Nordland and Troms Counties (*L. lutra*) and Sør-Trøndelag County (*V. lagopus*).

Description of sporulated oocyst: Unknown.

Description of sporocyst and sporozoites: Unknown.

Prevalence: Gjerde and Josefsen (2015) detected sarcocysts in 2/2 (100%) adult male otters from Norway, following their postmortem examinations in 1999 and 2000.

Sporulation: Unknown.

Prepatent and patent periods: Unknown.

Site of infection, definitive host: Unknown.

Site of infection, intermediate host: Skeletal muscle only, no sarcocysts in cardiac muscle.

Endogenous stages, definitive host: Unknown.

Endogenous stages, intermediate host: Sarcocysts were slender, spindle-shaped, L × W: 970 × 35–70, with a sarcocyst wall only ~0.5 thick and smooth with no visible projections.

Cross-transmission: None to date.

Pathology: Apparently none.

Materials deposited: Nucleotide sequences of the complete 18S rRNA gene (KM657769, KM657770), the partial 28S rRNA gene (KM657771, KM657772), the complete ITS-1 region (KM657773, KM657805), and the partial *cox1* (KM657808, KM657809) of *S. lutrae* are deposited in GenBank. Two partial *cox1* sequences obtained from an arctic fox in a previous study (Gjerde and Schulze, 2014), and originally deposited in GenBank (KF601326,

KF601327) under the species name *S. arctica*, now have been assigned to *S. lutrae* by Gjerde and Josefsen (2015). Histological sections of sarcocysts and DNA samples are deposited in the Department of Food Safety and Infection Biology, the Norwegian University of Life Sciences, Oslo, Norway.

Etymology: The name is derived from the Latin name of the type intermediate host, *L. lutra*.

Remarks: Gjerde and Josefsen (2015) took portions of unfixed diaphragm of both otters collected at their autopsies (1999, 2000) and froze them; they resumed their study about 14 years later in 2013. The thawed diaphragms were examined for sarcocysts, but none could be found so they extracted genomic DNA in small pieces of diaphragm from both otters, and the samples were found to contain DNA belonging to the Sarcocystidae. They used that DNA selectively for PCR amplification and sequencing of nuclear 18S and 28S ribosomal (r) RNA genes, and the ITS-1 region, as well as the mitochondrial cytochrome b (*cytb*) and cytochrome c oxidase subunit 1 (*cox1*) genes. Their sequence comparisons showed that both otters were infected by the same *Sarcocystis* species and with no genetic variation (100% identity) among sequenced isolates at the 18S and 28S rRNA genes (6 identical isolates at both loci) or at *cox1* (13 identical isolates).

Their PCR products comprising the ITS-1 region were cloned before sequencing because of intraspecific sequence variation. They sequenced 33 clones, and these sequences were most similar (93.7%–96.0%) to a sequence of *Sarcocystis kalvikus* from the wolverine in Canada, but their phylogenetic analyses placed all of them as a monophyletic sister group to *S. kalvikus*. Because they believed these differences represented a novel species, they named it *S. lutrae*. Sequence comparisons and phylogenetic analyses based on sequences of the 18S and 28S rRNA genes and *cox1*, for which little or no sequence data were available for

S. kalvikus, suggested to them that *S. lutrae* was most closely related to various *Sarcocystis* species using birds and/or carnivores as intermediate hosts. The *cox1* sequences of *S. lutrae* from the otters were identical to two sequences of a *Sarcocystis* species from an arctic fox, i.e., *S. arctica*, with high identity (99.4%) at this gene, and complete identity with *S. arctica* at three other loci. Additional PCR amplifications and sequencing of *cox1* (10 sequences) and the ITS-1 region (four sequences) using four DNA samples from this fox as templates, generated exclusively *cox1* sequences of *S. lutrae* but ITS-1 sequences of *S. arctica*; Gjerde and Josefsen (2015) believed this confirmed that the arctic fox was an intermediate host for both *S. arctica* and *S. lutrae*.

Gjerde and Josefsen (2015) also said that the sarcocysts of *S. lutrae* were morphologically similar to those of an unnamed *Sarcocystis* species in a Japanese marten (Kubo et al., 2009) and to those of the unnamed *Sarcocystis* species found in sea otters by Dubey et al. (2001c, 2003a). Gjerde and Josefsen (2015) also thought *S. lutrae* might be identical to the unnamed *Sarcocystis* species described by Wahlström et al. (1999) because the otter in the 1999 study originated from the same area of Norway as the infected otters in their 2015 study and had apparently become infected in that area, because no sarcocysts were found in 69 other otters they examined that originated from Sweden. They concluded that all other otters with muscular sarcocysts may have interacted with the same definitive host species within a limited geographical area.

SARCOCYSTIS SPECIES

There is at least one report of mature sarcocysts of a *Sarcocystis* being found in the skeletal muscles *L. lutra* in Norway, but no identification to species was made (see Chapter 19).

SUBFAMILY MUSTELINAE FISCHER, 1817

GENUS *GULO* PALLAS, 1780 (MONOTYPIC)

SARCOCYSTIS KALVIKUS DUBEY, REICHARD, TORRETTI, GARVON, SUNDAR, AND GRIGG, 2010b

For light and electron micrographs of tissue cysts and zoites of *S. kalvikus* see Figs. 1 and 2 in Dubey et al. (2010b).

Definitive type host: Unknown.

Type locality: North America: Canada: Nunavut, Kitikmeot Region, 67.41667°N, 115.0667°W.

Intermediate type host: *Gulo gulo* (L., 1758), Wolverine (No. 7, adult female).

Other intermediate hosts: Unknown.

Geographic distribution: North America: Canada.

Description of sporulated oocyst: Unknown.

Description of sporocyst and sporozoites: Unknown.

Prevalence: Dubey et al. (2010b) said sarcocysts of this species were found in 14/41 (34%) wolverine tongues, whereas 12/34 (29%) had this species and *S. kitikmeotensis*, and 33/41 (80%) of all tongues examined had sarcocysts representing *Sarcocystis* species.

Sporulation: Unknown.

Prepatent and patent periods: Unknown.

Site of infection, definitive host: Unknown.

Site of infection, intermediate host: Tongue muscle.

Endogenous stages, definitive host: Unknown.

Endogenous stages, intermediate host: Dubey et al. (2010b) found and described two structurally distinct types of sarcocysts. Their type A sarcocysts were L × W: 900 × 100 and had a thin wall, <1 thick. Ultrastructurally, the Pvm was wavy in outline and had minute undulations or blebs that had no stalk, lacked villar protrusions, and did not invaginate into the granular layer. Mature sarcocysts contained fully formed bradyzoites that were slender, ~5 × 1. Groups of bradyzoites were separated by septa.

Cross-transmission: None to date.

Pathology: Unknown.

Materials deposited: Histological sections stained with H&E from wolverine No. 7 (syntype specimen) in the USNPC, No. 102435 and voucher specimens of H&E sections from wolverine Nos. 2, 4, 5, 6, 8, 12, 20, 24, 25, 27, 32, 38, 39, 40 also deposited in the USNPC as Nos. 102437–102449.

Etymology: The species epitaph is for the host species, i.e., Kalvik, local language, Inuinnaqtun name for wolverine.

Remarks: The wolverine is the largest member of the Mustelinae, and is considered a top predator in circumpolar regions throughout North America and Eurasia. This is the first paper documenting a *Sarcocystis* species in the wolverine but as an intermediate host rather than as a definitive host. Dubey et al. (2010b) said that these sarcocysts were distinct from known species of *Sarcocystis* and possessed a novel 18S and ITS-1 sequence, sharing 98% and 78% sequence similarity with *S. canis*. Dubey et al. (2015a) listed this as a valid species (Tables 24.1 and 24.4).

SARCOCYSTIS KITIKMEOTENSIS DUBEY, REICHARD, TORRETTI, GARVON, SUNDAR, AND GRIGG, 2010b

For electron micrographs of tissue sarcocyst wall of *Sarcocystis kitikmeotensis* see Fig. 3 in Dubey et al. (2010b).

Definitive type host: Unknown.

Type locality: North America: Canada: Nunavut, Kitikmeot Region, 67.3333°N, 11.03333°W.

Intermediate type host: *Gulo gulo* (L., 1758), Wolverine (No. 19, adult male).

Other intermediate hosts: Unknown.

Geographic distribution: North America: Canada.

Description of sporulated oocyst: Unknown.

Description of sporocyst and sporozoites: Unknown.

Prevalence: Dubey et al. (2010b) said sarcocysts of this species were found in 7/41 (17%) wolverine tongues, whereas 12/34 (29%) of them had this species and *S. kalvikus* sarcocysts, and 33/41 (80%) of all tongues examined had sarcocysts representing *Sarcocystis* species.

Sporulation: Unknown.

Prepatent and patent periods: Unknown.

Site of infection, definitive host: Unknown.

Site of infection, intermediate host: Tongue muscle.

Endogenous stages, definitive host: Unknown.

Endogenous stages, intermediate host: Dubey et al. (2010b) found and described two structurally distinct types of sarcocysts. Their type B sarcocysts were L × W: 1,100 × 120, with a relatively thick wall, <2 thick. Ultrastructurally, the outer layer of the sarcocyst Pvm's wavy outline was "thrown in to straight to sloping up to 1 μm-long villar protrusions." The interior of the Pvm was lined by a 40 nm-thick electron-dense layer that thinned out at irregular distances. Mature sarcocysts containing fully formed bradyzoites were larger than those of *S. kalvikus* and measured L × W: 9–13 × 2–3. Groups of bradyzoites were separated by septa.

Cross-transmission: None to date.

Pathology: Unknown.

Materials deposited: Histological sections stained with H&E from wolverine No. 19 (syntype specimen) are in the USNPC as No. 102436 and voucher specimens of H&E-stained sections from wolverine Nos. 5, 14, 21, 31, 34, and 41 are deposited in the USNPC as Nos. 102450–102455. Additional vouchers of both this species and of *S. kalvikus* from wolverine Nos. 8, 15, 16, 17, 22, 23, 28, 30, 33, 35, 36, and 39 are also deposited as USNPC Nos. 102456–102467.

Etymology: The species epitaph is for the host geographic area, i.e., Kitikmeot, the westernmost region of Nunavut.

Remarks: Morphologically, sarcocysts from wolverines were distinct from known species of *Sarcocystis* in all other hosts. Dubey et al. (2010b) stated they were not aware of any previous reports of sarcocysts in wolverines, and neither are we. The sarcocyst wall of *S. kitikmeotensis* was distinctly different from those of other species of *Sarcocystis*, a fact further supported, according to the authors, by the unique ITS-1 sequence that had no homology with any published GenBank sequence. It did, however, share significant sequence identity in the 18S rDNA locus with numerous *Sarcocystis* species confirming that this parasite belongs in the Sarcocystidae. Dubey et al. (2010b) also emphasize that the 80% prevalence of sarcocysts in the wolverines examined indicates that this host is a true host of these parasites, even though carnivores are generally the definitive hosts for *Sarcocystis* species. Dubey et al. (2015a) listed this as a valid species (Tables 24.1 and 24.4) and provided additional information in other tables (Tables 1.2, 19.1, 23.1, and 23.2, 24.1, 24.4.), for those interested readers.

GENUS MARTES PINEL, 1792 (8 SPECIES)

SARCOCYSTIS NEURONA DUBEY, DAVIS, SPEER, BOWMAN, DE LAHUNTA, GRANSTROM, TOPPER, HAMIR, CUMMINGS, AND SUTER, 1991b

Definitive hosts: *Didelphis virginiana* Kerr, 1792, Virginia Opossum; *Didelphis albiventris* Lund, 1840, White-eared Opossum; *Didelphis marsupialis* L., 1758, Common Opossum.

Intermediate host: *Martes pennanti* (Erxleben, 1777), Fisher.

Geographic distribution: North America: Canada; USA.

Remarks: Gerhold et al. (2005) found a free-ranging, juvenile fisher with ataxia, lethargy, stupor, and intermittent whole-body tremors and found meningoencephalitis caused by *S. neurona*. Sarcocysts found in the skeletal muscles were negative for *S. neurona* by PCR but were morphologically similar to previous LM and TEM descriptions of *S. neurona* sarcocysts. For more complete information on *S. neurona*, see Genus *Procyon*, below, for the natural intermediate host, *P. lotor*.

SARCOCYSTIS SPECIES

There are at least four reports of *Sarcocystis* sarcocysts in muscles or sporocysts in the feces of *Martes* spp., but these were not *S. neurona*, and no specific identification was made (see Chapter 19).

GENUS MELES BRISSON, 1762 (3 SPECIES)

SARCOCYSTIS HOFMANNI ODENING, STOLTE, WALTER, AND BOCKHARDT, 1994b

For light and electron micrographs of tissue cysts and zoites of this species see Figs. 1–3 in Odening et al. (1994b).

Synonyms: *Sarcocystis* sp. "type Rh 1" of Bergmann and Kinder, 1976; *Sarcocystis* sp. "thick-walled cyst" of Schramlová and Blažek, 1978; *Sarcocystis* sp. of Erber et al., 1978; *Sarcocystis* sp. "type 1, 2, 3" of Entzeroth, 1982a; *Sarcocystis gracilis* in Entzeroth (1985) and Dubey et al. (1989b), *nec* Rátz, 1909.

Definitive type host: Unknown.

Type locality: Europe: Germany, ~70 km NNW of Berlin, near Fürstenberg.

Intermediate type host: *Meles meles* (L., 1758), European Badger.

Other intermediate host: *Procyon lotor* (L., 1758), Raccoon (?).

Geographic distribution: Asia: Japan (?); Europe: Germany.

Description of sporulated oocyst: Unknown.

Description of sporocyst and sporozoites: Unknown.

Prevalence: Odening et al. (1994b) said sarcocysts of this species were found in 1/9 (11%) badgers (No. 2, female) that were found as road kills between September 1992 and September 1993.

Sporulation: Unknown.

Prepatent and patent periods: Unknown.

Site of infection, definitive host: Unknown.

Site of infection, intermediate host: Heart muscle.

Endogenous stages, definitive host: Unknown.

Endogenous stages, intermediate host: Sarcocysts were 0.8–1.2 mm long when fresh and 78 μm wide in formalin-fixed histological sections. Bradyzoites in semithin sections under the LM were L × W: 9.3 × 2.3 (8–10 × 2–4); under TEM they were L × W: 9–12 × 2–4. The cyst wall was 0.7–0.9 wide; its surface had palisade- or finger-like protrusions and their diameter was 1.1–1.4 at their base and their length was 6.3–6.6. The distance between protrusions at their base was 0.2–0.3. The core of the protrusions was a granular substance streaked with numerous filaments. Protrusions arose from the sarcocyst wall surface and were rhombic to triangular in cross section.

Cross-transmission: None to date.

Pathology: Unknown.

Materials deposited: Holotype (Fig. 2, in Odening et al., 1994b) is part of a sarcocyst embedded in Epon and is stored in the Collection of Protozoa, Institute for Zoo Biology and Wildlife Research, Alfred-Kowalke-Str. 17, D-10315 Berlin, Germany, No. B 2/1993.

Etymology: The name was "a dedication to Professor Dr. Reinhold R. Hofmann, to whom wildlife biology is greatly indebted for his research work, namely in roe deer and European badger."

Remarks: Odening et al. (1994b) regarded the European badger as a "devious" intermediate host of a *Sarcocystis* species of the roe deer. They decided to name it as new because they said it had no valid name as a parasite of roe deer. According to these authors (Odening et al., 1994b), Rátz (1909) described a *Sarcocystis* species from roe deer as *S. gracilis*, but this name is connected with a complicated history, which follows. Babudieri (1932) (apparently) erroneously said the red deer (*Cervus elaphus*) was host to this species. As an outcome of this mistake, Matschoulsky (1947a,b) and Levchenko (1963) described new *Sarcocystis* species from roe deer (*Capreolus capreolus*) in Central Siberia (*S. sibirica*) and Kirghizia (*S. capreoli*), respectively, because they believed there were no *Sarcocystis* species yet described from *Capreolus*. The usage of the incorrect host name for *S. gracilis* was repeated by Kalyakin and Zasukhin (1975) and Levine and Tadros (1980) but was later corrected by Levine (1986, 1988).

Earlier, however, Erber et al. (1978) listed three species of *Sarcocystis* in roe deer in Europe that could be distinguished by LM alone; these were *S. gracilis*, *S. capreolicanis*, and a third species as just *Sarcocystsis* sp. because they could not determine the definitive host. Odening et al. (1994b) believed that the *S.* sp. of Erber et al. (1978) was morphologically indistinguishable from *S. hofmanni*, which is why they decided to give this "open nomenclature" for its name. Sedlaczek and Wesemeier (1995) examined sarcocysts from roe deer by both LM and TEM. They found the same three types of cysts as did Erber et al. (1978) and described the species with finger-like protrusions in good detail; Sedlaczek and Wesemeier (1995) referred to this species as *S.* cf. *hofmanni* because they thought the cysts resembled those of *S. hofmanni* from the European badger as described by Odening et al. (1994b). Odening (1998) also listed this form as one of the 189 *Sarcocystis* species in his review and pointed out how similar its descriptive features are to those of *S. tarandi, S. odoi, S. hemione,* and to the *Sarcocystis* type III of

Atkinson et al. (1993). Kutkienė (2001) also continued down this misleading path. When inserted between a genus and specific epitaph, "cf" (L., bring together or to confer) simply indicates that the sarcocysts seen in roe deer by Sedlaczek and Wesemeier (1995), and the others, *might be* the same species as *S. hofmanni* from European badgers because of their morphological similarity, but it does not *prove* that they are the same parasite. This becomes a dangerous assumption, for example, because in a later paper, Stolte et al. (1996a) actually confused *S. hofmanni* with cysts that had similar finger-like protrusions found in roe deer, and Stolte et al. (1996b) suggested its occurrence in the raccoon as well as in the badger. And Odening (1998), in a review of known *Sarcocystis* species in various hosts, listed *S. hofmanni* as a parasite of badgers and cervids, ignoring that several similar-looking species already had been named from various cervid hosts when the name *S. hofmanni* was proposed. Thus, the name gets embedded in the literature as a true parasite of the roe deer by default but not by real data. After spelling out this argument in much more historic detail than we have, Gjerde (2012) felt the name *S. hofmanni* should be restricted to the species described from the badger, unless and until it can be proven that the same species also occurs in unrelated intermediate hosts such as the roe deer. We concur with his view. Dubey et al. (2015a) listed this as a valid species and with additional information (their Tables 19.1, 24.1, and 24.4).

SARCOCYSTIS MELIS ODENING, STOLTE, WALTER, AND BOCKHARDT, 1994b

For light and electron micrographs of tissue cysts and zoites of this species see Figs. 6–9 in Odening et al. (1994b).

Synonym: *Sarcocystis* cf. *sebeki* of Odening et al. (1994b).

Definitive type host: Unknown.

Type locality: Europe: Germany, Berlin (Grunewald).

Intermediate type host: *Meles meles* (L., 1758), European Badger.

Other intermediate hosts: *Mustela nivalis* L., 1766, Least Weasel (?); *Procyon lotor* (L., 1758), Raccoon (?).

Geographic distribution: Europe: Germany.

Description of sporulated oocyst: Unknown.

Description of sporocyst and sporozoites: Unknown.

Prevalence: Odening et al. (1994b) said sarcocysts of this species were found in 1/9 (11%) badgers (No. 4, female) that were found as road kills between September 1992 and September 1993.

Sporulation: Unknown.

Prepatent and patent periods: Unknown.

Site of infection, definitive host: Unknown.

Site of infection, intermediate host: Muscles of the loin.

Endogenous stages, definitive host: Unknown.

Endogenous stages, intermediate host: Sarcocysts 2–5 mm long in fresh preparations and 51–71 μm wide in histological section. Sarcocyst compartments were polyhedral with a maximum 7 sides, 9.6 wide, and 11.6 deep (9.3–11.0 7.1–13.8). Bradyzoites were fusiform, 7.4 × 1.4 (6.9–8.2 × 0.8–1.7), and the sarcocyst wall was 0.4–0.6 wide, with small "elevations" and "fossule-like" invaginations of the primary cyst wall. Filiform protrusions arose from the surface in irregular, mostly greater (?), distances and were streaked with several parallel, longitudinally running fibrillar elements, which partially proceeded into the ground substance of the cyst wall (Odening et al., 1994b).

Cross-transmission: None to date.

Pathology: Unknown.

Materials deposited: Holotype (see Fig. 8, Odening et al., 1994b) is part of a sarcocyst embedded in Epon and is stored in the Collection of Protozoa, Institute for Zoo Biology and Wildlife Research, Alfred-Kowalke-Str. 17, D-10315 Berlin, Germany, No. B 3/1993.

Etymology: Genitive singular of *Meles* (L., for badger).

Remarks: Odening et al. (1994b) named this form as new because the sarcocyst wall "has an ultrastructure hitherto not described (cf. Dubey et al., 1989b)." Odening (1998) in his compilation of *Sarcocystis* named species, listed this as a valid species and noted that the sarcocyst was a TEM type 1 (cf. Dubey et al., 1989b) and may be identical with *S.* cf. *sebeki* of Odening et al. (1994b). In the same paper, Odening (1998) offered a contradiction and listed *S. sebeki* (Tadros and Laarman, 1976) Levine, 1978 as a valid *Sarcocystis* species. Dubey et al. (2015a) classified the sarcocyst as a TEM type 1f, and listed this as a valid species of *Sarcocystis*. In addition, Dubey et al. (2015a) listed *S. sebeki* as a valid species but of the tawny owl (*Strix aluco* L., 1758) as the possible definitive host (Table 19.1).

SARCOCYSTIS SPECIES

There are at least three reports of *Sarcocystis* sarcocysts in muscles of *Meles* spp.; these were not *S. neurona*, but no specific identifications were made (see Chapter 19).

GENUS MELLIVORA STORR, 1780 (MONOTYPIC)

SARCOCYSTIS SPECIES

There is at least one report of *Sarcocystis* sarcocysts in the muscles of *Mellivora capensis*, but no specific identification was made (see Chapter 19).

GENUS MELOGALE I. GEOFFROY SAINT-HILAIRE, 1831 (4 SPECIES)

SARCOCYSTIS SPECIES

There is at least one report of *Sarcocystis* sarcocysts in the muscles of *Melogale moschata*, but no specific identification was made (see Chapter 19).

GENUS MUSTELA L., 1758 (17 SPECIES)

SARCOCYSTIS CITELLIVULPES PAK, PERMINOVA, AND ESHTOKINA, 1979

Definitive host: *Mustela eversmanii* Lesson, 1827, Steppe Polecat.
Remarks: For more complete information on *S. citellivulpes*, see Genus *Vulpes*, above.

SARCOCYSTIS EVERSMANNI PAK, SKLYAROVA, AND DYMKOVA, 1991

Definitive type host: Unknown.
Intermediate type host: *Mustela eversmanni* Lesson, 1827, Steppe Polecat.
Geographic distribution: Asia: Kazakhstan (former USSR).
Remarks: Odening (1998) decided to consider as a valid named species this *Sarcocystis* named by Pak et al. (1991), even though the only information known from that publication is a brief description of the bradyzoites said to measure 7.0–8.4 × 2.8–3.0. We believe it might be best to keep this form as a *species inquirenda*; however, Dubey et al. (2015a) repeated the minimal mensural data from Pak et al. (1991) (their Table 19.1) and listed this form as a valid species of *Sarcocystis* (Tables 24.1 and 24.4).

SARCOCYSTIS MELIS ODENING, STOLTE, WALTER, BOCKHARDT, 1994b

Intermediate host: *Mustela nivalis* L., 1766, Least Weasel.
Remarks: For more complete information on *S. melis*, see Genus *Meles*, above.

SARCOCYSTIS PUTORII (RAILLIET AND LUCET, 1891) TADROS AND LAARMAN, 1978a

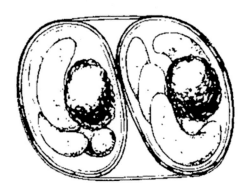

FIGURE 15.2   Line drawing of the sporulated oocyst of *Sarcocystis putorii*. *(Fig. 58) from Levine, N.D., Ivens, V., 1981. The Coccidian Parasites (Protozoa, Apicomplexa) of Carnivores. Illinois Biological Monograph No. 51. University of Illinois Press, Urbana, Illinois, USA. 249 p. The University of Illinois Press, Urbana, Illinois USA, has released the copyright.*

Synonyms: *Endorimospora putorii* (Railliet and Lucet, 1891) Tadros and Laarman, 1976; *Coccidium bigeminum* var. *putorii* Railliet and Lucet, 1891 *nomen nudum*; *Isospora putorii* (Railliet and Lucet, 1891) Becker, 1934 *nomen nudum*; *Lucetina putorii* (Railliet and Lucet, 1891) Henry and Leblois, 1926.

Definitive type host: *Mustela nivalis* L., 1766, Least Weasel.

Type locality: Europe: The Netherlands.

Other definitive hosts: *Mustela erminea* L., 1758, Ermine; *Mustela* (syn. *Putorius*) *putorius furo* (L., 1758), European Polecat/Domestic Ferret; *Neovison* (syn. *Mustela*) *vison* (Schreber, 1777), American Mink.

Intermediate type host: *Microtus arvalis* (Pallas, 1778), Common Vole.

Other intermediate host: *Microtus agrestis* (L., 1761), Short-tailed Vole.

Geographic distribution: Europe: The Netherlands, Switzerland; North America: USA: Illinois.

Description of sporulated oocyst: Oocyst shape: is typically sarcocystid-like and variable, with wall crenated around SPs; number of walls, 1; wall characteristics: colorless, thin; L × W: 12 × 9 (11–14 × 7–11); L/W ratio: 1.3; M, OR, PG: all absent (Levine, 1948; Tadros and Laarman, 1975). Distinctive features of oocyst: none as the one-layered wall is so thin and attached to the sporocysts as to be almost invisible.

Description of sporocyst and sporozoites: Sporocyst shape: ellipsoidal; L × W: 11 × 7; L/W ratio: 1.6; SB, SSB, PSB: all absent; SR: present; SR characteristics: a large spheroidal to ellipsoidal aggregation of granules; SZ: sausage-shaped. Distinctive features of sporocyst: none; a "typical" *Sarcocystis*-type SP, lacking SB, SSB, PSB and with a distinct, granular SR.

Prevalence: Tadros and Laarman (1975) found this species in 1/1 *Mu. nivalis* live-trapped in Holland. Frank (1978) said she found only sporocysts of this species in the jejunum of five *Mustela putorius* from "Illmitz in the European Soviet Union (probably Austria)."

Sporulation: Endogenous with sporulated, infective sporocysts shed in the feces of the definitive host.

Prepatent and patent periods: Prepatency can be from 7 to 13 DPI, and patency in the definitive host can last from 2 weeks up to 3 months.

Site of infection, definitive host: Lamina propria of the small intestine.

Site of infection, intermediate host: Meronts are known from the "liver and other visceral organs" (Levine and Ivens, 1981), and sarcocysts are found in the muscles of voles.

Endogenous stages, definitive host: Gamonts, gametocysts, zygotes, oocysts, and sporocysts in the small intestine's lamina propria.

Endogenous stages, intermediate host: Tadros and Laarman (1976) said the first generation meronts develop in the liver and other visceral organs, and the sarcocysts (last generation meronts) measured up to several centimeters long. Sarcocysts of this species are compartmentalized and contain both metrocytes and bradyzoites. The sarcocyst wall has a sparse scattering of villus-like projections up to three long, with numerous fibrils.

Cross-transmission: Tadros and Laarman (1975) found sporocysts of what was likely this species in the feces of *Mu. nivalis* in Holland and fed them to laboratory-bred *Mi. arvalis*. Six months later they found microscopic *Sarcocystis* sarcocysts, several millimeters long, in the skeletal muscles of one experimentally infected vole. This infected vole was then fed to a captive weasel kept on a rodent-free diet, and on the 7th DPI, it began to shed sporocysts in its feces. Completing Koch's postulates, these sporocysts were then fed to laboratory-bred *Mi. arvalis*, and 2 weeks later they killed the vole and found meronts, L × W: 15 × 12, in the spleen and lymph nodes. A second vole was killed on the 37th DPI, and they found numerous meronts in the liver and many sarcocysts in the musculature. Tadros and Laarman (1975) did not name the *Sarcocystis* species at that time, but it almost certainly was *S. putorii* (see Levine and Tadros, 1980). Tadros and Laarman (1976) found sporocysts of *S. putorii* in the feces of *Mu. nivalis*, fed them to a vole, *Mi. arvalis*, produced sarcocysts in it, and then used these muscle cysts to infect *Mu. erminea* (ermine), *Mu. putorius furo* (ferret) and *Mu. nivalis* (weasel).

Pathology: This species does not seem to exhibit any overt signs of pathogenicity in the definitive mustelid hosts, but heavy infections in voles result in loss of appetite, lethargy, excessive thirst, muscular weakness, and death (Tadros and Laarman, 1976). Frank (1978) said, "alterations of intestinal mucus or other harmful effects were not detectable."

Materials deposited: None.

Remarks: Tadros and Laarman (1975, 1976) measured sporocysts in *Mu. nivalis* that were L × W: 11–13 × 8–10, slightly larger than those measured earlier by Levine (1948). Frank (1978) said she found this species in *M. putorius* trapped near Lake Neusiedl, Austria, right on the border with Hungary, but she gave no morphological or prevalence data. Levine and Ivens (1981) suggested that this species is "probably the same organism that Galli-Valerio (1935)

called '*Isospora bigemina* var. *putorii*' in a *Mustela erminea* in Switzerland, and it may well be the '*Isospora bigemina*' that Levine (1948) found in the intestine of a fur-farm mink, *M. vison*, in Illinois." We see no reason to challenge their statement at this time. Levine (1986) named this as one of the valid *Sarcocystis* species in his list of 122. Odening (1998), in his compilation of 189 *Sarcocystis* names, listed this as a valid species, and added that it had a TEM type 9 or 10 sarcocyst wall (originally type 9, Dubey et al., 1989b). Dubey et al. (2015a) mentioned *S. putorii* multiple times. They said sarcocysts were macroscopic, several millimeters long, with a thin, bristly wall that resembled TEM type 9b (?), and they also listed it as a valid species of *Sarcocystis* (their Tables 21.3, 24.1, and 24.4).

SARCOCYSTIS SPECIES

There is at least one report of *Sarcocystis* sarcocysts in muscles of *Mu. nivalis*, but no specific identification was made (see Chapter 19).

GENUS NEOVISON BARYSHNIKOV AND ABRAMOV, 1997 (2 SPECIES)

SARCOCYSTIS PUTORII (RAILLIET AND LUCET, 1891), TADROS AND LAARMAN, 1978a

Definitive host: *Neovison* (syn. *Mustela*) *vison* (Schreber, 1777), American Mink.

Remarks: For more complete information on *S. putorii*, see Genus *Mustela*, above.

SARCOCYSTIS SPECIES

There is at least one report of *Sarcocystis*-type sarcocysts in muscles of *N. vison*, but no specific identification was made (see Chapter 19).

GENUS *TAXIDEA* WATERHOUSE, 1839 (MONOTYPIC)

SARCOCYSTIS CAMPESTRIS CAWTHORN, WOBESSER, AND GAJADAR, 1983

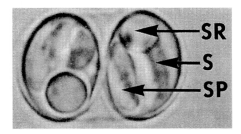

FIGURE 15.3 Photomicrograph of a sporulated oocyst of *Sarcocystis campestris*, with its two sporocysts (S) tightly bound together by the thin oocyst wall, taken from intestinal scraping of a naturally-infected badger. Note the large globular sporocyst residuum (SR) and sporozoite (SP). *From Cawthorn, R.J., Wobesser, G.A., Gajadhar, A.A., 1983. Description of* Sarcocystis campestris *sp. n. (Protozoa: Sarcocystidae): a parasite of the badger* Taxidea taxus *with experimental transmission to the Richardson's ground squirrel,* Spermophilus richardsonii. *Canadian Journal of Zoology 61 (2), 370–377, copyright 2008 Canadian Science Publishing or its licensors. Reproduced with their permission.*

Definitive host: *Taxidea taxus* (Schreber, 1777), American Badger.

Intermediate host: *Spermophilus richardsonii* (Sabine, 1822), Richardson's Ground Squirrel.

Geographic distribution: North America: Canada: Saskatchewan.

Remarks: Cawthorn et al. (1983) described this species from 4/4 (100%) wild-caught badgers in Canada. Sporocysts in these badger feces were L × W (n = 100): 10.2 × 8.0 (9–12 × 6–9.5), L/W ratio: 1.3 (1.1–1.7), and sporocysts in experimentally infected badgers were nearly identical in size, L × W (n = 100): 10.2 × 8.0 (9.5–12 × 6.5–9.5), L/W ratio: 1.3 (1.1–1.6). They inoculated 35 *S. richardsonii* with various numbers of sporocysts from badger feces. Of 14 squirrels inoculated with 1.5×10^3 sporocysts, 4 died on 11–13 DPI, before they could be necropsied to look for tissue stages. Apparently, all 35 squirrels in three different experiments became infected when inoculated with sporocysts, but one cat and one skunk did not become infected as no sporocysts were found in their feces for up to 25 DPI. For details on the tissue stages of *S. campestris* infection in ground squirrels see Cawthorn et al. (1983). Cawthorn et al. (1983) described the pathology of *S. campestris* infection in experimentally infected ground squirrels. Hepatitis and phlebitis of hepatic veins were present in squirrels killed 4–8 DPI, and meronts were found in endothelial cells in many tissues beginning on 9 DPI and were most numerous in the lungs. Four of 10 squirrels infected with only 1,500 sporocysts died between 11 and 13 DPI. In squirrels that survived, foci of inflammation were visible in the myocardium and the brain when they were killed 64 DPI (Cawthorn et al., 1983). Levine (1986) listed this species as one of the 122 names he considered as valid species of *Sarcocystis* at that time. Odening (1998) listed this species as one of the 189 valid species of *Sarcocystis* in his thorough review of the genus. Dubey et al.'s (2015a) review of the literature mentioned *S. campestris* 10 times and included life cycle and other information (their Tables 1.3, 21.5, 24.1 and 24.4); they also included four figures of this species (their Figs. 1.2, 1.10C, 1.40, and 1.45A).

OTARIIDAE GRAY, 1825

GENUS ARCTOCEPHALUS É. GEOFFROY SAINT-HILAIRE AND F.G. CUVIER (8 SPECIES)

SARCOCYSTIS NEURONA DUBEY, DAVIS, SPEER, BOWMAN, DE LAHUNTA, GRANSTROM, TOPPER, HAMIR, CUMMINGS, AND SUTER, 1991b

Definitive hosts: *Didelphis albiventris* Lund, 1840, White-eared Opossum; *Didelphis marsupialis* L., 1758, Common Opossum; *Didelphis virginiana* Kerr, 1792, Virginia Opossum.

Intermediate host: *Arctocephalus townsendi* Merriam, 1897, Guadalupe Fur Seal.

Remarks: Barbosa et al. (2015) sampled 227 marine mammals, most with clinical or pathological evidence of potential disease and, using a nested PCR assay, tested them for the presence of coccidian parasites. They found an overall prevalence of infection for *S. neurona* in 136/227 (60%) animals, including 11/25 (44%) Guadalupe fur seals. This parasite is an important cause of protozoal encephalitis among marine mammals in the northeastern Pacific Ocean, and their work identified a unique, new molecular signature (Ag type XIII MS type hh) to help identify *S. neurona* isolates responsible for fatal infections in marine mammals. All but one individual with single genotype XIII infections, and all with coinfections (with *T. gondii*) that included type XIII, had marked to severe protozoal encephalitis, and all died of protozoal disease, demonstrating that this genotype is highly pathogenic and is an important cause of mortality in marine mammals. Barbosa et al. (2015) pointed out that in recent decades, small mammals such as the Virginia opossum have been observed to shift their geographic ranges northward, both due to global warming of surface temperatures and the likely increased availability of food sources from human population expansions. They warned that as the range of the opossum expands, new *S. neurona* genotypes, such as type XIII, may emerge to cause infection in susceptible host species not previously exposed to these pathogens such as marine mammals. We think their warning is clear!

GENUS *CALLORHINUS* J.E. GRAY, 1859 (MONOTYPIC)

SARCOCYSTIS NEURONA DUBEY, DAVIS, SPEER, BOWMAN, DE LAHUNTA, GRANSTROM, TOPPER, HAMIR, CUMMINGS, AND SUTER, 1991b

Definitive hosts: *Didelphis albiventris* Lund, 1840, White-eared Opossum; *Didelphis marsupialis*

L., 1758, Common Opossum; *Didelphis virginiana* Kerr, 1792, Virginia Opossum.

Intermediate host: *Callorhinus ursinus* (L., 1758), Northern Fur Seal.

Remarks: Barbosa et al. (2015) sampled 227 marine mammals, most with clinical or pathological evidence of potential disease and, using a nested PCR assay, tested them for the presence of coccidian parasites. They found an overall prevalence of infection for *S. neurona* in 136/227 (60%) animals, including 1/5 (20%) northern fur seals. This parasite is an important cause of protozoal encephalitis among marine mammals in the northeastern Pacific Ocean.

SARCOCYSTIS SPECIES

There is at least one report of *Sarcocystis* sarcocysts in masseter muscle of *C. ursinus*, but no specific identification was made (see Chapter 19).

GENUS *EUMETOPIAS* GILL, 1866 (MONOTYPIC)

SARCOCYSTIS CANIS DUBEY AND SPEER, 1991

Intermediate host: *Eumetopias jubatus* (Schreber, 1776), Steller Sea Lion.

Remarks: Welsh et al. (1014) documented *S. canis* associated with hepatitis in a Steller sea lion, *E. jubatus* from Alaska, USA. For full description of *S. canis*, see Genus *Canis*, above.

SARCOCYSTIS NEURONA DUBEY, DAVIS, SPEER, BOWMAN, DE LAHUNTA, GRANSTROM, TOPPER, HAMIR, CUMMINGS, AND SUTER, 1991b

Definitive hosts: *Didelphis albiventris* Lund, 1840, White-eared Opossum; *Didelphis marsupialis* L.,

1758, Common Opossum; *Didelphis virginiana* Kerr, 1792, Virginia Opossum.

Intermediate host: *Eumetopias jubatus* (Schreber, 1776), Steller Sea Lion.

Remarks: Barbosa et al. (2015) sampled 227 marine mammals, most with clinical or pathological evidence of potential disease and, using a nested PCR assay, tested them for the presence of coccidian parasites. They found an overall prevalence of infection for *S. neurona* in 136/227 (60%) animals, including 3/8 (38%) Steller sea lions. This parasite is an important cause of protozoal encephalitis among marine mammals in the northeastern Pacific Ocean. For the remainder of our comments, see above under *A. townsendi*.

GENUS *ZALOPHUS* GILL, 1866 (3 SPECIES)

SARCOCYSTIS CANIS DUBEY AND SPEER, 1991

Intermediate host: *Zalophus californianus* (Lesson, 1828), California Sea Lion.

Remarks: Dubey et al. (2006) retrospectively examined *S. canis*-like meronts in the liver of a sea lion (*Z. californianus*) by sequencing both conserved (18S) and variable (ITS-1) portions of nuclear rDNA; they found a "genetic signature" that they said was "provisionally representative of *S. canis.*" For full description of *S. canis*, see Genus *Canis*, above.

SARCOCYSTIS HUETI (MOULÉ, 1888) LABBÉ, 1899

Synonym: *Miescheria hueti* (R. Blanchard, 1885) Moulé, 1888.

Definitive host: Unknown.

Intermediate host: *Zalophus californianus* (Lesson, 1828) (syn. *Otaria californiana* Lesson, 1828), California Sea Lion.

Geographic distribution: Unknown.

Remarks: Brumpt (1913) placed all sarcosporidia known in his time into the genus *Sarcocystis*, and listed this species as *S. hueti* R. Blanchard, 1885, and said that it was only found in the muscles of the California sea lion. Levine (1986) listed this species as *S. hueti* Blanchard, 1885, as one of the 122 names he considered as valid species of *Sarcocystis* at that time. Odening (1998) also listed this species in his systematic list of *Sarcocystis* species names but adjusted the authority as we have noted above. Dubey et al. (2015a) agreed with the authority change of Odening (1998) and provided what minimal mensural data are available on this species (their Table 18.3) and considered it a valid species name (their Tables 24.1 and 24.4). Sarcocysts can be up to 4 mm long and bradyzoites are only described as 4–5 long.

SARCOCYSTIS NEURONA DUBEY, DAVIS, SPEER, BOWMAN, DE LAHUNTA, GRANSTROM, TOPPER, HAMIR, CUMMINGS, AND SUTER, 1991b

Definitive hosts: *Didelphis virginiana* Kerr, 1792, Virginia Opossum; *Didelphis albiventris* Lund, 1840, White-eared Opossum; *Didelphis marsupialis* L., 1758, Common Opossum.

Intermediate host: *Zalophus californianus* (Lesson, 1828), California Sea Lion.

Geographic distribution: North America: Canada; USA.

Remarks: Gibson et al. (2011) screened tissues from 161 marine mammals identified as suspect protozoal encephalitis cases based on observed antemortem neurologic signs, animals on postmortem condition found dead, and stranded animals. Tissues included 12 *Z. californicus*, 10 of which were healthy. DNA was extracted and the ITS-1 and ITS-1_{500} were amplified to distinguish among closely related, and novel, species of tissue-encysting coccidian parasites including *T. gondii* and *S. neurona*. Size polymorphism in the ITS-1 region was used to readily distinguish between single *T. gondii*, *S. neurona*, and dual infections. Unfortunately, the authors did not present results for individual host species, but overall, 147/161 (91%) marine mammals tested positive for protozoal infection. Of the 10 healthy adult California sea lion males sampled from the Columbia River, all were infected with either *S. neurona* (n=8) or *T. gondii* (n=1) or coinfected with *T. gondii* and *S. neurona* (n=1); 121/151 (80%) of the remaining suspect protozoal cases were infected either with *S. neurona* (n=29) or *T. gondii* (n=31) or coinfected with *T. gondii* and *S. neurona* (n=61). Carlson-Bremer et al. (2012) diagnosed *S. neurona*-induced myositis in a free-ranging, adult female, California sea lion that became stranded on the California shore and was captured. The animal was lethargic and in poor body condition and active myositis was diagnosed on the basis of elevated activities of alanine aminotransferase and creatine kinase. Positive diagnosis of *S. neurona* was made on immunological staining and quantitative PCR on biopsy specimens from the diaphragm and muscles of the dorsal cervical region. Ponazuril (10 mg/kg PO, q 24 hours), continued for 28 days, and prednisone (0.2 mg/kg PO, q 12 hours) for 2 days and then every 24 hours for 5 days were both administered as treatment. The sea lion was clinically normal at the end of treatment and was released, about three months after being stranded. For more complete information on *S. neurona*, see Genus *Procyon*, below for the natural intermediate host, *P. lotor*. Barbosa et al. (2015) sampled 227 marine mammals, most with clinical or pathological evidence of potential disease and, using a nested PCR assay, tested them for the presence of coccidian parasites. They found an overall prevalence of infection for *S. neurona* in 136/227 (60%) animals, including 3/4 (75%) California sea lions. This parasite is an important cause of protozoal encephalitis among marine mammals in the northeastern Pacific Ocean. For the remainder of our comments, see above under *A. townsendi, the Guadalupe fur seal*.

SARCOCYSTIS SPECIES

There is at least one report of *Sarcocystis* sarcocysts in various tissues, including the liver of *Z. californianus*; the parasite may or may not be *S. neurona*, but no definitive identification was made at the time (see Chapter 19).

PHOCIDAE GRAY, 1821

GENUS *ERIGNATHUS* GILL, 1866 (MONOTYPIC)

SARCOCYSTIS SPECIES

There is at least one report of *Sarcocystis* sarcocysts in the skeletal muscle/tongue of one *Erignathus barbatus* in the Arctic, but no definitive identification was made at the time (see Chapter 19).

GENUS *HYDRURGA* GISTEL, 1848 (MONOTYPIC)

SARCOCYSTIS HYDRURGAE ODENING AND ZIPPER, 1986

Definitive type host: *Hydrurga leptonyx* (de Blainville, 1820), Leopard Seal (?) (this seems unlikely, see *Remarks*).

Type locality: Antarctica: South Shetland Islands, King George Island (62° 12′ S, 58° 54′ W).

Other definitive hosts: None known to date.

Intermediate type host: *Hydrurga leptonyx* (de Blainville, 1820), Leopard Seal.

Other intermediate hosts: None known to date.

Geographic distribution: Antarctica: South Shetland Islands.

Description of sporulated oocyst: Unknown. However, Odening (1984) and Odening and Zipper (1986) reported finding "presumably associated oocysts," likely unsporulated, which were roundish, 7.8–12.2 wide, with a clearly double-contoured hyaline wall.

Description of sporocyst and sporozoites: Unknown.

Prevalence: Odening and Zipper (1986) found sarcocysts in one *H. leptonyx* that was shot.

Sporulation: Unknown.

Prepatent and patent periods: Unknown.

Site of infection, definitive host: Unknown, except that Odening and Zipper (1986) said they found "presumed" unsporulated oocysts, which they suggested (unsupported by data) may be associated with this species name in the skeletal muscles associated with sarcocysts.

Site of infection, intermediate host: Skeletal muscles of the leopard seal.

Endogenous stages, definitive host: Unknown.

Endogenous stages, intermediate host: Odening and Zipper (1986) used both LM and TEM to examine the sarcocysts in muscles of the seal they examined. Only mature sarcocysts (without metrocytes) were seen in the skeletal muscles of *H. leptonyx*; septate sarcocysts were described to be L × W: 1.8–13.0 × 0.09–1.9 mm, with a thin primary cyst wall that formed a real boundary between itself and the host muscle cell fibers. There were short invaginations that gave the appearance of being coarsely granular, and they had a uniform electron-dense layer with a thickness of 0.11. There were distinct villi, about 0.73 long, but they did not contain fibrils or microtubules. A "cystic base substance" (Figs. 2 and 3 in Odening and Zipper, 1986) was included in the villous formation; thickness of the cyst base substance, without villi, was 0.83. Cystozoites (bradyzoites?) were disk-shaped, 6.1 × 2.2.

Cross-transmission: None to date.

Pathology: Not reported.

Materials deposited: One sarcocyst embedded in Epon was deposited in the Protozoan Collection, Research Center for Vertebrate Research (Am Tierpark 125, Berlin, DDR-1136) as No. B1/1984.

Remarks: Sarcocysts found in the skeletal muscles of *H. leptonyx* were first studied by Odening (1983) using LM; later, Odening (1984) reported that in addition to the sarcocysts, and unusually, occasional oocysts were seen. Thus, Odening and Zipper (1986) studied the ultrastructure of the material available to them, which is the information reported here. Their paper was published the same year as Levine's (1986) review paper so *S. hydrurgae* was not mentioned by Levine (1968). Odening's (1998) review of valid *Sarcocystis* binomials listed *S. hydrurgae*, and he noted that the sarcocyst is a type 1 (as per Dubey et al., 2015a) but added no additional data. Dubey et al. (2015a) also listed *S. hydrurgae* as a valid species name (Tables 24.1 and 24.4), but they added no additional data to what was presented in the original publication of Odening and Zipper (1986) other than the cyst type, when viewed by TEM, is a type 1e.

GENUS *LEPTONYCHOTES* GILL, 1872 (MONOTYPIC)

SARCOCYSTIS SPECIES

There is at least one report of *Sarcocystis* sarcocysts in the skeletal muscles of the chest, back, tongue, and esophagus of one *Leptonychotes weddelli* in the Antarctic, but no definitive identification was made at the time (see Chapter 19).

GENUS *LOBODON* GRAY, 1844 (MONOTYPIC)

SARCOCYSTIS SPECIES

There is at least one report of *Sarcocystis* sarcocysts in the skeletal muscles of the chest, back, tongue, and esophagus of one *Lobodon carcinophaga* in the Antarctic, but no definitive identification was made at the time (see Chapter 19).

GENUS MIROUNGA GRAY, 1827
(2 SPECIES)

SARCOCYSTIS NEURONA DUBEY, DAVIS, SPEER, BOWMAN, DE LAHUNTA, GRANSTROM, TOPPER, HAMIR, CUMMINGS, AND SUTER, 1991b

Definitive hosts: *Didelphis albiventris* Lund, 1840, White-eared Opossum; *Didelphis marsupialis* L., 1758, Common Opossum; *Didelphis virginiana* Kerr, 1792, Virginia Opossum.

Intermediate host: *Mirounga angustirostris* (Gill, 1866), Northern Elephant Seal.

Remarks: Barbosa et al. (2015) sampled 227 marine mammals, most with clinical or pathological evidence of potential disease and, using a nested PCR assay, tested them for the presence of coccidian parasites. They found an overall prevalence of infection for *S. neurona* in 136/227 (60%) animals, including 3/3 (100%) northern elephant seals. This parasite is an important cause of protozoal encephalitis among marine mammals in the northeastern Pacific Ocean, and their work identified a unique, new molecular signature (Ag type XIII MS type hh) to help identify *S. neurona* isolates responsible for fatal infections in marine mammals. All but one individual with single genotype XIII infections, and all with coinfections (with *T. gondii*) that included type XIII, had marked to severe protozoal encephalitis and all died of protozoal disease, demonstrating that this genotype is highly pathogenic and an important cause of mortality in marine mammals. Barbosa et al. (2015) pointed out that in recent decades, small mammals such as the Virginia opossum have shifted their geographic range northward, both due to global warming of surface temperatures and the likely increased food availability from human population expansions. They warned that as the range of the opossum expands, new *S. neurona* genotypes such as type XIII may emerge to

cause infection in susceptible host species not previously exposed to these pathogens such as marine mammals. We wonder if anyone will heed their warning!

SARCOCYSTIS SPECIES

There is at least one report of *Sarcocystis* sarcocysts in the skeletal muscles of the chest, back, tongue, and esophagus of one *Mirounga leonina* in the Antarctic, but no definitive identification was made at the time (see Chapter 19).

GENUS MONACHUS FLEMING, 1822 (3 SPECIES)

SARCOCYSTIS CANIS DUBEY AND SPEER, 1991

Intermediate host: *Monachus schauinslandi* Matschie, 1905, Hawaiian Monk Seal.

Remarks: Yantis et al. (2003) reported finding asexual stages of *S. canis* in the hepatocytes of *M. schauinslandi*. For full description of *S. canis*, see Genus *Canis*, above.

GENUS PHOCA L., 1758
(2 SPECIES)

SARCOCYSTIS NEURONA DUBEY, DAVIS, SPEER, BOWMAN, DE LAHUNTA, GRANSTROM, TOPPER, HAMIR, CUMMINGS, AND SUTER, 1991b

Definitive hosts: *Didelphis albiventris* Lund, 1840, White-eared Opossum; *Didelphis marsupialis* L., 1758, Common Opossum; *Didelphis virginiana* Kerr, 1792, Virginia Opossum.

Intermediate host: *Phoca vitulina* L., 1758 (syn. *Phoca richardii* (Gray, 1864)), Harbor Seal.

Remarks: Barbosa et al. (2015) sampled 227 marine mammals, most with clinical or pathological evidence of potential disease and, using a nested PCR assay, tested them for the presence of coccidian parasites. They found an overall prevalence of infection for *S. neurona* in 136/227 (60%) animals, including 76/121 (63%) Pacific harbor seals. This parasite is an important cause of protozoal encephalitis among marine mammals in the northeastern Pacific Ocean. For the remainder of our comments, see above under *M. angustirostris, the northern elephant seal*.

SARCOCYSTIS RICHARDII HADWEN, 1922

Definitive host: Unknown.

Intermediate host: *Phoca vitulina* L., 1758 (syn. *P. richardii* (Gray, 1864)), Harbor Seal.

Geographic distribution: North America: USA: Alaska.

Remarks: Hadwen (1922) published a lengthy paper on cyst-forming protozoa in reindeer and caribou and only briefly mentioned seeing sarcocysts in a harbor seal in Alaska, USA. Sarcocysts in the diaphragm muscles were over 2-cm long with a mean of 1.2 cm, and trophozoites (bradyzoites?) averaged 10 × 2.5. Some endogenous developmental stages (meronts) also were mentioned. Levine (1986) named this as one of the valid *Sarcocystis* species on his list of 122. Odening (1998), in his compilation of 189 *Sarcocystis* names, listed this as a valid species, but gave no other information. Dubey et al. (2015a) mentioned *S. richardii* only briefly, gave the minimal data noted above, and listed this as a valid binomial (their Tables 18.3, 24.1, and 24.4). Unfortunately, there is such little information available on *S. richardii*, and it has not been found since its original description, that we question if it is better considered a *species inquirenda* until more information is available.

SARCOCYSTIS SPECIES

There are at least two reports of *Sarcocystis* sarcocysts in the heart and/or esophagus muscles of *P. vitulina*, but no definitive identification was made at the time (see Chapter 19).

GENUS *PUSA* SCOPOLI, 1771 (3 SPECIES)

SARCOCYSTIS SPECIES

There are at least two reports of *Sarcocystis* sarcocysts in the heart and/or skeletal muscles of *Pusa capsica* and *Pusa hispida*, but no definitive identification was made at the time (see Chapter 19).

PROCYONIDAE GRAY, 1825

GENUS *NASUA* STORR, 1780 (2 SPECIES)

SARCOCYSTIS NEURONA DUBEY, DAVIS, SPEER, BOWMAN, DE LAHUNTA, GRANSTROM, TOPPER, HAMIR, CUMMINGS, AND SUTER, 1991b

Definitive hosts: *Didelphis albiventris* Lund, 1840, White-eared Opossum; *Didelphis marsupialis* L., 1758, Common Opossum; *Didelphis virginiana* Kerr, 1792, Virginia Opossum.

Intermediate host: *Nasua narica molaris* Merriam, 1902, White-nosed Coati.

Remarks: Dubey et al. (2017c) reported a case of highly disseminated sarcocystosis in a white-nosed coati (*Nasua narica*) that was resident in the Philadelphia Zoo, USA. A complete postmortem examination was done and tissues were prepared and examined microscopically (LM, TEM) and immunohistologically for *S. neurona*. DNA was extracted from lung tissue for amplification and sequencing, and multilocus PCR-DNA was identified with an *S. neurona* infection using 18S, 28S, and ITS-1 markers, and a novel genotype using primer pairs against antigenic surface proteins (SnSAG3, SnSAG4, SnSAG1-5-6) and microsatellite markers (MS, SN7, SN9). The genotype was similar to the type VI strain with a novel allele at SnSAG5, and different MS repeats at SN7 and SN9.

GENUS POTOS É. GEOFFROY SAINT-HILAIRE AND F.G. CUVIER, 1795 (MONOTYPIC)

SARCOCYSTIS SPECIES

There is at least one report of *Sarcocystis* sarcocysts in the heart and skeletal muscles of a kinkajou (*Potos* sp.) in Panama, but no definitive identification was made at the time (see Chapter 19).

GENUS PROCYON STORR, 1780 (3 SPECIES)

SARCOCYSTIS CRUZI (HASSELMANN, 1923) WENYON, 1926a

Definitive host: *Procyon lotor* (L., 1758), Raccoon.
Remarks: For more complete information on *S. cruzi*, see Genus *Canis*, above.

SARCOCYSTIS HOFMANNI ODENING, STOLTE, WALTER AND BOCKHARDT, 1994b

Intermediate host: *Procyon lotor* (L., 1758), Raccoon (?).
Remarks: For more complete information on *S. hofmanni*, see Genus *Meles*, above.

SARCOCYSTIS KIRKPATRICKI SNYDER, SANDERSON, TOIVIO-KINNUCAN, AND BLAGBURN, 1990

For light and electron micrographs of tissue cysts and zoites of this species see Figs. 1–3 in Snyder et al. (1990).

Definitive type host: Unknown.
Type locality: North America: USA: Illinois.
Other definitive hosts: Unknown.
Intermediate type host: *Procyon lotor* (L., 1758), Raccoon.
Other intermediate hosts: Unknown.
Geographic distribution: North America: USA: Florida, Illinois, Ohio, Pennsylvania.
Description of sporulated oocyst: Unknown.
Description of sporocyst and sporozoites: Unknown.
Prevalence: Sarcocysts of this species were found in 66/100 (66%) raccoons in Illinois and in 26/52 (50%) raccoons in Florida, Ohio, and Pennsylvania, USA (Kirkpatrick et al., 1987). Of the tissues examined from raccoons in Illinois, 61/100 (61%) had sarcocysts in their tongues, 42/90 (47%) in their diaphragms, 32/99 (32%) in their esophagus, and 2/99 (2%) in their heart muscles.
Sporulation: Unknown, but almost certainly endogenous with sporulated, infective sporocysts shed in the feces of the definitive host.
Prepatent and patent periods: Unknown.
Site of infection, definitive host: Unknown.
Site of infection, intermediate host: Sarcocysts were found in skeletal musculature of *P. lotor*, including the tongue, diaphragm, masseter, esophagus, and heart.
Endogenous stages, definitive host: Unknown.
Endogenous stages, intermediate host: Sarcocysts were similar in all muscle tissues in which they were found. Sarcocyst walls were 2–3 thick, and had fine, hair-like projections and indistinct interior septa. Sarcocyst cross sections (n=25) in muscles were 129 (71–169) thick and the longest

sarcocyst was 801 long. The primary cyst wall (n=10) was 50 nm (46–63) thick. It had a scalloped appearance and was folded into straight to sloping villar projections that were (n=10) 2.8 × 0.5 nm (2–4 × 0.46–0.57) nm. The cores of these villar projections contained longitudinal tubular filaments that extended from the tip to the base where they terminated in a granular electron-dense layer of the primary cyst wall. Bradyzoites within the sarcocyst measured L × W: 3.9–5.2 × 1.2–2.0.

Cross-transmission: Snyder et al. (1990) attempted to feed sarcocysts of *S. kirkpatricki* to three 16-month-old dogs and three domestic, mixed-breed cats; none of these animals discharged sporocysts in their feces up to 18 days after their last feeding of sarcocyst-infected raccoon muscle.

Pathology: Snyder et al. (1990) saw no histopathologic lesions associated with the presence of sarcocysts in the muscles of raccoons.

Materials deposited: Syntypes are deposited in the USNPC (now at the USNHM), No. 80999.

Etymology: This species was named for Dr. Carl E. Kirkpatrick, who made many significant contributions to the field of parasitology.

Remarks: The ultrastructural results of Snyder et al. (1990) were similar to those reported earlier by Kirkpatrick et al. (1987), which is why former authors concluded they were working with the same *Sarcocystis* species in *P. lotor* in the four USA states mentioned above. Snyder et al. (1990) made a couple of interesting observations. First, they suggested that the prevalence of sarcocysts in the raccoons they examined was probably higher than they observed because the examination of tissue sections is less sensitive than techniques such as muscle digestion to detect bradyzoites. The second observation was the significant age-related difference in infection rates found between juvenile (52/60, 87% infected) and adult raccoons (14/40, 35% infected). The mechanism(s) for the differences

recorded is unknown, but they speculated that immunity to reinfection and resorption of older sarcocysts may explain the decreased prevalence they found in adult raccoons. Odening (1998), in his compilation of *Sarcocystis* names, listed this as a valid species as did Dubey et al. (2015a).

SARCOCYSTIS LEPORUM CRAWLEY, 1914

Definitive hosts: *Felis catus* L., 1758, Domestic Cat; *Procyon lotor* (L., 1758), Raccoon.

Intermediate hosts: *Sylvilagus floridanus* (J.A. Allen, 1890), Eastern Cottontail; *Sylvilagus nuttalli* (Bachman, 1837), Mountain Cottontail; *Sylvilagus palustris* (Bachman, 1837), Marsh Rabbit.

Geographic distribution: North America: USA: probably wherever cottontails are found (see Duszynski and Couch, 2013); and Europe: Germany (Elwasila et al., 1984).

Remarks: Crawley (1914) examined a fresh arm and shoulder of a male rabbit shot near Bowie, Maryland, USA, on December, 1913. Unfortunately, he did not identify the rabbit, but it likely was the eastern cottontail, *S. floridanus*; he did mention, "there are four specimens of this parasite in the collection of the Zoological Division of the Bureau of Animal Industry, from four different states." Sarcocysts in the fresh tissues examined were 2 mm long by 200–250 μm thick. In tissue sections, Crawley (1914) reported the sarcocyst wall was 5–6 thick, with a typical striated appearance, under low power, but that he saw a great number of papilliform processes closely packed together on the wall under higher magnification. We mention this paper because of its historical significance, being the first published report of sarcocysts in any lagomorph species. Levine and Ivens (1981) summarized much of the information known then about prevalence, oocyst structure, merogony, pathogenicity, and cross-transmission studies. Levine (1986) named this one of the 122

Sarcocystis species he said were valid species. Odening (1998) in his compilation of *Sarcocystis* names, listed this as a valid species. Duszynski and Couch (2013) summarized the biology and most other information known about this species. Dubey et al. (2015a) provided structural and some life cycle data (their Tables 1.4, 15.2, 21.4, 24.1, and 24.4). Also see the cross-transmission studies by Fayer and Kradel (1977) and Crum and Prestwood (1977).

SARCOCYSTIS MELIS ODENING, STOLTE, WALTER, AND BOCKHARDT, 1994b

Intermediate host: *Procyon lotor* (L., 1758), Raccoon.

Remarks: For more complete information on *S. melis*, see Genus *Meles*, above.

SARCOCYSTIS MIESCHERIANA (KÜHN, 1865) LABBÉ, 1899

Definitive host: *Procyon lotor* (L., 1758), Raccoon.

Remarks: For more complete information on *S. miescheriana*, see Genus *Canis*, above.

SARCOCYSTIS NEURONA DUBEY, DAVIS, SPEER, BOWMAN, DE LAHUNTA, GRANSTROM, TOPPER, HAMIR, CUMMINGS, AND SUTER, 1991b

A photomicrograph of a sporulated oocyst of *S. neurona* from Dubey et al., 2000a (their Fig. F) is available in Duszynski, 2016 (p. 118, Fig. 7.8)

Definitive type host: *Didelphis virginiana* Kerr, 1792, Virginia Opossum.

Type locality: North America: USA: Illinois.

Other definitive hosts: *Didelphis albiventris* Lund, 1840, White-eared Opossum (Dubey et al., 2001a,b); *Didelphis marsupialis* L., 1758,

Common Opossum (Dubey et al., 2001a; Dubey et al., 2015a).

Intermediate carnivore type host: Duszynski (2016) listed the horse (*Equus caballus* L., 1758) as the intermediate type host but was unaware, at the time, of the opinions of Dubey et al. (2001d) and Stanek et al. (2002) that identified the raccoon, *Procyon lotor* (L., 1758), as a suitable candidate to be the "natural" intermediate type host (see *Endogenous stages intermediate host* and *Remarks*).

Other intermediate carnivore hosts: *Canis lupus familiaris* (syn. *C. familiaris*) L., 1758, Domestic Dog (natural, Dubey et al., 2014); *Enhydra lutris nereis* (Merriam, 1904), Sea Otter (natural, Dubey et al., 2001c; Lindsay et al., 2001a); *Felis catus* L., 1758, Domestic Cat (experimental and natural, Fenger et al., 1995; Dubey and Hamir, 2000; Dryburgh et al., 2015); *Lynx canadensis* Kerr, 1782, Canadian Lynx (Forest et al., 2001); *Martes pennanti* (Erxleben, 1777), Fisher; *Mephitis mephitis* (Schreber, 1776), Striped Skunk (experimental and natural, Fenger et al., 1995; Dubey et al., 1996; Cheadle et al., 2001); *Mustela* (syn. *Putorius*) *putorius furo* L., 1758, European Polecat/Domestic Ferret (Britton et al., 2010); *Neovison* (syn. *Mustela*) *vison* (Schreber, 1777), American Mink (Dubey and Hedstrom, 1993; Dubey and Hamir, 2000); *Phoca vitulina richardii* (Gray, 1864), Harbor Seal (Lapointe et al., 1998; Miller et al., 2001b); *Zalophus* (syn. *Otaria*) *californianus* (Lesson, 1828), California Sea Lion (Dubey et al., 2006; 2015).

Geographic distribution: Throughout North America (including Canada and the United States), South America and likely Central America.

Description of sporulated oocyst: Unknown.

Description of sporocyst and sporozoites: Sporocyst shape: ellipsoidal; L × W: 10.5–12 × 6.5–8; L/W ratio: unknown; SB, SSB, PSB: all absent; SR: present; SR characteristics: composed of large, hyaline granules that either are scattered or condensed at one end of the sporocyst even within the same oocyst; SZ: banana-shaped, without distinct RB or N visible (Dubey et al., 2000a). Distinctive features of sporocyst: none, this is a typical *Sarcocystis*-type sporocyst.

Prevalence: For prevalence in opossums, see Duszynski (2016). Sarcocysts of *S. neurona*, or an *S. neurona*-like form, have been found in many carnivores. Dubey et al. (1991d) found what was almost certainly *S. neurona* in the brain of one raccoon, *P. lotor*, in Ohio, USA. Dubey and Hamir (2000), using IHC, detected *S. neurona* in the brains of two minks from Oregon, USA, a cat from California, USA, two skunks, one from Massachusetts, the other from Oregon, USA, and two raccoons, one from Ohio, the other from New York, USA (Dubey et al., 1990b, 1996; Dubey and Hedstrom, 1993; Dubey et al., 1994; Dubey and Hamir, 2000). Lapointe et al. (1998) found seven Pacific harbor seals with meningo-encephalitis associated with *S. neurona*-like parasites. Forest et al. (2001) reported this species in a 13-year-old Canadian lynx that died after a short clinical illness and necropsy showed multifocal encephalitis with meronts in cerebral vascular endothelial cells. The meronts stained immunohistochemically with antiserum to *S. neurona*. Dubey et al. (2001c) found sarcocysts in 2/2 (100%) naturally-infected sea otters, *E. lutris*. The sarcocysts were characterized biologically (KO mice with γ-interferon gene), ultrastructurally, and genetically by PCR amplification followed by RFLP analysis and sequencing. Their (2001c) conclusion was that sea otters exposed to *S. neurona* sporocysts can support the development of mature sarcocysts that are infectious to competent definitive hosts (opossums). Between 1993 and 2000, Dubey et al. (2002c) collected sera from 502 domestic cats (*F. catus*) from São Paulo and Guarulhos cities, São Paulo State, Brazil and examined them for the presence of antibodies of *S. neurona* via the direct agglutination test with respective antigen; no antibodies to *S. neurona* were found in 1:50 dilution of any cat sera. This negative result suggested to them (2002c) that cats in São Paulo State were not exposed to *S. neurona* sporocysts in opossum feces. Dubey et al. (2002b) also reported *S. neurona* in 3/4 (75%) striped skunks from Oregon, USA.

Vashisht et al. (2005) also found sarcocysts in the skeletal muscles of one 6-year-old Labrador retriever; ultrastructurally, the cyst wall had villar protrusions consistent with sarcocysts and IHC with monoclonal *S. neurona* antibodies demonstrated positive labeling of zoites in the meronts. Finally, Dubey et al. (2014) reported *S. neurona* in a 9-week-old golden retriever from Mississippi, USA and their data suggested the dog was transplacentally-infected.

Sporulation: Endogenous with infective sporocysts shed in the feces of the definitive host (Dubey et al., 2000a).

Prepatent and patent periods: Two opossums fed sarcocyst-infected cat meat shed sporocysts at 11 and 13 days PI (Dubey et al., 2000a).

Site of infection, definitive host: Unknown, but likely the intestinal epithelium in opossums.

Site of infection, carnivore intermediate host: Dubey et al. (1991b) found meronts of what was almost certainly *S. neurona* in the brain of a raccoon from Ohio, USA. Parasites were located in the cytoplasm of macrophages, neurons, and multinucleated giant cells but were not surrounded by a **PV**. They divided by endopolygeny, leaving a residual body, and meronts were 5–35 × 5–20 with up to 35 merozoites that did not have **rhoptries.** In cats fed sporocysts from opossums, Dubey et al. (2000a) found muscle sarcocysts as early as 57 days PI in tongue, diaphragm, abdomen, legs, spine, and head, but these contained only metrocytes; even at 144 days, not all sarcocysts were mature. This suggested to Dubey et al. (2000a) a slow rate of maturation for *S. neurona* sarcocysts, at least in cats. Two raccoons (*P. lotor*) fed sporocysts of *S. neurona* from opossums developed clinical illness, and *S. neurona*-associated encephalomyelitis; they were killed 14 and 22 days postinfection, and meronts and merozoites were seen in encephalitic lesions (Dubey et al., 2001d).

Endogenous stages, definitive host: Unknown.

Endogenous stages, carnivore intermediate host: Only asexual stages are found in intermediate hosts, often within neural cells and leukocytes of the brain and spinal cord (Dubey et al.,

1991a,b,d); uniquely, the parasite locates in the host cell cytoplasm, does not have a PV, and divides by endopolygeny. Meronts measured L × W: 5–35 × 5–20 and contained 4–40 merozoites arranged in a rosette around a prominent residual body, but the meronts lacked rhoptries. The longest sarcocyst seen in muscle tissue sections in cats was 700 long, the widest one was 50 (Dubey et al., 2000a,b), and the sarcocyst wall was relatively thin with slender villar protrusions up to 2.5 long. Ultrastructurally, villar protrusions were seen to contain microtubules, and bradyzoites were slender, about 5–7 long (Dubey et al., 2000a). Stanek et al. (2002) were the first to report the complete development of *S. neurona* meronts and sarcocysts in *P. lotor*. Sporozoites were seen in sections of *P. lotor* intestines, 1–3 DPI with sporocysts from opossums. Young meront-like structures were seen in one raccoon 5 days after infection. Meronts varied in shape and size depending on the organ parasitized and age (days after infection). Meronts in the spinal cord and brain were smaller than those in the tongue. At 22 DPI with sporocysts, immature sarcocysts were L × W: 125 × 8–10, with a thin wall, <0.5 thick, and contained only metrocytes. By 37 DPI, sarcocysts were L × W: 270 × 50, and the wall was 1.5 thick with prominent villar protrusions. By 77 DPI, sarcocysts were mature, contained numerous slender bradyzoites, had numerous septa, and the sarcocyst wall was up to 2.5 thick with villar protrusions up to 2.5 long. The sarcocysts in the muscle of cats are similar to those in the muscles of raccoons (Stanek et al., 2002). Gerhold et al. (2005) found multiple, mature sarcocysts in skeletal muscle of a fisher and these cysts were not associated with inflammation. These cysts were L × W: 200 × 30, with a sarcocyst wall 1–3 thick. Metrocytes were primarily at the periphery of the sarcocyst with bradyzoites more centrally located. Bradyzoites in longitudinally-cut tissue sections were L × W (n = 4): 3.9–5.5 × 1.1–1.9 and contained organelles typical of *Sarcocystis* species bradyzoites. Gerhold et al. (2005) also found meronts in the cytoplasm

of neurons; developing merozoites contained micronemes but not rhoptries, and mature intra- and extracellular merozoites were also seen to have micronemes but no rhoptries. Dubey et al. (2006) also reported *S. neurona* meronts in the central nervous system, lungs, and kidneys of dogs. They also noted something interesting, i.e., no serological reactivity to *S. neurona* antibodies occurred when *S. canis*-like liver meronts were found in two dogs, a dolphin, a sea lion, a horse, a chinchilla, a black bear, and in two polar bears. In a dog thought to be infected transplacentally, Dubey et al. (2014) found lesions and parasite stages in the eyes, tongue, heart, liver, intestines, nasal turbinates, skeletal muscle, and brain, all of which acted intensely with *S. neurona* polyclonal antibodies.

Cross-transmission in carnivores: Cheadle et al. (2001) inoculated striped skunks with sporocysts collected from a naturally-infected Virginia opossum (*D. virginiana*); the skunks developed antibodies to *S. neurona*, and later developed sarcocysts in their muscles. Sarcocysts in skunk muscles were then fed to lab-reared opossums, which then shed sporulated sporocysts in their feces. Both sarcocysts from skunks and sporocysts from opossums fed infected skunk muscle were identified as *S. neurona* using PCR and DNA sequence analysis (Cheadle et al., 2001). Dryburgh et al. (2015) obtained (from colleagues in other labs) culture-derived merozoites of *S. neurona* strains from a raccoon, a sea otter, a cat, and a horse. Each of four 11-week-old raccoons was inoculated with 1×10^7 merozoites of one of these strains; each dose of merozoites was divided equally to inoculate raccoons by three routes: intravenous, intramuscular, and subcutaneous. At 75 DPI, raccoons were euthanized and their muscle tissues were fed to lab-raised opossums (*D. virginiana*), the definitive host of *S. neurona*. Intestinal scrapings showed sporocysts in opossums that received muscle tissue from raccoons inoculated with raccoon-derived and sea otter-derived isolates but not the cat or horse isolates.

Pathology in carnivores: In 1993, Dubey and Hedstrom (1993) were the first to report *Sarcocystis*-associated meningoencephalitis in mink. Two 1-month-old *M. vison* from near Corvalis, Oregon, USA were submitted for examination. The kits had come from a farm of ~15,500 mink; they were weak and comatose and died shortly after submission. At the time of submission, 50 other kits had died over a 2-week-period on the farm. Tissue sections were stained with antisera to *T. gondii*, *N. caninum*, and *S. cruzi*. Microscopically the cerebral cortex had extensive areas of severe necrosis and inflammation that often involved the entire gyrus. Sheets of inflammatory cells consisted primarily of neutrophils. There were multifocal abscesses throughout the remaining brain parenchyma, angiocentric accumulations of leukocytes, vasculitis, meningitis, and gliosis. Many tissue sections revealed immature and mature meronts. When examined by both LM and TEM, meronts were seen to locate in the cytoplasm of neurons, without a PV. Meronts were 5–25 wide, with up to 25 merozoites, each about 5–6 × 1–1.2. By TEM the merozoites were seen to contain organelles found in other *Sarcocystis* merozoites, but no rhoptries were found. The organisms reacted to anti-*Sarcocystis* serum but not to *T. gondii* and *N. caninum* antisera. These facts led Dubey and Hedstrom (1993) to conclude that the mink kits were infected with *S. neurona*. Later, Dubey et al. (1996) found a juvenile male striped skunk in Cape Cod, Massachusetts, USA with paresis and paralysis. On necropsy, they found multiple foci of encephalitis, characterized by perivascular infiltration of moderate numbers of mononuclear cells, glial nodules, and foci of necrosis, throughout the brain. Meronts and merozoites were eventually identified as *S. neurona*-like but definitely not *T. gondii* or *N. caninum*.

Lapointe et al. (1998) described meningoencephalitis due to this species in seven Pacific harbor seals found stranded over a stretch of central California coastline; all seals had marked to severe nonsuppurative meningoencephalitis,

most severe in the cerebellar cortex, and IHC for *S. neurona* antigens was positive on brain tissue in all cases and showed numerous merozoites and developing and mature meronts. Miller et al. (2001b) also reported meningoencephalomyelitis in a Pacific harbor seal from Monterey, California, USA and identified the causative agent as *S. neurona* using IHC and various molecular characterizations. This animal also was infected with *T. gondii*. Similarly, Lindsay et al. (2001a) reported a fatal dual infection of a northern sea otter (*E. lutris*) with both *S. neurona* and *T. gondii* found in the brain of the infected otter. Gerhold et al. (2005) reported meningoencephalitis caused by *S. neurona* in a free-ranging, juvenile fisher (*M. pennanti*), approximately 5–7-months-old, from Maryland, USA. Microscopically, the brain had multifocally extensive areas of necrosis and inflammation in the cerebrum, cerebellum, brainstem, and leptomeninges. The lesions were most severe in the thickened, inflamed leptomeninges and the gray matter of the cerebrum, especially the hippocampus. The inflamed areas varied from glial nodules to areas of necrosis infiltrated with numerous macrophages and fewer lymphocytes, plasma cells, and neutrophils. The cytoplasm of several neurons contained ovoidal meronts arranged either in a rosette or an irregular pattern. Organisms in the brain were immunopositive for *S. neurona*.

Cooley et al. (2007) reported the first protozoal myeloencephalitis case in a 1.5-year-old male Feist dog. Initially, the dog showed reluctance to stand on its hind legs and treatment with dexamethasone initially resulted in a favorable response. However, posterior paresis soon returned and progressed to recumbency, hyperesthesia, and attempts to bite its owner. On necropsy, multiple foci of encephalitis were found in the cerebrum and especially in the cerebellum. The parasite at the sites of intense inflammation and malacia was identified as *S. neurona* using both IHC, with polyclonal and monoclonal antibodies, and PCRs that were specific for *S. neurona*.

Britton et al. (2010) found rhinitis and disseminated disease in a naturally-infected ferret from British Columbia. The ferret exhibited severe rhinitis with intralesional *S. neurona* merozoites and meronts. Diagnosis of *S. neurona* was confirmed by staining with *S. neurona*-specific antibodies and by a phylogenetic analyses of conserved and variable portions of nuclear rDNA. The authors (2010) proposed an olfactory nerve pathway route of infection for *S. neurona* meningoencephalitis.

Gerhold et al. (2014) examined a basset hound–beagle mix that had progressive neurological impairment; on necropsy, the dog had multiple raised masses on the spinal cord between nerve roots. *Sarcocystis neurona* was detected in the central nervous system by IHC and PCR. Merozoites of *S. neurona* also have been identified in cerebrospinal fluid of a dog, and lesions of this parasite were identified in eyes, tongue, heart, liver, intestines, nasal turbinates, skeletal muscle, and brain of the infected dog (Dubey et al., 2014); these tissue stages reacted intensely with *S. neurona* polyclonal antibodies. In the same animal, mature sarcocysts were seen in the muscles, and the sarcocysts were ultrastructurally similar to those of *S. neurona* from experimentally-infected animals. These results led Dubey et al. (2014) to conclude that the domestic dog is another intermediate host for *S. neurona*.

Materials deposited: Syntypes from horse No. 1 of Dubey et al. (1974) are deposited in the USNM Helminthological Collection, USDA, Beltsville, Maryland as USNM Helminthological Collection No. 18450. Paratypes from a horse from Cornell University from which the organism was cultured *in vitro* were deposited as USNM Helminthological Collection No. 18451.

Etymology: The species name was derived from *neural* (Gk) and refers to the location of the parasite in the intermediate host.

Remarks: For a complete summary of the discovery of *S. neurona* and its pathology in horses and marsupials, see Duszynski (2016). This species is unusual in that opossums (*D. virginianus*, *D. albiventris*) are considered the primary definitive hosts whereas other carnivores (dogs, cats, raccoons, some marine mammals) and horses are intermediate hosts, in which most of the pathology is manifested. In horses, *S. neurona* causes a fatal disease, equine protozoa myeloencephalitis (EPM), and numerous reports of fatal EPM-like infections have been reported in other carnivore species but most often without central nervous system signs. These EMP-like infections always are associated with meront stages of this parasite. Raccoons are considered the most important intermediate host in the life cycle of *S. neurona* in the United States (Dryburgh et al., 2015). Fenger et al. (1995) compared a unique region they identified in the small subunit ribosomal RNA (18S rRNA) gene of *S. neurona* and developed a species-specific amplification primer. Using this primer in a PCR assay they tried to identify *S. neurona* in feces and intestinal digest of various wild mammals (cats, a coyote, opossums, raccoons, skunks). They successfully identified several opossum sporocyst samples using their specific primer in the PCR assay and confirmed the samples were *S. neurona*. These data suggested to them that the opossum is the definitive host of *S. neurona*.

Dubey et al. (1996) reported an *S. neurona*-like organism associated with encephalitis in a striped skunk (*M. mephitis*) in Massachusetts, USA. Dubey et al. (2000a,b) completed the life cycle of *S. neurona* experimentally in the lab and described sarcocysts in an experimental intermediate host (*F. catus*, domestic cat). Dubey and Hamir (2000) reported producing a high-titer *S. neurona*-specific serum in a rabbit using cultured merozoites; then, using that serum's specificity, they were able to confirm *S. neurona* infections in two raccoons, two minks, two skunks, and a cat. They also mentioned that other *S. neurona*-like infections were found in California harbor seals (*P. vitulina richardii*, see Lapointe et al.,

1998), and in sea otters (*E. lutris*, see Rosonke et al., 1999; Lindsay et al., 2000b; Dubey et al., 2001c). Structurally, meronts of *S. neurona* closely resemble those of other *Sarcocystis* species; however, the merozoites of *S. neurona* lack rhoptries, are located free in the host cell cytoplasm of cells in the brain and spinal cord, and they divide by endopolygeny. This suite of characters helps distinguish *S. neurona* from other species of *Sarcocystis* found, to date, in other domestic animals. Stanek et al. (2002) suggested that *P. lotor* is the natural intermediate host for *S. neurona* in the United States. As a terrestrially derived pathogen, *S. neurona* is associated with overland runoff events, which can impact the health of threatened marine wildlife such as sea otters, seals, and sea lions. Dubey et al. (2014) reported a fatal disseminated *S. neurona* infection in a 9-week-old golden retriever dog from Mississippi, USA (see *Pathology*, above). Diagnosticians should be aware of and vigilant for *Sarcocystis*-associated disease conditions in the animals brought to them for evaluation; and they need to be aware that encephalomyelitis may manifest in some animals (horses, raccoons, minks, dogs), whereas the disease only involves the livers in others (bears, sea lions, chinchilla) (Dubey and Speer, 1991; Mense et al., 1992; Rakich et al., 1992; Zeman et al., 1993).

Sarcocystis neurona is the best-known sarcocystid that has the capacity to undergo complete asexual development terminating in sarcocyst formation in some hosts, including many carnivores (e.g., cats, dogs, raccoons, sea otters, skunks), whereas asexual multiplication is limited to the presarcocyst meront stages, usually within the central nervous system in many other hosts, most characteristically horses, which many authors (Dubey et al., 2001a,b,c,d; Miller et al., 2009; Gjerde and Josefsen, 2015) consider as aberrant hosts rather than true intermediate hosts. Natural infections occur only in the Americas because the definitive hosts, opossums (*D. virginiana, D. albiventris, D. marsupialis*), are found there.

SARCOCYSTIS SPECIES

There are at least six reports of *Sarcocystis* sarcocysts in muscles or sporocysts in the feces of *P. lotor*, but no specific identification was made at the time of these surveys (see Chapter 19).

URSIDAE FISCHER DE WALDHEIM, 1817

GENUS *HELARCTOS* HORSFIELD, 1825 (MONOTYPIC)

SARCOCYSTIS SPECIES

There is a single report of *Sarcocystis* sarcocysts being found in the diaphragm, but not in the tongue, esophagus, heart, or skeletal muscles, of one *Helarctos malayanus* in a zoo in Korea, but no definitive identification was made at the time (see Chapter 19).

GENUS *URSUS* L., 1758 (4 SPECIES)

SARCOCYSTIS CANIS DUBEY AND SPEER, 1991

Intermediate hosts: *Ursus americanus* Pallas, 1780, American Black Bear; *Ursus maritimus* Phipps, 1774, Polar Bear.

Remarks: Dubey et al. (2006) retrospectively examined *S. canis*-like meronts in the liver of a black bear (*U. americanus*) and of two polar bears (*U. maritimus*) by sequencing both conserved (18S) and variable (ITS-1) portions of nuclear rDNA; they found a "genetic signature" that they said was "provisionally representative of *S. canis*."

SARCOCYSTIS URSUSI DUBEY, HUMPHREYS, AND FRITZ, 2008a

For light and electron micrographs of tissue cysts and zoites of this species see Figs. 1–3 in Dubey et al. (2008a).

Definitive type host: Unknown.

Type locality: North America: USA: Pennsylvania.

Intermediate type host: *Ursus americanus* Pallas, 1780, American Black Bear.

Other intermediate hosts: Unknown.

Geographic distribution: North America: USA: Pennsylvania.

Description of sporulated oocyst: Unknown.

Description of sporocyst and sporozoites: Unknown.

Prevalence: Sarcocysts of this species were found in 2/374 (~0.5%) black bears legally shot in Pennsylvania, but only one cyst was found in each bear.

Sporulation: Unknown, but almost certainly endogenous with sporulated, infective sporocysts shed in the feces of the definitive host.

Prepatent and patent periods: Unknown.

Site of infection, definitive host: Unknown.

Site of infection, intermediate host: Sarcocysts were found in skeletal musculature of *U. americanus* and only one sarcocyst was found in each of two bears.

Endogenous stages, definitive host: Unknown.

Endogenous stages, intermediate host: Sarcocysts were microscopic and contained only bradyzoites. The sarcocyst wall was thin (<0.5) and had minute serrations. Ultrastructurally, the serrations on the sarcocyst wall consisted of villar protrusions that were 0.5 long and had bundles of electron-dense microtubules that were as wide as long. The microtubules extended deep into the ground substance layer, a feature that distinguished this species from other unnamed sarcocysts from the black bear. Bradyzoites were 4.6–6.0 long.

Cross-transmission: None to date.

Pathology: Unknown.

Materials deposited: Two histological sections were deposited as syntypes for bears Nos. 1, 2 in the USNPC, Nos. 10101, 10102 and one slide of stained sections from bear No. 3 was deposited as a voucher specimen as USNPC No. 10103.

Remarks: Sarcocysts from the two black bears in this study were distinct from the unnamed species previously reported from black bears by Dubey et al. (1998b) in that its sarcocyst wall had villar protrusions that were about 2 long and lacked microtubules. Dubey et al. (2015a) listed this as a valid species (their Tables 24.1 and 24.4) and provided additional information (their Tables 1.2 and 19.1).

SARCOCYSTIS SPECIES

There are at least five reports of *Sarcocystis* sarcocysts in various muscles of both *U. americana* and *U. maritimus*, but no specific identifications was made at the time of these surveys (see Chapter 19).

SUBORDER FELIFORMIA KRETZOI, 1945

FELIDAE FISCHER DE WALDHEIM, 1817

SUBFAMILY FELINAE FISCHER DE WALDHEIM, 1817

GENUS ACINONYX BROOKES, 1828 (MONOTYPIC)

SARCOCYSTIS FELIS DUBEY, HAMIR, KIRKPATRICK, TODD, AND RUPPRECHT, 1992b

Intermediate host: *Acinonyx jubatus* (Schreber, 1775), Cheetah.

Remarks: For more complete information on *S. felis*, see Genus *Lynx*, below.

GENUS *FELIS* L., 1758
(7 SPECIES)

SARCOCYSTIS BOVIFELIS HEYDORN, GESTRICH, MEHLHORN, AND ROMMEL, 1975b

Definitive host: *Felis catus* L., 1758, Domestic Cat.

Intermediate hosts: *Bos frsontalis* Lambert, 1804, Gaur; *Bos javanicus* d'Alton, 1823, Banteng; *Bos taurus*, L., 1758, Aurochs; *Bison bonasus* (L., 1758), European Bison; *Bison bison* (L., 1758), American Bison.

Geographic distribution: Europe: Germany. Probably worldwide.

Remarks: Levine and Ivens (1981), Levine (1986), Odening (1998), and Dubey et al. (2015a) did not consider *S. bovifelis* to be a valid species name; rather, it is considered by most to be a junior synonym of *S. hirsuta*. However, Gjerde (2016a) did a thorough review of the literature, especially papers comprising TEM photomicrographs of thick-walled sarcocysts in cattle and found that (in the late 1980s) the cat-transmitted *S. bovifelis*, after having been renamed *S. hirsuta*, was erroneously synonymised with a second cat-transmitted species in cattle, allowing the name to slide into obscurity. Subsequently, *S. hirsuta* was used consistently for the second cat-transmitted taxon in cattle. In his literature review, Gjerde (2016a) discovered that *S. bovifelis* is morphologically indistinguishable from a species described from water buffalo as *S. sinensis* (Zuo et al., 1995) and that indistinguishable sarcocysts also have been found in cattle in New Zealand and Canada. For the sake of nomenclatural stability, Gjerde (2016a) suggested we should continue to use the name *S. hirsuta* for the taxon-forming macroscopic sarcocysts, and the name *S. bovifelis* for the species with microscopic cysts originally described from cattle by Gestrich et al. (1975) and Heydorn et al. (1975b), "as well as for morphologically indistinguishable taxa reported from cattle under the names *S. sinensis* (Moré et al., 2014) and *S. rommeli* (Dubey et al., 2016b)." Gjerde (2016a) concluded his argument by suggesting that *if* the *S. bovifelis*-like taxon in water buffalo is genetically different from *S. bovifelis*, then the name *S. sinensis* should be used for that taxon.

SARCOCYSTIS BUFFALONIS HUONG, DUBEY, NIKKILÄ, AND UGGLA, 1997a

A photomicrograph of a sporulated oocyst (Fig. 10) and an isolated sporocyst (Fig. 11) of *S. buffalonis*, along with LM (Figs. 1 and 2) and TEM micrographs (Figs. 3–9) of sarcocysts are found in Huong et al. (1997a,b).

Synonym: *Sarcocystis levinei* Dissanaike and Kan, 1978, *ex parte*.

Definitive type host: *Felis catus* L., 1758, Domestic Cat.

Other definitive hosts: Unknown.

Type locality: Asia: Vietnam, Ho Chi Minh City.

Intermediate type host: *Bubalus bubalis* (L., 1758), Water Buffalo.

Other intermediate hosts: Unknown.

Geographic distribution: Africa: Egypt; Asia: Vietnam; Middle East: Iran.

Description of sporulated oocyst: Oocyst shape: irregular, with one thin wall; L × W (n = 10, partially-sporulated): 16 × 13; L/W ratio, 1.2; M, OR, PG: all absent. Distinctive features of oocyst: typical thin-walled *Sarcocystis*-type, which usually breaks down releasing sporocysts into the intestinal lumen.

Description of sporocyst and sporozoites: Sporocyst shape: ellipsoidal; L × W: 13 × 8 (12.5–13.5 × 7.5–9.5); L/W ratio: 1.5; SB, SSB, PSB: all absent; SR: present; SR characteristics: subsphe-roidal mass of large granules that occupy about 50% of space in SP (Figs. 10 and 11 in Huong et al., 1997a); SZ: not described but appear to be sausage-shaped, about as long as SP. Distinctive features of sporocyst: none; a "typi-cal" *Sarcocystis*-type SP, lacking SB, SSB, PSB and with a distinct, granular SR.

Prevalence: Huong et al. (1997a) said sarco-cysts were found grossly in 68/647 (10.5%) adult water buffalo carcasses examined dur-ing 1992–95 at three abattoirs in Ho Chi Minh City, Vietnam, and Huong (1999) found this spe-cies in 131/396 (33%) water buffalo in Vietnam between 1996 and 1997. Oryan et al. (2010) found it in 3/100 (3%) water buffalo slaughtered in Khuzestan, Iran. Dubey et al. (2015a) also said this species was found in buffalo in Egypt.

Sporulation: Endogenous with sporulated, infective sporocysts shed in the feces of the definitive host.

Prepatent and patent periods: Prepatent period was 10 days in 2/7 (28.5%) cats fed isolated sar-cocysts of this species.

Site of infection, definitive host: Unknown, but likely the intestinal epithelium of the cat.

Site of infection, intermediate host: Sarcocysts were found in muscle tissues including scapular, cervical, abdominal, diaphragm, and esophagus and were found more often in skeletal muscles than in the esophagus, but they were never found in the tongue or heart (Huong et al., 1997a).

Endogenous stages, definitive host: Unknown.

Endogenous stages, intermediate host: Sarcocysts were L × W: 1–8 mm × 0.1–0.5 mm; under LM the cyst wall was 3–8 thick, and appeared radially-striated. With TEM the cyst wall had palisade-like villar protrusions up to 12 long, constricted at their base, expanded laterally in mid-section, and tapered distally. These protrusions contained microfilaments and dense granules. Bradyzoites were L × W: 10–13 × 2.6–3.2.

Cross-transmission: In their first experiment, Huong et al. (1997a) infected four cats and four dogs, all about 2-weeks-old, with 50 isolated sarcocysts of the type under investigation. One other cat was fed 250 sarcocysts, and feces from all animals were collected on the day after inoc-ulation and from 7 to 30 DPI. In their second experiment, two specific pathogen-free female cats were fed 260 isolated sarcocysts. Only 1/5 (20%) cats in experiment 1 shed sporulated oocysts and sporocysts of *Sarcocystis* 10 DPI; in the second experiment, 1/2 (50%) cats had oocysts and sporocysts of *Sarcocystis* in its intes-tines. None of the four dogs shed oocysts or sporocysts.

Pathology: Unknown.

Materials deposited: Histological sections of sarcocysts in the USNPC as No. 86878.

Remarks: Huong et al. (1997a) said that the low infectivity of *S. buffalonis* to cats is not surprising because this phenomenon is often observed with cat-borne species of *Sarcocystis* (Dubey et al., 1989b). Sarcocysts of this species were distinguished from those of *S. fusiformis* by their location, gross appearance, and struc-ture. These sarcocysts are up to 8 mm long and appear as white threads under the perimysial connective tissue along the longitudinal axis of the myocytes and they sometimes have a twisted or curved appearance when underlying muscle fibers contract postmortem. *Sarcocystis fusiformis* sarcocysts also were found by Huong et al. (1997a), but they were 3–38 mm long, appearing to resemble cucumber seeds, were common in the esophagus and less frequent in skeletal mus-cles, and were not embedded deeply into the host tissue. Odening (1998) believed this species was probably a synonym of *S. hirsuta* because of the similarity of its type 28 (Dubey et al., 1989a) sarcocysts. Dubey et al. (2015a) summarized some of the morphological and geographical data (their Tables 10.1 and 10.2). Natural infec-tions with *Sarcocystis* species in water buffalo are quite frequent.

SARCOCYSTIS CAPRIFELIS EL-RAFAII, ABDEL-BAKI, AND SELIM, 1980

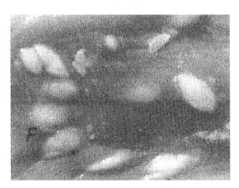

FIGURE 15.4 Photomicrograph of the large sarcocysts of *Sarcocystis caprifelis* in the esophagus of an Iraq goat. *From Barham, M., Stützer, H., Karanis, P., Latif, B.M., Neiss, W.F., 2005. Seasonal variation in* Sarcocystis *species infections in goats in northern Iraq. Parasitology 130 (2), 151–156, copyright by Parasitology, used with permission.*

Definitive host: *Felis catus* L., 1758, Domestic Cat.

Intermediate host: *Capra hircus* L., 1758, Goat.

Geographic distribution: Africa: Egypt; Middle East: Iraq.

Remarks: El-Rafaii et al. (1980) first reported sarcocysts in goats from Egypt. Levine (1986) listed this species as a parasite in which goats have sarcocysts in their muscles and cats are the definitive host. However, Dubey et al. (2014) said there are only three distinct species of *Sarcocystis* in goats, *S. capracanis* and *S. hircicanis* with canids as definitive hosts, and *S. moulei* with felids as definitive hosts. They reiterated this a year later (Dubey et al., 2015a) saying again that these are the only three species of *Sarcocystis* in domestic goats. *Sarcocysstis caprifelis* was not mentioned in either Odening (1998) or in Dubey et al. (2015a). Barham et al. (2005) presented the first photomicrographs of the large sarcocysts of *S. caprifelis* they found (mostly) in the esophagus of goats in Iraq. Barham et al. (2005) found this species in 278/826 (34%) goats slaughtered in

northern Iraq; the highest specificity of infection was 275/278 (99%) in the esophagus with similar cysts found in the skeletal muscles (12/278, 4%) and diaphragm (7/278, 2.5%) to a much lesser degree. These "fat" cysts measured L × W: 6.2 × 3.8 mm (2–17 × 2–7 mm) and were "fully-packed" with banana-shaped bradyzoites that were L × W: 14.1 × 4.5 (11–17 × 3–6).

SARCOCYSTIS CUNICULORUM (BRUMPT, 1913) ODENING, WESEMEIER, AND BOCKHARDT, 1996b

Synonym: *Sarcocystis cuniculi* Brumpt, 1913.

Definitive host: *Felis catus* L., 1758, Domestic Cat (experimental).

Intermediate hosts: *Oryctolagus cuniculus* (L., 1758), European (domestic) Rabbit; *Lepus europaeus* Pallas, 1778, European Hare; *Lepus timidus* L., 1758, Mountain Hare (?).

Geographic distribution: Probably worldwide.

Remarks: Brumpt (1913) placed all sarcosporidia then known into the genus *Sarcocystis* and listed *S. cuniculi* as the correct binomial of this species, whereas Levine (1986) said the correct binomial was *S. cuniculi* Brumpt, 1913 of Babudieri (1932). The former author said this species was found in the muscles of the domestic rabbit, *Lepus domesticus* (syn. *O. cuniculus*) and in *L. timidus*, the mountain hare, whereas Levine (1986) only listed *O. cuniculus* as an intermediate host. Levine and Ivens (1981) documented sporocyst structure from feces, and merogony in rabbit muscles as developing sarcocysts; they also reported that Tadros and Laarman (1977) were unable to infect a dog, a hand-reared fox, *V. vulpes*, a weasel, *Mu. nivalis*, or a kestrel, *Falco tinnunculus*, by feeding them sarcocysts in rabbit muscle. Levine (1986) named this one of the 122 *Sarcocystis* species he said were valid species, whereas Odening et al. (1996b) and Odening (1998) said that *S. cuniculi* was, in fact, a nomen nudum and corrected the name to *S. cuniculorum*. Duszynski and Couch (2013) summarized the biology and most other information known about this species (but using the name *S. cuniculi*), including the contribution by Černá et al. (1981), who found that 43/117 (37%) domestic rabbits in the Czech Republic had antibodies to *Sarcocystis* (using the indirect immunofluorescent antibody test) and did experimental cross-infection studies from rabbit to cat and back to rabbit to satisfy Koch's postulates. Dubey et al.'s (2015a) thorough review of the *Sarcocystis* literature mentioned *S. cuniculi* four separate times (their Tables 1.4, 15.2, and 21.4) summarizing intermediate host, sarcocyst size, and other limited knowledge about this species. However, they also pointed out that the species name with Brumpt, 1913 was invalid (Table 24.3) and that the mensural data available could only be attributed to an unnamed *Sarcocystis* species; however, the work by Odening et al. (1996b) seems to have resolved that problem.

SARCOCYSTIS CYMRUENSIS ASHFORD, 1978

Synonym: *Sarcocystis rodentifelis* Grikienienė Arnastauskienė and Kutkienė, 1993.

Definitive host: *Felis catus* L., 1758, Domestic Cat.

Intermediate hosts: *Bandicota indica* (Bechstein, 1800), Greater Bandicoot Rat; *Rattus norvegicus* (Berkenhout, 1769), Brown Rat; *Rattus rattus* (L., 1758), Roof Rat; *Rattus tanezumi* Temminck, 1844, (syn. *Rattus flavipectus* (Milne-Edwards, 1872)), Oriental House Rat; *Myodes glareolus* (Schreber, 1780) (syn. *Clethrionomys glareolus*), Bank Vole.

Geographic distribution: Asia: China; Southeast Asia: Thailand; Europe: United Kingdom: Wales. Probably worldwide in distribution.

Remarks: Ashford (1978) studied rats and parts of rats (e.g., hind legs preserved in formalin) from Wales in the United Kingdom. Muscles with sarcocysts were fed to laboratory cats, ferrets (*Mustela putorius*), and dogs. Ashford (1978) said sporulated sporocysts, L × W: 10.5 × 7.9,

with a distinct SR were passed in the feces of cats only but not the dog or the ferret. Atkinson (1978) reported finding sarcocysts of this species in 1/5 (20%) wild *R. novegicus*, also in Wales. Feeding infected flesh to a cat resulted in gametogony taking place in the cat intestine and oocysts, L × W: 15 × 11; L/W ratio: 1.4, and sporocysts, L × W: 11 × 9; L/W ratio: 1.2, being discharged in cat feces. Atkinson (1978) said he found "free zoites" in the blood of a rat 11–15 days after feeding it oocysts and meronts (L × W: ~25 × 12) in the liver and lungs of a rat killed at 12 DPI. Ashford (1978) said that 3 months postingesting oocysts, the sarcocysts in rat muscles were not visible to the naked eye, being only 0.5 mm long, but that by 9-months postfeeding, sarcocysts could be up to 5 cm long. Ashford (1978) also said the prepatent period in cats was four or more days, but that patency could last up to 100 days. Because relatively few sporocysts are found in cat feces after eating sarcocysts, Ashford (1978) speculated the domestic cat might not be the "normal definitive host." Unfortunately, Atkinson's (1978) contribution was only an abstract, and a full publication never resulted, to our knowledge. Levine and Ivens (1981) added more detailed information from the only two papers on this species (Ashford, 1978; Atkinson, 1978) prior to their work, and Levine (1986) considered it a valid species. Jäkel et al. (1997) identified this species, for the first time in Southeast Asia from muscle sarcocysts in 11/56 (20%) bandicoot rats and in 6/36 (17%) wild *R. norvegicus* in Thailand. Both rat species were captured near human habitation, and Jäkel et al. (1997) said the parasite was likely transmitted to rats via cats. Odening (1998) included this species in his summary of 189 valid *Sarcocystis* species names, but also included *S. rodentifelis* (see Grikienienė et al., 1993) as a valid *Sarcocystis* species. However, we agree with Dubey et al. (2015a) who synonymized the two forms based on their indistinguishable morphological and biological characteristics, and its presumed low intermediate host specificity; Dubey et al. (2015a) also summarized all of the recent experimental work done since Levine's list (1986). Hu et al. (2011) added another rat, *R. tunezumi* (syn. *R. flavipectus*) to the intermediate host list, but they were not the first to suggest that rats were both intermediate and definitive hosts for *S. cymruensis*. Šlapeta et al. (2001) summarized the work of Grikienienė et al. (1993) that an alternative development occurs during which the cat (normal definitive host) is eliminated from the life cycle, and its role is replaced by the development of cystozoites into gamonts and oocyst/sporocysts within the intestine of the rat, an alternative definitive host! Koudela and Modrý (2000) described a similar life cycle for *S. muris* in mice. According to Dubey et al. (2015a), a number of studies have indicated that both *R. norvegicus* and *M. glareolus* are capable of circulating *S. cymruensis* among themselves, without the participation of the definitive host, the cat (Arnastauskienė and Grikienienė, 1989; Grikienienė and Arnastauskienė, 1992; Grikienienė, 1993; Kutkienė and Grikienienė, 1993). How cool is this information and who will be the next to discover similar cycles in other *Sarcocystis* life histories? Or, maybe someone will discover new twists that these parasites have evolved to continue their development and success in their intermediate and definitive hosts that we still do not comprehend? And there is even more adventure.

It seems particularly interesting and certainly worth much more research that this species may be transmissible by cannibalism (Kutkienė and Grikienienė, 1995; 2003); for example, Kutkienė and Grikienienė (1998) said that they infected dams in their first or last week of pregnancy with rat muscle "heavily laden with sarcocysts," and their offspring were "found to harbour infections at 51% and 91%, respectively." However, Kutkienė and Grikienienė (2003), after further experimentation, said, "transplacental transmission of the parasite was not established," and Dubey et al. (2015a) cautioned that other evidence suggested transplacental transmission may not be a particularly viable or efficient mechanism of transmission. Grikienienė and Kutkienė (1998) suggested that Norway rats can

act as both definitive and intermediate hosts, at least under certain laboratory conditions. To wit, they (Grikienienė and Kutkienė, 1998) infected Wistar Norway lab rats by feeding them ground skeletal muscles of other lab rats with high levels of sarcocysts in them. Grikienienė and Kutkienė (1998) reported that from 8 to 47 DPI, fully sporulated oocysts, and from 10 to 70 days postinfection, typical *Sarcocystis* sporocysts were found in mucosal scrapings and in the rest of the small intestine wall in 23/26 (88%) infected rats! The oocysts and sporocysts they measured were L × W (n = 58): 14.6 × 11.0 (14–16 × 9–12.5); L/W ratio: 1.3; and L × W (n = 58): 10.6 × 7.3 (9–12 × 7–8.5); L/W ratio: 1.45, respectively. This is the first record, according to Grikienienė and Kutkienė (1998), of finding oocysts and sarcocysts of the same *Sarcocystis* species in a rodent.

There is certainly a lot of interesting follow-up work to be done and much more yet to learn about the life cycles of all *Sarcocystis* species in carnivores. Dubey et al. (2015a) added additional mensural and life history data in their tables (Tables 1.2, 1.4, 1.5, 15.2, 21.2, 24.1, and 24.4) for *S. cymruensis*.

SARCOCYSTIS FELIS DUBEY, HAMIR, KIRKPATRICK, TODD, AND RUPPRECHT, 1992b

Intermediate host: *Felis catus* L., 1758, Domestic Cat.

Remarks: For more complete information on *S. felis*, see Genus *Lynx*, below.

SARCOCYSTIS FUSIFORMIS (RAILLIET, 1897) BERNARD AND BAUCHE, 1912

Synonyms: *Balbiania fusiformis* Railliet, 1897; *Balbiania siamensis* von Linstow, 1903; *Sarcocystis blanchardi* Doflein, 1901; *Sarcocystis siamensis* (von Linstow, 1903); *Sarcocystis bubali* Willey, Chalmers and Philip, 1904; *Sarcocystis babuli*

(A)   **(B)**

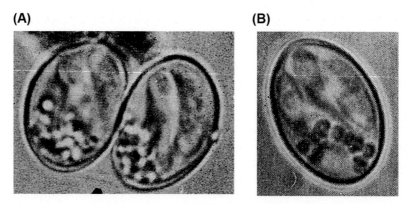

FIGURE 15.5   Photomicrographs of the (A) oocyst and (B) sporocyst, respectively, of *Sarcocystis fusiformis* in cat feces. *From Markus, M.B., Killick-Kendrick, R., Garnham, P.C.C., 1974b. The coccidial nature and life-cycle of* Sarcocystis. *Journal of Tropical Medicine and Hygiene 77 (11), 248–259, with permission of John Wiley and Sons, Inc., permission conveyed through the Copyright Clearance Center, Inc.*

Willey, Chalmers and Phillips, 1904 of Kalyakin and Zasuhin (1975) *lapsus calami*.

Definitive type host: *Felis catus* L., 1758, Domestic Cat.

Intermediate host: *Bubalus bubalis* (L., 1758), Water Buffalo.

Geographic distribution: Africa: Egypt; Asia: China; India; Philippines; Vietnam; Europe: Italy; Romania; Middle East: Iran; Turkey; South America: Brazil.

Remarks: Brumpt (1913) placed all sarcosporidia then known into the genus *Sarcocystis*, listed this species as *S. fusiformis* Railliet, 1897, and said that it was only found in the muscles of buffalo. Markus et al. (1974a) attempted infection of chimpanzees and cats with *Sarcocystis* of cattle. Levine and Ivens (1981) provided what information was known on oocyst and sporocyst structure and gamogony in the definitive host intestine and merogony and sarcocyst structure in the intermediate host muscles. They mentioned that the only cross-transmission study to that date (in a paper they apparently did not see) was by Dissanaike et al. (1977) who failed to infect four monkeys with sarcocysts from water buffalo. (Issues of the Southeast Asian Journal of Tropical Medicine and Public Health are available online, but

their archive only goes to December, 1991, Vol. 22, No. 4; thus, we also were unable to see the original published paper). Levine (1986) listed this species as one of the 122 names he considered as valid species of *Sarcocystis* at that time using the authorities given above, and Odening (1998) concurred. Dubey et al.'s (2015a) review of the literature mentioned *S. fusiformis* 39 times and summarized morphological, geographical, and other data (Tables 1.2, 1.4, 10.1, 10.2, 15.2, 23.1, 24.1, and 24.4). Natural infections with *Sarcocystis* species in water buffalo are quite frequent.

SARCOCYSTIS GIGANTEA (RAILLIET, 1886a,b) ASHFORD, 1977

Synonyms: *Balbiania gigantea* Railliet, 1886a,b; *Sarcocystis ovifelis* Heydorn, Gestrich, Melhlhorn, and Rommel, 1975b; *Sarcocystis tenella* (Railliet, 1886a,b) Moulé, 1886, *pro parte*; *Endorimospora tenella* (Railliet, 1886a,b) Tadros and Laarman, 1976 *pro parte*.

Definitive hosts: *Felis catus* L., 1758, Domestic Cat; *Vulpes vulpes* (L., 1758), Red or Silver Fox (experimental).

Intermediate hosts: *Ovis aries* L., 1758, Red Sheep; *Ovis canadensis* Shaw, 1804, Bighorn Sheep; *Capra hircus* L., 1758, Domestic Goat.

Geographic distribution: Australia: South Australia; Europe: Czech Republic; Slovakia; Spain; Middle East: Iran; Iraq; Jordan; Saudi Arabia; North America: USA: Michigan, Texas. Probably worldwide in its distribution.

Remarks: Ashford (1977) found macroscopic sarcocysts in the esophagi of naturally-infected sheep but did not examine the tissues histologically to determine if microscopic sarcocysts also were present. He fed these sheep esophagi to five live foxes trapped and collected from Wales and Exmoor and said that he successfully infected them eight times with sheep esophagi. Thus, he (Ashford, 1977) maintained that he was able to transmit *S. gigantea* to the red fox, but neither the domestic dog (Rommel et al., 1972) nor the laboratory rat (Aryeetey and Piekarski, 1976) can be infected with it. Levine and Ivens (1981) mentioned that the sexual stages occur in the lamina propria of villi of the small intestine of the cat and sarcocysts in the skeletal muscles of the wall of the sheep esophagus. This species is extremely common in sheep but rare in goats. Mehlhorn (1974), Mehlhorn and Scholtyseck (1973, 1974b), Porchet-Henneré and Ponchel (1994), Mehlhorn et al. (1976), and others have studied early merogony and the development and structure of the sarcocysts in sheep by both LM and TEM. Becker et al. (1979), Rommel et al. (1972, 1974), and Mehlhorn and Scholtyseck (1974a) described endogenous sexual stages in the cat and determined that the prepatent period is 11–12 DPI and patency can last 6–7 weeks, or longer. This species was listed in Levine's (1986) review of valid *Sarcocystis* species through 1985 and in Odening's (1998) list of valid species through 1997. Giannetto et al. (2005) used Dubey et al.'s (1989b) classification of 24 sarcocyst types to identify sarcocysts of this species (type 21) in 34/50 (68%) esophagus samples from sheep in Sicily, Italy. Dubey et al. (2015a) included sarcocyst structure, life cycle information known to date, and pathogenicity (mild).

SARCOCYSTIS HIRSUTA MOULÉ, 1888

Synonyms: *Endorimospora cruzi* (Hasselmann, 1926) Tadros and Laarman, 1976; *Miescheria cruzi* Hasselmann, 1923, *pro parte*; *Sarcocystis fusiformis* Railliet, 1897 of Babudieri (1932) and *auctores*, *pro parte*; *Sarcocystis marcovi* Vershinin, 1975 *pro parte*; *Sarcocystis bovifelis* Heydorn, Gestrich, Mehlhorn, and Rommel, 1975b; large form of *Isospora bigemina* of Gestrich, Mehlhorn, and Heydorn, 1975.

Definitive hosts: *Felis catus* L., 1758, Domestic Cat; *Felis silvestris* Schreber, 1777, Wildcat.

Intermediate hosts: *Bos frontalis* Lambert, 1804, Gaur; *Bos javanicus* d'Alton, 1823, Banteng; *Bos taurus*, L., 1758, Aurochs; *Bison bonasus* (L., 1758), European Bison; *Bison bison* (L., 1758), American Bison.

Geographic distribution: Africa: Egypt; Asia: India; Japan; Thailand; Vietnam; Europe: Belgium; Czech Republic; Germany; Italy; Lithuania; Middle East: Iran; Turkey; New Zealand; South America: Argentina; Brazil, Uruguay. Probably worldwide in its distribution.

Remarks: Brumpt (1913) placed all sarcosporidia then known into the genus *Sarcocystis* and listed this species as *S. hirsuta* Moulé, whereas Levine (1986) added the date to the authority. Brumpt (1913) said that the cysts were "in the connective tissue of the ox and buffalo and were probably identical to *S. blanchardi* Doflein, 1901 (now a synonym of *S. fusiformis*) and *S. bubali*" (did he mean *S. buvalis* Dogel, 1916 from *Alcelphus buselaphus* (Pallas, 1766), Coke's Hartebeest?). Dubey (1976) pointed out that *S. hirsuta* is nonpathogenic for cattle. Levine and Ivens (1981) reviewed most of the known biology on this species including oocyst structure and sporulation, prevalence in various surveys, merogony in the intermediate host, gamogony in the definitive host, prepatent and patent periods in the definitive host, pathogenicity in calves (slight), and cross-transmission studies done to that date (1981). Levine (1986) listed *S. hirsuta* as one of 122 valid species of *Sarcocystis* covered in his review. Odening (1998) also listed this form as one of the 189 *Sarcocystis* species in his review and he suggested that the European hare, *L. europaeus*, might be an accidental host from time to time. Dubey et al. (2015a) did a thorough review of the literature and covered much of what is known to date on the structure of sarcocysts in the intermediate host, the life cycle stages in the cat, and the pathogenicity in cattle. They also pointed out that because the sarcocysts are large and macroscopic, there is a large annual economic toll that results from the condemnation of carcasses during meat inspections, especially those intended for human consumption.

Fischer and Odening (1998) isolated sarcocysts of *S. hirsuta* from two cattle (*B. taurus*) and compared sequenced PCR products of their 18S rRNA genes; sequences of both isolates from the same host species always showed a very high, nearly complete identity to each other both within all or only the conserved overlapping nucleotides, verifying they were the same species. However, over the last decade, most of the relevant work using both morphological studies at all levels (LM, TEM, SEM), and molecular amplification of several gene sequences (18S rRNA, 28S rRNA, ITS-1, *cox1*) of *Sarcocystis* spp. sarcocysts in various wild and domesticated Artiodactyla species, has been done in Norway, and a few other countries, by Gjerde et al. (Gjerde, 2012; 2013, 2014a,b,c; Gjerde and Josefsen, 2015; Gjerde, 2016a,b; Gjerde et al., 2017). Regarding this species, Gjerde reiterated that a cat-transmitted species, with microscopic sarcocysts, was initially named *S. bovifelis* (by Heydorn et al., 1975b), but the name was changed to *S. hirsuta* because it was considered to be identical to that previously named species that had priority (but which had marcoscopic sarcocysts). After thoroughly reviewing the literature of papers comprising TEM photomicrographs of thick-walled sarcocysts in cattle, he determined that the species *S. bovifelis* Heydorn et al. (1975b), as described from cattle

in Germany, was *S. sinensis*-like and indistinguishable sarcocysts had been found in cattle in New Zealand and Canada in the 1980s. In the New Zealand study, small sarcocysts were erroneously thought to represent early developmental stages of a species with ultrastructurally similar, but macroscopic sarcocysts because the macroscopic cysts were infective for cats. Gjerde (2016a) concluded that since the late 1980s, the cat-transmitted *S. bovifelis*, after having been named *S. hirsuta*, was erroneously synonymized with a second cat-transmitted species in cattle, and then the name slid into obscurity until recently being rediscovered as an *S. sinensis*-like species of cattle. Because the name *S. hirsuta* has consistently been used for the species with macroscopic sarcocysts, Gjerde suggested this usage be continued (Gjerde, 2016a). Gjerde (2016b) excised 200 individual sarcocysts from 12 beef cattle samples from five countries (Argentina, Brazil, Germany, New Zealand, Uruguay) and genomic DNA was extracted from 147 of these sarcocysts. Using PCR amplification and sequencing of the partial *cox1* gene and three regions of nuclear ribosomal DNA (complete 18S rRNA, complete ITS-1 region, and partial 28S rRNA gene), he compared results with previous molecular identifications to evaluate the regions for species delimitations and phylogenetic inferences. Based on his molecular characterizations, and sarcocyst morphology, 56 macroscopic sarcocysts (3–8 × 0.5), with finger-like protrusions, were assigned to *S. hirsuta*; these sarcocysts of *S. hirsuta* came from beef samples from Argentina, Brazil, Germany, and New Zealand.

SARCOCYSTIS HORVATHI RÁTZ, 1908

Definitive host: *Felis catus* L., 1758, Domestic Cat (Golubkov, 1979) (?).

Remarks: For more complete information on *S. horvathi*, see Genus *Canis*, above.

SARCOCYSTIS MEDUSIFORMIS COLLINS, ATKINSON, AND CHARLESTON, 1979

Definitive host: *Felis catus* L., 1758, Domestic Cat.

Intermediate hosts: *Ovis aries* L., 1758, Red Sheep; *Ovis ammon* (L., 1758), Argali.

Geographic distribution: Australia: South Australia; Europe: Spain; Middle East: Iran; Jordan; New Zealand.

Remarks: Levine and Ivens (1981) did not include this species in their first treatise on the coccidian parasites of carnivores, but Levine (1986) listed *S. horvathi* as one of the valid named species of *Sarcocystis*. Odening (1998) in his compilation of *Sarcocystis* names also listed this as a valid species and noted that the sarcocyst was a TEM type 20 (as per Dubey et al., 1989b). Dubey et al. (2015a) noted that sheep have four universally recognized species of *Sarcocystis* in their muscles as sarcocysts: *S. tenella*, *S. arieticanis*, *S. medusiformis*, and *S. gigantea*. Of these, *S. tenella* and *S. arieticanis*, transmitted via canids, are pathogenic, whereas *S. gigantea* and *S. medusiformis*, transmitted via cats, are nonpathogenic. Dubey et al. (2015a) pointed out how little is really known about the biology and structure of *S. medusiformis*. The sarcocysts are relatively small, ~8 × 0.2 mm, with a very thin wall (<2 μm) and do not attain their maximum length (15 mm) in their hosts until they are approximately 4-years-old; thus, little is known about development in the intermediate host and nothing about the endogenous development in the definitive host except that after eating flesh with sarcocysts, cats will excrete sporocysts in 15–30 DPI (prepatent period).

SARCOCYSTIS MOULEI NEVEU-LEMAIRE, 1912

Synonym: *Sarcocystis orientalis* Matschoulsky and Miskaryan, 1958 (?).

Definitive host: *Felis catus* L., 1758, Domestic Cat.

Intermediate host: *Capra hircus* L., 1758, Goat.

Geographic distribution: Africa; Asia; Europe; Middle East: Iran.

Remarks: Brumpt (1913) placed all sarcosporidia then known into the genus *Sarcocystis*, listed this species as noted above, as did Levine (1986), and said that it was only found in muscles of the goat. Levine (1986) suggested that *S. orientalis* may be a synonym of this species, but he also said that the domestic dog, *C. l. familiaris*, was the definitive host, which it is not. Odening (1998) in his compilation of *Sarcocystis* names listed this as a valid species and noted that the sarcocyst was a TEM type 21 (cf. Dubey et al., 1989b); he also noted that this form was "similar to *S. gigantea* (sibling species), but separated from that species by intermediate host specificity and molecular genetic features." Dubey et al. (2015a) did their thorough review of the literature on this species and added good information on its structure and life history and its natural infection in goats. They (Dubey et al., 2015a) pointed out that when this species was originally described in Iran, there were two kinds of macroscopic sarcocysts found, fat sarcocysts only in the esophageal muscle and thin sarcocysts in the diaphragm and skeletal muscles; the former fat ones had slightly larger bradyzoites, L × W: 14.1 × 4.5 (11–17 × 3–6), than did the thinner sarcocysts, L × W: 12.2 × 2.9 (9–13 × 2–4). We believe it likely that these represent different species with the fat sarcocysts belonging to *S. moulei* and transmitted by cats.

SARCOCYSTIS MURIS (RAILLIET, 1886a) LABBÉ, 1899

Synonyms: *Miescheria muris* Blanchard, 1885; *Miescheria muris* Railliet, 1885 of *auctores*; *Coccidium bigeminum* var. *cati* Railliet and Lucet, 1891; *Sarcocystis muris* (Blanchard, 1885) Labbé, 1899; *Lucetina cati* (Railliet and Lucet, 1891) Henry and Leblois, 1926; *Endorimospora muris* (Blanchard, 1885) Tadros and Laarman, 1976;

Sarcocystis musculi Blanchard, 1885 of Kalyakin and Zasukhin (1975) *lapsus calami*; probably *Isospora cati* (Railliet and Lucet, 1891); possibly *Cryptosporiodium* (sic) sp. Dubey and Pande, 1963b from *Felis chaus* (Levine and Ivens, 1981).

Definitive hosts: *Felis catus* L., 1758, Domestic Cat; *Mustela* (syn. *Putorius*) *putorius furo* (L., 1758), European Polecat/Domestic Ferret; possibly *Felis chaus* Schreber, 1777, Jungle Cat (see Levine and Ivens, 1981, p. 122, regarding misidentification by Dubey and Pande, 1963b).

Intermediate host: *Mus musculus* L., 1758, House Mouse.

Geographic distribution: Africa: Egypt; Europe: France, Switzerland; Central America: Costa Rica. Probably distributed worldwide.

Remarks: This was the first species of *Sarcocystis* ever found when its sarcocysts were discovered in the muscles of mice caught in his home by Professor Friedrich Miescher in Basel, Switzerland (Miescher, 1843). Brumpt (1913) placed all sarcosporidia then known into the genus *Sarcocystis* and listed this species as *S. muris* R. Blanchard, 1885. He said it was a common muscle parasite in some mouse breeding (colonies?), was widespread in older animals, and could be found in wild or domestic mice and rats; the latter host still has not been verified to our knowledge. Ruiz and Frenkel (1976) were the first to take sarcocysts obtained from both lab and house mice and transmit the parasite experimentally to cats. They said that the bradyzoites from the sarcocyst developed directly into gametes in the intestinal mucosa of cats, and they defined the prepatent and patent periods in cats and the size of sporocysts shed in the feces, and they determined that sporozoites from infective sporocysts multiplied first in the livers and then in the skeletal muscles of mice and that in heavy infections sarcocysts could be seen to outline the major muscle groups of mice. Sarcocysts in mice required approximately 76 days of development before becoming infective for cats. Fayer and Frenkel (1979) inoculated either 50× or 120 × 10³ sporocysts of *S. muris* into

two calves, but calves remained normal even though one calf had an increase in antibody to *S. muris*. When calves were killed 76 and 91 DPI, and their tissues ground and fed to coccidiafree cats, the cats did not produce sporocysts. Levine and Ivens (1981) discussed the possibility of other intermediate hosts, but thought this unlikely, given the contradictory experimental evidence available (see Ruiz and Frenkel, 1976). McKenna and Charleston (1980b) found sarcocysts in the skeletal muscles of mice that had been inoculated with sporocysts they recovered from the feces of naturally-infected cats. Kittens fed these mice shed similar sporocysts that measured, L × W: 10.8 × 8.7; L/W ratio: 1.2. They then fed these sporocysts to mice and rats that resulted in the formation of sarcocysts in the muscles of mice, but not in rats. Levine and Ivens (1981) also summarized the knowledge known at that time on the endogenous stages in the lamina propria of the cat intestine, including the structure of oocysts and sporocysts, prepatent and patent period information regarding oocyst/sporocyst discharge, and merogony and sarcocyst development in mouse muscles, and noted that this species was not pathogenic for the cat but it was for the mouse. Woodmansee and Powell (1984) were unable to infect six meadow voles (*Microtus pennsylvanicus*) and six gerbils (*Meriones unguiculatus*) when they were fed 50 *S. muris* sporocysts. Entzeroth (1984) used electron microscopy to study the penetration mechanism of *S. muris* into cultured dog kidney cells and into intestinal epithelial cells of a young kitten. Entzeroth et al. (1985) fed sarcocysts in skeletal tissues of *M. musculus* to seven kittens, killed them at 7, 10, 14, 24, 30, 36, and 48 hours postinfection and described the gamogony of *S. muris* at the TEM level. Levine (1986) listed this species as one of the 122 names he considered as valid species of *Sarcocystis* at that time using the authorities given above. Odening (1998), in his compilation of *Sarcocystis* names, also listed this as a valid species and noted that the sarcocyst was a TEM type 1 (cf. Dubey et al.,

1989b). Dubey et al.'s (2015a) thorough review of the literature mentioned *S. muris* 112 times and provides information on: the structure of sarcocysts in mouse muscles; gametogenesis in the dog intestine; the ultrastructure and antigenic property of its bradyzoites; the experimental transmission of *S. muris* by ferrets (see Ruiz and Frenkel, 1976; Rommel, 1979); transmission to immunocompetent/immunocompromised mice (Al-Kappany et al., 2013); the four phases of infections that include sporozoite migration (2–10 DPI), merogony (11–17 DPI), merozoite migration (18–27 DPI), and sarcocyst formation (28–50 DPI); the value of *S. muris* as a laboratory model to study processes that may be applicable to other *Sarcocystis* species (Rommel et al., 1981); and the life cycle and timing of parasite development (merogony) in the mouse.

Perhaps the most interesting aspect of the life cycle work on this species is that by Koudela and Modrý (2000), who described a life cycle for *S. muris* in mice similar to that already noted for *S. cymruensis* (syn. *S. rodentifelis*) (above), that an alternative development occurs during which the cat (normal definitive host) is eliminated from the life cycle and its role is replaced by the development of cystozoites into gamonts and oocyst/sporocysts within the intestine of the mouse, an alternative definitive host! Various investigators have tried to transmit this species to the Norway rat (*Rattus norvegicus*), golden hamster (*Mesocricetus auratus*), guinea pigs (*Cavia porcellus*), meadow voles (*Microtus pennsylvanicus*), and Mongolian jirds (*Meriones unguiculatus*), all with negative results (Ruiz and Frenkel, 1976; McKenna and Charleston, 1980b; Woodmansee and Powell, 1984).

SARCOCYSTIS ODOI DUBEY AND LOZIER, 1983

A photomicrograph of a sporulated oocyst (Fig. 11), four LM sections of sarcocysts (Figs. 1–4), and six TEM photomicrographs of sarcocysts *S. odoi* (Figs. 5–10) are found in Dubey and Lozier (1983).

Definitive host: Felis catus L., 1758, Domestic Cat.

Intermediate host: Odocoileus virginianus (Zimmermann, 1780), White-tailed Deer.

Geographic distribution: North America: USA: Montana.

Remarks: Dubey and Lozier (1983) described sarcocysts infecting a white-tailed deer in Montana, USA and named it *S. odoi*. They diagnosed 27/36 (75%) *O. virginianus*, with two structurally distinct types of sarcocysts, one thin-walled and one thick-walled. They identified the thin-walled sarcocysts as *S. odocoileocanis* and named the thick-walled sarcocysts *S. odoi*. These sarcocysts measured L × W (n = 6): 655 × 137 (260–1,050 × 70–260); the thick sarcocyst wall measured 6.5 to 12 wide. A cat fed deer meat with both thin- and thick-walled sarcocysts shed oocysts and sporocysts 24 DPI; sporulated oocysts were L × W (n = 37): 18 × 14 (16–21 × 12.5–16), L/W ratio: 1.3; and sporocysts were L × W (n = 73): 13.3 × 9.6 (11–15 × 9–11), L/W ratio: 1.4, both measured from intestinal scrapings of the infected cat. Sporocysts found in the cat's feces were slightly smaller, L × W (n = 10): 12 × 9 (11–15 × 7–11); L/W ratio: 1.3. Levine (1986) listed *S. odoi* as one of 122 valid species of *Sarcocystis* covered in his review. Odening (1998), in his compilation of 189 *Sarcocystis* names, also listed this as a valid species; he noted that, initially, the sarcocyst was a TEM type 10 (cf. Dubey et al., 1989b), but as more information came to light he classified it as a TEM type 10/15/16. Odening (1998) also pointed out that *S. odoi* was similar to the *Sarcocystis* sp. of Dubey and Lozier (1983) with a TEM type 15, and to the *Sarcocystis* sp. type III of Atkinson et al. (1993), both from *O. virginianus*, as well as to *S. hemioni* and *S. youngi* from *O. hemionus* in North America, and to *S. hofmanni/S. tarandi* in the Palearctic. Dubey et al. (2015a) did a thorough review of the literature and listed the TEM wall as type 10a (their Table 1.2), and in their Fig. 1.45B, they mentioned that the *S. odoi* sarcocyst wall is type 10a, but similar to type 9a, with tightly packed villar protrusions. Bradyzoites measured, L × W: 9.5–12.5 × 2.4–3.5 (their Table 18.1). They (2015a) also listed this as a valid species (their Tables 24.1 and 24.4).

SARCOCYSTIS PECKAI ODENING, 1997

Definitive host: *Felis catus* L., 1758, Domestic Cat (?).

Remarks: For more complete information on *S. peckai*, see Genus *Canis*, above.

SARCOCYSTIS POEPHAGI WEI, CHANG, DONG, WANG, AND XIA, 1985

Definitive type host: *Felis catus* L., 1758, Domestic Cat.

Type locality: Asia: China.

Other definitive hosts: Unknown.

Intermediate type host: *Bos grunniens* L., 1766 (syn. *Poephagus grunniens* Gray, 1843), Yak.

Other intermediate hosts: Unknown.

Geographic distribution: Asia: China.

Description of sporulated oocyst: Not available.

Description of sporocyst and sporozoites: Sporocyst shape: spheroidal to ovoidal; L × W: 13.7 × 9.4 (9–16 × 7–13); L/W ratio: 1.5; SB, SSB, PSB: all absent; SR: present; SR characteristics: not mentioned; SZ: not mentioned. Distinctive features of sporocyst: none; a "typical" *Sarcocystis*-type SP, lacking SB, SSB, PSB and with a distinct, granular SR.

Prevalence: Unknown.

Sporulation: Unknown, but likely endogenous with sporulated, infective sporocysts shed in the feces of the definitive host.

Prepatent and patent periods: Prepatent period in kittens is 7–10 days and the patent period lasted for 8–12 days.

Site of infection, definitive host: Unknown.

Site of infection, intermediate host: Striated muscles.

Endogenous stages, definitive host: Unknown.

Endogenous stages, intermediate host: Sarcocysts were macroscopic, fusiform, with a wall ~4 mm thick and a secondary wall 7.4 μm wide; SEM showed that the sarcocyst wall had a tree bark–like appearance (Wei et al., 1985). Bradyzoites were not measured.

Cross-transmission: Wei et al. (1990) tried to infect 20 domestic puppies, *C. l. familiaris*, with 4,000 individual sarcocysts dissected from yaks, but the dogs never passed oocysts in their feces; on the other hand, they fed 4,000 individual sarcocysts dissected from yaks to 10 oocyst-free kittens and detected sporocysts in their feces. Wei et al. (1990) also experimentally infected white rats, mice, guinea pigs, domestic rabbits, and chicks with sarcocysts from yaks, but no sporocysts were ever detected in fecal examinations. Finally, they (1990) then infected all of the above animals with sporocysts (from their cats), but no sarcocysts were detected in the muscles of all animals in necropsy 90 DPI with the sporocysts.

Pathology: Unknown.

Materials deposited: None.

Remarks: Levine (1986) did not include this species in his list of valid *Sarcocystis* species. Odening (1998) listed this species name in his compilation of 189 *Sarcocystis* named species but did not know the cat had been implicated as the definitive host. Dubey et al. (2015a) cited it as a valid species from the cat and mentioned it five times (their Tables 1.4, 15.2, 18.2, 24.1, and 24.4). We had Wei et al.'s (1990) paper translated by colleagues in China, and the measurements of sporocysts in cat feces are those given above; however, Dubey et al. (2015a) listed sporocyst size for this species to be L × W: 20.8–25.7 × 15.9–22.4 (their Table 15.2) and then listed cat oocysts of this species to be L × W: 13.7 × 9.4 (their Table 18.2), which actually is the size of the sporocysts reported by Wei et al. (1990). Stojecki et al. (2012) listed 32 species of *Sarcocystis* from selected domesticated intermediate hosts (mostly mammals, two birds), selecting names from Tenter (1995) with modifications of Elsheikha and Mansfield (2007) and Olias et al. (2009); definitive hosts were listed when they were known. They listed *S. poephagi* as a valid species but apparently had missed the paper by Wei et al. (1990) because they said the definitive host was unknown.

SARCOCYSTIS PORCIFELIS DUBEY, 1976

Synonym: *Sarcocystis miescheriana* (Kühn, 1865) Labbé, 1899.

Definitive host: *Felis catus* L., 1758, Domestic Cat.

Intermediate host: *Sus scrofa* L., 1758, Wild Boar.

Geographic distribution: Asia: India (?); Japan; (former) USSR; Eastern Europe: Lithuania, Romania. Possibly worldwide (Levine and Ivens, 1981).

Remarks: This species was named by Dubey (1976), based on the findings of Golubkov et al. (1974). Levine and Ivens (1981) mentioned that, at the time of their book, this species only had been found in the former USSR (by Golubkov et al., 1974), but speculated that it likely was found worldwide. They also provided what little information was known, to that date, on location of gametes in the cat intestine and on the prepatent and patent periods but not much else. Levine (1986) named this as one of the valid *Sarcocystis* species on his list of 122. Odening (1998), in his compilation of 189 *Sarcocystis* names, also listed this as a valid species. Dubey et al. (2015a), however, cast some doubt on the validity of this species. Initially, Dubey et al. (2015a) noted that Golubkov et al. (1974) apparently completed **Koch's postulates** when they fed *Sarcocystis*-infected pig esophagi to four cats, the cats excreted sporulated oocysts in 5–10 days, sporocysts from these cats were fed to eight littermate pigs, all piglets became ill, and sarcocysts were found in their skeletal muscles and hearts.

The sporocysts discharged by cats were L × W: 13.5 × 7.6, L/W ratio: 1.8, with SZs measuring L × W: 9.5 × 3.8, but the structure of the sarcocysts in pigs never were described. Dubey et al. (2015a) then summarized isolated findings of sarcocysts in pigs in Romania (Suteu and Mircean, 1996), Lithuania (Arnastauskienė, 1989), Japan (Ohino et al., 1993), and India (Bhatia, 1996), which might be *S. porcifelis*, and in one of these reports (Romania) two cats were fed infected pig meat, and both discharged sporocysts in their feces 9–13 DPI; the sporocysts were L × W: 14.5 × 8.9; L/W ratio: 1.6. So far, so good. Then, inexplicably to us, they wrote: "Note: *Sarcocystis* sporocysts have *never* (emphasis is ours) been reported in feces of cats fed pork. In a US national survey for *Toxoplasma gondii* infection, 2,049 samples of pork were fed to cats and feces of cats were examined for oocysts (Dubey et al., 2005); *Sarcocystis* sporocysts were not found (unpublished)." In other investigations sporocysts were not found in feces of cats fed *Sarcocystis*-infected pork from domestic pigs (Dubey, 1979a) or from wild pigs (Barrows et al., 1981).

SARCOCYSTIS ROMMELI DUBEY, MORÉ, VAN WILPE, CALERO-BERNAL, VERMA, AND SCHARES, 2016b

See LM of a sarcocyst (Fig. 1A), three sporocysts (Figs. 1D and E), and TEMs of the sarcocyst wall and villar protrusions (Figs. 1B and C) in Hu et al. (2017).

Definitive host: *Felis catus* L., 1758, Domestic Cat.

Type locality: Asia: China, Kunming City, southwestern China.

Other definitive hosts: None to date.

Intermediate type host: *Bos taurus* L., 1758, Aurochs.

Other intermediate hosts: None to date.

Geographic distribution: Asia: China.

Description of sporulated oocyst: Oocyst shape: not stated, but presumably with one thin membrane (wall) stretched over the two SP; L × W (n = 30, *in situ*): 17.1 × 12.3 (17–18 × 11.5–13); L/W ratio: 1.4; M, OR, PG: all absent. Distinctive features of oocyst: typical thin-walled *Sarcocystis*-type, which usually breaks down releasing sporocysts into the intestinal lumen.

Description of sporocyst and sporozoites: Sporocyst shape: ellipsoidal; L × W (n = 40): 12.0 × 7.8 (11–13 × 7–8); L/W ratio: 1.5; SB, SSB, PSB: all absent; SR: present; SR characteristics: a number of large globules as an irregular mass, sometimes obscuring a few SZ; SZ: sausage-shaped, L × W (n = 27): 8.7 × 2.0 (8–10 × 1.8–2.4). Distinctive features of sporocyst: none, a "typical" *Sarcocystis*-type SP, lacking SB, SSB, PSB and with a distinct, granular SR.

Prevalence: Sarcocysts of *S. rommeli* were found in 6/34 (18%) cattle in China by Hu et al. (2017); in reality, they purchased skeletal muscle samples from a farmer's market and believed that each sample represented a different animal.

Sporulation: Unknown, but likely endogenous with sporulated, infective sporocysts shed in the feces of the definitive host.

Prepatent and patent periods: The prepatent period in two experimentally-infected domestic cats was 14 and 15 DPI. Oocysts and sporocysts were still being shed in the feces when the experiment ended on 30 DPI, so the patent period lasts at least 15–16 days.

Site of infection, definitive host: Oocysts and sporocysts were found in epithelial cells of the intestinal mucosa, mostly concentrated toward the tips of the villi.

Site of infection, intermediate host: Skeletal muscles.

Endogenous stages, definitive host: Unknown.

Endogenous stages, intermediate host: Under LM, sarcocysts appeared striated, had thick walls, and possessed numerous slightly sloping villar protrusions that measured L × W (n = 40): 8.3 × 4.6. Mature sarcocysts were L × W (n = 30): 480–1,130 × 72–110, had septa, and contained many bradyzoites that measured L × W (n = 45): 9.5–14.3 × 3.2–4.8. Under TEM, the sarcocyst wall contained numerous villar protrusions (Vp) that were L × W (n = 21): 4.7–5.2 × 0.2–0.3, each about 0.3–0.5 apart from each other. The interior of the Vp was filled with microtubules that were dispersed and extended from the tip of the Vp to the middle of the ground substance layer.

Cross-transmission: 2/2 cats fed cattle muscle containing only *S. rommeli* sarcocysts both excreted oocysts/sporocysts.

Pathology: Unknown.

Materials deposited: Two 18S rRNA nucleotide sequences from a single sarcocyst (KY120284, KY120285) were submitted to GenBank, as was one mitochondrial *cox1* nucleotide sequence, 1,085-bp long (KY120286). Six mitochondrial *cox1* clones amplified from oocysts/sporocysts (KY120287-KY120292) also were submitted to GenBank.

Remarks: This species name was initially proposed by Dubey et al. (2016b) for the thick-walled *S. sinensis*-like sarcocysts found in cattle muscle, based on their assumption that *Sarcocystis* species of cattle and water buffalo should be specific to the intermediate host, even though there was little molecular evidence, and the definitive host was unknown at that time. Hu et al. (2017) found sarcocysts they were able to identify with this species in six samples of cattle skeletal muscle in China. Using LM and TEM they were able to identify sarcocysts in the muscle, feed cats isolated sarcocysts, and photograph and measure oocysts and sporocysts. Then, using PCR amplification, cloning, and sequencing techniques they isolated the near full-length 18S rRNA and partial mitochondrial *cox1* sequences. A BLAST search revealed a 98.7% identity and 99.2% identity with sequences of *S. bovini*. Partial *cox1* sequences from oocysts/sporocysts shared 99.4% and 99.5% identity with *cox1* sequences of *S. rommeli* and *S. bovini* sarcocysts, respectively. Their phylogenetic analysis confirmed that *S. rommeli* formed a clade with *S. bovini* and was within the same group comprising species of *Sarcocystis* that cycled between ruminant intermediate hosts and felid definitive hosts; i.e., *S. bovifelis* and *S. hirsuta* in cattle, *S. buffalonis*, *S. fusiformis*, and *S. sinensis* in water buffalo, and *S. gigantea* in sheep. The sarcocysts reported by Hu et al. (2017) were identical to those of *S. rommeli* and using sarcocysts to infect cats, Hu et al. (2017) were the first to identify the definitive host of *S. rommeli* from cattle.

SARCOCYSTIS WENZELI ODENING, 1997

Definitive host: *Felis catus* L., 1758, Domestic Cat (?).

Remarks: For more complete information on *S. wenzeli*, see Genus *Canis*, above.

SARCOCYSTIS SPECIES

There are about 19 reports of *Sarcocystis* sarcocysts in various muscles or sporocysts in the feces of *Felis* spp., but no specific identifications were made at the time of these surveys (see Chapter 19). We are sure these represent just the tip of the iceberg of similar surveys that are published in journals throughout the world.

GENUS *LEOPARDUS* GRAY, 1842 (9 SPECIES)

SARCOCYSTIS FELIS DUBEY, HAMIR, KIRKPATRICK, TODD, AND RUPPRECHT, 1992b

Intermediate hosts: *Leopardus geoffroyi* (d'Orbigny and Gervais, 1844), Geoffroy's Cat; *Leopardus tigrinus* (Schreber, 1775) (syn. *Leopardus guttulus* (Hensel, 1872)), Oncilla; *Leopardus wiedii* (Schinz, 1821), Margay.

Remarks: For more complete information on *S. felis*, see Genus *Lynx*, next.

GENUS *LYNX* KERR, 1752 (4 SPECIES)

SARCOCYSTIS FELIS DUBEY, HAMIR, KIRKPATRICK, TODD, AND RUPPRECHT, 1992b

Definitive type host: Unknown.

Type locality: North America: USA: Arkansas.

Other definitive hosts: Unknown.

Intermediate type host: *Lynx* (syn. *Felis*) *rufus* (Schreber, 1777), Bobcat.

Other intermediate hosts: *Acinonyx jubatus* (Schreber, 1775), Cheetah; *Felis catus* L., 1758, Domestic Cat; *Leopardus colocolo* (Molina, 1782), Colocolo; *Leopardus geoffroyi* (d'Orbigny and Gervais, 1844), Geoffroy's Cat; *Leopardus tigrinus* (Schreber, 1775) (syn. *Leopardus guttulus* (Hensel, 1872)), Oncilla; *Leopardus wiedii* (Schinz, 1821), Margay; *Panthera leo* (L., 1758), Lion; *Puma* (syn. *Felis*) *concolor coryi* (Bangs, 1899), Florida Panther; *Puma* (syn. *Felis*) *concolor stanleyana* (Goldman, 1938), Cougar; *Puma yagouaroundi* (É. Geoffory Saint-Hilaire, 1803), Jaguarundi.

Geographic distribution: North America: USA: Arkansas, Florida, Georgia, Oregon; South America: Brazil.

Description of sporulated oocyst: Not available.

Description of sporocyst and sporozoites: Not available.

Prevalence: Dubey et al. (1992b) found sarcocysts representing this form in striated muscles of 4/6 (67%) bobcats from Arkansas, USA. Muscle sarcocysts in felids also have been found in 4/4 cougars and in 11/14 (79%) panthers (Greiner et al., 1989), and Dubey et al. (1992b) believed that they all represented *S. felis*. Briggs et al. (1993) recovered *S. felis* from 7/10 (70%) cheetahs at a captive-breeding colony in Winston, Oregon, USA. Using PCR amplification of the ITS-1 locus, Cañón-Franco et al. (2016) molecularly characterized *S. felis* from South American wild felids and found this species in 4/7 (57%) *L. colocolo*, in 8/22 (36%) *L. geoffroyi*, in 7/28 (25%) *L. tigrinus* (Schreber, 1775) (syn. *L. guttulus*), in

6/10 (60%) *L. wiedii*, and in 6/22 (27%) *P. yagoua-roundi*. Prior to the work by Cañón-Franco et al. (2016), *S. felis* was thought to be limited to cats in North America, namely, the continental United States; theirs was the first report of *S. felis* infections in wild felids from Brazil.

Sporulation: Unknown, but likely endogenous with sporulated, infective sporocysts shed in the feces of the definitive host.

Prepatent and patent periods: Unknown.

Site of infection, definitive host: Unknown.

Site of infection, intermediate host: Greiner et al. (1989) found sarcocysts most frequently in the tongue, followed by the skeletal muscles, and then the diaphragm and saw only one sarcocyst in heart muscle. Sarcocysts were found in the striated muscles of the tongue, heart, masseter, and esophagus by Dubey et al. (1992b).

Endogenous stages, definitive host: Unknown.

Endogenous stages, intermediate host: Sarcocysts were up to 2.1 mm long and up to 150 wide. The cyst wall was 1.0–1.5 thick with 0.4–1.2 long finger-like, villar projections. The Pvm of the primary cyst wall folded into short hobnail-like bumps, and villar projections were 0.6–1.2 long × 0.3–0.4 wide at uneven distances, and villi were without microtubules. The Pvm, including villi and hobnail bumps, was lined by a 66 nm-thick electron-dense layer. Septa were 0.1–0.2 thick, and bradyzoites were L × W: 7–10 × 1.5 (1.5–2.0); micronemes were seen in the apical one-third portion and the N in the rounded end of the bradyzoites (Dubey et al., 1992b). Greiner et al. (1989) said sarcocysts under LM were L × W: 966 × 28–93 and were filled with bradyzoites. The sarcocyst wall contained finger-like projections evenly distributed, were of equal length, and were septate. When viewed under TEM, Greiner et al. (1989) saw the primary cyst wall to be folded into short, rounded, 1.0 × 0.5 finger-like villi. The cyst wall consisted of a Pvm on the external surface, beneath which was a 60–80 nm thick electron-dense layer that was modified into "hobnail"-like protrusions over the surface of the sarcocyst at the base of and between the villi. The ground substance of the sarcocyst was about 500 nm thick, composed of fine granules and fibrils. The internal septa that divided the sarcocyst into compartments were continuous with the ground substance of the cyst wall. Briggs et al. (1993) used both LM and TEM to examine sarcocysts from seven cheetahs and found that the septate sarcocysts were strikingly similar to those described for *S. felis* (Dubey et al., 1992b).

Cross-transmission: Greiner et al. (1989) fed sarcocyst-infected muscle to two lab-reared, 6-month-old domestic cats that were killed 30 DPI. No oocysts or sporocysts were seen in the feces or in the intestinal digest of the scraped mucosa.

Pathology: Presumably none in the cat, because neither degeneration of myocardium nor inflammatory cell infiltration is associated with the sarcocysts in all of the muscles of the different cat species observed to date (Kirkpatrick et al., 1986; Everitt et al., 1987; Hill et al., 1988; Greiner et al., 1989; Dubey et al., 1992b; Briggs et al., 1993).

Materials deposited: Section of tongue from the bobcat deposited in the USNM, No. 82095.

Remarks: We think it useful to reconstruct the history of discovery of feline sarcocysts now attributed to this species. Kirkpatrick et al. (1986) found sarcocysts in muscles of 3/3 domestic cats. One had numerous sarcocysts in gastrocnemius and epaxial musculature and in the diaphragm but not in cardiac muscle. Sarcocysts had a thin, non-striated wall and measured L × W (n = 17): 282 × 73 (44–1,000 × 24–160); numerous bradyzoites were present in all sarcocysts and septa divided them into compartments. By TEM, the intact sarcocyst wall consisted of a Pvm that had small, 0.42 × 0.39, villar projections at irregular intervals; the Pvm was underlined by an interrupted electron-dense layer except in the villar projections. Just beneath the Pvm was a homogeneous layer of ground substance that continued into the villar projections and into the septa. Maximum thickness of sarcocyst wall, including villar projections and ground substance was 1.4. Bradyzoites contained a conoid, micronemes, and rhoptries at the anterior end, a N toward the rounded posterior end, and numerous intracytoplasmic polysaccharide granules. Their (Kirkpatrick et al., 1986) second cat had sarcocysts in the heart that were L × W: 60 × 40, but no cysts were found in tongue, and their third cat had sarcocysts only in muscle tissue dispersed within an adenocarcinoma tumor. They said sarcocysts found in all three cats were structurally similar. Nonetheless, they stated, "Taxonomy of *Sarcocystis* based only on sarcocyst structure is inexact and cross-transmission experiments are necessary. Since the cat is not a prey animal, it is unlikely that the cat is the normal intermediate host of any *Sarcocystis* sp."

Everitt et al. (1987) mentioned that domestic cats and other carnivores have been reported from time to time to have sarcocysts in striated muscles, citing Einstein and Innes (1956). Everitt et al. (1987) used LM and TEM to examine 12 domestic cats for sarcocysts and found sarcocysts in skeletal muscles of three cats, and in cardiac muscle of a fourth. Sarcocysts were round in cross section and in long section they were L × W: 198 × 38 (24–700 × 28–270). TEM showed cysts with numerous compartments filled with bradyzoites. An electron-dense primary cyst wall, 60 nm thick, had numerous, irregularly spaced villous protrusions that were 0.4–1.0 long × 0.3–0.6 wide. The primary cyst wall appeared serrated except at the regions capped with villous projections; serrations seemed to be due to numerous small pores. A zone of fine granular ground substance, ~1 thick, was below the primary cyst wall. This zone extended as septa into the cyst, dividing it into compartments. Bradyzoites were 0.7–1.3 wide, had numerous granules, a conoid, micronemes, anterior rhoptries, and a prominent N. Everitt et al. (1987) said this description closely corresponded to the one of Kirkpatrick et al. (1986) from cats.

Hill et al. (1988) found sarcocysts in skeletal muscle (1) and myocardium (1) of two cats in Georgia, USA. Sarcocysts in cat thigh skeletal muscle were L × W (n = 5): 280 × 53 and contained large numbers of bradyzoites, 8–10 long. They had a striated cyst wall associated with a wide homogeneous eosinophilic ground substance that was 1.5–2.0 thick. Sarcocysts in the myocardium of the second cat were similar in size to those in striated muscle of the first. Both cats were debilitated and immunocompromised, unlike the cats examined by Kirkpatrick et al. (1986) in which sarcocysts were found incidentally during examination of tissues; however, Kirkpatrick et al. (1986) also found sarcocysts in a third cat they examined. Sarcocyst size, wall striations, size of bradyzoites, and their compartmentalization by septa made these all seem like the same species.

Dubey et al. (1992b) maintained that the structure of the sarcocyst wall is usually considered a reliable criterion to help distinguish various *Sarcocystis* species, which differed from the statement by Kirkpatrick et al. (1986). Dubey et al. (1992b) applied the first binomial to a *Sarcocystis* species known only from sarcocysts in felid muscles; at the time, this phenomenon (sarcocysts in top predators) was considered to be rare. Bhatavdekar and Purohit (1963) may have been the first to document sarcocysts in felid muscles when they found, "a very thin hyaline capsule and the cavity was filled with numerous crescentic bodies" in sections of heart muscle from two zoo lions, presumably *Panthera leo* (L., 1758), that had died in India. Bhatavdekar and Purohit's (1963) cysts, examined only under LM, were L × W: 12.3 × 2.4 but did not have "discernible" septa, and they were found in both striated and cardiac muscle fibers and in the cells of Purkinje fibers. Because of the small size and lack of septa (?), Bhatavdekar and Purohit's form (1963) cannot be attributed to *S. felis* and can only be considered a *species inquirenda* (see Chapter 19). We mention it here both for its historical significance, and because Dubey et al. (1992b) suggested that felid sarcocysts may all represent the same species. Dubey et al. (1992b) said the sarcocysts they saw resembled sarcocysts from the domestic cat (Kirkpatrick et al., 1986; Everitt et al., 1987; Edwards et al., 1988; Fiori and Lowndes, 1988; Hill et al., 1988), from panthers and cougars (Greiner et al., 1989), and those from the Florida bobcats (Anderson et al., 1992); however, we see differences between these various descriptions that may or may not be substantive. Dubey et al. (1992b) believed that *Sarcocystis* species were generally host specific for their intermediate host, but this is not always the case and not necessarily true (see *Sarcocystis neurona*, above; Duszynski, 2016). Odening (1998) suggested that *S. felis* also might be found in the domestic dog. Dubey et al. (1992b), Greiner et al. (1989), and Anderson et al. (1992) showed that muscle sarcocysts in felids are not rare and likely are all the same species. This may or may not be true because none of these life cycles are known. Both careful cross-transmission work and additional gene sequencing data are needed on all the sarcocyst forms found in feline muscles to be able to confirm their true identity or identities.

Anderson et al. (1992) discussed a concept that may be worth testing. They (1992) noted that in many of the various cats in which sarcocysts have been found in their muscles, the individual animals might have been immunocompromised from feline parvovirus or feline immunodeficiency virus infection, or other disease entities, and that this immune suppression may be the cause for the "abnormal" presence of tissue sarcocysts. They also raised the issue presented by Matuschka and Bannert (1987) that some species of *Sarcocystis* may be monoxenous and, thus, pick up theirs or other feline sporocysts from the environment that result in their tissue sarcocysts. This is more interesting food for thought and illustrative of the great amount of work still needing to be accomplished. Dubey et al. (2015a) included much of the life cycle information known about *S. felis* (their Tables 1.2, 19.1, 23.1, and 23.2) and illustrated the TEM of a mature *S. felis* sarcocyst (their Fig. 15.1), and listed it as a valid *Sarcocystis* species (their Tables 24.1 and 24.4).

GENUS *PRIONAILURUS* SEVERTZOV, 1858 (5 SPECIES)

SARCOCYSTIS SPECIES

We know of only a single report from *Prionailurus bengalensis* in Japan, in which *Sarcocystis* sarcocysts were found in various muscles, but no specific identification was made at the time of the survey (see Chapter 19).

GENUS PUMA JARDINE, 1834 (2 SPECIES)

SARCOCYSTIS FELIS DUBEY, HAMIR, KIRKPATRICK, TODD, AND RUPPRECHT, 1992b

Intermediate hosts: *Puma* (syn. *Felis*) *concolor coryi* (Bangs, 1899), Florida Panther; *Puma* (syn. *Felis*) *concolor stanleyana* (Goldman, 1938), Cougar; *Puma yagouaroundi* (É. Geoffroy Saint-Hilaire, 1803), Jaguarundi.

Remarks: For more complete information on *S. felis*, see Genus *Lynx*, above.

SARCOCYSTIS SPECIES

We know of only two reports from *P. concolor*, one in which *Sarcocystis* sarcocysts were found in various muscles, and the other in which sporocysts were found in fecal samples, but no specific identifications were made at the time of these surveys (see Chapter 19).

SUBFAMILY PANTHERINAE POCOCK, 1917

GENUS PANTHERA (L., 1758) (4 SPECIES)

SARCOCYSTIS FELIS DUBEY, HAMIR, KIRKPATRICK, TODD, AND RUPPRECHT, 1992b

Intermediate host: *Panthera leo* (L., 1758), Lion.
Remarks: For more complete information on *S. felis*, see Genus *Lynx*, above.

SARCOCYSTIS SPECIES

There are at least eight reports of *Sarcocystis* sarcocysts in various muscles or sporocysts in the feces of *Panthera* spp., but no specific identifications were made at the time of these surveys (see Chapter 19). We are sure many similar surveys exist in the world's literature.

DISCUSSION AND SUMMARY

The Caniformia branch of the Carnivora consists of nine families composed of 72 genera with 165 species (Wilson and Reeder, 2005). There is at least one named *Sarcocystis* species in eight of the nine families, but none are reported yet in the monotypic walrus family Odobenidae. The only species in the other monotypic family, Ailuridae, the red panda, is known to harbor only *S. neurona* as an intermediate host. In the Canidae, 8/13 (61%) genera and 15/35 (43%) species have been documented to host 48 named *Sarcocystis* species, either as intermediate or as definitive hosts, or both. As an example of how species-rich these hosts can be, just four species in the genus *Canis* are known to host 34 different *Sarcocystis* species; likewise, just 4 of the 12 *Vulpes* species host 21 different *Sarcocystis* species, 12 of which are different from those in *Canis*. In the Mephitidae, only 1/4 (25%) genera and 1/12 (8%) species have been studied, but three *Sarcocystis* species have been identified just from *M. mephitis*, the striped skunk. In the Mustelidae, 10/22 (45%) genera and 14/59 (24%) species have been studied and found to play host to 11 different named *Sarcocystis* species, nine of which are unique to them. In the Otaridae, 4/7 (57%) genera and 4/16 (25%) species have been examined, and there are three known *Sarcocystis* species. In the Phocidae, 8/13 (61%) genera and 10/19 (53%) species have three known *Sarcocystis* species, two of which are unique to them. In the Procyonidae, 3/6 (50%) genera and 3/15 (20%) species are known to harbor seven *Sarcocystis* species, two of which are unique, whereas the other five are shared with other hosts ranging from bison to pigs to rabbits. In the Ursidae, 2/5 (40%) genera and 3/8 (37.5%) species have been examined for and documented to harbor *Sarcocystis* species, one of which is unique to *Ursus*. In total, we have knowledge that about 62 distinct species of *Sarcocystis* are known to be present in 8/9 (89%) families, 37/72 (51%) genera with 51/165 (31%) species in the Caniformia branch of the Carnivora.

The Feliformia branch of the Carnivora consists of six families composed of 54 genera with 121 species (Wilson and Reeder, 2005), but its members have not been as well studied for *Sarcocystis* species as have those in the Caniformia. There are no named *Sarcocystis* species in 43 genera and 76 species from five of the six families in this lineage. Only members of the Felidae have been studied to any extent for *Sarcocystis* species, and 7/14 (50%) genera including only 12/40 (30%) of their species have been found to harbor 19 named *Sarcocystis* species, of which at least 14 are unique to the group. Only two species in the genus *Felis* host all of these species. In total, we have knowledge that about 19 *Sarcocystis* species are known to be present in 1/6 (17%) families, 7/54 (13%) genera, and in 12/121 (10%) species in the Feliformia branch of the Carnivora.

To summarize for all Carnivora, with few exceptions (domestic and lab dogs and cats), only a few wild or zoo carnivore specimens have been examined in only 9/15 (60%) families, 44/126 (35%) genera, and 63/286 (22%) species. From these modest efforts, 78 named *Sarcocystis* species, and a lot of unnamed forms, have been described, to date, from the Carnivora, 58 in which they serve as definitive hosts and discharge sporocysts into the environment, 16 in which they serve as intermediate hosts in which sarcocysts occur in their muscles, and 4 in which either the same carnivore or two different carnivores serve as both definitive and intermediate hosts in the cycle; these latter 4 include,

Sarcocystis corsaci, S. erdmanae, S. hydrurgae, and *S. mephitisi.* Unfortunately, only a couple of sarcocysts found in carnivore muscles have been examined by molecular methods such that they can be reliably discriminated from other known *Sarcocyst* species via sequence comparisons and phylogenetic analyses (Gjerde and Josefsen, 2015).

These latter cycles and species are particularly interesting. The domestic dog, *C. l. familiaris,* serves as definitive host for *S. erdmanae,* and the stripped skunk, *M. mephitis,* as the intermediate host. The question must be asked, how often do *Canis* species attack, kill, and ingest skunk flesh in the wild for this cycle to exist, or do we just not know enough about this parasite to understand it correctly? The Corsac fox, *V. corsac,* serves as both the definitive and intermediate host for *S. corsaci.* Is cannibalism common among foxes or do they prey on sick or dead congeners in the wild to make this cycle work in nature? Clearly there is much yet to be done to assess biodiversity and illuminate the biology of these parasites in carnivores. *Sarcocystis hydrurgae* has been found only as sarcocysts in Antarctic leopard seals, *Hydrurga leptonyx.* How is that cycle completed in nature? And, finally, *S. mephitisi* is only known from sarcocysts found in four of five striped skunks (*M. mephitis*) in Oregon. This skunk is widespread throughout southern Canada, most of the continental United States and northern Mexico. It has a formidable musk spray to defend itself, so it has few natural enemies; however, predators may include cougars, coyotes, bobcats, badgers, larger foxes, and a few predatory birds such as golden and bald eagles and the great horned owl, but we do not know which, if any, of these may be involved in this life cycle. There is still so much more to learn and work to be done!

There is a long history of taxonomic issues involving *Sarcocystis.* Dubey (1976) published the first comprehensive review of *Sarcocystis* and other coccidia (*Besnoitia, Hammondia, Isospora*) from dogs and cats. While his manuscript was *in press,* Tadros and Laarman (1976) proposed a new classification system for the genus names of coccidians that discharged *Isospora*-like oocysts in their feces, depending on whether the oocysts sporulated within or outside their host. For the moment, we want to make this an important taxonomic point. Tadros and Laarman (1976) placed the genera *Sarcocystis* and *Frenkelia* into a new genus, *Endorimospora,* because sporulation occurred within the host. We strongly agree with Dubey (1977a,b), and others, that according to the International Code of Zoological Nomenclature (Ride et al., 1999), such well-established names as *Sarcocystis* cannot and should not be changed. Thus, we consider the name *Endorimospora* a nomen dubium (a name of doubtful application) or a *nomen oblitum* (a name that does not take precedence over a younger synonym in prevailing usage) as per the ICZN(Ride et al., 1999, p. 111).

More relevant to this chapter, studies on the taxonomy and biodiversity of *Sarcocystis* in carnivores will require systematic sampling of the other 78% of carnivore hosts not yet examined and studied to identify new parasite species and host records so we can begin to sort out the real taxonomy of *Sarcocystis* that infect carnivores. Existing species names need to be validated and cryptic species identified (also see Chapter 19). Given the hints on the biodiversity of *Sarcocystis* species in carnivores so far (e.g., 34+ species in four *Canis* spp., 19+ species in 2 *Felis* species), the real number of *Sarcocystis* species, i.e., those not yet discovered, described, or named, is likely to be in the hundreds, if not thousands! Consider not only the 224 current extant carnivores that still need to be sampled well as potential hosts (both in numbers and throughout their ranges), but also the major regions of the planet that need to be explored to collect them: Latin and South America, Africa, Asia, and the Arctic and Antarctic faunas, including birds of prey.

A key issue that has contributed to some taxonomic confusion is that many authors in the past used the fine structure of the sarcocyst wall to separate species. Dubey et al. (2015a) distinguished 42 *Sarcocystis* wall types, many of which have from 2 to 15 subtypes. However, the sarcocyst wall structure itself changes dramatically in some species as it ages (see Munday and Obendorf, 1984), and looking only at this one dimension, is not always useful to determine species. Odening (1998) argued that interpretation hinders the correct evaluation of this important feature. It is true that the characteristics of the cyst wall are only valid when the sarcocyst is mature (i.e., contains cystozoites) because, once mature, deforming changes that could impair differentiation and the species-diagnostic value of this feature no longer occur. Odening (1998), however, perhaps overstated the case when he wrote, "In case of doubt, the TEM picture is decisive." TEM results on sarcocysts are useful because frozen/thawed or formalin-fixed sarcocysts can be processed without any essential loss of structural definition. Odening (1998) did caution, however, that morphological classification cannot be based solely on sarcocyst structure because there are examples where sarcocysts are similar, but the sporocysts are distinct. There are cases where different sarcocyst species cannot be distinguished by TEM type and, with a growing knowledge base as new species are added, the number of TEM types will increase. On the other hand, the sarcocyst is an important morphological identifier because it is usually larger and easier to work with than are thin-walled oocysts and sporocyst, and they are suitable to use as holotypes as per the ICZN (2000, art. 72.5.1, 72.5.2).

Since the mid 1990s, molecular methods have been increasingly used for the specific identification of sarcocysts, in what we define as their intermediate hosts. Most of that time, sequences from the nuclear ribosomal (r)DNA unit, particularly of the 18S ribosomal RNA (rRNA) gene mainly were used to gain inferences of the phylogenetic relationships of different *Sarcocystis* species to each other and to members of other genera. In 2013, the mitochondrial *cox1* gene was introduced as an additional molecular marker

for species delimitation and phylogenetic inferences among *Sarcocystis* species (Gjerde, 2013), and follow-up work by Gjerde (2014c, 2016b) has demonstrated that the *cox1* marker is superior to the 18S rRNA gene in separating closely related *Sarcocystis* species in various ruminant intermediate hosts. Such closely related species share the same sarcocyst morphology and are probably sibling species that have diverged fairly recently from a common ancestor along with the divergence of their intermediate hosts (Gjerde et al., 2017).

Of the basic biology and life histories of *Sarcocystis* in carnivores we have a reasonable start in that we know at least one or more definitive and intermediate hosts for about 58 of the 78 named species, but for the remaining 20 *Sarcocystis* species, we know virtually nothing about their life cycles, and there are large numbers of reports of sarcocysts in many animal species without any attempts to name the species or determine the definitive host(s) (see Chapter 19). It is believed that most *Sarcocystis* species have a limited range of definitive and intermediate hosts and, for each species, there is usually a naturally-occurring predator/prey or scavenger/carrion relationship between the two host types. Hence, carnivores predominantly act as definitive hosts, but at least 16 named species act as intermediate hosts, harboring fully developed sarcocysts, but we have no knowledge about what their definitive hosts might me. It has also been thought that specificity for the intermediate host is stricter than for the definitive host, but findings in noncarnivore species suggest this is not true (Box and Duszynski, 1978; Box et al., 1984; Duszynski and Box, 1978). Thus, some *Sarcocystis* species either never managed to develop such specificity or they may have recently become adapted to relatives of their original host(s) due to human intervention during the past few centuries via habitat loss. Such thoughts led Gjerde et al. (2017) to write, "In fact, it may well be that the putative gradual development towards intermediate host-specific *Sarcocystis* species has now (nearly) ceased due to the ever-increasing human interference with different animals and their habitats and the consequent disruption/alteration of the previous opportunities of the established (natural, ancient) intermediate and definitive host of various *Sarcocystis* species to interact."

A fruitful area for research would be to look closer at some of the named species that share intermediate or definitive hosts. For example, Elwasila et al. (1984) compared the structure of sarcocysts of *S. cuniculi* and *S. leporum* by LM and TEM and found only minor differences. They suggested that cross-transmission studies were needed to determine the relationship between the two species and molecular markers of both forms would also be useful. Many bovid and cervid (Artiodactyla) species harbor multiple sarcocysts (e.g., microscopic and macroscopic; thin-walled and thick-walled) in their muscles and act as intermediate hosts for several *Sarcocystis* species of carnivore definitive hosts. LM, TEM, and SEM studies initially suggested that these "sarcocyst types" represented different *Sarcocystis* species in the different hosts. Recent molecular work, however, mostly using the 18S rRNA gene sequences of *Sarcocystis* species found in reindeer, moose, roe deer, and red deer in Norway (Dahlgren and Gjerde 2007, 2008, 2009, 2010a) suggests that the *Sarcocystis* species examined possess varying degrees of host specificity for their intermediate host(s). Thus, morphologically identical sarcocysts in different hosts may represent only one *Sarcocystis* species (e.g., *S. ovalis* in moose and red deer) or indistinguishable sarcocysts in one cervid species, such as the red deer, sometimes can represent multiple species (e.g., *S. hardangeri* and *S. ovalis*). Such observations led Gjerde (2012) to conclude, based on morphological and genetic comparisons and phylogenetic analyses,

that certain sarcocyst types may represent separate, but closely related, sibling species, each one having evolved with, and adapted to, one or more closely related cervid hosts.

Details on endogenous development in both intermediate and definitive hosts are sorely lacking. Once sporozoites excyst from their sporocysts and penetrate the gut wall of the intermediate host, they enter endothelial cells of blood vessels in many tissues where they undergo merogony, preceding the development of the sarcocysts in the muscles. The number of merogonous stages is not known for most species, but merozoites eventually reach and penetrate muscle cells, where sarcocysts begin to develop and grow as they mature. Two distinct regions are recognized within the sarcocyst proper. The most peripheral region contains globular-shaped metrocytes; metrocytes bud internally, a process called endodyogeny, forming two daughter cells, after several such divisions, the globular metrocytes give rise to banana-shaped bradyzoites. Bradyzoites are structurally similar to coccidian merozoites except they have many more micronemes. Metrocytes are structurally like bradyzoites except they lack rhoptries and micronemes. Early meronts and metrocytes are not infective to definitive hosts that may consume them. The definitive host only becomes infected by ingesting mature intramuscular sarcocysts containing bradyzoites from the proper intermediate host. Unfortunately, we know almost nothing about intramuscular sarcocyst development for most *Sarcocystis* species.

From the above discussion, it is clear there is great opportunity for a parasitologist or any other biologist, fascinated with taxonomy, biology, and parasite life histories, to spend a lifetime focused on *Sarcocystis* with a near limitless number of questions to be asked and answered.

Sarcocystidae: Toxoplasmatinae in the Carnivora

SARCOCYSTIDAE: TOXOPLASMATINAE IN THE CARNIVORA

INTRODUCTION

In Chapter 14, we covered the apicomplexans (*Cystoisospora* species) in the first subfamily, Cystoisosporinae Frenkel et al., 1987, of the Sarcocystidae that parasitize carnivores, and in Chapter 15, the second subfamily, Sarcocystinae Poche, 1913 (*Sarcocystis, Frankelia* species). In this chapter, there are four genera (*Besnoitia, Hammondia, Neospora,* and *Toxoplasma* species) within this third subfamily, Toxoplasmatinae, which infect carnivores. An overview of each genus is covered below.

***Besnoitia* Henry, 1913.** Jellison (1956) reviewed (most of) the older literature concerning this genus name, and the species name *B. besnoiti*, pointing out the unusual amount of confusion regarding the authorship of these names; some of this history is repeated here, briefly. Jellison (1956) missed the paper by Darling (1910), in Panama, who found unusual cysts in an opossum, *Didelphis marsupialis,* and named the parasite as a member of the genus

Sarcocystis, even though he was concerned with some of the features that separated his cysts from the defining characteristics of the genus. Besnoit and Robin (1912) found a protozoan causing cutaneous and internal lesions in cattle in France, associated with subspheroidal cysts; they also tentatively referred the organism to *Sarcocystis* but did not propose a binomial. Marotel (1912), unaware of Darling's (1910) paper, discussed Besnoit and Robin's (1912) work and wrote "nothing similar has been found in animals... and this is why I propose to designate their parasite with the name *Sarcocystis besnoiti*" (Jellison, 1956). Besnoit and Robin's (1912) paper was further discussed in detail in November, 1912, at a meeting of the Société des Sciences Vétérinaires de Lyon, and the remarks of several speakers were published in March, 1913 (see Bru, 1913). Later that year, Henry (1913) reexamined the characteristics of the organism, and the nomenclature assigned to it, and used the genus name *Besnoitia.* That early history regarding genus-switching (e.g., to *Gastrocystis* and later to *Globidium*) for these organisms can be found by the reader, if interested, in the published literature (Darling, 1910; Besnoit and Robin, 1912; Marotel, 1912; Bru,

© 2018 Donald W. Duszynski published by Elsevier Inc. All rights reserved.

1913; Henry, 1913; Jellison, 1956; Schneideer, 1967a,b; Levine, 1973; Dubey, 1977a,b,c; Frenkel, 1977; Smith and Frenkel, 1977). *Besnoitia* species are obligatorily heteroxenous coccidia, similar to that of *Sarcocystis* species, but they differ from *Sarcocystis* in three unique ways: (1) unsporulated oocysts are shed by their definitive hosts and have relatively thick walls; (2) the completion of the sexual cycle in the definitive host is dependent on ingestion of tissue cysts from a suitable intermediate host—i.e., the ability of oocysts to initiate gametogenesis in the definitive host has been lost; and (3) these species can be successfully propagated asexually by mechanical transmission from intermediate host to intermediate host by blood-sucking arthropods. Wallace and Frenkel (1975) were among the first to recognize the cyclic transmission of *Besnoitia* by cats, when Wallace isolated some unidentified *Isospora*-type oocysts in the feces of a stray cat in Hawaii, USA, and they inoculated these oocysts into laboratory mice and rats in which they produced *Besnoitia* cysts in the omentum and mesentery and on the serosal surface of their viscera. Other details, of what little we know about the life cycle of various *Besnoitia* species, have been summarized by Leighton and Gajadhar (2001), Dubey et al. (2003c), Houk et al. (2011), Charles et al. (2011) and Duszynski and Couch (2013). *Besnoitia* is the fifth apicomplexan to be a mammalian tissue parasite, along with *Cystoisospora, Hammondia, Sarcocystis,* and *Toxoplasma.* There are now approximately 10 valid species in this genus, but the definitive (carnivore) host, the domestic cat (*Felis silvestris catus*), is known only from four or five of them. Thus, since there are no *Besnoitia* species known from any other carnivores, the information on the four species with known life cycles will be covered under the genus *Felis* (below).

Finally, the life cycle of *Besnoitia* species has been described as "mysterious" (Jacquiet et al., 2010). Because the cat serves as (one of?) the definitive host for four *Besnoitia* species, it is presumed that domestic or wildcats, or another wild carnivore(s), always serve as its definitive hosts (Peteshev et al., 1974; Diesing et al., 1988; Basso et al., 2001), but this hypothesis is still unproven. For example, Diesing et al. (1988) found no oocysts in the feces of 23 carnivores belonging to 12 species (including domestic cats) fed with tissue containing *B. besnoiti* cysts. In a study by Basso et al. (2011), dogs and cats fed with *B. besnoiti* tachyzoites did not seroconvert, whereas cats fed with *B. besnoiti* tissue cysts did. And Millán et al. (2012), in a serosurvey for *B. besnoiti* in 205 free-roaming carnivores in Spain (16 wolves, *Canis lupus*; 41 red foxes, *Vulpes vulpes*; 21 pine martens, *Martes martes*; 8 stone martens, *M. foina*; 12 Eurasian badgers, *Meles meles*; 18 common genets, *Genetta genetta*; 5 Egyptian mongooses, *Herpestes ichneumon*; 28 European wildcats, *Felis silvestris silvestris*; 43 feral domestic cats, *Felis silvestris catus*; 1 least weasel, *Mustela nivalis*; 2 European polecats, *Mustela putorius*; 4 Eurasian otters, *Lutra lutra*; 1 American mink, *Neovison vison*; 3 Iberian lynx, *Lynx pardinus*; 1 South American coati, *Nasua nasua*; 1 northern raccoon, *Procyon lotor*) did not find any evidence to support their hypothesis that wild carnivores are implicated in the transmission of *B. besnoiti* in Spain. So, until further notice, the jury is still out on the principal carnivores in the life cycle of *Besnoitia* species.

***Hammondia* Frenkel, 1974.** First a bit of ancient history. As pointed out by Wenyon (1923), our knowledge of the coccidia of cats began with observations by Finch (1854) on changes that occurred in the intestinal epithelium of cats, while he studied the process of food absorption for his doctoral dissertation; he did not understand the true parasitic nature of the intracellular forms he described, and he called the structures he observed, *corpuscules geminés.* In fact, they were developmental stages of a coccidium. From that time, until the picture became somewhat clarified (by Wenyon, 1923), the stages of this form in the dog and cat were considered to be a single coccidium. Rivolta (1873, p. 382, see Wenyon, 1923), referring to the presence of psorosperms in domestic animals, confirmed that Finck's observations were made in the cat, as were those of Ercolani (1859). The parasite was studied in dogs by Rivolta (1874, 1878), who called it *Cytospermium millosum intestinalis canis*, and by Railliet and Lucet (1890), who also recognized it as a true coccidium, and called it *coccidia geminé*. Shortly after their 1890 publication, Stiles was working on coccidia in Balbiani's laboratory in Italy, and Railliet gave him some of his original material to study further. In a short time, Stiles reached the same results of Railliet and Lucet (1890), changed the French expression they used by referring this parasite into Latin, and renamed it in a preliminary note, based on the observations by Finch (1854) and the material of Railliet and Lucet (1890). His paper was to be read before the Société Zoologique de France, on June 9, 1891, but he was unable to prepare illustrations of the parasite because he received a cable to return immediately to the United States, before presenting his paper in person. Nonetheless, he did provide this parasite's first name, *Isospora bigeminum* Stiles, 1891, the "twin-coccida" parasite. He delayed publication of his figures, hoping to obtain more material from infected cats, but that did not happen, and since *I. bigeminum* already had appeared in several publications, he finally decided not to delay publication of the type figures, which he produced a year later (Stiles, 1892). Dobell (1919) inadvertently added confusion to the history when he referred to Finck's observations as having been made in the dog, instead of the cat. After Wenyon (1923) cleared some of the confusion on terminology of *Isospora*-type oocysts in cats and dogs, not much else was accomplished until the 1970s.

Regarding the nomenclature of this parasite (*Hammondia*), little was accomplished until the work of Wallace (1973b,c), in Hawaii, who inoculated mice with *Toxoplasma*-like oocysts from cat feces and produced what he thought were sarcocysts in mouse diaphragm, but which Frenkel (1974) distinguished as something completely different. But then a series of nomenclatural errors were made and this genus was named as new on three separate occasions by Frenkel. It was first named as new (Frenkel, 1974, p. 139 [Table 2], and p. 149) in the published form of a review paper he presented at the 3rd International Congress of Parasitology, held in Munich, earlier that year. In that published account (Frenkel, 1974), he defined the parameters of the Family Sarcocystidae Poche, 1913, and listed three established genera and their authorities (*Arthocystis* Levine et al., 1970, *Frenkelia* Biocca, 1968, *Sarcocystis* Lankester, 1882) and stated the defining characters of each genus. Then he listed a fourth genus in the family, "Genus *Hammondia* gen. nov.," and defined it. This was followed by his establishing the type species, "*Hammondia hammondi* nov. spec.," in which he defined it as his CR-4 oocyst isolate, and Wallace's WC-1170-A cyst isolate (see Wallace, 1973b); he followed by stating the size of the oocyst, its sporulation time, the size of muscle cysts, the final host (cat), and a list of experimental intermediate hosts (mouse, rat, hamster), but (unfortunately) added, "to be further described (Frenkel and Dubey, 1974)." In our opinion, and in the opinion of Markus (1979), this 1974 publication established the genus and species names, by satisfying Requirement (a) (i) of Article 13 (**Names published after 1930**…) of the International Code of Zoological Nomenclature (ICZN) and, thus, established the genus and authority as, *Hammondia* Frenkel, 1974, and the type species authority as *H. hammondi* Frenkel, 1974. This paper by Frenkel (1974) was important because it was one of the first synthetic compilations of the old phylum Sporozoa, at a time we were only beginning to understand the biology and life cycles of the heteroxenous (two-host) coccidia. Nonetheless, it just started the confusion. Unfortunately, this was not the first time the process of naming a new species was done without attention to the Code (see below, under *Neospora*, for a similar nomenclatural mistake).

The "further to be described by Frenkel and Dubey, 1974" paper was still in preparation when Frenkel (1974) mentioned it, but it was not published until 1975, with the title, "*Hammondia hammondia* gen. nov., sp. nov., from domestic cats..." (Frenkel and Dubey, 1975b); the second time these names were presented as new. And later in 1975 (Frenkel and Dubey, 1975a), it was named as new for the third time in their paper in *Science*. In Markus' (1979) short paper ("The authorship of *Hammondia hammondi*"), he characterized this situation as, "an undignified scramble among workers to establish priority as regards scientific names and in some instances the code of ethics set out in appendix A of the ICZN, adopted by the 15th International Congress of Zoology (International Commission on Zoological Nomenclature, 1964), has been violated." Finally (almost) Frenkel (1977) perpetuated the mistake when he listed the genus name as "*Hammondia* Frenkel and Dubey, 1975," which is incorrect, for reasons already stated, but this led almost every author in the past 40+ years to perpetuate the mistake! Thus, the date of its publication is 1974 (Article 10 of the Code) and, in the future, we hope that authors will make the correct citation: *Hammondia* Frenkel, 1974 and *H. hammondi* Frenkel, 1974. The Frenkel and Dubey (1975b) follow-up paper helped to better define both the genus and species as distinct from closely related forms and deposited type specimens to anchor their names.

The genus *Hammondia* is characterized by elongate cysts that conform to their host (skeletal) muscle cell or could be subspheroidal in the brain (rare), and these cysts have no septa or radial spines. The sexual cycle occurs in the definitive host (a carnivore), where enteroepithelial multiplication (merogony) occurs, followed by gamogony with unsporulated oocysts shed in the feces. Frenkel and Dubey (1975a) reiterated the biological and life cycle differences between *H. hammondi* and related genera such as *Isospora*, *Sarcocystis*, and *Toxoplasma*. *Hammondia hammondi* has a prepatent period of 5–7 days and mostly spheroidal oocysts averaging 11–13 wide that sporulate exogenously in 2–3 days. Muscle cysts are 100–340 long and 40–95 wide in their intermediate hosts, which include many species.

At about the same time, Heydorn and Rommel (1972) and Heydorn (1973) reported the isolation of small, unsporulated oocysts (along with sporocysts of a *Sarcocystis* species) from the feces of dogs that had fed on raw beef. After sporulation, these slightly subspheroidal, *Isospora*-like oocysts measured, $L \times W$: 11.9×11.1 ($10–15 \times 9–13$); L/W ratio: 1.1, similar in size to oocysts described by Wenyon (1926a) as the small form of *I. bigemina*, and they found the sexual endogenous stages in the epithelium, rather than the lamina propria, of the dog intestine. They called this form, *I. bigemina* isolate, Berlin-1971, and, in a series of experiments, Heydorn (1973), Heydorn et al. (1975b,c), Heydorn (unpublished, but see Heydorn and Mehlhorn, 2002) reported some important discoveries for Berlin-1971, including (1) differentiating it from *T. gondii* by firmly establishing the dog as the definitive host; (2) determining that it had an obligate heteroxenous life history; (3) demonstrating that these small oocysts were infective both for the definitive host (although dogs fed sporulated oocysts can become infected but not shed oocysts) and several intermediate hosts (calves, sheep, goats); (4) that oocysts seemed to be nonpathogenic in the hosts they can infect, but oocyst production was always very low in the dog; (5) oocysts were not infective for cats, rabbits and mice; and (6) although they could not detect tissue stages in dogs and calves, they could demonstrate the parasite's presence via feeding experiments. As a result of their work, Tadros and Laarman (1976) proposed a new name, *I. heydorni*, to replace *I. bigemina* small form (Berlin-1971). A year later, Dubey (1977a,b,c) transferred *I. heydorni* to the genus *Hammondia* because of its obligate heteroxenous life cycle, and the name *H. heydorni* (Tadros and Laarman, 1976) Dubey, 1977c, was accepted and established, and later studies demonstrated that guinea pigs, water buffaloes, camels, and moose also could serve as intermediate hosts. Further confusing the terminology, however, Levine (1978) named the small race of *I. bigemina* as *I. babiensis* based on a paper by de Moura Costa (1956), who reported oocysts that measured L×W: 13×11 (12.3–13.6×10.7–12.3); L/W ratio: 1.2, in one dog, and 11.4–13.6×10.7–12.3 in a second dog from Bahia, Brazil, and had named the parasite, *I. bigemina* var *bahiensis*. Levine (1978) should not have made this designation because the name *H. heydorni* (Tadros and Laarman, 1976) Dubey, 1977c, had priority. Information on the biology, endogenous development, prepatent and patent periods, and pathogenicity of *H. heydorni* can be found in Heydorn (1973), Dubey and Fayer (1976), and Levine and Ivens (1965, 1981). This may also represent the species found in 4/136 (3%) red foxes (*V. vulpes*) in Bulgaria but reported only from unsporulated oocysts.

To our knowledge, there are two other species of named *Hammondia*, but the literature on these is paltry. Hendricks et al. (1979) named *H. pardalis* found in a fecal sample of an ocelot, *Leopardus* (syn. *Felis*) *pardalis*, in a zoo on a US Air Force Base in the Panama Canal Zone. This species has been found on only two other occasions in the literature.

Ellis et al. (1999) examined the relationships among *Hammondia, Neospora,* and *Toxoplasma* by DNA sequence comparisons of the D2/D3 domain of the large subunit ribosomal DNA and the internal transcribed spacer 1 (ITA-1). Their results led them to reject the hypothesis that *N. caninum* and *H. heydorni* are the same species, and they showed that *H. hammondi* is probably the sister taxon to *T. gondii*, making the genus *Hammondi* **paraphyletic**. Heydorn and Mehlhorn (2002) suggested that almost everything that has been published on *H. heydorni*, but especially the nucleotide sequences (Ellis et al., 1999; Mugridge et al., 1999), might actually be, "descriptions of further separate coccidian species, which may be different from the original *I. bigemina* isolate of Heydorn (1973)." Perhaps this was prophetic! Gjerde and Dahlgren (2011) named the fourth species, *H. triffittae*, using genomic DNA to distinguish this species found in foxes, from *H. heydorni* found in domestic dogs and, later, Gjerde (2013) distinguished between *H. triffittae, H. heydorni, T. gondii,* and *N. caninum* using full-length mitochondrial copies and partial nuclear copies of their cytochrome b and cytochrome c oxidase subunit I genes.

***Neospora* Dubey, Carpenter, Speer, Topper, and Uggla, 1988a.** Probably the first case of fatal **encephalomyelitis** (EPM, in horses), attributed to an unknown protozoan, was reported in 1970, in the United States (Rooney et al., 1970). Over the intervening 15 years Fayer and Dubey (1987) estimated that probably >100 horses a year were being diagnosed with EPM in Florida, Ohio, and Texas, alone, with other cases reported in horses in California, Illinois, New Jersey, New York, Pennsylvania, USA, and Saskatchewan, Canada. The protozoan responsible was often misidentified as *T. gondii* (Dubey and Lindsay, 1996), until it was later determined to bear the greatest resemblance to the genus *Sarcocystis*, based on its mode of replication, staining characteristics, location in hosts' cells, serology, and epidemiology. Because the distribution of EPM was thought to be limited to North America, Fayer and Dubey (1987) suggested that attempts to identify the organism and its source, should focus on animal sources unique to that continent.

Dubey and Lindsay (1996, Table 1) and Dubey et al. (2017b, Table 1.2) gave a somewhat different summary of the history of *N. caninum* and neosporosis, from the viewpoint of the (dog) definitive host. Briefly, a neuromuscular syndrome in dogs, which simulated toxoplasmosis, was recognized and documented in Norway by three Norwegian veterinarians (Bjerkås et al., 1984), who reported a protozoan causing severe encephalomyelitis in six Norwegian pups, but which had no antibodies to *T. gondii*. All dogs originated from three litters from a single Boxer bitch. The pups appeared healthy until 2-months-old.

Five of these pups had neurological signs for several months, and all six were examined at necropsy and diagnosed with encephalitis and myositis with protozoa found in the lesions, including numerous tachyzoites and a few tissue cysts in their brains. Ultrastructurally, tachyzoites were like *T. gondii*, but with more rhoptries than seen in *T. gondii*. Thus, vertical transmission of neosporosis was first recognized in these successive litters from a bitch in Norway in 1984 (Bjerkås et al., 1984). In a retrospective study, a congenitally-infected German shorthaired Pointer bitch, from Ohio, USA, transmitted infection to its progeny in 1957, resulting in the description of the most severe outbreak of neosporosis identified to date (Dubey et al., 1990c).

Dubey was initially unable to secure microscope slides of the original material from Norway, so he examined tissue sections and case histories from all dogs and cats that had died of a *T. gondii*–like illness from 1952 to 1987 and were archived in the Angell Memorial Animal Hospital (AMAH), Boston, Massachusetts, USA, the largest hospital for dogs and cats in the United States, which keeps meticulous records of pathology cases. He and Dr. James Carpenter, a pathologist at AMAH, examined thousands of slides from dogs and cats and concluded that the syndrome recognized by Bjerkås et al. (1984) was not toxoplasmosis. In addition to neuromuscular clinical signs, dogs suffered severe disease involving the heart, lungs, liver, and skin (Dubey et al., 2017b).

Dubey et al. (1988a,c) found a similar parasite in formalin-fixed tissues from 10 dogs in the United States, and named a new genus, *Neospora*, and *N. caninum* Dubey, Carpenter, Speer, Topper, and Uggla, 1988a, became the type species. From our perspective as taxonomists, the authors of this paper were ill-informed about how to properly, and correctly, name and describe new genera and species to be in agreement with the ICZN. One cannot just plop down a name (or names) and leave it at that, without adhering to standard and acceptable procedures, not the least of which are to deposit type specimens, and to discriminate the new taxon from already described genera and species that seem to be most closely related to those receiving new names (see Heydorn and Mehlhorn, 2002 and their arguments summarized, briefly, below).

A decade later, McAllister et al. (1998a) finally established dogs as the definitive host of *N. caninum*. The genus definition, then, included at least the following: (1) tissue cysts in several cell types, primarily in the neural tissues; (2) tissue cyst wall up to 4 μm thick, (3) numerous bradyzoites, not separated by septa; (4) tachyzoites with numerous electron-dense rhoptries, some posterior to the N; (5) canids (dog, coyote, wolf) as definitive hosts, and many intermediate hosts, including dogs, cattle, horses, goats, deer, water buffaloes, coyotes, red foxes, and camels (see Dubey, 1999; Lindsay and Dubey, 2000); (6) tachyzoites and tissue cysts in both intermediate and definitive hosts; (7) oocysts discharged unsporulated in the feces; (8) transmission by carnivorism, transplacental, and fecal; and (9) tachyzoites, tissue cysts, and oocysts all infectious to both intermediate and definitive hosts.

The name *N. caninum* (Dubey et al., 1988a) initially aroused considerable scientific controversy because the original naming and "description" were inadequate, as pointed out by Mehlhorn and Heydorn (2000) and Heydorn and Mehlhorn (2002), because it was (1) based on parasites in tissue sections, and many scientists felt that it was likely a new species or strain of *Toxoplasma*; (2) the new genus and species were not sufficiently discriminated from already described, closely-related forms; (3) there were no type specimens identified in the original article or were any "types" deposited into an accredited museum; and (4) their review was based on 9 of 10 case histories by reexamining histological tissue sections, while the only "live" specimen was a dog with ulcerative cutaneous lesions, which were not seen in the other 9 cases. Heydorn and Mehlhorn (2002) criticized the basic science of the original description, pointed out contradictions in supporting descriptive parameters that were used by the original authors (e.g., presence/absence of a parasitophorous vacuole (PV), thickness of the cyst wall, size/shape of the tissue cysts, etc.), questioned the absence of a life cycle study, and had other criticisms that led them to conclude "The story of *N. caninum* is characterized by inconsistent observations, contradictory arguments and arbitrary statements" and, "Due to the nonfulfilment of the rules needed for the description and publication of new species and genera, the name *Neospora caninum* becomes invalid… and is a nomen nudum in relation to both genus and species."

To his great credit, and in collaboration with more than two dozen scientists around the world, Dubey et al. (2002a) redescribed the parasite, satisfied all of the criticisms presented by Heydorn and Mehlhorn (2002), and deposited live parasites in culture and wet and histological specimens into multiple museums (American Type Culture Collection; US National Parasite Collection). Interested readers may consult their original paper (Dubey et al., 2002a) to obtain the 13 various accession numbers for their vouchered specimens.

At least four characters now clearly separate *N. caninum* from *T. gondii*: (1) Paralysis, particularly of the hind limbs, was a syndrome not observed in other species diagnosed to have toxoplasmosis; (2) Tissue cysts of this parasite were morphologically distinct—they had thicker walls than those of *T. gondii* (1–4 *vs.* 0.5)—and seemed restricted to neural tissue and sometimes the skin (vs. *T. gondii*, found in many organs); (3) Antibodies to *T. gondii* were not present in these dogs, and the parasites did not react to *T. gondii* antibodies in immunohistochemical tests; and (4) They are biologically different: *N. caninum* causes a major disease in cattle, and canids are its definitive hosts, whereas *T. gondii* is a major public health problem (humans) and felids are its definitive host. Both parasites have

wide intermediate host ranges. Considerable progress in understanding the biology of neosporosis has been made in the last 30 years, resulting in more than 2,000 scientific publications, which we do not intend to cover here. For the interested reader, Dubey et al. (2017b) have produced a comprehensive, well-organized, easily read book on this subject and cover a good number of these references.

After *N. caninum* became established (Dubey et al., 1988a,c, 2002a,d), one of the questions asked was whether neosporosis is a new disease. In collaboration with Bjerkås and several other colleagues (Bjerkås and Dubey, 1991; Dubey et al., 1990c) Dubey reevaluated case histories of the original histological sections of the Norwegian dogs, and paraffin sections were stained with *N. caninum* antibodies. The presence of *N. caninum*, and not *T. gondii*, was confirmed in all six dogs, including thick-walled tissue cysts in the retina (Dubey et al., 1990c). Since then, numerous milestones have been achieved in helping to define and understand the biology and the importance of *N. caninum* as an ecological driver of disease in cattle and, perhaps, other animals. These include (1) isolating it in cell culture and mice (Dubey et al., 1988a,c; Lindsay and Dubey, 1989c); (2) development of the indirect fluorescent antibody test (IFAT) for serological diagnosis (Dubey et al., 1988a,c); (3) development of an immunohistochemical test to identify *N. caninum* in tissues of infected hosts (Lindsay and Dubey, 1989a); (4) *N. caninum* specifically identified as the cause of abortion in dry lot and dairy cattle (Anderson et al., 1991; Barr et al., 1991; Thilsted and Dubey, 1989); (5) the inducement of transplacental transmission of *N. caninum* in dogs, cats, cattle, and sheep (Dubey and Lindsay, 1989a,b; Dubey and Lindsay, 1990; Dubey et al., 1992c); (6) drug screening for chemotherapy of neosporosis (Lindsay and Dubey, 1989a,c; Lindsay and Dubey, 1990); and (7) development of an enzyme-linked immunosorbent assay (ELISA) test for diagnosis of neosporosis in dogs and cattle (Björkman et al., 1994;

Dubey et al., 1997; Paré et al., 1995) and others (Dubey et al., 2017b, see Table 1.2).

There are three infectious stages of *N. caninum*: tachyzoites, bradyzoites, and sporulated oocysts. **Tachyzoites** (Gk., tachos=speed) are a rapidly multiplying stage that can proliferate (repeated endodyogeny) in almost all cell types in the body, including neural cells, endothelial cells, dermal cells, retinal cells, macrophages, hepatocytes, and fibroblasts. Intracellular tachyzoites are located in the host cell cytoplasm within a **PV** surrounded by a parasitophorous vacuolar membrane (PVM). Often the PVM is so closely butted against host cytoplasm that it appears that the PVM is absent; each tachyzoite may contain 6–16 rhoptries. **Bradyzoites** (also called **cystozoites**) are the encysted, tissue cyst stage of the parasite. These cysts, without septa, remain intracellular and grow by endodyogeny; they vary in size, depending on the host, and the type of cell parasitized. Young tissue cysts are small (5 wide) and contain just a few bradyzoites, whereas older cysts may contain >200 bradyzoites. In the brain, they are round, up to 107 wide, with a wall 0.5–4 thick. Intramuscular cysts, more elongate, may be 100 long, and have a thin cyst wall, but these seem to be rare in other organs of naturally-infected animals. **Oocysts** represent the only unambiguous stage of *N. caninum* and are shed unsporulated in canid feces. Unsporulated oocysts are 10–11 μm wide, whereas sporulated oocysts are slightly larger, L×W: 11.7×11.3 (11–12×11–12), L/W ratio: 1.0. Oocyst wall is colorless, smooth, 0.6–0.8 thick. Sporocysts are, L×W: 8.4×6.1 (7–9×5.6–6.4), L/W ratio: 1.4. Sporozoites measure L×W: 6.5×2.0 (6–7×1.8–2.2). Developmental stages, merogony and gametogony, in the dog (type host) gut are unknown. Ingestion of sporulated oocysts is the only demonstrated mode for postnatal (horizontal) transmission in herbivores; thus, oocysts are the key in the epidemiology of neosporosis, even though the number of oocysts shed by dogs is usually small. Because *N. caninum* oocysts structurally resemble those of *Hammondia heydorni*, it is epidemiologically important to properly identify *N. caninum* oocysts (Schares et al., 2005; Šlapeta et al., 2002a,b; Soares et al., 2011).

Neospora caninum can be transmitted postnatally (horizontally, laterally) by ingestion of tissues with tachyzoite- or bradyzoite-containing tissue cysts (e.g., raw meat, infected intermediate hosts, or infected bovine placental tissue), by ingestion of food or drinking water contaminated by sporulated oocysts, or transplacentally (vertically, congenitally), from an infected dam to her fetus during pregnancy. Transplacental transmission occurs when tachyzoites multiply in the maternal part of the placenta, cross it, and then spread to invade fetal tissues; *N. caninum* usually parasitizes both definitive and intermediate hosts without producing overt clinical signs.

The number of viable *Neospora* in naturally-infected tissues is usually low and randomly distributed, especially in asymptomatic animals. Hematological and biochemical findings can be helpful, but they are nonspecific; for example, myositis commonly results in increased creatine kinase and aspartase aminotransferase activities, but these tests alone do not identify a *N. caninum* infection. Methods to specifically diagnose *N. caninum* include but are not limited to clinical signs; fecal flotation for oocysts; cytology; conventional histopathology; scanning (SEM) and transmission electron microscopy (TEM); immunohistochemical staining (IHC); mono- and polyclonal antibodies specific to *N. caninum* (both commercially available); ELISA; IFAT; immunoblot; direct *Neospora* agglutination test (NAT), direct agglutination test (DAT) kits with appropriate formalin-fixed antigen; latex agglutination test (LAT); bioassay in dogs; and polymerase chain reaction (PCR) detection of various loci (e.g., 18S rDNA, ITS-1). The random amplified polymorphic DNA PCR technique (RAPD) is able to differentiate between *N. caninum*, several *T. gondii* strains, and *Sarcocystis* species (Barber and Trees, 1996; Irwin, 2002; Dubey et al., 2015a,b).

Histopathology may confirm the presence of *N. caninum*, but owners of pets often decline invasive biopsy procedures, especially when the sensitivity is low and general anesthesia is necessary. Moreover, serology may yield controversial results. High antibody titers may be detected in healthy dogs, while some dogs with clinical neosporosis may be seronegative. Titer magnitudes do not correlate to the severity of clinical signs (Dijkstra et al., 2001; Lyon, 2010). Thus, diagnostic methods should provide the clinician with a guide, but he/she must exercise his/her clinical judgment and take all the data into account. If the diagnosis is not certain, a clinical strategy is to start treatment.

Neospora caninum is recognized as the cause of meningoencephalitis, polymyositis, polyradiculoneuritis, and dermatological diseases in dogs (definitive host), whereas cats and a variety of hoof-stock animals are natural intermediate hosts (Dubey and Beattie, 1988; Dubey, 2003; Sedlák and Bártová, 2006b). The natural host range for *N. caninum*, as detected by parasite isolation, DNA, antibody, and clinical confirmation of disease, includes herbivores/ omnivores and carnivores. At least the following *noncarnivores* are documented hosts of *N. caninum*: alpaca (*Vicugna pacos*), Axis deer (*Axis axis*), bank vole (*Myodes glareolus*), black rat (*Rattus rattus*), black-tailed deer (*Odocoileus hemionus columbianus*), capybara (*Hydrochaeris hydrochaeris*), cattle/aurochs (*Bos taurus*), common vole (*Microtus arvalis*), Eld's deer (*Panolia eldii*), equids (*Equus* spp.), European bison (*Bison bonasus*), field or wood mouse (*Apodemus sylvaticus*), goat (*Capra hircus*), harvest mouse (*Micromys minutus*), house mouse (*Mus musculus*), humans (*Homo sapiens*) and other primates, llama (*Lama glama*), Norway rat (*Rattus norvegicus*), Parma wallaby (*Macropus parma*), pig (*Sus scrofa domesticus*), rabbit (*Oryctolagus cuniculus*), rhinoceros (Rhinocerotidae), several avian species (e.g., *Gallus gallus domesticus*), sheep (*Ovis aureus*), shrew (*Sorex araneus*), squirrel (*Spermophilus variegates*), water buffalo (*Bubalus arnee*), water vole (*Arvicola terrestris*), white-tailed deer (*Odocoileus virginianus*), white-toothed shrew (*Crocidura russula*), and yellow-necked mouse (*Apodemus flavicollis*) (Tables 2.1, 2.2, Dubey et al. 2017b). *Neospora caninum* antibodies, confirmed clinical neosporosis, and/ or associated abortions have been detected in cattle in 62 countries worldwide and in 25 of 50 states in the United States (Tables 4.1, 4.2 Dubey et al., 2017b). The existence of a sylvatic cycle of *N. caninum* was suggested by Gondim et al. (2004a,b), who fed naturally-infected deer tissues to dogs, which then started to discharge oocysts, and by Almería et al. (2007), who recorded the presence of antibodies of *N. caninum* in noncarnivore wildlife hosts (deer, barbary sheep, and wild boars).

The "type" definitive host species for *N. caninum* is, of course, the domestic dog, *Canis lupus familiaris* L., 1758. Prevalence of *N. caninum*–like oocysts in dog feces have been documented in Argentina, Australia, Costa Rica, China, Czech Republic, Ethiopia, Germany, Iran, Italy, Portugal, Romania, Spain, Switzerland, the United Kingdom, and the United States (Table 2.3, Dubey et al., 2017b). Serological prevalence data indicate that *N. caninum* infections are common, but clinical disease is relatively rare. Why some dogs develop clinical neosporosis, whereas most do not develop symptoms is unknown.

Canine neosporosis has been isolated and verified in at least 15 countries: Australia, Austria, Belgium, Canada, Costa Rica, Finland, France, Germany, Israel, Italy, Japan, South Africa, Sweden, the United Kingdom (England, Ireland), and at least 5 states in the United States (Lindsay and Dubey, 2000). Four forms of canine neosporosis can be differentiated (Dubey, 2013; Kramer et al., 2000; Ruehlmann et al., 1995): (1) The most severe signs are in transplacentally-infected pups that develop progressive ascending rear limb paresis and paralysis, with atrophy and rigid contracture of the muscles of the pelvic limbs, often including muscle atrophy. (2) Adult dogs may suffer from a nongeneralized neosporosis and may develop a range of manifestations, predominantly including encephalitis, meningoencephalomyelitis, or polymyositis. Paraparesis and polymyositis are the most common neurological sign, but seizures, abnormal behavior, and vestibular dysfunction also can occur. Signs of myositis include stiff gait, weakness, and pain or atrophy of skeletal muscles. Almost any other organ can be involved, including the lungs, liver, spleen, eyes, and heart. (3) In some dogs a multifocal, systemic dissemination affecting a variable number of organs, other than the CNS, is observed. (4) In addition, there are several case reports on a polygranulomatous *N. caninum* dermatitis with or without a systemic dissemination of the parasite into other organs. Dermal neosporosis affects mainly adult dogs. Factors thought to affect clinical infections are age, breed, and tissues parasitized, and dogs rarely excrete large numbers of *N. caninum* oocysts (see Dubey et al., 2017b, for details, and Table 2.3). Because *N. caninum* oocysts are morphologically similar to those of *H. heydorni* and related parasites (e.g., *T. gondii* observed in dog feces most likely because of coprophagia) bioassay is the only safe way to confirm the identity of viable oocysts in canine feces (Schares et al., 2005). In addition, molecular tools can also discern the identity of the oocysts (Cavalcante et al., 2011; Hill et al., 2001; Schares et al., 2001b). Either the prevalence of *N. caninum* antibodies, clinical neosporosis, or the isolation of viable organisms has been found in domestic dogs in 49 countries worldwide including 35 states in the United States (Table 5.1, Dubey et al., 2017b).

Many wild canids, other than the domestic/lab dog, also are known to have been exposed to *N. caninum*, either by being seropositive, demonstrating oocysts in their feces, or exhibiting signs of neosporosis. Such instances have been documented in the following 21 countries: **Australia**: Australian dingo (*Canis lupus* [*familiaris*] *dingo*); **Argentina**: South American gray fox (*Lycalopex* [syn. *Dusicyon*] *griseus*), culpeo fox (*Lycalopex culpaeus*); **Austria**: red fox (*Vulpes*

vulpes); **Belgium**: red fox (*Vulpes vulpes*); **Brazil**: Azara's or gray fox (*Lycalopex gymnocercus*), crab-eating fox (*Cerdocyon thous*), hoary fox (*Lycalopex vetulus*); maned wolf (*Chrysocyon brachyurus*), bush dog (*Speothos venaticus*); **China**: blue fox (*Vulpes* [syn. *Alopex*] *lagopus*); **Chile**: Darwin's or Chiloé fox (*Lycalopex* [syn. *Pseudalopex*] *fulvipes*); **Canada**: coyote (*Canis latrans*), red fox (*Vulpes vulpes*); **Czech Republic**: Australian dingo (*Canis lupus* [*familiaris*] *dingo*), Eurasian wolf (*Canis lupus*), fennec fox (*Vulpes zerda*), red fox (*Vulpes vulpes*); maned wolf (*C. brachyurus*); **Germany**: red fox (*Vulpes vulpes*); **Hungary**: red fox (*Vulpes vulpes*); **Israel**: gray wolf (*Canis lupus*), golden jackal (*Canis aureus*), red fox (*Vulpes vulpes*); **Korea**: raccoon dog (*Nyctereutes procyonoides koreensis*); **Norway**: gray wolf (*Canis lupus*); **Poland**: red fox (*Vulpes vulpes*), silver fox (probably *Vulpes vulpes*); **Romania**: red fox (*Vulpes vulpes*); **Slovakia**: Eurasian wolf (*Canis lupus lupus*), fennec fox (*Vulpes zerda*), maned wolf (*Chrysocyon brachyurus*), red fox (*Vulpes vulpes*); **Sweden**: gray wolf (*Canis lupus*), red fox (*Vulpes vulpes*); **Spain**: gray wolf (*Canis lupus*), red fox (*Vulpes vulpes*); the **United Kingdom**: red fox (*Vulpes vulpes*); the **United States**: coyote (*Canis latrans*), gray wolf (*Canis lupus*), gray fox (*Urocyon cinereoargenteus*), red fox (*Vulpes vulpes*) (Dubey et al., 2017b, Tables 16.1, 16.4).

Many wild noncanid carnivores also are known to have been exposed to *N. caninum*, either by being seropositive, demonstrating oocysts in their feces, or exhibiting signs of neosporosis. Such instances have been documented in eight countries (see Dubey et al., 2017b, Tables 16.2, 16.3, 16.4, 17.1): **Czech Republic**: black bear (*Ursus americanus*), fisher (*Martes pennanti*), polar bear (*Ursus maritimus*), South American sea lion (*Otaria flavescens*); **Japan**: bearded seal (*Erignathus barbatus*), Kuril harbor seal (*Phoca vitulina stejnegeri*), ribbon seal (*Histriophoca* [syn. *Phoca*] *fasciata*), spotted seal (*Phoca largha*); **Kenya**: spotted hyena (*Crocuta crocuta*); **Senegal**: spotted hyena (*Crocuta crocuta*); **Slovakia**: black bear (*Ursus americanus*), brown bear (*Ursus arctos*), fisher (*Martes pennanti*), polar bear (*Ursus maritimus*), South American sea lion (*Otaria* *flavescens*); **Spain**: common genet (*Genetta genetta*), Egyptian mongoose (*Herpestes ichneumon*), Eurasian badger (*Meles meles*), pine martin (*Martes martes*), polecat (*Mustela putorius*), beach marten (*Martes foina*); the **United Kingdom**: American mink (*Neovison* [syn. *Mustela*] *vison*), European badger (*Meles meles*), Eurasian otter (*Lutra lutra*), domestic ferret (*Mustela* [syn. *Putorius*] *putorius furo*), pine martin (*Martes martes*), polecat (*Mustela putorius*), ermine (*Mustela erminea*); the **United States**: bearded seal (*Erignathus barbatus*), black bear (*Ursus americanus*), harbor seal (*Phoca vitulina*), North American river otter (*Lontra canadensis*), raccoon (*Procyon lotor*), ribbon seal (*Histriophoca* [syn. *Phoca*] *fasciata*), ringed seal (*Pusa* [syn. *Phoca*] *hispida*), California sea lion (*Zalophus californianus*), sea otter (*Enhydra lutris*), spotted seal (*Phoca largha*), and walrus (*Odobenus rosmarus*).

Special mention should be made about the role of domestic cats (*Felis catus*) and wild felidae in relation to *N. caninum*. Cats are not important intermediate hosts of *N. caninum* (McAllister et al., 1998a,b), and there is no evidence for clinical neosporosis in felids. Serological prevalence of *N. caninum* antibodies in domestic cats (*F. catus*) has been found in Albania, Brazil, Czech Republic, Hungary, Iran, Italy, and Thailand (Dubey et al., 2017b, see Tables 11.1 and 11.2).

Serological prevalence of *N. caninum* antibodies in wild felids has been found in seven countries, and here we mention a brief note of each finding: **Brazil**: André et al. (2010) found antibodies to *N. caninum* in the following captive neotropical and exotic wild felids: lion (*Panthera leo*), jaguar (*Panthera* [syn. *Puma*] *onca*), jaguarundi (*Puma yagouaroundi*), little-spotted cat (*Leopardus tigrinus*), ocelot (*Leopardus pardalis*), puma/cougar (*Puma concolor*), tiger (*Panthera tigris*), pampas cat (*Leopardus* [syn. *Oncifelis*] *colocolo*), caracal (*Caracal caracal*), serval (*Leptailurus serval*), and fishing cat (*Prionailurus viverrinus*); Onuma et al. (2014) also reported the presence of *N. caninum* in the jaguar in Brazil. **Czech Republic**: Sedlák and Bártová (2006a,b) examined zoo animals for

antibodies to *N. caninum* and found the following felids to be positive: Eurasian lynx (*Lynx lynx*), cheetah (*Acinonyx jubatus*), Indian lion (*Panthera leo goojratensis*), and jaguarundi (*P. yagouaroundi*). **Kenya**: Ferroglio et al. (2003) examined wild animals for antibodies to *N. caninum* and found both cheetahs (*Acinonyx jubatus*) and lion (*Panthera leo*) to be positive. **Senegal**: Kamga-Waladjo et al. (2009) found lions (*Panthera leo*) to be seropositive for both *N. caninum* and *T. gondii*. **South Africa**: Cheadle et al. (1999) looked as seroprevalence in nondomestic felids and found both the cheetah (*Acinonyx jubatus*) and lion (*Panthera leo*) to be positive for antibodies to *N. caninum*. **Spain**: Millán et al. (2009) did a seroprevalence study for *N. caninum* and *T. gondii* in feral cats in Majorca and found the Eurasian wildcat (*Felis silvestris*) to be positive for *N. caninum*; also in Spain, Sobrino et al. (2008) found antibodies for *N. caninum* in wild Iberian lynx (*Lynx pardinus*). the **United States**: Spencer et al. (2003) did a seroprevalence study for *N. caninum* and *T. gondii* in captive and free-ranging nondomestic felids and found the following species to be positive for *N. caninum*: Amur leopard (*Panthera pardus orientalis*), lion (*Panthera leo*), Geoffroy's cat (*Leopardus* [syn. *Oncifelis*] *geoffroyi*), puma/cougar (*Puma concolor*), tiger (*Panthera tigris*), clouded leopard (*Neofelis nebulosa*), and the snow leopard (*Uncia* [syn. *Panthera*] *unica*). The zoonotic potential of *N. caninum* is still unproven and has not been confirmed.

In 1998, a new species of *Neospora*, *N. hughesi*, was described from a horse in California, USA (Marsh et al., 1998); to date, *N. hughesi* has been reported only from horses, and the definitive host is still unknown so we need not mention it further in this chapter.

***Toxoplasma gondii* (Nicolle and Manceaux, 1908) Nicolle and Manceaux, 1090.** Although some have proposed as many as six named *Toxoplasma* species in poikilotherms (Duszynski and Upton, 2010), most parasitologists who work in this area believe there is only one species, *T. gondii*, in mammals, and this apicomplexan parasite has worldwide distribution. The complete life cycle of *T. gondii* was proposed in the early 1970s, nearly 50 years ago (see below). Since then, there have been numerous attempts to make the genus multispecific, but *Toxoplasma* consistently has been recognized by most investigators as monospecific. Levine and Ivens (1981) proposed naming two other *Toxoplasma* species, *T. hammondi* (Frenkel, 1974) Levine, 1977, from, the domestic cat, in place of *Hammondia hammondi* (Frenkel and Dubey, 1975a,b) Tadros and Laarman, 1976, and *T. pardalis* (Hendricks et al., 1979) Levine and Ivens, 1981, from the ocelot, in place of *Hammondia pardalis* Hendricks et al., 1979. Alan Johnson (1998) asked the question, "Is there more than one species in the genus *Toxoplasma*?" He reviewed recent studies on closely-related taxa, including *Neospora, Hammondia, Frenkelia, Isospora,* and *Sarcocystis,* noting they have convincingly showed the need for a reclassification of many of the species in these genera. He also summarized the work of several laboratories, including his own, which have used molecular techniques (e.g., isoenzyme electrophoresis, restriction fragment length polymorphism (RFLP) analyses, RAPD–PCR, comparisons of 18S rRNA, DNA polymerase alpha intron, and 70 kDa HSP gene nucleotide sequences) to investigate the genetic diversity among *T. gondii* strains. All of these results confirm that the strains of *Toxoplasma* comprise a limited number of clonal lineages directly correlated with their virulence in mice. After reviewing the molecular research to raise the hypothesis that there may be more than one species of *Toxoplasma*, with distinct and different life cycles, Johnson reached the conclusion that molecular data are consistent with the hypothesis that two clonal lineages of *Toxoplasma* (virulent vs. avirulent) are evolving to the point where they will eventually become two distinct, reproductively isolated, species; but, probably not in our lifetimes.

Prior to the early 1970s, it was thought that *T. gondii* might be transmitted by blood sucking arthropods. For example, Woke et al. (1953) summarized the results of an extensive series of experiments they did to test if 17 arthropod species (including mites, bedbugs, conenose bugs, flies, fleas, ticks, lice) could be possible vectors of the RH strain of *T. gondii*; rabbits, guinea pigs, hamsters, rats, mice, voles, chicks, and pigeons were used as recipient hosts. Their experiments did not incriminate any of the arthropods tested as effective vectors of toxoplasmosis. Then it was considered possible that dogs might be important in transmitting toxoplasmosis because of the close and long-standing relationship between humans and dogs. Jacobs et al. (1955) noted that under some circumstances *T. gondii* can cause severe disease in dogs, and that a prior survey reported anti-*Toxoplasma* antibodies in 30/51 (59) dogs. They attempted to judge the role of the dog in regard to the manner in which *T. gondii* might be transmitted to other animals and humans. All attempts to find transmission stages in feces or urine of infected dogs proved negative. Hutchison's work (Hutchison, 1965, 1967; Hutchison et al., 1968.), although later found to be incorrect, was important because it changed the focus of research from blood sucking arthropods and fecal transmission by dogs to fecal transmission by cats (see Frenkel et al., 1970; Sheffield and Melton, 1970; Dubey et al., 1970; Overdulve, 1970a,b for the earliest work identifying cats as definitive hosts; Frenkel, 1973, 1974, and Overdulve, 1978 for brief reviews).

We now realize that *T. gondii*, in fact, may be the most ubiquitous parasite on Earth because it can be transmitted directly (fecal/oral, including using arthropods as mechanical vectors), transplacentally, and by carnivorism (see Chapter 8, pp. 133–140, in Duszynski, 2016, for brief review). Clinical toxoplasmosis has been reported in virtually all species of warm-blooded animals, including humans, domestic, and wild animals (Dubey and Beattie, 1988; Dubey, 2010). It has an indirect life cycle with cats and other felids serving as definitive hosts in which the parasite goes through both asexual and sexual **endogenous development** in intestinal epithelial cells. Pelster and Piekarski (1971) did one of the first transmission electron microscope (TEM) studies on its endogenous development when they reported on the microgametogeny of *T. gondii*. They noted a peculiarity in that the microgametes developed in groups, one after the other, in contrast to what had been seen in the eimeriid coccidia in which microgametes seem to all develop simultaneously. Ultimately, very small (~10 μm), spheroidal, unsporulated oocysts are discharged into the cat's feces. Oocysts require 1–5 days outside the cat to reach infectivity (undergo **sporulation**), this process being dependent on temperature and aeration. Except for felids, all other vertebrate animals that ingest sporulated oocysts are susceptible to infection but, in them, *T. gondii* forms cysts in cells of virtually any tissue in the body. If these tissue cysts are eaten by another omnivore or nonfelid carnivore, the process can be repeated, with the development of tissue cysts in the new host. When felids consume an animal harboring mature tissue cysts, endogenous development in the gut can be initiated, depending on that host's immune status to *T. gondii* from a previous infection, and/or bradyzoites from the ingested cysts can go on to develop in the tissues of that felid, too. Dubey and Frenkel (1972a) outlined the sequence of events in the epithelial cells of cats inoculated orally with tissue cysts of *T. gondii* and found five new structural stages they designated as "types" A–D. Interestingly, the feeding of each of the three principal *T. gondii* stages to cats results in different prepatent periods. If chronically-infected mice (older tissue cysts with bradyzoites) are fed to cats, oocysts can be found in cat feces 3–5 DPI; cats fed acutely-infected mice (young tissue cysts with tachyzoites) would not shed unsporulated oocysts until 5–10 DPI, and cats fed sporulated oocysts usually do not begin to shed oocysts until at least 20–24 DPI. Wallace (1973a,b) looked at the ecology of these principal stages when he discussed the role of cats in the natural history of *T. gondii* in field observations (Wallace, 1973b), and also

began to determine the intermediate and transport hosts that were important in this natural history (Wallace, 1973a).

The mechanisms by which *T. gondii* is transmitted in nature to maintain its ubiquity as an infectious agent still are not completely understood because they are so highly varied. Mayer (1965), was one of the first to explore such mechanisms (even before the oocyst stage was recognized), when he fed *T. gondii* in a drop of infected lab mouse peritoneal exudate to American cockroaches (*Periplaneta americana*). The cockroaches were triturated at intervals after exposure and inoculated into lab mice; *T. gondii* reportedly survived at least 65 days in the cockroach. This demonstrated, at the least, that insects in nature could become infected and, if they were ingested by mammals or birds, could be important transport hosts. Wallace (1971) demonstrated the potential of both *Musca domestica* (common housefly) and *Chrysomya megacephala* (oriental latrine fly) to be able to transmit sporulated oocysts of *T. gondii* for at least 24 and 48 hours, respectively, and *P. americana* and *Rhyparobia maderae* (syn. *Leucophaea maderae*) (Madeira cockroach) for up to 12 DPI. However, to be of practical interest, it needed to be determined that cockroaches could ingest and excrete viable oocysts, and that some of the more prevalent cockroaches were prone to ingest cat feces. Chinchilla and Ruiz (1976) did just that, working with three of the most common cockroaches in Costa Rica, *P. americana*, *P. australasiae*, and *R. maderae*, by experimentally showing that both *Periplaneta* species ate cat feces even in the presence of common foods (e.g., dough, sugar, bread, cheese) found in most Costa Rican homes, and that *R. maderae* showed the greatest tendency to ingest cat feces. Their results led them to conclude that these insects are potential transport hosts for oocysts of *T. gondii* in cat feces. They also noted that these three cockroach species are the most common in city markets were cats also abound. Later, Smith and Frenkel (1978) found German cockroaches (*Blattella germanica*) in the same room as lab mice that had become infected "spontaneously" with muscle cysts of *Sarcocystis muris* from time to time. To assess the role of *B. germanica* and *P. americana* in transmission of parasite stages in cat feces, cockroaches were exposed to cat feces that contained oocysts of *S. muris*, *Isospora felis*, *I. rivolta*, and *T. gondii*. They found that *T. gondii* oocysts were transmitted to mice by *P. americana* for up to 10 days, but only intermittently by *B. germanica* postexposure to infected cat feces.

Oocysts of *T. gondii* also appear to weather well in the external environment. Frenkel and Dubey (1973) surveyed the early literature on oocyst survival and, using experimental laboratory conditions, determined that sporulated oocysts suffer little attrition after constant or intermittent freezing at −6°C, but greater attrition at −21°C, and that sporulated oocysts survive −20°C for 28 days indicating that freezing weather alone does not eliminate oocyst infectivity from soil contaminated by cat feces. Frenkel et al. (1975) looked at the effects of freezing and soil storage at various temperature regimes in Costa Rica and Kansas (USA); in Costa Rica infectivity persisted for 1 year in three shaded sites, two moist, and one relatively dry site in the soil, and in Kansas infectivity lasted up to 18 months, including two winters. Interestingly, Frenkel et al. (1975) recovered oocysts from the surface of one *Musca*, several soil isopods, and earthworms. These results led them to suggest that the persistence of *T. gondii* oocysts in soil supported the concept that infectivity in nature may be increased logarithmically by cats. Dubey (1998) looked at the survival of sporulated *T. gondii* oocysts under defined temperatures and then tested their infectivity by mouse bioassay. There was no marked loss of infectivity of oocysts stored at 10, 15, 20, and 25°C for 200 days; oocysts stored at 35°C were infective for 32 days, but not at 62 days, those at 40°C were infective for 9 days, but not 28 days, those at 45°C were infective for 1 day, but not for 2 days. Sporulated oocysts remained infective up to 54 months at 4°C, and no loss of infectivity was

seen in oocysts stored for 106 days at −5°C and −10°C, and for 13 months at 0°C.

There have been thousands of surveys around the world looking at cat feces (for oocysts), at blood (for antibodies in a variety of *in vitro* tests), and at tissues (for cysts) in many other vertebrates, including other carnivores. Dubey (1976) pointed out that even though >60% of cats in the United States, and elsewhere, have antibody to *T. gondii*, only about 1%, or less, shed unsporulated oocysts at any given time. Dubey (2007) and Duszynski (2016) have given overviews of the history and life cycle of *T. gondii*, so that information does not need to be repeated here, and Weiss and Kim (2007) contributed a definitive textbook on the perspectives and methods of *T. gondii* as a model apicomplexan. Our intent is to give a brief overview of the pertinent and more recent literature of carnivores that have been documented as hosts for *T. gondii*, and the other three related genera of apicomplexan parasites covered in this chapter.

SPECIES DESCRIPTIONS

SUBORDER CANIFORMIA KRETZOI, 1938

AILURIDAE GRAY, 1843

GENUS *AILURUS* F.G. CUVIER, 1825 (MONOTYPIC)

AILURUS FULGENS F.G. CUVIER, 1825, RED PANDA

Hammondia. No records in the literature, yet.

Neospora. Sedlák and Bártová (2006a) surveyed 87 carnivores in zoos in the Czech and the Slovak Republics for antibodies to *N. caninum* using the IFAT. They only examined one red panda, *A. fulgens*, and it was negative. Loeffler et al. (2007) surveyed eight red pandas from the

Chengdu Research Base of Giant Panda Breeding in Sichuan, China, using the indirect fluorescent antibody assay (IFA), all of them with negative results. Qin Qin et al. (2007) surveyed red pandas from 10 captive facilities in China, in 2004, and reported that 3/73 (4%) tested positive for *N. caninum* with the "IFA screen in this study (two at 1:40, one ≥1:80)."

Toxoplasma gondii. Zhang et al. (2000) examined the sera of "rare wild carnivores" in the Shanghai Zoological Gardens, using both the modified agglutination test (MAT) and an ELISA. They collected sera from 36 wild carnivores and 27/36 (75%) were positive for *T. gondii* antibodies; these included 3/4 *A. fulgens*, which was both ELISA-positive and MAT-positive. Sedlák and Bártová (2006b) surveyed 87 carnivores in zoos in the Czech and Slovak Republics for antibodies to *T. gondii* using the IFAT. They only examined 1 red panda, *A. fulgens*, and it was positive, with a titer of 1:2,560. Loeffler et al. (2007) surveyed 8 red pandas from the Chengdu Research Base of Giant Panda Breeding in Sichuan, China using the IFA, all of them with negative results. Qin Qin et al. (2007) surveyed 73 red pandas from 10 captive facilities in China in 2004. They neglected to mention which serological test they used, but wrote, "seropositive red pandas ranged from 33% to 94% in 4 of the 10 facilities," and, "of seropositive individuals, 52% had *T. gondii* titers of a magnitude consistent with clinical disease in domestic species."

CANIDAE FISCHER, 1817

GENUS CANIS L., 1758 (6 SPECIES)

CANIS AUREUS L., 1758, GOLDEN JACKAL

Hammondia. No records in the literature, yet.

Neospora. Steinman et al. (2006) evaluated the role of wild canids in the epidemiology of bovine neosporosis in Israel. They collected wild canids and tested them for antibodies to *N. caninum*; only 4/147 (<3%) were positive for *N. caninum* antibodies, and these included 2/114 (2%) golden jackals. They concluded that wild canids probably do not have an important role in the epidemiology of *N. caninum* in Israel.

Toxoplasma gondii. Dubey et al. (2010a) surveyed the sera of many carnivores at the Breeding Centre for Endangered Arabian Wildlife (BCEAW), Sharjah, United Arab Emirates (UAE), and demonstrated antibodies to *T. gondii* in 6/8 (75%) golden jackals. Takács et al. (2014) found *Toxoplasma*-like oocysts in the feces of 1/20 (5%) wild golden jackals in Hungary. Since they only looked at oocysts in the feces, and failed to mention if they looked at sporulated oocysts or just measured unsporulated oocysts, this record must be accepted with caution.

CANIS LATRANS SAY, 1823, COYOTE

Hammondia. Gompper et al. (2003) said they found oocysts of *H. heydorni* in 4/23 (19%) *C. latrans* collected from Black Rock Forest near Cornwall, New York; their identification was based on the size of oocysts in the feces, so it should be taken with caution. Gondim et al. (2004b) used PCR tests with captive-raised coyote pups for *H. heydorni*, but they were negative.

Neospora. Coyotes are considered important in the epidemiology of neosporosis in North America (Barling et al., 2000) and *N. caninum*–like oocysts were found in the feces of 2/185 (1%) coyotes in Canada, based on PCR. Gondim et al. (2004a) used the IFAT to detect IgG antibodies against *N. caninum* and found 12/113 (11%) coyotes in three states in the United States to be positive. Gondim et al. (2004b) had four captive-raised coyote pups consume tissues from *N. caninum*–infected calves and examined their feces from 4 days prior to ingestion until 28 DPI. One pup shed *N. caninum*–like oocysts, which tested positive for *N. caninum* but negative for *H. heydorni* using PCR tests. Coyotes are the second known definitive host of *N. caninum* (also see Gondim, 2006) although Zhang et al. (2007) maintained that viable *N. caninum* oocysts have not yet been identified in feces of naturally-infected coyotes. However, many wild canids are known to have been exposed to *N. caninum*, either by being seropositive, demonstrating oocysts in their feces, or exhibiting signs of neosporosis, including coyotes in Canada and the United States. Wapenaar et al. (2007) evaluated the performance and agreement of serological assays (ELISA, IFAT, *Neospora caninum* agglutination test [NAT] and immunoblot) using reference sera and field sera from foxes to estimate their *N. caninum* seroprevalence on Prince Edward Island (PEI), Canada. They collected serum from 201 coyotes, and the seroprevalence observed in the different assays ranged from 0.5% to 14% in coyotes. The seroprevalence, when taking more than one test positive as cutoff value was 3% for coyotes. Wapenaar et al. (2007) felt that positive agreement was moderate-to-poor among all assays utilized in their study. Although the seroprevalence observed was low, *N. caninum* antibodies were present in coyotes on PEI. Stieve et al. (2010) examined serum samples from *C. latrans* that had been collected by the Alaska Department of Fish and Game, and the Yukon Department of the Environment; samples were assayed for *N. caninum*–reactive antibodies by the IFAT, and they found 2/12 (17%) coyotes to be positive.

Toxoplasma gondii. Franti et al. (1976) tested 2,796 serum samples from wild and domestic mammals and birds in northern California for antibodies to *T. gondii* and found 16/58 (28%) coyotes to be positive. Quinn et al. (1976) surveyed the blood of a variety of wild carnivores in southern Ontario, for antibodies to *T. gondii*, using the Sabin–Feldman dye test; they found 123/158 (78%) *C. latrans* to be positive for antibodies. Tizard et al. (1976) surveyed the blood of a variety of wild carnivores in central Ontario for antibodies to *T. gondii*, also using the dye test,

and found 18/28 (64%) *C. latrans* to be positive for antibodies. Gondim et al. (2004a) used the IFAT to detect IgG antibodies against *T. gondii* and found 35/113 (31%) coyotes in three US states to be positive. In Alaska, Stieve et al. (2010) examined serum samples from *C. latrans* that had been collected by the Alaska Department of Fish and Game, and the Yukon Department of the Environment; samples were assayed for *T. gondii*–reactive antibodies with a MAT, and they found 2/2 coyotes to be negative.

CANIS LUPUS L., 1758, WOLF

Hammondia. No records in the literature, yet.
Neospora. Gray wolves are considered important hosts in the epidemiology of neosporosis in wildlife and free-range cattle in the United States. The existence of a sylvatic cycle of *N. caninum* was suggested by Gondim et al. (2004b), who fed naturally-infected deer tissues to dogs, which later discharged oocysts. Gondim et al. (2004a) also reported the presence of *N. caninum* antibodies in 25/164 (39%) wolves from Minnesota, by using the IFAT. During their serosurvey of wild animals in the United States, Dubey and Thulliez (2005) detected antibodies to *N. caninum* in 4/122 (3%) *C. lupus* from Alaska, using the NAT. Steinman et al. (2006) evaluated the role of wild canids in the epidemiology of bovine neosporosis in Israel. They collected wild canids and tested them for antibodies to *N. caninum*; only 4/147 (<3%) were positive for *N. caninum* antibodies, and these included 1/9 (11%) *C. lupus*. They concluded that wild canids probably do not play an important role in the epidemiology of *N. caninum* in Israel. Sedlák and Bártová (2006a,b) surveyed 87 carnivores in zoos in the Czech and Slovak Republics for antibodies to *N. caninum* using the IFAT; they reported that two *C. l. dingo* (dingo) were negative, but 2/10 (20%) *C. l. lupus* (Eurasian wolf) had positive titers. André et al. (2010) detected antibodies to *N. caninum* in wild captive carnivores in

zoos of São Paulo and Mato Grosso states, and the Federal District, Brazil. Serum antibodies were detected by the IFAT using tachyzoites of *N. caninum* NC-1 strain; André et al. (2010) found 2/3 (57%) European wolves to be seropositive for *N. caninum*. In Alaska, Stieve et al. (2010) examined serum samples from *C. lupus* collected by the Alaska Department of Fish and Game, and the Yukon Department of the Environment; samples were assayed for *N. caninum*–reactive antibodies by IFAT, and they found 29/324 (9%) wolves to be positive. Björkman et al. (2010) examined blood samples from wolves within the Scandinavia Wolf Project, Skandulv. Samples were analyzed by *N. caninum* iscom ELISA, and by immunoblotting, and only those positive with both tests were considered positive; 4/190 (<4%) wolves were positive indicating that the parasite was found in a few Scandinavian wolves, but the authors could not say how they might have acquired the infections. Finally, *Neospora caninum*–like oocysts were found in the feces of 3/73 (4%) wolves (Dubey et al., 2011), and oocysts from one of these samples proved to be *N. caninum* by bioassays in KO mice, propagation in cell culture, and by DNA characterization.

Toxoplasma gondii. Zhang et al. (2000) examined the sera of "rare wild carnivores" in the Shanghai Zoological Gardens using both the MAT and an ELISA. They collected sera from 36 wild carnivores, and *T. gondii* antibodies were found in 8/10 (80%) wolves; all 8 were ELISA-positive, whereas 6 were positive via the MAT. Sedlák and Bártová (2006a,b) surveyed 87 carnivores in zoos in the Czech and Slovak Republics for antibodies to *T. gondii* using the IFAT; they reported that 1/2 (50%) *C. l. dingo* (dingo) and 10/10 (100%) *C. l. lupus* (Eurasian wolf) had positive titers. A serosurvey of *T. gondii* in free-ranging carnivores in Spain was carried out by Sobrino et al. (2007). Serum samples from 282 wild carnivores from different regions were tested for antibodies, using the MAT (as per Dubey and Desmonts, 1987, cutoff ≥ 1:25);

antibodies to *T. gondii* were detected in 15/32 (47%) *C. lupus*.

Canine distemper virus predisposes dogs to a variety of secondary infections, particularly toxoplasmosis (Dubey et al., 2002a; Ehrensperger and Pospischil, 1989), and the canine distemper/toxoplasmosis synergism is well documented (Freitas-Girau, 2002). André et al. (2010) detected antibodies to *T. gondii* in wild captive carnivores in zoos of São Paulo and Mato Grosso states, and the Federal District, Brazil, using the IFAT with tachyzoites of *T. gondii* RH strain as antigen; they found 2/3 (57%) European wolves to be seropositive for *T. gondii*. Dubey et al. (2010a) surveyed the sera of many carnivores at the BCEAW, Sharjah, UAE, and demonstrated antibodies to *T. gondii* in 5/8 (62.5%) wolves, *Canis lupus arabs* Pocock, 1934. In Alaska, Stieve et al. (2010) examined serum samples from *C. lupus* that had been collected by the Alaska Department of Fish and Game, and the Yukon Department of the Environment; samples were assayed for *T. gondii*–reactive antibodies with a MAT, and they found 57/320 (18%) wolves to be positive.

CANIS LUPUS DINGO MEYER, 1793, AUSTRALIAN DINGO

Hammondia. No records in the literature, yet.

Neospora. King et al. (2010) looked at Australian dingoes as definitive hosts of *N. caninum*. Three dingo pups raised in captivity, and three domestic dogs, were fed tissue from calves infected with an Australian isolate of *N. caninum*. Oocysts of *N. caninum*, confirmed by species-specific PCR, were shed in small numbers by one dingo on 12–14 DPI, but not by domestic dogs. However, the blood from 2/3 (67%) dingoes tested positive for DNA of *N. caninum*, using PCR, on 14 and 28 DPI, and the blood of 2/3 domestic dogs also converted to seropositive, using ELISIA, on the 28th DPI. The authors suggested that the shedding of oocysts by one dingo demonstrated that dingoes are a definitive host of *N. caninum*, and horizontal transmission of the parasite from dingoes to farm animals and wildlife may occur in Australia. In a follow-up study, King et al. (2011) emphasized that dingoes in Australia, as top-order predator, suggested a potential sylvatic cycle of transmission between them and, as yet unknown, native wildlife and domestic animals, via domesticated dogs that have access to infected tissues on farms. They summarized all the literature in Australia, to that date, on serological and molecular identifications of *N. caninum*, showing that domestic dogs (via IFTA or PCR) had a prevalence ranging from 5% to 14% (depending on the state sampled). Dingoes are considered important in the epidemiology of neosporosis in Australia because wild dogs in aboriginal communities are most likely dingo/wild dog hybrids. In fact, Barber et al. (1997) did an IFAT seroprevalence survey of antibodies to *N. caninum* in canid populations from five countries on three continents. In New South Wales, Australia, 0/117 dingo/wild dog hybrids (they called them *C. familiaris dingo*) had antibodies to *N. caninum*, whereas 15/52 (29%) Queensland hybrid dingoes were seropositive with titers of 1:50 (n=4), 1:200 (n=4), 1:800 (n=3), and 1:3,200 (n=4), all considered low.

Toxoplasma gondii. Sedlák and Bártová (2006a) used the IFAT to try to detect antibodies to *T. gondii* in 556 zoo animals in the Chech and Slovak Republics. Only 1/2 (50%) dingoes had antibodies to *T. gondii*, with a titer of 1:640.

CANIS LUPUS FAMILIARIS L., 1758, DOMESTIC DOG

Hammondia. *Hammondia heydorni* represents and takes the place of, the small race of *I. bigemina* (see Introduction, above), which has gone by several names (e.g., *I. bigemina* var. *babiensis*, *I. babiensis*, *C. babiensis*). Wenyon and Sheather (1925) exhibited specimens illustrating an *I. bigemina* (small form) infection of dogs at a laboratory meeting held at the Royal Army Medical College, Millibank, London; there they described an acute infection in which the whole of the epithelial lining of the small intestine, from stomach to large intestine, was involved. They said, "Practically every villus in its distal portion had its epithelium crowded with schizonts, which produce eight small merozoites. Numbers of female gametocytes were also present." The oocysts passed by the dog had fairly thick walls, were unsporulated, and measured 11×10 in length. McKenna and Charleston (1980d), working on the North Island, New Zealand, examined fecal samples from domestic dogs and identified oocysts of *H. heydorni* in 13/481 (3%) samples. Matsui et al. (1981) infected guinea pigs, mice, rats, rabbits, hamsters, dogs, and cats with sporulated oocysts, which they called "small type of *Isospora bigemina*," but which were almost certainly *H. heydorni*. Their oocysts were $L \times W$: 12.4×11.2 (10.5–13.5×8.5–13); L/W ratio: 1.1 (1.0–1.3), with M, OR, PG: all absent; subspheroidal to ellipsoidal sporocysts were $L \times W$: 9.3×7.0 (7.5–11×5–8); L/W ratio: 1.3 (1.0–1.7) without SB, but with an SR. None of the animals inoculated with sporulated oocysts discharged fresh oocysts, but organs from a guinea pig and a dog fed sporulated oocysts were fed to two puppies and both discharged fresh, unsporulated oocysts on 7 and 8 DPI, respectively. A mouse, rat, rabbit, and a hamster were inoculated with sporulated oocysts and killed on various days from 60 to 107 DPI; their organs were each fed to one dog, but none of these dogs shed any oocysts. Later, Matsui et al. (1986, 1987), using oocysts they called *Isospora heydorni*–like (= *H. heydorni*), studied the endogenous stages in dog intestine after feeding them organs of guinea pigs that had been inoculated with oocysts. Endogenous stages were seen throughout the jejunum and ileum, and most were located in epithelial cells at the tips of the villi. Asexual development was both by binary and multiple fission (merogony) and meronts contained 2–15 merozoites. Microgametocytes and microgametes were observed, but not macrogametes (Matsui et al., 1986). Oocysts harvested from infected dogs were used to infect two 10-month-old Holstein calves that were killed between 43 and 53 DPI. When calf tissues (brain, small intestine, striated muscles, liver, mesenteric lymph nodes) were fed to dogs, all recipients began to shed unsporulated oocysts between 6 and 9 DPI. Haralabidis et al. (1988) took fecal samples from 232 healthy dogs in the area of Thessaloniki, Greece, and reported that only one (0.04%) passed oocysts of *H. heydorni*. Varga and Dubos-Kováca (1988) reported the first finding of *H. heydorni* in Hungary, when they collected oocysts from the feces of a 14-week-old dog and inoculated them into guinea pigs. The guinea pigs were killed 33 DPI, and skinned, minced carcasses fed to six puppies that began to shed unsporulated oocysts 8–10 DPI, and continued to shed oocysts from 1 to 6 days longer. Blagburn et al. (1988) helped further characterize the biology of *H. heydorni* with their cross-infection studies administering sporulated oocysts from a dog to three other dogs, five goats, a calf, and three guinea pigs, and then inoculating tissues from these into other coccidia-free dogs. Although dogs fed goat tissues infected with *H. heydorni* did excrete oocysts, no developmental stages were found in histological sections of the tissues from any of the animals in their experiments. Gothe and Reichler (1990) checked fecal samples of 100 randomly selected dog families in Germany; they reported that the "excretion extent of the litters and their mothers was 7% and 6% for *H. heydorni*." Shanker et al. (1991) pooled muscle samples from the esophagus and diaphragm of goats collected from slaughter houses in Haldwani and Pantnagar, India, and fed 250 g quantities to two pups for two consecutive days, after which they monitored their feces. Both pups started shedding unsporulated oocysts on 5 and 7 DPI and continued shedding oocysts for 7 and 8 more days, respectively. Oocysts sporulated in 2–3 days and measured L×W: 11–14×10.5–13; oocysts lacked M, PG, and OR, and sporocysts lacked a SB and SSB, but had a SR, which was a compact mass of granules. No clinical symptoms were noticed in either of the pups. Hilali et al. (1992) fed nine dogs pooled heart and esophagus muscle from

different numbers (15–30) of camels (*Camelus dromedarius*), and monitored their fecal output, via salt flotation, for 70 DPI. Two dogs began passing oocysts later identified (after sporulation) as those of *H. heydorni* on 3 and 13 DPI, patency lasted 2 and 9 days, respectively, and the small, subspheroidal oocysts (L×W: 12×11) sporulated after 72 hours at 27°C in 2.5% aqueous potassium dichromate ($K_2Cr_2O_7$) solution in Petri dishes (Hilali et al., 1992). Epe et al. (1993), in Germany, surveyed fecal samples from domestic dogs between 1984 and 1991 and found 7/3,329 (0.2%) pass *H. heydorni* oocysts. Bugg et al. (1999) examined fecal samples collected from urban dogs originating from four pet shops, three refuges, six breeding kennels, eight veterinary clinics, and two exercise areas in the Perth metropolitan area, Western Australia. Samples were processed by centrifugation–flotation in saturated zinc sulfate solution, and *H. heydorni* was detected in 7/421 (<2%) samples, mostly in dogs from refuges. Gennari et al. (1999) examined fecal samples of domestic dogs from São Paulo, Brazil, using sucrose flotation and water–ether centrifugation–sedimentation techniques; they found oocysts of *H. heydorni* in 3/353 (<1%) fecal samples.

Neospora. Transplacental infection of *N. caninum* was induced experimentally in dogs (Dubey and Lindsay, 1989b; Cole et al., 1995). Barber et al. (1997) did an IFAT seroprevalence survey for *N. caninum* in canid populations from five countries on three continents. In Australia, 42/451 (9%) domestic dogs had antibodies to *N. caninum*, but this varied by city: Melbourne, 11/207 (5%), Sydney, 18/150 (12%), Perth 13/94 (14%). In South America, Uruguay had 82/414 (20%) dogs positive with antibodies, but the Falkland Islands had only 1/500 (0.2%) domestic dogs positive for *N. caninum* antibodies. In Africa, Kenya had 0/140 dogs positive, whereas in Tanzania, 11/49 dogs (22%) had antibodies to *N. caninum* via the IFAT. Also using the IFAT, Patitucci et al. (2001) found 36/201 (18%) dogs positive for antibodies (≥1:50), with rural dogs (21/81, 26%) having a higher incidence of infection/exposure than urban dogs (34/120, 12.5%). Kim et al. (2003) studied antibodies to *N. caninum* among domesticated urban and rural dogs in Korea, using both the IFAT and the NAT; they found sera from 23/289 (8%) domestic urban dogs, and 33/51 (22%) dairy farm dogs, in Korea, to be positive for *N. caninum*. Dubey et al. (2006) found at least two dogs that had died of neosporosis. Their Dog No. 4 was reported to have produced one pup that died at 7-months-old of a *Neospora*-like disease; it had interstitial myocarditis and hepatitis and *N. caninum*–like tachyzoites in cardiac myosites. Their Dog No. 5 had numerous tachyzoites, and a few tissue cysts, in the brain and spinal cord that reacted with *N. caninum* monoclonal antibody, and this diagnosis was confirmed with retrospective staining of brain sections and spinal cord with polyclonal antibodies. Dubey et al. (2008b) looked at the prevalence of antibodies to *N. caninum* in the serum of dogs in Granada, West Indies, using the IFAT, and found only 2/107 (2%) to be positive; both dogs also had antibodies to *T. gondii*. Salb et al. (2008) examined blood sera of dogs from two remote northern Canadian communities (Fort Chipewyan, Alberta; Fort Resolution, Northwest Territories). Sera were screened for antibodies against *N. caninum* using the IFAT and *N. caninum* was detected, but the number of positive samples and further details were not provided.

King et al. (2012) conducted what was likely the first parasitological survey of wild dogs and Aboriginal community dogs in Australia. Wild dogs are those that are not dependent on humans for survival and include the dingo, feral domestic dog, and their hybrid genotypes. Aboriginal community dogs are dependent on humans, are domesticated and owned by a family, but roam with free-access throughout the community; they consist mostly of domestic dogs or domestic/dingo hybrids. King et al. (2012) examined 75 wild dogs and 299 Aboriginal dogs and used a combination of microscopic, molecular, and serological techniques to determine the extent of *N. caninum* infection in them. Serum (n=14), blood (n=4), and fecal (n=66) samples were

collected from 75 wild dogs in 8 rural areas of New South Wales and Queensland. Similarly, blood (n=37), serum (n=249), and fecal (n=66) samples were collected from 299 Aboriginal dogs in communities of the Northern Territory, Western Australia, northwestern New South Wales, and tropical north Queensland. Fecal samples (n=132) were examined for *N. caninum*–like oocysts via standard flotation techniques, serum samples (n=263) were screened for antibodies to *N. caninum* using a competitive ELISA (cELISA *N. caninum*) test kit, and 194 of these serum samples also were screened for *N. caninum* antibodies using an IFAT with *N. caninum* tachyzoites. Only 2/132 (1.5%) juvenile Aboriginal community dogs had small numbers of unsporulated oocysts (~10–11.5 wide) in their feces, and both samples contained *N. caninum* DNA using Nc5 and ITS-1 rDNA. Given the low sensitivity and moderate specificity of the cELISA, King et al. (2012) attempted to optimize the manufacturer's recommended percentage inhibition cutoff (>30%) using an IFAT to detect *N. caninum* in the 263 serum samples tested; they determined that the true prevalence of infection was 71/263 (27%). Of the 41 blood samples (34 adults, 6 juveniles) only 3/41 (7%) had detectable *N. caninum* DNA. This study found a relatively high seroprevalence of *N. caninum* in Australian dogs, with significantly more adult than juvenile dogs being infected, indicating that postnatal exposure to *N. caninum* is most likely occurring. This study also demonstrated that *N. caninum* in dogs is widespread throughout Australia, including the semiarid and arid regions of northwestern New South Wales, and the Northern Territory. Dubey et al. (2014) studied two *Sarcocystis* species in four domestic dogs, and one of their dogs (Dog D from British Columbia, Canada) was tested for antibodies to *T. gondii* (negative), but had a low (1:50) antibody titer to *N. caninum*.

Toxoplasma gondii. Sedlák and Bártová (2006b), using the IFAT, with both IgM and IgA antibodies, found IgM antibodies to *T. gondii* in 10/413 (2%) dogs and IgG antibodies in 107/413

(26%) dogs in the Czech Republic. In pet dogs, 10/250 (4%) had IgM titers and 82/250 (33%) had IgG titers, whereas antibody titers in police dogs were 0/115 and 25/115 (22%), respectively, for these antibodies. They found no statistically significant differences in antibody prevalence between clinically healthy (n=115) and diseased (n=80) pet dogs and concluded that even though *T. gondii* is common in domestic dogs, its clinical importance is low in the Czech Republic. Prior to their study (Sedlák and Bártová, 2006b), *T. gondii* had been reported in dogs in other European countries including Austria (63/242, 26%, Wanha et al., 2005), Czech Republic (501/1,002, 50%, Svoboda and Svobodová, 1987), Germany (58/200, 29%, Klein and Muller, 2001), Spain (17/139, 12%, Ortuno et al., 2002), and Sweden (70/303, 23%, Uggla et al., 1990). Suzán and Ceballos (2005) did a serosurvey of wildlife infections in two nature reserves within Mexico City limits and used a complement fixation test to find antibodies to *T. gondii*. They collected 16 blood samples from carnivores and found 2/3 (67%) *C. l. familiaris* to be positive for *T. gondii*. Dubey et al. (2008b) looked at the prevalence of antibodies to *T. gondii* and *N. caninum* in the serum of dogs in Granada, West Indies, using the MAT, and antibodies to *T. gondii* were found in 52/107 (48.5%) of the dogs sampled; their titers ranged widely: 1:25 in 17 dogs; 1:50 in 19 dogs; 1:100 in 7 dogs; 1:1,600 in 5 dogs; and 1:3,200 or higher in 4 dogs. Seroprevalence increased with age from 2% in dogs <6-months-old to 19% in dogs ≥2-years-old. Salb et al. (2008) examined sera of dogs from two remote northern Canadian communities (Fort Chipewyan, Alberta; Fort Resolution, Northwest Territories). Sera were screened for antibodies against *T. gondii* by a modified direct agglutination technique, and *T. gondii* was detected, but the number of positive samples and further details were not provided. Costa et al. (2012) did a serosurvey of domestic and wild animals in Fernando de Noronha, Brazil, looking for antibodies to *T. gondii* using the IFAT or the MAT, or both; overall, they found 36/91 (40%) domestic dogs demonstrated antibodies. Gerhold et al. (2014) examined a 2-year-old male basset hound-beagle mix, postmortem and found progressive neurological impairment; the dog had multiple raised masses on the spinal cord between nerve roots. Microscopically, Gerhold et al. (2014) diagnosed protozoal myeloencephalitis, and both *T. gondii* and *Sarcocystis neurona* were detected in the CNS by immunohistochemistry and PCR. This was the first report of dual *T. gondii* and *S. neurona* infections in a dog. Pomerantz et al. (2016) did a serosurvey of carnivores at Kirindy Mitea and Ankarafantsika National Parks in Madagascar and tested them for antibodies to five viral pathogens, as well as for *T. gondii* (by ELISA); samples included 51 *C. l. familiaris* from villages near the parks, and antibodies to *T. gondii* were detected in 14/16 (88%) domestic dogs. Scorza and Lappin (2017) examined blood sera of dogs on the Pine Ridge Indian Reservation, South Dakota, USA, for ELISA-specific antibodies against *T. gondii*; they reported 12/82 (15%) positive samples.

GENUS *CERDOCYON* C.H.E. SMITH, 1839 (MONOTYPIC)

CERDOCYON THOUS (L., 1766), CRAB-EATING FOX

Hammondia. Soares et al. (2009) demonstrated that *C. thous* can serve as a definitive host for *H. heydorni*. Infected masseter muscle and brain from two 2-year-old bovines were minced and pooled and fed to four *C. thous* on two consecutive days. Two foxes shed unsporulated, subspheroidal oocysts that were 10–15 wide, on 8 and 9 DPI. One of the foxes eliminated oocysts for 5 days and the other for 9 days. DNA samples of oocysts were collected on each DPI and their 18S rRNA and heat-shock protein 70 kDa genes were sequenced. Nucleotide sequences amplified from the oocysts shed by these foxes revealed 100% identity with homologous sequences of *H. heydorni* to demonstrate that *C. thous* is a good definitive host for *H. heydorni*.

Neospora. Cañón-Franco et al. (2004) utilized both the IFAT and the NAT to examine sera from three species of wild canids in Brazil for antibodies to *N. caninum.* They found 4/15 (27%) *C. thous* to test positive for *N. caninum.* André et al. (2010) detected antibodies to *N. caninum* and *T. gondii* in sera of wild captive carnivores from zoos of São Paulo and Mato Grosso states, and the Federal District, Brazil. Antibodies were detected by the IFAT using tachyzoites of *N. caninum* NC-1 strain antigen. André et al. (2010) found 13/39 (33%) *C. thous* to be seropositive for *N. caninum.*

Toxoplasma gondii. André et al. (2010) detected antibodies to *T. gondii* in wild captive carnivores in zoos of São Paulo and Mato Grosso states, and the Federal District, Brazil. Antibodies were detected by the IFAT using tachyzoites of *T. gondii* RH-strain as antigen; they found 14/39 (36%) *C. thous* were seropositive for *T. gondii.* Richini-Pereira et al. (2016) looked for the presence of *T. gondii* in tissue samples of 64 road-killed animals using PCR. Positive samples were then typed by PCR–RFLP using 7 specific markers (SAG1, 5′-3′ SAG2, SAG3, BTUB, c29-6, PK1, Apico). PCR–RFLP targeting the 18S rRNA gene was performed on all samples to detect other apicomplexan parasites; they detected *T. gondii* DNA in one road-killed *C. thous.* The amplified *T. gondii* 18S rRNA products (GenBank accession No. L37415.1) were confirmed by sequencing.

GENUS *CHRYSOCYON* C.H.E. SMITH, 1839 (MONOTYPIC)

CHRYSOCYON BRACHYURUS (ILLIGER, 1815), MANED WOLF

Hammondia. No records in the literature, yet.
Neospora. Vitaliano et al. (2004) obtained sera from captive maned wolves from six zoos and one ecological reserve in southeastern and midwestern Brazil and used the IFAT to determine the presence of *N. caninum;* they found 5/59 (8%) wolves had antibodies to *N. caninum.* Sedlák and Bártová (2006a,b) surveyed 87 carnivores in zoos in the Czech and the Slovak Republics for antibodies to *N. caninum* using the IFAT; they reported only 1/6 (17%) *C. brachyurus* had a positive titer. André et al. (2010) detected antibodies to *N. caninum* in wild captive carnivores in zoos of São Paulo and Mato Grosso states, and the Federal District, Brazil. Antibodies were detected by the IFAT, using tachyzoites of *N. caninum* NC-1 strain as antigen, and they found 5/21 (24%) maned wolves to be seropositive for *N. caninum.*

Toxoplasma gondii. Vitaliano et al. (2004) examined sera from captive maned wolves from six zoos and one ecological reserve in southeastern and midwestern Brazil and used an ELISA protocol to determine the presence of *T. gondii;* they found 44/59 (75%) wolves with antibodies to *T. gondii.* Sedlák and Bártová (2006a,b) surveyed 87 carnivores in zoos in the Czech and Slovak Republics for antibodies to *T. gondii* using the IFAT; they reported 6/6 (100%) *C. brachyurus* had positive titers. Using the IFAT with tachyzoites of *T. gondii* RH-strain as antigen, André et al. (2010) examined wild captive carnivores in zoos of São Paulo and Mato Grosso states, and the Federal District, Brazil, and found 11/21 (52%) maned wolves to be seropositive for *T. gondii.* Vitaliano et al. (2014) studied fragments of the brain and heart tissues of free-living and captive wild animals from Brazil to isolate and genotype *T. gondii;* all samples were submitted to mice bioassay and screened by PCR based on 18S rRNA sequences, and 15/226 (7%) *T. gondii* isolates were obtained, including the only maned wolf sampled. DNA from the isolates, from mice bioassay, and from the tissues of the wild animal, was genotyped by PCR–RFLP, using 12 genetic markers (SAG1, SAG2, alt. SAG2, SAG3, BTUB, GRA6, c22-8, c29-2, L258, PK1, CS3, and Apico). Vitaliano et al. (2014) identified 17 *T. gondii* genotypes, 13 for the first time, and 4 already reported in published literature, including the 1 from the maned wolf. From their study, and the work of others, it seems clear that Brazil has both high diversity and unique genotypes of *T. gondii.* Clearly, future studies on *T. gondii* from wildlife are needed to understand population genetics and structure of this parasite.

GENUS CUON HODGSON, 1838 (MONOTYPIC)

CUON ALPINUS (PALLAS, 1811), DHOLE

Hammondia. No records in the literature, yet.
Neospora. No records in the literature, yet.
Toxoplasma gondii. Zhang et al. (2000) examined one dhole that was kept in the Shanghai Zoological Garden and found it negative for antibodies to *T. gondii* by both ELISA and MAT.

GENUS *LYCALOPEX* BURMEISTER, 1854 (6 SPECIES)

LYCALOPEX (SYN. DUSICYON) CULPAEUS (MOLINA, 1782), CULPEO

Hammondia. No records in the literature, yet.
Neospora. Martino et al. (2004) did a serological survey in the Patagonia region of Argentina to estimate the prevalence of 9 disease agents in 28 free-ranging culpeos; using the IFAT (≥1:25), they found 17/28 (61%) culpeos to be positive for *N. caninum.*
Toxoplasma gondii. Thiermann (1962) examined one culpeo captured in Caleu, Santiago, Chile; its blood demonstrated antibodies to *T. gondii* by the Sabin–Feldman dye test (1:256) and by a compliment–fixation reaction (1:5). Muscle, liver, and heart tissues were macerated and injected intraperitoneally into mice, which later were positive for *T. gondii*, both by the dye test (1:1,000) and compliment fixation (1:160). In a second subtransplant to mice, Thiermann (1962) found numerous trophozoites of *T. gondii* in their peritoneal exudate. Martino et al. (2004) did a serological survey, in the Patagonia region of Argentina, to estimate the prevalence of nine disease agents in free-ranging culpeo. They used

the MAT to detect titers (≥1:32) for *T. gondii* and found 11/28 (36%) culpeos to be positive.

LYCALOPEX (SYN. PSEUDALOPEX) FULVIPES (MARTIN, 1837), DARWIN'S OR CHILOÉ FOX

Hammondia. No records in the literature, yet.
Neospora. Patitucci et al. (2001) used the NAT on sera they collected from two Chiloé foxes and both were positive (≥1:320); these animals are native of Chile, but they were owned by a local zoo.
Toxoplasma gondii. No records in the literature, yet.

LYCALOPEX (SYN. DUSICYON) GRISEUS (GRAY, 1837) SOUTH AMERICAN GRAY FOX

Hammondia. No records in the literature, yet.
Neospora. Martino et al. (2004), in the Patagonia region of Argentina, used the IFAT to find specific antibodies (≥1:25) for *N. caninum* and found 20/56 (36%) gray foxes to be positive.
Toxoplasma gondii. Martino et al. (2004) also used the modified DAT to detect titers (≥1:32) for *T. gondii* and found the sera of 19/56 (34%) gray foxes to be positive.

LYCALOPEX GYMNOCERCUS (G. FISCHER, 1814), PAMPAS OR AZARA'S FOX

Hammondia. No records in the literature, yet.
Neospora. Cañón-Franco et al. (2004) utilized the IFAT and the NAT to examine sera from three species of wild canids in Brazil for antibodies to *N. caninum.* They found 5/12 (42%) *L. gymnocercus* to test positive for *N. caninum.*
Toxoplasma gondii. No records in the literature, yet.

LYCALOPEX (SYN. PSEUDALOPEX) VETULUS (LUND, 1842), HOARY FOX

Hammondia. No records in the literature, yet.

Neospora. André et al. (2010) detected antibodies to *N. caninum* in wild captive carnivores in zoos of São Paulo and Mato Grosso states, and the Federal District, Brazil, by the IFAT using tachyzoites of *N. caninum* NC-1 strain, and found 4/7 (57%) hoary foxes to be seropositive for *N. caninum.* Nascimento et al. (2015) looked for the presence of *N. caninum* DNA in brain tissue samples from 49 hoary foxes, in Paraíba, Brazil. DNA was extracted and PCR performed using species-specific primers, and they found 6/49 (12%) foxes positive for *N. caninum.* The hoary fox is a wild canid native to Brazil and is commonly found in the semiarid northeastern area living in contact with cattle. Nascimento et al. (2015) demonstrated the presence of *N. caninum* DNA in free-ranging foxes in Brazil for the first time, confirming this species as an intermediate host.

Toxoplasma gondii. André et al. (2010) examined wild captive carnivores in zoos of São Paulo and Mato Grosso, and the Federal District, Brazil, by the IFAT using tachyzoites of *T. gondii* RH strain as antigen, and found 5/7 (71%) hoary foxes to be seropositive for *T. gondii.* Vitaliano et al. (2014) studied fragments of brain and heart tissues from free-living and captive wild animals from Brazil to isolate and genotype *T. gondii*; all samples were submitted to mice bioassay and screened by PCR based on 18S rRNA sequences; 15/226 (7%) *T. gondii* isolates were obtained, including samples from the only hoary fox examined. DNA from all isolates, from mice bioassay and from the tissues of the hoary fox, was genotyped by PCR–RFLP, using 12 genetic markers (SAG1, SAG2, alt. SAG2, SAG3, BTUB, GRA6, c22-8, c29-2, L258, PK1, CS3, and Apico). Vitaliano et al. (2014) identified 17 *T. gondii* genotypes, 13 for the first time including the one in the fox, and four already reported in published literature. From theirs, and the work of others, it is clear that Brazil has both high diversity and unique genotypes of *T. gondii.*

Nascimento et al. (2015) looked for the presence of *T. gondii* DNA in brain tissue from 49 hoary foxes, in Paraíba, Brazil. DNA was extracted and PCR was performed using primers specific for *T. gondii,* and 7/49 (14%) foxes were positive for *T. gondii.* Nascimento et al. (2015) demonstrated the presence of *T. gondii* DNA in free-ranging foxes in Brazil for the first time, confirming that this species is an important intermediate host.

GENUS LYCAON BROOKES, 1827 (MONOTYPIC)

LYCAON PICTUS (TEMMINCK, 1820), AFRICAN WILD DOG

Hammondia. No records in the literature, yet.

Neospora. Sedlák and Bártová (2006a,b) surveyed 87 carnivores in zoos in the Czech and Slovak Republics for antibodies to *N. caninum* using the IFAT; they reported that all nine *L. pictus* tested were negative.

Toxoplasma gondii. Sedlák and Bártová (2006a,b) surveyed 87 carnivores in zoos in the Czech and Slovak Republics for antibodies to *T. gondii* using the IFAT; they reported that 6/9 (67%) *L. pictus* had positive titers for *T. gondii.*

GENUS NYCTEREUTES TEMMINCK, 1838 (MONOTYPIC)

NYCTEREUTES PROCYONOIDES KOREENSIS MORI, 1922, KOREAN RACCOON DOG

Hammondia. No records in the literature, yet.

Neospora. Kim et al. (2003) studied antibodies to *N. caninum* in dogs and raccoon dogs in Korea, using both the IFAT and the NAT. They found the sera from 6/26 (23%) Korean raccoon dogs to be positive for *N. caninum.*

Toxoplasma gondii. No records in the literature, yet.

NYCTEREUTES PROCYONOIDES VIVERRINUS TEMMINC, 1838, KOREAN RACCOON DOG

Hammondia. No records in the literature, yet.
Neospora. No records in the literature, yet.
Toxoplasma gondii. Murasugi et al. (1996) used latex fixation tests for mainland raccoon dogs, all of which were kept in the Kanazawa Zoo, Yokohama City, Kanagawa Prefecture, Japan, to measure levels of *T. gondii* antibodies; they found 20/109 (18%) raccoon dogs were positive, verifying that *T. gondii* infection exists in the *N. p. viverrinus* population in Kanagawa Prefecture, and that it could be a source of infection as a zoonotic disease agent.

GENUS *SPEOTHOS* LUND, 1839 (MONOTYPIC)

SPEOTHOS VENATICUS (LUND, 1842), BUSH DOG

Hammondia. No records in the literature, yet.
Neospora. Sedlák and Bártová (2006a,b) surveyed 87 carnivores in zoos in the Czech and Slovak Republics for antibodies to *N. caninum* using the IFAT; they reported that the three bush dogs they tested were negative. Mattos et al. (2008) demonstrated for the first time the presence of antibodies to *N. caninum* in 2/6 (33%) *S. venaticus* from Brazil. André et al. (2010) drew blood from 258 wild captive carnivores in zoos of São Paulo and Mato Grosso states, and the Federal District, Brazil, to detect antibodies by the IFAT using tachyzoites of *N. caninum* NC-1 strain as antigen. They (2010) found 16/27 (59%) bush dogs to be seropositive for *N. caninum*.

Toxoplasma gondii. Sedlák and Bártová (2006a,b) surveyed 87 carnivores in zoos in the Czech and Slovak Republics for antibodies to *T. gondii* using the IFAT; they reported that 3/3 (100%) *S. venaticus* had positive titers. André et al. (2010) examined the blood of wild captive carnivores in zoos of São Paulo and Mato Grosso states, and the Federal District, Brazil; using the IFAT with tachyzoites of *T. gondii* RH strain as antigen, they found 17/27 (63%) bush dogs to be seropositive for *T. gondii*.

GENUS UROCYON BAIRD, 1857 (2 SPECIES)

UROCYON LITTORALIS (BAIRD, 1858), ISLAND FOX

Hammondia. No records in the literature, yet.
Neospora. No records in the literature, yet.
Toxoplasma gondii. Clifford et al. (2006) surveyed island fox populations on six California Channel Islands for a variety of pathogens, including *T. gondii* and *N. caninum* using the IFAT with a fluorescence titer of ≥1:640 considered to be positive. They found: on San Miguel Island, 0/16 wild- (8) and captive-born (8) foxes with antibodies; on Santa Rosa Island, 2/14 (14%) wild-born foxes had antibodies, but none of 28 captive-born foxes did; on Santa Cruz Island, 1/43 (2%) wild foxes had antibodies, but none of 5 captive-born foxes did; on Santa Catalina Island, 3/58 (5%) wild foxes had antibodies; on San Clemente Island, 12/78 (15%) wild foxes had antibodies; and on San Nicolas Island, none of 70 wild foxes sampled had antibodies to *T. gondii*.

UROCYON CINEREOARGENTEUS (SCHREBER, 1775), GRAY FOX

Hammondia. No records in the literature, yet.
Neospora. Lindsay et al. (2001c) determined the prevalence of antibodies to *N. caninum* in a population of gray foxes from a nonagricultural setting in South Carolina. Antibody levels were measured in DATs using *N. caninum* formalin-fixed tachyzoites as antigen; they found 4/26 (15%) gray foxes had titers to *N. caninum*.
Toxoplasma gondii. Franti et al. (1976) tested 2,796 serum samples from wild and domestic

mammals and birds in northern California for antibodies to *T. gondii* and found 7/26 (7%) gray foxes to be positive. Lindsay et al. (2001c) examined blood samples in a population of gray foxes in South Carolina by DATs using *T. gondii* formalin-fixed tachyzoites as antigen; they found 16/26 (61.5%) foxes had titers to *T. gondii*. Results of this study indicated that gray foxes have more exposure to *T. gondii* than to *N. caninum* in this environment.

GENUS *VULPES* FRISCH, 1775 (12 SPECIES)

VULPES CANA BLANFORD, 1877, BLANFORD'S FOX

Hammondia. No records in the literature, yet.

Neospora. No records in the literature, yet.

Toxoplasma gondii. Dubey and Pas (2008) diagnosed fatal toxoplasmosis in a *V. cana* fox from the UAE. They found tachyzoites associated with the intestine, spleen, liver, kidneys, lungs, skeletal muscles, brain, and heart. The tachyzoites they found reacted positively by the latex agglutination (LA) or the modified DAT with *T. gondii*–specific polyclonal antibodies. Also, they detected antibodies in 10/12 (83%) *V. cana* kept at the BCEAW, Sharjah, UAE. Dubey et al. (2010a) also surveyed the sera of many carnivores at the BCEAW and demonstrated antibodies to *T. gondii* in 8/14 (57%) Blanford's foxes.

VULPES (SYN. *ALOPEX*) *LAGOPUS* (L., 1758), ARCTIC OR BLUE FOX

Hammondia. Dubey (1982b) surveyed feces of wild carnivores in Montana for coccidia. He reported *Hammondia heydorni*–like oocysts in the feces of 1/198 (17%) *V. lagopus*. Gjerde and Dhalgren (2011) found a *Hammondia* species in moose muscle, fed the infected flesh to arctic and red foxes, and they shed unsporulated oocysts in

their feces 6–7 DPI. The oocysts measured, 10–12 in diameter. Using isolates from foxes examined by PCR and sequence analysis of six loci, they found consistent genetic differences between the dog and fox isolates at the ITA-2 region, the lsu rRNA gene, the alpha-insulin gene, and the HSP70 gene. They also established that dogs were unsuitable as definitive hosts for the *Hammondia* sp. of foxes (*H. triffittae*), and the form from wolf-like canids (*H. heydorni*) was unsuitable for and unable to infect foxes (*V. lagopus, V. vulpes*).

Neospora. Antibodies to *N. caninum* were found in blue foxes in China (Dubey et al., 2017b, Table 16.1) and *N. caninum* tissue cysts were reported in histological sections of kidneys and brain of five blue foxes with an undiagnosed illness (Yu et al., 2009). A blue fox inoculated IM with *N. caninum*–infected dog brain developed encephalitis and tachyzoites were found in tissue lesions (Bjerkås et al., 1984).

Toxoplasma gondii: Prestrud et al. (2007) sampled blood or tissue fluid from 594 Arctic foxes from Svalbard, Norway, and assayed them for antibodies against *T. gondii* using a DAT; they found 255/594 (43%) foxes were positive for antibodies to *T. gondii*.

VULPES RUEPPELLII (SCHINZ, 1825), RÜPPELL'S FOX

Hammondia. No records in the literature, yet.

Neospora. No records in the literature, yet.

Toxoplasma gondii. A small group of Rüppell's foxes are kept at the BCEAW, Sharjah, UAE. In December, 2005, three pups were born to a dam that also had raised three pups the previous year. A few days after the pups were 6-weeks-old, one of the two males was found dead with its head bitten off, presumably by one of the parents; the other two pups remained healthy. Pas and Dubey (2008) were able to examine tissues from the dead pup and found *T. gondii*–like tachyzoites associated with necrosis in the intestine, spleen, liver, pancreas, lungs, mesenteric lymph nodes and heart and these tachyzoites reacted positively with *T.*

gondii–specific polyclonal antibodies. Serum samples from eight captive *V. rueppellii* were banked frozen at −20°C a year earlier and were retrospectively tested for *T. gondii* antibodies via the MAT; all eight demonstrated exposure to *T. gondii* with titers of 1:800 or higher (Pas and Dubey, 2008). Dubey et al. (2010a) later surveyed the sera of many carnivores at the BCEAW and demonstrated antibodies to *T. gondii* in 3/3 (100%) *V. rueppellii*.

VULPES VULPES (L., 1758), RED OR SILVER FOX

Hammondia. During an investigation to determine the definitive host(s) of *Sarcocystis* species infecting Arabian gazelles (*Gazella gazella* Pallas) in Saudi Arabia, Mohammed et al. (2003) found unsporulated oocysts in the feces of a *V. vulpes arabica* cub between 6 and 8 days after it had fed on meat from *G. gazella*. The oocysts sporulated in 8 days at room temperature (25±2°C) and were, L×W: 10.9×10.1, L/W ratio: 1.1, and sporocysts were, L×W: 6.0×4.7, L/W ratio: 1.1. Using molecular and standard morphological techniques, they identified the oocysts as *H. heydorni* and concluded that the Arabian red fox and mountain gazelle in Saudi Arabia are now definitive and intermediate hosts for *H. heydorni*. However, Abel et al. (2006) sequenced the ITS-1 for rDNA obtained from dog oocysts and from fox oocysts, previously thought to be *H. heydorni*, and found that they contained identical ITS-1 sequences, but differed by the presence/absence of a 9 bp insertion/deletion within intron 1 of the alpha-tubulin gene, and this difference was conserved across a number of different oocyst populations from the two different host species. A PCR assay was established that takes advantage of this insertion/deletion and was able to differentiate between the fox and dog oocyst populations. Thus, Abel et al. (2006) concluded that the *H. heydorni* oocysts from dogs and foxes represent two distinct genetic lineages that "might" suggest the existence of another *Hammondia* species, but admitting that

further research should focus on establishing the biological, ecological, and epidemiological differences (if any) between them. Dahlgren and Gjerde (2010b) found a *Hammondia* species tissue cyst in moose muscle; they fed infected flesh to eight red foxes, which began shedding unsporulated oocysts in their feces 6–7 DPI. The oocysts measured 10–12 wide, but no other information was given. This led them (Gjerde and Dahlgren, 2011) to look more carefully at the genomic DNA from three oocyst isolates of *Hammondia* from foxes (*V. vulpes, V. lagopus*) and one oocyst isolate of *H. heydorni* from a dog, by PCR and sequence analysis of six loci, to determine if the isolates were conspecific. They found consistent genetic differences between the fox and dog isolates at the ITS-2 region, the lus rRNA gene, the alpha-tubulin gene, and the JSP70 gene (but not at the ssu rRNA gene or ITS-1 locus). Their infection experiments showed that dogs were unsuitable as definitive hosts for the *Hammondia* form from foxes, and this led them to name *H. triffittae* as the fourth know species in the genus. Reindeer, moose, sheep, goats, foxes, and rabbits act as intermediate hosts for *H. triffittae*. Sporulated oocysts were, L×W: 12.5×10.9, L/W ratio:1.1. They also suggested the lsu rRNA gene and the alpha-tubulin gene were the most suitable genetic markers to distinguish between *H. heydorni* and *H. triffittae*. Gjerde (2013) extracted genomic DNA from three oocyst isolates of *H. triffittae* from foxes, two oocyst isolates of *H. heydorni* from dogs, from cell-culture tachyzoites of *T. gondii* (RH strain) and *N. caninum* (NC-Liverpool strain), and examined by PCR with primers targeting cytochrome b (*cytb*) and cytochrome c oxidase subunit I (*cox1*) genes. Pairwise sequence comparisons based on either *cytb* or *cox1* clearly separated *T. gondii* from *N. caninum*, and both of these species from the two *Hammondia* species. The two *Hammondia* species were 100% identical at *cytb* but shared 99.3% identity at *cox1*. Nonetheless, Gjerde (2013) maintained there were species-specific differences in the nucleotide composition of the nuclear gene fragments, identical to the differences in the mitochondrial genes that allowed the separation of the two *Hammondia* species, *H. heydorni* and *H. triffittae*.

Neospora. Almería et al. (2002) studied red foxes in Spain to determine if they are natural intermediate and/or definitive hosts for *N. caninum* using both fecal and brain tissues of foxes from 21 rural areas of Catalonia. For PCR-based diagnosis of *N. caninum* in brains, the specific genomic Nc5 region was their target sequence for DNA amplification; to control for PCR failure and facilitate identification of truly negative samples, the competitor pNc5C molecule was added to all negative samples in a second round of PCR reactions. They found 13/122 (11%) fox brains to be positive by PCR for *N. caninum*, although signal intensities of all positives were relatively weak. None of the 122 fecal samples demonstrated oocysts compatible with *N. caninum*. They concluded, "Detection of stages of *N. caninum* in brain from naturally infected red foxes demonstrated that they are a natural intermediate host for *N. caninum*." Oocysts also were not found in fox feces in Ireland (Wolfe et al., 2001) or Germany (Constantin et al., 2011), and red foxes that were experimentally fed *N. caninum*–infected tissues did not excrete oocysts (Schares et al., 2002). However, *N. caninum*–like oocysts were reported in feces of 2/271 (0.7%) foxes in Canada based on PCR testing (Wapenaar et al., 2006). A few studies suggest red foxes are important intermediate hosts (Almería et al., 2002; Schares et al., 2001b) and seroprevalence of *N. caninum* antibodies in free-ranging red foxes has been reported in many European countries, including Austria (Wanha et al., 2005), Belgium (Buxton et al., 1997), Germany (Schares et al., 2001a,b), Hungary (Jakubek et al., 2007), Poland (Śmielewska-Łoś et al., 2003), Spain (Marco et al., 2008), Sweden (Jakubek et al., 2001), and the United Kingdom (Barber et al., 1997; Hamilton et al., 2005; Murphy et al., 2007; Simpson et al., 1997; Wolfe et al., 2001). In the Belgium study, Buxton et al. (1997) collected serum samples from 121 red foxes as part of a rabies control program and tested them by IFAT for IgG antibody

to *N. caninum* and *T. gondii*. The foxes included 116 from rural areas of Luxembourg Province and five from a suburb of Brussels. Antibody titers to *N. caninum* (>1:64) were detected in 21/121 (17%) foxes; all 21 samples with *N. caninum* titers also had *T. gondii* titers (>1:128), indicating no significant cross-reaction between the two tests. Śmielewska-Łoś et al. (2003) collected serum samples, in Poland, from 105 adult farmed silver foxes, and wildlife red foxes (both *V. vulpes*), and tested them for IgG antibodies to *N. caninum* by the IFAT. Antibody titers to *N. caninum* were detected in low titers in 2/45 (4%) red foxes and in 1/60 (2%) farmed silver foxes. This was the first report on *N. caninum* in canids from Poland. Hamilton et al. (2005) studied the prevalence of IgG antibodies to *N. caninum* in lung samples of red foxes collected in the United Kingdom using the IFAT; only 5/549 (<1%) red foxes tested were seropositive for *N. caninum* indicating that red foxes in the United Kingdom have minimal exposure in their environment. DNA of *N. caninum* was detected in the brains of 7/152 (5%) red foxes in the Czech Republic (Hůrková and Modrý, 2006) by PCR-based diagnosis of *N. caninum* using the specific genomic Nc5 region as the target sequence for DNA amplification with primers Np21-plus and Np6-plus. Hůrková and Modrý (2006) stressed that the red fox is known to serve only as an intermediate host, although the route of infection is unknown, and that domestic dogs are, so far, the only known definitive host. Steinman et al. (2006) evaluated the role of wild canids in the epidemiology of bovine neosporosis in Israel, by collecting sera of wild canids and testing them for antibodies to *N. caninum*; only 4/147 (<3%) samples were positive for *N. caninum*, including 1/24 (2%) red foxes. They concluded that wild canids probably do not have an important role in the epidemiology of *N. caninum* in Israel. Murphy et al. (2007) tested thoracic fluid samples from foxes for *N. caninum* antibodies using an IFAT, with a titer of ≥1:100 being indicative of infection; they found only 6/220 (3%) foxes had antibodies to *N. caninum*. Murphy et al. (2007)

also examined the brains of foxes for histological lesions, and pathological changes suggestive of parasitic encephalitis were observed in 33/148 (22%); one fox had antibodies to both *T. gondii* and *N. caninum*, but PCR assays on DNA from the 33 brains with lesions were negative for *N. caninum*. Jakubek et al. (2007) investigated the seroprevalence of *N caninum* in *V. vulpes* from 16 (of 19) counties in Hungary. Antibodies to *N. caninum* were detected in an indirect iscom ELISA; they found only 5/337 (1.5%) positive for *N. caninum*. Latent infections of red foxes with *N. caninum* in Hungary do not seem to be common. Wapenaar et al. (2007) evaluated the performance and agreement of serological assays (ELISA, IFAT, NAT, and immunoblot) using reference sera and field sera from foxes to estimate their *N. caninum* seroprevalence on PEI, Canada. They collected serum from 271 foxes and the seroprevalence observed in the different assays ranged from 1% to 35% in foxes. The seroprevalence, when taking more than one test positive as cutoff value was 1% for foxes. They felt that positive agreement was moderate to poor among all assays utilized in their study. Although the seroprevalence observed was low, *N. caninum* antibodies are present in foxes on PEI. de Craeye et al. (2011) examined brain samples from Belgian red foxes for the presence of *N. caninum* DNA using multiplex real-time PCR. They detected *N. caninum* in 20/304 (7%) of the red foxes. In Ireland, Stuart et al. (2012) studied a bank of serum, fecal, and brain materials that included varying samples from 101 *V. vulpes*. Serum samples were tested for antibodies to *N. caninum* using a commercial IFAT. Only 1/101 (1%) *V. vulpes* had antibodies against *N. caninum*. Both LM and a PCR extraction technique were used to look for *N. caninum* oocysts, or DNA, respectively in fecal samples; all 91 fox fecal samples were negative for *N. caninum*. Stuart et al. (2012) also examined brain samples by a nested PCR for *N. caninum* DNA targeting the ITS-1 region; 9/151 (6%) fox brains were positive for *N. caninum*, whereas 50 badger, 33 stoat, and 8 pine marten brain samples all were negative.

Bartley et al. (2013) examined the brain and other tissues from red foxes in Great Britain by extracting DNA and testing by specific nested ITS-1 PCR for *N. caninum*. They reported 4/83 (5%) to be positive for *Neospora*-specific DNA. The levels of infection with *N. caninum* observed in red foxes by PCR are generally low, as seen in almost all the studies cited here, and by Almería (2013). However, Marco et al. (2008), using the NAT, observed red foxes in the Pyrenees of Catalonia (NE Spain) that had a high prevalence of antibodies at dilutions of ≥1:40 (70%), ≥1:80 (47%) and ≥1:160 (7.5%), indicating a localized area of high endemicity.

Toxoplasma gondii. Quinn et al. (1976) surveyed the blood of a variety of wild carnivores in southern Ontario for antibodies to *T. gondii*, using the Sabin–Feldman dye test, and found 84/158 (53%) *V. vulpes* to be positive. Tizard et al. (1976) surveyed the blood of a variety of wild carnivores in central Ontario for antibodies to *T. gondii*, also using the dye test, and found 81/96 (84%) *V. vulpes* to be positive. Dubey (1983a) used five littermates of 6-week-old *V. vulpes*, three species of *Sarcocystis* that previously had been isolated from and identified in their intermediate hosts (cattle, sheep, goats) in Montana, and oocysts and tissue cysts of *T. gondii* to conduct a series of cross-transmission experiments. Two foxes (Nos. 1, 2) each was fed two mice infected with the TC-1 strain of *T. gondii*, and two foxes (Nos. 3, 4) each was fed 350 sporulated oocysts of the GT-1 strain of *T. gondii*. Foxes were killed between 36 and 55 DPI. At necropsy, portions of numerous organs were removed, digested, washed, and the homogenate inoculated subcutaneously; six mice received an inoculation from each of six tissues. Foxes remained clinically normal throughout Dubey's (1983a) study, and *T. gondii* was recovered from one to six of the six mice inoculated with each of the six tissues. However, neither *T. gondii* nor *T. gondii* lesions were found in tissue sections of any of the four foxes. This demonstrated that *V. vulpes* can harbor mouse-virulent *T. gondii* without any ill effects. It should be noted that while the foxes were infected with *T. gondii* they also were used in various combinations to ingest sarcocyst-infected flesh of calves (*S. cruzi*), goats (*S. capracanis*), or sheep (*S. tenella*), and all produced sporocysts in their feces. Once these experiments were completed (see Chapter 15), the foxes were killed to complete the study with *T. gondii*. Buxton et al. (1997) collected serum samples collected from red foxes as part of a rabies control program and tested them by IFAT for IgG antibody to *T. gondii* (and *N. caninum*). The foxes included 116 from rural areas of Luxembourg Province and 5 from a suburb of Brussels. Antibody titers to *T. gondii* (>1:128) were detected in 119/121 (98%) foxes; their results suggested the widespread occurrence of *Toxoplasma* in the food supply of the foxes but indicated that *N. caninum* does not infect wild foxes in Belgium to any significant degree. Śmielewska-Loś et al. (2003) collected serum samples, in Poland, from 105 adult farmed silver foxes, and wildlife red foxes (both *V. vulpes*), and tested them for IgG antibodies to *T. gondii* by the IFAT. Antibody titers to *T. gondii* (≥1:20) were found in 22/60 (37%) farm foxes and in 15/45 (33%) red foxes. Hamilton et al. (2005) studied the prevalence of IgG antibodies to *T. gondii* in lung samples of red foxes collected in the United Kingdom using the IFAT; 111/549 (20%) red foxes tested were seropositive for *T. gondii* indicating that red foxes in the United Kingdom have significant exposure to *T. gondii* in their environment. Hůrková and Modrý (2006), in the Czech Republic, examined 240 brains of wild Canidae and Mustelidae by PCR-based diagnosis of *T. gondii*. For *T. gondii* diagnosis, a fragment of the B1 gene was amplified using primers TM1 and TM2. They found *T. gondii* DNA in 2/152 (1%) red foxes. Sobrino et al. (2007) did a serosurvey for *T. gondii* in free-ranging wild carnivores in different regions of Spain using the MAT (as per Dubey and Desmonts, 1987, cutoff value, 1:25) to test for antibodies to *T. gondii* and found 66/102 (65%) *V. vulpes* to demonstrate antibodies. Murphy et al. (2007) tested thoracic fluid (pleural fluid and clotted blood) from *V. vulpes* for antibodies to *T. gondii* using an IFAT (titer of ≥1:100 considered positive) and found 115/206 (56%)

foxes had antibodies to *T. gondii*. Jakubek et al. (2007) investigated the seroprevalence of *T. gondii* in *V. vulpes* from 16 (of 19) counties in Hungary. Antibodies to *T. gondii* were detected using a commercial DAT and they found 228/337 (68%) foxes positive for *T. gondii*. The high prevalence of foxes positive for *T. gondii* in Hungary might be explained by the widespread occurrence of the parasite in the diet of foxes. Murphy et al. (2007) also examined the brains of foxes for histological lesions, and pathological changes suggestive of parasitic encephalitis were observed in 33/148 (22%); 22/33 (67%) of these foxes had antibodies to *T. gondii*, and one had antibodies to both *T. gondii* and *N. caninum*. However, PCR assays on DNA from the 33 brains with lesions showed that only one of the brains was positive for *T. gondii*. Dubey et al. (2010a,b,c) surveyed the sera of many carnivores at the BCEAW, Sharjah, UAE, and demonstrated antibodies to *T. gondii* in 9/15 (60%) *V. v. arabica* Thomas, 1902. de Craeye et al. (2011) examined brain samples from red foxes for the presence of *T. gondii* using multiplex real-time PCR. They detected *T. gondii* in 57/304 (19%) of the red foxes sampled; 26 of the *T. gondii*–positive DNA extracts from the fox samples were genotyped: 25 were type II and only 1 was type III. Burrells et al. (2013) extracted DNA from tissues of 390 carnivores in the United Kingdom and detected parasite DNA using a nested ITS-1 PCR-specific for *T. gondii*. They tested brain tissue of *V. vulpes* and found 5/83 (6%) to be positive for *T. gondii* DNA; their fox samples were collected from the University of Edinburgh and the Moredun Research Institute, Scotland.

VULPES ZERDA (ZIMMERMANN, 1780), FENNEC FOX

Hammondia. No records in the literature, yet.

Neospora. Sedlák and Bártová (2006a,b) surveyed 87 carnivores in zoos in the Czech and Slovak Republics for antibodies to *N. caninum* using the IFAT; they reported that 2/2 (100%) *V. zerda* sampled had positive titers.

Toxoplasma gondii. Sedlák and Bártová (2006a,b) surveyed 87 carnivores in zoos in the Czech and Slovak Republics for antibodies to *T. gondii* using the IFAT and said that both of the *V. zerda* tested had positive titers.

MEPHITIDAE BONAPARTE, 1845

GENUS *MEPHITIS* É. GEOFFROY SAINT-HILAIRE AND F.G. CUVIER, 1795 (2 SPECIES)

MEPHITIS MEPHITIS (SCHREBER, 1776), STRIPED SKUNK

Hammondia. No records in the literature, yet.
Neospora. No records in the literature, yet.
Toxoplasma gondii. Franti et al. (1976) tested 2,796 serum samples from wild and domestic mammals and birds in northern California for antibodies to *T. gondii* and found 7/32 (22%) *M. mephitis* to be positive. Quinn et al. (1976) surveyed the blood of a variety of wild carnivores in southern Ontario for antibodies to *T. gondii*, using the Sabin–Feldman dye test, and found 88/158 (56%) *M. mephitis* to be positive. Tizard et al. (1976) also surveyed the blood of wild carnivores in central Ontario for antibodies to *T. gondii*, also used the dye test, and found 19/62 (31%) *M. mephitis* to be positive. Dubey et al. (2002a) found a *Toxoplasma*-like tissue cyst, 45×30, in the tongue of 1/4 (25%) striped skunks collected near Corvallis, Oregon, USA.

GENUS *SPILOGALE* GRAY, 1865 (4 SPECIES)

SPILOGALE GRACILIS MERRIAM, 1890, WESTERN SPOTTED SKUNK

Hammondia. No records in the literature, yet.
Neospora. No records in the literature, yet.

Toxoplasma gondii. Suzán and Ceballos (2005) did a serosurvey of wildlife infections in two nature reserves within Mexico City limits and used a complement-fixation test to find antibodies to *T. gondii*. They collected 16 blood samples from carnivores and found 3/6 (50%) *S. gracilis* to be positive for *T. gondii*.

MUSTELIDAE FISCHER, 1817

SUBFAMILY LUTRINAE BONAPARTE, 1838

GENUS *ENHYDRA* FLEMMING, 1822 (MONOTYPIC)

ENHYDRA LUTRIS (L., 1758), SEA OTTER

Hammondia. No records in the literature, yet.
Neospora. Dubey et al. (2003d) looked for evidence of infections by *Neospora*, *Sarcocystis*, and *Toxoplasma* species in a variety of marine mammals. For *N. caninum*, sera were diluted 1:40, 1:80, 1:160, and 1:320 and examined with the NAT using mouse-derived tachyzoites. NAT antibodies to *N. caninum* were found in 28/145 (19%) *E. lutris*. This was the first report of *N. caninum* antibodies in any marine mammals.

Toxoplasma gondii. Lindsay et al. (2001a) documented *T. gondii* in a male sea otter found stranded and convulsed along the beach in Grays Harbor, California, USA. The otter was diagnosed with **meningoencephalomyelitis**, thought to be due mainly to *Sarcocystis neurona*, which the sea otter also was infected with. However, histological sections of brain using antisera specific to *T. gondii* suggested that the sea otter was suffering from reactivated toxoplasmosis. Isolates of *T. gondii* were made from mice inoculated with brain tissue from this otter, and a cat fed infected mouse brain tissue excreted oocysts of *T. gondii*, which were infective for mice. This apparently is the first report of dual

S. neurona and *T. gondii* in a marine mammal. Miller et al. (2002) did an epidemiological study to determine the seroprevalence of *T. gondii* in southern sea otters along the California, USA, coast from 1997 to 2001. They found antibodies in 49/116 (42%) live and in 66/107 (62%) dead sea otters and determined that the risk factors positively associated with *T. gondii* seropositivity included being an older male. Otters sampled from the Morro Bay region of California, particularly otters sampled near areas of maximal freshwater runoff, were three times more likely to be seropositive than otters sampled in areas of low flow. This led Miller et al. (2002) to conclude an association among anthropogenic environmental disturbance, pathogen pollution of the marine ecosystem, and the emergence of infectious diseases in these sea otters. Dubey et al. (2003d) looked for evidence of infections by *Neospora, Sarcocystis*, and *Toxoplasma* species in a variety of marine mammals. For *T. gondii*, sera were diluted 1:25, 1:50, and 1:500 and assayed in the MAT; antibodies to *T. gondii* (MAT≥1:25) were found in 89/115 (77%) dead, and in 18/30 (60%) apparently healthy *E. lutris*. Conrad et al. (2005) examined seroprevalence samples of the endangered southern sea otters (*E. l. nereis*) along the California, USA, coast from 1998 to 2004; they found 159/305 (52%) freshly dead, beachcast otters, and 98/257 (38%) live sea otters were infected with *T. gondii*. The areas with high exposure were predominantly sandy bays near urban areas with freshwater runoff. They concluded that otters can serve as sentinels of protozoal pathogen flow into the marine environment because otters share the environment and consume some of the same food as humans. Miller et al. (2004) noted that *T. gondii*–associated meningoencephalitis is responsible for about 16% of all mortality in beachcast carcasses of *E. lutris nereis*. They studied *T. gondii* isolated in 35 California otters necropsied between 1998 and 2002 using multilocus PCR–RFLP and DNA sequencing of 18S rDNA and ITA-1 (conserved), and B1, SAG1, SAG3, and GRA6 (polymorphic)

genes and identified two distinct genotypes, type II and a novel genotype, which they called type x because it possessed distinct alleles at three of the four polymorphic loci sequenced. They reported that 9/12 (75%) otters that had *T. gondii*–associated meningoencephalitis as a primary cause of death were infected with type x parasites. Thomas et al. (2007) used histopathology and immunohistochemistry to study naturally-occurring cases of meningoencephalitis in *E. lutris* due to *T. gondii* and/or *Sarcocystis neurona* along the California and Washington, USA, coastlines from 1985 to 2004. Overall, 39/344 (11%) of the sea otters were positive for one or both protist parasites, including 5/39 (13%) infected sea otters with *T. gondii*, 22/39 (56%) infected otters with *S. neurona*, and 12/39 (31%) with concurrent infections. Thomas et al. (2007) pointed out that protozoal meningoencephalitis was more frequent in the expanding population of Washington otters (10/31, 32%) than in the declining California population (29/313, 9%); they also noted that otters with neurological signs prior to death had active *S. neurona* encephalitis supporting that *S. neurona* (not *T. gondii*) is the most significant protist pathogen in the CNS of sea otters.

GENUS LONTRA GRAY, 1843 (4 SPECIES)

LONTRA CANADENSIS (SCHREBER, 1777), NORTH AMERICAN RIVER OTTER

Hammondia. No records in the literature, yet.

Neospora. Many wild noncanid carnivores are known to have been exposed to *N. caninum*, either by being seropositive, demonstrating oocysts in their feces, or exhibiting signs of neosporosis, including the North American river otter in the United States. Gaydos et al. (2007a,b, see below) tested the sera of 40 *L. canadensis* for antibodies to *N. caninum*, but all were negative.

Toxoplasma gondii. Gaydos et al. (2007a) did a survey to examine whether the proximity of humans affects the disease exposure in marine-foraging river otters to *T. gondii* and other infectious agents. Serum samples were collected from 55 otters, 35 captured in Prince Edward Sound, Alaska (low human density), and 20 from the San Juan Islands, Washington state, USA (high human density). Of the river otters tested by IFAT, 7/40 (17.5%) otters were positive for antibodies to *T. gondii*, all from Washington state, but none of the 15 tested sera from Alaska were positive. This suggested to Gaydos et al. (2007a) that living proximal to higher human density, and its associated agricultural activities, domestic animals, and rodent populations, could enhance river otter exposure to pathogens endemic to humans and their companion animals.

GENUS *LUTRA* BRISSON, 1762 (3 SPECIES)

LUTRA LUTRA (L., 1758), EUROPEAN OTTER

Hammondia. No records in the literature, yet.

Neospora. In Ireland, Stuart et al. (2012) studied a bank of serum, fecal, and brain materials that included varying samples from 30 *L. lutra.* Serum samples were tested for antibodies to *N. caninum* using a commercial IFAT, but none of 30 serum samples from otters demonstrated exposure to the parasite. Both LM and a PCR extraction technique were used to look for *N. caninum* oocysts, or DNA, respectively, in fecal samples, but all 25 otter fecal samples were negative for *N. caninum.* Stuart et al. (2012) also examined brain samples by a nested PCR for *N. caninum* DNA targeting the ITS-1 region; 1/24 (4%) otter brains was positive for *N. caninum*, whereas 50 badger, 33 stoat, and 8 pine marten brain samples were all negative. Santoro et al. (2017) examined fecal samples of six road-killed carcasses of *L. lutra*

from southern Italy, using standard sedimentation and flotation methods. Tissue samples (heart and brain) were screened by PCR amplification of the 16S rRNA gene and *N. caninum* was not detected in any of the samples.

Toxoplasma gondii. Sobrino et al. (2007) did a serosurvey of free ranging carnivores from different regions of Spain to detect *T. gondii*, using the MAT (as per Dubey and Desmonts, 1987, with a cutoff value of 1:25). Sobrino et al. (2007) detected antibodies to *T. gondii* in 6/6 (100%) *L. lutra.* Gjerde and Josefsen (2015) examined muscle samples from two adult male otters via PCR amplification and sequencing of the entire ITS-1 region (five isolates) and/or partial cytb (eight isolates), and *cox1* (one isolate), and found them both to harbor *T. gondii* because these sequences were identical to several previous sequences of *T. gondii* in GenBank. Thus, both otters had a dual infection with *Sarcocystis lutrae*, which they named as new (see Chapter 15), and *T. gondii.*

SUBFAMILY MUSTELINAE FISCHER, 1817

GENUS *EIRA* C.E.H. SMITH, 1842 (MONOTYPIC)

EIRA BARBARA (L., 1758), TAYRA

Hammondia. No records in the literature, yet.

Neospora. No records in the literature, yet.

Toxoplasma gondii. Frenkel and Sousa (1983) tested serum samples from 180 mammals representing 22 species in Panama for antibodies and found 2/2 (100%) tayras to be positive for *T. gondii.* de Thoisy et al. (2003) did a serosurvey for *T. gondii* in 18 forest mammal species in French Guiana, using a DAT, and found 5/7 (72%) *E. barbara* and coatis (*N. nasua*) positive. They did not provide sample sizes and prevalences for the two species separately.

GENUS MARTES PINEL, 1792 (8 SPECIES)

MARTES FOINA (ERXLEBEN, 1777), BEECH MARTEN

Hammondia. No records in the literature, yet.

Neospora. Sobrino et al. (2008), did a serosurvey of carnivores from different regions of Spain, used the c-ELISA, NAT, and/or IFAT, and detected antibodies to *N. caninum* in 5/14 (36%) beech martens. Many wild noncanid carnivores are known to have been exposed to *N. caninum*, either by being seropositive, demonstrating oocysts in their feces, or exhibiting signs of neosporosis, including *M. foina* in the Spain.

Toxoplasma gondii. Hůrková and Modrý (2006), in the Czech Republic, examined 240 brains of wild Canidae and Mustelidae by PCR-based diagnosis of *T. gondii* using a fragment of the B1 gene amplified with primers TM1 and TM2. They confirmed the presence of *T. gondii* in 3/61 (5%) *M. foina*. A serosurvey by Sobrino et al. (2007) to detect *T. gondii* in free-ranging carnivores from different regions of Spain, using the MAT (as per Dubey and Desmonts, 1987, cutoff value, 1:25) detected antibodies to *T. gondii* in 17/20 (85%) *M. foina*.

MARTES MARTES (L., 1758), EUROPEAN PINE MARTIN

Hammondia. No records in the literature, yet.

Neospora. The serosurvey of Sobrino et al. (2008) for carnivores from Spain, found 3/3 (100%) pine martens with antibodies to *N. caninum*.

Toxoplasma gondii. Tizard et al. (1976) surveyed the blood of a variety of wild carnivores in Central Ontario for antibodies to *T. gondii*, using the Sabin–Feldman dye test. They found 15/139 (11%) *M. martes* to be positive. The blood survey of Sobrino et al. (2007) in different regions of Spain detected antibodies to *T. gondii* in 4/4 (100%) pine martens.

MARTES PENNANTI (ERXLEBEN, 1777), FISHER

Hammondia. No records in the literature, yet.

Neospora. Sedlák and Bártová (2006a) examined carnivores in zoos in the Czech and Slovak Republics using the IFAT and found antibodies to *N. caninum* in 1/2 (50%) fishers.

Toxoplasma gondii. Tizard et al. (1976) surveyed the blood of wild carnivores in Central Ontario for antibodies to *T. gondii* and found 157/379 (41%) *M. pennanti* to be positive for antibodies. Sedlák and Bártová (2006a) examined carnivores in zoos in the Czech and Slovak Republics and found antibodies to *T. gondii* in 2/2 (100%) fishers tested. Larkin et al. (2011) examined fishers in Pennsylvania, USA, for *Sarcocystis* spp. and *T. gondii*. Using the MAT (≥1:25) and an IFAT (≥1:128), they found antibodies to *T. gondii* in all 38 of the fishers tested by MAT and in 32/45 (71%) of the fishers tested by IFAT.

GENUS MELES BRISSON, 1762 (3 SPECIES)

MELES MELES (L., 1758), EUROPEAN BADGER

Hammondia. No records in the literature, yet.

Neospora. Sobrino et al. (2008) serosurveyed carnivores from Spain, using the c-ELISA, NAT, and/or IFAT to detect antibodies to *N. caninum*; they found 6/31 (19%) *M. meles* seroconverted. Bartley et al. (2013) examined the brain and other tissues from European badgers in Great Britain by extracting DNA and testing by specific nested ITS-1 PCR for *N. caninum*; they reported 7/64 (11%) *M. meles* to be positive for *Neospora*-specific DNA.

Toxoplasma gondii. Sobrino et al. (2007) recorded antibodies to *T. gondii* in the sera of 26/37 (70%) *M. meles* in Spain. Burrells et al. (2013) extracted DNA from 390 carnivores in the

United Kingdom, using a nested ITS-1 PCR specific for *T. gondii*. They tested the brain, tongue, heart, lung, liver, kidney spleen, spinal cord, clotted blood, submandibular lymph node, neck muscle, and hind leg muscle tissues and found 16/64 (23%) *M. meles* positive for *T. gondii* DNA; their badger samples were collected at the Moredun Research Institute, Scotland.

GENUS *MUSTELA* L., 1758 (17 SPECIES)

MUSTELA ERMINEA L., 1758, ERMINE OR STOAT

Hammondia. No records in the literature, yet.

Neospora. Bartley et al. (2013) examined the brain and other tissues from nine stoats in Great Britain by extracting DNA and testing by specific nested ITS-1 PCR for *N. caninum*; they reported all nine were negative for *Neospora*-specific DNA.

Toxoplasma gondii. Burrells et al. (2013) extracted DNA from 390 carnivores in the United Kindgom and used a nested ITS-1 PCR specific for *T. gondii*. They tested the brain, tongue, heart, lung, liver, kidney, spleen, clotted blood, neck muscle, and hind leg muscles of *M. erminea* and found 4/9 (44%) positive for *T. gondii* DNA; all nine stoats were collected on the Moredun Research Institute, Scotland.

MUSTELA NIGRIPES (AUDUBON AND BACHMAN, 1851), BLACK-FOOTED FERRET

Hammondia. No records in the literature, yet.

Neospora. No records in the literature, yet.

Toxoplasma gondii. Black-footed ferrets can be highly susceptible to toxoplasmosis. Burns et al. (1993) documented a serious outbreak with the disease at the Louisville Zoo, Kentucky, USA. The source of the infections was not determined but was thought to be associated with rabbit meat used in the diet of these ferrets. The disease did

not reoccur, it has not been found in other captive breeding facilities, and there is no current clinical evidence of transmission from dams to their offspring. This outbreak served to highlight several points about the disease and maintenance of captive, endangered species; namely, that some species may have a heightened degree of susceptibility by virtue of their degree of inbreeding, the stresses of captivity, and exposure to immunosuppressive agents that heighten their susceptibility (Williams and Thorne, 1996).

MUSTELA PUTORIUS L., 1758, EUROPEAN POLECAT

Hammondia. No records in the literature, yet.

Neospora. Sobrino et al. (2008) did a serosurvey of carnivores from different regions of Spain to detect antibodies to *N. caninum*; they found 1/2 (50%) *M. putorius* seroconverted. Bartley et al. (2013) examined the brain and other tissues from 70 European polecats in Great Britain by extracting DNA and testing it by specific nested ITS-1 PCR for *N. caninum*. They reported 13/70 (19%) to be positive for *Neospora*-specific DNA.

Toxoplasma gondii. Sobrino et al. (2007) did a serosurvey of free-ranging carnivores from different regions of Spain using the MAT (≥1:25) and detected antibodies to *T. gondii* in 4/4 (100%) *M. putorius*. Burrells et al. (2013) extracted DNA from tissues of carnivores in the United Kingdom, using a nested ITS-1 PCR; they tested brain tissue of *M. putorius* and found 22/70 (31%) to be positive for *T. gondii* DNA. Their polecat samples were collected in England, Scotland, and Wales.

MUSTELA (SYN. *PUTORIUS*) *PUTORIUS FURO*, DOMESTIC FERRET

Hammondia. No records in the literature, yet.

Neospora. Bartley et al. (2013) examined the brain and other tissues from ferrets in Great

Britain by extracting DNA and testing by specific nested ITS-1 PCR for *N. caninum*. They reported 10/99 (10%) to be positive for *Neospora*-specific DNA.

Toxoplasma gondii. Sobrino et al. (2007, see above) detected antibodies to *T. gondii* in the blood of the only domestic ferret they tested. Burrells et al. (2013) extracted DNA from tissues of 390 carnivores in the United Kingdom, using a nested ITS-1 PCR specific for *T. gondii*. They tested brain tissue of *M. (putorius) furo* and found 23/99 (23%) to be positive for *T. gondii* DNA; all domestic ferrets were collected on the Moredun Research Institute, Scotland.

GENUS NEOVISON BARYSHNIKOV AND ABRAMOV, 1997 (2 SPECIES)

NEOVISON VISON (SCHREBER, 1777) (SYN. MUSTELA VISON SCHREBER, 1777), AMERICAN MINK

Hammondia. Dubey (1982b) surveyed feces for coccidians from wild carnivores in Montana. He reported *Hammondia heydorni*–like oocysts in the feces of 1/4 (25%) mink.

Neospora. In Ireland, Stuart et al. (2012) studied serum, fecal, and brain materials from American mink and other wild carnivores. Serum samples were tested for antibodies using a commercial IFAT, but only 1/114 (1%) mink had antibodies against *N. caninum*. Both LM and a PCR extraction technique looked for *N. caninum* oocysts, or DNA, respectively, in fecal samples, but all 82 mink fecal samples were negative. Stuart et al. (2012) also examined brain samples by a nested PCR for *N. caninum* DNA, targeting the ITS-1 region; 6/197 (3%) mink brains were positive for *N. caninum*, whereas 50 badger, 33 stoat, and 8 pine marten brain samples were all negative. Bartley et al. (2013) examined brain tissues from 65 American mink in Great Britain by extracting DNA, and testing by specific nested

ITS-1 PCR for *N. caninum*, and found 3/65 (5%) to be positive for *Neospora*-specific DNA.

Toxoplasma gondii. Franti et al. (1976) tested 2,796 serum samples from wild and domestic mammals and birds in northern California for antibodies to *T. gondii* and found the only *N. vison* they examined to be positive. Tizard et al. (1976) surveyed the blood of wild carnivores in Central Ontario for antibodies to *T. gondii*, using the Sabin–Feldman dye test. They found 55/100 (55%) *N. vison* to be positive for antibodies. Burrells et al. (2013) extracted DNA from mink samples collected from the Food and Environment Research Agency, Scotland, and detected parasite DNA using a nested ITS-1 PCR specific for *T. gondii*. They tested brain, tongue, and neck muscle tissue of *N. vison* and found 19/65 (29%) to be positive for *T. gondii* DNA.

ODOBENIDAE ALLEN, 1880

ODOBENUS ROSMARUS (L., 1758), WALRUS

Hammondia. No records in the literature, yet.

Neospora. Dubey et al. (2003d) looked for evidence of infections by *Neospora, Sarcocystis*, and *Toxoplasma* species in a variety of marine mammals. For *N. caninum*, sera were diluted 1:40, 1:80, 1:160, and 1:320 and examined with NAT using mouse-derived tachyzoites. NAT antibodies to *N. caninum* were found in 3/53 (6%) walruses. Theirs was the first report of *N. caninum* antibodies in walruses.

Toxoplasma gondii. In the marine mammal survey by Dubey et al. (2003d, above) sera were diluted 1:25, 1:50, and 1:500 and assayed for *T. gondii* in the MAT; antibodies to *T. gondii* (MAT ≥ 1:25) were found in 3/53 (6%) apparently healthy walruses. Prestrud et al. (2007) sampled blood or tissue fluid from walruses from Svalbard, Norway, and assayed them for antibodies against *T. gondii* using a DAT; they found 1/17 (6%) walruses positive for antibodies to *T. gondii*. Dubey et al. (2009) looked for infections with *T. gondii* in marine mammals because such infections would be indicative of contamination of the ocean environment and coastal waters with oocysts of this parasite. They also found one captive walrus at a sea aquarium in Canada with antibodies to *T. gondii*. Their PCR–RFLP typing using 11 markers (B1, SAG1, SAG2, SAG3, BTUB, GRA6, c22-8, c29-2, L358, PK1, and Apico) identified a Type II strain of this parasite. The DNA sequencing of B1 and SAG1 alleles amplified from TgDoCA1 and directly from the brain of the walrus showed archetypal alleles consistent with infection by a Type II strain. No unique polymorphisms were detected. This is apparently the first report of isolation of *T. gondii* from a marine mammal in Canada.

OTARIIDAE GRAY, 1825

GENUS ARCTOCEPHALUS É GEOFFROY SAINT-HILAIRE AND F.G. CUVIER, 1862 (8 SPECIES)

ARCTOCEPHALUS AUSTRALIS (ZIMMERMANN, 1783), SOUTH AMERICAN FUR SEAL

Hammondia. No records in the literature, yet.
Neospora. No records in the literature, yet.
Toxoplasma gondii. von Hänichen et al. (1991) reported *T. gondii* as the cause of perinatal death of a South American fur seal using electron-optical and immunohistochemical tools. They reported foci of necrotizing placentitis with *T. gondii* cysts on histological examination of the fur seal pup immediately after apparently normal parturition. Pulpy hyperplasia of the spleen was the only additional postmortem finding. The authors speculated that contaminated shoes of animal attendants might have played the role of a vector for infection, presumably oocysts from a cat.

ARCTOCEPHALUS FORSTERI (LESSON, 1828), AUSTRALIAN FUR SEAL

Hammondia. No records in the literature, yet.
Neospora. No records in the literature, yet.
Toxoplasma gondii. Donahoe et al. (2014) reported a confirmed case of toxoplasmosis in an Australian pinniped when they detected *T. gondii* DNA in the brain of a free-ranging subadult New Zealand seal, with nonsuppurative meningoencephalitis, hypophysitis, posterior uveitis, retrobulbar cellulitis, and myocarditis associated with cysts and tachyzoites. The seal was emaciated and moribund when it stranded on a beach in northern Sydney, New South Wales. Histopathology, immunohistochemistry, and PCR assays confirmed the presence of *T. gondii* (NZfs8825) as a type II (ToxoDB PCR–RFLP genotype #1), based on the direct sequencing and virtual RFLP of multilocus DNA markers (SAG1, 5′- and 3′-SAG2, alt. SAG2, SAG3, BTUB, GRA6, c22-8, c29-2, L358, PK1, and Apico). Their 2014 study suggested that *T. gondii* oocysts originated from mainland Australia, which has a large population of feral cats that may act as a disease threat to native marine fauna. The type II-like lineage is active and causes disease in Australian and Southern Ocean waters.

ARCTOCEPHALUS GAZELLA (PETERS, 1875), ANTARCTIC FUR SEAL

Hammondia. No records in the literature, yet.
Neospora. No records in the literature, yet.
Toxoplasma gondii. From 2007 to 2011, Rengifo-Herrera et al. (2012) collected sera from five species of pinnipeds from different locations in the South Shetland Islands and Antarctic Peninsula and analyzed them for *T. gondii*, with a commercially-available agglutination test kit. In all, 28/211 (13%) samples were positive for *T. gondii*, including 4/165 (2%) *A. gazella*. Jensen et al. (2012) collected blood samples from 102 Antarctic pinnipeds and assayed the serum, also using a

commercial DAT kit, to determine if antibodies to *T. gondii* were present. They found antibodies (≥1:40) to *T. gondii* in 12/21 (57%) *A. gazelle* from Bird Island, South Georgia. The 1:40 cutoff used on samples from terrestrial animals has not been validated for seals, but it is commonly used. These two reports are the first reports documenting *T. gondii* antibodies in Antarctic marine mammals.

GENUS *CALLORHINUS* J.E. GRAY, 1859 (MONOTYPIC)

CALLORHINUS URSINUS (L., 1758), NORTHERN FUR SEAL

Hammondia. No records in the literature, yet.
Neospora. No records in the literature, yet.
Toxoplasma gondii. Holshuh et al. (1985) found a mature female *C. ursinus* in poor condition and stranded on the coast of California, USA; the seal died a month after capture. At necropsy, sections of cerebral cortex, brain stem, cerebellum, and spinal cord were infiltrated with mixed inflammatory cells, with prominent perivascular cuffing, focal malacia, and numerous *T. gondii* cysts. Severe suppurative necrotizing myocarditis was seen in both ventricles. Marked nonsuppurative adrenalitis with numerous *T. gondii* cysts was seen. Sections of the brain stained specifically with *T. gondii* antibody (peroxidase–antiperoxidase technique) revealed numerous protozoal cysts throughout the brain tissue.

GENUS *OTARIA* PÉRON, 1816 (MONOTYPIC)

OTARIA FLAVESCENS (SHAW, 1800) (SYN. *OTARIA BYRONIA* [DE BLAINVILLE, 1820]), SOUTH AMERICAN SEA LION

Hammondia. Iskander (1984) reported finding oocysts in the feces and gamonts in columnar epithelial cells of gut scrapings, which he identified as *I. bigemina*, in a dead male 5-year-old sea lion at the Giza Zoological Garden, Egypt. We now know that the small form of *I. bigemina* is *H. heydorni* (see above), but we do not know if Iskander's (1984) identification was correct, or not, since he did not sporulate the oocysts. The spheroidal to ovoidal unsporulated oocyts measured, L×W: 20–25×17–20, and the gametocytes were 7.5 wide.

Neospora. Sedlák and Bártová (2006a,b) examined carnivores in zoos in the Czech and Slovak Republics using the IFAT and found no antibodies to *N. caninum* in two sea lions.

Toxoplasma gondii. Sedlák and Bártová (2006a), using the IFAT, did not detect antibodies to *T. gondii* in the two sea lions they examined. Sepúlveda et al. (2015) did postmortem examinations on four *O. flavescens* from an urban colony in Valdivia, Chile. They also analyzed blood samples from three of them for antibodies to *T. gondii* and found 1/3 (33%) to be serologically positive. No other information was given.

GENUS *PHOCARCTOS* PETERS, 1866 (MONOTYPIC)

PHOCARCTOS HOOKERI (GRAY, 1844), NEW ZEALAND SEA LION

Hammondia. No records in the literature, yet.
Neospora. No records in the literature, yet.
Toxoplasma gondii. Michael et al. (2016) examined archived serum samples of *P. hookeri* from two recolonizing mainland populations, Otago Peninsula (n=15) and Stewart Island (n=12), and from a declining population at Enderby Island (n=28) for *T. gondii* using a commercially-available ELISA test. They found 5/27 (18.5%) mainland sea lions, but none of the Stewart Island sea lions, positive for *T. gondii*, and concluded that *T. gondii* was unlikely to be a major contributor to poor reproductive success in New Zealand sea lions. Roe et al. (2017) examined a 1-year-old female *P. hookeri* that had been observed for about 11 months in the Otago Region, always dragging her hind flippers.

When the sea lion was found dead, they did a postmortem examination and found meningo-encephalomyelitis, radiculomyelitis of the cauda equina, myocarditis, and myositis and detected organisms identified as *T. gondii* following immu-nohistochemistry in the brain, spinal cord, spinal nerves, and pelvic muscles. In addition, nested PCR analysis and sequencing, confirmed the presence of *T. gondii* DNA in uterine and lung tissues. Using multilocus PCR–RFLP analysis, they identified the organism as a variant type II *T. gondii* genotype. Roe et al. (2017) suggested that toxoplasmosis could play an important role in morbidity and mortality in this endangered marine mammal, particularly in mainland popu-lations that are close to feline sources and *T. gon-dii* oocysts.

GENUS *ZALOPHUS* GILL, 1866 (3 SPECIES)

ZALOPHUS CALIFORNIANUS (LESSON, 1828), CALIFORNIA SEA LION

Hammondia. No records in the literature, yet.
Neospora. Dubey et al. (2003d) looked for protozoan infections in a variety of marine mammals by examining blood samples. For *N. caninum*, the sera were diluted 1:40, 1:80, 1:160, and 1:320 and examined with the NAT using mouse-derived tachyzoites. NAT anti-bodies to *N. caninum* were found in 1/27 (4%) *Z. californianus*.
Toxoplasma gondii. Ratcliffe and Worth (1951) were the first to report that toxoplasmosis was a cause of death in one 10-day-old *Z. califor-nianus*. Microparasites were found in histologi-cal sections in the liver, heart, and lungs. Migaki et al. (1977) reported a case of toxoplasmosis in one *Z. californianus*; parasites were observed in necroses in heart and in the stomach. Dubey et al. (2003d) looked for evidence of infections by *Neospora*, *Sarcocystis*, and *Toxoplasma* species in a variety of marine mammals. For *T. gondii*,

their sera were diluted 1:25, 1:50, and 1:500 and assayed in the MAT; antibodies to *T. gondii* (MAT ≥ 1:25) were found in 19/45 (42%) appar-ently healthy *Z. californianus*.

FAMILY PHOCIDAE GRAY, 1821

GENUS *CYSTOPHORA* NILSSON, 1820 (MONOTYPIC)

CYSTOPHORA CRISTATA (ERXLEBEN, 1777), HOODED SEAL

Hammondia. No records in the literature, yet.
Neospora. No records in the literature, yet.
Toxoplasma gondii. Measures et al. (2004) collected sera from Canadian phocids from 1995 to 1997 and tested them by a MAT for *T. gondii* with titers ≥1:25 considered evidence of exposure. Only 1/60 (2%) hooded seals tested were positive for exposure to *T. gondii*. Measures et al. (2004) speculated that finding *T. gondii* in marine mammals might indicate natural infections that are unknown because of the lack of study or might indicate recent con-tamination of the marine environment from terrestrial environments by natural or anthro-pogenic activities.

GENUS *ERIGNATHUS* GILL, 1866 (MONOTYPIC)

ERIGNATHUS BARBATUS (ERXLEBEN, 1777), BEARDED SEAL

Hammondia. No records in the literature, yet.
Neospora. Dubey et al. (2003d) looked in a variety of marine mammals for evidence of *N. caninum* infection with the NAT using mouse-derived tachyzoites; they found only 1/8 (12.5%) bearded seals with NAT antibodies to *N. caninum*. This was one of the first reports

of *N. caninum* antibodies in any marine mammals. Fujii et al. (2007) did a serological survey to detect antibodies to *N. caninum* in seals in Hokkaido, Japan. They collected serum from a single *E. barbatus* at Nosappu and used recombinant surface antigen of *N. caninum* (NcSAG1t) in an ELISA to detect antibodies, but their only bearded seal had no antibodies to *N. caninum*.

Toxoplasma gondii. Dubey et al. (2003d) looked at the sera of a variety of marine mammals for *T. gondii*, using the MAT; antibodies to *T. gondii* (MAT ≥ 1:25) were found in 4/8 (50%) apparently healthy bearded seals. Fujii et al. (2007), using the same blood from one *E. barbatus*, as above, tried to detect antibodies to *T. gondii* using recombinant surface antigen of *T. gondii* (SAG2t) as antigen with an ELISA test, but their one bearded seal did not display antibodies to *T. gondii*. Jensen et al. (2010) examined the blood of bearded seals from Svalbard, Norway, for antibodies to *T. gondii*. In their study, 10/80 (12.5%) seals were positive for antibodies.

GENUS *HALICHOERUS* NILSSON, 1820 (MONOTYPIC)

HALICHOERUA GRYPUS (FABRICIUS, 1791), GRAY SEAL

Hammondia. No records in the literature, yet.
Neospora. No records in the literature, yet.
Toxoplasma gondii. Measures et al. (2004) collected sera from Canadian phocids from 1995 to 1997 and tested it by a MAT for antibodies to *T. gondii*; titers ≥1:25 were considered evidence of exposure. Of the gray seals tested, 11/122 (9%) were positive for exposure to *T. gondii*. Probable maternal antibody transfer was observed in one gray seal pup at 14 days of age. They speculated that finding *T. gondii* in marine mammals might indicate natural infections that are unknown because of the lack of study or might indicate recent contamination of the marine environment from

terrestrial environments by natural or anthropogenic activities. Gajadhar et al. (2004) used lab-reared gray seals to assess their susceptibility to *T. gondii*. They inoculated four of them with 100 or 10,000 sporulated oocysts of *T. gondii* and noted that occasionally, mild behavioral changes occurred in all inoculated seals, but not in uninoculated seals. A MAT demonstrated antibodies to *T. gondii* in all inoculated animals. However, no evidence of *T. gondii* was found on extensive histological examination of seal tissues although IHC of tissue sections revealed a single cyst in one seal. Cats fed brain and muscle tissue from inoculated seals passed *T. gondii* oocysts in their feces; this demonstrated to the authors that *T. gondii* can establish viable infections in seals and that marine mammals can acquire infections from oocysts in surface water runoff and sewage discharge. Cabezón et al. (2011) assayed the blood of harbor and gray seals from the Atlantic coasts of Scotland and France, between 1998 and 2004, and used the MAT to look for antibodies to *T. gondii*. They found 11/47 (23%) gray seals from four locations to have antibodies to *T. gondii*. No significant infection differences were found between age, sex, or geographic locations of the gray seals. Cabezón et al. (2011) said their results show natural exposure of gray seals to *T. gondii* oocysts in the Atlantic Ocean.

GENUS *HISTRIOPHOCA* GILL, 1873 (MONOTYPIC)

HISTRIOPHOCA (SYN. PHOCA) FASCIATA (ZIMMERMAN, 1783) RIBBON SEAL

Hammondia. No records in the literature, yet.
Neospora. Fujii et al. (2007) did a serological survey to detect antibodies to *N. caninum* in seals in Hokkaido, Japan. They collected serum from four *H.* (syn. *Phoca) fasciata* at Nosappu, between 1998 and 2006. Recombinant surface antigen of

N. caninum (NcSAG1t) was used as antigen for an ELISA to detect antibodies. They found that none of the four *P. fasciata* were infected with *N. caninum*.

Toxoplasma gondii. Fujii et al. (2007) did a serological survey to detect antibodies to *T. gondii* in seals in Hokkaido, Japan. They collected serum from four *H.* (syn. *Phoca*) *fasciata* at Nosappu, between 1998 and 2006. Recombinant surface antigen of *T. gondii* (SAG2t) was used as antigen for an ELISA to detect antibodies. They found that none of the four *P. fasciata* were infected with *T. gondii*.

GENUS *LEPTONYCHOTES* GILL, 1872 (MONOTYPIC)

LEPTONYCHOTES WEDDELLII (LESSON, 1826), WEDDELL SEAL

Hammondia. No records in the literature, yet.
Neospora. No records in the literature, yet.
Toxoplasma gondii. From 2007 to 2011, Rengifo-Herrera et al. (2012) collected sera from five species of pinnipeds from different locations in the South Shetland Islands and Antarctic Peninsula and analyzed them with a commercially available agglutination test kit for antibodies to *T. gondii*. In all, 28/211 (13%) serum samples were positive for *T. gondii* antibodies, including 13/31 (42%) Weddell seals. Jensen et al. (2012) collected fresh blood samples from 102 Antarctic pinnipeds and assayed the serum samples using a commercial DAT kit, according to the manufacturer's instructions, to determine if antibodies to *T. gondii* were present. They found antibodies (≥1:40) to *T. gondii* in 17/33 (51.5%) *L. weddellii*, from Hutton Cliffs, East Antarctica. The 1:40 cutoff used on samples from terrestrial animals has not been validated for seals, but it is commonly used. These two serosurveys are the first reports on the detection of *T. gondii* antibodies in Antarctic marine mammals.

GENUS *LOBODON* GRAY, 1844 (MONOTYPIC)

LOBODON CARCINOPHAGA (HOMBRON AND JACQUINOT, 1842), CRABEATER SEAL

Hammondia. No records in the literature, yet.
Neospora. No records in the literature, yet.
Toxoplasma gondii. Rengifo-Herrera et al. (2012) collected sera from five species of pinnipeds from different locations in the South Shetland Islands and Antarctic Peninsula, from 2007 to 2011, and analyzed them with a commercially-available agglutination test kit for antibodies to *T. gondii*. In all, 28/211 (13%) serum samples were positive for *T. gondii* antibodies, including 1/2 (50%) crabeater seals. Theirs may be the first report on the detection of *T. gondii* antibodies in Antarctic marine mammals.

GENUS *MIROUNGA* GRAY, 1827 (2 SPECIES)

MIROUNGA ANGUSTIROSTRIS (GILL, 1866), NORTHERN ELEPHANT SEAL

Hammondia. No records in the literature, yet.
Neospora. No records in the literature, yet.
Toxoplasma gondii. Dubey et al. (2004a) identified *T. gondii* in one elephant seal that had encephalitis. Tissue cysts were found in sections of cerebrum and the positive identification of *T. gondii* was confirmed by IHC with *T. gondii*–specific polyclonal rabbit serum. This was the first (and only) report of *T. gondii* in an elephant seal.

MIROUNGA LEONINA (L., 1758), SOUTHERN ELEPHANT SEAL

Hammondia. No records in the literature, yet.
Neospora. No records in the literature, yet.

Toxoplasma gondii. From 2007 to 2011, Rengifo-Herrera et al. (2012) collected sera of pinnipeds from different locations in the South Shetland Islands and Antarctic Peninsula and analyzed them with a commercially available agglutination test kit for antibodies to *T. gondii*. In all, 10/13 (77%) Southern elephant seals were positive for *T. gondii* antibodies. Jensen et al. (2012) collected blood samples from 102 Antarctic pinnipeds, and assayed the serum using a commercial DAT kit, to determine if antibodies to *T. gondii* were present. They found antibodies (≥1:40) to *T. gondii* in 11/48 (23%) *M. leonina* from Macquarie Island, the Pacific Ocean, and South Georgia (south Atlantic). For the southern elephant seals, 11 (23%) showed agglutination at the 1:40 dilution, and three (6%) remained positive at the 1:80 dilution. The 1:40 cutoff used on samples from terrestrial animals has not been validated for seals, but it is commonly used. These two serosurvey reports are the first ones on the detection of *T. gondii* in Antarctic marine mammals.

GENUS MONACHUS FLEMING, 1822 (3 SPECIES)

MONACHUS SCHAUINSLANDI MATSCHIE, 1905, HAWAIIAN MONK SEAL

Hammondia. No records in the literature, yet.
Neospora. No records in the literature, yet.
Toxoplasma gondii. Honnold et al. (2005) identified *T. gondii* in a Hawaiian monk seal that had visceral and cerebral lesions. Tachyzoites were found in the lymph nodes, spleen, diaphragm, heart, adrenal glands, and brain. A few tissue cysts were found in sections of the cerebrum. Their diagnosis was confirmed serologically by IHC with *T. gondii*–specific polyclonal rabbit serum and by the detection of *T. gondii* DNA. This particular *T. gondii* genotype was determined to be type III by RFLP of the SAG2 gene. This was the first report of *T. gondii* infection in a Hawaiian monk seal. Infection of monk seals indicates contamination of the ocean environment with oocysts from cats.

GENUS PHOCA L., 1758 (2 SPECIES)

PHOCA LARGHA PALLAS, 1811, SPOTTED SEAL

Hammondia. No records in the literature, yet.
Neospora. Fujii et al. (2007) did a survey to detect *N. caninum* in seals in Hokkaido, Japan, by collecting serum from *P. largha* at Nosappu, Erimo, Yagishiri Island, Hamamasu, and Syakotan, from 1998 to 2006. Recombinant surface antigen of *N. caninum* (NcSAG1t) was used in an ELISA to detect antibodies. They found 2/46 (4%) *P. largha* infected with *N. caninum*.
Toxoplasma gondii. Dubey et al. (2003d) looked at sera from a variety of marine mammals for *T. gondii*, in a MAT; antibodies to *T. gondii* (MAT ≥ 1:25) were found in 1/9 (11%) apparently healthy spotted seals. Fujii et al. (2007) did a survey of seals in Hokkaido, Japan; they collected serum from *P. largha* at Nosappu, Erimo, Yagishiri Island, Hamamasu, and Syakotan, between 1998 and 2006. Recombinant surface antigen of *T. gondii* (SAG2t) was used in an ELISA to detect antibodies, but they found that none of the 46 *P. largha* tested were infected with *T. gondii*.

PHOCA VITULINA L., 1758, HARBOR SEAL

Hammondia. No records in the litereature, yet.
Neospora. Dubey et al. (2003d) looked at the sera of a variety of marine mammals for *N. caninum* with the NAT using mouse-derived

tachyzoites. NAT antibodies to *N. caninum* were found in 11/311 (3.5%) *P. vitulina*. Theirs was one of the first reports of *N. caninum* antibodies in marine mammals.

Toxoplasma gondii. Van Pelt and Dieterich (1973) reported a case of toxoplasmosis in one 23-day-old *P. v. vichardii* as a complication of a septic cutaneous infection with *Staphylococcus*. Cysts and trophozoites of *T. gondii* were found both inside and around necrotic loci in the entire liver parenchyma. Lambourn et al. (2001) worked with the Puget Sound Ambient Monitoring Program of the Washington Department of Fish and Wildlife by examining the blood of harbor seals for antibodies to *T. gondii*. Using a modified MAT that incorporated formalin-fixed tachyzoites, they were able to detect antibodies to *T. gondii* in 29/380 (8%) *P. vitulina*. They said that their results indicate natural exposure of the seals to *T. gondii*. Dubey et al. (2003d) looked at blood of a variety of marine mammals for *T. gondii*, assayed in the MAT; antibodies to *T. gondii* (MAT ≥ 1:25) were found in 51/311 (16%) apparently healthy *P. vitulina*. Measures et al. (2004) collected sera from Canadian phocids from 1995 to 1997 and tested it by a MAT for antibodies to *T. gondii* (titers ≥1:25 were considered evidence of exposure). Only 3/34 (9%) *P. vitulina* tested were positive for exposure to *T. gondii*. Probable maternal antibody transfer was observed in one harbor seal pup at 10 days of age. Measures et al. (2004) speculated that finding *T. gondii* in marine mammals might indicate natural infections that are unknown because of the lack of study or might indicate recent contamination of the marine environment from terrestrial environments by natural or anthropogenic activities. Fujii et al. (2007) also surveyed seals in Hokkaido, Japan, by collecting serum from *P. v. stejnegeri* at Nosappu, Akkeshi, and Erimo, Japan, from 1998 to 2006. Recombinant surface antigen of *T. gondii* (SAG2t) was used in an ELISA to detect antibodies, but only 3/322 (<1%) *P. v. stejnegeri* demonstrated antibodies

for *T. gondii*. Cabezón et al. (2011) assayed the blood of harbor and gray seals from the Atlantic coasts of Scotland and France, between 1998 and 2004, and used the MAT for detecting antibodies to *T. gondii*; they found that 3/36 (5%) harbor seals from four locations had antibodies to *T. gondii*. No significant infection differences were found between age, sex, or geographic locations of these seals, which let them to say that they had found natural exposure of European harbor seals to *T. gondii* oocysts in the Atlantic Ocean.

PHOCA VITULINA RICHARDSI (GRAY, 1864), PACIFIC HARBOR SEAL

Hammondia. No records in the literature, yet.

Neospora. No records in the literature, yet.

Toxoplasma gondii. Miller et al. (2001b) documented *T. gondii* in a female Pacific harbor seal found depressed, seizuring, and unresponsive in northwest Monterey, California, USA. The seal was diagnosed with meningoencephalomyelitis, which was thought to be due mainly to *Sarcocystis neurona*, with which the seal also was infected. However, purified zoites from a second isolate reacted positively with *T. gondii* polyclonal antiserum (1:81,920) and with the harbor seal's own serum (1:640).

PHOCA VITULINA STEJNEGERI (J.A. ALLEN, 1902), KURIL HARBOR SEAL

Hammondia. No records in the literature, yet.

Neospora. Many wild noncanid carnivores are known to have been exposed to *N. caninum*, either by being seropositive, demonstrating oocysts in their feces, or exhibiting signs of neosporosis, including the Kuril harbor seal in Japan. Fujii et al. (2007) surveyed seals in Hokkaido, Japan, by collecting serum from

Kuril harbor seals, *P. v. stejnegeri*, from 1998 to 2006. Recombinant surface antigen of *N. caninum* (NcSAG1t) was used in an ELISA to detect antibodies, and they found 13/322 (4%) Kuril harbor seals were infected with *N. caninum*.

Toxoplasma gondii. No records in the literature, yet.

GENUS *PUSA* SCOPOLI, 1771 (3 SPECIES)

PUSA (SYN. *PHOCA*) *HISPIDA* (SCHREBER, 1775), RINGED SEAL

Hammondia. No records in the literature, yet.

Neospora. Dubey et al. (2003d) looked at sera from a variety of marine mammals to determine infection rates with a variety of protists. Using the NAT with mouse-derived tachyzoites, antibodies to *N. caninum* were found in 4/32 (12.5%) ringed seals.

Toxoplasma gondii. Dubey et al. (2003d) looked for evidence of infections by *Neospora*, *Sarcocystis*, and *Toxoplasma* species in a variety of marine mammals. For *T. gondii*, sera were diluted 1:25, 1:50, and 1:500 and assayed in the MAT; *T. gondii* (MAT≥1:25) was found in 5/32 (16%) apparently healthy ringed seals. Jensen et al. (2010) examined the blood of ringed seals from Svalbard, Norway, for antibodies to *T. gondii*. In their study, 49/262 (19%) seals were positive for antibodies to *T. gondii*.

PROCYONIDAE GRAY, 1825

GENUS *BASSARICUS* J.A. ALLEN, 1876 (5 SPECIES)

BASSARISCUS ASTUTUS (LICHTENSTEIN, 1830), CIVET OR RINGTAIL CAT

Hammondia. No records in the literature, yet.

Neospora. No records in the literature, yet.

Toxoplasma gondii. Franti et al. (1976) tested 2,796 serum samples from wild and domestic mammals and birds in northern California for antibodies to *T. gondii* and found the only civet cat they examined to be positive.

GENUS *NASUA* STORR, 1780 (2 SPECIES)

NASUA NASUA (L., 1766), SOUTH AMERICAN COATI

Hammondia. No records in the literature, yet.

Neospora. No records in the literature, yet.

Toxoplasma. Frenkel and Sousa (1983) tested serum samples from 180 mammals representing 22 species in Panama for antibodies to *Toxoplasma gondii* and found 2/4 (50%) coatis to be positive. de Thoisy et al. (2003) serosurveyed 18 forest mammal species in French Guiana using a DAT and found 5/7 (72%) coatis and tayras (*Eira barbara*) positive for antibodies to *T. gondii*, but they did not provide sample sizes and prevalences for the two species separately.

GENUS *POTOS* É. GEOFFROYI SAINT-HILAIRE AND F.G. CUVIER, 1795 (MONOTYPIC)

POTOS FLAVUS (SCHREBER, 1774), KINKAJOU

Hammondia. No records in the literature, yet.

Neospora. No records in the literature, yet.

Toxoplasma. Frenkel and Sousa (1983) serosurveyed 180 mammals from 22 species in Panama for antibodies and found none of their nine kinkajou samples to be positive. de Thoisy et al. (2003) did a serosurvey for *Toxoplasma gondii* in 18 forest mammal species in French Guiana, using a DAT, and found 1/10 (10%) kinkajous positive.

GENUS PROCYON STORR, 1780 (3 SPECIES)

PROCYON CANCRIVORUS (G. [BARON] CUVIER, 1798), CRAB-EATING RACCOON

Hammondia. No records in the literature, yet.

Neospora. No records in the literature, yet.

Toxoplasma gondii. Richini-Pereira et al. (2016) looked for the presence of *T. gondii* in tissue samples of 64 road-killed animals using PCR. Positive samples were then typed by PCR–RFLP, with seven specific markers (SAG1, 5'-3' SAG2, SAG3, BTUB, c29-6, PK1, Apico). PCR–RFLP targeting the 18S rRNA genes was performed on all samples to detect other apicomplexan parasites. They detected *T. gondii* DNA in one road-killed *P. cancrivorus*. The amplified *T. gondii* (GenBank accession No. L37415.1) 18S rRNA products were confirmed by sequencing.

PROCYON LOTOR (L., 1758), RACCOON

Hammondia. Lemberger et al. (2005) (see below) extracted DNA from the brain of a raccoon in Illinois, USA, and used specific PCR to look for the presence of *H. hammondi*, but the results were negative.

Neospora. Lindsay et al. (2001b) examined sera from raccoons in Florida, Massachusetts, New Jersey, and Pennsylvania, USA, for the prevalence of agglutinating antibodies to *N. caninum* that employed formalin-fixed tachyzoites. They found 10/99 (10%) raccoons to have antibodies for *N. caninum* including 1/24 (4%) in Florida, 3/25 (12%) in Massachusetts, 3/25 (12%) in New Jersey, and 3/25 (12%) in Pennsylvania. Lemberger et al. (2005) found a juvenile, female raccoon in Illinois, USA, suffering from seizures; the animal was killed and necropsied. Sections of its cerebellum stained immunohistochemically for *N. caninum* and showed a round to

ovoidal cyst, ~40 wide, which had a cyst wall, 2–3 thick, and was filled with round to ovoidal bradyzoites. PCR results were positive for *N. caninum* using DNA extracted from the brain.

Toxoplasma gondii. Franti et al. (1976) tested 2,796 serum samples from wild and domestic mammals and birds in northern California for antibodies to *T. gondii* and found 12/48 (25%) raccoons to be positive. Tizard et al. (1976) surveyed blood of wild carnivores in Central Ontario, using the Sabin–Feldman dye test, and found 19/105 (18%) *P. lotor* to be positive for antibodies. Lindsay et al. (2001b,c) examined sera from raccoons in Florida, Massachusetts, New Jersey, and Pennsylvania, USA, for agglutinating antibodies to *T. gondii* that employed formalin-fixed tachyzoites, and found 46/99 (46%) raccoons to be positive for *T. gondii* including, 7/24 (29%) in Florida, 23/25 (92%) in Massachusetts, 10/25 (40%) in New Jersey, and 6/25 (24%) in Pennsylvania. Matoba et al. (2002), in Japan, surveyed 260 feral raccoons for oocysts (see Chapters 8 and 14); they also examined sera for antibodies to *T. gondii* in 33 raccoons from Nopporo Forest Park (Sapporo), and 171 raccoons from Naoi Hills (Hokkaido), Japan. They found 6/33 (18%) on Sapporo and 28/171 (16%) on Hokkaido to demonstrate antibody titers to *T. gondii*, but they did not mention the antibody test they used. There was no statistical difference in positive samples between localities or between juveniles and adults. Also in Japan, Sato et al. (2011) studied the seroprevalence of *T. gondii* in feral raccoons using the LAT (LAT, ≥1:64) and found seropositivity varied by geographic region, season, and host weight. Overall, 92/929 (10%) feral raccoons were positive for antibodies to *T. gondii*; in northern Japan (Hokkaido), 39/492 (8%) raccoons were seropositive, in central (Honshu, Kanagawa, and Chiba Prefectures) Japan, 47/285 (16.5%) raccoons were positive, and in western areas (Honshu, Wakayama Prefecture), 6/152 (4%) were positive. Seroprevalence by season varied from 13/153 (8.5%) in the spring to 14/74 (19%) in the winter, significantly higher than the other seasons. These authors suggested that the raccoon may serve as a useful indicator for the distribution of *T. gondii* in peridomestic environments in Japan. Lemberger et al. (2005) also used DNA from the brain of a raccoon in Illinois, USA (above), to look for the presence of *T. gondii* via specific PCR, but the results were negative.

PROCYON PYGMAEUS (MERRIAM, 1901), PYGMY RACCOON

Hammondia. No records in the literature, yet.
Neospora. No records in the literature, yet.
Toxoplasma gondii. McFadden et al. (2005) tested blood samples of critically endangered pygmy raccoons on Cozumel Island, Mexico, and found antibodies to *T. gondii* in 3/28 (11%) samples including two adult females and one adult male. McFadden et al. (2005) suggested that the presence of *T. gondii* in the pygmy raccoon, one of the three endemic carnivore species on the Island was due to the introduction of domestic cats.

URSIDAE FISCHER DE WALDHEIM, 1817

GENUS AILUROPODA MILNE-EDWARDS, 1870 (MONOTYPIC)

AILUROPODA MELANOLEUCA (DAVID, 1869), GIANT PANDA

Hammondia. No records in the literature, yet.
Neospora. Loeffler et al. (2007) surveyed 19 giant pandas from the Chengdu Research Base of Giant Panda Breeding, Sichuan, China, using the IFA test, all with negative results.
Toxoplasma gondii. Loeffler et al. (2007) surveyed giant pandas from the Chengdu Research Base of Giant Panda Breeding, Sichuan, China, using the IFA assay, and found antibodies to *T. gondii* in 6/19 (32%) pandas. Ma et al. (2015) reported a fatal case of toxoplasmosis in a giant panda at the Zhengzhou Zoo, Henan Province, China.

GENUS URSUS L., 1758 (4 SPECIES)

URSUS AMERICANUS PALLAS, 1780, AMERICAN BLACK BEAR

Hammondia. No records in the literature, yet.
Neospora. During a serosurvey of wild animals in the United States using the NAT, Dubey, and Thulliez (2005) did not detect antibodies to *N. caninum* in 64 *U. americanus* from North Carolina nor in 133 *U. americanus* from Alaska. However, these animals were highly seropositive for *T. gondii*. Sedlák and Bártová (2006a) examined carnivores in zoos in the Czech and Slovak Republics using the IFAT and found no antibodies to *N. caninum* in three *U. americanus*. The absence of *N. caninum* antibodies in black bears suggests they are not suitable hosts for this parasite, and that there is no cross-reactivity between the *N. caninum* and *T. gondii* agglutination tests.
Toxoplasma gondii. Quinn et al. (1976) did a serosurvey of wild carnivores in southern Ontario for antibodies to *T. gondii*, using the Sabin–Feldman dye test, and found 52/158 (33%) *U. americanus* positive. Tizard et al. (1976) also surveyed blood of wild carnivores in central Ontario, using the Sabin–Feldman dye test and found 7/16 (44%) *U. americanus* positive for *T. gondii*. Binninger et al. (1980) sampled blood of black bears in Idaho, USA, using the IHA test with the RH strain of *T. gondii* and found 23/303 (8%) with positive titers, and positive males had a significantly higher mean age (7.7 years, n = 18) than did negative males (4.9 years, n = 15). Older bears having a greater prevalence of *T. gondii* could be due to their longer potential exposure time and their extensive home ranges (Binninger et al., 1980). Ruppanner et al. (1982) surveyed black bears from three areas of California, USA, also using IHA, but with the California 76 strain of *T. gondii* as antigen; 40/149 (27%) bears tested were positive for *T. gondii*, substantially higher than they found in rodents (14/559, 2.5%), but less than half that found in bobcats (59/86, 69%) in an earlier

survey in northern California (Franti et al., 1976). Chomel et al. (1995) did a serosurvey of black bears in interior Alaska from 1988–91. Using a commercial latex aggulutination test (LAT) they detected antibodies to *T. gondii* (≥64) in 6/40 (15%) *U. americana*. Nutter et al. (1998) serosurveyed black bears killed in eastern North Carolina, USA, using the MAT, and found 120/143 (84%) positive for antibodies to *T. gondii*. Females and older animals had significantly higher titers than males or the young. Sedlák and Bártová (2006a) examined carnivores in zoos in the Czech and Slovak Republics using the IFAT and found 3/3 (100%) bears with antibodies to *T. gondii*. Chambers et al. (2012) serosurveyed wild black bears in Florida and found 13/29 (45%) positive for *T. gondii*. Dubey et al. (2016a) conducted a seroepidemiological study of black bears in Pennsylvania, USA, and found 206/235 (88%) positive for *T. gondii* antibodies (MAT, cutoff 1:25). Another serosurvey of wild black bears in the central Appalachian Mountains, USA, by Cox et al. (2017) found 33/53 (62%) positive for *T. gondii*.

URSUS ARCTOS L., 1758, BROWN (OR GRIZZLY) BEAR

Hammondia. No records in the literature, yet.

Neospora. Čobádiová et al. (2013) examined tissue samples (muscle, liver, spleen) from 45 brown bears in different locations of Central Slovakia, using the PCR amplification of Nc-5 and ITS-1 rRNA genes. They detected DNA of *N. caninum* in 11/45 (24%) bears (9 from the liver, 2 from the spleen). This was the first molecular evidence of *N. caninum* in European brown bears in Slovakia. The authors suggested various possibilities of how the bears acquired their infections such as predation of infected deer or rodents, transplacental transmission, infection with oocysts from a contaminated environment, and dissemination of the oocysts by dairy farm dogs.

Toxoplasma gondii. Kiupel et al. (1987) used TEM to examine tissues of the cubs of breeding grizzly bears in the Rostock Zoological Garden, Germany, from 1971 to 1985; they diagnosed various stages of *T. gondii* in 16/21 (76%) cubs that were 114–356-days-old and reported that toxoplasmosis was the sole principle cause of death in nine animals. In acute cases they found interstitial pneumonia with alveolar proliferation and desquamation, general lymph node dilation with extensive necrosis, and lymphoblastic eruption, liver necrosis (1 animal), encephalitic lymphocytopenia with focal glial cell proliferation, ulcerative leukocyte infiltration, focal pyocarditis, catarrhal enteritis ulceration, and necrotizing pseudocystitis. Chomel et al. (1995) did a serosurvey of *U. arctos* in Alaska from 1988–91. Using a commercial LAT they detected antibodies to *T. gondii* (≥64) in 87/480 (18%) grizzly bears and Zarnke et al. (1997) found 220/887 (25%) *U. arctos* from Alaska with antibodies to *T. gondii* (≥25) with a MAT. Zhang et al. (2000) examined the sera of "rare wild carnivores" in the Shanghai Zoological Gardens using both the MAT and an ELISA, and 27/36 (75%) samples were positive for *T. gondii* antibodies, including the only *U. arctos lasiotus*, which was both ELISA- and MAT-positive.

URSUS MARITIMUS PHIPPS, 1774, POLAR BEAR

Hammondia. No records in the literature, yet.

Neospora. Sedlák and Bártová (2006a) examined carnivores in zoos in the Czech and Slovak Republics using the IFAT and found no antibodies to *N. caninum* in the only polar bear they were able to examine.

Toxoplasma gondii. Rah et al. (2005) surveyed polar bears captured in the Beaufort and Chukchi Seas, using the LAT, and detected *T. gondii* in 30/500 (6%) samples. Sedlák and Bártová (2006a) tested the same polar bear they examined for *N. caninum*, to detect *T. gondii*, and found it to have a positive titer of 1:320. Oksanen et al. (2009) examined serum from polar bears from Svalbard and the Barents Sea (collected 1990–2000) and from East Greenland (collected 1999–2004) and assayed them for *T. gondii* using a MAT; they found 86/419 (20.5%) polar bears of all ages (<2- to >15-years-old) from Svalbard were positive for *T. gondii*, while only 12/198 (6%) polar bears of all ages from East Greenland were positive for *T. gondii*. Jensen et al. (2010) also examined polar bear blood from Svalbard, Norway, for antibodies to *T. gondii*, and found 104/228 (46%) samples to be positive for to *T. gondii*. The prevalence was significantly higher in males than in females, but the most surprising aspect of their study was the overall prevalence was double the rate reported earlier by Oksanen et al. (2009) and almost eight times higher that reported by Rah et al. (2005), just 5 years earlier.

SUBORDER FELIFORMIA KRETZOI, 1945

EUPLERIDAE CHENU, 1850

SUBFAMILY EUPLERINAE CHENU, 1850

GENUS CRYPTOPROCTA BENNETT, 1833 (MONOTYPIC)

CRYPTOPROCTA FEROX BENNETT, 1833, FOSSA

Hammondia. No records in the literature, yet.

Neospora. Sedlák and Bártová (2006a) sero-surveyed zoo animals in the Czech and Slovak Republics for the occurrence of *N. caninum* antibodies using the IFAT, but they found no antibodies to *N. caninum* in two *C. ferox*.

Toxoplasma gondii. Sedlák and Bártová (2006a) also looked for antibodies to *T. gondii* using the IFAT and found 2/2 *C. ferox* to have positive tires. Corpa et al. (2013) reported *T. gondii* infection in one *C. ferox*, a Madagascar endemic. A 7-year-old captive-bred female fossa, born at a German zoo and then transferred to the zoo in Valencia, Spain, was fed exclusively on a frozen commercial meat diet and later was diagnosed with *T. gondii*. The

animal exhibited neurologic signs (ataxia), atrophy of hind limb muscles, weight loss, and progressive wasting before dying 12 months after the onset of clinical signs. PCR from the EDTA-blood was positive for *T. gondii*, but negative for *Neospora*, *Ehrlichia*, and *Rickettsia* species. At necropsy, Corpa et al. (2013) found a moderate, multifocal, nonsuppurative encephalomyelitis. Occasionally, *T. gondii*–like tissue cysts, surrounded by a thin wall and containing numerous bradyzoites, were detected in lesions in the gray matter of the brain, and in the white matter of the thoracic spinal cord. Immunohistochemistry on the cysts was positive for *T. gondii* but negative for *N. caninum* and *S. neurona*. The source of infection was not determined but was thought to be associated with oocysts, discharged by feral cats, which may have contaminated the feed. Pomerantz et al. (2016) did a serosurvey of carnivore species at Kirindy Mitea and Ankarafantsika National Parks, Madagascar, and tested them for antibodies to five viral pathogens and for *T. gondii* (by ELISA); antibodies to *T. gondii* were detected in 42/45 (93%) fossa, of which 33 had high titers (≥1:1,024) suggestive of a recent or active infection. The only known definitive hosts of *T. gondii* are domestic and wild felids, which shed oocysts in their feces. Madagascar has no endemic felids, and the presence of *T. gondii* in free-ranging fossa indicates parasite "spillover" from an introduced cat species, either *F. catus* or *F. silvestris*. Presence of antibodies to *T. gondii* in fossa was significantly higher in adults than in immatures (juveniles, subadults) suggesting horizontal transmission, likely through ingestion of intermediate hosts. The diet of free-ranging fossa consists of a wide range of animals, including the black rat, *Rattus rattus*, a potential intermediate host of *T. gondii*. Fossa not only are solitary, **cathemeral** carnivores found at low densities mainly in forested areas, but also are known to visit villages and prey on poultry (Hawkins and Racey, 2005; Kotschwar Logan et al., 2015). These raids into villages may facilitate interactions with domestic animals and transmission of pathogens across species. In a captive fossa noted earlier by Corpa et al. (2013),

T. gondii caused encephalomyelitis resulting in ataxia, muscular atrophy, and eventually death. However, the high prevalence of antibodies to *T. gondii* reported by Pomerantz et al. (2016) in free-ranging fossa suggests that *Toxoplasma* infection may not be universally lethal in fossa.

SUBFAMILY GALIDIINAE CHENU, 1850

GENUS *MUNGOTICTIS* POCOCK, 1915 (MONOTYPIC)

MUNGOTICTIS DECEMLINEATA (GRANDIDIER, 1867), NARROW-STRIPED MONGOOSE

Hammondia. No records in the literature, yet.

Neospora. No records in the literature, yet.

Toxoplasma gondii. Pomerantz et al. (2016) did a serosurvey of carnivores at Kirindy Mitea and Ankarafantsika National Parks in Madagascar and tested them for antibodies to five viral pathogens and for *T. gondii* (by ELISA); the samples included six narrow-striped mongooses and antibodies to *T. gondii* were detected in 1/6 (17%) *M. decemlineata*.

FELIDAE FISCHER DE WALDHEIM, 1817

SUBFAMILY FELINAE FISCHER DE WALDHEIM, 1817

GENUS ACINONYX BROOKES, 1828 (MONOTYPIC)

ACINONYX JUBATUS (SCHREBER, 1775), CHEETAH

Hammondia. No records in the literature, yet.

Neospora. Cheadle et al. (1999) did a seroprevalence study of nondomestic felids in South Africa and found antibodies in the cheetah, as did Ferroglio et al. (2003) in Kenya, who examined wild animals for antibodies and found 1/5 (20%) *A. jubatus* to be positive using the NAT. Sedlák and Bártová (2006a) serosurveyed zoo animals in the Czech and Slovak Republics for *N. caninum* antibodies by the IFAT and found 2/15 (13%) *A. jubatus* had antibodies to *N. caninum*.

Toxoplasma gondii. Polomoshnov (1979) reported finding a cheetah infected with *T. gondii*. Van Rensburg and Silkstone (1984) caught three littermate cheetahs, and all died from feline infectious peritonitis (FIP) after about 9 weeks in captivity. Only one cheetah was necropsied, and the postmortem examination showed typical signs of FIP and lesions in the liver and brain of a concomitant *T. gondii* infection. Lappin et al. (1991) collected serum from nondomestic felids and evaluated them for antibodies to *T. gondii* using a LA kit, an IHA kit, and an ELISA for IgM (IgM–ELISA), IgG (IgG–ELISA), and for antigen (AG–ELISA) to define optimal diagnostic procedures. Antigen to *T. gondii* was detected in 25/33 (76%) cheetahs using IgG ELISA, in 20/33 (61%) using the LA test, and in 19/33 (58%) using the IHA test. Positive titers (≥1:128) were found in 8/8 *A. jubatus* at White Oaks Plantation, Yulee, Florida. Sedlák and Bártová (2006a) serosurveyed zoo animals in the Czech and Slovak Republics for *T. gondii* antibodies by the IFAT and found 13/15 (87%) *A. jubatus* were positive. de Camps et al. (2008) were interested in *T. gondii* infections in zoo cats, marsupials, and prosimians because many captive animals die of clinical toxoplasmosis and because of the potential risk of exposure that oocysts from zoo and feral cats may pose to children and the elderly. They used the MAT to test for antibodies (titer ≥1:25 indicative of exposure) to *T. gondii*. Blood samples were collected from wild zoo felids in eight zoos in the midwestern United States and antibodies to *T. gondii* were found in 6/22 (27%) *A. j. jubatus*. Dubey et al. (2010a,b,c) surveyed the sera of many carnivores at the BCEAW, Sharjah, UAE, and demonstrated antibodies to *T. gondii* in 31/34 (91%) *A. j. soemmerringii* (Fitzinger,

1855); they (2010) also surveyed the sera of carnivores at the Al Wabra Wildlife Preservation (AWWP) facility in Qatar and found antibodies to *T. gondii* in 5/5 *A. j. soemmerringii*, and in 1/1 king cheetah, *A. j. rex* Pocock, 1927.

GENUS CARACAL GRAY, 1843 (MONOTYPIC)

CARACAL CARACAL (SCHREBER, 1776), CARACAL

Hammondia. No records in the literature, yet.

Neospora. André et al. (2010) did a serological survey of captive neotropical and exotic wild felids in Brazil and found antibodies to *N. caninum* in the only caracal they surveyed.

Toxoplasma gondii. de Camps et al. (2008) looked for *T. gondii* infections in zoo cats, using the (MAT) to test for antibodies (titer ≥1:25 indicative of exposure) to *T. gondii*. Blood samples were taken from felids in eight zoos in the midwestern United States, and antibodies to *T. gondii* were found in 2/4 (50%) caracals sampled. Dubey et al. (2010a) surveyed the sera of carnivores at the BCEAW, Sharjah, UAE, and found antibodies to *T. gondii* in 5/6 (83%) *C. c. schmitzi* (Matschie, 1912) and in 1/1 African caracal, *C. c. alegria* (Wagner, 1841).

GENUS CATOPUMA SEVERTZOV, 1858 (2 SPECIES)

CATOPUMA TEMMINCKII (VIGORS AND HORSFIELD, 1827), ASIAN GOLDEN CAT

Hammondia. No records in the literature, yet.

Neospora. No records in the literature, yet.

Toxoplasma gondii. Zhang et al. (2000) examined the sera of "rare wild carnivores" in the Shanghai Zoological Gardens, using both the MAT, and an ELISA, and they found 27/36 (75%)

were positive for *T. gondii* antibodies, including 5/6 (83%) *C.* (syn. *Felis*) *temminckii*, which were both ELISA-positive and MAT-positive.

GENUS FELIS L., 1758 (7 SPECIES)

FELIS CATUS L., 1758, DOMESTIC CAT

Besnoitia. There are now about five *Besnoitia* species for which the carnivore definitive host has been identified, and all (or most) use the domestic cat, as far as we currently know.

Besnoitia besnoiti **(Marotel, 1912) Henry, 1913.** Peteshev et al. (1974) first demonstrated that cats are the definitive host for *B. besnoiti* in Kazakhstan, but others have not yet been able to repeat or confirm this work. Levine and Ivens (1981, pp. 142–148) summarized what was known to that time about definitive and intermediate hosts, geographic distribution, location of endogenous stages in felids, a few prevalence studies, sporulation time, prepatent and patent periods, immunity, cultivation, and known pathogenicity in its intermediate hosts. More recently, Kiehl et al. (2010) did a comprehensive phylogenetic study of the ITS-1 and ITA-2 regions and 18S rDNA gene sequences of *B. besnoiti* tissue cysts, from an outbreak in cattle in Germany, and found almost identical sequence alignments when compared with previously sequenced *B. besnoiti* isolates from Israel and Spain. Nonetheless, no one has yet reproduced the work of Peteshev et al. (1974) to verify that this species does, indeed, use cats as definitive hosts, and Dubey et al. (2003c) expressed their conviction the definitive host is not a felid.

Besnoitia darlingi **(Brumpt, 1913) Mandour, 1965.** Smith and Frenkel (1977) demonstrated that tissue cysts of *B. darlingi* in two road-killed opossums, *Didelphis marsupialis*, when inoculated into mice and hamsters, resulted in acute, lethal infections, and that when these cysts were fed to cats resulted in the shedding of isosporid-type oocysts 11–14 DPI; these oocysts sporulated in 48–72 hours, and measured L×W (n=20): 12.0×10.3 (11–13×10–11), L/W ratio: 1.2, and they lacked a M, OR, and PG. Sporocysts of *B. darlingi* were, L×W (n=20): 7.9×5.4 (6–9×5–6), L/W ratio: 1.5, and had a diffuse granular SR, but no SB, SSB, or PSB. Levine and Ivens (1981, pp. 150–152) summarized what was known to that time about definitive and intermediate hosts, geographic distribution, location and structure of endogenous stages in felids, prevalence, oocyst structure, sporulation time, prepatent and patent periods, immunity, cross-transmission work, and known pathogenicity in its intermediate hosts. Houk et al. (2011) did a serological survey of cats in Virginia and in Pennsylvania, USA, by developing an IFAT to examine IgG antibodies to tachyzoites of *B. darlingi*. Antibodies to *B. darlingi* were detected in 32/232 (14%) cats in Virginia and in 4/209 (2%) cats in Pennsylvania.

***Besnoitia neotomofelis* Dubey and Yabsley, 2010.** Dubey and Yabsley (2010) detected this parasite by bioassay of woodrat (*Neotoma micropus*) tissues in lab mice, while trying to isolate *T. gondii*. Tachyzoites were successfully cultured *in vitro* in bovine monocytes and African green monkey kidney cells and then *in vivo* in mice. Tissue cysts were microscopic, up to 210 long, and were infective orally to mice. Cats fed tissue cysts shed unsporulated oocysts that were 14×13. Enteroepithelial meronts and gamonts were found in cats fed tissue cysts. First-generation meronts were 50×40 and developed in the lamina propria of the cat small intestine. Second-generation meronts, ~8 wide, contained 4–8 merozoites. Gamonts and oocysts were seen in goblet cells of the small intestine epithelium, and tachyzoites were present in mesenteric lymph nodes of cats. Phylogenetic analysis showed that *B. neotomofelis* was related to other *Besnoitia* from rodents, rabbits, and opossums; this species was also found in 1/55 (<2%) southern plains woodrats (*N. micropus*) in Texas, USA,

by Charles et al. (2011). In *N. micropus*, cysts were found in the tongue, facial region, musculature of the limbs, and subcutis of the dorsum and flanks, and little or no inflammation was noted around these tissue cysts. Houk et al. (2011) did a serological survey of cats in Virginia and Pennsylvania, USA, by developing an IFAT to examine IgG antibodies to tachyzoites of *B. neotomofelis*. Antibodies to *B. neotomofelis* were detected in 12/232 (5%) cats in Virginia and in 8/209 (4%) cats in Pennsylvania. One of the 232 cats from Pennsylvania demonstrated positive antibodies to both *B. darlingi* and *B. neotomofelis*.

***Besnoitia oryctofelisi* Dubey, Sreekumar, Lindsay, Hill, Rosenthal, Venturini, Venturini and Greiner, 2003c.** One of the coauthors who named this species found tissue cysts of a *Besnoitia* species in a naturally-infected rabbit (*Oryctolagus cuniculus*) on a farm in La Plata, Argentina (Venturini et al., 2002). The cysts were fed to a 2-month-old kitten in La Plata, and it shed oocysts in its feces 13 DPI. The oocysts were separated from fecal debris, washed, suspended in 2.5% aqueous potassium dichromate for 1 week at room temperature, and shipped by air to the laboratory in Beltsville, Maryland, USA. There, Dubey et al. (2003c) described the life cycle, and its biology, in both intermediate and definitive hosts, and provided molecular and protein data to substantiate the validity of their new species. They experimentally propagated the parasite in mice, gerbils, rabbits, cats, and cell culture. Rabbits developed tissue cysts that were fed to cats, which shed oocysts 9–13 DPI. After sporulation, these oocysts were infective orally to gerbils and cats. They were able to cultivate and maintain tachyzoites successfully in bovine monocytes and African green monkey kidney cells. After infecting cats with tissue cysts, they documented that meronts were present in mesenteric lymph nodes, liver, and other extraintestinal organs. Discharged oocysts were L×W: 10–14×10–13. They noted that this rabbit-derived form resembled *B. darlingi* from the opossum (*D. viriginiana*), but it was not transmissible to opossums, and *B. darlingi* from opossums was not transmissible to rabbits. Based on their comprehensive effort, they named the Argentina species from a rabbit as a new species (Dubey et al., 2003c).

***Besnoitia wallacei* (Wallace and Frenkel, 1975) Frenkel, 1977 N. Comb.** Wallace and Frenkel (1975) were the first to solidly establish the experimental groundwork for our understanding of the cyclic transmission of a *Besnoitia* species between felids and their prey. In their seminal paper, they used oocysts from a stray cat on Oahu, Hawaii, to infect laboratory mice and rats, but they did not name it. Dubey (1977b), in his review chapter on *Toxoplasma, Hammondia, Besnoitia, Sarcocystis,* and other tissue cyst-forming coccidia (Table VII, p. 201), cited the work of Tadros and Laarman (1976), without explanation, detail, or valid species description or descriptors, and created the name "*B. wallacei* (Tadros and Laarman, 1976) Dubey, 1977," which is how many authors cite this species in the literature when using the name. Unfortunately, Dubey (1977b) did not follow any of the tenents (principles) of the ICZN regarding the naming of a species (also see Bandoni and Duszynski, 1988). Frenkel (1977) also used the name *Besnoitia wallacei,* but without an authority. We believe that Frenkel (1977), not Dubey (1977b) is the correct authority for this name and that, in the future, it should be cited as we indicate, above.

In their original descriptive information (Wallace and Frenkel, 1975), the oocysts were L×W: 16×13, and when inoculated into mice and rats, tissue cysts were produced in the omentum and mesentery; these cysts were then fed to 23 cats, 17 of which developed patent infections, discharging unsporulated oocysts 11–13 DPI, and with a patent period that lasted ~11 (5–12) days. Oocysts placed in 1%–2% aqueous sulfuric acid sporulated in 48–96 hours when maintained at 24°C and exposed to air. The sporulated oocysts produced were, L×W (n=100): 16×13 (15–18×12–15), L/W ratio: 1.2, and they lacked a M, OR, and PG. Their sporocysts were, L×W (n=50): 11×8 (10–11×7–8), L/W ratio: 1.4, and had a diffuse granular SR, but no SB, SSB, or PSB. Later Frenkel (1977) named this species *B. wallacei,* gave detailed information that includes the description of oocysts along with their mensural data and type specimens (photosyntypes, see Duszynski, 1999), and life cycle details including asexual tissue stages in mice and sexual stages in epithelial cells of the cat ileum. Frenkel (1977) also offered the first reclassification of the known cyst-forming isosporid coccidians, including creating the genus name *Cystoisospora.* Ito et al. (1978), in Japan, studied the life cycle of what they called "the large type of *Isospora bigemina* of the cat," but which we think could be *B. wallacei.* Sporulated oocysts were nearly identical in size to those described as *B. wallacei,* and they were not directly infective for cats. Rats (*Rattus norvegicus*), mice (*Mus musculus*), voles (*Microtus montebelli*), domestic rabbits (*Oryctolagus cuniculus*), and Mongolian gerbils (*Meriones unguiculatus*) were susceptible to infection via sporulated oocysts by developing mature *Besnoitia*-type cysts by 27 DPI or more, but hamsters did not become infected. Fayer and Frenkel (1979) fed sporulated oocysts of *B. wallacei* to calves, to look for clinical signs of infection, for 26–115 DPI, but neither gross lesions, microscopic lesions, nor parasites were found in any of the experimentally-infected calves. When a mixture of organs from each calf was fed back to cats they did not establish patent infections. Mason (1980) reported the first detection of *B. wallacei* in Australia, when he found cysts in free-living rats (*Rattus norvegicus, R. rattus*), fed them to cats, and those that were fed tissues of *R. norvegicus* passed unsporulated oocysts 14 DPI. These oocysts sporulated in 5–14 days, at room temperature, in 2% aqueous potassium dichromate solution. Sporulated oocysts were, L×W (n=30): 17.0×14.9 (15–18×13–16), L/W ratio: 1.1, and sporocysts measured, L×W (n=58): 11.5×7.8 (9–14×6–11), L/W ratio: 1.5. Sporulated oocysts from cats were administered orally and intraperitoneally to mice, rats, and a guinea pig;

only the mice and rats became infected, but not the guinea pig. McKenna and Charleston (1980c) dosed rats with isosporan oocysts recovered from the feces of a feral cat. Later, they found macroscopically visible, spheroidal cysts up to 260 wide that looked to them like a *Besnoitia* species. Kittens were fed the infected rats, and 11–12 DPI they shed similar oocysts, L×W: 16.9×14.6 in their feces. These sporulated oocysts were fed to mice, rats, rabbits, and guinea pigs and McKenna and Charleston (1980c) said that they later found *Besnoitia* cysts in all experimentally-infected hosts except the guinea pigs. Although they did not attempt to name their organism, we think it likely that they were looking at *B. wallacei*. Levine and Ivens (1981, pp. 148–150) summarized what was known to that time about definitive and intermediate hosts, geographic distribution, location and structure of endogenous stages in felids, oocyst structure, sporulation time, prepatent and patent periods, immunity, cultivation, and known pathogenicity in its intermediate hosts. Ito and Shimura (1986) followed up their previous work (Ito et al., 1978) by comparing various life cycle parameters between *I. bigemina* large type and *B. wallacei* and concluded that they represented the same species. There is one experimental infection utilizing cats (and dogs) worth mentioning. Dubey et al. (2004b) redescribed *B. tarandi*, known to cause pathology in reindeer (*Rangifer tarandus*), from tissue cysts found in naturally-infected reindeer from Finland. They fed tissue cysts to four cats and two dogs, but none of them excreted oocysts in their feces, which were examined daily for 30 days postinoculation.

Finally, the early history of discovery of *Besnoitia* species suggested they were non-pathogenic for the majority of their hosts. However, this seems to be true principally in the carnivore definitive host, while infections in intermediate hosts are usually recognized as important pathogens. *Besnoitia besnoiti* of domestic cattle and wild bovids, *B. bennetti* of horses, *B. caprae* of caprids, *B. tarandi* of caribou, and *B. darlingi* of opossums (Charles et al., 2011 from Ellis, unpub. obs.) are known to cause disease and economic loss due to pathogenesis that includes induction of poor body condition, edema, thickened skin, hair loss, blindness, vascular obstruction, severe inflammation of affected internal organs, and secondary infections (Leighton and Gajadhar, 2001; Elsheikha et al., 2003; Charles et al., 2011). With the exception of *B. darlingi*, none of the definitive hosts for these species are known.

Hammondia. Dubey (1975a) fed *H. hammondi* oocysts to 8 dogs and tissue cysts (from mice) to 4 dogs; none of the 12 dogs shed oocysts within 16 days. At postmortem, the extraintestinal tissues from these dogs were pooled and fed to *Hammondia*-free cats. Two of these cats that ingested tissues from dogs that received oocysts per os 16 and 38 days previously shed unsporulated *H. hammondi* oocysts, one on 8 and one on 10 DPI, but no cats fed extraintestinal tissues from dogs that ingested (mouse) tissue cysts discharged oocysts. Dubey (1975a) did not find lesions in any of the internal organs of the 12 experimental dogs. His results indicated that dogs are poor hosts for *H. hammondi*. Dubey and Streitel (1976a) infected 66 mice with sporulated oocysts of *H. hammondi* from cats. On 1 DPI, and continuing through 11 DPI, six mice were killed each day and fed to a different cat. The nine cats, fed six mice each on 1–9 DPI, did not discharge oocysts for 50 days. However, the cats fed mice on 10 and 11 DPI discharged oocysts of *H. hammondi* after 6 DPI, indicating to the authors that tachyzoites are not infectious to cats, but the cysts that developed in mice by 10 DPI are infective and lead to the production of oocysts. Rommel and Seyerl (1976) were the first to isolate unsporulated oocysts of *H. hammondi* from the feces of a cat in Germany; the oocysts measured, L×W: 13.8 × 12.2 (12–17.5 × 10–15); L/W ratio: 1.1, and sporulation was complete in 203 days. Infecting mice per os with these oocysts led to the formation of large tissue cysts in the muscles that measured, 44–100 × 32–45, but the days PI when these cysts were measured was not stated

(Rommel and Seyerl, 1976) and they were unable to transfer the infection from mouse-to-mouse by intraperitoneal injection of cystozoites. From March 1974 to April 1975, Christie et al. (1977) examined the feces of 1,000 cats killed by a county Humane Society, Columbus, Ohio. Only two of the 1,000 fecal samples were determined to have unsporulated oocysts of *H. hammondi*. Eydelloth (1977) inoculated two canine and six feline species with mouse tissue infected with cysts of *H. hammondi*; none of the five domestic dogs (*C. familiaris*), two European foxes (*Vulpes vulpes*), two lions (*Panthera leo*), two tigers (*Panthera tigris*), two pumas (*Felis concolor*), two bobcats (*Lynx rufus*) and two jungle cats (*Felis chaus*) excreted oocysts during the 3 weeks their feces were examined for oocysts of *H. hammondi*. However, Eydelloth (1977) reported that sexual stages developed in one European wildcat (*F. silvestris*), resulting in the discharge of unsporulated oocysts of *H. hammondi* in its feces, with a prepatent period of 11 days, and a patent period of 16 days. Eydelloth (1977) also reported feeding sporulated oocysts to a variety of rodent and domestic animal species, killing them 28–258 DPI, and feeding the pooled tissues from each potential intermediate host species to two cats; he said that either one or both of the cats fed musculature from the following intermediate hosts, excreted *H. hammondi* oocysts with prepatent periods ranging from six to 17 days: two bank voles (*Clethrionomys glareolus*), two common European voles (*Microtus arvalis*), two field voles (*Microtus agrestis*), two long-tailed field mice (*Apodemus sylvaticus*), one yellow-necked field mouse (*Apodemus flavicollis*), one common hamster (*Cricetus cricetus*), two of three rabbits (*Oryctolagus cuniculus*), and one of the four pigs (*Sus scrofa*). Mason (1978) said that he detected *H. hammondi* for the first time in Australia in the feces of a cat that was fed only commercially-prepared cat food and free-living rats (*Rattus norvegicus, R. rattus*). Mice dosed with these oocysts developed small, thin-walled cysts, 35–90 × 9–40, containing bradyzoites in their striated muscles and the cysts resembled (to him) those of *H. hammondi*. He concluded that the source of *H. hammondi* was *R. rattus*, but this work needs to be examined again, but more carefully.

Fayer and Frenkel (1979) fed sporulated oocysts of *H. hammondi* to calves to look for clinical signs of infection from 26 to 115 DPI, but neither gross lesions, microscopic lesions, nor parasites were found in any of the experimentally-infected calves. When a mixture of organs from each calf was fed back to cats, they did not establish patent infections. Shimura and Ito (1986) fed muscles from a goat to a cat, which shed *Toxoplasma*-like oocysts 43 days after feeding. These sporulated oocysts were, L × W: 13.0 × 11.4, and 10^5 sporulated oocysts were inoculated per os into mice; 1–15 DPI, tachyzoites were found in their kidneys, lungs, mesenteric lymph nodes, small intestines and spleens, as well as in the brain and various muscles. Cysts measured 25–224 × 20–80 in skeletal muscle and 35 × 35 in the brain on 181 DPI. Bradyzoites were not infectious for other mice and *Toxoplasma* antibody was found in some mouse sera, but the titer was always low. Cats that received bradyzoites in mouse tissues began to discharge oocysts from 7–8 DPI, but cats inoculated with 10^5 oocysts did not shed oocysts. These life cycle features convinced Shimura and Ito (1986) that they had discovered the first isolate of *H. hammondi* in Japan. In São Paulo, Brazil, Ogassawara et al. (1986) examined fecal samples of domestic cats from different areas of the city using flotation in saturated sugar solution and centrifugation in water–ether. They reported finding oocysts of *H. hammondi* in 2/215 (<1%) fecal samples, contending that their form was distinguished from *T. gondii* both morphologically and serologically.

Abbitt et al. (1993) reported finding another species, *H. pardalis*, in a dry lot dairy confinement of about 800 Holstein cows located in northeastern Mexico. The herdsman at this facility estimated there were 300 cats (*F. catus*) living in the facility, the progeny of several cats introduced in 1979, to control rodents. Abbitt et al. (1993) isolated 11 domestic cats in separate cages and collected feces daily for 14 days to determine that they were coccidia-free. Eight of these cats were fed fresh tissue from lactating cows slaughtered within 2 days of aborting; these cats all shed unsporulated oocysts with a prepatent period of 6–11 days and a patent period of 5–11 days. Sporulated oocysts were ovoidal and measured, L×W (n=100): 40.2×29.3, L/W ratio: 1.4, and were said to have a M at each end (?). Sporulation was completed in 7 days in 2.5% potassium dichromate solution maintained at ~22°C. Sporocysts were L×W (n=100): 26.8×21.3, L/W ratio: 1.3 (Abbitt et al., 1993, p. 445) or 22.2×16.4, L/W ratio: 1.35 (p. 447). Two other domestic cats were inoculated with 3,000 sporulated oocysts but did not shed oocysts in the next 14 DPI. The same two cats were fed mice that had been given 5,000 sporulated oocysts per os (length of time before inoculation with oocysts not stated) and these cats began shedding unsporulated oocysts on 6 and 7 DPI. In looking at all the protists known to infect cats that discharge oocysts, Abbitt et al. (1993) concluded their oocysts were similar in size only to *I. felis* and *H. pardalis* but because their oocysts were not infective for cats, as *I. felis* is known to be, they concluded they were dealing with *H. pardalis* described first from an ocelot in Panama. Suzán and Ceballos (2005) did a serosurvey of wildlife infections in two nature reserves within Mexico City limits and used a complement fixation test to find antibodies to *T. gondii*. They collected blood samples and found 4/6 (67%) *F. catus* to be positive for *T. gondii*. Dubey et al. (2013) used both molecular and biological parameters to document the first isolates of *H. hammondi* in 2/6 (33%) feral cats (*F. catus*) from Addis Ababa, Ethiopia. Sporulated oocysts were infective for mice, which developed tissue cysts, and when infected mouse tissue was fed to laboratory-raised cats they shed oocysts 5 DPI. DNA extracted from sporulated oocysts reacted with *H. hammondi*–specific primers and sequences were deposited into GenBank.

Neospora. Dubey and Lindsay (1989a) studied transplacental transmission in two pregnant cats. Cat 1 was inoculated subcutaneously with cell culture–derived tachyzoites on day 47 of her gestation. She gave birth to one full-term kitten 17 DPI and the kitten died when 2-days-old of a generalized *N. caninum* infection. Cat 1 was killed three days after parturition and had a macertaed kitten her uterus, severe placentitis, metritis, hepatitis, and nephritis due to an *N. caninum* infection. Cat 2 was fed *N. caninum* tissues cysts and mated 111 days later. She gave birth to three healthy full-term kittens; the kittens were killed at 2-, 22-, and 30-days-old. *Neospora* was found in the tissues of one of the three kittens. These results indicated that *N. caninum* is transplacentally transmitted in cats during both acute and chronic stages if infection. Dubey and Lindsay (1989a) also demonstrated *N. caninum*–specific IgG antibodies in the sera of both nursing cats and kittens.

Between 1993 and 2000, Dubey et al. (2002d) collected sera from domestic cats from São Paulo and Guarulhos cities, São Paulo State, Brazil, and examined them for the presence of antibodies to *N. caninum* via the DAT with respective antigen; 60/502 (12%) cat sera demonstrated antibodies to *N. caninum* with titers of 1:40 dilution in 36 cats, 1:80 in 18 cats, 1:160 in 5 cats, and 1:800 in 1 cat using the NAT. Antibodies to *N. caninum* were confirmed by Western blotting the sera of 10 positive cats, suggesting that at least 10 cats had *N. caninum*–specific antibodies confirmed by these two tests. Theirs was the first documentation of natural exposure of cats to *N. caninum*. Serological prevalence of *N. caninum* antibodies in domestic cats now has been found in at least seven countries, Albania, Brazil, Czech Republic, Hungary, Iran, Italy, and Thailand (Dubey et al., 2017b, see Tables 11.1, 11.2).

Toxoplasma gondii. Chessum (1972) found that a latent infection of *T. gondii* in a cat was reactivated by administration of 1×10^5 sporulated oocysts of *Isospora felis*, with oocysts of both species being released in the feces concurrently. Dubey (1973) surveyed the serum of house cats in Kansas City, Missouri, and stray cats in Iowa and Missouri, using the Sabin–Feldman dye test. In Kansas City, 26/302 (9%) kittens (4½–10-weeks-old) were positive, while 13/80 (16%) young cats (11–26-weeks-old), and 48/128 (37.5%) adult cats (>6-months-old) were infected. Antibody titer in stray cats from Iowa and Missouri was higher with 91/157 (58%) demonstrating antibodies to *T. gondii*. Iseki et al. (1974) studied 100 stray cats in Osaka, Japan by autopsy and fecal examination via flotation/centrifugation. The sera of the cats were examined via a hemagglutination test and 59/98 (60%) were positive for antibodies, but *T. gondii* oocysts were not found in any of the 100 samples of cat feces examined. Dubey et al. (1977a) examined the feces of cats killed by a county Humane Society, Columbus, Ohio, but only 7/1,000 (0.7%) samples had unsporulated oocysts of *T. gondii* which, after sporulation, were infectious for mice. Fayer and Frenkel (1979) fed sporulated oocysts of three strains of *T. gondii* (T-1, Jacobs' and Melton's strain; T-2, from a brown wooly monkey; T-37, from a naturally-infected Costa Rican cat) to uninfected calves. All three strains were infectious, but pathogenicity varied with the strain. Symptoms produced in calves from the two most pathogenic strains (T-2, T-37) were diarrhea, anorexia, poor weight gain, depression, weakness, fever, and dyspnea. Cats fed organs from these *T. gondii*–infected calves all shed *T. gondii* oocysts from 7 to 14 DPI. McKenna and Charleston (1980a) working on the North Island, New Zealand, examined fecal samples from domestic cats and identified oocysts of *T. gondii* in 51/508 (1%) samples. Ruiz and Frenkel (1980) studied domestic cats in seven localities in Costa Rica and tested the blood for *T. gondii* antibodies by the Sabin–Feldman dye test and/or searching the feces for oocysts that were injected into mice. *Toxoplasma* oocysts were isolated from 55/237 (23%) cats and antibody in blood samples

was found in 109/237 (46%); overall, 142/237 (60%) of the cats sampled were infected as shown by antibody or oocyst shedding. Coman et al. (1981) examined fecal samples of mostly adult feral cats and blood sera of cats from three habitat types: national parks/wildlife reserves; remote mountainous areas; and miscellaneous sites (e.g., rubbish piles, picnic reserves, camp grounds) in southeastern Australia (Victoria, Western New South Wales). Oocysts of *T. gondii* were recovered in 6/300 (2%) fecal samples by flotation and specific antibodies against *T. gondii* were detected in 15/75 (20%) sera samples by an IHA test with a commercial Tox HA test kit. Specific antibodies to feline panleukopenia virus (79%), feline calicivirus (77%), and feline herpes virus (11%) were concurrently detected in the examined cats. Nichol et al. (1981a,b) neither did they observe *T. gondii* oocysts in 69 feral cat fecal samples from London and Sheffield, England, nor did they find any in 947 domestic cats from London, using salt flotation. Lappin et al. (1989) did a serological study to determine the prevalence of *T. gondii* using an ELISA test detecting IgM, IgG, and circulating *T. gondii* antigens in 81 healthy cats, and 107 cats with clinical signs indicating toxoplasmosis, in Athens, Georgia, USA. The prevalence of infection (all three assays) was 44/81 (54%) healthy cats, and 70/107 (65%) clinically-ill cats. Shastri (1990) reported *T. gondii* oocysts in the feces of a domestic kitten in Parbhani, Maharashtra, India. Oocysts were of two sizes, 11.4–14.3 × 10.5–12.4 (smaller) and 15.2–19.0 × 11.4–15.2 (larger), with both OR and PG present and sporocysts had an SR, but lacked SBs. Sporulated oocysts were given per os to two rabbits and two guinea pigs; 3 and 4.5 months PI, their tissues were fed to kittens. All the cats discharged oocysts of the same morphology as the original isolate, with a patent period of 3–5 days and prepatent period 11 days in kittens fed with the rabbit tissues and 5–7 days in kittens fed with the guinea pig tissues. Dubey and Carpenter (1991) reported *T. gondii*–like meronts, in PVs, in the tracheal epithelium of an 8-year-old male cat.

Meloni et al. (1993) examined fecal samples of cats from eight Aboriginal communities in the tropics of the west Kimberley region, Western Australia, and detected *T. gondii* in 6/33 (18%) samples by direct smears and zinc sulfate flotation. Milstein and Goldsmid (1997) surveyed feral cats in southern Tasmania and tested blood sera for *T. gondii* by a LAT (Toxocell, Biokit Immunodiagnostics, Australia) and reported 9/18 (50%) blood samples to be positive, suggesting to them a high exposure rate and a potential risk to humans and other animals. Nutter et al. (2004) surveyed feces and blood of feral cats (47 females, 53 males) and healthy pet cats (39 females, 37 males; mostly of stray/shelter origin) in rural Randolph County, North Carolina, USA. Sera were tested for antibodies against *T. gondii* by a MAT for IgG (sensitivity 83%, specificity 90%); they found 63/100 (63%) feral and 26/76 (34%) pet cats had antibodies (titer ≥1:25) to *T. gondii*; this difference between feral and pet cats was statistically significant. Cirak and Bauer (2004) examined fecal samples of cats from three animal shelters in central Germany, primarily to compare the effectivity of conventional coproscopical methods and a commercial coproantigen ELISA kit to detect *Cryptosporidium*. All cats were without diarrhea. Oocysts of *T. gondii* were found in 2/100 (2%) cats using $ZnCl_2$–NaCl flotation. Clifford et al. (2006) did a serosurvey of island fox populations on six California Channel Islands for a variety of pathogens, including *T. gondii*; they found foxes on four islands to have antibodies. Three of those islands had significant feral cat populations, so they surveyed the blood of 92 cats on three islands using the IFA test with a fluorescence titer ≥1:640. Santa Catalina Island had 28/63 (44%) feral cats with antibodies; San Clemente Island had 1/21 (5%) wildcats with antibodies; and San Nicolas Island had 2/8 (25%) wildcats with antibodies to *T. gondii*. Sedlák and Bártová (2006b), used the IFAT with both IgM and IgA, and found IgA antibodies to *T. gondii* in 8/286 (3%) and IgG antibodies in 126/286 (44%) pet cats in the Czech Republic. They concluded

that although *T. gondii* is a common parasite of cats in the Czech Republic, its clinical importance is low. Prior to their study (2006b), *T. gondii* had been reported in pet cats in other European countries, including the Czech Republic (219/357, 61%, Svobodová et al., 1998), Germany (138/306, 45%, Tenter et al., 1994; 6/1,147, 0.5%, Epe et al., 1993), Spain (187/585, 32%, Ortuno et al., 2002), and Sweden (102/244, 42%, Uggla et al., 1990). In general, cats kept indoors had a lower prevalence of infection than farm and stray cats. Alvarado-Esquivel et al. (2007) did a serosurvey of the prevalence of antibodies to *T. gondii*, using a MAT on sera of domestic cats from Durango City, Mexico; they found antibodies in 22/105 (21%) cats with titers of 1:25 (3 cats), 1:50 (4 cats), 1:200 (5 cats), 1:400 (2 cats), 1:800 (2 cats), 1:1,600 (4 cats), and ≥1:3,200 (2 cats). Older cats (>1 year) had a significantly higher frequency of infection than younger cats. Alvarado-Esquivel et al. (2007) noted that the seroprevalence of *T. gondii* antibodies in cats in Durango City was much lower compared with those reported in other countries. de Camps et al. (2008) did a serosurvey of zoo cats using the MAT to test for antibodies to *T. gondii* (titer ≥1:25, indicative of exposure). Blood samples were taken from wild felids from eight zoos in the midwestern United States, and from domestic feral cats trapped in three of the zoos; antibodies to *T. gondii* were found in 10/34 (29%) feral cats in/near zoos, but not in any of 78 fecal samples from wild and domestic cats not associated with zoos. From 1997 to 2007, Gates and Nolan (2009) surveyed fecal samples of cats in Philadelphia, USA, for endoparasites and examined them by zinc sulfate centrifugation and, in some cases, supplemented by formalin–ethyl acetate. Oocysts of *T. gondii* were detected in only 1/1,566 (≪1%) samples tested. Dubey et al. (2010a) surveyed the sera of many carnivores at the BCEAW, Sharjah, UAE, and found antibodies to *T. gondii* in 1/4 (25%) feral domestic cats. Costa et al. (2012) did a serosurvey of domestic and wild animals in Fernando de Noronha, Brazil, using the IFAT or the MAT, or both; they found

70/118 (59%) *F. catus* to have antibodies, including 32/48 (67%) feral cats and 38/70 (54%) domestic cats. Mancianti et al. (2015) surveyed feces of privately owned, healthy pet European shorthair cats in Tuscany and Liguria (Pisa, Florence, and Genoa Provinces). Nested PCR amplification of the B1 region, followed by genotyping via multiplex multilocus PCR–RFLP for 12 genetic markers, detected *T. gondii* in 15/146 (10%) samples; genotype I was present in seven samples, genotype II in one sample, and genotype III in seven samples. Microscopic examination of feces was negative for *T. gondii* oocysts in all samples. Pomerantz et al. (2016) did a serosurvey of carnivores at Kirindy Mitea and Ankarafantsika National Parks on Madagascar and tested them for antibodies to five viral pathogens and for *T. gondii* (by ELISA); the samples included domestic cats from the villages near the parks. Antibodies to *T. gondii* were detected in 4/18 (22%) domestic cats. Nyambura Njuguna et al. (2017) surveyed fecal samples of indoor and outdoor household cats for the prevalence of gastrointestinal parasites in the Thika region, Kiambu county, central Kenya; they detected *T. gondii* oocysts in 8/103 (8%) cats by sugar flotation, which was further confirmed by mouse bioassay (using the BALB/c mice), followed by nested PCR of the repetitive 529 bp DNA fragment in mouse brain tissue to detect tissue cysts. Scorza and Lappin (2017) examined sera of cats on the Pine Ridge Indian Reservation, South Dakota, USA, for ELISA-specific antibodies against *T. gondii*; they reported 2/32 (6%) positive samples.

FELIS MANUL (PALLAS, 1776), PALLAS'S CAT

Hammondia. No records in the literature, yet.
Neospora. Sedlák and Bártová (2006a) serosurveyed zoo animals in the Czech and Slovak Republics for the occurrence of *N. caninum*

antibodies using the IFA test, but the two Pallas's cats they sampled were both negative.

Toxoplasma gondii. Riemann et al. (1974) studied one male and two female Pallas's cats from a zoo in California, USA, that all had unusually high serum antibody titers to *T. gondii*, as tested by a microtiter IHA test using commercial antigen. The male cat (No. 1) had a steady increase in IHA antibody to a high of 1:131,072, but with no signs of illness. The female cat (No. 2) became pregnant and her antibody titer reached a peak of 1:16,777,216; she never gave birth as the fetuses either were aborted and eaten or resorbed. Female cat (No. 3) also became pregnant and gave birth to three kittens that were apparently in good health, until 6 weeks of age, when they became ill with central nervous system involvement and head tilt; all kittens died 2–3 days later. Necropsy and histopathology of two of the kittens showed multiple foci of hepatic necrosis, hepatitis, severe interstitial pneumonia, interstitial nephritis, reticuloendothelial hyperplasia in spleen and lymph nodes, myocardial necrosis, and meningitis with *Toxoplasma* organisms evident in sections of the liver, lung, kidney, brain, and spinal cord. Polomoshnov (1979) reported fecal oocysts, and Dubey et al. (1988b) recorded pathology and fatality in a 6-year-old Pallas wildcat kept in an enclosed exhibit in the Milwaukee, Wisconsin County Zoo; the cat died of acute, overwhelming toxoplasmosis with necrotic enteritis, multifocal necrotizing granulomatous hepatitis, and pneumonia and meronts (types D and E), gamonts, and oocysts were present in the epithelium of the small intestine. Sedlák and Bártová (2006a) serosurveyed zoo animals in the Czech and Slovak Republics for the occurrence of *T. gondii* antibodies using the IFAT, and found antibodies in both of the two Pallas's cats they sampled. de Camps et al. (2008) used the MAT to test for antibodies (titer ≥1:25 indicative of exposure) to *T. gondii*; blood samples were taken from wild zoo felids from eight zoos in the midwestern United States and antibodies to *T. gondii* were found in 1/5 (20%) Pallas's cats.

FELIS MARGARITA LOCHE, 1858, SAND CAT

Hammondia. No records in the literature, yet.

Neospora. No records in the literature, yet.

Toxoplasma gondii. Dubey et al. (2010a,b,c) studied sand cats in a captive breeding program at the BCEAW, Sharjah, UAE, because they had experienced high newborn mortality rates, and congenital toxoplasmosis was recognized as one of the causes of mortality. Dubey et al. (2010a) found *T. gondii* in histological tissue sections that reacted with polyclonal antibodies by immunohistochemistry, and *T. gondii* DNA was found by PCR in liver and lung tissues of an 18-month-old sand cat that had died. They also identified *T. gondii* using the MAT, and a bioassay in mice for the cat that died and two others at the BCEAW, and in another sand cat at the AWWP facility in Qatar, which had died of visceral toxoplasmosis. The genotype from the cat from AWWP was a genetic Type II strain with a Type I allele at locus Apico. This was the first report of genetic characterization of *T. gondii* isolates from Middle East. Dubey et al. (2010a) also demonstrated antibodies to *T. gondii* at the AWWP in 14/21 (67%) Arabian sand cats, *F. m. harrisoni* Hemmer, Grubb, and Groves, 1976.

FELIS SILVESTRIS SCHREBER, 1777, WILDCAT

Hammondia. No records in the literature, yet.

Neospora. Sobrino et al. (2008) used the c-ELISA, NAT, and/or IFAT to detect antibodies to *N. caninum* in 1/6 (17%) *F. silvestris* in Spain. Millán et al. (2009) did a seroprevalence study for *N. caninum* and *T. gondii* in feral cats in Majorca, Spain, and found *F. silvestris* to be positive for *N. caninum*. Millán et al. (2009) assayed serum samples from feral cats (*F. s. catus*) in Majorca, Balearic Islands, Spain, for antibodies to *N. caninum* by cELISA (VMRD), and confirmed by an IFA test, and found 4/59 (7%) cats to be seropositive.

Toxoplasma gondii. Polomoshnov (1979) said he found oocysts of *T. gondii* in the feces of what he called *Felis lybica* Foster, 1780, the African wildcat (now a junior synonym of *F. silvestris*). Lukešová and Literák (1998) found oocysts of *T. gondii* in 14/175 (8%) fecal samples examined from zoos in the Czech Republic. Sobrino et al. (2007) looked at free-ranging carnivores in Spain using the MAT (as per Dubey and Desmonts, 1987) and detected the antibodies to *T. gondii* in 3/6 (50%) *F. silvestris*. Millán et al. (2009) assayed serum samples from feral cats (*F. s. catus*) in Majorca, Balearic Islands, Spain, by the MAT and found 50/59 (85%) cats had positive titers (≥1:25), with seroprevalence significantly higher in adults (95%) than in juveniles (<6-months-old; 40%). The prevalence of *T. gondii* observed in wildcats in Majorca is one of the highest reported worldwide, and the highest observed in Europe to date. The results suggest that feral cats in Majorca have a high rate of *T. gondii* infection with important implications for public health on the island because the seropositive cats are likely to have already shed *T. gondii* oocysts in the environment. Dubey et al. (2010a) surveyed the sera of many carnivores at the BCEAW, Sharjah, UAE, and demonstrated antibodies to *T. gondii* in 5/5 (100%) Gordon's wildcats (*F. s. gordoni* Harrison, 1968). Dubey et al. (2010a) also surveyed the sera of carnivores at the AWWP facility in Qatar and found antibodies to *T. gondii* in 1/1 African wildcat, *F. s. gordoni*. Herrmann et al. (2013) examined carcasses of 12 dead *F. s. silvestris* from the German Federal State of Saxony-Anhalt and analyzed their brains and lungs for the presence of *T. gondii* by specific PCR; 4/12 (33%) tested positive for *T. gondii* DNA. That DNA was analyzed further by PCR–RFLP typing using nine markers (nSAG2, SAG3, BTUB, GRA6, c22-8, c29-2, L358, PK1, and Apico) to characterize the genetic strain of *T. gondii*. Their results indicated that type II *T. gondii* is the most common genotype infecting wildcats in Germany. Pomerantz et al. (2016) did a serosurvey of carnivores at Kirindy Mitea and

Ankarafantsika National Parks in Madagascar and tested them for antibodies to five viral pathogens, and for *T. gondii* (by ELISA) and 3/8 (38%) wildcats had antibodies to *T. gondii*.

GENUS *LEOPARDUS* GRAY, 1842 (9 SPECIES)

LEOPARDUS (SYN. ONCIFELIS) COLOCOLO (MOLINA, 1782), COLOCOLO OR PAMPAS CAT

Hammondia. No records in the literature, yet.

Neospora. André et al. (2010) drew blood from 258 wild captive carnivores in zoos of São Paulo and Mato Grosso states, and the Federal District, Brazil, to detect antibodies to *N. caninum* and *T. gondii*. Antibodies in the serum of each animal were detected by the IFAT using either tachyzoites of *N. caninum* NC-1 strain or tachyzoites of *T. gondii* RH strain as antigens, respectively. They (2010) found 3/3 (100%) colocolos seropositive for *N. caninum*.

Toxoplasma gondii. Pizzi et al. (1978) said they found *T. gondii* in the colocolo from the province of Cordoba in Argentina. André et al. (2010), in the study noted above found 1/3 (33%) colocolos seropositive for *T. gondii*. Cañón-Franco et al. (2013) examined tissue samples from free-ranging, wild, small Neotropical felids from Rio Grande do Sul, Brazil, and amplified the ITS-1 marker to detect *T. gondii*; 31/90 (34%) samples were positive including 1/7 (14%) *L. colocolo*. Multilocus PCR–RFLP genotyping of 11 felids using molecular markers SAG1, 5′3′SAG2, alt. SAG2, SAG3, BTUB, GRA6, c22-8, c29-2, L358, PK1, Apico, and CS3 allowed them to partially characterization eight *T. gondii* genotypes. This study was the first detection and genotypic characterization of *T. gondii* in free-ranging felids in Brazil, demonstrating the occurrence of the parasite in wild populations, and suggesting its potential transmissibility to humans and other domestic and wild animals.

LEOPARDUS (SYN. ONCIFELIS) GEOFFROYI (D'ORBIGNY AND GERVAIS, 1844), GEOFFROY'S CAT

Hammondia. No records in the literature, yet.

Neospora. Spencer et al. (2003) did a seroprevalence study in captive and free-ranging nondomestic felids in the United States and found *L. geoffroyi* to be positive for *N. caninum*.

Toxoplasma gondii. Pizzi et al. (1978) reported *T. gondii* in *L. geoffroy* from the Province of Cordoba, Argentina. Lukešová and Literák (1998) found oocysts of *T. gondii* in 4/39 (10%) fecal samples they examined from zoos in the Czech Republic; however, they identified the host as *Oncifelis geoffroyi*, which is now considered a synonym of *L. geoffroyi*. Cañón-Franco et al. (2013) examined tissue samples from 90 free-ranging, wild, small Neotropical felids from Rio Grande do Sul, Brazil, and amplified the ITS-1 marker to detect *T. gondii*; 6/22 (27%) *L. geoffroyi* were positive. Multilocus PCR–RFLP genotyping of 11 felids using molecular markers SAG1, 5′3′SAG2, alt. SAG2, SAG3, BTUB, GRA6, c22-8, c29-2, L358, PK1, Apico, and CS3 allowed them to partially characterization eight *T. gondii* genotypes. This study was the first detection and genotypic characterization of *T. gondii* in free-ranging felids in Brazil, demonstrating the occurrence of the parasite in wild populations and suggesting its potential transmissibility to humans and other domestic and wild animals.

LEOPARDUS PARDALIS (L., 1758), OCELOT

Hammondia. Hendricks et al. (1979) found unsporulated oocysts resembling *Isospora felis* in a fecal sample of an ocelot housed at a US Air Force base zoo in the Panama Canal Zone. They described it as an obligate heteroxenous coccidian, with felids as the definitive host and laboratory mice as the experimental intermediate host. Oocysts were shed unsporulated by cats and, when sporulated (after 1 week in 2.5% potassium dichromate solution kept at room temperature), they were infective only for mice (*M. musculus*), but not for cats. Sporulated oocysts were, L×W: 40.8×28.5 (36–46×25–35), L/W ratio: 1.4. Mice were fed 5×10^4 sporulated oocysts and at 15 DPI were found to have small intracellular cysts, 13–16×10–15, in their mesenteric lymph nodes, lungs, and intestinal submucosa; meronts in these early cysts were 6×3. When infected mice were fed to felids, the prepatent period was reported as 5–8 days and patency was 5–13 days. Hendricks et al. (1979) said they were successfully able to infect 6/6 laboratory-reared kittens, 5/5 ocelots and 1/1 jaguarundi feeding them infected mice. However, neither of four raccoons (*P. lotor*) became infected when fed infected mice nor did three lab-reared cats become infected after ingesting 1×10^5 sporulated oocysts. We are unable to determine whether the form identified by Hendricks et al. (1979) was a *Hammondia* or a *Cystoisospora* species. Patton et al. (1986) did a fecal survey of parasites of wild neotropical Felidae from the Cockscomb Basin, Belize, Central America, and said they found oocysts of an *H. pardalis* in 1/8 (12.5%) fecal samples from ocelots.

Neospora. Sedlák and Bártová (2006a) serosurveyed zoo animals in the Czech and Slovak Republics using the IFAT and found no antibodies to *N. caninum* in the only *L. pardalis* they sampled. André et al. (2010) tried to detect antibodies in wild captive carnivores in zoos of São Paulo and Mato Grosso states, and the Federal District, Brazil, by the IFAT using tachyzoites of *N. caninum* NC-1 strain as antigens; they found 30/42 (71%) ocelots sampled seropositive for *N. caninum*.

Toxoplasma gondii. Oocysts of *T. gondii* were isolated from the feces of two *F. pardalis*, which initially lacked antibody to *T. gondii*, and established for the first time that other members of the Felidae can spread *Toxoplasma* via their feces (Jewell et al., 1972). Patton et al. (1986) did a fecal survey of neotropical felids in Belize and found

Toxoplasma-like oocyst in the feces of 2/8 (25%) ocelots. Sedlák and Bártová (2006a) serosurveyed zoo animals in the Czech and Slovak Republics using the IFAT and found antibodies to *T. gondii* in the only *L. pardalis* they sampled. André et al. (2010) detected antibodies in wild captive carnivores in zoos of São Paulo and Mato Grosso states, and the Federal District, Brazil, using the IFAT with tachyzoites of *T. gondii* RH strain as antigen; they found 28/42 (67%) ocelots sampled seropositive for *T. gondii*. Cañón-Franco et al. (2013) examined tissue samples from free-ranging, wild, small Neotropical felids from Rio Grande do Sul, Brazil, and amplified the ITS-1 marker to detect *T. gondii*; they found *T. gondii* in the only ocelot they sampled. Multilocus PCR–RFLP genotyping of 11 felids using molecular markers SAG1, 5′3′SAG2, alt. SAG2, SAG3, BTUB, GRA6, c22-8, c29-2, L358, PK1, Apico, and CS3 allowed them to partially characterization eight *T. gondii* genotypes.

LEOPARDUS TIGRINUS (SCHREBER, 1775), ONCILLA OR LITTLE SPOTTED CAT

Hammondia. No records in the literature, yet.

Neospora. Sedlák and Bártová (2006a) serosurveyed zoo animals in the Czech and Slovak Republics for the occurrence of *N. caninum* antibodies using the IFAT but found no antibodies in the only *L. tigrinus* they sampled. André et al. (2010) studied sera from wild captive carnivores in zoos of São Paulo and Mato Grosso states, and the Federal District, Brazil, by the IFAT using tachyzoites of *N. caninum* NC-1 strain as antigen; they found 11/35 (31%) little spotted cats seropositive for *N. caninum*.

Toxoplasma gondii. Sedlák and Bártová (2006a) serosurveyed zoo animals in the Czech and Slovak Republics using the IFAT and found antibodies to *T. gondii* in the only *L. tigrinus* they sampled. André et al. (2010) studied antibodies in wild captive carnivores in zoos of São Paulo and Mato Grosso states, and the Federal District,

Brazil, using the IFAT with tachyzoites of *T. gondii* RH strain as antigen; they found 22/35 (63%) little spotted cats sampled seropositive for *T. gondii*. Cañón-Franco et al. (2013) examined tissue samples from free-ranging, wild, Neotropical felids from Rio Grande do Sul, Brazil, and amplified the ITS-1 marker to detect *T. gondii*; 8/28 (29%) oncilla tested positive. Multilocus PCR–RFLP genotyping of 11 felids using molecular markers SAG1, 5'3'SAG2, alt. SAG2, SAG3, BTUB, GRA6, c22-8, c29-2, L358, PK1, Apico, and CS3 allowed Cañón-Franco et al. (2013) to partially characterization 8 *T. gondii* genotypes. This study demonstrated the occurrence of *T. gondii* in wild populations and suggested its potential transmissibility to humans and other domestic and wild animals. Vitaliano et al. (2014) studied fragments of brain and heart tissues from free-living and captive wild animals from Brazil with the intention to isolate and genotype *T. gondii*. All samples were submitted to mice bioassay and screened by PCR based on 18S rRNA sequences, and 15/226 (7%) *T. gondii* isolates were obtained, including a sample from one *L. tigrinus*. DNA of the isolates, from mice bioassay and from the tissues of the wild animal, was genotyped by PCR–RFLP, using 12 genetic markers (SAG1, SAG2, alt. SAG2, SAG3, BTUB, GRA6, c22-8, c29-2, L258, PK1, CS3, and Apico). Vitaliano et al. (2014) identified 17 *T. gondii* genotypes, 13 for the first time including the one in the oncilla, and four already reported in published literature. From theirs and the work of others, it seems clear that Brazil has both high diversity and unique genotypes of *T. gondii*. Clearly, future studies on *T. gondii* from wildlife are needed to understand population genetics and structure of this parasite.

LEOPARDUS WIEDII (SCHINZ, 1775), MARGAY

Hammondia. No records in the literature, yet.
Neospora. André et al. (2010) found none of four margays sampled to be seropositive for *N. caninum* in Brazil (see below).

Toxoplasma gondii. Sedlák and Bártová (2006a) serosurveyed zoo animals in the Czech and Slovak Republics using the IFAT and found antibodies to *T. gondii* in the only *L. tigrinus* they sampled. André et al. (2010) detected antibodies in wild captive carnivores in zoos of São Paulo and Mato Grosso states, and the Federal District, Brazil, by the IFAT, using tachyzoites of *T. gondii* RH strain as antigen, and found 4/4 (100%) margays seropositive for *T. gondii*. Cañón-Franco et al. (2013) examined tissues from free-ranging, wild, small Neotropical felids from Rio Grande do Sul, Brazil, and amplified the ITS-1 marker; 6/10 (60%) margays sampled were positive. Multilocus PCR–RFLP genotyping of 11 felids using molecular markers SAG1, 5'3'SAG2, alt. SAG2, SAG3, BTUB, GRA6, c22-8, c29-2, L358, PK1, Apico, and CS3 allowed them to partially characterization 8 *T. gondii* genotypes.

GENUS *LEPTAILURUS* SEVERTZOV, 1858 (MONOTYPIC)

LEPTAILURUS SERVAL (SCHREBER, 1776), SERVAL

Hammondia. No records in the literature, yet.
Neospora. Sedlák and Bártová (2006a) serosurveyed zoo animals in the Czech and Slovak Republics using the IFAT and found no antibodies in the only *L. serval* they sampled. André et al. (2010) studied wild captive carnivores in zoos of São Paulo and Mato Grosso states, and the Federal District, Brazil, using the IFAT, with tachyzoites of *N. caninum* NC-1 strain as antigen, and found the only serval sampled to be seropositive for *N. caninum*.
Toxoplasma gondii. Lappin et al. (1991) collected serum from nondomestic felids to evaluate them using a LA kit, an IHA kit, and ELISA for IgM (IgM–ELISA), IgG (IgG–ELISA), and for antigen (AG–ELISA) to define optimal diagnostic procedures. Antigen to *T. gondii* was detected in 25/33 (76%) samples using IgG–ELISA, in 20/33 (61%) using the LA test, and in 19/33 (58%)

using the IHA test. Positive titers (≥1:128) were found in 1/2 (50%) *L. serval* from Central Florida Zoological Park, Lake Monroe, Florida. No nondomestic felid had detectable IgM antibodies. Sedlák and Bártová (2006a) serosurveyed zoo animals in the Czech and Slovak Republics using the IFAT and found antibodies to *T. gondii* in the only *L. serval* they sampled. André et al. (2010) also were able to survey the blood of only one serval in Brazil and found it to be seropositive for *T. gondii*.

GENUS *LYNX* KERR, 1752 (4 SPECIES)

LYNX LYNX (L., 1758), EURASIAN LYNX

Hammondia. No records in the literature, yet.
Neospora. Sedlák and Bártová (2006a) serosurveyed zoo animals in the Czech and Slovak Republics using the IFAT and found antibodies in 1/2 (50%) *L. lynx* they sampled.
Toxoplasma gondii. Sedlák and Bártová (2006a) serosurveyed zoo animals in the Czech and Slovak Republics using the IFAT and found antibodies to *T. gondii* in 2/2 *L. lynx* sampled.

LYNX PARDINUS (TEMMINCK, 1827), IBERIAN LYNX

Hammondia. No records in the literature, yet.
Neospora. Sobrino et al. (2008), and used the c-ELISA, NAT, and/or IFAT, and detected antibodies to *N. caninum* in 5/25 (20%) Iberian lynx.
Toxoplasma gondii. Sobrino et al. (2007) looked at free-ranging carnivores from Spain using the MAT and detected antibodies to *T. gondii* in 22/27 (81.5%) *L. pardinus*. The high seroprevalence in Iberian lynx and the European wildcat (see above) may be of epidemiologic significance because seropositive cats might have shed significant numbers of oocysts into their surrounding environments.

LYNX RUFUS (SCHREBER, 1777), BOBCAT

Hammondia. No records in the literature, yet.
Neospora. No records in the literature, yet.
Toxoplasma gondii. One of the seven *L. rufus*, from Texas, fed sporulated oocysts of *T. gondii* collected from house cats, shed oocysts in its feces 3–14 DPI (Miller et al., 1972), whereas the other six bobcats, four from Kansas and two from Oklahoma, did not shed oocysts after inoculation with sporulated oocysts. Oertly and Walls (1980) examined bobcats from Georgia and West Virginia for *T. gondii* antibodies by the IHA test, and found 27/150 (18%) to be positive, with titers ≥1:16, but no *T. gondii* oocysts were seen in any of their fecal samples. Dubey et al. (1987) found *T. gondii* in the tissues of a captive 1-week-old bobcat from Ronan, Montana, USA, which died of myocarditis, hepatitis, and encephalitis. They thought the infection was congenitally-acquired from the mother, which probably became infected by ingesting horsemeat and chickens in her diet. Dreesen (1990) found 27/150 (18%) bobcats from the southeastern United States to be seropositive for *T. gondii*.

GENUS *PRIONAILURUS* SEVERTZOV, 1858 (5 SPECIES)

PRIONAILURUS BENGALENSIS (KERR, 1792), LEOPARD CAT

Hammondia. No records in the literature, yet.
Neospora. No records in the literature, yet.
Toxoplasma gondii. Two *P. bengalensis*, fed sporulated oocysts of *T. gondii* collected from house cats, shed oocysts in their feces 3–7 DPI (Miller et al., 1972). Janitschke and Werner (1972) infected two leopard cats and seven other carnivores orally with tissue cysts and/or oocysts of *T. gondii*, but only leopard cats excreted oocysts of *T. gondii* in their feces. Lukešová and Literák (1998) found oocysts of *T. gondii* in 5/133 (4%)

fecal samples they examined from zoos in the Czech Republic, however, they identified the host as *Felis euptilurus* (Elliot, 1871), amur leopard cat, which is now considered a junior synonym of *P. bengalensis*.

PRIONAILURUS IRIOMOTENSIS IMAIZUMI, 1967, IRIOMOTE CAT

Hammondia. No records in the literature, yet.

Neospora. No records in the literature, yet.

Toxoplasma gondii. Akuzawam et al. (1987) looked at the blood (n=19) and stools (n=45) of *P. iriomotensis* from Iriomote-jima Island, Japan. Using the passive HAT they found 4/16 (25%) serum samples to be positive (titer >1:256) for *T. gondii*. They also found *T. gondii* oocysts, 12×9–11, in 2/45 (4%) fecal samples, and the oocysts were fed to mice and serum antibodies to *T. gondii* were detected in the blood of infected mice 30 DPI. However, they did not mention if either of the two cats passing oocysts was 1 of the 16 cats tested by the passive hemagglutination test. They also said they found larger oocysts, 35–37 × 30–32, which they identified as *I.* (=*C.*) *felis*, in 6/45 (13%) fecal samples examined from *P. iriomotensis*.

PRIONAILURUS VIVERRINUS (BENNET, 1833), FISHING CAT

Hammondia. No records in the literature, yet.

Neospora. André et al. (2010) serosurveyed wild captive carnivores in zoos of São Paulo and Mato Grosso states and Federal District, Brazil, by the IFAT using tachyzoites of *N. caninum* NC-1 strain as antigen, and found the only fishing cat examined to be seropositive for *N. caninum*, but not for *T. gondii* (with tachyzoites of the RH strain of *T. gondii*).

Toxoplasma gondii. de Camps et al. (2008) used the MAT to test for antibodies (titer ≥1:25 indicative of exposure) to *T. gondii*; they took blood samples of wild zoo felids from eight zoos in the midwestern United States and demonstrated antibodies to *T. gondii* in 1/4 (25%) *P. viverrinus* they sampled.

GENUS *PUMA* JARDINE, 1834 (2 SPECIES)

PUMA CONCOLOR (L., 1771), COUGAR

Hammondia. Patton et al. (1986) did a fecal survey of neotropical felids from the Cockscomb Basin, Belize, Central America; they said they found oocysts of *H. pardalis* in the feces of 1/4 (25%) cougars.

Neospora. Spencer et al. (2003) did a seroprevalence study for *N. caninum* and *T. gondii* in captive and free-ranging nondomestic felids in the United States and found *N. caninum* antibodies in cougars. André et al. (2010) did a serosurvey of wild captive carnivores in zoos of São Paulo and Mato Grosso states, and the Federal District, Brazil, using the IFAT with tachyzoites of *N. caninum* NC-1 strain as antigen; they found 5/18 (28%) pumas sampled to be seropositive for *N. caninum*.

Toxoplasma gondii. Miller et al. (1972) demonstrated that one cougar shed *T. gondii* oocysts after ingestion of sporulated oocysts derived from house cats. Pizzi et al. (1978) said that they found *T. gondii* in a cougar from Cordoba Province, Argentina. Lappin et al. (1991) collected serum from nondomestic felids to evaluate for antibodies to *T. gondii* using a LA kit, an IHA kit, and ELISA for IgM (IgM–ELISA), IgG (IgG–ELISA), and for antigen (AG–ELISA) to define optimal diagnostic procedures. Antigen to *T. gondii* was detected in 25/33 (76%) using IgG–ELISA, in 20/33 (61%) using the LA test, and in 19/33 (58%) using the IHA test. Positive titers (≥1:128) were found in 5/6 (83%) *P. concolor* from the Central Florida Zoological Park, Lake Monroe, Florida, and in 2/3 (67%) cougars from the White Oaks

Plantation, Yulee, Florida. Aramini et al. (1998) necropsied 12 *P. c. vancouverensis* from Vancouver Island, British Columbia, Canada, and one additional fecal sample from the Victoria watershed environment. One of the 12 (8%) necropsied cougars had *T. gondii* oocysts in its feces, as confirmed by passage in mice. Eleven of the 12 (92%) had antibodies to *T. gondii* by the MAT with titers of 1:50 (8 cougars) and 1:500 (3 cougars). The fecal sample from the Victoria watershed cougar also contained oocysts of *T. gondii*. de Camps et al. (2008) used the MAT to test for antibodies (titer ≥1:25 indicative of exposure) to *T. gondii*; antibodies to *T. gondii* were found in 3/6 (50%) *P. concolor*, and in 2/2 Texas pumas, *P. c. stanleyana*, sampled. André et al. (2010) did a serosurvey of wild captive carnivores in zoos of São Paulo and Mato Grosso states and Federal District, Brazil, using the IFAT with tachyzoites of *T. gondii* RH strain as antigen, and found 14/18 (78%) pumas sampled seropositive for *T. gondii*.

PUMA YAGOUAROUNDI (É. GEOFFORY SAINT-HILAIRE, 1803), JAGUARUNDI

Hammondia. No records in the literature, yet.

Neospora. Sedlák and Bártová (2006a) serosurveyed zoo animals in the Czech and Slovak Republics using the IFAT and found antibodies to *N. caninum* in the only *P. yagouaroundi* they sampled. In Brazil, André et al. (2010) did a serosurvey of wild captive carnivores in zoos of São Paulo and Mato Grosso states, and the Federal District, Brazil, using the IFAT with tachyzoites of *N. caninum* NC-1 strain as antigen and found 5/25 (20%) jaguarundis seropositive for *N. caninum*. Onuma et al. (2014) also found antibodies to *N. caninum* in the jaguarundi in Brazil.

Toxoplasma gondii. Oocysts of *T. gondii* were isolated from the feces of one *P. yagouaroundi*, which initially lacked antibody to *T. gondii*, helping establish that not only domestic cats but also other members of the Felidae can spread

Toxoplasma via their feces (Jewell et al., 1972). Pizzi et al. (1978) said they found *T. gondii* in the jaguarundi from Cordoba Province, Argentina. Lukešová and Literák (1998) did not find oocysts in the feces of 13 *P. yagouaroundi* in zoos in the Czech Republic, but Sedlák and Bártová (2006a), also in the Czech and Slovak Republics, used the IFAT, and found antibodies to *T. gondii* in the only *P. yagouaroundi* they sampled. André et al. (2010) studied wild captive carnivores in zoos of São Paulo and Mato Grosso states, and the Federal District, Brazil, by the IFAT using tachyzoites of *T. gondii* RH strain as antigen and found 10/25 (40%) jaguarundis seropositive for *T. gondii*. Cañón-Franco et al. (2013) examined tissue samples from free-ranging, small Neotropical felids from Rio Grande do Sul, Brazil, amplified the ITS-1 marker to detect *T. gondii*, and found 9/22 (41%) jaguarundi samples positive. Multilocus PCR–RFLP genotyping of 11 felids using molecular markers SAG1, 5′3′SAG2, alt. SAG2, SAG3, BTUB, GRA6, c22-8, c29-2, L358, PK1, Apico, and CS3 allowed them to partially characterization 8 *T. gondii* genotypes. This study demonstrated the occurrence of *T. gondii* in wild populations and suggested its potential transmissibility to humans and other domestic and wild animals Cañón-Franco et al. (2013).

SUBFAMILY PANTHERINAE POCOCK, 1917

GENUS NEOFELIS GRAY, 1867 (MONOTYPIC)

NEOFELIS NEBULOSA (GRIFFITH, 1821), CLOUDED LEOPARD

Hammondia. No records in the literature, yet.

Neospora. Sedlák and Bártová (2006a) serosurveyed zoo animals in the Czech and Slovak Republics using the IFAT and found no antibodies in the only *N. nebulosa* they sampled. Spencer et al. (2003) also did a seroprevalence study of captive and free-ranging nondomestic felids in the United States and found antibodies to *N. caninum* in the clouded leopard.

Toxoplasma gondii. Sedlák and Bártová (2006a) serosurveyed zoo animals in the Czech and Slovak Republics using the IFAT but found no antibodies in the only *N. nebulosa* they sampled. de Camps et al. (2008) used the MAT to test for antibodies (titer ≥1:25 indicative of exposure) to *T. gondii*. Blood samples were taken from wild zoo felids from eight zoos in the midwestern United States and *T. gondii* was found in 1/7 (14%) clouded leopards sampled.

GENUS PANTHERA (L., 1758) (4 SPECIES)

PANTHERA LEO (L., 1758), LION

Hammondia. No records in the literature, yet.

Neospora. Cheadle et al. (1999) looked at seroprevalence in nondomestic felids in South Africa and found *P. leo* to be positive for antibodies to *N. caninum*. Spencer et al. (2003) did a seroprevalence study for *N. caninum* in captive and free-ranging nondomestic felids in the United States and also found antibodies to *N. caninum* in the lion. In Kenya, Ferroglio et al. (2003) examined wild animals for antibodies to *N. caninum* and found 5/18 (30%) of the lions (*P. leo*) sampled to be positive using the NAT. Sedlák and Bártová (2006a) serosurveyed zoo animals in the Czech and Slovak Republics for the occurrence of *N. caninum* antibodies using the IFAT and found no antibodies in the two *P. leo* they sampled, but did find antibodies in 1/2 (50%) Indian lions (*P. l. goojratensis*) sampled. Kamga-Waladjo et al. (2009) found lions (*P. leo*) from Senegal to be seropositive for both *N. caninum* and *T. gondii*. André et al. (2010) did a serosurvey of wild captive carnivores in zoos of São Paulo and Mato Grosso states and Federal District, Brazil, using the IFAT and tachyzoites of *N. caninum* NC-1

strain as antigen and found 1/9 (11%) lions surveyed to be seropositive for *N. caninum*.

Toxoplasma gondii. Polomoshnov (1979) and Ocholi et al. (1989) reported finding African lions infected with *T. gondii*. Lappin et al. (1991) collected serum from nondomestic felids and used an LA kit, an IHA kit, and ELISA for IgM (IgM–ELISA), IgG (IgG–ELISA), and for antigen (AG–ELISA) to define optimal diagnostic procedures. Antigen to *T. gondii* was detected in 25/33 (76%) felids using IgG–ELISA, in 20/33 (61%) using the LA test, and in 19/33 (58%) using the IHA test, with positive titers (≥1:128) found in 2/2 *P. leo* from Central Florida Zoological Park, Lake Monroe, Florida. Sedlák and Bártová (2006a) serosurveyed zoo animals in the Czech and Slovak Republics using the IFAT and found antibodies in 2/2 *P. leo* and in 2/2 of the Indian lions (*P. l. goojratensis*). de Camps et al. (2008) looked at captive zoo cats using the MAT (titer ≥1:25 indicative of exposure) to find antibodies to *T. gondii*; blood samples were taken from wild zoo felids from eight zoos in the midwestern United States, and antibodies to *T. gondii* were found in 12/22 (54.5%) lions sampled. André et al. (2010) did a serosurvey of captive carnivores in zoos of São Paulo and Mato Grosso states, and the Federal District, Brazil, using the IFAT with tachyzoites of the *T. gondii* RH strain as antigen, and found 5/9 (55.5%) lions seropositive. Moudgil (2015) reported the sera of two lions in India positive for antibodies to *T. gondii* using iELISA test kits.

PANTHERA (SYN. PUMA) ONCA (L., 1758), JAGUAR

Hammondia. Patton et al. (1986) examined the feces of neotropical felidae from the Cockscomb Basin, Belize, Central America, and reported that 3/23 (13%) jaguars had oocysts of *H. pardalis* in their feces.

Neospora. Sedlák and Bártová (2006a) serosurveyed zoo animals in the Czech and Slovak

Republics using the IFAT and found no antibodies in the only *P. onca* they sampled. André et al. (2010) did a serological survey of captive neotropical and exotic felids in Brazil and reported antibodies to *N. caninum* in 8/13 (61.5%) jaguars sampled. Onuma et al. (2014) also reported antibodies to *N. caninum* in jaguars in Brazil.

Toxoplasma gondii. Patton et al. (1986) did a fecal survey of neotropical felids in Belize and reported *Toxoplasma*-like oocyst in the feces of 1/25 (4%) jaguars. Sedlák and Bártová (2006a) serosurveyed zoo animals in the Czech and Slovak Republics using the IFAT and found antibodies in the only *P. onca* sampled. de Camps et al. (2008) used the MAT (titer ≥1:25 indicative of exposure) to test blood samples from zoo felids from eight zoos in the midwestern United States, and antibodies to *T. gondii* were found in the only jaguar they sampled. André et al. (2010) did a serosurvey of captive carnivores in zoos of São Paulo and Mato Grosso states and Federal District, Brazil, using IFAT with tachyzoites of the *T. gondii* RH strain as antigen, and found 11/18 (85%) jaguars seropositive for *T. gondii*.

PANTHERA PARDUS (L., 1758), LEOPARD

Hammondia. No records in the literature, yet.

Neospora. Spencer et al. (2003) did a seroprevalence study of captive and free-ranging nondomestic felids in the United States and found the Amur leopard to have antibodies to *N. caninum*. Sedlák and Bártová (2006a) serosurveyed zoo animals in the Czech and Slovak Republics for the occurrence of *N. caninum* antibodies using the IFAT and found no antibodies in three Amur leopards (*P. pardus orientalis*) they sampled.

Toxoplasma gondii. Lappin et al. (1991) collected serum from nondomestic felids and using an LA kit, an IHA kit, and ELISA for IgM (IgM–ELISA), IgG (IgG–ELISA), and for antigen (AG–ELISA), they detected *T. gondii* in 25/33 (76%) felids using IgG ELISA, in 20/33 (61%)

using the LA test, and in 19/33 (58%) using the IHA test and positive titers (≥1:128) were found in 2/3 (67%) *P. pardus* from Central Florida Zoological Park, Lake Monroe, Florida. Patton and Rabinowitz (1994) examined fecal material from leopards in Thailand and said 1/54 (<2%) had *Toxoplasma*-like oocysts; unfortunately, the fecal samples had been previously preserved in 10% formalin, so the identification was tentative. Zhang et al. (2000) collected sera from wild carnivores in the Shanghai Zoological Gardens, and using both the MAT and an ELISA reported that 27/36 (75%) were positive for *T. gondii* antibodies, including 1/1 *P. pardus* and 1/1 *P. p. sakicolor*, which were both ELISA-positive and MAT-positive. Sedlák and Bártová (2006a) serosurveyed zoo animals in the Czech and Slovak Republics using the IFAT and found antibodies in all three Amur leopards (*P. pardus orientalis*) they sampled. André et al. (2010) did a serosurvey of captive carnivores in zoos of São Paulo and Mato Grosso states, and the Federal District, Brazil, and using the IFAT, with tachyzoites of *T. gondii* RH strain as antigen, found the only tiger they sampled to be seropositive for *T. gondii*. Dubey et al. (2010a) surveyed the sera of many carnivores at the BCEAW, Sharjah, UAE, and demonstrated antibodies to *T. gondii* in 6/7 (86%) Arabian leopards, *P. p. nimr* (Hemprich and Ehrenberg, 1833).

PANTHERA TIGRIS (L., 1758), TIGER

Hammondia. No records in the literature, yet.

Neospora. Spencer et al. (2003) did a seroprevalence study of captive and free-ranging nondomestic felids in the United States and found antibodies to *N. caninum* in the tiger. Sedlák and Bártová (2006a) serosurveyed zoo animals in the Czech and Slovak Republics using the IFAT and found no antibodies to *N. caninum* in two Siberian tigers (*P. tigris altaica*), six Sumatran tigers (*P. t. sumatrae*), or in the one

Bengal tiger (*P. t. tigris*) they sampled. André et al. (2010) surveyed captive neotropical and exotic wild felids in Brazil and found antibodies to *N. caninum* in 4/6 (67%) of the tigers they sampled.

Toxoplasma gondii. Dorny and Fransen (1989) reported a case of toxoplasmosis in the Siberian tiger (*P. t. altaica*). Lappin et al. (1991) collected serum from nondomestic felids and evaluated them for antibodies to *T. gondii* using an LA kit, an IHA kit, and ELISA for IgM (IgM–ELISA), IgG (IgG–ELISA), and for antigen (AG–ELISA); positive titers (≥1:128) were found in 4/6 (67%) *P. tigris* that included 3/4 (75%) from Central Florida Zoological Park, Lake Monroe, Florida, and 1/2 (50%) from White Oaks Plantation, Yulee, Florida. Zhang et al. (2000) examined the sera of wild carnivores in the Shanghai Zoological Gardens, using both the MAT and an ELISA, and found 27/36 (75%) to be positive for *T. gondii* antibodies, including 6/7 (86%) *P. tigris amoyensis*, which were both ELISA- and MAT-positive, and 2/2 *P. t. tigris*, which also were both ELISA- and MAT-positive. Sedlák and Bártová (2006a) serosurveyed zoo animals in the Czech and Slovak Republics using the IFAT and reported antibodies in both Siberian tigers (*P. t. tigris*), in six Sumatran tigers (*P. t. sumatrae*), and in the one Bengal tiger (*P. t. tigris*) they sampled. de Camps et al. (2008) used the MAT to test for antibodies (titer ≥1:25 indicative of exposure) to *T. gondii*. Blood samples were taken from wild zoo felids from eight zoos in the midwestern United States and antibodies to *T. gondii* were found in 5/18 (28%) of the Amur tigers (*P. t. altaica*) sampled. André et al. (2010) serostudied captive carnivores in zoos of São Paulo and Mato Grosso states, and the Federal District, Brazil, using the IFAT and tachyzoites of the RH strain of *T. gondii* as antigen, and found 4/6 (67%) tigers sampled seropositive for *T. gondii*. Moudgil (2015) reported finding the sera of three tigers in India positive for antibodies to *T. gondii* using iELISA test kits.

GENUS *UNCIA* GRAY, 1854 (MONOTYPIC)

UNCIA UNCIA (SCHREBER, 1775), SNOW LEOPARD

Hammondia. No records in the literature, yet.

Neospora. Spencer et al. (2003) did a seroprevalence study for *N. caninum* and *T. gondii* in captive and free-ranging nondomestic felids in the United States and found antibodies to *N. caninum* in the endangered snow leopard.

Toxoplasma gondii. Ratcliffe and Worth (1951) examined 13 mammal species that died between 1940 and 1950 in the Philadelphia Zoological Gardens, including one snow leopard that died February 26, 1940. The leopard had been on exhibit for 21 months when it became ill and it died 2 weeks later. Ratcliffe and Worth (1951) said that *Toxoplasma* was recognized in the lungs, liver, abdominal lymph nodes, and in the serous surface of the adrenal glands. de Camps et al. (2008) used the MAT to test for antibodies (titer ≥1:25 indicative of exposure) to *T. gondii*; blood samples were taken from wild zoo felids from eight zoos in the midwestern United States, and antibodies to *T. gondii* were found in 5/14 (36%) snow leopards sampled.

HERPESTIDAE BONAPARTE, 1845

GENUS *HERPESTES* ILLIGER, 1811 (10 SPECIES)

HERPESTES EDWARDSI (E. GEOFFROY SAINT-HILAIRE, 1818), INDIAN GRAY MONGOOSE

Hammondia. No records in the literature, yet.

Neospora. No records in the literature, yet.

Toxoplasma gondii. Dubey et al. (2010a,b,c) surveyed the sera of many carnivores at the

BCEAW, Sharjah, UAE, and demonstrated antibodies to *T. gondii* in the only *H. edwardsi* they examined.

HERPESTES ICHNEUMON (L., 1758), EGYPTIAN MONGOOSE

Hammondia. No records in the literature, yet.
Neospora. Sobrino et al. (2008) serosurveyed carnivores from different regions of Spain using the c-ELISA, NAT, and/or the IFAT, and detected antibodies to *N. caninum* in 3/23 (13%) Egyptian mongooses.
Toxoplasma gondii. Sobrino et al. (2007) used the MAT (as per Dubey and Desmonts, 1987), with a cutoff value of 1:25, on free-ranging carnivores from different regions of Spain and detected the antibodies to *T. gondii* in 13/22 (59%) *H. ichneumon.*

HERPESTES JAVANICUS (É. GEOFFROY SAINT-HILAIRE, 1818) (SYN. HERPESTES AUROPUNCTATUS [HODGSON, 1836]), SMALL ASIAN MONGOOSE

Hammondia. No records in the literature, yet.
Neospora. No records in the literature, yet.
Toxoplasma gondii. Janitschke and Werner (1972) infected three *H. javanicus* orally with tissue cysts and/or oocysts of *T. gondii*, but they were never able to find oocysts of *T. gondii* in their feces.

GENUS ICHNEUMIA I. GEOFFROY SAINT-HILAIRE, 1837 (MONOTYPIC)

ICHNEUMIA ALBICAUDA (G. [BARON] COUVIER, 1829), WHITE-TAILED MONGOOSE

Hammondia. No records in the literature, yet.
Neospora. No records in the literature, yet.

Toxoplasma gondii. Dubey et al. (2010a) surveyed the sera of many carnivores at the BCEAW, Sharjah, UAE, and found antibodies to *T. gondii* in 2/2 *I. albicauda*.

GENUS SURICATA DESMAREST, 1804 (MONOTYPIC)

SURICATA SURICATTA (SCHREBER, 1776), MEERKAT

Hammondia. No records in the literature, yet.
Neospora. No records in the literature, yet.
Toxoplasma gondii. Juan-Sallés et al. (1997) diagnosed fatal disseminated toxoplasmosis in seven captive slender-tailed meerkats in the Barcelona Zoo, Spain, from 1992 to 1995. Respiratory distress and insufficiency and incoordination were the most consistent clinical signs although 2/7 (28.5%) died unexpectedly. At necropsy, they found parasites in the lungs, lymph nodes, spleen, and pericardium as the most commonly-infected organs. Their work, along with that of Basso et al. (2009), indicated that meerkats may be highly susceptible to toxoplasmosis. Basso et al. (2009) diagnosed three captive slender-tailed meerkats that had died in the Zoo of La Plata, Argentina, and reported on the *in vitro* isolation and molecular characterization of *T. gondii* as the cause of fatal disseminated toxoplasmosis. Prior to death, the meerkats showed depression, dyspnea, and hypothermia and died within 1–5 days from the onset of symptoms. Histopathology showed interstitial pneumonia, nonsuppurative inflammatory changes, and focal necrosis in liver, spleen, kidney and brain, and tachyzoites or tissue cysts were found in lung, liver, spleen, brain, striated muscle, kidney, intestine and mesenteric lymph node sections, and stained strongly with *T. gondii* antiserum in immunohistochemical analysis. Basso et al. (2009) cryopreserved their isolate and named it, TG-Suricata-1. PCR–RFLP analysis of markers based in the loci 3′-SAG2,

5′-SAG2, BTUB, GRA6, SAG3, c22-8, L358, PK1, c29-2, and Apico of *T. gondii* produced patterns corresponding to the clonal type III; interestingly, this strain possesses little or no virulence in the mouse model. This was the first report of isolation and genotyping of *T. gondii* from *S. suricatta*.

HYAENIDAE GRAY, 1821

GENUS CROCUTA KAUP, 1828 (MONOTYPIC)

CROCUTA CROCUTA (ERXLEBEN, 1777), SPOTTED HYENA

Hammondia. No records in the literature, yet.

Neospora. Many wild, noncanid carnivores are known to have been exposed to *N. caninum*, either by being seropositive, demonstrating oocysts in their feces, or exhibiting signs of neosporosis, including the spotted hyenas in Kenya and Senegal. In Kenya, Ferroglio et al. (2003) examined wild animals for antibodies to *N. caninum* and found 1/3 (33%) *C. crocuta* to be positive using the NAT.

Toxoplasma gondii. Wait et al. (2015) screened *C. crocuta* for *T. gondii* antibody titers. Felids are the closest domestic relation of hyenas, so *T. gondii* antibody titers were first compared in 26 feral cats with specific or nonspecific fluorophore-labeled secondary reagents, i.e., anticat IgG or protein A. Substitution of anticat IgG with protein A caused a statistically significant drop in titer measurements in cats ($P = .01$) with a reduction of the geometric mean titer equivalent to one doubling-dilution. The same procedures were then applied to captive spotted hyenas. Titers measured in 9 of 10 hyenas were identical whether anticat IgG or protein A was used as the secondary reagent: 5 had titers <1:16, 2 had titers 1:16, and 2 had titers 1:32.

One hyena had maximum titers of 1:64 or 1:32 when anticat IgG or protein A was used, respectively. The use of protein A as the secondary reagent in serologic assays can be applied to a range of mammalian species and seems unlikely to affect test specificity; however, the use of protein A may reduce test sensitivity, as suggested in this study using cats. Despite a control program, Wait et al. (2015) said some exposure to *T. gondii* had occurred in the Zoo's spotted hyenas.

GENUS *HYAENA* BRISSON, 1762 (2 SPECIES)

HYAENA BRUNNEA THUNBERG, 1820 (SYN. PARAHYAENA BRUNNEA WERDELIN AND SOLOUNIAS, 1991), BROWN HYENA

Hammondia. No records in the literature, yet.

Neospora. Sedlák and Bártová (2006a) examined carnivores in zoos in the Czech and Slovak Republics using the IFAT and did not find antibodies to *N. caninum* in three brown hyenas (which they called *P. brunnea*) they examined.

Toxoplasma gondii. Sedlák and Bártová (2006a) examined carnivores in zoos in the Czech and Slovak Republics using the IFAT and found antibodies to *T. gondii* in 3/3 (100%) brown hyenas sampled.

HYAENA HYAENA (L., 1758), STRIPED HYENA

Hammondia. No records in the literature, yet.

Neospora. No records in the literature, yet.

Toxoplasma gondii. Dubey et al. (2010a) surveyed the sera of many carnivores at the BCEAW, Sharjah, UAE, and found antibodies to *T. gondii* in 3/6 (50%) striped hyenas.

VIVERRIDAE GRAY, 1821

SUBFAMILY PARADOXURINAE GRAY, 1865

GENUS *ARCTICTIS* TEMMINCK, 1824 (MONOTYPIC)

ARCTICTIS BINTURONG (RAFFLES, 1821), BINTURONG

Hammondia. No records in the literature, yet.
Neospora. No records in the literature, yet.
Toxoplasma gondii. Oronan et al. (2013) tested blood of captive civets in the Protected Areas and Wildlife Bureau, Wildlife Rescue Center, Quezon City, Philippines, for antibodies to *T. gondii*, using the Immunocomb ELISA Feline *Toxoplasma* and *Chlamydophila* test kit and found that 3/4 (75%) *A. binturong whitei* J.A. Allan, 1910, had antibody titers (1:16 or 1:32) for *T. gondii*. The presence of these antibodies does not mean that the civets had clinical disease, but they did confirm the presence of, or exposure to, *T. gondii* in the wildlife facility, and the authors cautioned that the zoonotic potential of *T. gondii* should be investigated and that management within the Rescue Center should try to minimize its occurrence or transmission.

GENUS *PAGUMA* GRAY, 1831 (MONOTYPIC)

PAGUMA LARVATA (C.E.H. SMITH, 1827), MASKED PALM CIVET

Hammondia. No records in the literature, yet.
Neospora. No records in the literature, yet.
Toxoplasma gondii. Janitschke and Werner (1972) infected two masked palm civets, orally with tissue cysts and/or oocysts of *T. gondii*, but they were never able to recover oocysts of *T. gondii*

in their feces. Huo et al. (2016) did seroprevalence and genotyping for *T. gondii* in masked palm civets in China. They examined 500 serum samples from 5 administrative farms in tropical China, and assayed each for *T. gondii* antibodies by the MAT; also, brain samples of 20 aborted fetuses were examined by seminested PCR, and positive aborted fetuses (50%) were necropsied to collect the brain tissue for molecular and bioassay examinations. Genomic DNA was extracted from 29 brain tissues of infected mice, and the *T. gondii* B1 gene was amplified using multilocus PCR–RFLP. Huo et al. (2016) reported that 140/500 (28%) civets tested positive for *T. gondii* antibodies. Their results indicated that Toxo DB Genotype #9 has a distribution in masked palm civet that could be potential reservoirs for *T. gondii* transmission, and which may pose a threat to human health.

GENUS *PARADOXURUS* F.G. CUVIER, 1821 (3 SPECIES)

PARADOXURUS HERMAPHRODITUS (PALLAS, 1777), ASIAN PALM CIVET

Hammondia. No records in the literature, yet.
Neospora. No records in the literature, yet.
Toxoplasma gondii. Oronan et al. (2013) tested the blood of captive civets in the Protected Areas and Wildlife Bureau, Wildlife Rescue Center, Quezon City, Philippines, using the Immunocomb ELISA Feline *Toxoplasma* and *Chlamydophila* test kit, and found 1/6 (17%) *P. hermaphroditus* had an antibody titer (1:16) for *T. gondii*. The presence of antibodies does not mean that the civet had clinical disease but did confirm the presence of, or exposure to, *T. gondii* in the wildlife facility, and Oronan et al. (2013) cautioned that the zoonotic potential of *T. gondii* should be investigated and that management within the Rescue Center should be reviewed to minimize its occurrence or transmission.

SUBFAMILY VIVERRINAE GRAY, 1821

GENUS *GENETTA* F.G. COUVIER, 1816 (14 SPECIES)

GENETTA GENETTA (L., 1758), COMMON GENET

Hammondia. No records in the literature, yet.

Neospora. Sobrino et al. (2008) serosurveyed carnivores from different regions of Spain, using the c-ELISA, NAT, and/or the IFAT, and detected antibodies to *N. caninum* in 1/19 (5%) common genets, *G. genetta* via the c-ELISA test.

Toxoplasma gondii. Sobrino et al. (2007) used the MAT (as per Dubey and Desmonts, 1987), with a cutoff value of 1:25, on free-ranging carnivores from different regions of Spain, and detected the antibodies to *T. gondii* in 13/21 (62%) common genets. André et al. (2010) surveyed only one genetta in Brazil and found it to be seropositive for *T. gondii*, but not for *N. caninum*. Dubey et al. (2010a) surveyed the sera of many carnivores at the BCEAW, Sharjah, UAE, and demonstrated antibodies to *T. gondii* in 1/1 *G. genetta*.

GENUS *VIVERRA* L., 1758 (4 SPECIES)

VIVERRA TANGALUNGA GRAY, 1832, MALAYAN CIVET

Hammondia. No records in the literature, yet.

Neospora. No records in the literature, yet.

Toxoplasma gondii. Oronan et al. (2013) tested blood of captive civets in the Protected Areas and Wildlife Bureau, Wildlife Rescue Center, Quezon City, Philippines, using the Immunocomb ELISA Feline *Toxoplasma* and *Chlamydophila* test kit, and found 1/2 (50%) *V. tangalunga* had an antibody titer (1:16) for *T. gondii*. Thus confirming the presence of, or exposure

to, *T. gondii* in the facility; Oronan et al. (2013) cautioned that the zoonotic potential of *T. gondii* should be investigated and that management within the Rescue Center should be reviewed to minimize its occurrence or transmission.

VIVERRA ZIBETHA, L., 1758, LARGE INDIAN CIVET

Hammondia. No records in the literature, yet.

Neospora. No records in the literature, yet.

Toxoplasma gondii. Janitschke and Werner (1972) orally infected two *V. zibetha* with tissue cysts and/or oocysts of *T. gondii*, but neither could be demonstrated to shed oocysts of *T. gondii* in their feces.

GENUS *VIVERRICULA* HODGSON, 1838 (MONOTYPIC)

VIVERRICULA INDICA (É. GEOFFROY SAINT-HILAIRE, 1803), SMALL INDIAN CIVET

Hammondia. No records in the literature, yet.

Neospora. No records in the literature, yet.

Toxoplasma gondii. Pomerantz et al. (2016) did a serosurvey of carnivores at Kirindy Mitea and Ankarafantsika National Parks in Madagascar and tested them for antibodies to five viral pathogens, including *T. gondii* (by ELISA); the samples included one *V. indica*, but no antibodies to *T. gondii* were detected in the only Indian civet examined.

DISCUSSION AND SUMMARY

The Caniformia consists of 9 families, 72 genera, and 165 species (Wilson and Reeder, 2005) and at least 1 of the 4 genera in the Toxoplasmatinae has been found to parasitize all nine families, including the only species in each monotypic family, Ailuridae and Odobenidae. Within the Canidae, 9/13 (69%) genera and 24/35 (69%) species have been documented to host one or more toxoplasmatinae species. In the Mephitidae, 2/4 (50%) genera and 2/12 (17%) species are known to host these species. In the Mustelidae, 8/22 (36%) genera and 13/59 (22%) species act as hosts, and in the Otariidae, 5/7 (%) genera and 7/16 (44%) species are infected by them. In the Phocidae, 10/13 (77%) genera and 14/19 (74%) species act as hosts. In the Procyonidae, 4/6 (67%) genera and 6/15 (40%) species act as hosts. In the Ursidae, 2/5 (40%) genera and 4/8 (50%) species have been examined and documented to harbor one or more species in the toxoplasmatinae. In total, we have knowledge that one or more species in the four genera of the Toxoplasmatinae are known to parasitize at least one species in all nine families and can be found in 42/72 (58%) genera with 72/165 (44%) species in the Caniformia branch of the Carnivora.

The Feliformia group of carnivores consists of 6 families with 54 genera, and 121 species (Wilson and Reeder, 2005), but its members have not been as well studied for Toxoplasmatinae genera and species as have those in the Caniformia. There are neither known Toxoplasmatinae genera/species in the only monotypic family (genus), Nandiniidae (*Nandinia*) nor are there any in 29 genera and 42 species from the other 5 families in this lineage. In the Eupleridae, 2/7 (28.5%) genera and 2/8 (25%) species have been examined and both are documented to harbor *T. gondii* while *C. ferox* also is known to be a host to *N. caninum*. The Felidae is where the action has been; 12/14 (86%) genera and 27/40 (67.5%) of their species harbor one or more of the four genera in the Toxoplasmatinae. In five of the felid's seven monotypic genera, each has their only species (*A. jubatus*, *C. caracal*, *L. serval*, *N. nebulosi*, *U. uncia*) documented to serve as hosts to *N. caninum* and *T. gondii*, whereas the other two monotypic genera (*Pardofelis*, *Profelis*) have not yet been examined for these

apicomplexan parasites. Only *F. catus* is host to five *Besnoitia* species, *H. hammondi*, *N. caninum*, and *T. gondii*, and only *Panthera* has had all its (four) species examined and documented to host at least two genera of the Toxoplasmatinae. In the Herpestidae, 3/14 (21%) genera and 5/33 (15%) species are known to host protists in the Toxoplasmatinae. In the Hyaenidae, 2/3 (67%) genera and 2/4 (50%) species have been examined and found to host Toxoplasmatinae species, whereas in the Viverridae, 6/15 (%) genera and 7/35 (20%) species have been examined and found to have Toxoplasmatinae species. In total, we now know that one or more species in the four genera of the Toxoplasmatinae infect 5/6 (83%) families, 25/54 (46%) genera, and 43/121 (35.5%) species in the Feliformia branch of the Carnivora.

To summarize for all Carnivora, a relatively healthy number of species in this mammalian order have been examined for parasites in the Toxoplasmatinae, certainly more than in any other parasite group summarized in this book. Domestic and lab dogs and cats, of course, have been well studied because of their utility as lab animals and their availability as pets and companion animals, traits that lend them to closer and more careful examination because of our human ties to them. In all, 14/15 (93%) families, 67/126 (53%) genera, and 115/286 (40%) species of the Carnivora, have been found to harbor *Besnoitia*, *Hammondia*, *Neospora*, and/or *Toxoplasma* species and, often, the incidence of infection is high. But what about the other half of the carnivores for which no species yet have been identified? In most cases, it's because we have not looked, and the reason is, "Size matters!" The transmission propagules of the parasites in this subfamily of the Sarcocystidae, those of the previous subfamily (Sarcocystinae, Chapter 15), and, to a lesser extent, those in the Cryptosporidiae (Chapter 17) are very small, have few structural features that can be measured and/or used to distinguish one from the other with an LM, and they have cryptic species that now are being identified as genetic strains evolving closely with their host(s), determinations that only can be made with laboratories well-equipped with the tools and reagents to do molecular and genetic determinations. We believe that fewer parasitologists are being trained in this area, and those who are trained do not seem to be encouraged to sample large vertebrate species groups in time and space to fill in the missing pieces of this enormous puzzle, even when the financial hurdles of molecular labs can be overcome.

The taxonomy of this lineage of parasites, along with those in the two previous chapters (Cystoisosporinae, Sarcocystinae), has been both confused and confusing. Characters that traditionally and historically were used to define genera or families of apicomplexans—namely oocyst structure and life history developmental stages—have become fluid. Historically, all coccidia that had oocysts with two sporocysts, each sporocyst having four sporozoites (disporic, tetrazoic) were placed in the genus *Isospora*, which had been classified in the family Eimeriidae. Early on, it was believed that all members of the family had a homoxenous life cycle, with merogony and gamogony occurring in host epithelial cells, and sporogony occurring outside the host in the external environment. Beginning in the early 1970s, however, the apicomplexan world began to change dramatically when studies on the genera *Sarcocystis* and *Toxoplasma* began to show that these parasitic protists had heteroxenous life cycles in which asexual developmental stages resulted in forming cysts in various tissues of an intermediate host and that these stages were linked to a sexual stage of development in the intestine of the definitive host, a carnivore/omnivore. In the mid-1970s, work on well-studied *Isospora* species of dogs and cats started to reveal similar trends, involving intermediate hosts (Chapter 14). We encourage our readers to study the introductory sections in our three chapters in which we have tried to trace the historical sequence of discoveries that

have led us to our current understanding of this very interesting and formerly enigmatic group of parasites. We now know that all these parasites are closely related, based on our relatively new knowledge of the sequencing of some of their genes (e.g., Carreno et al., 1998 and many others).

All of the molecular work that has begun to clear the fog about just what is an isospora-type oocyst also has resulted in different hypotheses regarding who begat whom. One hypothesis suggests that the cyst-forming (heteroxenous) coccidia evolved from homoxenous coccidia because of the tendency of some early homoxenous species to invade deeper tissues of the intestine, eventually reaching other tissues (e.g., liver) or the blood, where they could become available to secondary hosts. The alternative hypothesis is that homoxenous coccidia of the vertebrate intestine evolved after being introduced there from heteroxenous species. The purview of this book is to present what is presently known about the apicomplexan coccidia in the Carnivora, not to debate competing hypotheses. We encourage interested readers to seek out this information elsewhere (Barta, 1989; Landau, 1982; Tadros and Laarman, 1982; Tenter and Johnson, 1997; Carreno et al., 1998) so they can draw their own conclusions.

There are many narratives regarding the toxoplasmatinae coccidia that can be elaborated upon. One that seems increasingly important to us is the increasing prevalence of these parasites, and the pathology they cause, in pinnipeds and other marine carnivores in the families Otariidae and Phocidae. Marine mammals in these lineages are increasingly becoming infected by the protist parasites of our closest terrestrial companions, dogs and cats. We know, for example (see sections above), that many marine species are becoming infected with both *T. gondii*, and to a lesser degree with *N. caninum*; and these parasites cause morbidity and mortality in their new hosts. Infections have been recorded in both wild and captive animals that include, but are not limited to, walruses, monk seals, ringed seals, Antarctic, Northern, South American, and New Zealand fur seals, elephant seals, sea lions, bearded seals, and many others. This is not just happening along the California coast, but infected marine carnivores are being found from the Arctic to south of the equator and everywhere in-between, where coastal waters are becoming heavily contaminated by oocysts from pet and feral cats and dogs and other anthropogenic activities. Some infected animals seem normal, but others get sick, and some die. The pathology caused can include enlarged spleen, meningoencephalitis, myocarditis, inflammatory foci in the central nervous system, myositis, uncoordinated flipper flapping, and death. Cats fed infected tissues from affected marine animals pass *T. gondii* oocysts in their feces, demonstrating that *T. gondii* can establish viable infections in marine mammals that acquire oocysts in surface water runoff and sewage discharge. Roe et al. (2017) suggested that toxoplasmosis could play an important role in morbidity and mortality in endangered marine mammals, particularly in mainland populations that are close to feline sources and their *T. gondii* oocysts.

A third carnivore family, Mustelidae, contains an important (and cute) clade of otters that include both marine and freshwater forms that also have been impacted by at least *T. gondii*. There is good evidence of an emergence and increasing prevalence of *T. gondii* in the members of this group, especially the sea otters, and this has been proposed as a contributing factor in their population decline. Miller et al. (2002) found 66 of 106 (62%) dead Southern sea otters along the central California coast to be seropositive for *T. gondii*, and because dead otters, when compared with live otters, were more than twice as likely to be seropositive, they proposed that the higher seropositivity for dead otters might be attributed to increased risk of mortality from *T. gondii*. Other studies have supported that *Toxoplasma* encephalitis is a significant cause of sea otter mortality (Thomas and Cole, 1996).

Bears (Ursidae) are another narrative worth mentioning. Their territories stretch from the Arctic to south of the equator, and their eight members include Earth's largest predators. They are thought to be the most recent carnivore lineage to evolve, splitting from the main canid line only about 20–25 MYA. Although only four of the eight living ursid species have been examined for these parasites, all four are susceptible, and highly seropositive, for *Toxoplasma*. The monotypic family, Ailuridae, has a single species, the red panda (*A. fulgens*), thought by some authorities to be an intermediate form between the Ursidae and the Procyonidae. The red panda also is known to harbor *T. gondii*. Of the eight ursid species, polar bears are true carnivores, six of the others are omnivores, and the giant panda is 99% a bamboo herbivore. Four of these ursid species have been serotested and all of them are documented to acquire *T. gondii*. Loeffler et al. (2007) surveyed giant pandas (*A. melanoleuca*) in China and found antibodies to *T. gondii* in 32%, and Ma et al. (2015) reported a fatal case of toxoplasmosis in a giant panda in a zoo in China. The American black bear (*U. americanus*) from Alaska is known to be highly seropositive for *T. gondii*, with prevalence ranging from 27% to 88% in various surveys that included over 600 bears; these are prevalences higher than those found in rodents in the United States. The brown or grizzly bear (*U. arctos*) also seems to acquire *T. gondii* easily, at prevalence rates equal to or higher than those found in black bears. Kiupel et al. (1987) diagnosed various stages of *T. gondii* in 76% of grizzly cubs, and Zhang et al. (2000) found 75% of their blood samples positive for *T. gondii* antibodies. In addition to *T. gondii*, grizzly bears also have been documented to harbor *N. caninum* in their livers and spleens (see Čobádiová et al., 2013), so theirs is a double whammy. Even polar bears (*U. maritimus*) are susceptible. In various recent serosurveys their prevalences of infection range from 6% to 21% to 46% so they seem to be less susceptible (for whatever ecological reasons) than grizzly and black bears;

however, their overall prevalence rates seem to be increasing through time. In one instance, "almost eight times higher than reported... just five years earlier." The mechanisms of how all bears acquire their infections still need to be investigated because their feeding habits are all different; contributing factors include predation of infected large (e.g., deer) and small (rodents) animals, scavenging dead carcasses, feeding on berries, grasses, and roots, transplacental transmission, overlapping habitats with coyotes, foxes, bobcats, dogs, and cats that may expose them to certain canine and feline parasites, and direct contact with oocysts from companion animals of humans.

Neospora caninum, apparently and fortunately, is not common in bears, and we know little about its pathogenic potential, unlike *T. gondii*, which is known to cause a variety of disease conditions (e.g., pneumonia, liver necrosis, etc.) and even death (see Ursidae, above). Interestingly, bears are the only mammals with significant amounts of ursodeoxycholic acid (UDCA), which is produced in their liver and stored in their gallbladder. When concentrated, UDCA is used to treat gallstones and some chronic liver diseases. Thus, bears are harvested, often illegally, to support popular "traditional medicine" in East Asia. Bears also are threatened by climate change because shifting temperatures change entire food webs that make them change their natural diets as migration routes change and fruits ripen early. Six of eight living bear species are now listed as "Vulnerable" on the IUCN Red List of Threatened Species. Poaching, climate change, habitat loss, and now *Toxoplasma*, all contribute their part to this tragedy in the making. How long will most of them last? We saw a quote from senior editor, Gemma Tarlach, at *Discover*, which seems most appropriate: "A future without them (bears) would be, well, unbearable."

A fourth narrative could be thoroughly developed and expanded, but we will keep it short. Black-footed ferrets are listed as "Endangered" on the IUCN Red List of Threatened Species, and

they can be highly susceptible to toxoplasmosis. Serious outbreaks have been documented, but their source(s) of infection have not been determined. Speculation by various authors includes being associated with certain meat used in their diet, or contamination by a handler due to lack of strict sanitation and/or maintenance in the breeding facilities in which they were housed. The maintenance of captive, endangered species may exacerbate their degree of susceptibility by virtue of their inbreeding, the stresses of captivity, and exposure via caretakers and unsanitary facilities.

Finally, there is no coccidian, and perhaps no parasitic organism, which has received more study than *T. gondii*. With this parasite's ability to infect an amazingly broad range of intermediate hosts, it has been the focus of wide ranging studies and spawned a diverse community of research specialists focusing on various aspects of its effects on host physiology, immunology, development, neurology, animal behavior, and ecology/epidemiology. The studies on *T. gondii* in humans are voluminous, with tens of thousands of published research papers available to any interested reader. But our focus here must remain only on the Carnivora, so we will focus on these final observations. In studies of parasite–host coevolution, *T. gondii* has been used as a two-host parasite model to test the hypothesis that parasites are capable of altering host behavior to enhance transmission, so as to facilitate completion of their life cycle. Berdoy et al. (2000) reported that *T. gondii* alters the behavior of rodent intermediate hosts to increase the probability they will be predated on by cats, thus facilitating transmission from intermediate to definitive host, and completion of their life cycle. They also found that *T. gondii* manipulated an infected rat's behavior to alter its perception of the risk of cat predation and changed its innate avoidance of feline predators into an impudent attraction! Thus, *T. gondii* subtly alters the brain of its intermediate host to enhance predation rate, while leaving other behaviors of the rodent and its general health intact. A variety of other behavioral and neurological impacts of *T. gondii* infection on intermediate hosts have been studied, including infections contributing to progression of schizophrenia and Huntington's disease (Torrey and Yolken, 2003; Donley et al., 2016), increased sexual attraction to cat odors by rodents (House et al., 2011), and behavioral changes in humans including altered personality, IQ decline, and changes in psychomotor activity (Flegr, 2013). For example, Stepanova et al. (2017) reported a statistically significant relationship for seropositive versus seronegative chronic *T. gondii* infection with chronically infected drivers 2.4 times more likely to be involved in an accident than uninfected drivers in Moscow, Russia. How *T. gondii* might impact wild carnivore behaviors in ways that make them more susceptible to harm or death can only be speculated about. Apparent increases in marine mammal strandings, human-aggressive bear encounters, road fatalities, etc., could all be partly attributable to chronic *T. gondii* infections and altered host behavior. We just do not know. Yet!

17

Cryptosporidiidae in the Carnivora

CRYPTOSPORIDIIDAE IN THE CARNIVORA

INTRODUCTION

The genus *Cryptosporidium* was discovered and described by Tyzzer in 1907. Its taxonomy has changed considerably since then because it possesses features of both coccidians and gregarines. It was initially classified with the Coccidia, but it was found later to be phylogenetically more closely related to Gregarinasina (Carreno et al., 1999; Barta and Thompson, 2006; Kuo et al., 2008). Currently, it is a distinct group of the Conoidasida, on equal status with the Coccidia and the Gregarinasina (Adl et al., 2012). Formerly, it was thought to be a monospecific genus (Tzipori et al., 1980; Tzipori and Campbell, 1981) because of its presumed lack of host specificity, nearly identical life cycle developmental stages (both exogenous and endogenous), and their shared antigenicity. However, with the advent of gene sequencing and other molecular innovations that can tease apart subtle genetic differences, it is now believed that there may be at least 30 valid species and over 50 genotypes, many of which may be mostly adapted to a narrow spectrum of hosts (Lucio-Forster et al., 2010; Osman et al., 2015; L. Xiao, pers. comm.). However, this area of study is still a work in progress and no definitive documentation exists yet regarding the exact number of *Cryptosporidium* species

(Plutzer and Karanis, 2000; Fayer et al., 2010); many isolates have been classified as "genotypes," without species definitions (Fayer, 2010), and may simply represent cryptic species.

Cryptosporidium species are obligate, monoxenous, intracellular, but extracytoplasmic, parasites. They have been found to infect a wide variety of vertebrate species worldwide, including humans, their domestic food and companion animals, and many species of wild and laboratory animals, including many carnivores. Since recognition of the seeming ubiquity of *Cryptosporidium* oocysts in host feces, searching for them has historically followed two paths. First, their oocysts are intentionally sought out in cases of chronic or acute clinical illness, especially in our domesticated and companion animals. Second, general, noninvasive surveys of larger sample sizes of various vertebrate populations have been conducted worldwide to determine prevalence. But prevalence studies rely principally on morphology of the oocysts found and therein lies the problem. Oocysts are so small, nondescript, difficult to find, and they lack in mensural characters such that they are virtually impossible to use to identify species. At present, fecal flotation, several staining procedures, and immunofluorescence assays (IFAs) of fecal samples are the most commonly-used laboratory techniques for diagnosing *Cryptosporidium*. Thus, light microscopy (LM) is routinely used for diagnostics; however, it does not allow the identification of species

© 2018 Donald W. Duszynski published by Elsevier Inc. All rights reserved.

because of the morphological uniformity of the oocysts. Moreover, LM suffers from low sensitivity because the oocysts (1) may be shed in small numbers, often under detectable levels; (2) are translucent and small (measuring ~4–7 μm); and (3) may be confused with yeasts, fungal spores, and/or other structures in fecal samples. Thus, examination under LM requires a trained technician because the oocysts may be overlooked easily or may be misdiagnosed and leads to false-positive or to false-negative diagnoses. Moreover, because oocysts are shed intermittently, one negative fecal exam may not necessarily mean that the host individual is not parasitized. Therefore, repeated fecal exams should be undertaken when possible.

Due to their small size, intermittent shedding, and limited morphological variation, only molecular and immunological methods can begin to tease apart the subtle sequence/genetic differences between *Cryptosporidium* species and genotypes. Of particular relevance in evaluating, detecting, resolving, and differentiating the identity of *Cryptosporidium* species, the following diagnostic and genotyping methods are particularly useful: polymerase chain reaction (PCR), real-time PCR (q-PCR), nested PCR–restriction fragment length polymorphism (RFLP), immunomagnetic separation-qPCR, qPCR-melting curve analysis assay, enzyme immunoassays, and sequencing of specific genes or regions (Jiang and Xiao, 2003; Lindergard et al., 2003; Xiao et al., 2004; Leoni et al., 2006; Feng et al., 2009; Homem et al., 2012; Gao et al., 2013; Lalonde et al., 2013; Silva et al., 2013). In the case of *Cryptosporidium* species, several markers/loci are now commonly employed to determine species/genotype differences including, but not limited to, partial and full sequences of 18S rRNA, *Cryptosporidium* oocyst wall protein (COWP), 70-kDa heat shock protein (HSP70), 60-kDa glycoprotein (gp60), and actin genes, with partial 18S rRNA gene sequences being the most commonly used marker. Clearly, combining as many of these techniques as possible is much more sensitive in detecting *Cryptosporidium*-positive fecal samples (Morgan and Thompson,

1998; McGlade et al., 2003; Scorza et al., 2003; Fayer et al., 2006; others) than could be expected under only LM. However, a positive PCR does not provide information on the viability and infectivity of the pathogen. Thus, a combination of methods (LM, transmission electron microscopy (TEM), molecular detection, and immunological methods) is recommended and vital, especially in cases where only a few oocysts are present in the feces or when any doubts are raised regarding the diagnosis, especially in the isolates involved in human outbreaks and/or epidemiological studies.

Oocysts already are sporulated when passed, thus immediately infective. They remain stable and infective in the environment for a long period of time, are resistant to most common disinfectants, and are also able to survive routine wastewater treatment (Fayer et al., 2000; Ryan and Power, 2012). Only 10% (w/v) aqueous formalin or 5% (w/v) aqueous ammonia solutions are effective in destroying the oocysts (Barr, 1997). The most common environmental and alimentary sources of *Cryptosporidium* are water treatment facilities, raw sewage discharge, especially into rivers, wells, ditches, and oceans, where molluscs, oysters, and vegetables become exposed (Meireles, 2010). When sporulated oocysts have been ingested by a suitable host, the infection is usually self-limiting in immunocompetent individuals but may become acute leading to morbidity and mortality in the immunocompromised ones (e.g., dogs with distemper virus). Therefore, *Cryptosporidium* species can and do have a great influence on public health.

By our count, there are 10 valid, named *Cryptosporidium* species/genotypes identified in carnivores. By this, we mean *Cryptosporidium* species that are "polyphasically characterized" (as per Egyed et al., 2003), including morphological, biological, and genetic information, and following the recommendations and guidelines of Xiao et al. (2004) and Jirků et al. (2008). These species include *C. andersoni*, *C. canis*, *C. felis*, *C. hominis*, *C. meleagridis*, *C. muris*, *C. parvum*, *C. ryanae*, *C. scrofarum*, and *C. ubiquitum*. Only these named *Cryptosporidium* species are included in this chapter, each under its appropriate carnivore host. Two of these species, *C. canis* and *C. felis*, were described from our companion carnivores, dogs and cats, and their complete species descriptions are included, similar to the full species descriptions of eimeriid Coccidia in previous chapters. The other eight cryptosporidians were described from "type hosts" that are noncarnivore, but lacking strict host specificity, they have been reported in a variety of carnivore hosts, and we have tried to update these references to the best of our ability. Finally, hundreds of surveys examine only fecal material for various parasite groups and many of these have found and reported *Cryptosporidium* oocysts in carnivore feces (i.e., "*Cryptosporidium* species"); these are mentioned briefly under that carnivore species, along with the citing author, and the reader is referred to Chapter 19 (*species inquirendae*) for more detailed information in each *Remarks* section pertaining to that carnivore genus/species.

SPECIES DESCRIPTIONS

SUBORDER CANIFORMIA KRETZOI, 1938

FAMILY AILURIDAE GRAY, 1843

GENUS *AILURUS* F.G. CUVIER, 1825 (MONOTYPIC)

AILURUS FULGENS F.G. CUVIER, 1825, RED PANDA

CRYPTOSPORIDIUM ANDERSONI LINDSAY, UPTON, OWENS, MORGAN, MEAD, AND BLACKBURN, 2000

Type host: *Bos taurus* L., 1758, Aurochs.
Remarks: Wang et al. (2015b) surveyed fecal samples of 110 captive red pandas, *A. fulgens*, from 5 areas throughout China, which represented approximately one-third of China's captive population. Their feces were examined for the presence of *Cryptosporidium* using PCR, sequencing and analyses of the 18S rRNA gene. Wang et al. (2015b) found that 7/110 (7%) pandas were positive for *C. andersoni*. All the positive samples originated from Sichuan and Chongqing provinces. Given that *C. andersoni* can infect humans under certain circumstances, the infections in captive red pandas should be considered a public health concern, particularly for breeders, veterinarians, and zoo workers.

CRYPTOSPORIDIUM PARVUM TYZZER, 1912

Type host: *Mus musculus* (L., 1758), House Mouse.
Remarks: Karanis et al. (2007) reported the presence of *Cryptosporidium* oocysts in the feces of *A. fulgens*, in the Xining Zoo, China. Using the immunofluorescence test, nested PCR, and sequencing of the partial 18S rRNA gene, the oocysts were determined as *Cryptosporidium parvum* mouse genotype. Neither the number of examined pandas nor their origin was given.

FAMILY CANIDAE FISCHER, 1817

GENUS *CANIS* L., 1758 (6 SPECIES)

CANIS LATRANS SAY, 1823, COYOTE

Thompson et al. (2009) examined the feces of coyotes (*C. latrans*), collected in Prairie regions of southern Alberta and Saskatchewan, Canada, by sucrose flotation, immunofluorescence of monoclonal antibodies (MAbs) specific for *Cryptosporidium* (Crypt-a-Glo), and PCR amplification with subsequent sequencing and phylogenetic analyses of 18S rRNA and HSP70 genes.

Cryptosporidium was detected in 8/70 (11%) samples, all collected in winter; none of the samples collected in summer were positive. This may be because the coyotes were in poor condition and nutritionally compromised in the winter, so stress may have made them more susceptible to infection. Only 2/8 (25%) positive samples were successfully amplified and both 18S rRNA and HSP70 sequences, and phylogenetic analyses, identified them as *C. canis*.

CANIS LUPUS FAMILIARIS (SYN. C. FAMILIARIS) L., 1758, DOMESTIC DOG

CRYPTOSPORIDIUM CANIS FAYER, TROUT, XIAO, MORGAN, LAL, AND DUBEY, 2001

For photomicrographs of sporulated oocysts, molecular ladder lanes of their PCR-RFLP analysis, and other supporting figures including phylogenetic trees see Figs. 1–6 in Fayer et al., 2001, *Journal of Parasitology* 87 (6), 1415–1422.

Synonym: Cryptosporidium parvum Tyzzer, 1912 (of many early authors).

Type host: Canis lupus familiaris (syn. *C. familiaris*) L., 1758, Domestic Dog.

Type locality: North America: USA: Maryland.

Other hosts: Bos taurus L., 1758, Domestic Cow (experimental); *Homo sapiens* L., 1758, Human (HIV-infected); *Nyctereutes procyonoides* (Gray, 1834), Raccoon Dog.

Geographic distribution: Asia: China: Heilongjiang Prefecture, suburban Harbin (Zhang et al., 2016b); Japan: Saitama Prefecture (Yamamoto et al., 2009); Australia; North America: USA: Georgia, Maryland, Ohio; South America: Peru (from Fayer et al., 2001).

Description of sporulated oocyst: Oocyst shape: nearly spheroidal; number of walls, undetermined; wall characteristics: thin, smooth, colorless, with no protrusions on its surface

(Figs. 1–3, Fayer et al., 2001); L×W (n=200): 4.95×4.71 (3.68–5.88×3.68–5.88); L/W ratio: 1.05 (1.04–1.06); M: absent; OR or PG: present as a distinct, prominent eccentric granule or as a central globule. Distinctive features of oocyst: a typical *Cryptosporidium* oocyst, small size, no sporocysts, containing four SZ, apparently without a longitudinal suture, and with an eccentric granule or central globular body among the SZ.

Description of sporozoites: Could not be easily seen within the oocysts studied (see Figs. 1–3, Fayer et al., 2001).

Prevalence: Found naturally in the feces of one 25-kg, 16-month-old, female, mixed-breed dog, and in 1 HIV-infected adult male from Peru (as per Fayer et al., 2001). Yamamoto et al. (2009) surveyed fecal samples of dogs in public animal shelters in the Saitama Prefecture, Japan. Microscopic examination revealed the presence of *C. canis* oocysts in 8/906 (<1%) of the samples. Scorza and Lappin (2017) examined fecal samples of dogs on the Pine Ridge Indian Reservation, South Dakota, USA. Samples were examined by centrifugation–flotation in Sheather's sucrose solution and by commercial IFA for *Cryptosporidium* (Merifluor *Crypto/Giardia* kit). PCR amplification of the HSP70 gene was performed with immunofluorescence-positive samples. *Cryptosporidium* was detected in 6/84 (7%) samples, 4 of which were successfully sequenced and determined to be *C. canis*. Tangtrongsup et al. (2017) examined fecal samples of dogs from a variety of locations and lifestyles in the Chiang Mai province, Thailand. Samples were examined by IFA (Merifluor *Crypto/Giardia* kit) and by PCR amplification of HSP70 and 18S rRNA genes. They found *Cryptosporidium* in 34/109 (31%) samples, mostly in dogs <1-year-old, and were able to generate 22 gene sequences, of which 15 represented *C. canis*. Simonato et al. (2017) examined canine fecal samples collected not from dogs but in public green (270 samples) and urban (435 samples) areas, Padua municipality, Veneto region, northern Italy. Samples were screened by sedimentation–flotation, followed by nested PCR amplification and sequencing of the 18S rRNA gene. Samples concurrently positive for *Giardia* favored amplification of giardial DNA over the *Cryptosporidium* DNA, so these samples were also examined by a touchdown real-time PCR of the COWP gene. In all, 12/705 (2%) samples were positive for *Cryptosporidium*, but only 1/12 (8%) positives were identified as *C. canis*. Yu et al. (2017) examined wet-mount fecal samples of pet dogs with diarrhea from regions in Beijing, China. Samples then were examined by nested PCR amplification of the 18S rRNA gene. *Cryptosporidium* was detected in 24/485 (5%) samples, mainly in poodles and border collies, and 20/24 (83%) were determined to represent only *C. canis*.

Sporulation: Sporulation occurred endogenously, releasing sporulated oocysts in the feces.

Prepatent and patent period: Unknown.

Site of infection: Unknown.

Endogenous stages: Unknown.

Cross-transmission: Fayer et al. (2001) were able to use oocysts from the dog to infect 1 calf, but they were unable to infect from 4 to 10, 3- to 5-day-old BALB/c or from 4 to 10, 8-week-old C57b16/N (C57) mice.

Pathology: The dog infected with *C. canis* did not show any clinical signs of diarrhea or debilitation (Fayer et al., 2001). Miller et al. (2003) reported a case of gastrointestinal cryptosporidiosis and a concurrent infection with *Isospora* spp. in an 8-week-old female Yorkshire terrier puppy in Georgia, USA. The puppy suffered from weakness, diarrhea, and intestinal isosporiasis. Histology revealed severe gastric and intestinal cryptosporidiosis, severe intestinal isosporiasis, and thymic atrophy with lymphoid depletion. Mild-to-moderate gastric cryptitis was observed. Numerous "round unicellular organisms," 3–5 wide, loosely attached to the surface, were detected in the gastric crypts. Small numbers of "organisms" also were associated with the gastric surface epithelium and the villus border of the small intestine. Organisms were not observed in the bile ducts. Numerous sexual and asexual stages of *Isospora* spp. were recorded in the luminal and crypt epithelial cells of the small intestine. Neither histology nor isolation proved the presence of viruses. PCR amplification of the 18S rRNA and actin genes revealed the presence of *Cryptosporidium*. Subsequent sequencing of the actin gene and phylogenetic analysis identified the species as *C. canis*. This was the first report of gastric cryptosporidiosis in a canine. All previous reports have described only intestinal invasions.

Materials deposited: Phototypes were deposited in the U.S. National Parasite Collection, Beltsville, Maryland, USNPC No. 90587.

Etymology: The parasite is named for the domestic dog because the type specimens were based on genetic sequences obtained from oocysts that were repeatedly isolated from the domestic dog.

Remarks: For a quick history, Tzipori and Campbell (1981) first reported a *Cryptosporidium* infection (species/strain/genotype undetermined) in dogs in which they found serum antibodies in 16/20 (80%) dogs in Scotland, using the indirect immunofluorescence procedure. Wilson and Holscher (1983) described the first case of clinical cryptosporidiosis in a 1-week-old Pomeranian pup with acute diarrhea and labored breathing. They found numerous round to oval basophilic stages, 2–3 mm wide, covering the microvillous border of the tips of intestinal and crypt epithelium. TEM showed the presence of stages corresponding to developing trophozoites or maturing merozoites, attached to the microvillus border of intestinal epithelium, and mild villus atrophy was observed in the small intestine. However, the species/strains/genotypes were unresolved because the method(s) to make such determination was/were unavailable at that time.

Oocysts of *C. canis* are morphologically indistinguishable from, and possess surface antigens in common with, those of the human and bovine genotypes of *C. parvum*. However, unlike the bovine genotype of *C. parvum*, oocysts of *C. canis* are not infective for normal or immunosuppressed mice, and unlike the human genotype of *C. parvum*, oocysts of *C. canis* are infectious for cattle. In addition, *C. canis* differs markedly at the molecular level from all known species of *Cryptosporidium* based on sequence data for the 18S rDNA and the HSP70 gene. Analysis by PCR-RFLP of the 18S rRNA gene showed the *C. canis* oocysts from dogs had *ssp*I and *Vsp*I restriction patterns different from *C. parvum* but identical to the genotype previously described from dog-derived oocysts (Morgan et al., 1999c, 2000b; Xiao et al., 1999a,b).

Below, we summarize much of the current literature, immediately preceding and following the description by Fayer et al. (2001), in which various hosts (mostly canids) are now known to be hosts for *C. canis*. Morgan et al. (2000b) did a genetic and phylogenetic analysis of eight dog-derived *Cryptosporidium* isolates from Australia and the United States; two of the three Australian dogs were immunosuppressed (one by parvovirus, the second by immunomediated thrombocytopenia) and both shed small numbers of *Cryptosporidium* oocysts in their feces, whereas all six US dogs were asymptomatic. *Cryptosporidium* was initially identified by malachite green negative staining and PBS–ether sedimentation, together with Ficoll gradient centrifugation. PCR amplification and sequencing of 18S rRNA and HSP70 genes were followed by phylogenetic analyses. All HSP70 sequences were identical to each other but genetically distant from other genotypes of *C. parvum*, whereas 18S rDNA sequences were also identical to each other but clustered with *C. parvum*, *C. felis*, and *C. wrairi*. Their study preceded that by Fayer et al. (2001) and strongly suggested that a distinct "dog genotype" was conserved across geographic areas and indicated it may represent a valid new species.

Morgan-Ryan et al. (2002) experimentally transmitted their newly named *C. hominis* to various hosts, including 6 mixed-breed, 2-month-old dogs in Calgary, Canada, with no history of *Cryptosporidium*; the puppies were deemed to be negative after they were screened, prior to infection, by both PCR and LM. They were inoculated with 2 human-derived isolates and their feces were collected/examined by both LM and PCR daily until 16 days postinoculation (DPI). Two of the dogs started to shed oocysts 7–8 and 4–10 DPI, but genetic analysis showed the presence of *C. canis* in all their samples. Morgan-Ryan et al. (2002) suggested the dogs might have had a latent *C. canis* infection that relapsed, possibly from the stress of captivity and handling.

Giangaspero et al. (2006) examined fecal samples of 240 dogs (120 kenneled, 120 privately-owned) in the Abruzzo region of Teramo province, central Italy. Samples were examined by PCR amplification of the COWP gene. Only 1 of 240 samples, a privately-owned dog, was found to be positive for *C. canis*. Huber et al. (2007) examined fecal samples of four puppies in an animal shelter in Nova Iguaçu, Rio de Janeiro state, Brazil, using centrifugation–flotation, followed by nested PCR of 18S rDNA, subsequent RFLP analysis of the secondary PCR products, and phylogenetic analyses. They found 1/4 (25%) dogs to be positive for *C. canis*, the identity by phylogenetic analyses using the NJ (Neighbor Joining), MP (Maximum Parsimony), and ML (Maximum Likelihood) approaches. Thomaz et al. (2007), also in Brazil, examined dog fecal samples in different municipalities (São Paulo, São Bernardo do Campo, Jundiaí, Santo André, Taubaté, Araçatuba) of São Paulo. Unfortunately, they did not state the total number of dogs examined. Samples were examined by flotation–concentration in sucrose solution, and nine dogs were positive for *Cryptosporidium* oocysts. The oocysts were small and subspheroidal, ~5 wide. Nested PCR amplification of the 18S rRNA gene identified all nine isolates as *C. canis*. Palmer et al. (2008b) surveyed 1,400 fecal samples of dogs from both urban and rural areas across Australia, which were collected from 59 veterinary clinics (810 samples) and 26 refuges (590 samples). Samples initially were examined by saturated salt and D-glucose centrifugation–flotation method and malachite green staining. Microscopy-positive samples were further analyzed by the nested PCR amplification of the actin gene. Of the eight samples microscopically positive for *Cryptosporidium*, four of them were successfully sequenced, and all were identified as *C. canis*. Yamamoto et al. (2009) examined fecal samples of dogs in public animal shelters, Saitama Prefecture, Japan. LM examination revealed the presence of *Cryptosporidium* in 8/906 (<1%) of the samples, and molecular analysis confirmed the presence of *C. canis*.

Sevá et al. (2010) examined fecal samples of 28 pet dogs from 21 rural properties surrounding Atlantic dry forest fragments, Teodoro Sampaio municipality, São Paulo state, southeastern Brazil. Samples were inspected by conventional sucrose flotation, followed by genotyping based on nested PCR amplification of the 18S rRNA gene and subsequent phylogenetic analysis; they found 3/28 (11%) samples positive for *Cryptosporidium*, all determined as *C. canis* (100% identity). In Japan, Yoshiuchi et al. (2010) collected 77 fecal samples from privately-owned dogs in Osaka city. Samples were examined by centrifugal sucrose flotation and the direct IFA (Merifluor *Cryptosporidium*/*Giardia* commercial kit), followed by PCR amplification of 18S rRNA and COWP genes. *Cryptosporidium* was detected in 3/77 (4%) samples, all identified as *C. canis*. All positive dogs were without diarrhea. Duration of the oocyst excretion varied from 21 to 88 days, but it was unknown when these animals became infected.

Uehlinger et al. (2013) examined fecal samples of dogs <1-year-old on Prince Edward Island, Canada. Dogs originated from a local animal shelter (62 samples), private veterinary clinics (78 samples), and a pet store (69 samples). Samples were examined by centrifugation–flotation in zinc sulfate solution and sucrose gradient centrifugation, followed by direct antibody immunofluorescence microscopy for *Cryptosporidium* and nested PCR amplification of the HSP70 gene. *Cryptosporidium* was detected in 5/62 (8%) samples from the shelter and in 8/78 (10%) samples from the veterinary clinics; 4 of the samples were successfully sequenced and identified as *C. canis*. Koompapong et al. (2014) collected feces of dogs in central Thailand, 111 samples were collected from 105 dairy cattle farms and 95 samples from a temple in Ban Na District, Nakhon Nayok province. Samples were tested using the molecular identification of a fragment of the 18S rRNA gene. Koompapong et al. (2014) estimated that ~1,000 dogs live around the temple area and are fed by monks and volunteers. Samples from the farms were collected directly from the rectum, and samples from the temple were collected from the ground. Oocysts of *C. canis* were detected in 2/95 (2%) samples from the temple, but no *Cryptosporidium* was detected in the 111 samples from the dairy farms.

In China, Gu et al. (2015) collected 315 fresh fecal samples from pet dogs in Anhui and Zhejiang provinces; they used the nested PCR amplification of the 18S rRNA gene and subsequent sequencing to detect *Cryptosporidium* in 5/315 (2%) samples, mostly from dogs ≤12-months-old, and all positive samples were determined to be *C. canis*. Li et al. (2015), in Heilongjiang province, China, collected fecal samples from dogs; these included 108 from a pet market in Harbin, 39 from 3 pet hospitals in Harbin, 50 from 3 pet hospitals in Daqing, and 52 from 1 pet hospital in Qiqihar, all in southwestern Heilongjiang province. Samples were examined by the nested PCR amplification and by sequencing of the 18S rRNA gene. *Cryptosporidium* was detected in 6/267 (2%) samples; 5 samples were *C. canis* and 1 was identified to be *C. ubiquitum*. Market dogs had a significantly higher infection rate than the in-hospital dogs.

Osman et al. (2015) examined fecal samples of household dogs in the Lyons, France, using a standard semiquantitative flotation technique with saturated zinc sulfate solution and nested PCR amplification of the 18S rRNA gene. *Cryptosporidium* was detected in 3/116 (3%) dogs and genetically determined to be *C. canis*. All 3 dogs were puppies <15-weeks-old, all were concurrently infected with *Giardia*, and 1 was concurrently infected with a *Cystoisospora* sp.

Paoletti et al. (2011) examined fecal samples of dogs (117 kenneled in rescue shelters, 385 privately-owned) in central Italy. Samples were examined by flotation in a sodium nitrate solution, Baermann's technique, and fecal smears stained with cold Ziehl–Neelsen stain. *Cryptosporidium* oocysts were found in 1/502 (0.2%) samples, from a privately-owned dog, and determined by PCR amplification of the COWP gene to be *C. canis*.

Xu et al. (2016) examined fecal samples of dogs in urban areas of Shanghai, China: 102 from household dogs, 61 from dogs in a veterinary clinic, and 322 from dogs in pet shops. Samples were examined by PCR amplification and sequencing of the 18S rRNA gene. *Cryptosporidium* was detected in 39/485 (8%) samples; all positive samples were determined to be *C. canis*. Dogs in the clinic (8/61, 13%) and pet shops (31/322, 10%) had a significantly higher infection rate than household dogs, none of which were infected, and 13/39 (33%) *Cryptosporidium*-positive dogs were concurrently infected with *Giardia duodenalis* and one with *G. duodenalis* and *Enterocytozoon bieneusi*.

de Lucio et al. (2017) examined fecal samples of pet dogs from Álava province, Basque Country, northern Spain; each sample was examined by direct fluorescence microscopy (DFAT), followed by nested PCR targeting the 18S rRNA gene, and *Cryptosporidium* was detected in 3/55 (5%) samples, 2 of which were identified as *C. canis*. Gil et al. (2017), also in Álava province, Spain, examined fecal samples of dogs, oocysts of *Cryptosporidium* were detected by the DFAT, and species were identified by nested PCR amplification of the 18S rRNA gene. *Cryptosporidium* was confirmed in 8/194 (4%) samples; 5 positive samples were determined to represent *C. canis*, and 1 sample was *C. hominis*.

On the island of Crete, southern Greece, Kostopoulou et al. (2017) collected fecal samples from dogs, including 529 in private households, 278 from 11 shelters, and 72 shepherd dog samples from 29 sheep and goat farms. Fecal samples were examined by a sedimentation–flotation method and by the quantitative direct IFA with the commercial Merifluor *Cryptosporidium/Giardia* kit. Samples positive for *Cryptosporidium* then were identified by the PCR amplification and subsequent sequencing of the 18S rRNA and HSP70 genes. *Cryptosporidium* was detected in 52/879 (6%) samples; 2 samples were determined to contain *C. canis* and 1 sample was identified as *C. scrofarum*. If the latter identification is correct, it is the first report of a pig-specific *Cryptosporidium* in a dog. Shelter dogs were significantly more infected than household dogs; however, household dogs shed more oocysts than infected shelter dogs.

CRYPTOSPORIDIUM MELEAGRIDIS SLAVIN, 1955

Type host: *Meleagris gallopavo* L., 1758, Common Turkey.

Type locality: Europe: United Kingdom, Scotland, Lasswade.

Other hosts: Numerous (see Duszynski and Couch, 2013); carnivore hosts: *Canis lupus familiaris* (syn. *C. familiaris*) L., 1758, Domestic Dog.

Geographic distribution: Cosmopolitan.

Remarks: Hajdušek et al. (2004) examined fecal samples of two dogs for *Cryptosporidium* in the Czech Republic. Using LM, amplification of the 18S rRNA and COWP genes, and subsequent phylogenetic analyses, they identified *C. meleagridis* in one sample and *C. parvum* "cattle" genotype in the other. They reported that the oocysts of both species measured L×W: 4.7×4.3. This was the first record of *C. meleagridis* in a dog; however, it was obvious from both phylogenetic trees (i.e., the 18S rDNA and the COWP trees) that the sequences were not 100% homologous with *C. meleagridis* described from turkeys. Yang et al. (2017) examined fecal samples of 7- to 8-year-old, clinically healthy, "foxes" (genus/species not given) from the Heilongjiang, Jilin, and Liaoning provinces, northeastern China. Samples were examined by nested PCR amplification of 18S rRNA gene, and positive samples then subtyped by nested PCR amplification of the gp60 gene; 12/213 (6%) "fox" feces were positive for *Cryptosporidium*, and 1/12 (8%), from Jilin province, was identified as *C. meleagridis*, a species generally known to have low host specificity. This was its first record in a fox, further expanding the host range of *C. meleagridis*.

CRYPTOSPORIDIUM MURIS (TYZZER, 1907) TYZZER, 1910

Type host: *Mus musculus* L., 1758, House Mouse.

Remarks: Lupo et al. (2008) examined fecal samples of asymptomatic, kenneled hound dogs, 1- to 3-year-old, housed in 56 cages in Huntsville, Texas, USA. Samples were examined by EIA (ProSpecT *Cryptosporidium* Microplate Assay) for the detection of *Cryptosporidium* antigen. The EIA detected 49/70 (70%) samples as positive, originating from 40/56 (71%) cages. Six randomly-selected antigen-positive samples were analyzed by indirect IFA and by the nested PCR amplification of the 18S rRNA gene, followed by RFLP analysis. All six samples were determined as *C. muris* by RFLP, a sequence of one sample also identified the parasite as *C. muris*, and the IFA showed oocysts morphologically consistent with those of *C. muris*. This was the first report of a naturally-occurring *C. muris* infection in a canine host.

CRYPTOSPORIDIUM PARVUM TYZZER, 1912

Type host: *Mus musculus* (L., 1758), House Mouse.

Remarks: Lloyd and Smith (1997) infected six 6-week-old beagle dogs, with 2×10^6 of *C. parvum* oocysts of calf origin. The dogs were *Cryptosporidium* negative but *Toxocara canis* positive before the inoculation. Dogs were examined daily for 21 days and then 3 times/week for 80 days, using 5 different diagnostic methods. All 6 dogs started to shed oocysts in their feces from 1 DPI, but in low numbers. A cyclical nature of oocyst excretion was observed, with most of the oocysts being shed between 3 and 9 DPI, with two more peaks up to 32 DPI, and then in decreasing numbers after 32 DPI; 5 of 6 dogs passed oocysts for at least 80 days. None of the dogs displayed any clinical signs. The Weber concentration method followed by staining with immunofluorescent antibody and sediment staining with a modified Ziehl–Neelsen were the most sensitive methods to detect these *C. parvum* oocysts.

Morgan et al. (2000b) did a genetic/phylogenetic study of eight dog-derived *Cryptosporidium* isolates from Australia and the United States; two of three Australian dogs were immunosuppressed (one by parvovirus, one by immuno-mediated thrombocytopenia) and shed small numbers of oocysts in their feces, whereas all six US dogs were asymptomatic. *Cryptosporidium* was initially identified by a malachite green negative staining, and PBS–ether sedimentation together with Ficoll gradient centrifugation. PCR amplification and sequencing of 18S rRNA and HSP70 genes and subsequent phylogenetic analyses were then performed. All HSP70 sequences were identical to each other, but genetically distant from other genotypes of *C. parvum*, whereas 18S rDNA sequences were also identical to each other but clustered with *C. parvum*, *C. felis*, and *C. wrairi*. The study supported that the distinct "dog" genotype was conserved across geographic areas and indicated it may represent a valid species.

Denholm et al. (2001) reported a 9-week-old, male Bullmastiff puppy in Australia, with acute parvoviral gastroenteritis and a concurrent active infection with *C. parvum*. The puppy was vomiting, lethargic, dehydrated, and had a fever lasting for 24 hours. At 5 weeks of age it was inoculated with a modified-live vaccine containing canine parvovirus (CPV), distemper, and adenovirus. During the period of treatment, the puppy underwent intensive therapy and was administered a wide variety of chemotherapeutics (lactated Ringer's solution, metoclopramide, amoxicillin–clavulanate, crystalloids, Dextran, butorphanol, ranitidine syrup, amoxicillin, metronidazole, gentamicin, polymeric liquid diet, plasma transfusion, trimethoprim, sulfadoxine, metronidazole, cisapride). Fecal samples were initially negative for parvovirus by TEM, and fecal flotation did not show stages of any intestinal parasites. Ultrasonography revealed dilation of the entire intestines, reduced peristalsis, and multiple enlarged mesenteric lymph nodes. Histological examination demonstrated severe ileal crypt damage with hyperplasia, dilation, and villous atrophy. Numerous spheroidal organisms ≤1 wide were located on the surface of the cryptal epithelium. Later, and concurrently with histological findings, *Cryptosporidium* oocysts were identified in fresh feces stained with a malachite green. PCR amplification and subsequent sequencing of the 18S rRNA gene revealed a sequence that was identical to an isolate obtained from a dog in the United States and not previously recorded in Australia. A serum neutralization test to assess the CPV antibodies showed an increasing nature of high titers, which corresponded to a recent CPV infection. Fecal samples of the owners and veterinary staff were negative. The puppy continued to recover. The cause of gastroenteritis in this case was a CPV infection, exacerbated by a concurrent *Cryptosporidium* infection. *Cryptosporidium* of identical sequence was isolated also from another dog presented to the same veterinary hospital and undergoing immunosuppressive therapy.

Giangaspero et al. (2006) examined fecal samples of dogs (120 kenneled, 120 privately owned) in the Abruzzo region of Teramo province, central Italy. Samples were examined by PCR amplification of the COWP gene. Only 6/240 (2.5%) kenneled dogs were positive for *C. parvum*, whereas no privately-owned dogs tested positive for this parasite. Scorza et al. (2011) examined fecal samples of dogs owned by local people in San Isidro de El General, San Jose province, Costa Rica. Samples were collected directly from the rectum and examined by Sheather's sugar flotation followed by microscopy and IFA (Merifluor *Crypto/Giardia* kit); *Cryptosporidium*-positive samples were genotyped by PCR amplification and sequencing of 18S rDNA and *C. parvum* was detected in 1/60 (2%) samples. Sotiriadou et al. (2013) examined fresh feces of 81 domestic dogs for *Cryptosporidium* in Ludwigsburg, Germany. Samples were examined by sedimentation–flotation followed by nested PCR amplification of the 18S rRNA gene. *Cryptosporidium parvum* was detected in only one sample.

Simonato et al. (2017) examined canine fecal samples collected not from dogs, but in public green (270 samples) and urban (435 samples) areas, Padua municipality, Veneto region, northern Italy. Samples were screened by sedimentation–flotation, followed by nested PCR amplification and sequencing of the 18S rRNA gene. Samples concurrently positive for *Giardia* favored amplification of giardial DNA over the *Cryptosporidium* DNA, so these samples were also examined by a touchdown real-time PCR of the COWP gene. In all, 12/705 (2%) samples were positive for *Cryptosporidium*, 11 identified as "*C. parvum* species complex." Tangtrongsup et al. (2017) examined fecal samples of dogs from a variety of locations and lifestyles in the Chiang Mai province, Thailand. Samples were examined by IFA (Merifluor *Crypto/Giardia* kit) and by PCR amplification of HSP70 and 18S rRNA genes. They found *Cryptosporidium* in 34/109 (31%) samples, mostly in dogs <1-year-old, and were able to generate 22 gene sequences, of which 7 represented *C. parvum*.

CRYPTOSPORIDIUM SCROFARUM KVÁČ, KESTŘÁNOVÁ, PINKOVÁ, KVĚTOŇOVÁ, KALINOVÁ, WAGNEROVÁ, KOTKOVÁ, VÍTOVEC, DITRICH, MCEVOY, STENGER, AND SAK, 2013

Type host: *Sus scrofa* L., 1758, Wild Boar.
Type locality: Europe: Czech Republic, České Budějovice.
Other hosts: *Canis lupus familiaris* (syn. *C. familiaris*) L., 1758, Domestic Dog.
Geographic distribution: Europe: Czech Republic, but may be cosmopolitan.
Remarks: Kváč et al. (2013) described morphological, biological, and molecular characteristics of a *Cryptosporidium* pig genotype II and named it *C. scrofarum* saying it was prevalent in adult pigs worldwide. Its oocysts are nearly identical to those of *C. parvum*, measuring L×W (n=400): 5.2×4.8 (5–6×4–5); L/W ratio: 1.1. Oocysts of *C. scrofarum* obtained from a naturally-infected pig were infectious for 8-week-old pigs (but not 4-week-old pigs) and had a prepatent period of 4–6 days and patency lasted >30 days. Infected pigs showed no clinical signs of cryptosporidiosis. This species was not infective for adult SCID mice, adult BALB/c mice, Mongolian gerbils (*Meriones unguiculatus*), southern multimammate mice (*Mastomys coucha*), yellow-necked mice (*Apodemus flavicollis*), or guinea pigs (*Cavia porcellus*), but Kostopoulou et al. (2017), in Greece (see above), detected *C. scrofarum* in one domestic dog. Kváč et al. (2013) said that their phylogenetic analyses based on 18S rRNA, actin, and HSP70 gene sequences showed *C. scrofarum* to be genetically distinct from all known *Cryptosporidium* species.

CRYPTOSPORIDIUM SPP.

A number of surveys have identified *Cryptosporidium* spp. in the feces of *Canis* spp. (see Chapter 19).

GENUS CHRYSOCYON C.E.H. SMITH, 1839 (MONOTYPIC)

Cryptosporidium oocysts have been found in one maned wolf, *C. brachyurus*, but there was no attempt to name or identify it (see Chapter 19).

GENUS NYCTEREUTES TEMMINCK, 1838 (MONOTYPIC)

NYCTEREUTES PROCYONOIDES (GRAY, 1834), RACCOON DOG

CRYPTOSPORIDIUM CANIS FAYER, TROUT, XIAO, MORGAN, LAL, AND DUBEY, 2001

Type host: *Canis lupus familiaris* (syn. *C. familiaris*) L., 1758, Domestic Dog.
Remarks: Zhang et al. (2016b) examined fresh fecal samples of *N. procyonoides* on a farm in suburban Harbin, northeast China. Amplification and sequencing of the 18S rRNA gene was used to identify the presence of *Cryptosporidium* and the gp60 gene for the genotype determination. *Cryptosporidium canis* was detected in 17/162 (10.5%) samples.

CRYPTOSPORIDIUM PARVUM TYZZER, 1912

Type host: *Mus musculus* (L., 1758), House Mouse.
Remarks: Matsubayashi et al. (2004) examined a fecal sample from an injured wild raccoon dog, *N. p. viverrinus* Temminck, 1838,

hospitalized in the Osaka Municipal Tennoji Zoological Gardens, Japan. Light microscopy and immunofluorescence antibody tests (IFATs) showed the presence of *Cryptosporidium* oocysts. Amplification and sequencing of 18S rRNA, COWP, and HSP70 genes identified these oocysts as *C. parvum* "cattle" genotype. This was the first record of *Cryptosporidium* in a raccoon dog. Later, Matsubayashi et al. (2004) used this isolate for a subsequent "subgenotype" analysis. Sequencing of the gp60 gene demonstrated that this isolate did not correspond to any of the other described cattle subgenotypes, to date.

CRYPTOSPORIDIUM SPP.

A number of surveys have identified *Cryptosporidium* spp. in the feces of *Nyctereutes* spp. (see Chapter 19).

GENUS *VULPES* FRISCH, 1775 (12 SPECIES)

VULPES SPP.

CRYPTOSPORIDIUM CANIS FAYER, TROUT, XIAO, MORGAN, LAL, AND DUBEY, 2001

Type host: *Canis lupus familiaris* (syn. *C. familiaris*) L., 1758, Domestic Dog.

Remarks: Zhou et al. (2004) collected fecal samples from "wild foxes" (presumably *Vulpes*, but the host genus/species was not given) in Maryland, USA, and examined them for *Cryptosporidium* using the RFLP PCR of the 18S rRNA gene and subsequent sequencing. Animals ranged in age from 12-36-months. They said that 6/76 (8%) were positive for *Cryptosporidium*, 4 for *C. canis* fox genotype, 1 individual for *C. canis* dog genotype, and 1 individual for the *Cryptosporidium* muskrat genotype I.

Zhang et al. (2016a) collected fresh fecal samples of farmed *V. lagopus* from farms in northern China (91 from Jilin province, 70 from Heilongjiang province, and 141 from Hebei province). All foxes were asymptomatic for intestinal disease when sampled. Feces were examined by nested PCR amplification and sequencing of the 18S rRNA gene. *Cryptosporidium* was detected in 48/302 (16%) samples including 18/139 (13%) males and 30/163 (18%) females. All 48 positive isolates represented *C. canis*. This was the first report of *C. canis* in *V. lagopus* in China. Zhang et al. (2016a) collected fresh fecal samples from *V. vulpes* on a farm in suburban Harbin, northeast China. Amplification and sequencing of 18S rRNA gene was used for species identification of *Cryptosporidium* and gp60 gene for the genotype determination. *Cryptosporidium canis* was detected in 3/191 (2%) samples.

Mateo et al. (2017) collected fecal samples of *V. vulpes* in four autonomous regions of Spain (Andalusia, Basque Country, Castilla-La Mancha, and Extremadura). They were examined by nested PCR targeting the 18S rRNA gene, followed by genotyping based on the gp60 gene. *Cryptosporidium* was detected in 7/87 (8%) samples; two samples were determined to be *C. canis*. Yang et al. (2017) examined fecal samples of 7- to 8-year-old, clinically healthy, "foxes" (genus/species not given) from the Heilongjiang, Jilin, and Liaoning provinces, northeastern China. Samples were examined by nested PCR amplification of the 18S rRNA gene, and positive samples then subtyped by nested PCR amplification of the gp60 gene; 12/213 (6%) "fox" feces were positive for *Cryptosporidium* and 11 from the Heilongjiang province were all identified as *C. canis*.

CRYPTOSPORIDIUM FELIS ISEKI, 1979

Type host: *Felis catus* L., 1758, Domestic Cat.

Remarks: Mateo et al. (2017) collected fecal samples of *V. vulpes* in four autonomous regions of Spain (Andalusia, Basque Country,

Castilla-La Mancha, and Extremadura). They were examined by the nested PCR targeting the 18S rRNA gene, followed by genotyping based on the gp60 gene. *Cryptosporidium* was detected in 7/87 (8%) samples; 1 sample was determined to be *C. felis*. This was the first molecular finding of *C. felis* in a red fox.

CRYPTOSPORIDIUM PARVUM TYZZER, 1912

Type host: *Mus musculus* (L., 1758), House Mouse.

Remarks: Sturdee et al. (1999) collected fecal samples on the ground, purportedly from wild *V. vulpes*, in Warwickshire, central Britain. Samples were subjected to formol–ether sedimentation, followed by staining in multiwell microscope slides with an anti-*Cryptosporidium* fluorescein isothiocyanate-conjugated MAb and with modified Ziehl–Neelsen stain. They reported finding *C. parvum* in 2/23 (9%) samples and said the median shedding intensity was 3,000 oocysts/g feces. Nagano et al. (2007) collected rectal contents from captured *V. vulpes* in 19 counties in Ireland. Smears were stained with modified Ziehl–Neelsen, examined by LM, and presumptive positive specimens were examined by immunofluorescence microscopy. *Cryptosporidium* was detected in 10/124 (8%) samples, which were genotyped using a nested PCR-RFLP, targeting the 18S rRNA gene; only 2/10 (20%) positive samples were confirmed as *C. parvum*. These two samples were subgenotyped using a nested PCR of the gp60 gene, which identified the presence of *C. parvum* types Ic and II. Mateo et al. (2017) collected fecal samples from *V. vulpes* in four autonomous regions of Spain (Andalusia, Basque Country, Castilla-La Mancha, and Extremadura). They were examined by the nested PCR targeting the 18S rRNA gene, followed by genotyping based on the gp60 gene. *Cryptosporidium* was detected in 7/87 (8%) samples; 3 samples were determined as *C. parvum*.

CRYPTOSPORIDIUM UBIQUITUM FAYER, SANTÍN, AND MACARISN, 2010

Type host: *Coendou prehensilis* (L., 1758), Brazilian Porcupine.

Remarks: Mateo et al. (2017) collected fecal samples of *V. vulpes* in four autonomous regions of Spain (Andalusia, Basque Country, Castilla-La Mancha, and Extremadura). They were examined by the nested PCR targeting the 18S rRNA gene, followed by genotyping based on the gp60 gene. *Cryptosporidium* was detected in 7/87 (8%) samples; 1 sample was determined to be *C. ubiquitum*. This was the first molecular finding of *C. ubiquitum* in a red fox.

CRYPTOSPORIDIUM SPP.

A number of surveys have identified *Cryptosporidium* spp. in the feces of *Vulpes* spp. (see Chapter 19).

FAMILY MEPHITIDAE BONAPARTE, 1845

GENUS MEPHITIS É. GEOFFROY SAINT-HILAIRE AND F.G. CUVIER, 1795 (2 SPECIES)

MEPHITIS MEPHITIS (SCHREBER, 1776), STRIPED SKUNK

CRYPTOSPORIDIUM PARVUM TYZZER, 1912

Type host: *Mus musculus* (L., 1758), House Mouse.

Remarks: Perz and Le Blancq (2001) examined fecal samples of two wild, striped skunks, *M. mephitis*, collected at the Louis Calder Center field station of Fordham University, New York state, USA. Using the amplification of a fragment of the 18S rRNA gene, followed by Southern analysis, they found one individual positive for *C. parvum*. This was the first report of *Cryptosporidium* in a striped skunk.

CRYPTOSPORIDIUM SPP.

A number of surveys have identified *Cryptosporidium* spp. in the feces of *Mephitis* spp. (see Chapter 19).

FAMILY MUSTELIDAE FISCHER, 1817

SUBFAMILY LUTRINAE BONAPARTE, 1838

GENUS LONTRA GRAY, 1843 (4 SPECIES)

LONTRA CANADENSIS (SCHREBER, 1777), NORTH AMERICAN RIVER OTTER

CRYPTOSPORIDIUM PARVUM TYZZER, 1912

Type host: *Mus musculus* (L., 1758), House Mouse.
Remarks: Feng et al. (2007) collected fecal samples from eight wild North American river otters, *L. canadensis*, from the watershed of the New York City drinking water supply (NYCDEP), USA, and examined them for the presence of *Cryptosporidium*. Using RFLP analysis of the 18S rRNA gene, with subsequent sequencing, they detected *Cryptosporidium* skunk genotype W13 in 1/8 (12.5%) samples.

CRYPTOSPORIDIUM SPP.

At least one survey has identified *Cryptosporidium* spp. in the feces of *Lontra* spp. (see Chapter 19).

GENUS LUTRA BRISSON, 1762 (3 SPECIES)

CRYPTOSPORIDIUM SPP.

There are several records of *Cryptosporidium* reported from *Lutra*, but none of them have been identified to species (see Chapter 19).

SUBFAMILY MUSTELINAE FISCHER, 1817

GENUS MARTES PINEL, 1792 (8 SPECIES)

MARTES FOINA (ERXLEBEN, 1777), BEECH MARTEN

CRYPTOSPORIDIUM PARVUM TYZZER, 1912

Type host: *Mus musculus* (L., 1758), House Mouse.
Remarks: Rademacher et al. (1999) reported episodes of diarrhea in four captive beech martens, *M. foina*, one male and three females that were not related to each other. They said they saw numerous *Cryptosporidium* oocysts in the fecal samples that they detected by flotation and in smear preparations that were acid-fast-stained by Ziehl–Neelsen and safranin. Their oocysts (n=30) were L×W: 3.6×3.1 (3–4×3–4); L/W ratio: 1.2, which led them to identify their parasite as *C. parvum*. They also saw a few *Cystoisospora* sp. oocysts in one marten and, therefore, could not say whether the diarrhea was caused by *Cryptosporidium* or by *Cystoisospora*, or both (or neither). Their animals were treated with a 25% solution of sodium sulfamethoxypyridazine and drops of a preparation of vitamins A, D, and E. Diarrhea significantly decreased after 3 days of treatment and disappeared by the end of the treatment period. This was the first record of *Cryptosporidium* in beech martens.

CRYPTOSPORIDIUM SPP.

There are several records of *Cryptosporidium* reported from *Martes*, but none of them have been identified to species (see Chapter 19).

GENUS *MELES* BRISSON, 1762 (3 SPECIES)

MELES MELES (L., 1758), EUROPEAN BADGER

CRYPTOSPORIDIUM HOMINIS MORGAN-RYAN, FALL, WARD, HIJJAWI, SULAIMAN, FAYER, THOMPSON, AND OLSON, 2002

Type host: *Homo sapiens* L., 1758, Humans.
Type locality: Australia: Western Australia: Perth.
Remarks: Mateo et al. (2017) collected fecal samples from *M. meles*, in the Asturias and Castilla-La Mancha regions of Spain, and examined them by the nested PCR targeting the 18S rRNA gene, followed by genotyping based on the gp60 gene. *Cryptosporidium* was detected in 2/70 (3%) samples, both originated from Asturias; 1 was determined to be *C. hominis*. This was the first record of *C. hominis* from a badger.

CRYPTOSPORIDIUM PARVUM TYZZER, 1912

Type host: *Mus musculus* (L., 1758), House Mouse.
Remarks: Sturdee et al. (1999) collected fecal samples from the ground that presumably were deposited by wild European badgers, *M. meles*, in Warwickshire, Britain. Samples were examined using formol–ether sedimentation followed by staining in multiwell microscope slides with an anti-*Cryptosporidium* fluorescein isothiocyanate-conjugated MAb and with modified Ziehl–Neelsen stain. They detected *C. parvum* in 4/26 (15%) samples and said that the

median shedding intensity was 3,000 oocysts/g feces. Mateo et al. (2017) collected fecal samples from *M. meles*, in the Asturias and Castilla-La Mancha regions of Spain, and examined them by the nested PCR targeting the 18S rRNA gene, followed by genotyping based on the gp60 gene. *Cryptosporidium* was detected in 2/70 (3%) samples, both originated from Asturias; 1 was determined to be *C. parvum*.

GENUS *MUSTELA* L., 1758 (17 SPECIES)

MUSTELA PUTORIUS FURO L., 1758, DOMESTIC FERRET

CRYPTOSPORIDIUM PARVUM TYZZER, 1912

Type host: *Mus musculus* (L., 1758), House Mouse.
Remarks: Abe and Iseki (2003) examined the genotypes of *C. parvum* isolates obtained from three ferrets in a pet shop in Kanazawa, Japan. They PCR-amplified and directly sequenced the COWP and HSP70 genes. Their sequences clustered within the *C. parvum* ferret genotype. The ferrets did not show any visible clinical symptoms of infection.

MUSTELA ERMINEA L., 1758, ERMINE

CRYPTOSPORIDIUM PARVUM TYZZER, 1912

Type host: *Mus musculus* (L., 1758), House Mouse.
Remarks: Feng et al. (2007) examined a fecal sample of one ermine, *M. erminea* from the watershed of the NYCDEP, USA, for *Cryptosporidium* spp. Using the 18S rDNA and RFLP analysis followed by sequencing, they detected the presence of *Cryptosporidium parvum* ermine genotype (syn. genotype W18) in the sample.

CRYPTOSPORIDIUM SPP.

There are several records of *Cryptosporidium* reported from *Mustela*, but none of them have been identified to species (see Chapter 19).

GENUS NEOVISON BARYSHNIKOV AND ABRAMOV, 1997 (2 SPECIES)

NEOVISON VISON (SCHREBER, 1777), AMERICAN MINK

CRYPTOSPORIDIUM ANDERSONI LINDSAY, UPTON, OWENS, MORGAN, MEAD, AND BLACKBURN, 2000

Type host: *Bos taurus* L., 1758, Aurochs.
Remarks: Stuart et al. (2013) collected fecal samples from *N. vison* from Ireland and used nested PCR (according to Xiao et al., 1999a,b, 2001) to type the *Cryptosporidium* species found. *Cryptosporidium* was detected in 5/81 (6%) samples: 4 corresponded to *C. andersoni*, 1 to *Cryptosporidium* (*parvum*?) mink genotype, and amplification of 1 sample failed.

CRYPTOSPORIDIUM CANIS FAYER, TROUT, XIAO, MORGAN, LAL, AND DUBEY, 2001

Type host: *Canis lupus familiaris* (syn. *C. familiaris*) L., 1758, Domestic Dog.
Remarks: Zhang et al. (2016b) saved fresh fecal samples of *N. vison* on a farm in suburban Harbin, northeast China. Amplification and sequencing of the 18S rRNA gene was used to identify *Cryptosporidium* and the gp60 gene for the genotype determination. *Cryptosporidium* was detected in 48/162 (30%) samples, all originating from young minks aged 5- to 6-month-old,

and *C. canis*, *C. meleagridis*, and 3 novel subtype families (Xb, Xc, and Xd) of the *Cryptosporidium* mink genotype were recorded. Yang et al. (2017) also examined fecal samples of "minks" (again, genus/species not given) from the same provinces and 8/114 (7%) minks from Jilin province were positive for *Cryptosporidium*; 6/8 (75%) were identified as *C. canis*.

CRYPTOSPORIDIUM MELEAGRIDIS SLAVIN, 1955

Type host: *Meleagris gallopavo* L., 1758, Common Turkey.
Remarks: Zhang et al. (2016b) collected fresh fecal samples of 162 *N. vison* on a farm in suburban Harbin, northeast China; they were processed, as above, and *C. meleagridis* was one of the species identified in their samples.

CRYPTOSPORIDIUM PARVUM TYZZER, 1912

Type host: *Mus musculus* (L., 1758), House Mouse.
Remarks: Feng et al. (2007) collected fecal samples from four American minks from the watershed of the NYCDEP, USA, and examined them for the presence of *Cryptosporidium*. Using the 18S rDNA and RFLP analysis with subsequent sequencing, they detected *Cryptosporidium* in 1/4 (25%) samples, which they said represented a new genotype, the mink genotype. Gómez-Couso et al. (2007) harvested fecal samples of wild and farmed *N. vison* in Galicia, Spain: 33 samples at 2 farms in Coruña, Galicia, Spain, and 18 samples of wild individuals from river and stream banks in Galicia. They said 8/33 (24%) of the farmed animals were positive for *Cryptosporidium* oocysts by the direct IFAT and these oocysts measured 4.5–5.5. PCR-RFLP followed by sequencing of the COWP gene revealed that their form was most

closely related to *C. parvum* "ferret" genotype, differing only in one nucleotide. The positive animals were healthy, not showing any clinical symptoms. *Cryptosporidium* was not detected in any of the samples from wild animals. Wang et al. (2008) collected fecal samples from 469 *N. vison* on a farm in Hebei province in China. Using flotation/centrifugation, eight samples were *Cryptosporidium* positive. Six of the eight positive samples were successfully amplified and sequenced for 18S rRNA, HSP70, COWP, and actin genes. *Cryptosporidium* mink genotype was detected in all six samples. The authors suggested that the "ferret genotype" identified in Spain, by Gómez-Couso et al. (2007) may, in fact, also represent the *Cryptosporidium* mink genotype. Yang et al. (2017) also examined fecal samples of "minks" (again, genus/species not given) from the same provinces in China (see under *C. canis*), and 8/114 (7%) minks from Jilin province were positive for *Cryptosporidium*; 2/8 (25%) were identified as "*Cryptosporidium* mink genotype."

CRYPTOSPORIDIUM UBIQUITUM FAYER, SANTÍN, AND MACARISN, 2010

Type host: *Coendou prehensilis* (L., 1758), Brazilian Porcupine.

Remarks: Kellnerová et al. (2017) collected fecal samples of 300 farmed, adult *N. vison* in the Czech Republic and Poland; the minks originated from six farms, four in the Czech Republic and two in Poland, and all animals were in good health. Fecal samples were examined using the aniline–carbol–methyl violet staining method, followed by nested PCR of the 18S rRNA and actin genes, and subtyping by the gp60 gene. No oocysts were found microscopically, but three samples were positive by their molecular methods and identified as *C. ubiquitum* XIIa subtype family, which was previously restricted only to humans and ruminants.

This was the first description of this subtype in farmed fur animals.

CRYPTOSPORIDIUM SPP.

There are several records of *Cryptosporidium* reported from *Neovison*, but none of them have been identified to species (see Chapter 19).

FAMILY OTARIIDAE GRAY, 1825

GENUS ARCTOCEPHALUS É. GEOFFROY SAINT-HILAIRE AND F.G. CUVIER, 1826 (8 SPECIES)

ARCTOCEPHALUS GAZELLA (PETERS, 1875), ANTARCTIC FUR SEALS

Several attempts have been made to find *Cryptosporidium* in the feces of Antarctic fur seals, *A. gazella*, from the Antarctic Peninsula, but all 276 samples examined in two studies did not detect any *Cryptosporidium* using a variety of microscopic and molecular techniques (Rengifo-Herrera et al., 2011, 2013).

GENUS NEOPHOCA GRAY, 1866 (MONOTYPIC)

NEOPHOCA CINEREA (PÉRON, 1816), AUSTRALIAN SEA LIONS

Using nested PCR amplification of the 18S rRNA gene, Delport et al. (2014) tried to find *Cryptosporidium* in 290 fecal samples of endangered Australian sea lions, *N. cinerea*, in both wild and captive populations of Australia, but the parasite was not detected.

GENUS *OTARIA* PÉRON, 1816 (MONOTYPIC)

OTARIA FLAVESCENS (SHAW, 1800), SOUTH AMERICAN SEA LION

Cryptosporidium sp. has been identified from 10 *O. flavescens*, but no species determination was made (see Chapter 19).

GENUS *ZALOPHUS* GILL, 1866 (3 SPECIES)

ZALOPHUS CALIFORNIANUS (LESSON, 1828), CALIFORNIA SEA LION

CRYPTOSPORIDIUM PARVUM TYZZER, 1912

Type host: *Mus musculus* (L., 1758), House Mouse.

Remarks: Deng et al. (2000) examined fecal samples of California sea lions in northern California, USA, and detected *Cryptosporidium* oocysts, morphologically indistinguishable from those of *C. parvum*, in 3/6 (50%) individuals from Humboldt Bay. The *Cryptosporidium* oocysts were recognized by indirect IFA and confirmed by direct IFA. Genetically, the oocysts had 98% identity with sequences of *C. parvum* isolated from calves. Thus, based on morphological, immunological, and genetic characterization, they identified it as *C. parvum* and the first report of *Cryptosporidium* in a pinniped.

CRYPTOSPORIDIUM SPP.

There are several records of *Cryptosporidium* reported from *Zalophus*, but none of them have been identified to species (see Chapter 19).

FAMILY PHOCIDAE GRAY, 1821

GENUS *CYSTOPHORA* NILSSON, 1820 (MONOTYPIC)

CYSTOPHORA CRISTATA (ERXLEBEN, 1777), HOODED SEALS

Appelbee et al. (2010) screened feces and small intestine tissues of 10 hooded seals, *C. cristata*, from the Gulf of St. Lawrence, Québec, Canada, and used nested PCR to amplify the HSP70 gene, but *Cryptosporidium* was not detected in any samples. However, Bass et al. (2012) did identify oocysts in one hooded seal (see Chapter 19).

GENUS *ERIGNATHUS* GILL, 1866 (MONOTYPIC)

ERIGNATHUS BARBATUS (ERXLEBEN, 1777), BEARDED SEALS

Hughes-Hanks et al. (2005) examined fecal samples of 22 bearded seals, *E. barbatus*, from northern Alaska near Barrow, using the IFA, Santín et al. (2005) examined intestinal contents of 5 *E. barbatus* from Nunavik, Québec, Canada, and Dixon (2008) examined gut samples from 4 *E. barbatus*, also from Nunavik, but none of these authors were able to detect *Cryptosporidium* in any of the samples.

GENUS *HALICHOERUS* NILSSON, 1820 (MONOTYPIC)

HALICHOERUS GRYPUS (FABRICIUS, 1791), GRAY SEALS

Bass et al. (2012) examined fecal samples of two gray seals, *H. grypus*, from Biddeford, Maine, USA, using a nested PCR amplification and sequencing the 18S rRNA and HSP70 genes, but could not detect *Cryptosporidium* in either sample.

GENUS *HYDRURGA* GISTEL, 1848 (MONOTYPIC)

HYDRURGA LEPTONYX (DE BLAINVILLE, 1820), LEOPARD SEALS

Rengifo-Herrera et al. (2011) examined feces from four leopard seals, *H. leptonyx*, from the Antarctic Peninsula, using immunofluorescence microscopy and PCR amplification of the 18S rRNA and HSP70 genes, but could not detect *Cryptosporidium* in any of them.

GENUS *LEPTONYCHOTES* GILL, 1872 (MONOTYPIC)

LEPTONYCHOTES WEDDELLII (LESSON, 1826), WEDDELL SEALS

Rengifo-Herrera et al. (2011) examined fecal samples of 31 Weddell seals, *L. weddellii*, from the Antarctic Peninsula, using immunofluorescence microscopy and PCR amplification of the 18S rRNA and HSP70 genes, but could not detect *Cryptosporidium* in any of the samples. Later, Rengifo-Herrera et al. (2013) did identify some oocysts in two Weddell seals (see Chapter 19).

GENUS *LOBODON* GRAY, 1844 (MONOTYPIC)

LOBODON CARCINOPHAGA (HOMBRON AND JACKQUINOT, 1842), CRABEATER SEALS

Rengifo-Herrera et al. (2011) examined fecal samples of two crabeater seals, *L. carcinophaga*, from the Antarctic Peninsula, using immunofluorescence microscopy and PCR amplification of the 18S rRNA and HSP70 genes, but could not detect *Cryptosporidium* in either of the samples.

GENUS *MIROUNGA* GRAY, 1827 (2 SPECIES)

MIROUNGA ANGUSTIROSTRIS (GILL, 1866), NORTHERN ELEPHANT SEALS

Deng et al. (2000) examined fecal samples of eight northern elephant seals, *M. angustirostris*, in the northern California coastal area, USA. Using an indirect IFA, *Cryptosporidium* was not detected in any of the samples.

CRYPTOSPORIDIUM SPP.

There are several records of *Cryptosporidium* reported from *Mirounga*, but none of them have been identified to species (see Chapter 19).

GENUS *PAGOPHILUS* GRAY, 1844 (MONOTYPIC)

PAGOPHILUS GROENLANDICUS (ERXLEBEN, 1777), HARP SEALS

Appelbee et al. (2010) screened feces and small intestine tissues of 58 harp seals, *P. groenlandicus*, from the Gulf of St. Lawrence, Québec, Canada. Fecal samples were examined by microscopy and immunofluorescent staining. Tissues from the small intestine (duodenum, jejunum, and ileum) of 38 adult harp seals were examined using the nested PCR technique amplifying the HSP70. *Cryptosporidium* was not detected in any of the samples.

CRYPTOSPORIDIUM SPP.

There are several records of *Cryptosporidium* reported from *Pagophilus*, but none of them have been identified to species (see Chapter 19).

GENUS PHOCA L., 1758
(2 SPECIES)

PHOCA HISPIDA (SCHREBER, 1775), RINGED SEALS

Dixon et al. (2008) reported a *Cryptosporidium* sp. in 2/42 (5%) ringed seals, *P. hispida*, in northern Québec, Canada, but no further identification was made.

PHOCA VITULINA RICHARDII (GRAY, 1864), PACIFIC HARBOR SEALS

Deng et al. (2000) examined fecal samples of 13 Pacific harbor seals, *P. v. richardii*, on the northern California coast, Gaydos et al. (2008) examined fecal samples of 97 harbor seals from Washington state's inland marine waters, and Hueffer et al. (2011) examined fecal samples of 33 *P. vitulina* in Glacier Bay National Park (John Hopkins Inlet and Spider Reef), Alaska, USA, using various techniques; *Cryptosporidium* was not detected in any of their samples.

CRYPTOSPORIDIUM SPP.

There are several records of *Cryptosporidium* reported from *Phoca*, but none of them have been identified to species (see Chapter 19).

GENUS PUSA SCOPOLI, 1771
(3 SPECIES)

PUSA HISPIDA (SCHREBER, 1775), RINGED SEAL

CRYPTOSPORIDIUM MURIS (TYZZER, 1907) TYZZER, 1910

Type host: *Mus musculus* L., 1758, House Mouse.
Remarks: Santín et al. (2005) examined intestinal contents of 55 *P. hispida* from Nunavik,

Québec, Canada. Using PCR amplification of fragments of the 18S rRNA gene, they detected 10/55 (18%) seals positive for *Cryptosporidium*. PCR amplification of fragments of the HSP70 and actin genes showed four and two seals, respectively, positive for *Cryptosporidium*. They reported that three distinct genotypes were present: *C. muris*, *Cryptosporidium* sp. seal-1, and *Cryptosporidium* sp. seal-2. Years earlier, Olson et al. (1997) had sampled feces from 15 ringed seals in the western Arctic region of Canada, but they did not detect *Cryptosporidium* in their samples.

CRYPTOSPORIDIUM SPP.

There are several records of *Cryptosporidium* reported from *Pusa*, but none of them have been identified to species (see Chapter 19).

FAMILY PROCYONIDAE GRAY, 1825

GENUS PROCYON STORR, 1780
(3 SPECIES)

PROCYON LOTOR (L., 1758), RACCOON

CRYPTOSPORIDIUM PARVUM TYZZER, 1912

Type host: *Mus musculus* (L., 1758), House Mouse.
Remarks: Snyder (1988) surveyed fecal samples from 100 wild *P. lotor* in Central Illinois, USA, using an indirect immunofluorescent detection procedure and reported 13/100 (13%) had oocysts of *C. parvum*, all from juveniles. Perz and Le Blancq (2001) examined five fecal samples of *P. lotor*, collected at the Louis Calder Center field station, Fordham University, New York state, USA. They amplified a fragment of the 18S rRNA gene

and reported 1/5 (20%) to be infected with *C. parvum*. Chavez et al. (2012) examined fecal samples of 44 *P. lotor* in eastern Colorado, USA, using the direct fluorescent antibody detection and found *Cryptosporidium* in 11/44 (25%) samples. Sequencing the 18S rRNA gene was successful in only 6 of the 11 positive samples: 5 were homologous with *Cryptosporidium* skunk genotype and 1 with *C. parvum*.

CRYPTOSPORIDIUM SPP.

There are several records of *Cryptosporidium* reported from *Procyon*, but none of them have been identified to species (see Chapter 19).

FAMILY URSIDAE FISCHER DE WALDHEIM, 1817

GENUS *AILUROPODA* MILNE-EDWARDS, 1870 (MONOTYPIC)

AILUROPODA MELANOLEUCA (DAVID, 1869), GIANT PANDA

CRYPTOSPORIDIUM ANDERSONI LINDSAY, UPTON, OWENS, MORGAN, MEAD, AND BLACKBURN, 2000

Type host: *Bos taurus* L., 1758, Aurochs.

Remarks: Wang et al. (2015a) examined fecal samples of 322 giant pandas, *A. melanoleuca*, (122 captive, 200 free-ranging) from 4 habitats in Sichuan, China, for the presence of *Cryptosporidium*. Feces were examined using PCR and sequencing and analyses of the 18S rRNA gene. They found 19/122 (16%) of the captive and 1/200 (0.5%) of the wild-living pandas to be positive for *C. andersoni*. It was found across all gender and age groups in the captive pandas, being more frequent

in females (15/73; 20.5%) than males (4/49; 8%). This was the first report of *C. andersoni* in the giant panda. Given the fact that *C. andersoni* can infect humans under certain circumstances, the infections in captive pandas should be considered as a public health concern, particularly for breeders, veterinarians, and zoo workers.

CRYPTOSPORIDIUM SPP.

There are several records of *Cryptosporidium* reported from *Ailuropoda*, but none of them have been identified to species (see Chapter 19).

GENUS *HELARCTOS* HORSFIELD, 1825 (MONOTYPIC)

An unidentified *Cryptosporidium* species was found in two sun bears in Taiwan and in one sun bear in Egypt (see Chapter 19), but not in two *H. malayanus* in Japan (see Matsubayashi et al., 2005).

GENUS *URSUS* L., 1758 (4 SPECIES)

URSUS AMERICANUS PALLAS, 1780, AMERICAN BLACK BEAR

CRYPTOSPORIDIUM PARVUM TYZZER, 1912

Type host: *Mus musculus* (L., 1758), House Mouse.

Remarks: Duncan et al. (1999) examined a male American black bear cub, *U. americanus*, found dead in Rockingham County, Virginia, USA. Selected tissue samples were fixed in 10% buffered formalin and processed for histology.

In several sections, small round basophilic bodies, ~2–3 wide, were seen on the apical surfaces of enterocytes in the intestine and were identified as *C. parvum*. Other sections of small intestine were examined using rabbit anti-*C. parvum* antisera (1:500 dilution) and the avidin–biotin peroxidase complex immunohistological test. Stages in the bear's intestine reacted positively with the rabbit anti-*C. parvum* rabbit serum, which confirmed their identification; *Cryptosporidium* stages were not seen in hepatic lesions. The bear cub was infected with other parasites (nematodes) and was dehydrated due to a secondary bacterial-induced colitis; the authors regarded cryptosporidiosis as incidental. A year later, Xiao et al. (2000) characterized the isolate of Duncan et al. (1999) genetically using the sequences of 18S rRNA and HSP70 genes. They discovered that this parasite represented a new genotype of *C. parvum*, which was related to the *C. parvum* dog genotype, to support the hypothesis of the presence of several distinct host-adapted strains of *C. parvum*. Because *C. parvum* dog genotype has already been found in humans, it is important to consider the role of bears as reservoirs of *Cryptosporidium* and their zoonotic potential. Feng et al. (2007) and Ziegler et al. (2007) examined six fecal samples of wild *U. americanus* from New York City, USA, but *Cryptosporidium* was not detected. *Cryptosporidium* also was not detected in the fecal samples from three polar bears, *Ursus maritimus* Phipps, 1774, in a zoo in Osaka, Japan (Matsubayashi et al., 2005), but a *Cryptosporidium* sp. was reported from a polar bear in a zoo in Egypt (Siam et al., 1994, see Chapter 19).

CRYPTOSPORIDIUM SPP.

There are several other records of *Cryptosporidium* reported from *Ursus*, but none of them have been identified to species (see Chapter 19).

SUBORDER FELIFORMIA KRETZOI, 1945

FAMILY FELIDAE FISCHER DE WALDHEIM, 1817

SUBFAMILY FELINAE FISCHER DE WALDHEIM, 1817

GENUS ACINONYX BROOKES, 1828 (MONOTYPIC)

Siam et al. (1994) is the only report we know of that documents a *Cryptosporidium* sp. from a cheetah, *A. jubatus*, in a zoo in Egypt (see Chapter 19).

GENUS *FELIS* L., 1758 (7 SPECIES)

FELIS CATUS L., 1758, DOMESTIC CAT

CRYPTOSPORIDIUM FELIS ISEKI, 1979

Type host: *Felis catus* L., 1758, Domestic Cat.
Type locality: Asia: Japan: Osaka City.
Other hosts: *Homo sapiens* L., 1758, Humans (Lewis et al., 1985 and many others, see references under *Geographic distribution*); *Equus caballus* L., 1758, Horses (Guo et al., 2014); *Bos taurus* L., 1758, Aurochs (Bornay-Llinares et al. 1999; Cardona et al., 2015); *Vulpes vulpes* (L., 1758), Red Fox; *Mytilus* spp., Mussels (Miller et al., 2005).
Geographic distribution: Africa: Ethiopia; Kenya; Nigeria; Asia: China; India; Indonesia; Japan; Malaysia; Taiwan; Thailand; Australia; Eastern Europe: Czech Republic; Poland; Caribbean: Haiti; Jamaica; Western Europe: France; Portugal; Spain; Sweden; Switzerland; The Netherlands; The United Kingdom (England, Wales); North America: USA: California; South America: Brazil;

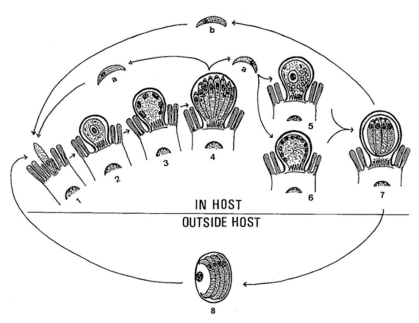

FIGURE 17.1   Line drawing of the life cycle of *Cryptosporidium felis*. *Fig. 1 from Iseki, M.M., 1979*. Cryptosporidium felis *sp. n. (Protozoa: Eimeriorina) from the domestic cat. Japanese Journal of Parasitology 28 (5), 285–307, with permission of JJP, copyright holder. 1. Zoite penetrating intestinal epithelial cell; 2. Fully grown trophozoite; 3. Meront with 6 N; 4. Mature meront with 8 merozoites; 5. Young microgametocyte; 6. Young macrogametocyte; 7. Mature oocyst with 4 SZ; 8. Oocyst in feces; a. Merozoites; b. SZ released from mature oocyst.*

Peru (Pieniazek et al., 1999; Morgan et al., 2000a; Alves et al., 2001; Guyot et al., 2001; Xiao et al., 2001; Gatei et al., 2002, 2006, 2007, 2008; Tiangtip and Jongwutiwes, 2002; Cama et al., 2003, 2006, 2007, 2008; Ryan et al., 2003; Matos et al., 2004; Das et al., 2006; Leoni et al., 2006; Llorente et al., 2006, 2007; Muthusamy et al., 2006; Priest et al., 2006; Raccurt et al., 2006; Ajjampur et al., 2007; Hung et al., 2007; Raccurt, 2007; Wielinga et al., 2008; Chalmers et al., 2009, 2011; Lucca et al., 2009; Lim et al., 2011; Wang et al., 2011; Cieloszyk et al., 2012; Elwin et al., 2012; Gherasim et al., 2012; Akinbo et al., 2013; Insulander et al., 2013; Kurniawan et al., 2013; Abal-Fabeiro et al., 2014; Adamu et al., 2014; Asma et al., 2015; Ebner et al., 2015; Mbae et al., 2015; de Lucio et al., 2016; Ukwah et al., 2017).

Description of sporulated oocyst: Oocyst shape: ellipsoidal; number of walls, 1; wall characteristics: thin, smooth, colorless, with no protrusions on its surface; L×W: 5×4.5; L/W ratio: 1.1;

M: absent; OR: round, ~1 wide, not granular; PG (?): an electron-dense, crystalline inclusion of nearly equilateral triangle was reported in the residual cytoplasm of the developing oocyst (Iseki, 1979). Distinctive features of oocyst: a typical cryptosporidial oocyst, small size, no sporocysts, containing four SZ, apparently without a longitudinal suture, but with an electron-dense crystalline body among the SZ.

Description of sporozoites: Four C-shaped or banana-shaped SZs occur within each oocyst; L×W: 4–5×1, each with a prominent N in the anterior or posterior portion; the line drawing showed SZ lined up next to each other along one side of oocyst, tightly enclosing the OR (Fig. 1, Iseki, 1979).

Prevalence: Iseki (1979) found this species in 5/13 (38%) domestic cats living with their owners in Osaka, Japan. Three of the infected cats were 1-month-old littermates and the other two were adults; all of the noninfected cats were adults and were later used for transmission experiments. Palmer et al. (2008a) surveyed fecal samples of cats from both urban and rural areas across Australia, which were collected from 59 veterinary clinics (572 samples) and 26 refuges (491 samples). Samples were examined by saturated salt and D-glucose centrifugation–flotation methods and malachite green staining. *Cryptosporidium* was detected in 23/1,063 (2%) cats, mostly from refuges. Yamamoto et al. (2009) surveyed fecal samples of cats in public animal shelters in Saitama Prefecture, Japan. Microscopic examination revealed the presence of *C. felis* oocysts in 30/1,079 (3%) of the samples. Ito et al. (2017) surveyed fecal samples of household cats in different regions in Japan (Hokkaido/Tohoku, Kanto, Kinki, Kyushu/Okinawa) and kittens from four pet shops in Kanto and Tohoku, Japan. Samples were examined by the nested PCR amplification of the 18S rRNA gene and subsequent sequencing; 7/357 (2%) household and 1/329 (0.3%) pet shop cats were positive for *Cryptosporidium*, all identified as *C. felis* (99%–100% similarity). Most positive cats were <1-year-old, without diarrhea, and lived outdoors.

Sporulation: Sporulation occurred endogenously, releasing sporulated oocysts in the feces. Iseki (1979) pointed out that oocyst formation and sporogony both take place in the parasitophorous vacuole (PV) within the microvillus.

Prepatent and patent period: Prepatency was reported to be 5–6 days and patency 7–10 days (Iseki, 1979).

Site of infection: Intracellular, but extracytoplasmic within the microvilli of intestinal epithelial cells and goblet cells. Although the parasites were distributed all over the surface of intestinal villi, they seemed to be more prevalent in and near the tips. They were neither found in the lamina propria or in the crypts in the small intestine nor were they ever found in cells of the stomach, cecum, and colon.

Endogenous stages: These were found throughout the small intestine, but meronts and oocysts were more numerous in the lower levels than in the upper and middle levels. Trophozoites (both SZ and merozoites) became an ovoidal or spheroidal body, $\sim 2 \times 1$, with a conspicuous N, within the PV after invading the microvillus of an epithelial cell. Shortly after penetrating the microvillus layer, the sporozoites or merozoites formed an attachment organ composed of many membranous folds at the site on which the parasite came in contact with the host cell cytoplasm. Mature meronts, 4–5 wide, were spheroidal and contained 8 banana-shaped merozoites, each $\sim 5 \times 1$, which were formed by external budding. Merozoites released from the microvilli then invaded other microvilli to form other meronts. The number of times this can be repeated is unknown, but in one of Iseki's naturally-infected cats, oocysts were observed in the feces for at least 5 months, although later in very small numbers and shedding was discontinuous. Developing macrogametes were ~ 4–5 wide, with a large number of refractile granules in their cytoplasm. Microgametocytes also were 4–5 wide and produced ~ 14–16 microgametes, which had no recognizable flagella. After fertilization both oocyst formation and sporulation occurred in the PV of the microvillus. Iseki (1979) also stated that SZ were sometimes seen escaping from mature oocysts in the microvilli, and these could lead to autoinfection in the small intestine.

Cross-transmission: Iseki (1979) infected 4 adult cats (Nos. 1–4) with 5×10^5 oocysts; 3/4 (75%) (Nos. 2–4) discharged oocysts, whereas 3/4 (Nos. 1–3) had endogenous stages in their small intestines. Iseki (1979) also fed mucosal scrapings from infected cats to two other adult cats (Nos. 5, 6); cat No. 6 discharged oocysts in its feces and both cats had endogenous stages of *C. felis* in their small intestines when killed. Iseki (1979) also infected three mice (ICR strain, 7-week-old females) and three guinea pigs (Hartley strain, 180–200 g in weight males) with 5×10^4 oocysts, but none of them discharged oocysts nor could Iseki find endogenous stages in their intestines when each of the three mice and guinea pigs was sacrificed at 7, 14, and 21 DPI.

Pathology: The cats infected with *C. felis* did not show any clinical signs of diarrhea or debilitation (Iseki, 1979).

Materials deposited: The holotype and paratype specimens were provisionally preserved in the laboratory at the Department of Medical Zoology, Osaka City University Medical School, Osaka, Japan, but no accession numbers were given by Iseki (1979).

Remarks: Iseki (1979), in Japan, first described the oocysts, endogenous stages, host specificity, and pathogenicity of a *Cryptosporidium* in cats and named it *C. felis*. Sporulated oocysts did not infect mice, rats, guinea pigs, or dogs, but they did infect cats, and a cow was infected, based on oocyst gene sequence data (Bornay-Llinares et al., 1999), from the same laboratory that reported the feline genotype (Sargent et al., 1998). Oocysts with the same genotype also were identified as *C. felis* (Morgan et al., 1998), helping to validate the species. Although the validity of the species continued to be discussed for several years, molecular characterization of several markers (18S rRNA, ITS1, HSP70, COWP, actin) conclusively supported its designation as a legitimate species (Sargent et al., 1998; Morgan et al., 1998; Xiao et al., 2004; Plutzer and Karanis, 2009; Fayer, 2010). Here we will reconstruct some of the early history of *C. felis* after it was named by Iseki (1979).

Bennett et al. (1985) found three 4- to 6-month-old cats, in Neston, England, to be positive for *Cryptosporidium*. One cat had a history of diarrhea, inappetence, weight loss, and dehydration and had to be euthanized, the second cat was asymptomatic, and the third was hospitalized with persistent diarrhea. Oocysts of *Cryptosporidium* were detected by flotation in modified Sheather's sucrose/phenol solution, in fecal smears stained with safranin and methylene blue, and by histology or biopsy that revealed endogenous stages of *Cryptosporidium* in the small intestine. One diarrheic cat was concurrently infected with *Feline calicivirus* the second with *Campylobacter*. The owner of the asymptomatic cat, a boy undergoing an immunosuppressive treatment for leukemia,

also discharged *Cryptosporidium* oocysts in his feces; however, it was impossible to conclude whether one infected the other or if both got infected from a common source. Lewis et al. (1985) described a mild case of recurring cryptosporidiosis in a 5.5-year-old boy on immunosuppressive maintenance treatment for acute lymphoblastic leukemia. While on treatment, and in hematological remission, the boy suffered from diarrhea, nausea, and anorexia. Similar symptoms appeared in both parents and a sister; although symptoms rapidly resolved in family members, they continued in the boy for 4 weeks, with profuse diarrhea, intermittent vomiting, and >10% weight loss. Bacterial and viral stool cultures of all family members were negative, but the boy's stool samples, stained with safranin–methylene blue, revealed *Cryptosporidium* oocysts. Jejunal biopsy showed *Cryptosporidium* trophozoites in both LM of Giemsa-stained sections and via TEM. The family had obtained a kitten, 2 weeks before the onset of symptoms, and the kitten suffered from occasional diarrhea; *Cryptosporidium* oocysts were found in its feces. Immunosuppressive drugs were discontinued in the boy, and when he was treated with nalidixic acid (quinolone antibiotic), symptoms resolved, and no oocysts were found in his stools 45 days after diagnosis. However, after restarting immunosuppressive treatment, a second episode of watery diarrhea occurred, and *Cryptosporidium* oocysts again were detected in his stools. Improvement, with the subsequent disappearance of oocysts, was detected again after discontinuation of the immunosuppressive treatment and beginning nalidixic acid treatment. The kitten also discharged *Cryptosporidium* oocysts again in its feces, so it was removed from the home. It is likely the boy became infected from the family kitten, and that the parasite was likely *C. felis*.

Sargent et al. (1998) surveyed fecal samples of domestic cats in the metropolitan area of Perth, Western Australia. Samples were examined by a malachite green background staining, PCR amplification of the 18S rRNA gene, and phylogenetic analyses. *Cryptosporidium* was detected in 2/162 (1%) samples by both LM and PCR. Both infected cats were females <1.5-year-old, and both were asymptomatic. Oocysts were L×W (n=40): 4.6×4.0 (3–5×3–4); L/W: 1.1 and were significantly smaller than those isolated from human samples (L×W: 5.0×4.5). Sequences from both samples were identical, and significantly different from those previously sequenced from humans and calves in 17bp positions, an 8% sequence divergence. Phylogenetic analyses placed both sequences obtained from cats into a distinct group separated from *C. parvum* isolates and other *Cryptosporidium* species. Sargent et al. (1998) suggested this *Cryptosporidium* to be a cat-adapted strain or species, but at that time, they doubted the validity of *C. felis* as a distinct species. Morgan et al. (1998), at Murdoch University, Australia, found *Cryptosporidium* oocysts in a 2-year-old male longhair cat with a history of diarrhea. Its feces were examined by PBS–ether sedimentation and Ficoll gradient centrifugation, followed by PCR amplification of the 18S rRNA gene with subsequent sequencing and phylogenetic analysis. Oocysts were similar in size and of an identical sequence to the isolates by Sargent et al. (1998). The cat was feline immunodeficiency virus (FIV) positive and, thus, immunosuppressed. Fecal samples of the owners, a second cat and a dog in the household, were negative for *Cryptosporidium* both by LM and PCR. Experimental inoculation of oocysts from the cat to 6-day-old nude mice failed. Later, fecal samples of three other domestic cats with bloody diarrhea, presented to the Veterinary Clinic at Murdoch University, were examined and identical sequences of *Cryptosporidium* were recorded. Thus, all 18S rRNA sequences obtained by Morgan et al. (1998) from cats were identical, distinctly different from other *Cryptosporidium* species, and all likely were *C. felis*. Later, Morgan et al. (2000a) reported the presence of *C. felis* in stool samples of HIV-infected people (three in Zurich, Switzerland, three from the United States) based on amplification and sequencing of

the 18S rRNA and HSP70 genes. All the patients suffered from chronic diarrhea and had very low CD4 lymphocyte counts; 3/6 (50%) *C. felis*-positive individuals had cats as a pet. Thus, they may have acquired their infection from their cats.

In Portugal, Alves et al. (2001) surveyed isolates from HIV-infected patients and 20 animals including 1 cat, for the presence of *Cryptosporidium*. Isolates were examined by water–ether sedimentation and by nested PCR-RFLP of 18S rRNA, COWP, thrombospondin-related adhesive protein of *Cryptosporidium*-1, and dihydrofolate reductase genes; *C. felis* was detected in the only cat tested. Ryan et al. (2003) examined fecal samples of humans and other animals in the Czech Republic, during a survey on *Cryptosporidium* species and genotypes and their host ranges. Using routine coprological methods, nested PCR, and sequencing of 18S rRNA and HSP70 genes, followed by phylogenetic analyses, they found *C. felis* in fecal samples of two domestic cats, but they did not give the total number of cats examined. Hajdušek et al. (2004) examined one cat fecal sample for *Cryptosporidium* in the Czech Republic. Using LM, amplification of the 18S rRNA, and COWP genes, and subsequent phylogenetic analyses, they identified *C. felis* in the sample; the oocysts measured L×W: 4.6×4.2; L/W ratio: 1.1.

Fayer et al. (2006) examined fecal samples of 18 mixed-breed, 3- to 6-month-old domestic cats in a closed cat colony; each cat was housed in a separate cage. Feces of each cat were examined daily via sucrose flotation. After 4 weeks, oocysts of *Cryptosporidium* were detected in two cats by LM. For the next 21 days, feces of each cat were examined daily using flotation, immunofluorescence microscopy, and nested PCR of 18S rDNA; 18/18 cats (100%) were infected with *C. felis* and excreted oocysts for 6–18 days. In addition, 8/18 (44%) cats were concurrently infected with *G. duodenalis* (Assemblage F), which is host-specific to cats. All 18 cats were asymptomatic, without diarrhea or any other clinical signs, during the entire study. In Bogota, Colombia, near Engativa,

Santín et al. (2006) examined rectal fecal samples and scrapings of duodenal and ileal mucosa of euthanized domestic or stray cats. Samples were examined by nested PCR of the 18S rRNA gene. *Cryptosporidium* was detected in the feces and in duodenal/ileal mucosal samples from 6/46 (13%) cats; 5 samples were identified as *C. felis*. This, presumably, was the first report of *Cryptosporidium* in cats in Colombia.

Huber et al. (2007) examined fecal samples of stray cats in Nova Iguaçu, Rio de Janeiro state, Brazil, by flotation, followed by nested PCR of 18S rDNA, subsequent RFLP analysis of the secondary PCR products, and phylogenetic analyses; 9/30 (30%) were positive for *Cryptosporidium*, and 3 were successfully amplified and determined to be *C. felis*, and phylogenetic analyses using neighbor joining, maximum parsimony, and maximum likelihood further confirmed the support. Thomaz et al. (2007), in São Paulo, Brazil, examined fecal samples of domestic cats (number not given) by the standard sucrose flotation; seven cats were positive for *Cryptosporidium* oocysts that were morphologically *C. parvum*-like, measuring L × W: ~5 × 5, but nested PCR amplification of the 18S rRNA gene identified all seven isolates as *C. felis*.

Palmer et al. (2008a) surveyed fecal samples of cats from both urban and rural areas across Australia (see *Prevalence*, above). Microscopy-positive samples were further analyzed by nested PCR amplification of the actin gene, 18 of them were successfully sequenced, and all 18 were identified as *C. felis* (Palmer et al., 2008b). Ballweber et al. (2009) surveyed fresh fecal samples of indoor and outdoor cats, both with and without diarrhea, from 159 households in Northeastern Mississippi and Northwestern Alabama, USA. Samples were examined by centrifugal concentration, followed by an IFA. They found that 30/250 (12%) samples, from 19 households, were positive for *Cryptosporidium*, mostly from indoor cats. Oocysts of 12 samples were successfully genotyped using the partial sequence of the 18S rRNA gene, and all were

identified as *C. felis* (strain C8). Twenty-five of the *Cryptosporidium*-positive samples also had *Giardia* sp., and five discharged other coccidian oocysts that were not differentiated.

Yamamoto et al. (2009) surveyed fecal samples of cats in public animal shelters in Saitama Prefecture, Japan, and found *Cryptosporidium* in 30/1,079 (3%) samples, and molecular analysis confirmed the presence of *C. felis*. Yoshiuchi et al. (2010) surveyed fecal samples of privately-owned Japanese domestic cats in Osaka, Japan. Samples were collected from the rectum and examined by centrifugal sucrose flotation and direct IFA (Merifluor *Cryptosporidium/Giardia* commercial kit), followed by PCR amplification of 18S rRNA and COWP genes. *Cryptosporidium* was detected in 7/55 (13%) samples, all determined to be *C. felis*, and 5/7 (71%) positive cats were without diarrhea. Duration of oocyst excretion varied from 48 to 116 days, but it was unknown when these animals became infected.

Koompapong et al. (2014) examined (presumed) cat feces from the ground for *Cryptosporidium* using the molecular identification of a fragment of the 18S rRNA gene. Samples were collected from a temple in Ban Na District, Nakhon Nayok province, central Thailand. About 500 cats live around the temple area, and they are fed by monks and volunteers. *Cryptosporidium felis* was detected in 2/80 (2.5%) ground samples. In the United Kingdom, Scorza et al. (2014) examined fecal samples of pedigree *F. catus* that attended a show, using the commercial IFA (Merifluor *Cryptosporidium/Giardia*). *Cryptosporidium* was detected in 25/145 (17%) samples and amplification and sequencing of 18S rRNA and HSP70 genes was performed on the IFA-positive samples. The 18S rDNA sequence only was able to identify *Cryptosporidium*; however, the HSP70 gene determined 9/25 (36%) positive samples as *C. felis*.

Beser et al. (2015) reported a case study of a zoonotic transmission of *C. felis* from a cat to a human in Sweden. A male Maine Coon cat had watery diarrhea and, as its health worsened, it was hospitalized; examination of its feces showed it to be infected with *Cryptosporidium*, so it was treated with tylosin. Several months later, its owner, a 37-year-old immunocompetent woman, had watery, nonbloody diarrhea, fever, and arthralgia in her legs. Fecal samples of both the cat and woman were examined by LM of Ziehl–Neelsen stained slides and/or staining with an anti-*Cryptosporidium* fluorescein isothiocyanate-conjugated MAb, followed by PCR, RFLP analyses, and sequencing. The presence of identical *C. felis* 18S rRNA, COWP, and HSP70 gene sequences were recorded in both hosts. After 2 years, the feces of the cat were examined again and were still positive for *C. felis* oocysts, both by LM and PCR, although the cat was without clinical signs.

Hinney et al. (2015) examined cat fecal samples from 56 private households (71), 15 catteries (121), and 2 animal shelters (98) in eastern Austria. Samples were examined by flotation/centrifugation, with saturated sucrose solution, and those positive for *Cryptosporidium* were genotyped by the nested PCR amplification of the 18S rRNA gene. *Cryptosporidium* was detected in 5/290 (2%) samples and determined to be *C. felis*. Most of the cats had no diarrhea. Cats from shelters were significantly more infected than privately-owned cats, probably due to overcrowding, which may lead to an increased infection risk. Li et al. (2015) examined fecal samples of cats from a pet market in urban Harbin, southwestern Heilongjiang province, China. Cats were without diarrhea. Samples were examined by nested PCR amplification and sequencing of the 18S rRNA gene. *Cryptosporidium* was detected in 2/52 (4%) samples and 1 was determined to be *C. felis*. Mancianti et al. (2015) surveyed fecal samples of privately-owned, healthy, pet European shorthair cats in Tuscany and Liguria, in the provinces of Pisa, Florence, and Genoa, Italy. Samples were examined by centrifugation–flotation using $ZnCl_2$ and NaCl, followed by nested PCR amplification of 18S rDNA, then genotyped with PCR-RFLP and confirmed by sequencing; *C. felis* was detected in 3/146 (2%) samples.

Yang et al. (2015) examined fecal samples of cats, both kittens and adults, of different breeds from Perth, Western Australia. Cats originated from a cat refuge center (179), three pet shops (29), a breeding establishment (10), and private owners (127); none of the cats showed any clinical symptoms. Samples were examined by nested PCR amplification and sequencing of the 18S rRNA gene. *Cryptosporidium* was detected in 34/345 (10%) samples; 8 positive samples were identified as *C. felis*, and the highest prevalence, 23/179 (13%), was detected in cats from the refuge center. Ito et al. (2016) examined fresh fecal samples of cats from seven breeding facilities in Japan (Nagano, Saitama, Aichi, Gifu, and Miyagi Prefectures). Samples were examined first using sucrose gradient flotation/centrifugation, and those found to be positive for *Cryptosporidium* oocysts were analyzed by nested PCR amplification of the 18S rRNA gene. *Cryptosporidium* was detected in 4/286 (1%) cats from 2 facilities, and all 4 were identified as *C. felis*.

Xu et al. (2016) examined fecal samples of *F. catus* in urban Shanghai, China; 120 specimens originated from pet shops and 40 from an animal shelter. Samples were examined by PCR amplification and sequencing of the 18S rRNA gene. *Cryptosporidium* was detected in 6/160 (4%) samples; all positive samples were identified as *C. felis*. One cat was concurrently infected with *C. felis* and *Enterocytozoon bieneusi*. de Lucio et al. (2017) examined 34 fecal samples of pet cats and 179 humans from 63 households in Álava province, Basque Country, northern Spain. Their interest was in the potential transmission among humans and domestic dogs and/or cats sharing the same spatial and temporal setting in rural and urban areas. Specimens were examined by DFAT, followed by nested PCR targeting the 18S rRNA gene. *Cryptosporidium* was detected in 3/34 (9%) samples from the pet cats; 1 sample was identified as *C. felis*. Gil et al. (2017) collected fresh fecal samples from *F. catus* in Álava province, northern Spain. Oocysts of *Cryptosporidium* were detected by DFAT and the species identified by nested PCR amplification of the 18S rRNA gene. *Cryptosporidium* was found in 3/65 (5%) samples; 1 sample was determined to be *C. felis*. Kostopoulou et al. (2017) collected fecal samples of cats from private households (205) and shelters (59) on Crete Island, southern Greece. Some cats had diarrhea, some did not. Samples were examined by sedimentation/flotation and by quantitative direct IFA using the commercial Merifluor *Cryptosporidium/Giardia* kit. Samples positive for *Cryptosporidium* were identified by PCR amplification and sequencing of the 18S rRNA and HSP70 genes. *Cryptosporidium* was detected in 18/264 (7%) samples, and 4/18 (22%) samples were *C. felis*.

Finally, oocysts of *C. felis* have been used together with other *Cryptosporidium* species to evaluate the detectability, resolution, differentiation, specificity, and sensitivity of various diagnostic and genotyping methods such as different types of staining methods, PCR, real-time PCR, nested PCR-RFLP, single-strand conformation polymorphism, enzyme immunoassays, sequencing of specific genes or regions, phylogenetic analyses, and others (Xiao et al., 1999a,b, 2000, 2004; Sulaiman et al., 2000, 2002; Carreno et al., 2001; Gasser et al., 2001; Guyot et al., 2002; Jiang and Xiao, 2003; Leoni et al., 2003, 2006; Lindergard et al., 2003; Nichols et al., 2003, 2006; Werner et al., 2004; Coupe et al., 2005; Feng et al., 2009; Tosini et al., 2010; Chalmers et al., 2011; Lalonde and Gajadhar, 2011; Ruecker et al., 2011; Silva et al., 2013).

CRYPTOSPORIDIUM MURIS (TYZZER, 1907) TYZZER, 1910

Type host: *Mus musculus* L., 1758, House Mouse.
Remarks: McGlade et al. (2003) examined multiple fecal samples from 125 domestic cats from various sources in metropolitan Perth, Western Australia. Samples were examined by two salt flotation techniques, followed by malachite green staining, and 40 randomly-selected samples also were screened by nested PCR of the 18S rRNA gene. None of the 418 fecal samples were positive by microscopy, but 4/40 (10%) PCR-examined samples were positive for *Cryptosporidium*, and one successfully-sequenced PCR product "most closely resembled" *C. muris*.

In Bogota, Colombia, near Engativa, Santín et al. (2006) examined fecal samples and scrapings of duodenal and ileal mucosa of euthanized domestic and stray cats by nested PCR of the 18S rRNA gene. *Cryptosporidium* was detected in the feces and in duodenal/ileal mucosal samples from 6/46 (13%) cats and 1 was identified as *C. muris*. In Prague, Czech Republic, Pavlásek and Ryan (2007) examined 6 fecal samples of a 3.5-month-old British, shorthair cat, suffering from gastroenteritis and vomiting by a flotation method; 5/6 (83%) samples were positive for *Cryptosporidium*, and the oocysts resembled *C. muris* in shape and size (L × W: 8.0 × 4.8). Five 35-day-old mice were inoculated per os with oocysts to verify identity with *C. muris*. Fecal samples of the inoculated mice were examined daily, 5–15 DPI, and then at 2- to 4-day intervals until 70 DPI; cryptosporidial oocysts started to be discharged by mice on 11 DPI and the patent period lasted for 42 days. Nested PCR amplifying the 18S rRNA gene of *Cryptosporidium* was performed on samples from both cat and mice, and all were identical with *C. muris* (100% homology). Pavlásek and Ryan (2007) stated that this was the first report of a natural infection of *C. muris* in a cat; however, they probably overlooked the publication by Santín et al. (2006) who reported *C. muris* in a cat in Colombia.

Fitzgerald et al. (2011) reported a 2-year-old, neutered male, longhaired cat that suffered from persistent diarrhea for >13 months, despite medical interventions that included dietary modification, metronidazole, fenbendazole, and amoxycillin–clavulanate. Tests for FIV and feline leukemia virus were negative, but fecal samples examined by malachite green staining revealed the presence of *Cryptosporidium* oocysts of two sizes: large oocysts (n = 30) that resembled *C. muris* (L × W: 8.0 × 5.8; L/W ratio: 1.4) and smaller oocysts (n = 20) that resembled

C. felis (L × W: 4.6 × 4.0; L/W ratio: 1.15). Stomach biopsy showed numerous *Cryptosporidium* stages within the gastric pits and the lumina of fundic glands; duodenal biopsy detected *Cryptosporidium* stages associated with the apical surface of enterocytes, and both findings were confirmed by *in situ* hybridization and immunohistochemistry. Nested PCR and subsequent amplification of 18S rRNA and actin genes confirmed the presence of *C. muris* in the stomach and *C. felis* in duodenum. Because tylosin was not available at that time, azithromycin along with a novel protein diet was used to treat the cat, but it was unsuccessful in resolving diarrhea. Fecal examination after 12 months still revealed *C. muris* oocysts in feces, but the smaller *C. felis* oocysts had disappeared. Yang et al. (2015) examined fecal samples of both kittens and adult cats, of different breeds from Perth, Western Australia. Cats originated from a cat refuge center (179), three pet shops (29), a breeding establishment (10), and private owners (127); none of the cats showed any clinical symptoms. Samples were examined by nested PCR amplification and sequencing of the 18S rRNA gene. *Cryptosporidium* was detected in 34/345 (10%) samples; only 1 of the positive samples was identified as *C. muris*.

CRYPTOSPORIDIUM PARVUM TYZZER, 1912

Type host: *Mus musculus* (L., 1758), House Mouse.
Remarks: Katsumata et al. (1998) did a community-based study of stool samples of people and their cats (and dogs) in eight villages in Surabaya, Indonesia, where neither the piped water nor artesian well water were potable, such that people were forced to boil their water for drinking. Fecal samples of cats were examined by Sheather's sucrose flotation and stained with a modified Kinyoun's acid-fast stain. Katsumata et al. (1998) said they detected oocysts of *C. parvum* in 13/532 (2%) cats and in 49/4,368 (1%) people, more frequently in children with diarrhea and

exclusively during the rainy season. The study suggested that contact with cats, rain, floods, and crowded living conditions were significant risk factors for *C. parvum*. Gennari et al. (1999) examined fecal samples of household cats from different areas of São Paulo, Brazil, via sucrose flotation and/or sedimentation in water–ether. They detected *C. parvum* in 27/187 (14%) samples. McReynolds et al. (1999) screened serum samples of domestic cats for antibodies to *C. parvum* in the continental United States, by an indirect enzyme-linked immunosorbent assay, which had minimal cross reactivity with other gastrointestinal parasites; they found that 50/600 (8%) samples were seropositive for *C. parvum*-specific IgG, throughout the United States. Seropositivity was most frequently detected in *T. gondii*-IgG seropositive cats, outdoor cats, and cats with gastrointestinal symptoms and was highest in cats >10-year-old, probably due to the increased risk of exposure over time. It is unknown how long cats infected with *C. parvum* maintain positive antibody titers; they may persist months to years after clinical resolution of the disease.

Scorza et al. (2003) orally inoculated eight *C. parvum*-naive adult, shorthaired cats from a commercial breeder with 1×10^6 oocysts of a *C. parvum* human isolate (Ohio strain). Fecal samples were examined daily until 30 DPI and then twice weekly until 126 DPI, using the MAb-based IFA and PCR. All infected cats tested positive for *C. parvum*. The first PCR detection was recorded on 2 DPI, whereas the first IFA detection was on 7 DPI; the majority of positive samples were recorded between 5–13 and 95–115 DPI. Scorza et al. (2003) said that PCR was more sensitive than IFA, detecting infection in 101/353 (29%) samples, whereas IFA detected only 52/353 (15%) of the samples as positive.

Scorza et al. (2011) examined fecal samples of pet cats in San Jose province, Costa Rica, by Sheather's sugar flotation and an IFA (Merifluor *Cryptosporidium*/*Giardia* kit); *Cryptosporidium*-positive samples were genotyped by PCR amplification and sequencing of 18S rDNA, and *C. parvum* was detected in 1/9 (11%) samples.

Sotiriadou et al. (2013), in Ludwigsburg, Germany, examined fresh feces of clinically ill domestic cats by sedimentation–flotation, followed by nested PCR amplification of the 18S rRNA gene; *C. parvum* was detected in 1/19 (5%) samples.

Li et al. (2015) examined fecal samples of cats from a pet market in urban Harbin, southwestern Heilongjiang province, China. Cats were without diarrhea. Samples were examined by nested PCR amplification and sequencing of the 18S rRNA gene. *Cryptosporidium* was detected in 2/52 (4%) samples, 1 of which was determined to be *C. parvum*.

CRYPTOSPORIDIUM RYANAE FAYER, SANTÍN, AND TROUT, 2008

Type host: *Bos taurus* L., 1758, Aurochs.

Remarks: Yang et al. (2015) examined fecal samples of both kittens and adult cats, of different breeds, from Perth, Western Australia. Cats originated from a cat refuge center (179), three pet shops (29), a breeding establishment (10), and private owners (127); none of the cats showed any clinical symptoms. Samples were examined by nested PCR amplification and sequencing of the 18S rRNA gene. *Cryptosporidium* was detected in 34/345 (10%) samples; only 1 sample was identified as *C. ryanae*, and this was the first report of *C. ryanae* in cats.

CRYPTOSPORIDIUM SPP.

There are many other records of *Cryptosporidium* oocysts reported from *Felis*, but none of them have been identified to species (see Chapter 19).

GENUS *LEOPARDUS* GRAY, 1842 (9 SPECIES)

An unidentified *Cryptosporidium* species was found in two oncillas, *L. tigrinus*, in Brazil (see Chapter 19).

GENUS *LYNX* KERR, 1752 (4 SPECIES)

An unidentified *Cryptosporidium* species was found in some bobcats in California and/or Colorado (see Chapter 19), but not in one *L. rufus* from Maine (Bass et al., 2012), nor in six Iberian lynx, *L. pardinus*, in Spain (Mateo et al., 2017).

CRYPTOSPORIDIUM SPP.

There are several records of *Cryptosporidium* oocysts reported from *Lynx*, but none of them have been identified to species (see Chapter 19).

GENUS *PUMA* JARDINE, 1834 (2 SPECIES)

Matsubayashi et al. (2005) examined fecal samples of two cougars, *P. concolor* (L., 1771), in Osaka, Japan, but *Cryptosporidium* was not detected in either. To our knowledge, there are no *Cryptosporidium* species yet reported from this genus.

SUBFAMILY PANTHERINAE POCOCK, 1917

GENUS *PANTHERA* (L., 1758) (4 SPECIES)

Matsubayashi et al. (2005) examined three fecal samples of lions, *Panthera leo* (L., 1758), two of jaguars, *Panthera onca* (L., 1758), and two of leopards, *Panthera pardus* (L., 1758), in Osaka, Japan, but they could not detect oocysts of *Cryptosporidium*. Karanis et al. (2007) also did not find *Cryptosporidium* oocysts in *P. leo* in China, but did not say how many lions were examined. Lim et al. (2008) reported *Cryptosporidium* from 3 subspecies of *P. tigris* in Malaysia, and Wang and Liew (1990) reported *Cryptosporidium* oocysts in a "leopard" in Taiwan (see Chapter 19).

CRYPTOSPORIDIUM SPP.

There are several records of *Cryptosporidium* oocysts reported from *Panthera*, but none of them have been identified to species (see Chapter 19).

FAMILY HERPESTIDAE BONAPARTE, 1845

GENUS *HERPESTES* ILLIGER, 1811 (10 SPECIES)

HERPESTES ICHNEUMON (L., 1758), EGYPTIAN MONGOOSE

CRYPTOSPORIDIUM CANIS FAYER, TROUT, XIAO, MORGAN, LAL, AND DUBEY, 2001

Type host: *Canis lupus familiaris* (syn. *C. familiaris*) L., 1758, Domestic Dog.

Remarks: Mateo et al. (2017) examined fecal samples of two Egyptian mongooses from the Extremadura Autonomous region of Spain, by nested PCR targeting the 18S rRNA gene, followed by genotyping based on the gp60 gene. *Cryptosporidium* was detected in 1/2 (50%) samples and identified as *C. canis*.

GENUS *MUNGOS* É. GEOFFROY SAINT-HILAIRE AND F.G. CUVIER, 1795 (2 SPECIES)

MUNGOS MUNGO (GMELIN, 1788), BANDED MONGOOSE

CRYPTOSPORIDIUM PARVUM TYZZER, 1912

Type host: *Mus musculus* (L., 1758), House Mouse.

Remarks: Abe et al. (2004) reported *Cryptosporidium* in a fecal sample of one banded mongoose, which was brought from Tanzania to the Osaka Zoo, Japan. The oocysts were 4–5 wide and were indistinguishable from those of *C. parvum*. According to partial 18S rRNA and HSP70 gene sequences, Abe et al. (2004) suggested that this represented a new, host-adapted genotype, closely related to the *Cryptosporidium* bear genotype. A year later, Matsubayashi et al. (2005) examined fecal samples of seven *M. mungo* at the same zoo in Osaka, and all samples were negative for *Cryptosporidium*.

FAMILY HYAENIDAE GRAY, 1821

GENUS *HYAENA* BRISSON, 1762 (2 SPECIES)

Only Matsubayashi et al. (2005) examined fecal samples of two hyenas, *Hyaena hyaena* (L., 1758), in a zoo in Osaka, Japan, but they did not detect *Cryptosporidium* in either sample. Thus, to our knowledge, there are no *Cryptosporidium* species reported from this genus.

FAMILY VIVERRIDAE GRAY, 1821

SUBFAMILY VIVERRINAE GRAY, 1821

GENUS *GENETTA* F.G. COUVIER, 1816 (14 SPECIES)

Mateo et al. (2017) examined fecal samples of six common genets, *G. genetta*, in Spain, and one was infected with *Cryptosporidium*, but not identified further (see Chapter 19). To our knowledge, there are no other reports of *Cryptosporidium* species from this genus.

DISCUSSION AND SUMMARY

The Caniformia branch of the Carnivora consists of 9 families composed of 72 genera with 165 species (Wilson and Reeder, 2005). There is at least one named *Cryptosporidium* species in 8 of the 9 families, but none yet are reported in the monotypic walrus family Odobenidae. Two *Cryptosporidium* species, *C. andersoni* and *C. parvum*, have been reported in the other monotypic family, Ailuridae, the red panda, in China. In the Canidae, 3/13 (23%) genera, and only 5/35 (14%) species have been documented to host 6 named *Cryptosporidium* species. In the Mephitidae, only 1/4 (25%) genera and 1/12 (8%) species have been studied, and only *C. parvum* has been identified from *M. mephitis*, the striped skunk. In the Mustelidae, 5/22 (23%) genera and 5/59 (8%) species play host to 6 different named *Cryptosporidium* species. In the Otariidae, only *C. parvum* and *C.* sp. are known from *Z. californianus*; thus, only 1/7 (14%) genera and 1/16 (6%) species in this family is known to have a named species of *Cryptosporidium*. In the Phocidae, 1/13 (8%) genera and 1/19 (5%) species is now known to have a valid, named *Cryptosporidium* species, *C. muris*, identified in *Pusa hispida*. In the Procyonidae, 1/6 (17%) genera and 1/15 (7%) species, *P. lotor*, is known to harbor *C. parvum* and a *C.* sp.; no other species in the family has ever been examined for these parasites. In the Ursidae, 2/5 (40%) genera and 2/8 (25%) species have been examined for and documented to harbor 2 *Cryptosporidium* species, *C. andersoni* and *C. parvum* dog genotype. In total, we have knowledge that about 9 distinct species of *Cryptosporidium* are known to be present in 8/9 (89%) families, 15/72 (21%) genera with 17/165 (10%) species in the Caniformia branch of the Carnivora. In addition, there are 22 genera and 29 species in the Caniformia from which *C.* sp. have been reported, most based only on oocysts in the feces (see Table 1).

The Feliformia branch of the Carnivora consists of 6 families composed of 54 genera with 121 species (Wilson and Reeder, 2005), but its members have not been as well studied for *Cryptosporidium* species as have those in the Caniformia. There are no named *Cryptosporidium* species in 4/6 (67%) Feliformia families, nor in 51/54 (94%) of their genera including 118/121 (97.5%) species in this lineage. Only *F. catus* (4), *H. ichneumon* (1), and *M. mungo* (1) are hosts for known, named *Cryptosporidium* species, whereas *A. jubatus* (cheetah), *F. catus* (domestic cat), *F. chaus* (jungle cat), *Leo. pardalis* (ocelot), *Leo. tigrinus* (oncilla), *Ly. rufus* (bobcat), *Pan. pardus* (leopard), *Pan. tigris* (tiger), and *G. genetta* (common genet) have been identified to harbor at least one *C.* sp., but that is all the information available. In total, we have knowledge that 5 *Cryptosporidium* species are known to be present in 2/6 (33%) families, 6/54 (11%) genera, and in 3/121 (2%) species, and *C.* sp. has been found in an additional 5 genera and species in the Feliformia branch of the Carnivora.

By our count, there are 10 valid, named *Cryptosporidium* species described, to date, from all Carnivora species: *C. andersoni*, *C. canis*, *C. felis*, *C. hominis*, *C. meleagridis*, *C. muris*, *C. parvum*, *C. ryanae*, *C. scrofarum*, and *C. ubiquitum*; and oocysts of *Cryptosporidium* sp. have been named many times. In total, then, various cryptosporidia (named and "sp.") are reported in 10/15 (67%) of the families, but only 21/126 (17%) of the genera and only 20/281 (7%) of the species in the Carnivora.

As we can see from the entries above, cryptosporidia in carnivores have been most often surveyed and detected in dogs and cats. In many countries worldwide, both stray and domesticated dogs and cats are documented to harbor *Cryptosporidium*, although most often such identifications are not identified to species. *Cryptosporidium canis* and *C. felis* are the most frequently identified species in our pets, although small numbers of zoonotic *C. parvum* and *C. muris* also have been detected in them. Both *C. canis* and *C. felis* are considered potentially zoonotic, particularly in children, those people who are immunocompromised, and/or elderly people, and because so many mammalian species can be infected with *C. parvum*, a large potential zoonotic reservoir exists in wild, domestic, and companion animals. Each of these 3 species deserves special concern.

Originally, a mouse species, *C. parvum*, was reported to infect dogs and cats (Scorza et al., 2011; Sotiriadou et al., 2013; Li et al., 2015) and other carnivores (e.g., Snyder, 1988; Duncan et al., 1999; Rademacher et al., 1999; Sturdee et al., 1999; Deng et al., 2000; Xiao et al., 2000; Perz and Le Blancq, 2001; Abe and Iseki, 2003; Gómez-Couso et al., 2007; Karanis et al., 2007; Chavez et al., 2012; Mateo et al., 2017), but it tends to be asymptomatic in carnivores. There are now >152 mammal species reported to have been infected with *C. parvum*-like parasites, and at least 8 genotypes of *C. parvum* have been identified in primates, artiodactyls, marsupials, rodents, and carnivores (Morgan et al., 1999a,b, 2000b; Fayer et al., 2000, 2001; Xiao et al., 1999a). Numerous studies have demonstrated/correlated transmission of *C. parvum* from various other animals to humans, especially to children, and such cases usually involve direct exposure to infected animals or their feces or exposure to contaminated raw milk, food, or water (Duszynski and Upton, 2010). Infection with *C. parvum* is of concern for humans because ingestion of even small numbers of oocysts can cause severe diarrhea in people (Angus, 1987). The oocysts survive well outside the host and are resistant to chlorination levels used for disinfection of tap water. Because so many wild mammals, including carnivores, have been identified as reservoirs of *C. parvum*, the oocysts shed in their feces may pose a threat to human health in urban and rural environments.

Cryptosporidium felis is the main species in cats, and *C. canis* is the main one in dogs; both may cause diarrhea in kittens and puppies. However, in dogs and cats, clinical signs of cryptosporidiosis (diarrhea, nausea, vomiting, dehydration, abdominal pain, fever, general malaise, weight loss, malnutrition, and malabsorption) often are absent, and their infections are subclinical. These companion animals, and increasingly pet ferrets, may act as natural reservoirs of a large number of zoonotic pathogens, and, therefore, may represent a significant source of infection to humans around the world. Some species and genotypes of *Cryptosporidium* are more likely to cause human illness than others and may be related to specific forms of pathogenicity, but we know so little about these parasites that it is difficult to make such broad generalizations. On the reverse side of that coin, Lucio-Forster et al. (2010) suggested that the risk of zoonotic transmission of *Cryptosporidium* spp. from pet dogs and cats is low. In most cases, dogs and cats harbor host-specific strains of *C. canis* and *C. felis*, respectively, and most human cases of cryptosporidiosis have been reported to be caused by *C. hominis* and *C. parvum*. Lucio-Forster et al. (2010) seem to suggest that *C. canis* and *C. felis* play only a minor role in a small number of human cases, usually in children and/or immunocompromised people (Goh et al., 2004; Gatei et al., 2008; Xiao and Feng, 2008; Lucio-Forster et al., 2010; Overgaauw et al., 2009; Beser et al., 2015). However, *C. canis*, in particular, may indeed pose a health risk to humans. It has been found in water samples from the main/primary rivers in western Romania (Imre et al., 2017), in human samples in England and Wales (Chalmers et al., 2009; Elwin et al., 2012), in symptomatic individuals and in people with gastrointestinal disorders in England (Leoni et al., 2006), in children (nondiarrheic and diarrheic) in Jordan, Peru, Mexico, Cambodia, Kenya, and Nigeria (Gatei et al., 2006; Cama et al., 2008; Hijjawi et al., 2010; Molloy et al., 2010; González-Díaz et al., 2016; Moore et al., 2016), in immunoincompetent and HIV-infected persons in France, Brazil, Jamaica, Peru, and Thailand (Gatei et al., 2002, 2008; Cama et al., 2003, 2006, 2007; Lucca et al., 2009; ANOPHEL Cryptosporidium National Network 2010), and in HIV/AIDS patients in Ethiopia (Adamu et al., 2014) and elsewhere.

And, it is now becoming evident that a *Cryptosporidium* sp. can be an important parasite of captive black-footed ferret (*M. nigripes*) kits and a few adults, in which it causes ill-thrift and mucoid diarrhea. However, it is not known whether the parasite occurs naturally in black-footed ferrets prior to their capture or whether the ferrets acquire the parasite in captivity where it can be introduced through food, contact with human carriers, or water (Williams and Thorne, 1996).

Persons who are in close direct and/or indirect contacts with mammals, such as breeders, farmers, children visiting farms, animal caretakers, workers in the animal and/or fur industry, and veterinarians and veterinary students, are at a high risk of the potential zoonotic transmission of *Cryptosporidium* infection. In addition, numerous outbreaks of cryptosporidiosis are related to waterborne or foodborne transmission; however, the source(s) of these outbreaks mostly remain(s) unknown. Improved management systems are needed to prevent the occurrence of cross-transmission and reinfection of *Cryptosporidium* among our domesticated animals and to reduce environmental contamination from animal manure.

Cryptosporidium infections in canines and felines are typically associated with low and intermittent excretion of small, but steady, numbers of oocysts, but almost no clinical signs in the animals discharging these oocysts. Exacerbating this environmental contamination issue is that laboratory detection via LM is difficult, and it does not enable identification of species because of the morphological uniformity of the oocysts. Intermittent oocyst shedding is known to vary markedly from day-to-day and week-to-week, both in companion animals and human patients. Thus, environmental prevalence may be markedly underestimated because in most cases only a single sample from each animal is examined. One negative fecal examination does not mean necessarily that the individual is *Cryptosporidium* negative. This fact underscores the value of performing more than one fecal examination and observing many fields at high magnification, when attempting to diagnose cryptosporidial infections, if only by LM. PCR-based techniques and sequencing now are the methods of choice to identify *Cryptosporidium* species and genotypes. However, a positive PCR does not provide information on the viability and infectivity of the oocysts. Thus, a combination of diagnostic methods (LM, TEM, molecular detection, and immunological methods) is recommended and vital.

Without molecular/genetic analysis it is impossible to accurately determine host specificity and/or the infection potential of any *Cryptosporidium* isolate, genotype, or species. Thus, our ability to identify and understand the epidemiology of the seemingly myriad of *Cryptosporidium* forms is limited, at present, to the tools available to the individual investigators, but we should try to heed the advice of Fayer et al. (2001), "In an effort to bring clarity to an increasingly complex subject, it is prudent to identify as clearly as possible each genetically and biologically unique member of this genus."

Treatment and Drug Therapies of Coccidiosis in Carnivora

TREATMENT AND DRUG THERAPIES OF COCCIDIOSIS IN THE CARNIVORA

INTRODUCTION

Treatment and therapy of coccidiosis in Carnivora, caused by various coccidian genera, is difficult because the anticoccidials have not been tested and/or registered for the majority of the carnivore genera. Therefore, their use is often only experimental and off-label. Moreover, in many cases (i.e., *Cryptosporidium*, *Cystoisospora*, *Eimeria*), infections are often self-limiting in immunocompetent individuals, and they resolve spontaneously without any medical intervention. Hosts also may develop a total or partial immunity against subsequent reinfections by the same parasite species. Complicating the transmission picture is that once coccidian oocysts are shed into the environment via the hosts' feces, most seem to be unusually resistant, remaining infective in the environment for a long period of time; thus, preventive measures are even more important than the therapy itself. Preventive measures include cage and house cleaning to decrease the number of oocysts in the environment and prevent reinfections, and the proper use of appropriate household and clinic disinfectants (e.g., bleach,

quaternary ammonium compounds, dry heat) for effective decontamination of the environment.

In this chapter, we provide a review of what has been published on treatment of coccidiosis in carnivores that is caused by specific coccidian genera and then the basic characteristics of the most often used chemotherapeutics. Acridines, antibiotics with antiprotozoal effect, carbanilide derivatives, diaminopyrimidines, nitrobenzamides, quinolone derivatives, sulfonamides, thiamine analogues, and triazines are the most often used drug classes in the treatment of coccidial infections in carnivores. However, it is necessary to point out that many antiprotozoal drugs are active only against a restricted range of coccidian genera, and, for many infections, treatment may not result in a complete parasitological cure. Moreover, resistance to antiprotozoal drugs is a growing problem among the myriad of apicomplexan parasites.

TREATMENT/DRUG THERAPY: CRYPTOSPORIDIUM IN CARNIVORA

So far, there is no effective treatment for cryptosporidiosis. Although a wide variety of potentially active agents have been tested to control cryptosporidiosis in immunocompromised

© 2018 Donald W. Duszynski published by Elsevier Inc. All rights reserved.

humans, none have proven satisfactory (Irwin, 2002; Robertson and Thompson, 2002; Armson et al., 2003). Most of the chemotherapeutic agents that have been shown to be effective in controlling coccidiosis in cattle, pigs, and poultry caused by *Eimeria* species have limited or no efficacy against cryptosporidiosis, which emphasizes the noncoccidian features of *Cryptosporidium* (Barta and Thompson, 2006; Thompson et al., 2008). Thus, early diagnosis is important, and clinical intervention is required to treat just the effects of infection. In carnivores, the situation is further complicated by the fact that they may have a concurrent immunosuppressing viral infection, such as distemper, parvovirus enteritis, feline leukemia virus, or feline immunodeficiency virus (Fukushima and Helman, 1984; Monticello et al., 1987; Turnwald et al., 1988; Goodwin and Barsanti, 1990; Mtambo et al., 1991; Barr, 1997; Morgan et al., 2000b; Denholm et al., 2001; Irwin, 2002). Thus, it is difficult for the veterinary clinician to assess whether a *Cryptosporidium* infection is actually causing the diarrhea or if other gastrointestinal disorders are at play in a pet that has been presented for treatment. No treatment is registered in the United States for *Cryptosporidium* in small mammals (Lucio-Forster et al., 2010). A limited anticryptosporidial effect of paromomycin, a broad-spectrum aminoglycoside antibiotic, has been described, although the mechanism has not yet been determined. Paromomycin has demonstrated efficacy, both in humans and other animals, in reduction of oocyst excretion and inhibition of the development of intracellular stages (Armitage et al., 1992; Fayer and Ellis, 1993a,b; Fichtenbaum et al., 1993; Verdon et al., 1994; White et al., 1994; Healey et al., 1995). It also was successfully tried in several dogs and cats and stopped oocyst shedding within 5 days of treatment (Barr et al., 1994a,b; Barr, 1997; Lappin, 2005). However, reports of acute renal failure attributed to intestinal absorption of paromomycin in four cats raised a question about the safety of this drug in individual cats

with severe gastrointestinal pathology (Gookin et al., 1999). Likewise, nitazoxanide, which is registered for children, reduced oocyst shedding in cats. Tylosin, a macrolide antibiotic, also has been successfully used in cats but requires a long period of administration (Lappin, 2005; Barr and Bowman, 2006; Lucio-Forster et al., 2010). Thus, current recommendations for treating cryptosporidiosis in carnivores are focused on treating symptoms, such as fluid therapy against dehydration and/or antibiotic therapy to prevent or treat secondary bacterial infections (Thompson et al., 2008).

Vaccination has been proposed as an additional potential method to control cryptosporidiosis in various animals. Whole oocyst preparations, subunit vaccines, and DNA vaccines have been manufactured and tested in mice and calves. Results of experimental trials showed reduction of clinical signs, but these vaccines neither eliminated nor reduced oocyst shedding (Harp et al., 1989; Harp and Goff, 1998; de Graaf et al., 1999; Perryman et al., 1999; Jenkins, 2001; Thompson et al., 2008). Passive immune protection by vaccination of dams, which will then produce a protective hyperimmune colostrum, represents another option for future study (Harp and Goff, 1998; Thompson et al., 2008).

Case Reports

Lewis et al. (1985) reported the positive effect of nalidixic acid (quinolone antibiotic) in treating recurring cryptosporidiosis that was diagnosed in a 5.5-year-old boy on immunosuppressive maintenance therapy for acute lymphoblastic leukemia; it was believed the boy probably got infected with *Cryptosporidium* oocysts from the family kitten. Lewis et al. (1985) reported that after discontinuing the immunosuppressive treatment and beginning of therapy with nalidixic acid, the clinical symptoms of cryptosporidiosis (diarrhea, vomiting, nausea, anorexia) resolved, and no oocysts were found in the child's stool for 45 days after diagnosis. However, after restarting immunosuppressive treatment, a second episode of *Cryptosporidium* infection and symptoms occurred, which again was improved and resolved after another therapy with nalidixic acid. Quinolones have not been previously used in cryptosporidiosis, and although the patient improved after treatment with nalidixic acid, the improvement could be attributed to concurrent withdrawal of the immunosuppressive maintenance treatment.

Barr et al. (1994b) reported a positive effect of paromomycin in treatment of cryptosporidiosis that was diagnosed in a 6-month-old, spayed, domestic short-hair cat suffering from persistent diarrhea for 2 months. The cat had been properly vaccinated and was both FeLV and FIV negative. Flotation in Sheather's sucrose solution revealed *Cryptosporidium* oocysts and *Toxocara cati* eggs in the cat's fecal sample. The cat was administered pyrantel pamoate 25 mg/kg body weight (BW) per os (p.o.) against *Toxocara*, metronidazole 20 mg/kg BW p.o. once daily (s.i.d.) for 6 days (against protozoans), and a special diet (Hill's c/d®). However, after 14 days the cat still suffered from diarrhea and still shed *Cryptosporidium* oocysts in its feces. It was then administered paromomycin, 165 mg/kg p.o. twice daily (b.i.d.), for 5 days, and on days 1, 8, and 34 after completing treatment, *Cryptosporidium* oocysts were not detected in its feces. On days 1 and 8, the diarrhea was still observed; however, by day 34, the feces were non-diarrheic about 80% of the time and no signs of toxicosis were observed. Thus, paromomycin stopped oocyst shedding in the feces following the treatment.

Similarly, Barr et al. (1994a) administered paromomycin at a dose 125–165 mg/kg BW, p.o., b.i.d., for 5 days to three cats and two dogs suffering from diarrhea and diagnosed with cryptosporidiosis based on the presence of *Cryptosporidium* oocysts in their feces. The oocysts ceased to be discharged and were not observed in feces, within 1 day of the last dose in all animals, and no signs of toxicity were observed. The diarrhea resolved within 5 days of the last dose in two cats and two dogs, and within 30 days in the third cat.

Rademacher et al. (1999) reported temporary episodes of diarrhea in four captive beech martens, *Martes foina*, one male and three females, that were not related to each other. Numerous *Cryptosporidium* oocysts were detected in fecal samples by flotation and in smear preparations that were acid-fast-stained by the Ziehl–Neelsen procedure and safranin, and all oocysts seen corresponded morphologically to *C. parvum*. The source of the infection was unknown, but furthermore, a few *Cystoisospora* sp. oocysts were found in one animal. The animals were treated with a 25% solution of sodium sulfamethoxypyridazin, 60 mg/kg BW, p.o., s.i.d., for 7 days, and with drops of vitamin ADE preparation, 0.5 mg/kg BW, p.o., s.i.d. Diarrhea significantly decreased after 3 days of treatment, and disappeared by the end of the treatment period. However, it was unknown whether the diarrhea was caused by *Cryptosporidium* or by *Cystoisospora*.

Denholm et al. (2001) reported a case of a concurrent active infection of canine parvovirus (CPV) and *C. parvum* in a puppy suffering from acute severe gastroenteritis in Australia. The puppy was treated with a wide variety of chemotherapeutics. This 9-week-old male Bullmastiff puppy was presented to a veterinary hospital with vomiting, lethargy, dehydration, and fever lasting for 24 hours. At 5 weeks of age it was inoculated with a modified live vaccine containing CPV, distemper, and adenovirus. First, the puppy was treated with lactated Ringers solution intravenously (i.v.), metoclopramide i.v., and amoxicillin–clavulanate 15 mg/kg BW subcutaneously (s.c.) once daily. After initial improvement, deterioration and vomiting began again after 24 hours. Fecal samples were negative for parvovirus by electron microscopy, and fecal flotation did not reveal any intestinal parasites. Ultrasonography showed dilation of the entire intestine, reduced peristalsis, and multiple enlarged mesenteric lymph nodes. The puppy was then treated with crystalloids i.v., Dextran i.v., butorphanol 0.15 mg/kg BW, s.c., and ranitidine syrup 2 mg/kg BW, p.o., b.i.d. On day 4, its stomach became distended and painful, so the treatment was changed to amoxicillin 10 mg/kg BW, i.v., four times daily + metronidazole 25 mg/kg BW, b.i.d. + gentamicin 2 mg/kg BW, i.v., b.i.d. Over the next few days, a polymeric liquid diet in a continuous i.v. infusion and a plasma transfusion were administered, the puppy improved, and the vomiting ceased by day 8. The therapy was changed to trimethoprim 20 mg, s.c., b.i.d. + sulfadoxine, 100 mg, s.c., b.i.d. + metronidazole 100 mg, p.o., b.i.d. + amoxicillin, 50 mg, p.o., t.i.d. (thrice daily) via a jejunostomy tube. The puppy continued to recover, so the tube feeding was discontinued and replaced by oral food. Cisapride, 0.4 mg/kg, p.o., was administered b.i.d. Histological examination revealed severe ileal crypt damage with hyperplasia, dilation, and villous atrophy. "Numerous spherical organisms ≤1 μm in diameter" were located on the surface of the cryptal epithelium. Concurrently, *Cryptosporidium* oocysts were identified in fresh feces stained with malachite green. Polymerase chain reaction (PCR) amplification and subsequent sequencing of the 18S rRNA gene disclosed a sequence that was identical to an isolate obtained from a dog in the United States, and not previously recorded in Australia. Serum neutralization testing to assess the CPV antibodies revealed a high titer that corresponded to a recent CPV infection. Fecal samples of the owners and veterinary staff were negative. The puppy continued to recover, and the cause of its gastroenteritis was determined to be a CPV infection, exacerbated by a concurrent *Cryptosporidium* infection. The CPV caused immunosuppression, leading to increased susceptibility to the cryptosporidial infection. *Cryptosporidium* of identical sequence also was isolated from another dog presented to the same veterinary hospital and undergoing immunosuppressive therapy.

Fitzgerald et al. (2011) reported a case of a natural mixed infection with *C. muris* and *C. felis* in a cat, which they confirmed by morphological, histopathological, and genetic characterization. A 2-year-old domestic, neutered, male long-haired cat suffered from chronic diarrhea for more than 13 months, with intermittent vomiting. Several trials of symptomatic therapy (high-fiber diet, cobalamin 200 mg/kg BW, s.c., weekly for 6 weeks, metronidazole 9.4 mg/kg BW, b.i.d., for 10 days, fenbendazole 50 mg/kg BW, p.o., s.i.d., for 5 days, amoxicillin–clavulanate 13.9 mg/kg BW, p.o., b.i.d.) were not successful, and FIV and FeLV tests were negative. Fecal samples examined by malachite green staining discovered the presence of *Cryptosporidium* sp. oocysts of two different sizes. In shape and size, large oocysts resembled *C. muris*, and smaller oocysts resembled *C. felis*. Because tylosin (a commonly recommended treatment of cryptosporidiosis) was not available at that time, the cat was treated with azithromycin 5.3 mg/kg BW, p.o., b.i.d., for 2 weeks, together with a novel protein diet. The vomiting ceased, and the diarrhea improved, but persisted. Fecal examination after 12 months still revealed *C. muris* oocysts in feces, but the smaller *C. felis* oocysts were no longer found.

TREATMENT/DRUG THERAPY: CYSTOISOSPORA AND *EIMERIA* IN CARNIVORA

For infections with *Cystoisospora* and *Eimeria*, no treatment is usually advised unless the infected animals exhibit signs of gastrointestinal disease. Clinical coccidiosis mainly affects cubs, young animals, and immunocompromised individuals, with watery, sometimes hemorrhagic diarrhea, vomiting, and abdominal discomfort. Depending on the animal's age, its immune status, and the parasite burden, severe dehydration and even death may occur (Daugschies et al., 2000; Lappin, 2010; Altreuther et al., 2011a). However, these infections often take a subclinical course. Increasing age and immunocompetence decrease the likelihood of these infections and, thus, the need for medication. When necessary, toltrazuril is the drug of choice against eimerians and cystoisosporans in carnivores. In such cases, it is advisable to treat all animals within a group where infection is suspected. Depending on the severity of clinical signs, additional treatment such as fluid therapy against dehydration, or antibiotic therapy to prevent or treat secondary bacterial infections, may be indicated. The genus *Cystoisospora* is the main causative agent of coccidiosis in canines and felines.

Drugs other than toltrazuril are listed in recommendations by the Companion Animal Parasite Council (CAPC, 2013) for treatment of *Cystoisospora* spp. in dogs and cats; however, the use of all of them, except sulfadimethoxine, are off-label: amprolium, amprolium + sulfadimethoxine, diclazuril, furazolidone, ponazuril, quinacrine, sulfadimethoxine + ormethoprim, and sulfa-guanidine.

Case Reports

In the report noted above (Rademacher et al., 1999) under *Cryptosporidium*, a few *Cystoisospora* sp. oocysts were found in one captive beech marten (*M. foina*). The animals were treated with a 25% solution of sodium sulfamethoxypyridazin 60 mg/kg BW, p.o., s.i.d., for 7 days, and drops of vitamin ADE preparation 0.5 mg/kg BW, p.o., s.i.d. Diarrhea significantly decreased after 3 days of treatment and disappeared by the end of the treatment period. However, it was unknown whether the diarrhea was caused by *Cryptosporidium* or by *Cystoisospora*.

Daugschies et al. (2000) studied the efficacy of toltrazuril treatment under experimental and field conditions, and 24 puppies were experimentally inoculated with 4×10^4 oocysts of *C. ohioensis*-complex. On 3 DPI, groups of 6 puppies were administered a single oral treatment with 5% toltrazuril suspension: 6 puppies

were administered a dose of 10 mg/kg BW, 6 puppies 20 mg/kg BW, 6 puppies 30 mg/kg BW, and 6 puppies served as a non-treated control group. Neither oocyst shedding nor diarrhea was observed in any of the treated groups, irrespective of the dose. Non-treated puppies started to discharge oocysts at 6 DPI and suffered from catarrhalic- to hemorrhagic diarrhea; on 12 DPI, 4 of 6 untreated puppies died, and 3- to 4-week-old naturally-infected puppies, diagnosed via coprological findings, were treated with a single oral application of toltrazuril suspension or **microgranulate** in a dose of 10–20 mg/kg BW, which also completely stopped oocyst shedding.

Altreuther et al. (2011a) performed randomized, blind, placebo-controlled studies to evaluate the efficacy of Procox® (emodepside, a nematocidal compound, plus toltrazuril, a coccidiocidal compound) oral suspension for dogs against *C. canis* and *C. ohioensis*-complex. Unweaned, 3- to 5-week-old puppies were experimentally infected with sporulated oocysts of *C. canis* and/or *C. ohioensis*-complex. The first group was treated with Procox® 2–4 DPI (i.e., during prepatency), the second group after the onset of patency, and the third group served as a control group treated with placebo at 2–4 DPI. A minimum therapeutic dose of 0.45 mg/kg BW emodepside, and 9 mg/kg BW toltrazuril, was administered in both treatment trials. Individual fecal samples were examined daily from 5 DPI until the end of the study, and consistency of feces was evaluated. Significantly lower oocyst counts were observed in both groups of the treated dogs compared to the control group, and there was a significantly lower frequency of diarrhea in treated dogs during the prepatent infection. However, no differences were observed between the treated and the control group during the patent infection. No adverse drug reactions were observed.

Similarly, Altreuther et al. (2011b) performed randomized, blind, and controlled field studies to evaluate the efficacy of Procox® oral suspension for dogs against naturally-acquired infections in dogs. First, one group of dogs naturally-infected with gastrointestinal nematodes and/or *Cystoisospora* spp. was treated with Procox®, and the second group was treated with a reference product (sulfadimethoxine [Kokzidiol SD®]). Second, efficacy of Procox® against prepatent *Cystoisospora* spp. infections compared with an untreated control group was tested in *Cystoisospora*-negative dogs at risk. A dose of 0.45 mg/kg BW emodepside, and 9 mg/kg BW toltrazuril, was administered in the treatment trials. In all studies, a markedly significant reduction of fecal egg counts and fecal oocyst counts was observed with Procox® treatment, compared with the reference product and the untreated control group. No adverse drug reactions were observed in any of the dogs. Thus, Procox®, developed to provide a treatment option for dogs with mixed infection with roundworms and coccidia, was shown to be a safe and highly efficient coccidiocide (and nematocide) for dogs, both experimentally and under field conditions.

TREATMENT/DRUG THERAPY: HEPATOZOON IN CARNIVORA

Hepatozoonosis, caused by *Hepatozoon canis* and other species (see Chapter 13), is among the most widespread of tick-borne diseases in dogs, and some of these parasites also can infect other carnivores (e.g., cats, foxes). *Hepatozoon canis* is transmitted via ingestion of an infected tick, primarily *Rhipicephalus sanguineus*, containing mature *H. canis* oocysts. Treatment is recommended for all infected dogs with *H. canis* because parasitemia increases over time and develops into a severe infection.

Although there is no "standard" treatment for canine hepatozoonosis, imidocarb dipropionate is the drug of choice against *H. canis* infection in dogs, in a dose of 5–6 mg/kg BW, s.c.

or intramuscularly (i.m.) twice a month for at least 2 months. It is often used in combination with doxycycline monohydrate administered 10 mg/kg BW, p.o., for 21 days, primarily to treat other possible tick-borne infections such as *Ehrlichia canis* or *Anaplasma* spp. It is also used in combination with toltrazuril and/or clindamycin (e.g., Elias and Homans, 1988; Krampitz and Haberkorn, 1988; Baneth et al., 1995; de Tommasi et al., 2014).

Case Reports

Sasanelli et al. (2010) studied the effect of different doses of imidocarb dipropionate in three adult asymptomatic dogs naturally-infected with *H. canis*. The dogs were treated repeatedly over 8 months at the Veterinary Hospital, University of Bari, Italy. Blood counts, **parasitemia** levels in their blood, parasites in concentrated buffy-coat smears, and PCR of blood all were monitored. First, Sasanelli et al. (2010) used an initial dose of 3 mg/kg BW (i.e., lower than recommended), s.c., twice a month; however, parasitemia persisted after 5 treatments. Because this dose was evidently insufficient, they continued with the standard (regular) dose of 6 mg/kg BW; parasitemia then disappeared only in 1 dog. Combined therapy with doxycycline monohydrate 10 mg/kg BW, p.o., s.i.d., for 4 weeks also failed. The authors (2010) reported that all the dogs treated with the regular dosage of imidocarb alone or imidocarb combined with doxycycline still remained *Hepatozoon*-PCR-positive, although parasitemia was not microscopically detected in the blood, and buffy-coat smears also were negative. They pointed out that PCR is the most sensitive method for detection, whereas buffy-coat smears and detecting parasitemia in blood smears are not reliable markers to assess the efficacy of the treatment.

Pasa et al. (2011) evaluated the effect of a combination therapy of imidocarb dipropionate (Imizol®) with toltrazuril (Baycox®) to determine if toltrazuril has a synergistic effect;

in other words, is it able to potentiate the effect of imidocarb? Twelve mixed-breed dogs from a shelter in Selcuk, Turkey, naturally-infected with *H. canis*, were included in their study; three dogs had a concomitant infection with *Ehrlichia canis*. Six dogs received monotherapy of 6 mg/kg BW of imidocarb dipropionate, s.c., twice in 14 days, and the other 6 dogs received 6 mg/kg BW of imidocarb dipropionate, s.c., twice in 14 days plus 10 mg/kg BW, p.o., s.i.d., of toltrazuril for the first 5 days. Clinical status, blood counts, and parasitemia levels in blood smears were monitored before the trial and then 14, 28, and 56 days after treatment. A complete clinical recovery was recorded in 4/6 dogs on monotherapy and in 5/6 dogs on combination therapy. Decrease of body temperature was detected in both groups. However, 5/6 dogs on monotherapy and 4/6 dogs on combination therapy had persisting *H. canis* gametocytes in blood smears at the end of the study. Thus, a combination therapy of imidocarb with toltrazuril provided better clinical response than the monotherapy; however, none of the tested therapies eliminated the parasite.

de Tommasi et al. (2014) evaluated the efficacy of two therapeutic protocols: (1) imidocarb dipropionate administered 5–6 mg/kg BW, s.c., once/week for 6 weeks, and (2) a combination of toltrazuril/emodepside (Procox®) (15 mg/kg BW, s.i.d., for 6 days) with clindamycin (15 mg/kg BW, s.i.d., for 21 days) in 32 dogs naturally-infected with *H. canis*. The dogs originated from a private shelter in the municipality of Putignano, Bari province, Italy. Cytology on buffy-coat, and PCR on blood, were done weekly for 18 weeks. After 18 weeks, the infection still persisted in both groups of treated dogs (and in the control group), diagnosed in 72% via cytology and 100% by PCR. Thus, both tested protocols failed.

Because imidocarb dipropionate and other chemotherapeutics studied thus far have not proved effective, research for new drugs is necessary for the treatment of infections with *Hepatozoon* spp.

TREATMENT/DRUG THERAPY: NEOSPORA IN CARNIVORA

Neosporosis, caused by *Neospora caninum*, may represent a serious disease in cattle and dogs worldwide. In cattle it usually causes repeated abortions, stillbirths, and severe economic losses. In dogs it causes **meningoencephalitis**, **polymyositis**, and **polyradiculoneuritis**. Although *N. caninum* is morphologically and phylogenetically related to *Toxoplasma gondii*, it varies in life cycle and pathogenicity, so the therapy is different.

Several drugs and substances have been screened for anti-*N. caninum* activity both *in vitro* in cell culture or *in vivo* using mouse models: these include amprolium (Lindsay and Dubey, 1990), artemether (Qian et al., 2015), artemisinin (Kim et al., 2002), artemisone (Mazuz et al., 2012), arylimidamide (Debache et al., 2011), atrazine (Qian et al., 2015), bumped kinase inhibitors (Ojo et al., 2014), curcumin (Qian et al., 2015), cyclophosphamide (Qian et al., 2015), diminazene aceturate (Qian et al., 2015), glyphosate (Qian et al., 2015), miltefosine (Debache and Hemphill, 2012), organometallic ruthenium complexes (Barna et al., 2013), ponazuril (Darius et al., 2004; Qian et al., 2015), praziquantel (Qian et al., 2015), thiazolide nitazoxanide (Esposito et al., 2005, 2007; Debache et al., 2011), and toltrazuril (Gottstein et al., 2001, 2005; Darius et al., 2004; Strohbusch et al., 2009; Qian et al., 2015).

Some of these represent promising drug candidates. For example, Qian et al. (2015) recorded a significant inhibitory activity *in vitro* (human foreskin fibroblast cultures) in parasite growth and replication in response to treatment with artemether, atrazine, curcumin, ponazuril, and toltrazuril; moreover, curcumin also was effective against host cell invasion but was ineffective *in vivo* (using 6-week-old BALB/c mice). Cyclophosphamide, diminazene aceturate, glyphosate, and praziquantel were ineffective both *in vitro* and *in vivo*. Müller et al. (2015) studied efficacy of buparvaquone, a hydroxynaphthoquinone that is registered against **theileriosis** and is in common use; they showed that it is highly active against *N. caninum* both *in vitro* and *in vivo*. *In vitro*, it inhibited tachyzoite replication but acted slowly, and only for a short period; *in vivo* (100 mg/kg buparvaquone i.p. and p.o.), it prevented acute neosporosis in mice. High numbers of parasites still remained in the central nervous system (CNS) but not in other organs of mice. Therefore, buparvaquone represents an interesting lead with the potential to diminish fetal infection during pregnancy.

Despite the efficacy of several substances mentioned above, clindamycin hydrochloride, trimethoprim–sulfadiazine, and pyrimethamine, alone or in combination, are still the most commonly used and recommended drugs for the treatment of neosporosis in dogs, although they often have a limited efficacy and significant side effects and do not eliminate *N. caninum* from the body (Lappin, 2000; Ordeix et al., 2002; Crookshanks et al., 2007; Lyon, 2010; Qian et al., 2015). Recommended doses and duration of treatment are provided in Table 3 (according to Lyon, 2010). In the case of myositis and dermatitis, clindamycin is the most efficient therapy. For neurological signs, trimethoprim–sulfadiazine or pyrimethamine + sulfadiazine are better treatment options because of more efficient penetration into the CNS. In addition to medical therapy, physiotherapy can also be beneficial to recovery. The prognosis improves if therapy is started early. However, dogs with untreated clinical neosporosis usually die, and the prognosis with treatment is variable, especially in puppies and dogs with severe neurological signs. Clinical improvement is unlikely if muscle contracture or rapidly ascending paralysis is present. To reduce the chance of illness, all puppies in a litter should be treated as soon as the diagnosis has been made in any puppy (Mayhew et al., 1991; Dubey and Lappin, 2006; Crookshanks et al., 2007). It has been demonstrated that administration of glucocorticoids,

other immunosuppressive drugs, and modified live vaccines may activate bradyzoites and result in clinical illness or worsen clinical disease, in dogs with neosporosis (Ordeix et al., 2002; Fry et al., 2009; Lyon, 2010).

Vaccination has been proposed as an additional potential method to control neosporosis in animals. So far, vaccines (both live and inactivated) have been designed against bovine neosporosis and may provide at least a partial protection in cattle, with overall efficacy ranging from 5% to 54% (Heuer et al., 2004; Romero et al., 2004; Dubey et al., 2007). Vaccination against bovine neosporosis in cattle is based on the finding that some *N. caninum*-infected cows can develop a degree of protective immunity against abortion and transmission. However, currently, available vaccines do not allow serological discrimination between the vaccinated and infected cattle; thus, vaccinated cattle cannot be introduced into a *Neospora*-free herd. Moreover, the absence of prions of bovine spongiform encephalopathy must be confirmed for the *N. caninum* isolates derived from bovine tissues or from dogs fed with bovine material (Dubey et al., 2007).

Case Reports

Poli et al. (1998) reported that a 5-year-old male Bernese cattle dog was presented to the veterinary clinic in Pistoia, Italy, with nodular dermatitis (cutaneous ulcerative lesion, 2–3 cm wide, in the skin of the tarsal region). Blood parameters were normal. Histopathology revealed diffuse necrotic dermatitis with a dense infiltrate of neutrophils and macrophages. Numerous tachyzoites of *N. caninum* were scattered in the lesions, and protozoans also were present within macrophages, neutrophils, fibroblasts, and endothelial cells. Specific immunohistochemical staining was positive for *N. caninum* but negative for *T. gondii* and *Leishmania*. A high serum antibody titer (1:640) to *N. caninum* was recorded by IFAT. Transmission electron microscopy (TEM) revealed numerous tachyzoites in the host cell cytoplasm measuring, 3.5–5 × 1.5–2.5, all located in parasitophorous vacuoles. The dog was diagnosed with cutaneous neosporosis, and the lesion was surgically excised; however, new small nodules reappeared after 4 weeks. The dog was treated with clindamycin hydrochloride, 7.5 mg/kg BW, for 3 weeks. After 21 days, the new nodules completely resolved. Dubey et al. (1995b) also described efficacy of clindamycin in treatment of canine cutaneous neosporosis, when the lesions resolved 30 days after the therapy.

Ordeix et al. (2002) reported a 4-year-old male Rottweiler that was presented to the veterinary hospital in Barcelona, Spain, with a 10-day history of papulonodular dermatitis without pruritus or pain. The dog was administered immunosuppressive treatment (prednisone + azathioprine) for pemphigus foliaceus for 9 months. Blood parameters were normal. Histopathology revealed periadnexal pyogranulomatous dermatitis and intraluminal folliculitis. "Numerous small intracellular basophilic round bodies resembling protozoal tachyzoites were present in the cytoplasm of dermal macrophages." Specific immunohistochemical staining was positive for *N. caninum* but negative for *T. gondii* and *Leishmania*. The dog was diagnosed with cutaneous neosporosis. A high serum antibody titer (1:1600) to *N. caninum* was recorded by *Neospora* agglutination test and TEM demonstrated numerous *N. caninum* tachyzoites within keratinocytes and macrophages; these measured 2.3–4 × 1.7–2.8, all located in parasitophorous vacuoles. It was treated with clindamycin hydrochloride (Dalacin®) 12.5 mg/kg BW, b.i.d., and the immunosuppressive medication was withdrawn. A surprisingly prolonged clinical remission was observed in the dog both for neosporosis and pemphigus foliaceus (10 months after the clindamycin therapy was discontinued, and 1 year after the withdrawal of the immunosuppressive therapy).

Crookshanks et al. (2007) reported a case of canine pediatric *N. caninum* myositis in a 7-week-old female Irish wolfhound puppy in Canada, which was referred to a veterinary college for an abnormal hind limb posture and gait lasting for 3 weeks. Seven puppies from the same litter and a bitch were asymptomatic. The palpation was painless, and the orthopedic examination, radiography, cerebrospinal fluid, and myelogram were normal. Neurological examination revealed severe bilateral atrophy of the quadriceps muscles and bilateral absence of patellar reflexes. Biochemically, creatine kinase activity was elevated. Electromyography revealed bilateral spontaneous depolarization of quadriceps, pectineus, and gracilis muscles, suggesting a myopathy or neuropathy. Histology of muscle biopsies revealed multiple focal infiltrates of lymphocytes, plasma cells, and macrophages, indicating a multifocal myositis. Cerebrospinal fluid and serum were negative for *T. gondii* antibodies by hemagglutination test. However, the serum examined by indirect immunoperoxidase testing contained a high titer (≥1:800) of IgG antibodies against *Neospora*, suggesting an active infection; IgM antibodies were not present. Immunohistochemistry of biopsies of the quadriceps muscle were negative for *T. gondii* but positive for *Neospora* sp. The bitch was also *Neospora* seropositive (>1:50) but asymptomatic. Thus, the puppy most likely was infected transplacentally. The puppy was treated with clindamycin hydrochloride (Antirobe®) at a dosage of 12 mg/kg BW, p.o., every 8 hours for 18 weeks, with physiotherapy and massage. Improvement occurred after 4 weeks of treatment, and its gait was 90% normal after 1 year.

Fry et al. (2009) reported a case of a fatal protozoal hepatitis, an uncommon manifestation of neosporosis, in a dog. A 4-year-old female spayed standard poodle was diagnosed with an idiopathic immune-mediated hemolytic anemia (IMHA) based on regenerative anemia with autoagglutination and spherocytosis, low hemoglobin concentration 69–76 g/L (reference range 120–180 g/L), and low PCV 24% (ref. range 37%–55%). The dog was weak, lethargic, with pale mucous membranes. Biochemistry revealed slightly increased creatine kinase, aspartate aminotransferase, bilirubin, and amylase. **Hepatosplenomegaly** was observed ultrasonographically. Other examinations were normal. The dog was treated with prednisone 2 mg/kg BW, p.o., b.i.d., but not seeing improvement, it was referred to a specialized veterinary department, where additional immunosuppressive therapy was continued with azathioprine 1 mg/kg BW, p.o. + cyclosporin 10 mg/kg BW, p.o. + aspirin 0.5 mg/kg BW, p.o., s.i.d. The dog responded well, and all treatment was discontinued after 1 year. However, the IMHA relapsed, so the dog was administered the same immunosuppressive therapy again; its hepatic enzymes and bilirubin were markedly elevated, and its hemoglobin and PCV were low. No improvement was observed despite the immunosuppressive therapy, so the dog was administered metronidazole, enrofloxacin, amoxicillin–clavulanic acid, clindamycin, fluid therapy, and plasma transfusion, but it died after 36 hours (probably due to the combination of drugs and/or the toxic level of cyclosporin). Histology of the hepatic parenchyma disclosed multifocal hepatocytes containing "numerous (20–100) basophilic globular to ovoid bodies 2–3 μm in diameter, resembling tachyzoites of *N. caninum* or *T. gondii*." Immunohistochemistry for *T. gondii* was negative, but PCR amplification of DNA isolated from the liver identified the presence of *N. caninum*. However, a full necropsy was not carried out; thus, the possibility of a more disseminated infection could not be ruled out. In this dog, either a subclinical infection was activated or the patient acquired the infection during the immunosuppressive therapy.

TREATMENT/DRUG THERAPY: TOXOPLASMA IN CARNIVORA

Carnivores may get infected with *T. gondii* by ingesting tissue cysts from raw meat in their food or prey or by ingesting food or water contaminated with oocysts from feces of infected feline definitive hosts. Tissue cysts of *T. gondii* are killed by freezing and cooking, but the oocysts are highly resistant and can survive in the environment for months. Although *T. gondii* is morphologically and phylogenetically related to *N. caninum*, it varies in life cycle and pathogenicity.

Clindamycin, azithromycin, and spiramycin were reported to be active against *T. gondii*, although the exact mechanism is still unknown (Araujo and Remington, 1974; Araujo et al., 1991; Pfefferkorn et al., 1992; Blais et al., 1993; Pfefferkorn and Borotz, 1994). Because of the existence of partial or complete cross-resistance to these antibiotics in selected resistant mutants, it is presumed that they share a common target in *T. gondii*; the most commonly accepted hypothesis is that they inhibit *T. gondii* by blocking protein biosynthesis in the apicomplexan organelle that contains a 35-kb genome (Pfefferkorn and Borotz, 1994). Clindamycin + pyrimethamine, and sulfadiazine + pyrimethamine also have been demonstrated to have anti-*Toxoplasma* activity, especially in patients with AIDS (Katlama, 1991; Dannemann et al., 1992).

Dubey and Thayer (1994) and Dubey et al. (1996a,b) found that sporulated oocysts and tissue cysts of *T. gondii* treated with various doses of ^{137}Cs gamma-irradiation were inactivated by low dosages of gamma-irradiation (0.3 kGy for the oocysts, and 0.4 kGy for the tissue cysts). Temperature during the irradiation had no marked effect on the viability of tissue cysts. Later, Dubey et al. (1998a) studied sporulation and viability of unsporulated and sporulated oocysts and tissue cysts of *T. gondii* in mice, and on raspberries experimentally contaminated with sporulated oocysts of *T. gondii*, after the treatment with various doses of ^{137}Cs gamma-irradiation. They found that the effect of irradiation differed with respect to the stage of the parasite irradiated and recommended a dosage level for killing oocysts is 0.5 **kGy**, which also kills tissue cysts of *T. gondii*. Thus, gamma-irradiation proved to be effective in inactivation of oocysts and tissue cysts of *T. gondii*.

Vaccination has been proposed as an additional approach to control toxoplasmosis in animals, and a live vaccine has been developed for sheep to prevent abortions caused by *T. gondii*. The vaccine was prepared by multiple passage of *T. gondii* through a mouse host, which caused an inability to produce tissue cysts (Meeusen et al., 2007).

TREATMENT, PREVENTION, AND CONTROL: CHEMOTHERAPEUTICS USED FOR CARNIVORES (LISTED ALPHABETICALLY)

Acridines

Quinacrine (Acriquine®, Atabrine®, Atebrin®, Mepacrine®) is an acridine derivative formerly widely used as an antimalarial drug, but superseded by safer and more effective agents (e.g., chloroquine). Later, it was used as an anthelmintic (mainly against cestodes), antiprotozoal (mainly against giardiasis and cutaneous leishmaniasis), antineoplastic agent (to treat certain types of malignant tumors), and antirheumatic. The exact mechanism of its antiparasitic action is unknown. It is supposed to act against a protozoan's cell membrane, but its effect against coccidia is questionable. Quinacrine concentrates in liver, spleen, lungs, and adrenal glands and is excreted in feces, urine, bile, sweat, and saliva. It is contraindicated in pregnant females (crosses the placenta and reaches fetus) and in individuals with impaired hepatic functions. Quinacrine is rapidly absorbed from the gastrointestinal tract and is commercially available in formulations for oral administration (tablets). Its use for the treatment of cystoisosporiasis in cats (10 mg/kg BW, s.i.d. for 5 days) is only off-label (CAPC, 2013).

Antibiotics With Antiprotozoal Effect

Azithromycin (Zithromax®) is a semisynthetic macrolide antibiotic, a derivative of erythromycin, belonging to azalides or "advanced-generation macrolides." It has a bacteriostatic effect, inhibiting protein biosynthesis in bacteria by binding to the P site of the 50S ribosomal subunit. It is stable in acid environments and displays an antimicrobial activity against Gram+ cocci and rods (*Streptococcus*, *Clostridium*, *Listeria*, *Mycobacterium*), some Gram− bacteria (*Actinobacillus*, *Aeromonas*, *Chlamydia*, *Bartonella*) and also against protozoans such as *Babesia* and *T. gondii*. Certain effects also have been recorded against *Cryptosporidium*. Azithromycin is more popular than erythromycin in the treatment of dogs and cats because of its longer half-life and better absorption by both species. Its distribution is mainly provided by the recipients' phagocytes, and it reaches high concentrations in tissues but binds to proteins minimally. The prolonged, high concentration of azithromycin at the site of infection permits once a day dosing and may allow for a shorter duration of treatment. Azithromycin interacts with, and is contraindicated in use with, other macrolides, oral antacids, cisapride, and drugs metabolized by cytochrome P450. In companion animal medicine, it is used mainly for treatment of respiratory, urogenital, and dermatological infections. For dogs and cats, azithromycin is commercially available in formulations for oral administration (tablets, powder). The recommended therapeutically effective dosage in dogs and cats is 5.3 mg/kg BW, p.o., b.i.d. for 2 weeks.

Clindamycin (Antirobe®, Clindamycin®, Dalacin®) is a semisynthetic lincosamide antibiotic, widely used in human and small animal medicine, displaying antimicrobial activity not only against Gram+ aerobes (cocci and rods) and anaerobic bacteria but also against some protozoans such as *T. gondii*, *N. caninum*, *Babesia microti*, and *Plasmodium falciparum* (Wittner et al., 1982; el Wakeel et al., 1985; Lindsay et al., 1994; Pfefferkorn and Borotz, 1994; Prescott, 2000; Schaumann et al., 2000; Batzias et al., 2005). It inhibits protein biosynthesis in bacteria by binding to the 23S rRNA of the 50S ribosomal subunit; in *T. gondii* the target site is another RNA molecule, encoded by a 35-kb circular extrachromosomal genome (Pfefferkorn and Borotz, 1994; Prescott, 2000; Batzias et al., 2005). For a long time, clindamycin was thought to be bacteriostatic, but several reports suggested that it displays concentration-independent bactericidal activity (Dow, 1988; Xue et al., 1996; Lewis et al., 1999; Batzias et al., 2005). It is widely and well-distributed in all tissues and body fluids and soluble in lipids, so it easily pervades barriers and cell membranes. It is able to achieve higher concentrations in leukocytes, via which it is distributed, and then reaches higher levels in the foci of infection. It undergoes hepatic biotransformation, and its parent compound and metabolites are excreted in the feces and urine. It induces a neuromuscular blockade that can be eliminated by calcium. However, resistance to clindamycin is common in bacteria (resistance of the MLS type and mutations). Clindamycin is practically nontoxic for dogs and cats, but contraindicated in individuals with impaired renal and hepatic functions, and in pregnant females. In companion animal medicine, it is used mainly for treatment of superficial or deep pyoderma, osteomyelitis, infections of the oral cavity, anaerobic infections, toxoplasmosis, and neosporosis (Boothe, 1990; Prescott, 2000; Ordeix et al., 2002; Batzias et al., 2005). Clindamycin hydrochloride (e.g., Antirobe®) is commercially available in formulations for oral administration (capsules, tablets, oral solution), and clindamycin phosphate (containing the phosphate ester) has injectable formulations for s.c., i.m., or i.v. administration. In dogs, pharmacokinetics was studied after p.o., s.c., i.m., and i.v. administration, and in cats after p.o. administration (Brown et al., 1989, 1990; Budsberg et al., 1992; Lavy et al., 1999). Absorption after p.o. administration is quite fast, with the maximum concentration (C_{max}) achieved at 1 hour, which is comparable to s.c. and i.m. administration. However, the bioavailability is significantly lower than that after the s.c. or i.m. administration. Based on serum clindamycin concentrations, the recommended therapeutically effective dosage in dogs

is 5.5–11 mg/kg BW, p.o., s.i.d., and for less susceptible bacteria b.i.d., and 11 mg/kg BW, i.m., s.i.d. or b.i.d. Although clindamycin is registered for dogs, the studies on its p.o. administration in cats at the same dosage as in dogs did not demonstrate any clinical signs of drug intoxication (Brown et al., 1989).

Doxycycline monohydrate (VibraVet®) is a semisynthetic second-generation tetracycline antibiotic, prepared from oxytetracycline, and possessing the depot effect for release of active antibiotic. It is widely used in human and small animal medicine, displaying bacteriostatic antimicrobial activity against a wide number of both Gram+ and Gram− bacteria, especially against *Bartonella*, *Borrelia*, *Brucella*, *Chlamydia*, *Clostridium*, *Haemophilus*, and *Mycoplasma*. However, acquired plasmid-encoded resistance to doxycycline is common in bacteria. Doxycycline inhibits protein biosynthesis in bacteria by binding to the proteins of the 30S ribosomal subunit, thus preventing the contact of the transfer RNA with ribosomes. It displays affinity to polyvalent cations and results in the formation of barely soluble chelates that negatively influence resorption. It undergoes an enterohepatic circulation, with high concentrations present in liver and bile, kidneys, spleen, and lungs. It does not undergo any biotransformation, so it is excreted in an active form in feces and urine. Doxycycline monohydrate is contraindicated in dysphagia and vomiting, in pregnant females, and in young, while their teeth are developing. In companion animal medicine, it is used mainly for treatment of skin, respiratory and gastrointestinal infections, and infections such as chlamydiosis or rickettsiosis, where other antibiotics are not efficient. In humans, it is also used for malaria prophylaxis. Doxycycline monohydrate is commercially available in formulations for oral administration (tablets, paste). The recommended therapeutically effective dosage is a single initial loading dose of 5 mg/kg BW, p.o. in both dogs and cats, followed by 2 doses of 2.5 mg/kg BW, p.o., b.i.d., and then a maintenance dose of 2.5 mg/kg BW, p.o., s.i.d. for 5 days.

Furazolidone (Dependal-M®, Furoxone®) is a nitrofuran antibiotic, acting as an inhibitor of monoamine oxidase. It displays antimicrobial activity not only against Gram+ (streptococci, staphylococci, *Clostridium*) and several Gram– bacteria (*E. coli*, *Salmonella*) but also against protozoans such as *Giardia*, *Histomonas*, and *Eimeria* species. It is used mainly for treatment of infections of the gastrointestinal tract. Furazolidone may cause very serious side effects when taken with certain food, beverages, and other medicine, as it seriously interacts with many drugs. Furthermore, it is recognized by the US Food and Drug Administration (FDA) as a mutagen/carcinogen, thus its use was discontinued in 1991, and it is no longer available in the United States. It is still commercially available in some countries, in formulations for oral administration (tablets, suspension) and is recommended to be administered 4 times a day for 7–10 days. Its use in dogs and cats (8–20 mg/kg BW, s.i.d. or b.i.d., for 5 days) is only off-label (CAPC, 2013).

Paromomycin (Humatin®) is a broad-spectrum aminoglycoside antibiotic produced by *Streptomyces rimosus* var. *paromomycinus*, and displaying bactericide antimicrobial activity not only against a wide range of both Gram+ and, especially, Gram– bacteria, but also against some protozoans such as *Giardia*, *Leishmania*, and *Entamoeba histolytica*. It is poorly absorbed from the gastrointestinal tract after oral administration, and almost entirely recoverable in the feces. Paromomycin has been shown to have anticryptosporidial activity for mice, calves, dogs, cats, and humans with AIDS (Armitage et al., 1992; Fayer and Ellis, 1993a,b; Fichtenbaum et al., 1993; Barr et al., 1994a,b; Sykes and Papich, 2014). Few specific data on toxicity for cats are available (Gookin et al., 1999; Sykes and Papich, 2014), but the extremely high LD_{50} dose (~15,000 mg/kg BW, p.o.) in mice and its poor absorption from the gastrointestinal tract suggest low toxicity.

It is also used in combination with other medicines to manage a serious complication of liver disease (hepatic coma). However, the acquired plasmid-encoded resistance, restricting the penetration of aminoglycoside into the bacterial cell, may arise in bacteria. Paromomycin affects protein biosynthesis in bacteria by binding to the ribosomes during translation, but it does not inhibit protein biosynthesis itself and forms the "nonsense-proteins" that clog the cytoplasm and kill bacterial cells. Barr et al. (1994a,b) successfully used it to treat cryptosporidiosis in dogs and cats with the dosage of 125–165 mg/kg BW, p.o., b.i.d., for 5 days.

Spiramycin (Provamicina®, Rovamycine®) is a first-generation macrolide antibiotic, isolated from *Streptomyces ambofaciens*. It inhibits protein biosynthesis in bacteria at the 27S or 50S ribosomal subunits, damaging the target structures. It not only has a bacteriostatic effect, displaying antimicrobial activity against a large number of bacteria including streptococci, *Mycoplasma*, *Chlamydia*, and *Legionella* but also has good antiprotozoal activity against *T. gondii* and *Entamoeba*. It is used mainly for treatment of infections of the respiratory and gastrointestinal tract and mastitis. Spiramycin is well resorbed, reaches high concentrations in saliva, lymph, and parenchyma, and is excreted in bile. Its metabolism has not been well studied, but it is thought to be metabolized in the liver to active metabolites. Because of its high concentrations in saliva, spiramycin often is used in combination with metronidazole (Stomorgyl®) to treat stomatitis in dogs. It is commercially available in formulations for oral administration (tablets, capsules), rectal administration (suppository), and in injectable formulations for i.m. or i.v. administration. The recommended therapeutically effective dosage in dogs and cats is 10–12 mg/kg BW, i.m., s.i.d., and 75,000 international units/kg BW, p.o., s.i.d. (however, even higher doses administered p.o. are not toxic).

Tylosin (Tylan®) is a first-generation macrolide antibiotic, isolated from *Streptomyces fradiae*, and used exclusively in veterinary medicine. It inhibits the initial phase of protein biosynthesis on bacterial ribosomes by binding to the proteins of the peptidyl transferase center, which causes the inhibition of release of polypeptides, prolongation of their chains, and their transfer. It has a bacteriostatic effect, displaying antimicrobial activity mainly against *Mycoplasma*, Gram+ cocci, and some other Gram+ and Gram– anaerobic bacteria. It was also reported to possess a certain anticryptosporidial effect in cats but required a long period of administration (Barr and Bowman, 2006; Lucio-Forster et al., 2010). Tylosin is well absorbed from the gastrointestinal tract and is eliminated in the urine and bile apparently in unchanged form. It is used mainly for treatment of infections of the respiratory and gastrointestinal tract, metritis, and mastitis. It does not have impact on efficacy of other antibiotics, is relatively nontoxic, non-hepatotoxic, and is effective in relatively low dosages. Tylosin is commercially available in formulations for oral administration (powder, oral liquid) and in injectable formulations for i.m. administration. The powder form is not FDA-approved for use in companion animals, but it is a common off-label practice for veterinarians. The recommended therapeutically effective dosage in dogs and cats is 10 mg/kg BW, i.m., b.i.d., and 5–15 mg/kg BW, p.o., every 6–8 hours. Oral treatment in dogs has been administered for several months with apparent safety. However, tylosin is contraindicated and even fatal for horses.

Carbanilide Derivatives

Imidocarb dipropionate (Carbesia®, Carbésia®, Forray®, Imidox®, Imizol®) is a carbanilide derivative with antiprotozoal activity, marketed only for veterinary use. It is the most commonly used drug against *Hepatozoon* infections, and it also is used for the treatment of *Trypanosoma brucei* and *Babesia ovis*. Its mode of action is uncertain, but it has been suggested that it acts against *T. brucei* by interfering with polyamine production, and

against *B. ovis* by blocking the entrance of inositol into erythrocytes (Bacchi et al., 1981; McHardy et al., 1986; Sasanelli et al., 2010). Imidocarb dipropionate is eliminated via urine and feces. It may display severe adverse effects, from pain at the site of infection, vomiting, diarrhea, agitation, lethargy, periorbital swelling, and acute renal tubular necrosis or hepatic necrosis (Sykes and Papich, 2014). It is usually administered as the dipropionate salt and is commercially available in injectable formulations for s.c. or i.m. administration. It is often used in combination with doxycycline monohydrate administered 10 mg/kg BW, p.o., for 21 days, primarily to treat other (possible) tick-borne infections such as *Ehrlichia canis*, *Rickettsia*, or *Anaplasma* species. It is also used in combination with toltrazuril and/or clindamycin (e.g., Elias and Homans, 1988; Krampitz and Haberkorn, 1988; Baneth et al., 1995; de Tommasi et al., 2014). However, no control studies or PCR-based methods have been employed to monitor the response to treatment (Baneth, 2006). Sasanelli et al. (2010) discovered that all dogs treated with the regular dosage of imidocarb alone, or imidocarb combined with doxycycline, remained *Hepatozoon*-PCR-positive, although parasitemia was not microscopically detected in their blood, and buffy-coat smears also were negative. Therefore, there is a need for new drugs to be developed for the treatment of *Hepatozoon* infections. Standard (regular) dosage in dogs calls for 5–6 mg/kg BW s.c. or i.m. twice a month at least for 8 weeks.

Diaminopyrimidines

Pyrimethamine (Daraprim®) was discovered in 1952 and introduced to the market in 1953. It is a synthetic derivative of ethyl pyrimidine, belonging to the diaminopyrimidines and antimalarials. It is a folic acid antagonist, acting as a competitive inhibitor of dihydrofolate reductase (DHFR), thus blocking biosynthesis of purines and pyrimidines. It is used to treat acute malaria, and in combination with sulfonamides (sulfadoxine, Fansidar®, or sulfadiazine) or antibiotics (azithromycin, clindamycin) to treat toxoplasmosis and neosporosis. It also was used for the treatment of cystoisosporiasis in humans. It may be used for the prevention of malaria in areas nonresistant to pyrimethamine; however, in humans, resistance to pyrimethamine is prevalent worldwide, so the drug alone is no longer recommended by the US Centers for Disease Control and Prevention or other experts for prevention of malaria. Pyrimethamine is distributed mainly to the kidneys, liver, spleen, and lungs and is well absorbed from the gastrointestinal tract. It is contraindicated in individuals with impaired renal and hepatic functions, with megaloblastic anemia caused by folate deficiency, and in pregnant females. In veterinary medicine, it has been successfully used for treatment of hepatozoonosis, leishmaniasis, neosporosis, sarcocystosis, and toxoplasmosis. For the treatment of neosporosis in dogs, it has a limited efficacy and does not entirely eliminate *N. caninum* from the body. For neurological signs of neosporosis, a combination of pyrimethamine with sulfadiazine is the best treatment option because of its more efficient penetration into the CNS. Pyrimethamine is commercially available in formulations for oral administration (tablets). Dosage of pyrimethamine required for the treatment of toxoplasmosis approaches the toxic level, so the recommended dosages should not be exceeded. In humans, the adult initial dose is 50–75 mg/day, together with 1–4 g/day of a sulfonamide (e.g., sulfadoxine) for 1–3 weeks. The dosage may then be reduced to about one-half that previously given for each drug and continued for an additional 4–5 weeks. Concurrent administration of folinic acid is recommended. A recommended dosage 1 mg/kg BW pyrimethamine, p.o., s.i.d. + 20 mg/kg BW sulfadiazine, p.o., s.i.d., for dogs and cats is only off-label (Sykes and Papich, 2014) but widely used by small animal veterinarians.

Trimethoprim (Primsol®, Proloprim®, Trimethoprim®, Trimpex®) is a basic substance to potentiate the effect of sulfonamides. Similar to diaminopyrimidines, it is a folic acid antagonist, acting as a competitive inhibitor of DHFR; it displays antimicrobial activity against Gram+ and Gram− bacteria. It also possesses anticoccidial and antimalarial effects; however, it is no longer used as an antimalarial because of its high toxicity. Trimethoprim is well absorbed from the gastrointestinal tract, is 90% metabolized, and the metabolites are excreted via kidneys and milk. It is contraindicated in individuals with impaired renal and hematopoietic functions and mainly is used in combination with sulfonamides (e.g., Amphoprim®, Avemix®, Coli Mix Plus®, Septotryl®, Sulfatrim®) primarily to treat toxoplasmosis, neosporosis, and intestinal coccidiosis in dogs and cats, which is safer and more effective than trimethoprim alone.

Nitrobenzamides

Nitazoxanide (Alinia®, Givotan®, Navigator®, Zoxanid®) is a promising drug now labeled for use in humans for treating *Cryptosporidium*. Nitazoxanide (2-acetyloxy-N-[5-nitro-2-thiazolyl] benzamide) is a synthetic antiprotozoal and anthelmintic agent for oral use, displaying activity against *Campylobacter jejuni*, *Cryptosporidium* spp., *Giardia duodenalis*, *Helicobacter* spp., *Sarcocystis neurona*, and some anaerobic bacteria. Following oral administration in humans, it is rapidly hydrolyzed to an active metabolite, tizoxanide (desacetyl-nitazoxanide). Tizoxanide then undergoes conjugation, primarily by hepatic glucuronidation, and then it is excreted via urine and bile. The antiprotozoal activity of nitazoxanide is believed to be due to interference with the pyruvate ferredoxin/ flavodoxin (PFOR) enzyme-dependent electron transfer reaction, which is essential to anaerobic energy metabolism (Sykes and Papich, 2014). Studies have shown that the PFOR enzyme from another intestinal parasitic protist, *Giardia duodenalis*, directly reduces nitazoxanide by transfer of electrons in the absence of ferredoxin;

the DNA-derived PFOR protein sequence of *C. parvum* appears to be similar to that of *G. duodenalis*. Dosage in humans calls for 500 mg b.i.d. for 14 days, 300 mg t.i.d. for 7 days, or 1 g b.i.d. for 7 days; the dosages tested in people were always accompanied with 20 mg of omeprazole (Prilosec®), for heartburn. Nitazoxanide has been sold as Navigator® for veterinary use to treat equine protozoal myeloencephalitis (EPM) caused by *Sarcocystis neurona*. Published papers about its use in cats and calves for cryptosporidiosis reported efficacy that seemed remarkable; administration of nitazoxanide stopped the shedding of oocysts; however, the infection was not fully eliminated, and adverse effects such as vomiting occurred frequently (e.g., Gookin et al., 2001). Li et al. (2003) reported that 50, 100, or 200 mg/kg BW, s.i.d. for 7 days, inhibited oocyst shedding in a dose-dependent manner in immunosuppressed rats and that shedding inhibition was unchanged 7 days after discontinuation of therapy.

Quinolone Derivatives

Decoquinate (Deccox®), a 4-hydroxyquinoline, is a synthetic coccidiostat used in veterinary medicine for poultry and cattle as a feed additive against *Eimeria* species. It inhibits mitochondrial respiration and electron transport in *Eimeria* (Fry and Williams, 1984; Sykes and Papich, 2014) and is supposed to act "by arresting the development of sporozoites following their penetration of the gut epithelium." However, the development of resistance to decoquinate is likely in *Eimeria*. It is also used to treat *Sarcocystis* spp. myositis in dogs and to prevent relapses in dogs chronically infected with *Hepatozoon americanum*. After absorption, decoquinate is rapidly eliminated via bile and feces and to a lesser extent also in the urine. Its target tissues are skin and fat, and metabolic equilibrium in these tissues is reached after 3 days. It is practically nontoxic, and it is commercially available in formulations for oral administration (suspension, powder, capsules). Although

decoquinate has been tested in dogs, its mechanism of action in dogs is unknown, and its recommended dosage for dogs (10–20 mg/kg BW p.o. s.i.d. or b.i.d.) and domestic ferrets (0.5 mg/kg BW, s.i.d. for 2 weeks or longer) is only off-label (CAPC, 2013; Sykes and Papich, 2014).

Sulfonamides

Sulfonamides were first introduced to medical practice about 10 years before antibiotics and, at the time, represented a new era in therapy of bacterial infections. They display antimicrobial activity not only against Gram+ cocci (streptococci, staphylococci) but also against Gram+ rods, Gram– cocci (*Neisseria*), and rods (*Haemophilus*, *Bacteroides*) and against some protozoans such as *T. gondii* and members of the Eimeriorina. They have a bacteriostatic effect, inhibiting the synthesis of folic acid, which is important for the development and reproduction of microbes, by blocking the enzyme dihydropteroate synthetase. They also have an antipyretic effect. In coccidia, they possess coccidiostatic effect at low doses and coccidiocidal effect at higher doses. They have activity against the first- and second-generation meronts, and likely also against the sexual stages (Mehlhorn and Aspöck, 2008). Acquired plasmid-encoded resistance to sulfonamides is frequent in bacteria, and resistance also has been reported in *Eimeria* species. Binding to plasma proteins varies depending on the particular sulfonamide and animal. Sulfonamides are widely and well distributed in tissues and organs and are able to pervade barriers, exudates, and transudates. They are excreted in urine, tears, and milk. In animals, they have practically no side effects but are contraindicated in individuals with impaired renal and hepatic functions. Sulfonamides are used mainly for treatment of septicemia, pyemia, infections in young, and coccidia. They are often used in combination with diaminopyrimidines, such as trimethoprim, which act on other stages of folate biosynthesis. Sulfonamides are commercially available in formulations for oral administration and in injectable formulations for parenteral (s.c., i.m., i.v.) administration. Parenteral administration is usually painful, and i.m. applications may cause prolonged changes including necroses. Generally, the recommended therapeutically effective dosage of sulfonamides in dogs and cats is 1.2–1.5 g/10 kg BW, p.o., per 24 hours, and 0.6–0.75 g/10 kg BW, when administered parenterally.

- *Sulfadiazine* belongs to the so-called "classic sulfonamides," has a strong effect, and is used mainly in combination with trimethoprim as a "sulfonamide with potentiated effect" (cotrimazine; Cotrimazin®).
- *Sulfadimethoxine* (Kokzidiol SD®) belongs to "sulfonamides with a protracted effect" (i.e., lasting longer than in classic sulfonamides). In coccidia, it has a coccidiostatic effect. In dogs it is highly (~95%) bound to plasma proteins, is well-resorbed after p.o. administration, and is practically nontoxic. However, it is contraindicated in individuals with impaired renal and hepatic functions and in newborns. Sulfadimethoxine is commercially available in formulations for p.o. administration (powder). The recommended therapeutically effective dosage in dogs and cats is 20–60 mg/kg BW, p.o., s.i.d. for 5–7 (up to 20) days, and for domestic ferrets 300 mg/kg BW in drinking water for 2 weeks or longer. It is used alone, or in combination with trimethoprim.
- *Sulfaguanidine* belongs to "classic sulfonamides" with good anticoccidial activity because of its limited resorption from the gastrointestinal tract (only about 40% is absorbed after p.o. administration). Its use in dogs and cats (150–200 mg/kg BW, s.i.d. for 6 days, or 100–200 mg/kg BW, every 8 hours for 5 days) is only off-label (CAPC, 2013).

- *Sulfamethoxypyridazin* (e.g., Vetkelfizina®) was introduced to the market as the first "sulfonamide with a protracted effect." It displayed significant side effects in people but not in companion animals, even when administered in high doses. It is commercially available in formulations for s.c., i.m., and i.v. administration. The recommended therapeutically effective dosage in dogs and cats is 25–50 mg/kg BW, s.i.d. only i.m. In veterinary medicine, it is also often combined with trimethoprim (Amphoprim®, Avemix®, Coli Mix Plus®, Septotryl®, Sulfatrim®).

Several other sulfonamides are also described to have an anticoccidial effect; however, they are not registered/used to treat carnivores (e.g., sulfaclozine, sulfadimidine, sulfathiazole, formosulfathiazole).

Thiamine Analogues

<u>Amprolium</u> (Amprol®, Amprolium®, Ampromed®, Amprosid®, Amprosol®, Amprovine®) is a quaternized derivative of pyrimidine that interferes with thiamine metabolism. It is a thiamine antagonist, blocking the thiamine receptors, thus preventing carbohydrate synthesis. It has a coccidiostatic effect at lower doses and coccidiocidal at higher doses. It is used to prevent and treat intestinal coccidiosis by blocking the thiamine transporter of *Eimeria* spp. meronts, which results in disruption of cell metabolism. It inhibits the development of merozoites and formation of second-generation meronts. It also has some activity against the sexual stages and oocyst sporulation (and possibly inhibits development of sporozoites) (Mehlhorn and Aspöck, 2008; Clarke et al., 2014). Amprolium is rapidly (within hours) eliminated from the organism via kidneys. It is commercially available in formulations for oral administration (oral solution for administration to drinking water). It has no adverse effects and is considered one of the

safest anticoccidial drugs. Amprolium is marketed only for veterinary use, sold alone or in combination with a substituted aminobenzoic methyl ester (ethopabate, a p-aminobenzoic acid analogue, which interferes with folic acid biosynthesis), or in combination with sulfonamides or pyrimethamine. It is used in poultry and cattle. Its use in dogs (300–400 mg total for 5 days, or 110–200 mg s.i.d. for 7–12 days), cats (60–100 mg/kg BW, s.i.d. for 7 days), and domestic ferrets (19 mg/kg BW, s.i.d. for 2 weeks or longer) is only off-label (CAPC, 2013).

Triazines

Diclazuril (Clinacox®, Protazil®, Vecoxan®) was originally developed for its activity against chicken *Eimeria* to control coccidiosis in poultry. It is a synthetic benzenacetonitrile derivative, belonging to the "asymmetric triazines." Its mode of action is not precisely known, however, it interrupts the life cycle of eimerians. Diclazuril is of low toxicity, and is commercially available in formulations for oral administration. It is registered for broilers and for oral use in lambs. Its use in cats (25 mg/kg BW for one dose) is only off-label (CAPC, 2013).

Ponazuril (Marquis®) was originally developed for its activity against *Sarcocystis neurona*, which causes EPM in horses; its great advantage against *S. neurona* is that it crosses the blood/brain barrier to reach the CNS where it kills the parasite. It belongs to the "symmetric triazines," is a derivative of toltrazuril, and is similar to toltrazuril; ponazuril acts against coccidia at several stages of their life cycle. Its efficacy was demonstrated both *in vitro* and *in vivo* (in mice and calves) against tachyzoites of *N. caninum* (Kritzner et al., 2002; Darius et al., 2004; Gottstein et al., 2005; Haerdi et al., 2006). It also has been used by veterinarians to treat the cryptosporidial infections, mostly in mammals and birds. It is commercially available in formulations for oral administration (paste). In clinical efficacy trials conducted at equine referral clinics,

Marquis® was effective at the recommended dose level (http://www.bayerdvm.com/), but this product is not for use in animals intended for food (Mehlhorn et al., 1984; Haberkorn and Stoltefuss, 1987; Bohrmann, 1991; Furr et al., 2001, 2006; Stafford et al., 1994; Lindsay et al., 2000a). The pharmacokinetics in dogs has not been reported, however, the recommended therapeutically effective dosage in dogs and cats to treat *Cystoisospora* infections is 20 mg/kg BW, p.o., s.i.d. for 1–5 days (CAPC, 2013; Sykes and Papich, 2014).

Toltrazuril (Baycox®) was first produced by Bayer in the 1980s and belongs to the class of "symmetric triazines." It was introduced to the market in 1986, and because it affects all intracellular developmental stages of various genera of coccidia, mainly *Eimeria, Isospora, Cystoisospora, Sarcocystis, T. gondii,* and *Hepatozoon* spp. (Mehlhorn and Aspöck, 2008; Sykes and Papich, 2014), it has been used with excellent results to combat coccidiosis in various animal species, mostly birds and mammals (primarily pigs) since its launch. It is not registered for use in the United States, but it is registered and commonly used in Europe, Australia, and Canada, where some veterinarians consider it the most effective treatment/control for coccidia. It is commercially available in formulations for oral administration (suspension, microgranulate). It is also available in combination with the anthelmintic emodepside (Procox® Oral Suspension for Dogs) to treat isosporiasis and roundworm infections in puppies over 2 weeks of age. Toltrazuril affects meronts, micro-, and macrogametes but not the tissue cells of host animals, as documented by both LM and TEM studies (Bayer Animal Health Studies, http://www.baycox.com/17/Mode_of_Action.htm). These findings suggest that toltrazuril interferes with the division of the parasite's nucleus and with the activity of mitochondria, which is responsible for the respiratory metabolism of coccidia. In the macrogamonts, toltrazuril damages the wall-forming bodies. In all intracellular developmental stages, severe vacuolization occurs due to inflation of the endoplasmic reticulum (Haberkorn and Stoltefuss, 1987; Harder and Haberkorn, 1989; Altreuther et al., 2011a). Toltrazuril, thus, has a coccidiocidal mode of action, which results in the following advantages: (1) It acts against all intracellular developmental stages; (2) It does not interfere with the development of immunity; (3) Follow-up treatment usually is not necessary; (4) Even an advanced infection (of 3–5 days; gametogony) can still be treated successfully; (5) Its efficacy is independent of the severity of infection; and (6) Because of its specific activity against apicomplexan parasites, it is practically nontoxic for mammal hosts. Also, because of its efficacy in birds and mammals, some veterinarians have used it with a degree of success in reptiles. Toltrazuril also is used for the treatment of hepatozoonosis, however, with conflicting results. For example, it was not effective in treatment of *H. canis* in dogs (Beaufils et al., 1996; Pasa et al., 2011), whereas it prevented death in voles experimentally infected with *H. erhardovae* but did not eliminate the parasite from the body (Krampitz and Haberkorn, 1988). It was reported to cause only a short-term remission (for several months) of clinical signs in dogs (Macintire et al., 1997). On the other hand, Perez Tort et al. (2007) reported its efficacy in dogs infected with *H. canis* in a dose of 14 mg/kg BW, s.i.d. for 7 days, and Voyvoda et al. (2004) reported a positive effect of combination of 10 mg/kg BW, toltrazuril p.o., s.i.d. for 5 days with trimethoprim sulfamethoxazole in treatment of a dog with severe *H. canis* infection. To treat cystoisosporiasis in dogs, the recommended therapeutically effective dosage is 10–30 mg/kg BW, p.o., s.i.d. for 1–3 days. For domestic ferrets, the recommended therapeutically effective dosage is 20 mg/kg BW (CAPC, 2013).

DISCUSSION AND SUMMARY

It is obvious from the above-mentioned text and case reports, that therapy of coccidiosis is rather complicated in carnivores. Despite the facts that the available drugs and/or substances are active only against a restricted range of coccidian genera, and, for many infections, the treatment often does not result in a complete elimination of the parasite, most of the anticoccidials are used off-label in carnivores. Another emerging problem is a growing resistance of coccidian parasites to antiprotozoal drugs. Therefore, prevention of infection via good husbandry plays a crucial role. Proper sanitation of indoor areas and objects (cages, cage tops, beddings, water bowls, gloves, shoes, cleaning tools, and other utensils) is essential for reducing the intensity of coccidia because defecation immediately contaminates the environment and outer surface of the animal itself. Care also must be used by animal handlers to prevent contamination with coccidia. Simply touching an infected animal or contaminated surface, and then handling other animals, cages, bedding, water bowls, or other items can transmit oocysts and, thus, the infection when they sporulate. Use of the same gloves when cleaning different cages is an ideal way to contaminate the work place. Indirect contamination of a third surface, such as telephones, computer keyboards, door knobs, light switches, and drawer handles, are other ways oocysts may, in time, find their way into a susceptible host. Flies, cockroaches, dung beetles, other arthropods, and even earthworms may carry infective oocysts, transporting them either on their surface or within their intestinal tract. Although prevention is the optimal means of dealing with coccidia, some animals will inevitably ingest infective oocysts and develop coccidiosis. At this stage, intervention may be required and the use of therapeutics may be needed. When the carnivores live outdoors or are free-ranging, ingestion of oocysts from the environment, tissue cysts in prey items, or infestation by ectoparasites (especially ticks and fleas) that may expose them to *Hepatozoon*, is likely, so these animals may need treatment with appropriate chemotherapeutics outlined above.

Species Inquirendae in the Carnivora

SPECIES INQUIRENDAE AND NOMENA NUDA IN CARNIVORA

INTRODUCTION

Surveys of various animal and plant species or populations are on-going events that occur worldwide on a regular basis by biologists of every persuasion (entomologists, marine biologists, botanists, mammalogists, ornithologists, herpetologists, etc.). Historically, however, collecting parasites or even some parasite stages (e.g., surface organisms or fecal stages) have **not** been part of this survey equation, and parasitic faunas got ignored. However, in recent decades parasites have achieved recognition as important and abundant components of ecosystems, and whole organism surveys now often make at least cursory attempts to determine the presence and identification of some of the parasites of a particular host plant or animal species. In this vein, fecal material is often collected from captured hosts and later examined for parasite transmission stages (cysts, eggs, oocysts) that allow biologists to make either superficial identifications (to parasite genus) from distinctive propagules or in many cases to identify new morphological forms (from oocysts) that can result in new species descriptions. In the former instances, parasite stages may be identified quite superficially

(an amoeba, a ciliate, a sporozoan) or they may be more specifically characterized (a *Toxocara* egg, an eimerian, an *Isospora* sp., a *Sarcocystis* sporocyst, etc.). It is these species "identifications" that, under certain circumstances, can provide useful information, but only in a general way; the forms with these kinds of names are listed in this chapter because no full specific identifications were made.

We now know that at least four genera covered in our book (*Besnoitia*, *Cystoisospora*, *Sarcocystis*, *Toxoplasma*) produce developmental stages in hosts that may be prey items of carnivores. For example, some *Sarcocystis* species from omnivorous and/or herbivorous hosts that usually employ carnivores as definitive host (e.g., roe deer, *Capreolus capreolus*), but in which there is no mention of a possible carnivore host, will not be mentioned here because there is no way to connect them to any member of the Carnivora, even though the association may have strong circumstantial evidence (e.g., López et al., 2003).

SPECIES INQUIRENDAE (481)

The International Code of Zoological Nomenclature uses this designation for "a species of doubtful identity needing further investigation." Implicit in this definition for the coccidia is that the taxonomic "species" has been

© 2018 Donald W. Duszynski published by Elsevier Inc. All rights reserved.

named in a published document, but without the existence of a "type specimen" of any kind (e.g., line drawing, photosyntype, stages in tissue sections, oocysts in preservative, etc.) and without quantitative and qualitative data on the most widely available stage in the life cycle, the sporulated oocyst, to distinguish it from other similar morphotypes or perhaps closely-related species. All the forms that we include in this chapter have lots of missing data that prevent them from having valid binomial designations.

SUBORDER CANIFORMIA KRETZOI, 1938

FAMILY AILURIDAE GRAY, 1843

GENUS *AILURUS* F.G. CUVIER, 1825 (MONOTYPIC)

SARCOCYSTIS NEURONA/ SARCOCYSTIS DASYPI OF ZOLL, NEEDLE, FRENCH, LIM, BOLIN, LANGOHR, AND AGNEW, 2015

Definitive host: Unknown.
Intermediate host: *Ailurus fulgens* F.G. Cuvier, 1825, Red Panda.
Remarks: Two neonatal male red panda littermates were submitted for necropsy. One animal was found dead with no prior signs of illness; the other had a brief history of labored breathing. Postmortem examination revealed disseminated protozoal infection. To characterize the causative agent, transmission electron microscopy (TEM), immunohistochemistry (IHC), polymerase chain reaction (PCR) and amplification, and nucleic acid sequencing were performed. IHC was negative for *Toxoplasma gondii* and *Neospora caninum* but was positive for *Sarcocystis* spp. TEM of cardiac muscle and lung revealed numerous intracellular apicomplexan protozoa within parasitophorous vacuoles (PV). PCR and nucleic acid sequencing of partial 18S rRNA and the internal transcribed

spacer (ITS-1) region confirmed a *Sarcocystis* sp. that shared 99% sequence homology to *S. neurona* and *S. dasypi*. This was the first report of sarcocystosis in red pandas. Zoll et al. (2015) believed that their histopathological, immunohistochemical, molecular, and ultrastructural findings support vertical transmission resulting in fatal disseminated disease, but they did not assign a binomial name to the parasite of the red panda, so it must be considered a *species inquirenda*, at least for now.

FAMILY CANIDAE FISCHER, 1817

GENUS *CANIS* L., 1758 (6 SPECIES)

COCCIDIA-LIKE ORGANISM OF SHELTON, KINTNER, AND MACKINTOSH, 1968 AND OF SANGSTER, STYER, AND HALL, 1985

Original host: *Canis lupus familiaris* (syn. *C. familiaris*) L., 1758, Domestic Dog.
Remarks: Shelton et al. (1968) found what they described as subcutaneous nodules and a nonfebrile wasting illness in a 6-month-old border collie in Gallatin, Missouri, USA. Nodules were 10–12 mm wide and located on the lateral surface of the right maxilla. One lump was excised and prepared for standard H & E histological examination. Frequently, trophozoites, meronts with mature merozoites, and micro- and macrogametocytes were all discovered in the same host cell. Mature meronts were 11–20 in fixed tissue, and merozoites appeared to be arranged radially from a nuclear remnant of the meront. Merozoites in tissues were 5.5–6 × 2.0, crescent-shaped with one end thicker and blunter than the other, and a thick basophilic N was near the center of each merozoite. There were 16–20, sometimes 30, merozoites per meront. Microgametocytes were

spheroidal, 8.5–11.5 wide. Spheroidal macrogametocytes, 8–9 wide, were the most prevalent structures seen, and each had a pale N with a distinct, centrally-located karyosome. Levine and Ivens (1981) thought these meronts appeared to be more like *Besnoitia* than any other genus, but they were unaware at the time that *Caryospora bigenetica* from rattlesnakes could produce similar infections in some mammals (see Chapter 4).

COCCIDIA SPP. OF BRAUN AND THAYER, 1962

Original host: *Canis lupus familiaris* (syn. *C. familiaris*) L., 1758, Domestic Dog.

Remarks: Braun and Thayer (1962) examined fecal samples of dogs in Iowa City, USA. All dogs were >6-months-old, and without clinical signs. "Coccidia spp." were detected in 18/224 (8%) dogs. No other information was given.

COCCIDIA OF FOK, SZATMÁRI, BUSÁK, AND ROZGONYI, 2001

Original host: *Canis lupus familiaris* (syn. *C. familiaris*) L., 1758, Domestic Dog.

Remarks: Fok et al. (2001) examined 490 fecal samples of dogs from various locations in eastern and northern regions of Hungary. The authors reported a prevalence of "Coccidia" in 3.5%, but only in their abstract. In their Table 1 (p. 97), *Isospora* spp. was reported in 17 dogs, and they placed *Eimeria* spp., into "spurious parasites," that they found in 18 dogs from a country town and a village. No other details were mentioned.

COCCIDIA OF JOFFE, VAN NIEKERK, GAGNÉ, GILLEARD, KUTZ, AND LOBINGIER, 2011

Original host: *Canis lupus familiaris* (syn. *C. familiaris*) L., 1758, Domestic Dog.

Remarks: Joffe et al. (2011) examined fecal samples of 477 household and 142 sheltered dogs in the Calgary, Alberta, Canada, by centrifugation/flotation in zinc sulfate solution. "Low coccidian oocyst prevalence was found." No more information was given.

COCCIDIA OF PONCE-MACOTELA, PERALTA-ABARCA, AND MARTÍNEZ-GORDILLO, 2005

Original host: *Canis lupus familiaris* (syn. *C. familiaris*) L., 1758, Domestic Dog.

Remarks: Ponce-Macotela et al. (2005) examined small intestinal contents of dogs from the "Centro de Control Canino Culhuacan" in southern Mexico City; they surveyed 100 dogs during the "cold" season, and another 100 dogs during the "warm" season and reported a presence of "Coccidia" in their Fig. 1 (p. 3), but no other details were given.

COCCIDIA OF STRONEN, SALLOWS, FORBES, WAGNER, AND PAQUET, 2011

Original host: *Canis lupus* L., 1758, Wolf.

Remarks: In the course of 2001–05, Stronen et al. (2011) surveyed fecal samples of gray wolves (*C. lupus*) from the Riding Mountain National Park region in southwestern Manitoba, Canada. "Coccidia (*Isospora* sp. or *Eimeria* sp.)" were detected in 10/601 (2%) samples, but no other information was given.

COCCIDIA OF VISCO, CORWIN, AND SELBY, 1977

Original host: *Canis lupus familiaris* (syn. *C. familiaris*) L., 1758, Domestic Dog.

Remarks: Visco et al. (1977) examined fecal samples of pet dogs in Missouri, USA and said,

"Coccidia" were detected in 56/1,468 (4%) dogs, mostly in those <6-months-old (32 dogs). No other information was given.

COCCIDIUM OF FARIAS, CHRISTOVÃO, AND STOBBE, 1995

Original host: *Canis lupus familiaris* (syn. *C. familiaris*) L., 1758, Domestic Dog.

Remarks: Farias et al. (1995) examined fecal samples of dogs in the Araçatuba Region, São Paulo, Brazil. Oocysts of "coccidia" were found in 3/314 (<1%) samples, but no other information was given.

COCCIDIUM OF LIPSCOMB, DUBEY, PLETCHER, AND ALTMAN, 1989

Original host: *Canis lupus familiaris* (syn. *C. familiaris*) L., 1758, Domestic Dog.

Remarks: Lipscomb et al. (1989) reported cholangiohepatitis associated with the presence of a coccidium they found by LM and TEM, within intrahepatic biliary epithelial cells of a male Doberman pinscher that had intermittent diarrhea for 3–4 weeks. The dog was treated with metronidazole, trimethoprim, and sulfamethoxazole, but its condition deteriorated, and he eventually died. Lipscomb et al. (1989) found only meronts present in intact biliary epithelial cells and all stages of merogony from uninucleate to fully mature meronts with multinucleate merozoites. They mentioned that six genera of coccidia are known to infect dogs: *Cryptosporidium*, *Hammondia*, *Isospora*, *Neospora*, *Sarcocystis*, and *Toxoplasma*, but none has been described in the biliary epithelium of dogs, and none share the peculiar location and morphology of the parasite they documented. It still remains a mystery to this day.

Yet it serves as another project for an interested reader and has more questions that need to be answered.

COCCIDIUM OF NUNES, 1993

Original host: *Canis lupus familiaris* (syn. *C. familiaris*) L., 1758, Domestic Dog.

Remarks: Nunes (1993) examined fecal samples of dogs in São Paulo, Brazil; oocysts of "coccidia" were found in 141/3,222 (4%) samples but were not identified further.

CRYPTOSPORIDIUM SP. OF ABARCA, LÓPEZ, PEÑA, AND LÓPEZ, 2011

Original host: *Canis lupus familiaris* (syn. *C. familiaris*) L., 1758, Domestic Dog.

Remarks: In Santiago, Chile, Abarca et al. (2011) surveyed feces of pet dogs maintained in families with immunocompromised children (oncology patients, HIV-positive, or patients after transplantations) in two hospitals. *Cryptosporidium* sp. oocysts were detected in 2/41 (5%) dogs, but feces of the two immunocompromised children maintaining the positive dogs were negative.

CRYPTOSPORIDIUM SPP. OF AWADALLAH AND SALEM, 2015

Original host: *Canis lupus familiaris* (syn. *C. familiaris*) L., 1758, Domestic Dog.

Remarks: Awadallah and Salem (2015) surveyed fecal samples from military dogs (40 samples), nomadic dogs (30), and household dogs (60) in Sharkia and Qalyubia provinces, Egypt. *Cryptosporidium* was detected in 7/130 (5%) samples, 4 from nomadic, 2 from a rural household, and 1 from upscale household dogs but none in military dogs.

CRYPTOSPORIDIUM SP. OF BARR, GUILFORD, JAMROSZ, HORNBUCKLE, AND BOWMAN, 1994a

Original host: *Canis lupus familiaris* (syn. *C. familiaris*) L., 1758, Domestic Dog.

Remarks: Barr et al. (1994a) diagnosed cryptosporidiosis in two dogs suffering from diarrhea, based on the presence of *Cryptosporidium* oocysts in their feces. The dogs were administered paromomycin for 5 days, and the diarrhea resolved 5 days after the last dose in both dogs. No other information was given.

CRYPTOSPORIDIUM SPP. OF BATCHELOR, TZANNES, GRAHAM, WASTLING, PINCHBECK, AND GERMAN, 2007

Original host: *Canis lupus familiaris* (syn. *C. familiaris*) L., 1758, Domestic Dog.

Remarks: Between 2003 and 2005, Batchelor et al. (2007) examined fecal samples of domestic pet dogs, with clinical gastrointestinal signs (usually diarrhea), from all parts of the United Kingdom. *Cryptosporidium* oocysts were detected in 29/4,526 (0.6%) samples, with a higher prevalence of shedding in winter months. No other information was given.

CRYPTOSPORIDIUM/SARCOCYSTIS SP. OF BEARUP, 1954

Original host: *Canis lupus dingo* Meyer, 1793, Dingo.

Remarks: Bearup (1954), in Sydney, Australia, found "oocysts" measuring 17×11, four SZ, ~11×2, and a prominent RB, 7 wide, in 1/4 (25%) dingos, and identified them as *Cryptosporidium*. The dingo was concurrently infected with *Cystoisospora rivolta* and *Eimeria canis* (?). Because these oocysts

were morphologically consistent with the detached sporocysts of *Cystoisospora* and were not noticed until the oocysts of *C. rivolta* developed to the sporozoite stage, Bearup (1954) suggested it was possible they were the released sporocysts from the ruptured oocyst of *Cystoisospora* instead of a *Cryptosporidium* species. Dubey (2009) stated they were probably sporocysts of a *Sarcocystis* sp. based on size. We will never know.

CRYPTOSPORIDIUM SP. OF CAUSAPÉ, QUÍLEZ, SÁNCHEZ-ACEDO, AND DEL CACHO, 1996

Original host: *Canis lupus familiaris* (syn. *C. familiaris*) L., 1758, Domestic Dog.

Remarks: Causapé et al. (1996) examined fresh fecal samples of 37 domestic and 44 stray dogs in an animal shelter in Zaragoza, Spain, and reported oocysts of *C. parvum* (?) in 6/81 (7%) samples, which included 3/37 (8%) from domestic and 3/44 (7%) from stray dogs; all of them shed only a few oocysts. Three of the positive dogs suffered from diarrhea, but two were concurrently infected with *Isospora* spp. and one with *Toxocara canis*. Thus, the role of *Cryptosporidium* in diarrhea remained uncertain. Given that dogs can be host to at least 10 named *Cryptosporidium* species, their identification as *C. parvum* is equivocal.

CRYPTOSPORIDIUM SP. OF CIRAK AND BAUER, 2004

Original host: *Canis lupus familiaris* (syn. *C. familiaris*) L., 1758, Domestic Dog.

Remarks: Cirask and Bauer (2004) examined fecal samples of dogs from three animal shelters in central Germany to detect *Cryptosporidium*. Direct fecal smears, fast-stained with carbol fuchsin, found 1/270 (0.4%) fecal samples to have *Cryptosporidium*, whereas the enzyme-linked immunosorbent assay (ELISA) test kit (ProSpecT

Cryptosporidium Microplate Assay) detected it in 62/270 (23%) samples. However, because the fecal samples containing *Isospora burrowsi/ I. ohioensis* were significantly more often positive by ELISA, which may reflect a false-positive or possible cross-reactions, ELISA should not be uncritically used for detection of *Cryptosporidium* in dogs and cats and should be confirmed with other detection methods. Identification of the *Cryptosporidium* species was not done.

CRYPTOSPORIDIUM SP. OF COX, GRIFFITH, ANGLES, DEERE, AND FERGUSON, 2005

Original host: *Canis lupus familiaris* (syn. *C. familiaris*) L., 1758, Domestic Dog.

Remarks: Cox et al. (2005) examined fecal samples of various domestic, native, and feral animals during a survey for protozoal, bacterial, and viral pathogens in four semiprotected drinking-water watersheds (Wollondilly, Braidwood, Upper Cox's, Wingcarribee) in Sydney, New South Wales. Fecal samples were fluorescence-stained and examined with an epifluorescence microscope. Oocysts of *Cryptosporidium* were detected in 2/8 (25%) of the samples examined from domestic dogs. No attempt was made to identify the species.

CRYPTOSPORIDIUM SP. OF DADO, IZQUIERDO, VERA, MONTOYA, MATEO, FENOY, GALVÁN, GARCÍA, GARCÍA, ARÁNGUEZ, LÓPEZ, DEL ÁGUILA, AND MIRÓ, 2012

Original hosts: *Canis lupus familiaris* (syn. *C. familiaris*) L., 1758, Domestic Dog; *Felis catus* L., 1758, Domestic Cat.

Remarks: Dado et al. (2012) examined 625 soil samples and 79 fecal samples ("presumably from dogs and cats") from playgrounds and public parks in southeastern Madrid, Spain, and examined them using the modified Telemann and MIF (merthiolate–iodine–formalin) methods,

and modified Ziehl-Neelsen staining followed by a rapid immunochromatographic assay. *Cryptosporidium* was not detected in any of the soil samples, but 7/79 (9%) fecal samples from four parks contained *Cryptosporidium* sp.

CRYPTOSPORIDIUM SPP. OF DUBNÁ, LANGROVÁ, NÁPRAVNÍK, JANKOVSKÁ, VADLEJCH, PEKÁR, AND FECHTNER, 2007

Original host: *Canis lupus familiaris* (syn. *C. familiaris*) L., 1758, Domestic Dog.

Remarks: From 1998 to 2000, Dubná et al. (2007) surveyed canine fecal samples from two animal shelters in Prague and from rural areas in central Bohemia, Czech Republic. Fecal samples were collected from streets, grass strips, and parks, but some were not collected directly from the animals, so their origin (canine or other host) is unknown. *Cryptosporidium*-like oocysts were detected in 52/3,780 (<2%) samples. Of 524 fecal samples collected directly from stray dogs in two animal shelters, *Cryptosporidium* oocysts were detected in some samples, but neither the number of infected dogs nor the prevalence was given; they only stated, "the prevalence increased sevenfold after a stay in the shelter over the time of admittance to the shelter." In their samples from rural areas in central Bohemia (one-third from dogs, two-third from "soil or street," so their origin is unknown), *Cryptosporidium* spp. was detected in 11/540 (2%) samples. Dubná et al. (2007) said that *Cryptosporidium* was more prevalent in dogs in rural areas.

CRYPTOSPORIDIUM SPP. OF EL-AHRAF, TACAL, SOBIH, AMIN, LAWRENCE, AND WILCKE, 1991

Original host: *Canis lupus familiaris* (syn. *C. familiaris*) L., 1758.

Remarks: El-Ahraf et al. (1991) collected feces from impounded stray dogs in San Bernardino, California USA, and screened for

Cryptosporidium oocysts. Only 4/200 (2%) dogs were passing cryptosporidial oocysts, but they were not identified to species.

CRYPTOSPORIDIUM SPP. OF FERREIRA, PENA, AZEVEDO, LABRUNA, AND GENNARI, 2016

Original hosts: *Canis lupus familiaris* (syn. *C. familiaris*) L., 1758, Domestic Dog; *Felis catus* L., 1758, Domestic Cat.

Remarks: Ferreira et al. (2016) surveyed fecal samples of pet dogs from the metropolitan region of São Paulo, Brazil. *Cryptosporidium* spp. were detected in 28/3,099 (1%) samples, mostly in younger dogs.

CRYPTOSPORIDIUM SP. OF FONTANARROSA, VEZZANI, BASABE, AND EIRAS, 2006

Original host: *Canis lupus familiaris* (syn. *C. familiaris*) L., 1758, Domestic Dog.

Remarks: Fontanarrosa et al. (2006) surveyed fecal samples of dogs in southern Buenos Aires, Argentina. Oocysts of *Cryptosporidium* were detected in 5/2,193 (0.2%) samples.

CRYPTOSPORIDIUM SP. OF FUKUSHIMA AND HELMAN, 1984

Original host: *Canis lupus familiaris* (syn. *C. familiaris*) L., 1758, Domestic Dog.

Remarks: Fukushima and Helman (1984) reported a pup in Tennessee, USA, with a concurrent infection of *Cryptosporidium* and canine distemper. Formalin-fixed tissues stained with H & E showed the presence of intranuclear and intracytoplasmic acidophilic inclusion bodies in epithelial cells of the biliary tract, stomach, lymphoid cells of the spleen, astrocytes, choroid plexus epithelial cells, and ependymal cells. In the jejunum, numerous extracellular oocysts of *Cryptosporidium*, 2–3 wide, were attached to villous epithelial cells, occasionally also in the crypts of Lieberkühn. TEM showed a *Cryptosporidium* sp. attached to the intestinal villous epithelial cells. The authors stated this was "the first report of cryptosporidiosis in a domesticated dog (*Canis familiaris*);" however, they were unaware of the work by Tzipori and Campbell (1981) and Wilson and Holscher (1983) that previously had recorded *Cryptosporidium* in domesticated dogs.

CRYPTOSPORIDIUM SP. OF FUNADA, PENA, SOARES, AMAKU, AND GENNARI, 2007

Original host: *Canis lupus familiaris* (syn. *C. familiaris*) L., 1758, Domestic Dog.

Remarks: Funada et al. (2007) examined fecal samples of domestic dogs in São Paulo, Brazil. *Cryptosporidium* oocysts were found in 43/1,755 (2.5%) samples, mostly in dogs <1-year-old.

CRYPTOSPORIDIUM SP. OF GENNARI, KASAI, PENA, AND CORTEZ, 1999

Original host: *Canis lupus familiaris* (syn. *C. familiaris*) L., 1758, Domestic Dog.

Remarks: Gennari et al. (1999) examined fecal samples of household dogs from different areas of São Paulo, Brazil and reported finding oocysts of *C. parvum* in 10/353 (3%) samples. However, because dogs can be host to a number of *Cryptosporidium* species, their identification as *C. parvum* was equivocal.

CRYPTOSPORIDIUM SP. OF GHAREKHANI, 2014

Original host: *Canis lupus familiaris* (syn. *C. familiaris*) L., 1758, Domestic Dog.

Remarks: Gharekhani (2014) examined smears and flotations of fecal samples, from asymptomatic pet dogs in Hamedan, Iran, and found oocysts of *Cryptosporidium* in 8/210 (4%) samples.

CRYPTOSPORIDIUM SP. OF GINGRICH, SCORZA, CLIFFORD, OLEA-POPELKA, AND LAPPIN, 2010

Original host: *Canis lupus familiaris* (syn. *C. familiaris*) L., 1758, Domestic Dog.

Remarks: Gingrich et al. (2010) studied fecal samples of privately-owned domestic dogs from Santa Cruz (51 dogs), San Cristobal (17 dogs), and Isabela (29 dogs) Islands of the Galápagos Archipelago; none of the dogs had diarrhea. *Cryptosporidium* oocysts were seen in only one dog from Santa Cruz Island.

CRYPTOSPORIDIUM SPP. OF HACKETT AND LAPPIN, 2003

Original host: *Canis lupus familiaris* (syn. *C. familiaris*) L., 1758, Domestic Dog.

Remarks: Hackett and Lappin (2003) examined fecal samples of pet dogs (59 healthy, 71 with acute diarrhea) in north-central Colorado, USA. *Cryptosporidium* oocysts were detected in 5/130 (4%) samples by IFA, but in none of the samples by flotation; four positive samples were from diarrheic dogs.

CRYPTOSPORIDIUM SP. OF HAMNES, GJERDE, AND ROBERTSON, 2007b

Original host: *Canis lupus familiaris* (syn. *C. familiaris*) L., 1758, Domestic Dog.

Remarks: In Norway, Hamnes et al. (2007b) studied the occurrence of *Cryptosporidium* in dogs by repeated sampling of their feces between 1- and 12-months-old. Fecal samples of pure-bred, privately-owned household dogs in 57 litters, 75 pooled samples from 43 litters, and 69 samples from their 41 mother bitches were examined by flotation/concentration and immunofluorescent staining; 128/290 (44%) dogs were positive for *Cryptosporidium*, mostly animals 3–4-months-old. The occurrence was higher in winter, when 35 of the positive dogs were concurrently infected with *Giardia*. Only 1/40 (2.5%) litters of 1-month-old pups but none of the 39 bitches were positive for *Cryptosporidium*. Of the 2-months-old pup litters, 8/35 (23%) and 1/29 (3%) bitches were positive for *Cryptosporidium*. Significant differences were observed in prevalence between different regions in Norway, being highest in eastern Norway and lowest in northern Norway (where density of dogs is the lowest). Genotyping of the cryptosporidia was not performed so no specific identity was available.

CRYPTOSPORIDIUM SPP. OF HERMOSILLA, KLEINERTZ, SILVA, HIRZMANN, HUBER, KUSAK, AND TAUBERT, 2017

Original host: *Canis lupus* L., 1758, Wolf.

Remarks: Hermosilla et al. (2017) collected fecal samples from wild European wolves in mountainous areas of Croatia. Samples were examined by a sodium acetate–acetic acid–formalin technique, *Cryptosporidium* coproantigen-ELISA (ProSpecT), and fecal smears stained with carbol fuchsin. *Cryptosporidium* oocysts were detected in 7/400 (2%) samples, only by ELISA.

CRYPTOSPORIDIUM SPP. OF HIMSWORTH, SKINNER, CHABAN, JENKINS, WAGNER, HARMS, LEIGHTON, THOMPSON, AND HILL, 2010

Original host: *Canis lupus familiaris* (syn. *C. familiaris*) L., 1758, Domestic Dog.

Remarks: Himsworth et al. (2010) collected fecal samples of free-roaming dogs from the environment around a remote indigenous community in northern Saskatchewan, Canada, to detect oocysts of *Cryptosporidium*; 5/155 (3%) samples had oocysts, but they were not identified to species. The authors admitted that multiple samples may have originated from a single dog, so their prevalence finding was probably distorted.

CRYPTOSPORIDIUM SP. OF HUBER, BOMFIM, AND GOMES, 2005

Original host: *Canis lupus familiaris* (syn. *C. familiaris*) L., 1758, Domestic Dog.

Remarks: Huber et al. (2005) surveyed fecal samples of stray dogs in an animal shelter and household pet dogs from the West Zone of Rio de Janeiro, to compare the natural infections with *Cryptosporidium* sp. between the two different environments; all dogs were clinically healthy. *Cryptosporidium* sp. was detected in 4/166 (2%) dogs that included 2/94 (2%) shelter dogs and 2/72 (3%) pet dogs. No attempt was made to identify the species of *Cryptosporidium*.

CRYPTOSPORIDIUM SPP. OF KATAGIRI AND OLIVEIRA-SEQUEIRA, 2008

Original host: *Canis lupus familiaris* (syn. *C. familiaris*) L., 1758, Domestic Dog.

Remarks: Katagiri and Oliveira-Sequeira (2008) examined fecal samples of dogs (129 stray from kennels, 125 household) from urban areas of Botucatu, São Paulo State, Brazil. *Cryptosporidium* was detected in 8/254 (3%) samples, 3 from strays and 5 from household dogs.

CRYPTOSPORIDIUM SPP. OF KIM, WEE, AND LEE 1998

Original host: *Canis lupus familiaris* (syn. *C. familiaris*) L., 1758, Domestic Dog.

Remarks: Kim et al. (1998) examined fecal samples of dogs (companion, farm, and watch dogs) from four areas in Korea (Chunchon, Kwachan, Sangju, Songnam) by an immunofluorescence assay using the commercial *Cryptosporidium* diagnostic kit (Meridian Diagnostics). Oocysts of *Cryptosporidium* were detected in 25/257 (10%) samples, mostly from the companion dogs from Kwachan and Chunchon areas. The average oocyst size was $4.7 \pm 0.5 \times 4.4 \pm 0.6\,\mu m$, which suggested their form was *C. parvum*.

CRYPTOSPORIDIUM SPP. OF MIRZAEI, 2012, AND MIRZAEI AND FOOLADI, 2013

Original host: *Canis lupus familiaris* (syn. *C. familiaris*) L., 1758, Domestic Dog.

Remarks: Mirzaei (2012) collected fecal samples from companion and stray dogs near Kerman, southeastern Iran. *Cryptosporidium* oocysts were found in 11/548 (2%) samples, including 4/98 (4%) strays, and 7/450 (1.5%) companion dogs. The oocysts seen were 5.4×4.5 and were said to be morphologically similar to those of *C. parvum*. The oocysts were in dogs <1-year-old, four of which suffered from diarrhea. Mirzaei and Fooladi (2013) surveyed pet dogs in Kerman City, Iran, and *Cryptosporidium* oocysts were seen in 3/100 (3%) dogs.

CRYPTOSPORIDIUM SPP. OF MUNDIM, ROSA, HORTÊNCIO, FARIA, RODRIGUES, AND CRY, 2007

Original host: *Canis lupus familiaris* (syn. *C. familiaris*) L., 1758, Domestic Dog.

Remarks: Mundim et al. (2007) surveyed fecal samples of dogs under different living conditions (89 strays in shelters, 199 kenneled, 145 household pet) in Minais Gerais State, Uberlândia, an urban district of Brazil. Oocysts of *Cryptosporidium* were found in

6/433 (1%) fecal samples, mostly in the stray dogs from shelters.

CRYPTOSPORIDIUM SPP. OF OVERGAAUW, VAN ZUTPHEN, HOEK, YAYA, ROELFSEMA, PINELLI, VAN KNAPEN, AND KORTBEEK, 2009

Original host: Canis lupus familiaris (syn. *C. familiaris*) L., 1758, Domestic Dog.

Remarks: Overgaauw et al. (2009) collected fecal samples from healthy household dogs in the Netherlands. *Cryptosporidium* sp. was detected in 8/92 (9%) samples. Genotyping based on PCR of 18S rDNA failed; therefore the species/genotype remained unknown.

CRYPTOSPORIDIUM SPP. OF PALMER, THOMPSON, TRAUB, REES, AND ROBERTSON, 2008a

Original host: Canis lupus familiaris (syn. *C. familiaris*) L., 1758, Domestic Dog.

Remarks: Palmer et al. (2008a) surveyed fecal samples of dogs from both urban and rural areas across Australia, which were collected from 59 veterinary clinics (810 samples) and 26 refuges (590 samples). *Cryptosporidium* was detected, but not identified, in 8/1,400 (0.6%) of the dogs.

CRYPTOSPORIDIUM SPP. OF PAPAZAHARIADOU, FOUNTA, PAPADOPOULOS, CHLIOUNAKIS, ANTONIADOU-SOTIRIADOU, AND THEODORIDES, 2007

Original host: Canis lupus familiaris (syn. *C. familiaris*) L., 1758, Domestic Dog.

Remarks: Papazahariadou et al. (2007) examined fecal samples of privately-owned dogs (117 shepherd dogs, 164 hunting dogs) from the Serres prefecture in northern Greece. *Cryptosporidium* was detected in 8/281 (3%) samples, 5 from shepherds and 3 from hunting dogs.

CRYPTOSPORIDIUM SPP. OF RINALDI, MAURELLI, MUSELLA, VENEZIANO, CARBONE, DI SARNO, PAONE, AND CRINGOLI, 2008

Original host: Canis lupus familiaris (syn. *C. familiaris*) L., 1758, Domestic Dog.

Remarks: Rinaldi et al. (2008) examined canine fecal samples in urban Naples, Campania region, southern Italy. Samples were examined by a commercial ELISA kit (ProSpecT® *Cryptosporidium* Microplate Assay) for the presence of coproantigen of *Cryptosporidium*; 7/415 (2%) samples were positive, but the species/genotype was not identified, and because samples were collected from the ground, we will never know whether they were really canine or not.

CRYPTOSPORIDIUM SPP. OF SCORZA AND LAPPIN, 2017

Original host: Canis lupus familiaris (syn. *C. familiaris*) L., 1758, Domestic Dog.

Remarks: During their survey on gastrointestinal parasites in dogs and cats, Scorza and Lappin (2017) examined fecal samples of dogs on the Pine Ridge Indian Reservation, South Dakota, USA. Samples were examined by centrifugation–flotation, and by a commercial immunofluorescence assay for *Cryptosporidium* (Merifluor Crypto/Giardia kit). PCR amplification of the HSP70 gene was performed with immunofluorescence-positive samples. *Cryptosporidium* was detected in 6/84 (7%) samples, 2 of which could not be identified further (the other 4 were *C. canis*).

CRYPTOSPORIDIUM SPP. OF SHUKLA, GIRALDO, KRALIZ, FINNIGAN, AND SANCHEZ, 2006

Original host: *Canis lupus familiaris* (syn. *C. familiaris*) L., 1758, Domestic Dog.

Remarks: Shukla et al. (2006) examined fecal samples of domestic dogs in the Niagara region, Ontario, Canada, by a fecal concentration method, acid-fast staining, and *Cryptosporidium* enzyme immunoassay (EIA) using the ProSpecT *Cryptosporidum* Microplate Assay. All samples were from dogs in one veterinary clinic; *Cryptosporidium* was detected in 5/68 (7%) samples, and all were found by the EIA test; neither of the other two methods detected *Cryptosporidium*.

CRYPTOSPORIDIUM SPP. OF SIMONATO, DI REGALBONO, CASSINI, TRAVERSA, TESSARIN, DI CESARE, AND PIETROBELLI, 2017

Original host: *Canis lupus familiaris* (syn. *C. familiaris*) L., 1758, Domestic Dog.

Remarks: Simonato et al. (2017) examined canine fecal samples from public green (270 samples) and urban (435 samples) areas, Padua municipality, Veneto region, northern Italy. Samples were examined by sedimentation–flotation, followed by nested PCR amplification and subsequent sequencing of 18S rRNA gene. For some reason, samples concurrently positive for *Giardia* favored amplification of giardial DNA over the cryptosporidial DNA, so these samples also were examined by a touch-down real-time PCR of the COWP gene. Simonato et al. (2017) said that 12/705 (<2%) samples were positive for *Cryptosporidium* spp., 1 sample identified as *C. canis*, and the other 11 as "*C. parvum* species complex." However, because the samples were collected from the ground, one may never know whether they were really canine or not.

CRYPTOSPORIDIUM SP. OF SISK, GOSSER, AND STYER, 1984

Original host: *Canis lupus familiaris* (syn. *C. familiaris*) L., 1758, Domestic Dog.

Remarks: Sisk et al. (1984) described intestinal cryptosporidiosis in two pups in Georgia, USA. A 6-week-old mixed-breed female was "in a weak, semicomatose condition" and died within 12 hours. It was negative for parvovirus, adenovirus, and herpesvirus. Necropsy revealed mild hyperemia of the small intestinal serosa, mild interstitial pneumonia, and numerous "oval to spherical, dense basophilic bodies 3–4 μm in diameter" in the ileum, attached to the enterocytes, or free in the lumen of the small intestine. "Organisms morphologically consistent with *Cryptosporidium*," including meronts, merozoites, and trophozoites were observed in the ileum by TEM. The second pup that had suffered seizures was a 6-week-old, mixed-breed, from a cattle farm. It was negative for viral and bacterial agents, but dilated crypts with cellular debris were observed in the small and large intestines, and "sparse coccoid bodies 3–4 μm in diameter" were attached to the surface of enterocytes in the ileum. "Organisms morphologically consistent with *Cryptosporidium*," also were observed in the ileum by TEM, but the pup likely died of intoxication because 7.0 ppm of the pesticide toxaphene was detected in its liver.

CRYPTOSPORIDIUM SP. OF SORIANO, PIERANGELI, ROCCIA, BERGAGNA, LAZZARINI, CELESCINCO, SAIZ, KOSSMAN, CONTRERAS, ARIAS, AND BASUALDO, 2010

Original host: *Canis lupus familiaris* (syn. *C. familiaris*) L., 1758, Domestic Dog.

Remarks: Soriano et al. (2010) surveyed 1,944 dog fecal samples collected in urban

(646 samples) and rural (1,298 samples) areas in the Province of Neuquén, Patagonia, Argentina. A subset of 100 samples were screened using a modified Ziehl-Neelsen staining for the detection of *Cryptosporidium*. Only 1/100 (1%) samples (an urban dog) was positive for *Cryptosporidium*.

CRYPTOSPORIDIUM SPP. OF STRONEN, SALLOWS, FORBES, WAGNER, AND PAQUET, 2011

Original host: *Canis lupus* L., 1758, Wolf.
Remarks: From 2001 to 2005, Stronen et al. (2011) collected fecal samples from gray wolves in Riding Mountain National Park, Manitoba, Canada, and examined them by immunofluorescence. *Cryptosporidium* was detected in 7/601 (1%) samples.

CRYPTOSPORIDIUM SPP. OF TANGTRONGSUP, SCORZA, REIF, BALLWEBER, LAPPIN, AND SALMAN, 2017

Original host: *Canis lupus familiaris* (syn. *C. familiaris*) L., 1758, Domestic Dog.
Remarks: Tangtrongsup et al. (2017) examined fecal samples of dogs in the Chiang Mai province, Thailand; 36 from the Small Animal Hospital, Chiang Mai University, 9 from private clinics, 15 from shelters, and 49 from breeders. Samples were examined by immunofluorescence assay (Merifluor *Crypto/Giardia* kit) and by PCR amplification of HSP70 and 18S rRNA genes. The overall prevalence of *Cryptosporidium*-positive samples was 34/109 (31%), mostly in dogs <1-year-old; 14 dogs (13%) were positive by immunofluorescence, and 21 dogs (19%) by either/both of the PCR assays, and 18/109 (16.5%) were concurrently infected with *G. duodenalis*.

CRYPTOSPORIDIUM SPP. OF THOMPSON, COLWELL, SHURY, APPELBEE, READ, NJIRU, AND OLSON, 2009

Original host: *Canis latrans* Say, 1823, Coyote.
Remarks: Thompson et al. (2009) examined coyotes in southern Alberta and Saskatchewan, Canada, by sucrose flotation, immunofluorescence of monoclonal antibodies specific for *Cryptosporidium* (Crypt-a-Glo™), and PCR amplification with subsequent sequencing and phylogenetic analyses of 18S rRNA and HSP70 genes. *Cryptosporidium* was detected in 8/70 (11%) samples, all collected in winter, whereas no samples collected in summer were positive. This may be because in winter the coyotes were in poor condition and nutritionally compromised; 6/8 (75%) positive samples could not be successfully amplified by PCR.

CRYPTOSPORIDIUM SP. OF TRALDI, 1990

Original host: *Canis lupus familiaris* (syn. *C. familiaris*) L., 1758, Domestic Dog.
Remarks: Traldi (1990) reported oocysts of a *Cryptosporidium* sp. in the feces of a 6-year-old, male Pyrenean Shepherd. The dog suffered from recurrent episodes of diarrhea that stopped spontaneously ~12 days after diagnosis, and follow-up examinations were negative. The oocysts were inoculated *per os* into a 2-day-old mouse that was killed and dissected 7 DPI; both its feces and histological sections of intestine were diagnosed positive for cryptosporidia, but no other information was given.

CRYPTOSPORIDIUM SPP. OF UGA, MATSUMURA, ISHIBASHI, YODA, YATOMI, AND KATAOKA, 1989

Original host: *Canis lupus familiaris* (syn. *C. familiaris*) L., 1758, Domestic Dog.

Remarks: Uga et al. (1989) examined rectal contents of stray dogs captured in Hyogo Prefecture, Japan, by centrifugation–flotation. Oocysts of *Cryptosporidium* were detected in 3/213 (1%) dogs, mostly in those with normal fecal consistency and ≤6-months-old.

CRYPTOSPORIDIUM SPP. OF YU, RUAN, ZHOU, CHEN, ZHANG, WANG, ZHU, AND YU, 2017

Original host: *Canis lupus familiaris* (syn. *C. familiaris*) L., 1758, Domestic Dog.

Remarks: Yu et al. (2017) examined fecal samples of pet dogs with diarrhea from various regions in Beijing, China, by LM of wet mounts, and nested PCR amplification of 18S rRNA gene. *Cryptosporidium* was detected in 24/485 (5%) samples, mainly in poodles and border collies, but 4/20 (20%) positive samples could not be successfully identified using the PCR amplification.

CRYPTOSPORIDIUM SPP. OF ZIEGLER, WADE, SCHAAF, STERN, NADARESKI, AND MOHAMMED, 2007

Original host: *Canis latrans* Say, 1823, Coyote.

Remarks: Ziegler et al. (2007) examined fecal samples from coyotes live-trapped in a New York City Watershed in southeastern New York state, USA. Samples were concentrated by flotation and examined by LM and by polyclonal *Cryptosporidium* antigen capture ELISA (positive with an optical density ≥0.05). They found *Cryptosporidium* in 5/19 (26%) samples.

CYCLOSPORA CAYETANENSIS OF AWADALLAH AND SALEM, 2015

Original host: *Canis lupus familiaris* (syn. *C. familiaris*) L., 1758, Domestic Dog.

Remarks: *Cyclospora cayetanensis* Ortega, Gioman, and Sterling, 1994 is a parasite of humans and most closely related to *Eimeria*. Awadallah and Salem (2015) surveyed fecal samples from military (40 samples), nomadic (30 samples), and household dogs (60 samples) in Sharkia and Qalyubia provinces, Egypt. Samples were examined by centrifugation–flotation. Awadallah and Salem (2015) reported finding some *C. cayetanensis* oocysts in 1/130 (<1%) samples from a nomadic dog. Their photomicrograph is blurred, and the oocyst shown does not resemble a *Cyclospora* oocyst (in our opinion). Knowing that dogs are coprophagous, we suspect this is a spurious finding of an oocyst passing through the dog's gut after ingesting infected human feces.

CYCLOSPORA SP. OF YAI, BAUAB, HIRSCHFELD, DE OLIVEIRA, AND DAMACENO, 1997

Original host: *Canis lupus familiaris* (syn. *C. familiaris*) L., 1758, Domestic Dog.

Remarks: Yai et al. (1997) reported an infection with *Cyclospora* sp. in each of two dogs from São Paulo, Brazil, 1 Siberian husky and 1 Rottweiler. Both dogs had a history or watery diarrhea, weight loss, and lethargy. However, their photomicrographs of (presumably) sporulated oocysts of *Cyclospora* were not convincing.

CYSTOISOSPORA OHIOENSIS COMPLEX OF PALMER, THOMPSON, TRAUB, REES, AND ROBERTSON, 2008a

Original host: *Canis lupus familiaris* (syn. *C. familiaris*) L., 1758, Domestic Dog.

Intermediate host: Unknown.

Remarks: Palmer et al. (2008a) surveyed fecal samples of dogs from both urban and rural areas across Australia, which were collected from 59 veterinary clinics (810 samples) and 26 refuges (590 samples). Samples were examined by centrifugation–flotation. "*I.* (=*C.*) *ohioensis* complex" was detected in 49/1,400 (3.5%) dogs, mostly from refuges.

CYSTOISOSPORA OHIOENSIS-LIKE OF GATES AND NOLAN, 2009

Original host: *Canis lupus familiaris* (syn. *C. familiaris*) L., 1758, Domestic Dog.

Intermediate host: Unknown.

Remarks: Between 1997 and 2007, Gates and Nolan (2009) surveyed fecal samples of dogs in Pennsylvania, USA, for the prevalence of endoparasite infections. Samples were examined mostly by zinc sulfate centrifugation. "*Cystoisospora ohioensis*-like" was detected in 129/6,555 (2%) samples, mostly in dogs <1-year-old.

CYSTOISOSPORA SPP. OF BARUTZKI AND SCHAPER, 2003

Original host: *Canis lupus familiaris* (syn. *C. familiaris*) L., 1758, Domestic Dog.

Intermediate host: Unknown.

Remarks: Barutzki and Schaper (2003) examined fecal samples of dogs in Freiburg, Germany. Each sample was examined by five standard, nonmolecular methods. *Cystoisospora* oocysts were detected in 1,881/8,438 (22%) samples, and the infection was higher in dogs up to 1-year-old.

CYSTOISOSPORA SPP. OF DUBNÁ, LANGROVÁ, NÁPRAVNÍK, JANKOVSKÁ, VADLEJCH, PEKÁR, AND FECHTNER, 2007

Original host: *Canis lupus familiaris* (syn. *C. familiaris*) L., 1758, Domestic Dog.

Intermediate host: Unknown.

Remarks: From 1998 to 2000, Dubná et al. (2007) surveyed canine fecal samples from the metropolitan area of Prague's city center animal shelters and from rural areas of central Bohemia, Czech Republic. Oocysts of *Cystoisospora* spp. were detected in 92/3,780 (2%) samples, mainly from Prague 1 and Prague 2 (city center districts). Fecal samples of 23/524 (4%) stray dogs in two animal shelters were positive for *Cystoisospora* spp. at their admittance. Surprisingly, the prevalence increased fourfold after a stay in the shelter from the time of admittance to the shelter. Of fecal samples collected from rural areas of central Bohemia (one-third from dogs, two-third from "soil or street"), *Cystoisospora* spp. was detected in 43/540 (8%) samples. Dubná et al. (2007) said that *Cystoisospora* was more prevalent in rural dogs.

CYSTOISOSPORA SPP. OF FERREIRA, PENA, AZEVEDO, LABRUNA, AND GENNARI, 2016

Original host: *Canis lupus familiaris* (syn. *C. familiaris*) L., 1758, Domestic Dog.

Intermediate host: Unknown.

Remarks: Ferreira et al. (2016) surveyed fecal samples of pet dogs at the University of São Paulo, from metropolitan São Paulo, Brazil. Oocysts of *Cystoisospora* were detected in 46/3,099 (1.5%) samples, mostly in younger dogs.

CYSTOISOSPORA SPP. OF FUNADA, PENA, SOARES, AMAKU, AND GENNARI, 2007

Original host: *Canis lupus familaris* (syn. *C. familiaris*) L., 1758, Domestic Dog.

Intermediate host: Unknown.

Remarks: Funada et al. (2007) examined fecal samples of domestic dogs in São Paulo, Brazil. Samples were examined by various standard concentration techniques. Oocysts of *Cystoisospora* were detected in 77/1,755 (4%) samples.

CYSTOISOSPORA SPP. OF GENNARI, KASAI, PENA, AND CORTEZ, 1999

Original host: *Canis lupus familiaris* (syn. *C. familiaris*) L., 1758, Domestic Dog.

Intermediate host: Unknown.

Remarks: Gennari et al. (1999) examined fecal samples of domestic dogs from different areas of São Paulo, Brazil. Samples were examined by flotation and oocysts of *Cystoisospora* sp. were detected in 9/353 (2.5%) samples.

CYSTOISOSPORA SPP. OF GILL, SINGH, VADEHRA, AND SETHI, 1978

Definitive host: *Canis lupus familiaris* (syn. *C. familiaris*) L., 1758, Domestic Dog.
Intermediate host: Unknown.
Remarks: Gill et al. (1978) found unsporulated *Isospora* oocysts in the feces of dogs that were fed diaphragm from water buffalo (*Bubalus bubalis*) naturally-infected with macroscopic sarcocysts of *S. fusiformis* (but they did not examine the diaphragm for microscopic cysts). Four dogs that had never been fed meat each were fed 25 g of buffalo diaphragm, and all four dogs started shedding unsporulated oocysts on 9 (three dogs) or 10 DPI (one dog), and the infected dogs continued shedding oocysts daily for 15, 18, 23, and 25 days. Sporulation was completed in 8–16 hours at room temperature. Sporulated oocysts were L×W (n=25): 18.2×13.3 (17.5–24×16–19), L/W ratio: 1.1 (1.0–1.3), and M, OR, PG: all absent. Sporocysts were L×W (n=25): 13.3×9.8 (11–16×9–11), L/W ratio: 1.4 (1.1–1.6), and SB, SSB, PSB: all absent, but with a large SR. Gill et al. (1978) said that these oocysts either were *Hammondia* or *Isospora* but neglected to assign their form to either. Levine and Ivens (1981, pp. 49–50) suggested this may be a *Toxoplasma* species, even though the sporulated oocysts are about the same size as those of *C. burrowsi* and *C. ohioensis*, but gave no reason to support calling it *Toxoplasma* sp.

CYSTOISOSPORA SPP. OF HUBER, BOMFIM, AND GOMES, 2005

Original host: *Canis lupus familiaris* (syn. *C. familiaris*) L., 1758, Domestic Dog.

Intermediate host: Unknown.
Remarks: Huber et al. (2005) surveyed fecal samples of 94 stray dogs from an animal shelter and 72 household pet dogs from the West Zone of Rio de Janeiro, Brazil. All the dogs were clinically healthy. Oocysts of *Cystoisospora* were detected in "some samples"; however, the number of positive samples was not given.

CYSTOISOSPORA SPP. OF LITTLE, JOHNSON, LEWIS, JAKLITSCH, PAYTON, BLAGBURN, BOWMAN, MOROFF, TAMS, RICH, AND AUCOIN, 2009

Original host: *Canis lupus familiaris* (syn. *C. familiaris*) L., 1758, Domestic Dog.
Intermediate host: Unknown.
Remarks: Little et al. (2009) reported a scale study of fecal samples of 1,199,293 pet dogs presented to veterinary clinics throughout the United States. The samples were submitted to Antech Diagnostics (national service laboratories), for examination; *Cystoisospora* spp. was detected in 53,176 (4%) dogs, mostly <6-months-old and originated mostly from the West (Arizona, Oregon; 16,113 dogs) and Midwest (Illinois, Nebraska; 11,377 dogs).

CYSTOISOSPORA SP. OF MUNDIM, ROSA, HORTÊNCIO, FARIA, RODRIGUES, AND CRY, 2007

Original host: *Canis lupus familiaris* (syn. *C. familiaris*) L., 1758, Domestic Dog.
Intermediate host: Unknown.
Remarks: Mundim et al. (2007) surveyed fecal samples of 89 stray dogs in shelters, 199 kenneled, and 145 household pets in Uberlândia, state of Minais Gerais, Brazil. Oocysts of *Cystoisospora* sp. were detected in 12/433 (3%) samples.

CYSTOISOSPORA SPP. OF PAPAZAHARIADOU, FOUNTA, PAPADOPOULOS, CHLIOUNAKIS, ANTONIADOU-SOTIRIADOU, AND THEODORIDES, 2007

Original host: *Canis lupus familiaris* (syn. *C. familiaris*) L., 1758, Domestic Dog.

Intermediate host: Unknown.

Remarks: Papazahariadou et al. (2007) examined fecal samples of privately-owned shepherd (117) and hunting (164) dogs from the Serres prefecture, northern Greece. *Cystoisospora* oocysts were detected in 11/281 (4%) samples, 5 from shepherds and 6 from hunting dogs, and prevalence was significantly higher in young dogs.

CYSTOISOSPORA SPP. OF SALB, BARKEMA, ELKIN, THOMPSON, WHITESIDE, BLACK, DUBEY, AND KUTZ, 2008

Original host: *Canis lupus familiaris* (syn. *C. familiaris*) L., 1758, Domestic Dog.

Intermediate host: Unknown.

Remarks: Salb et al. (2008) examined fresh fecal samples of dogs from two remote northern Canadian communities (Fort Chipewyan, Alberta; Fort Resolution, Northwest territories). The authors detected *Cystoisospora*-like oocysts, but the number of positive samples was not given.

CYSTOISOSPORA SPP. OF SIMONATO, DI REGALBONO, CASSINI, TRAVERSA, BERALDO, TESSARIN, AND PIETROBELLI, 2015

Original host: *Canis lupus familiaris* (syn. *C. familiaris*) L., 1758, Domestic Dog.

Intermediate host: Unknown.

Remarks: Simonato et al. (2015) examined canine fecal samples collected from dogs kept in eight rescue shelters in northeastern Italy (seven in Veneto region and one in Friuli-Venezia Giulia region). Oocysts of *Cystoisospora* were detected in 18/318 (6%) samples, 9 from each region.

CYSTOISOSPORA SPP. OF YU, RUAN, ZHOU, CHEN, ZHANG, WANG, ZHU, AND YU, 2017

Original host: *Canis lupus familiaris* (syn. *C. familiaris*) L., 1758, Domestic Dog.

Intermediate host: Unknown.

Remarks: Yu et al. (2017) examined fecal samples of pet dogs with diarrhea from various regions in Beijing, China. Samples were examined by LM of wet fecal smears, and *Cystoisospora* oocysts were detected in 21/485 (4%) samples, mainly in poodles and golden retrievers, but the parasites were not further identified to the species.

EIMERIA RAYII OF RAO AND BHATAVDEKAR, 1957

Original host: *Canis lupus familiaris* (syn. *C. familiaris*) L., 1758, Domestic Dog.

Remarks: Rao and Bhatavdekar (1957) described ovoidal to ellipsoidal oocysts from a dog in Bombay, India, which were L×W (n=50): 26.8×19.8 (22–29×18–22); L/W ratio: 1.35. The oocysts had a MC and a M, the former was 5.8 (4–7) and the latter was 1.7 (1–4) wide. Unfortunately, the oocysts were unsporulated so sporocyst numbers and size were not recorded. Levine and Ivens (1981) believe these oocysts resemble those of *E. arloingi* from goats merely passing through the gut of the dog. Whatever they were, they were not a parasite of the dog and thus can only be relegated to *species inquirenda*.

EIMERIA SPP. OF FOK, SZATMÁRI, BUSÁK, AND ROZGONYI, 2001

Original host: *Canis lupus familiaris* (syn. *C. familiaris*) L., 1758, Domestic Dog.

Remarks: Fok et al. (2001) examined fecal samples of dogs in eastern and northern Hungary and reported a presence of *Eimeria* spp., which they called "spurious parasites" (Table 1, p. 97), in 18/490 (4%) dogs from a country town and a village, but gave no details.

EIMERIA SP. OF STREITEL AND DUBEY, 1976

Original host: *Canis lupus familiaris* (syn. *C. familiaris*) L., 1758, Domestic Dog.

Remarks: Streitel and Dubey (1976) surveyed feces from stray dogs in a humane shelter in Ohio, USA and reported 2/500 (0.5%) samples to have oocysts of an *Eimeria* species. After sporulating the oocysts, they were inoculated via stomach tube, into one coccidia-free, 1-month-old lab-reared pup. The feces of the pup were monitored for 30 DPI, but no additional oocysts were ever found. Although there are several *Eimeria* species described from dogs, they suggested that, "*Eimeria* are probably accidental 'parasites' of dogs because the *Eimeria* sp. found in this survey was not infectious to a dog."

EIMERIA STIEDAE OF GUILLEBEAU, 1916

Original host: *Canis lupus familiaris* (syn. *C. familiaris*) L., 1758, Domestic Dog.

Remarks: Guillebeau (1916) described a small coccidium that he identified as *E. stiedae* in the liver cells of dogs, even though the oocysts only measured L × W: 12 × 7, far too small to be those of *E. stiedai* found in the liver of rabbits. Coccidial developmental stages in the liver of dogs would be an unusual finding, indeed, given all of the domestic dogs that have been examined worldwide in the last 100 years! Guillebeau's (1916) figures do not help in deciding even the nature of the organism at which he was looking; thus, another *species inquirenda*.

HAMMONDIA-LIKE OOCYSTS OF CIRAK AND BAUER, 2004

Original host: *Canis lupus familiaris* (syn. *C. familiaris*) L., 1758, Domestic Dog.

Remarks: Cirak and Bauer (2004) examined fecal samples of healthy dogs from animal shelters in Germany to compare conventional coproscopical methods versus a commercial coproantigen ELISA kit, to best detect *Cryptosporidium*. *Hammondia*-like oocysts were found in 2/270 (<1%) dogs using the $ZnCl_2$–NaCl flotation method.

HAMMONDIA–NEOSPORA OF BARUTZKI AND SCHAPER, 2003

Original host: *Canis lupus familiaris* (syn. *C. familiaris*) L., 1758, Domestic Dog.

Remarks: Barutzki and Schaper (2003) examined fecal samples of dogs in Freiburg, Germany. Each sample was examined by 4–5 standard isolation techniques; *Hammondia–Neospora*-like oocysts were detected in 143/8,438 (<2%) samples.

HAMMONDIA–NEOSPORA SPP. OF DUBNÁ, LANGROVÁ, NÁPRAVNÍK, JANKOVSKÁ, VADLEJCH, PEKÁR, AND FECHTNER, 2007

Original host: *Canis lupus familiaris* (syn. *C. familiaris*) L., 1758, Domestic Dog.

Remarks: Dubná et al. (2007) reported on their survey of canine and ground-collected fecal samples from various areas in and around Prague and from rural areas in central Bohemia, Czech Republic. They reported *Neospora/Hammondia* spp. in 19/3,780 (0.5%) samples.

HAMMONDIA–NEOSPORA OF EPE, COATI, AND SCHNIEDER, 2004

Original host: *Canis lupus familiaris* (syn. *C. familiaris*) L., 1758, Domestic Dog.

Remarks: In northern Germany, Epe et al. (2004) surveyed fecal samples of dogs from 1998 to 2002 and found 3/1,281 (0.2%) to pass *Hammondia*-like oocysts. Based on only the oocyst morphology, however, it was impossible to differentiate between the oocysts of *Hammondia* and *Neospora*.

HAMMONDIA–NEOSPORA OF FERREIRA, PENA, AZEVEDO, LABRUNA, AND GENNARI, 2016

Original host: *Canis lupus familiaris* (syn. *C. familiaris*) L., 1758, Domestic Dog.

Remarks: Ferreira et al. (2016) surveyed fecal samples of pet dogs in São Paulo, Brazil. Oocysts of *Hammondia/Neospora* were detected in 2/3,099 dogs, both ≥1-year-old. Based only on oocyst morphology, it was impossible to differentiate between genera or species.

HAMMONDIA–NEOSPORA OF FONTANARROSA, VEZZANI, BASABE, AND EIRAS, 2006

Original host: *Canis lupus familiaris* (syn. *C. familiaris*) L., 1758, Domestic Dog.

Remarks: Fontanarrosa et al. (2006) surveyed fecal samples of dogs in southern Buenos Aires, Argentina. Oocysts they identified as *Hammondia–Neospora* were detected in 66/2,193 (3%) samples, mostly in young dogs 0–6-months-old.

HAMMONDIA–NEOSPORA OF FUNADA, PENA, SOARES, AMAKU, AND GENNARI, 2007

Original host: *Canis lupus familiaris* (syn. *C. familiaris*) L., 1758, Domestic Dog.

Remarks: Funada et al. (2007) examined fecal samples of domestic dogs also in São Paulo, Brazil. Samples were examined by several concentration techniques. *Hammondia–Neospora*-like oocysts were detected in 7/1,755 (0.4%) samples.

HAMMONDIA–NEOSPORA OF HERMOSILLA, KLEINERTZ, SILVA, HIRZMANN, HUBER, KUSAK, AND TAUBERT, 2017

Original host: Canis lupus L., 1758, Wolf.

Remarks: Hermosilla et al. (2017) surveyed fecal samples of wild European wolves in mountainous areas of the Gorski Kotar Region, Croatia. *Hammondia/Neospora*-like oocysts were detected in 10/400 (3%) samples. Based on the morphology, it was not possible to identify these oocysts beyond these genera.

HEPATOZOON SP. OF DAVIS, ROBINSON, AND CRAIG, 1978

Original host: Canis latrans Say, 1823, Coyote.

Remarks: Davis et al. (1978) reported a naturally-occurring case of hepatozoonosis in a coyote in Austwell, Aransas county, Texas, USA. Meronts of *Hepatozoon* were found in the myocardium of an adult coyote that had been shot in Aransas National Wildlife Refuge. They said this was, "the first time hepatozoonosis has been recorded in Canidae in the Western Hemisphere." There was no attempt to reach a species identity.

HEPATOZOON SP. OF MATJILA, LEISEWITZ, JONGEIAN, BERTSCHINGER, AND PENZHORN, 2008

Original host: Canis lupus (syn. *C. familiaris*) L., 1758, Domestic Dog.

Remarks: Matjila et al. (2008) collected blood samples from wild dogs at the De Wildt Cheetah and Wildlife Centre, Pretoria, and five game reserves (four in the North-West province, one in Limpopo province), South Africa. Specimens were screened for *Babesia*, *Theileria*, *Hepatozoon*, and *Ehrlichia/Anaplasma* species using PCR and reverse line blot assays. Two dogs were positive for *Hepatozoon* sp.

HEPATOZOON SPP. OF MCCULLY, BASSON, BIGALKE, DE VOS, AND YOUNG, 1975

Original hosts: *Canis adustus* Sundevall, 1878, Side-striped Jackal; and Lions, Cheetahs, Hyaenas, and Leopards.

Remarks: McCully et al. (1975) studied hepatozoonosis in hyaenas, lions, jackals, cheetahs, and one leopard in the Kruger National Park, to compare possible symptoms with those seen in some dogs in South Africa. Meronts of *Hepatozoon* were found in many wild carnivores and they illustrated the progressive development of microschizonts. They reported meronts in the lung, myocardium, and skeletal muscle, and sometimes also in the spleen, liver, and lymph nodes. Gametocytes were present in leukocytes, but they saw very little of a host response to the presence of *Hepatozoon* infection, and there was no attempt to determine the species. Sporogony in ticks was reported in *Rhipicephalus simus* females removed from an infected hyaena and *R. sanguineus* adults fed on an infected jackal in the nymphal stage. Attempts to transmit *Hepatozoon* from a jackal to domestic dogs by means of ticks gave "inconclusive results."

HEPATOZOON SP. OF MERCER, JONES, RAPPOLE, TWEDT, LAACK, AND CRAIG, 1988

Original host: *Canis latrans* Say, 1823, Coyote.
Remarks: Mercer et al. (1988) collected skeletal and/or cardiac muscle samples from coyotes trapped in Robertson, Brazoria, Refugio, Wharton, and Calhoun counties, Texas, USA; the authors found that 12/59 (20%) were infected with a *Hepatozoon* species. They made no attempt to name or identify the species.

HOAREOSPORIDIUM PELLERDYI OF PANDE, BHATIA, AND CHAUHAN, 1972

Original host: *Canis lupus* (syn. *C. familiaris*) L., 1758, Domestic Dog.

Remarks: Pande et al. (1972) reported an unusual coccidium in the rectal contents of four pups slaughtered in India. It was similar to *Cryptosporidium* because of its asporous, tetrazoic oocysts, which they saw in fresh scrapings of the jejunum; however, it was intracellular in epithelial and subepithelial cells of the villi, rather than in the intracellular, but extracytoplasmic, location typical for *Cryptosporidium* species, so they decided to create a new genus for their organism. They measured their "oocysts" both extracellularly and intracellularly. Fresh "oocysts" were L×W (n=50): 14.8×9.1 (12–17×8.5–10.5), L/W ratio: 1.6 (1.2–1.8); the OR was a prominent mass of large-sized granules, and sausage-shaped SZ were 9.3×2.7 (9–10.5×2.6–3). Intracellular "oocysts" were L×W (n=25): 14.2×8.8 (12–17×7–10); L/W ratio: 1.6, and SZ were 8.2×2.4 (6–10.5×2–2.5). They said, "though the dimensions given for the oocysts in *V. vulpis* Wetzel, 1938 (from common red fox) are well within the range encountered in our material, the oocysts in this species, according to Pellérdy, could possibly be the freshly-shed sporocysts of some known or as yet unknown isosporan species." We are convinced that what Pande et al. (1972) reported actually were sporocysts of some *Sarcocystis* species developing in the dog's jejunal epithelial cells, which they mistook for oocysts of their new *Hoareosporidium pellerdyi*. We must conclude that this form can only be regarded as a *species inquirenda*.

ISOSPORA BIGEMINA (STILES, 1891) OF LÜHE, 1906

Synonyms: *Cystospermium villorum intestinalium canis* Rivolta, 1878, *nomen nudum*; *Coccidium rivolta* Grassi, 1879, *pro parte*; *Coccidium rivoltae* Leuckart, 1886, *pro parte*; *Coccidium bigemina* Stiles, 1891, *pro parte*; *Coccidium bigeminum* var. *canis* Railliet and Lucet, 1891; *Diplospora bigemina* Martin, 1909; *Coccidium bigeminum* Wigdor, 1918, *pro parte*; *Isospora cati* Marotel, 1922, *pro parte*; *Lucetina bigemina* (Stiles, 1891) Henry and Leblois, 1926; *Isospora bigemina* Gousseff, 1933, *lapsus*; *Isospora bigemina* var. *bahiensis* de Moura Costa, 1956; and others.

Type host: *Canis lupus familiaris* (syn. *C. familiaris*) L., 1758, Domestic Dog.

Remarks: Stiles (1891) found some parasites developing in the lamina propria of the domestic dog and called it *Coccidium bigemina*; Lindsay et al. (1997) suggested that he was likely looking at a *Sarcocystis* species because oocysts and sporocysts were seen to develop in the gut tissue and we agree. This organism was placed in the genus *Isospora* by Lühe (1906) and 2 decades later, Wenyon (1926a) suggested there were two "races" of *I. bigemina*, a large and a small race. The larger race, which was excreted as sporocysts and sporulated oocysts was a *Sarcocystis* species, and the smaller race, excreted as unsporulated oocysts, is now known to be *Hammondia heydorni*, an obligatory heteroxenous parasite (Heydorn et al., 1975c; Lindsay et al., 1997). Nukerbaeva and Svanbaev (1974, 1977) collected oocysts from domestic dogs, which they identified as *I. bigemina*. They tried to transmit their oocysts to one 40-day-old Arctic fox (*V. lagopus*), and two 1-year-old minks (*N. vison*), but none of these animals became infected. They were successful in transmitting their oocysts to a control dog, which shed oocysts in its feces on the 8th DPI.

ISOSPORA BIGEMINA FREE SPOROCYSTS OF GASSNER, 1940

Original host: *Canis lupus familiaris* (syn. *C. familiaris*) L., 1758, Domestic Dog.

Remarks: In Fort Collins, Colorado, USA, Gassner (1940) examined dogs and said that 253/320 (79%) dogs were infected with the small form of *Isospora bigemina* and discharged either sporocysts or oocysts in their feces; Because free sporocysts and sporulated oocysts were being discharged in the feces, we now know Gassner (1940) was seeing a species of *Sarcocystis*.

ISOSPORA BURROWSI/ISOSPORA OHIOENSIS-LIKE OF CIRAK AND BAUER, 2004

Original host: *Canis lupus familiaris* (syn. *C. familiaris*) L., 1758, Domestic Dog.

Remarks: Cirak and Bauer (2004) examined fecal samples of healthy dogs with normal stools in central Germany; oocysts of *Isospora burrowsi*/*Isospora ohioensis* were found in 3/270 (1%) dogs. They were unable to determine identity beyond that general observation.

ISOSPORA OHIOENSIS COMPLEX OF FONTANARROSA, VEZZANI, BASABE, AND EIRAS, 2006

Original host: *Canis lupus familiaris* (syn. *C. familiaris*) L., 1758, Domestic Dog.

Remarks: Fontanarrosa et al. (2006) surveyed fecal samples of dogs in southern Buenos Aires, Argentina. They detected an "*Isospora ohioensis* complex" of oocysts in 263/2,193 (12%) samples, mostly in young dogs 0–6-months-old.

ISOSPORA SPP. OF BLAZIUS, EMERICK, PROPHIRO, ROMÃO, AND DA SILVA, 2005

Original host: *Canis lupus familiaris* (syn. *C. familiaris*) L., 1758, Domestic Dog.

Remarks: Blazius et al. (2005) examined fecal samples of stray dogs in Itapema City, Santa Catarina, Brazil, and found *Isospora* oocysts they did not identify to species in 10/158 (6%) samples.

ISOSPORA SPP. OF CAUSAPÉ, QUÍLEZ, SÁNCHEZ-ACEDO, AND DEL CACHO, 1996

Original host: *Canis lupus familiaris* (syn. *C. familiaris*) L., 1758, Domestic Dog.

Remarks: Causapé et al. (1996) examined fresh fecal samples of 37 domestic and 44 stray dogs in Zaragoza, Aragón, Spain; oocysts of *Isospora* spp. were detected in 8/81 (10%) samples, including 7/37 (19%) domestic and 1/44 (2%) stray dogs.

ISOSPORA SPP. OF COLLINS, EMSLIE, FARROW, AND WATSON, 1983

Original host: *Canis lupus* (syn. *C. familiaris*) L., 1758, Domestic Dog.

Remarks: Collins et al. (1983) reported *Isospora* spp. in 6/110 (5.5%) fecal samples from dogs in Sydney, Australia, which were examined for "sporozoa." No other information was given.

ISOSPORA SPP. OF DE OLIVEIRA, DA SILVA, PARREIRA, RIBEIRO, AND GOMES, 1990

Original host: *Canis lupus familiaris* (syn. *C. familiaris*) L., 1758, Domestic Dog.

Remarks: de Oliveira et al. (1990) examined fecal samples of 11,563 dogs from Uberlândia, Minas Gerais, Brazil and found *Isospora* oocysts in 148/3,202 (5%) samples but did not identify them to species.

ISOSPORA SP. OF DUBEY, WEISBRODE, AND ROGERS, 1978b

Original host: *Canis lupus familiaris* (syn. *C. familiaris*) L., 1758, Domestic Dog.

Remarks: Dubey et al. (1978b) found a coccidium in the villar epithelium, lamina propria, and intestinal glands in the distal half of the ileum, cecum, and colon of a 10-week-old puppy that apparently died from the infection in Ohio, USA. They said that sporulation was exogenous and oocysts were L × W: 19 × 16 (16–23 × 14–20) in fecal smears and 13 × 11.5 (12–17 × 10–13) in tissue sections and speculated that the infection might be a mixture of *I. neorivolta* and *I. ohioensis*, but had to conclude that they could not identify the parasite because the culture was "inadvertently discarded." They also reported at least two structurally different meronts and three different-sized merozoites in tissue stages of the pup. For more descriptive information on these various stages, see either Dubey et al. (1978b) or Levine and Ivens (1981, p. 22).

ISOSPORA SPP. OF EPE, COATI, AND SCHNIEDER, 2004

Original host: *Canis lupus familiaris* (syn. *C. familiaris*) L., 1758, Domestic Dog.

Remarks: In northern Germany, Epe et al. (2004) surveyed fecal samples of domestic dogs between 1998 and 2002 and found 29/1,281 (2%) passing *Isospora* oocysts, which were not identified to species.

ISOSPORA SPP. OF EPE, ISING-VOLMER, AND STOYE, 1993

Original host: Canis lupus familiaris (syn. *C. familiaris*) L., 1758, Domestic Dog.

Remarks: Epe et al. (1993), in Germany, surveyed fecal samples from dogs between 1984 and 1991 and found 140/3,329 (4%) passing *Isospora* oocysts, which were not identified to species.

ISOSPORA SPP. OF FOK, SZATMÁRI, BUSÁK, AND ROZGONYI, 2001

Original host: Canis lupus familiaris (syn. *C. familiaris*) L., 1758, Domestic Dog.

Remarks: Fok et al. (2001) examined fecal samples of dogs in eastern and northern Hungary and reported a presence of *Isospora* spp. in 17/490 (3%) dogs (their Table 1, p. 97).

ISOSPORA SPP. OF HACKETT AND LAPPIN, 2003

Original host: Canis lupus familiaris (syn. *C. familiaris*) L., 1758, Domestic Dog.

Remarks: Hackett and Lappin (2003) examined fecal samples of 59 clinically healthy pet dogs and an additional 71 with acute diarrhea in north-central Colorado, USA. Oocysts of *Isospora* were detected in 3/130 (2%) samples, all in diarrheic dogs.

ISOSPORA SPP. OF INPANKAEW, TRAUB, THOMPSON, AND SUKTHANA, 2007

Original host: Canis lupus familiaris (syn. *C. familiaris*) L., 1758, Domestic Dog.

Remarks: Inpankaew et al. (2007) examined fecal samples of dogs from 20 different temples and their surrounding communities in Bangkok, Thailand. *Isospora* oocysts were detected in 23/229 (10%) samples.

ISOSPORA SPP. OF JASKOSKI, BARR, AND BORGES, 1982

Original host: Canis lupus familiaris (syn. *C. familiaris*) L., 1758, Domestic Dog.

Remarks: Jaskoski et al. (1982) reported collecting fecal samples from public areas (streets, parks, etc.) in Edgewater and Rogers Park, Chicago, Illinois, USA, areas where pet dogs were kept inside and leashed when outside. In 1970, 14/846 (<2%) samples had *Isospora* oocysts, but during 1979–1980, only 1/806 (0.1%) samples was found with *Isospora*-type oocysts. Unfortunately, fecal samples were not collected directly from dogs, so whether they all were canine was highly probable, but unknown for certain.

ISOSPORA SPP. OF JORDAN, MULLINS, AND STEBBINS, 1993

Original host: Canis lupus familiaris (syn. *C. familiaris*) L., 1758, Domestic Dog.

Remarks: Jordan et al. (1993) examined 12,515 canine fecal samples in Stillwater, Oklahoma, USA; they stated that *Isospora* spp. were found in "low prevalence (<5%) in the routine fecal examinations."

ISOSPORA SPP. OF ITOH, KANAI, HORI, HOSHI, AND HIGUCHI, 2009

Original host: Canis lupus familiaris (syn. *C. familiaris*) L., 1758, Domestic Dog.

Remarks: Itoh et al. (2009) surveyed fecal samples of household dogs in the Hachinohe area, Tohoku region, Aomori province, Japan, in 1997 (420 samples), 2002 (350 samples), and 2007 (335 samples). Oocysts of *Isospora* spp. were detected in 40/420 (9.5%) samples in 1997, 26/350 (7%) samples in 2002, and 15/335 (4%) samples in 2007; most infected dogs were <1-year-old, kept indoors, and originated from pet shops or breeding kennels.

ISOSPORA SPP. OF KATAGIRI AND OLIVEIRA-SEQUEIRA, 2008

Original host: *Canis lupus familiaris* (syn. *C. familiaris*) L., 1758, Domestic Dog.

Remarks: Katagiri and Oliveira-Sequeira (2008) examined fresh fecal samples of 129 stray, and 125 household dogs from urban areas of Botucatu, São Paulo State, Brazil. Samples were examined by multiple techniques. *Isospora* oocysts were found in 9/254 (3.5%) samples including 5/129 (4%) from stray and 4/125 (3%) from household dogs, but not identified to species.

ISOSPORA SPP. OF LORENZINI, TASCA, AND CARLI, 2007

Original host: *Canis lupus familiaris* (syn. *C. familiaris*) L., 1758, Domestic Dog.

Remarks: Lorenzini et al. (2007) examined fecal samples of dogs from different neighborhoods in Porto Alegre, Rio Grande do Sul, Brazil. They said that *Ancylostoma*, *Toxocara*, *Isospora*, and *Giardia* spp. were the most frequent parasites encountered. Dogs <6-months-old showed a high infection rate with 582/1,473 (39.5%) dogs demonstrating parasite stages in their feces, and the highest infection rates with *Isospora* and *Toxocara* spp. Summer was the season with the highest prevalence rate.

ISOSPORA SPP. OF MALLOY AND EMBIL, 1978

Original host: *Canis lupus familiaris* (syn. *C. familiaris*) L., 1758, Domestic Dog.

Remarks: Malloy and Embil (1978) examined fecal samples of stray dogs in Halifax, Nova Scotia, Canada; oocysts of *Isospora* spp. were detected in 14/474 (3%) dogs, mostly young dogs up to 2-years-old.

ISOSPORA SP. OF MECH AND KURTZ, 1999

Original host: *Canis lupus* L., 1758, Wolf.

Remarks: Mech and Kurtz (1999) found three 4-month-old *C. lupus* pups in the Superior National Forest of Minnesota, USA, which died in August/September, 1997, apparently of coccidiosis. Two of the pups had hemorrhagic feces and the third had a severely autolyzed intestine. The intestinal mucosa of two pups had many developmental stages in both enterocytes and in the lamina propria, which the authors attributed to an *Isospora* (probably *Cystoisospora*) species. No other information was provided.

ISOSPORA SP. OF MELONI, THOMPSON, HOPKINS, REYNOLDS, AND GRACEY, 1993

Original host: *Canis lupus familiaris* (syn. *C. familiaris*) L., 1758, Domestic Dog.

Remarks: Meloni et al. (1993) examined fecal samples of dogs from eight Aboriginal communities in the tropics of the western Kimberley region, Western Australia. Oocysts of what was presumably a single *Isospora* sp. were detected in 4/182 (2%) samples.

ISOSPORA SPP. OF MILLER, LIGGETT, RADI, AND BRANCH, 2003

Original host: *Canis lupus familiaris* (syn. *C. familiaris*) L., 1758, Domestic Dog.

Remarks: Miller et al. (2003) reported a concurrent infection with *Cryptosporidium canis* and *Isospora* spp. in an 8-week-old female Yorkshire terrier puppy in Tifton, Georgia, USA.

The puppy suffered weakness and diarrhea. Histology revealed severe gastric and intestinal cryptosporidiosis, severe intestinal isosporiasis, and thymic atrophy with lymphoid depletion. Numerous sexual and asexual stages of *Isospora* spp. were observed in the luminal and crypt epithelial cells of the small intestine.

ISOSPORA SP. OF NIESCHULZ, 1925

Original host: *Canis lupus familiaris* (syn. *C. familiaris*) L., 1758, Domestic Dog.

Remarks: Nieschulz (1925) discussed *Isospora* infections in dogs and cats in the Netherlands; in addition to brief descriptions of *I.* (=*C.*) *rivolta* and *I.* (=*C.*) *felis*, he said he saw "free sporocysts (not whole oocysts) of an *Isospora* species in intestinal material of a young dog," which were ellipsoidal, L×W: 15.5×9.2 (14–17×8–10). Clearly, he saw and measured sporocysts of a *Sarcocystis* species.

ISOSPORA SPP. OF RAMÍREZ-BARRIOS, BARBOZA-MENA, MUÑOZ, ANGULO-CUBILLÁN, HERNÁNDEZ, GONZÁLEZ, AND ESCALONA, 2004

Original host: *Canis lupus familiaris* (syn. *C. familiaris*) L., 1758, Domestic Dog.

Remarks: Ramírez-Barrios et al. (2004) examined fecal samples of pet dogs in Maracaibo, Zulia state, Venezuela. Oocysts of *Isospora* spp. were detected in 50/614 (8%) dogs, mostly in (39) dogs younger than 6-months-old.

ISOSPORA SPP. OF SORIANO, PIERANGELI, ROCCIA, BERGAGNA, LAZZARINI, CELESCINCO, SAIZ, KOSSMAN, CONTRERAS, ARIAS, AND BASUALDO, 2010

Original host: *Canis lupus familiaris* (syn. *C. familiaris*) L., 1758, Domestic Dog.

Remarks: Soriano et al. (2010) studied dog fecal samples collected in urban streets, parks, squares (646 samples), and in peridomicile and farm settings (1,298 samples) of the Province of Neuquén, Patagonia, Argentina. Oocysts of *Isospora* spp. were detected in 19/1,944 (1%) samples, mostly from rural areas (18 of 19 samples).

ISOSPORA SP. OF STEHR-GREEN, MURRAY, SCHANTZ, AND WAHLQUIST, 1987

Original host: *Canis lupus familiaris* (syn. *C. familiaris*) L., 1758, Domestic Dog.

Remarks: Stehr-Green et al. (1987) examined fecal samples of pups from 14 pet stores in metropolitan Atlanta, Georgia, USA and detected an *Isospora* sp. in 13/143 (9%) samples.

ISOSPORA SPP. OF UEHLINGER, GREENWOOD, MCCLURE, CONBOY, O'HANDLEY, AND BARKEMA, 2013

Original host: *Canis lupus familiaris* (syn. *C. familiaris*) L., 1758, Domestic Dog.

Remarks: Uehlinger et al. (2013) examined fecal samples of dogs <1-year-old on Prince Edward Island, Canada. Dogs originated from a local animal shelter, private veterinary clinics, and a pet store. *Isospora* spp. oocysts were detected in 4/62 (6%) samples from the shelter, 10/78 (13%) samples from veterinary clinics, and 34/69 (49%) samples from the pet store.

ISOSPORA THEILERI OF YAKIMOFF AND LEWKOWITSCH, 1932

Original host: *Canis aureus* L., 1758, Golden Jackal.

Remarks: Yakimoff and Lewkowitsch (1932) reported finding oocysts in one golden jackal in Azerbaijan (former USSR). Their oocysts were spheroidal or slightly ovoidal, L×W: 21.2×17.1–18.0, and had ellipsoidal sporocysts that were 16×11 (sic) (13–16×9–11); oocysts lacked a M, OR, and PG, and sporocysts lacked SB, SSB, PSB but were illustrated to have a granular SR. They said that sporocysts were found free in the intestine, which suggests they had seen a *Sarcocystis* sp., and that during transportation to Leningrad almost all of the oocysts' walls broke and disappeared, which would support this idea. Yakimoff and Lewkowitsch (1932) failed to transmit this form to the domestic dog with sporulated oocysts. Glebezdin (1978) surveyed wild mammals in southwestern Turkmenistan from 1974 to 1977; he reported finding, in *C. aureus*, ellipsoidal oocysts of *I. theileri* that measured L×W: 23.0×17.5 (22–25×17–20), L/W ratio: 1.3; sporocysts were L×W: 11.6×9.1 (11–14×8–11). Levine and Ivens (1981, p. 51) hoped that someone will find this form again and suggested, "it too should be restudied if it is ever rediscovered." The data available are so sketchy and tentative, that we strongly agree.

OOCYSTS OF CARLSLAKE, HILL, SJÖLANDER, HII, PRATTLEY, AND ACKE, 2017

Original host: *Canis lupus familiaris* (syn. *C. familiaris*) L., 1758, Domestic Dog.

Remarks: Carlslake et al. (2017) examined dog fecal samples in Samoa, South Pacific. All dogs were mixed-breed and free-roaming, and Carlslake et al. (2017) reported the presence of "oocysts" in 9/204 (4%) dogs.

SARCOCYSTIS CAPREOLI OF LEVCHENKO, 1963

Synonym: *Sarcocystis capreolicanis* Erber, Boch, and Barth, 1978.

Definitive hosts: *Canis lupus familiaris* (syn. *C. familiaris*) L., 1758, Domestic Dog; *Vulpes vulpes* (L., 1758), Red Fox.

Intermediate host: *Capreolus capreolus* (L., 1758), European Roe Deer.

Remarks: The relationship of this species to *S. gracilis* and *S. sibirica* is unknown, but we can find no other information on this species that was listed as a valid species by Levine (1986). Levine and Ivens (1981) did not mention this species nor did Dubey et al. (2015a). Sedlaczek and Wesemeier (1995) examined 66 roe deer in Germany and Poland to compare the ultrastructure of their sarcocysts. They identified three distinct species, and when defining one of them, *S. capreolicanis* Erber et al. (1978), they said that Levchenko's (1963) "species" is not recognizable in its original description and, therefore, should be a *species inquirenda*. We agree.

SARCOCYSTIS FUSIFORMIS OF MEHLHORN, SENAUD, HEYDORN, AND GESTRICH, 1975a

Definitive hosts: *Canis lupus familiaris* (syn. *C. familiaris*) L., 1758, Domestic Dog; *Felis catus* L., 1758, Domestic Cat.

Intermediate host: *Bos taurus* L., 1758, Aurochs.

Remarks: Mehlhorn et al. (1975b) published a paper in which they tried to compare the ultrastructure of sarcocysts of (what they called) *S. fusiformis* in the muscles of naturally-infected cows with sarcocysts in cow muscle after experimental infection by sporocysts of *I. hominis* and sporocysts of the large forms of *I. bigemina* from the dog and cat. In naturally-infected cows they found two kinds of sarcocysts, probably *S. fusiformis* from cats and *S. cruzi* from dogs, but in their defense, these life cycles were still unknown at the time. They concluded that one type of sarcocyst in cows was produced by the large form of *I. bigemina* from dogs and the second type of sarcocysts "were caused by infection with *I. hominis* and the large form of *I. bigemina* from the cat."

SARCOCYSTIS MIESCHERIANA OF FARMER, HERBERT, PARTRIDGE, AND EDWARDS, 1978

Definitive host: *Canis lupus familiaris* (syn. *C. familiaris*) L., 1758, Domestic Dog.

Intermediate host: Unknown.

Remarks: Farmer et al. (1978) surveyed feces from 123 working sheepdogs in Gwynedd, 33 greyhounds from the London area, and 41 red foxes killed on Anglesey or in the Bangor area of England. They found sporocysts of *Sarcocystis* spp. in 35/123 (28%) sheepdogs, 8/33 (24%) greyhounds, and 7/41 (17%) red foxes (their Table 1, p. 79). Based only on sporocyst dimensions, they said that *S. porcifelis* (syn. their *S. miescheriana*) sporocysts were identified in 11/47 (23%) sheepdogs and 2/8 (25%) greyhound samples they measured (their Table 3, p. 79). At that early stage in time, when we knew little about the true identity and life cycles of most *Sarcocystis* species, using only sporocyst measurements to place them into the correct species diagnosis was a bit risky; and we now know that *S. porcifelis* (syn. their *S. miescheriana*) seems to only be transmitted by felids so we must relegate their form to a *species inquirenda*.

SARCOCYSTIS SP. OF ABARCA, LÓPEZ, PEÑA, AND LÓPEZ, 2011

Definitive hosts: *Canis lupus familiaris* (syn. *C. familiaris*) L., 1758, Domestic Dog.

Intermediate host: Unknown.

Remarks: Abarca et al. (2011) surveyed feces of dogs maintained as pets of families with immunocompromised children (oncology patients, HIV-positive, or patients after transplantations) in Santiago, Chile. A *Sarcocystis* sp. was detected in 1/41 (2%) dogs.

SARCOCYSTIS SPP. OF BARHAM, STÜTZER, KARANIS, LATIF, AND NEISS, 2005

Definitive host: *Canis lupus familiaris* (syn. *C. familiaris*) L., 1758, Domestic Dog.

Intermediate host: *Capra hircus* L., 1758, Goat.

Remarks: Barham et al. (2005) surveyed goats slaughtered in the winter in northern Iraq and found three morphologically distinct types of sarcocysts, macrocysts (both fat and thin), and microcysts; macrocysts occurred in 281/826 (34%) goats, but these were not identified.

SARCOCYSTIS SPP. OF BARUTZKI AND SCHAPER, 2003

Definitive host: *Canis lupus familiaris* (syn. *C. familiaris*) L., 1758, Domestic Dog.

Intermediate host: Unknown.

Remarks: During a coprological survey of dogs and cats in Germany, Barutzki and Schaper (2003) examined feces from both hosts in Freiburg, Germany; sarcocysts of *Sarcocystis* spp. were detected in 759/8,438 (9%) samples.

SARCOCYSTIS SP. OF BLAGBURN, BRAUND, AMLING, AND TOIVIO-KINNUCAN, 1989

Definitive host: Unknown.

Intermediate host: *Canis lupus familiaris* (syn. *C. familiaris*) L., 1758, Domestic Dog.

Remarks: Blagburn et al. (1989) found a single sarcocyst in the biceps femoris muscle of a dog in Alabama, USA. The sarcocyst was spheroidal to ovoidal and measured 52 × 47 with a wall thickness of ~2.3. Sarcocyst wall projections were barely visible with the LM, but under TEM they appeared as irregularly-spaced electron-dense projections that were 1.5 × 0.9. Septa were visible in the sarcocyst and contained numerous, irregularly arranged bradyzoites, but no metrocytes were seen. The sarcocyst did not elicit an inflammatory response in the adjacent muscle tissue.

SARCOCYSTIS SPP. OF BUGG, ROBERTSON, ELLIOT, AND THOMPSON, 1999

Definitive host: Unknown.

Intermediate host: *Canis lupus familiaris* (syn. *C. familiaris*) L., 1758, Domestic Dog.

Remarks: Bugg et al. (1999) examined fecal samples of urban dogs from four pet shops, three refuges, six breeding kennels, eight veterinary clinics, and two exercise areas in Perth, Western Australia. *Sarcocystis* sporocysts were detected in 26/421 (6%) samples, mostly in puppies from refuges.

SARCOCYSTIS SP. OF CARLSLAKE, HILL, SJÖLANDER, HII, PRATTLEY, AND ACKE, 2017

Original host: *Canis lupus familiaris* (syn. *C. familiaris*) L., 1758, Domestic Dog.

Remarks: Carlslake et al. (2017) examined fecal samples from mixed-breed, free-roaming dogs in Samoa, South Pacific. Sporocysts of a *Sarcocystis* spp. were detected in 1/204 (0.5%) dogs.

SARCOCYSTIS SP. OF CAUSAPÉ, QUÍLEZ, SÁNCHEZ-ACEDO, AND DEL CACHO, 1996

Definitive host: Unknown.

Intermediate host: *Canis lupus familiaris* (syn. *C. familiaris*) L., 1758, Domestic Dog.

Remarks: Causapé et al. (1996) examined fecal samples of 37 domestic and 44 stray dogs in

shelters in Zaragoza, Aragón, Spain. *Sarcocystis* sporocysts were found in 1/81 (1%) dogs, a stray.

SARCOCYSTIS SPP. OF CHHABRA, MAHAJAN, GUPTA, AND GAUTAM, 1984

Definitive host: *Canis lupus familiaris* (syn. *C. familiaris*) L., 1758, Domestic Dog.

Intermediate host: Unknown.

Remarks: Chhabra et al. (1984) examined fecal samples of domestic dogs from North India (Delhi, Rishikesh, and Lucknow). Sporocysts of *Sarcocystis* were detected in 2/118 (2%) samples.

SARCOCYSTIS SPP. OF CIRAK AND BAUER, 2004

Definitive host: *Canis lupus familiaris* (syn. *C. familiaris*) L., 1758, Domestic Dog.

Intermediate host: Unknown.

Remarks: Cirak and Bauer (2004) examined fecal samples of dogs from three animal shelters in central Germany; all dogs were without diarrhea. *Sarcocystis* sporocysts were found in 4/270 (1.5%) dogs.

SARCOCYSTIS SP. OF CRUM, FAYER, AND PRESTWOOD, 1981

Definitive host: *Canis lupus familiaris* (syn. *C. familiaris*) L., 1758, Domestic Dog.

Intermediate host: *Odocoileus virginianus* (Zimmermann, 1780), White-tailed Deer.

Remarks: Crum et al. (1981) described *S. odocoileocanis* from sarcocysts in the white-tailed deer and determined that the dog was the definitive host. However, one cat fed sarcocysts from a wild-caught *O. virginianus* from West Virginia, USA, began to shed sporocysts 14 DPI, and sporocysts were detected intermittently between 14 and 38 DPI. These sporocysts measured L×W (n = 35): 11.5 × 8.1 (11–13 × 7). No one to our knowledge has yet named this species so it must remain a *species inquirenda*.

SARCOCYSTIS SPP. OF DUBEY, 1980a

Definitive hosts: *Canis latrans* Say, 1823, Coyote; *Canis lupus familiaris* (syn. *C. familiaris*) L., 1758, Domestic Dog.

Intermediate hosts: *Ovis aries* L., 1758, Red Sheep; *Capra hircus* L., 1758, Goat; *Bos taurus* L., 1758, Aurochs; *Alces alces* (L., 1758), Eurasian Elk, Moose; *Bison bison* (L., 1758), American Bison; *Cervus elaphus* L., 1758 (syn. *Cervus canadensis* Erxleben, 1777), Red Deer, Elk, Wapiti.

Remarks: Dubey (1980a) fed 1 kg of tissues from bison, cattle, elk, goats, moose, and sheep to different *Sarcocystis*-free coyotes, and all 12 coyotes shed sporocysts of *Sarcocystis* in their feces with prepatent periods of 9–15 DPI. Dubey (1980a,b) said that sporocysts in coyote feces fed infected musculature of cattle, sheep, goats, and elk were all structurally similar and that this was the first report of the completion of the life cycle of *Sarcocystis* species in moose and bison. One other cross-transmission experiment indicated that one goat *Sarcocystis* species completed its life cycle in both the dog and coyote and that ovine *Sarcocystis* is not transmissible to goats. None of the *Sarcocystis* species were identified, thus all must remain *species inquirendae*.

SARCOCYSTIS SPP. OF DUBEY, CALERO-BERNAL, ROSENTHAL, SPEER, AND FAYER, 2015a

Definitive host: Unknown.
Intermediate hosts: Cattle, Wild Ruminants.
Remarks: Dubey et al. (2015a) listed various *Sarcocystis species inquirendae* from cattle and wild ruminants (27 species) in their Table 24.3. Some of those indeterminant species/forms are

listed here, others are not. The interested reader is referred to their work.

SARCOCYSTIS SPP. OF DUBEY, CALERO-BERNAL, ROSENTHAL, SPEER, AND FAYER, 2015a

Definitive host: Unknown.
Intermediate hosts: Marine carnivores.
Remarks: Dubey et al. (2015a) listed five *Sarcocystis species inquirendae* from a sea lion, bearded seal, ringed seal, northern fur seal, and sea otter in their Table 24.3. Some of those indeterminant species are listed here, others are not. The interested reader is referred to their work.

SARCOCYSTIS SPP. OF DUBEY, CALERO-BERNAL, ROSENTHAL, SPEER, AND FAYER, 2015a

Definitive hosts: Wild carnivores.
Intermediate hosts: Wild carnivores.
Remarks: Dubey et al. (2015a) listed 18 *Sarcocystis species inquirendae* from a variety of wild carnivores (e.g., jackals, otters, raccoons, red foxes, others) in their Table 24.3. Some of those indeterminant species are listed here, others are not. The interested reader is referred to their work.

SARCOCYSTIS SPP. OF DUBEY, CALERO-BERNAL, ROSENTHAL, SPEER, AND FAYER, 2015a

Definitive host: Unknown.
Intermediate hosts: Small mammals.
Remarks: Dubey et al. (2015a) listed 15 *Sarcocystis species inquirendae* from a variety of small mammals (e.g., rabbits, rats, squirrels, others) in their Table 24.3. In most, the definitive hosts are unknown so they are not covered in this book, but a few of those species in which the

definitive host is/may be known are listed here. The interested reader is referred to their work.

SARCOCYSTIS SP. OF DUBEY, COSENZA, LIPSCOMB, TOPPER, SPEER, HOBAN, DAVIS, KINCAID, SEELY, AND MARRS, JR., 1991a

Definitive host: Unknown.

Intermediate host: *Canis lupus familiaris* (syn. *C. familiaris*) L., 1758, Domestic Dog.

Remarks: Dubey et al. (1991a) examined a litter of eight dogs born to a primiparous 2-year-old Rottweiler in Maryland, USA. All of the pups had medical issues, but one (dog 1), at 7-weeks-old, was listless and anorectic with mild anemia after surgery for entropion. It was killed 2 days later and specimens of liver and small intestine were examined histologically. Protozoan meronts were seen free in the cytoplasm of hepatocytes adjacent to necrotic foci; the parasites were without a PV, divided by merogony, and resembled *Sarcocystis* structurally and antigenically, as it reacted with *Sarcocystis* antiserum. It was uncertain how the pup became infected, but was noteworthy to find *Sarcocystis* in the visceral tissues of dogs. There was no way to know what species they saw so this must be considered as another *species inquirenda*.

SARCOCYSTIS SP. OF DUBEY, DUNCAN, SPEER, AND BROWN, 1992a

Definitive host: Unknown.

Intermediate host: *Canis lupus familiaris* (syn. *C. familiaris*) L., 1758, Domestic Dog.

Remarks: Dubey et al. (1992a) examined paraffin-embedded tissue samples of liver, spleen, lungs, and kidneys of a 2-day-old female bullmastiff puppy that died 2½ days after birth. Initially deparaffinized tissues reacted with antisera to *T. gondii*, *N. caninum*, and *S. cruzi*.

To better identify the protozoan, they studied tissue sections for developmental stages, documented some of the pathology, and isolated meronts to find whether they reacted with *S. cruzi* antiserum, but not with antisera to *T. gondii* or *N. caninum*. Lesions were seen in all tissues examined. The main lung lesion was interstitial pneumonia characterized by infiltration of mononuclear cells and neutrophils in the alveolar wall and alveolar hemorrhage and necrosis due to numerous meronts in the vascular endothelium. Hepatic lesions included necrosis of hepatocytes, moderate perivascular infiltration of mononuclear cells, and the presence of meronts and merozoites in hepatocytes and Kupffer cells. Renal lesions showed necrosis of glomeruli associated with all developmental stages of meronts, and multifocal areas of necrosis were present. Mature meronts with merozoites were L × W (n = 13): 14–20 × 10–20, contained 12–28 merozoites, and they are divided by endopolygeny. They were located in the host cell cytoplasm without a PV. The authors said, "The parasite was antigenically and structurally identical to the newly named protozoan *Sarcocystis canis* from Rottweiler dogs (Dubey and Speer, 1991)," but they declined to say that *Sarcocystis* found in this Louisiana puppy was *S. canis*.

SARCOCYSTIS SP. OF DUBEY, SLIFE, SPEER, LIPSCOMB, AND TOPPER, 1991c

Definitive host: Unknown.

Intermediate host: *Canis lupus familiaris* (syn. *C. familiaris*) L., 1758, Domestic Dog.

Remarks: Dubey et al. (1991c) examined a 10-month-old Rottweiler from Illinois, USA that had multiple cutaneous abscesses over its body, particularly in its hind limbs that were swollen, hot, and painful. The dog died shortly after a few biopsies were taken, so portions of skin, liver, lungs, kidney, and lymph nodes were processed for examination. *Toxoplasma gondii*, *N. caninum*, and *Caryospora* species are parasites that can cause dermatitis and disseminated infection in dogs, but these were all eliminated by not reacting with the appropriate antisera and/or physical structure of the protozoan stages found. Dubey et al. (1991c) concluded, "the present case resembles the *Sarcocystis* parasite that causes fatal encephalomyelitis in horses, cattle, and sheep. Although the central nervous system in the infected dog was not examined, its littermate died of protozoan encephalomyelitis."

SARCOCYSTIS SPP. OF DUBEY AND STREITEL, 1976c

Definitive host: *Canis lupus familiaris* (syn. *C. familiaris*) L., 1758, Domestic Dog.

Intermediate hosts: *Ovis aries* L., 1758, Red Sheep; *Bos taurus* L., 1758, Aurochs.

Remarks: Dubey and Streitel (1976c) did cross-infections between dogs, cats, sheep, pigs, and cattle from Iowa or Ohio, USA. Two dogs fed 100 sheep esophagi and hearts from Iowa shed sporocysts, but cats did not. Sporocysts were L×W (n=11): 14.0×9.2 (13–15×9–10), L/W ratio: 1.5 and were shed for >8 days. Dogs shed large numbers of sporocysts and sporulated oocysts for >8 days after ingesting bovine tissue; sporocysts were L×W (n=27): 15.0×9.5 (14–17×8–10), L/W ratio: 1.6. Because cats also shed sporocysts when fed bovine tissues, Dubey and Streitel (1976c) suggested that separate species of *Sarcocystis* parasitize cattle in different areas of the United States, but they did not suggest a name for any of these *Sarcocystis* species.

SARCOCYSTIS SPP. OF DUBNÁ, LANGROVÁ, NÁPRAVNÍK, JANKOVSKÁ, VADLEJCH, PEKÁR, AND FECHTNER, 2007

Original host: *Canis lupus familiaris* (syn. *C. familiaris*) L., 1758, Domestic Dog.

Remarks: Dubná et al. (2007) reported on a survey of canine and ground-collected fecal samples from various areas in and around Prague, and from rural areas in central Bohemia, Czech Republic. Sporocysts of *Sarcocystis* spp. were detected in 24/3,780 (<1%) samples.

SARCOCYSTIS SP. OF ENTZEROTH, 1982b

Definitive host: *Canis lupus familiaris* (syn. *C. familiaris*) L., 1758, Domestic Dog.

Intermediate host: *Capreolus capreolus* (L., 1758), European Roe Deer.

Remarks: Entzeroth (1982b) studied the ultrastructure of gamonts and gametes and fertilization of a *Sarcocystis* species in dogs after they were fed sarcocysts from roe deer in Germany. Unfortunately, he did not attempt to name the species. He may have been dealing with the same species seen by Erber (1978) 4 years earlier (below) and both may have been working with *S. gracilis*, which is now known from the European roe deer. Nonetheless, we can only call it a *species inquirenda* based on the information provided by Entzeroth (1982b).

SARCOCYSTIS SPP. OF ENTZEROTH, SCHOLTYSECK, AND GREUEL, 1978

Definitive host: *Canis lupus familiaris* (syn. *C. familiaris*) L., 1758, Domestic Dog.

Intermediate host: *Capreolus capreolus* (L., 1758), European Roe Deer.

Remarks: In Germany, Entzeroth et al. (1978) fed muscles of roe deer infected with sarcocysts to a coccidia-free fox, dog, and cat (species not stated). After a prepatency of 8 DPI, the fox shed sporulated sporocysts in its feces that were L×W: 14.5×8.5, and after the 11th day, unsporulated oocysts discharged by the fox were 13.1 × 11.6 and "resembled the small form of *Isospora bigemina* (*Hammondia*)." The dog shed sporulated sporocysts that were L×W: 15.6×10, with a prepatent period of 10–14 days, and sporocysts continued to be discharged for 51 days. The cat fed sarcocyst-infected deer meat shed unsporulated oocysts on the 8th DPI that were L×W: 12.2×10.9. The small isosporan oocysts from the fox and the cat were inoculated into mice; Entzeroth et al. (1978) reported they found typical *Toxoplasma* cysts in the brain of the mice and cysts typical of *Hammondia hammondi* in the muscle of the mice with oocysts from the cat but that "oocysts from the fox did not cause any visible infection in mice." When they (Entzeroth et al., 1978) examined the muscle sarcocysts in roe deer with the TEM, they said there were three types of sarcosporidian cysts, but nothing else. Thus, more *species inquirendae*.

SARCOCYSTIS SP. OF ENTZEROTH, STUHT, CHOBOTAR, AND SCHOLTYSECK, 1982b

Definitive host: *Canis lupus familiaris* (syn. *C. familiaris*) L., 1758, Domestic Dog.

Intermediate host: *Odocoileus virginianus* (Zimmermann, 1780), White-tailed Deer.

Remarks: Entzeroth et al. (1982b) found 14/48 (29%) white-tailed deer infected with *Sarcocystis*, with a preference in location for the tongue. This was only about 4 months after Crum et al. (1981) named a species with sarcocysts in white-tailed deer tissue (especially tongue), and dogs as definitive hosts that discharged sporocysts as *S. odocoileocanis*. Entzeroth et al. (1982b) said their sarcocysts were spindle-shaped and measured 300–620×60–120, had a thin wall, and were divided into compartments by septa. They fed a lab-reared dog infected venison flesh and on 14 DPI the dog began to discharge sporulated sporocysts that were L×W: 14.9×10.6 (13.5–16.5×9–11); patency lasted at least 10 days, after which no fecal samples were checked. This deer/dog cycle is remarkably similar to that described by Crum et al. (1981), and their sporocyst size, prepatent and patent periods also overlap, but the sarcocysts in the Michigan deer were larger than those reported by Crum et al. (1981) in deer from several southeastern

states (e.g., 264×40 (150–536×30–51) versus 300–620×60–120). Unfortunately, Entzeroth et al. (1982b) were unaware of the paper published by Crum et al. (1981) and they chose not to name their species "until additional details of the life cycle are known." Thus, their form can only be considered a *species inquirenda*.

SARCOCYSTIS SPP. OF EPE, ISING-VOLMER, AND STOYE, 1993

Definitive host: *Canis lupus familiaris* (syn. *C. familiaris*) L., 1758, Domestic Dog.

Intermediate host: Unknown.

Remarks: Epe et al. (1993), in Germany, surveyed 3,329 fecal samples from dogs between 1984 and 1991 and found 100 (3%) to pass *Sarcocystis* spp. sporocysts, which were not identified to species.

SARCOCYSTIS SPP. OF ERBER, 1978

Definitive host: *Canis lupus familiaris* (syn. *C. familiaris*) L., 1758, Domestic Dog.

Intermediate host: *Capreolus capreolus* (L., 1758), European Roe Deer.

Remarks: Erber (1978) reported three types of sarcocysts in the tongues and abdominal musculature of 391/421 (93%) *C. capreolus*, in West Germany. He fed raw muscles infected with his type 1 and type 2 sarcocysts to dogs, foxes, and cats. On 10–11 DPI, the dogs and foxes shed sporocysts in their feces that were L×W: 16–18×9–12, and the patent period lasted 50 days. The cats did not shed oocysts (Levine and Ivens, 1981). To our knowledge, these forms were never studied again.

SARCOCYSTIS SPP. OF FERREIRA, PENA, AZEVEDO, LABRUNA, AND GENNARI, 2016

Definitive host: *Canis lupus familiaris* (syn. *C. familiaris*) L., 1758, Domestic Dog.

Intermediate host: Unknown.

Remarks: Ferreira et al. (2016) surveyed fecal samples of pet dogs from the metropolitan region of São Paulo, Brazil. *Sarcocystis* sporocysts were detected in 16/3,099 (0.5%) samples, mostly in dogs ≥1-year-old.

SARCOCYSTIS SPP. OF FONTANARROSA, VEZZANI, BASABE, AND EIRAS, 2006

Definitive host: *Canis lupus familiaris* (syn. *C. familiaris*) L., 1758, Domestic Dog.

Intermediate host: Unknown.

Remarks: Fontanarrosa et al. (2006) surveyed fecal samples of dogs in southern Buenos Aires, Argentina and detected sporocysts of *Sarcocystis* in 219/2,193 (10%) samples, mostly in young dogs 0–11-months-old, and its prevalence decreased with increasing age.

SARCOCYSTIS SPP. OF FUNADA, PENA, SOARES, AMAKU, AND GENNARI, 2007

Definitive host: *Canis lupus familiaris* (syn. *C. familiaris*) L., 1758, Domestic Dog.

Intermediate host: Unknown.

Remarks: Funada et al. (2007) examined fecal samples of domestic dogs in the city of São Paulo, Brazil. *Sarcocystis* sporocysts were detected in 25/1,755 (1%) samples.

SARCOCYSTIS SPP. OF GATES AND NOLAN, 2009

Definitive host: *Canis lupus familiaris* (syn. *C. familiaris*) L., 1758, Domestic Dog.

Intermediate host: Unknown.

Remarks: From 1997 to 2007, Gates and Nolan (2009) studied fecal samples of dogs in Philadelphia, Pennsylvania, USA, and *Sarcocystis* sporocysts were seen in only 5/6,555 (<0.1%) samples.

SARCOCYSTIS SPP. OF GENNARI, KASAI, PENA, AND CORTEZ, 1999

Definitive host: *Canis lupus familiaris* (syn. *C. familiaris*) L., 1758, Domestic Dog.

Intermediate host: Unknown.

Remarks: Gennari et al. (1999) examined fecal samples of domestic dogs from São Paulo, Brazil. *Sarcocystis* sporocysts were found in 6/353 (2%) samples.

SARCOCYSTIS SP. OF GOMPPER, GOODMAN, KAYS, RAY, FIORELLO, AND WADE, 2003

Definitive host: *Canis latrans* Say, 1823, Coyote.

Intermediate host: Unknown.

Remarks: Gompper et al. (2003) said they found sporocysts of a *Sarcocystis* sp. in 3/23 (12.5%) *C. latrans* collected from Black Rock Forest near Cornwall, New York, USA; their identification was based on finding some sporocysts in the feces, so it should be taken with caution.

SARCOCYSTIS SPP. OF HERMOSILLA, KLEINERTZ, SILVA, HIRZMANN, HUBER, KUSAK, AND TAUBERT, 2017

Definitive host: *Canis lupus* L., 1758, Wolf.

Intermediate host: Unknown.

Remarks: Hermosilla et al. (2017) surveyed fecal samples of wild European wolves in mountainous areas of the Gorski Kotar region, Croatia. *Sarcocystis* sporocysts were seen in 76/400 (19%) samples.

SARCOCYSTIS SP. OF HILL, CHAPMAN, JR., AND PRESTWOOD, 1988

Definitive host: Unknown.

Intermediate host: *Canis lupus familiaris* (syn. *C. familiaris*) L., 1758, Domestic Dog.

Remarks: Hill et al. (1988) saw sarcocysts in the myocardium of a 2-year-old, spayed, female

Doberman pinscher in Georgia, USA and said the dog's sarcocysts were similar in size and structure to sarcocysts they found in two cats, when examined by LM and TEM. The minor difference in sarcocysts from the dog (vs. cat sarcocysts) were a thinner layer of ground substance associated with the cyst wall and slightly larger bradyzoites. The cyst wall of both the dog and cats had striations, septa for compartmentalization, and fairly large bradyzoites.

SARCOCYSTIS SPP. OF JANITSCHKE, PROTZ, AND WERNER, 1976

Definitive host: *Canis lupus familiaris* (syn. *C. familiaris*) L., 1758, Domestic Dog.

Intermediate host: *Nanger granti* (Brooke, 1872) (syn. *Gazella granti*), Grant's Gazelle.

Remarks: Janitschke et al. (1976) found sarcocysts in Grant's gazelle in Tanzania, fed infected flesh to both cats and dogs, and reported finding sporocysts and sporulated oocysts in the feces of both. Sporocysts shed by the dog were L×W: 16×11 (13–18×8–12), L/W ratio, 1.45; the prepatent period in the dog was 10 days, and patency lasted 42 days. They thought they were dealing with two *Sarcocystis* species, but without further infection and/or molecular studies, it is not possible to determine which-was-which. Therefore, these must remain *species inquirendae* until they can be differentiated and named. There are at least three *Sarcocystis* species that have been named from gazelles, but only from sarcocysts in their muscle tissues. All three, *S. gazellae* Balfour, 1913, *S. mongolica* Matschoulsky, 1947, and *S. woodhousei* Dogel, 1916, are mentioned in Levine (1986) and in Dubey et al. (2015a), but the carnivore definitive host is not known for any of them. Clearly a lot of work still needs to be done in sorting out the various *Sarcocystis* species in gazelles.

SARCOCYSTIS SPP. OF KATAGIRI AND OLIVEIRA-SEQUEIRA, 2008

Definitive host: Unknown.

Intermediate host: *Canis lupus familiaris* (syn. *C. familiaris*) L., 1758, Domestic Dog.

Remarks: Katagiri and Oliveira-Sequeira (2008) examined fecal samples of 129 stray and 125 pet dogs from urban Botucatu, São Paulo State, Brazil. Samples were examined by multiple techniques. *Sarcocystis* sporocysts were found in 7/254 (3%) samples, 4 from strays and 3 from household dogs.

SARCOCYSTIS SPP. OF KING, BROWN, JENKINS, ELLIS, FLEMING, WINDSOR, AND ŠLAPETA, 2012

Definitive host: *Canis lupus familiaris* (syn. *C. familiaris*) L., 1758, Domestic Dog.

Intermediate host: Unknown.

Remarks: King et al. (2012) mentioned briefly in the discussion of their paper on the presence of *N. caninum* in Australian Aboriginal dogs that they had seen "*Sarcocystis* spp. sporocysts in many of the dog feces examined," but gave no other information.

SARCOCYSTIS SPP. OF MCKENNA AND CHARLESTON, 1980d

Definitive host: *Canis lupus familiaris* (syn. *C. familiaris*) L., 1758, Domestic Dog.

Intermediate host: Unknown.

Remarks: McKenna and Charleston (1980d) examined fecal samples from domestic dogs on the North Island of New Zealand and found 283/481 (59%) samples had oocysts/sporocysts they identified as *Sarcocystis* spp.

SARCOCYSTIS SPP. OF MELONI, THOMPSON, HOPKINS, REYNOLDS, AND GRACEY, 1993

Definitive host: *Canis lupus familiaris* (syn. *C. familiaris*) L., 1758, Domestic Dog.

Intermediate host: Unknown.

Remarks: Meloni et al. (1993) examined fecal samples of dogs from eight Aboriginal communities located in the tropical west Kimberley region, Western Australia. Fecal samples were examined by direct stool microscopy and zinc sulfate flotation. *Sarcocystis* sporocysts were seen in 8/182 (4%) samples.

SARCOCYSTIS SPP. OF PALMER, THOMPSON, TRAUB, REES, AND ROBERTSON, 2008a

Definitive host: *Canis lupus familiaris* (syn. *C. familiaris*) L., 1758, Domestic Dog.
Intermediate host: Unknown.
Remarks: Palmer et al. (2008a) surveyed fecal samples of dogs from urban and rural areas across Australia, including 810 samples (59 veterinary clinics) and 590 samples (26 refuges). *Sarcocystis* sporocysts were found in 50/1,400 (4%) dogs, mostly from vet clinics.

SARCOCYSTIS SP. OF PECKA, 1990

Definitive host: *Canis lupus familiaris* (syn. *C. familiaris*) L., 1758, Domestic Dog.
Intermediate host: *Phasianus colchicus* L., 1758, Common or Ring-necked Pheasant.
Remarks: Pecka (1990) found 3/90 (3%) pheasants, from two pheasant farms in the Czech Republic, infected with a *Sarcocystis* species with banana-shaped cystozoites, 6×2, and 46/90 (51%) were infected with a *Sarcocystis* species with lancet-shaped cystozoites, 14–16×2–3. A dog was infected experimentally with the latter species and pheasants were successfully reinfected, presumably with sporocysts from the dog, but this was not stated. Pecka (1990) said he suspected foxes to be the main final host for the pheasant species. No other information was given.

SARCOCYSTIS SP. OF SAHASRABUDHE AND SHAH, 1966

Definitive host: Unknown.
Intermediate host: *Canis lupus familiaris* (syn. *C. familiaris*) L., 1758, Domestic Dog.
Remarks: Sahasrabudhe and Shah (1966) reported finding sarcocysts in the muscles of an esophageal nodule of a dog in India. These sarcocysts had no septa, were 110–250 wide, and contained thousands of crescent-shaped merozoites, 4–5×1.5. They said that theirs was the first report of a *Sarcocystis* species from a domestic carnivore.

SARCOCYSTIS SPP. OF SALB, BARKEMA, ELKIN, THOMPSON, WHITESIDE, BLACK, DUBEY, AND KUTZ, 2008

Definitive host: *Canis lupus familiaris* (syn. *C. familiaris*) L., 1758, Domestic Dog.
Intermediate host: Unknown.
Remarks: Salb et al. (2008) examined fresh fecal samples of dogs presented to veterinary clinics from two remote northern Canadian communities (Fort Chipewyan, Alberta, Fort Resolution, Northwest Territories). The authors detected *Sarcocystis* sporocysts, but the number of positive samples and further details were not provided.

SARCOCYSTIS SPP. OF SORIANO, PIERANGELI, ROCCIA, BERGAGNA, LAZZARINI, CELESCINCO, SAIZ, KOSSMAN, CONTRERAS, ARIAS, AND BASUALDO, 2010

Definitive host: *Canis lupus familiaris* (syn. *C. familiaris*) L., 1758, Domestic Dog.
Intermediate host: Unknown.

Remarks: Soriano et al. (2010) surveyed dog fecal samples in urban (646 samples) and rural (1,298 samples) areas of Neuquén province, Patagonia, Argentina. *Sarcocystis* sporocysts were found in 110/1,944 (6%) samples, mostly from rural areas (99 of 110 samples).

SARCOCYSTIS SPP. OF STREITEL AND DUBEY, 1976

Definitive host: Canis lupus familiaris (syn. *C. familiaris*) L., 1758, Domestic Dog.
Intermediate host: Unknown.
Remarks: Streitel and Dubey (1976) surveyed feces from stray dogs in a humane shelter in Ohio, USA and found only 9/500 (2%) samples to have sporocysts of a *Sarcocystis* species. The sporocysts measured L × W: 13.5–16.2 × 8–11, but the species was neither identified nor was there an attempt to transmit it to another animal; thus, another *species inquirenda*.

SARCOCYSTIS SPP. OF STRONEN, SALLOWS, FORBES, WAGNER, AND PAQUET, 2011

Definitive host: Canis lupus L., 1758, Wolf.
Intermediate host: Unknown.
Remarks: From 2001 to 2005, Stronen et al. (2011) surveyed fecal samples of gray wolves from Riding Mountain National Park, southwestern Manitoba, Canada. *Sarcocystis* sporocysts were seen in 224/601 (37%) samples.

SARCOCYSTIS SPP. OF WEI, CHANG, DUONG, WANG, AND XIA, 1985

Definitive hosts: Canis lupus familiaris (syn. *C. familiaris*) L., 1758, Domestic Dog; or *Felis catus* L., 1758, Domestic Cat.

Intermediate host: Bos grunniens L., 1766 (syn. *Poephagus grunniens* Gray, 1843), Yak.
Remarks: Wei et al. (1985) named two species of *Sarcocystis* from yaks, using LM, TEM, and SEM to distinguish between their sarcocysts, *S. peophagi* and *S. poephagicanis*. Wei et al. (1989) then examined 23 3–5-month-old fetuses taken from slaughtered yaks in Gan Su province, China and examined their tissues (heart, liver, kidney, mesenteric lymph nodes, femoral and diaphragm muscles, intestines) histologically for sarcocysts. They detected sarcocysts in 6/23 (26%) fetuses, three in diaphragm and three in myocardium and found meronts, but not clear merozoites. They did not name the species of *Sarcocystis*, even though they had named the only two known species in yaks (Wei et al., 1985) and did cross-transmission work with both species a year later (Wei et al., 1990). This was not the first time that various stages of sarcocyst development were seen in fetal tissue; earlier, Munday and Black (1976) had reported *Sarcocystis* spp. in brain tissue of two aborted bovine fetuses, and Hong et al. (1982) found the vascular epithelium over all body parts contained immature and mature meronts of *Sarcocystis* in aborted bovine fetuses. These two studies, and their own work (Wei et al., 1985), led them to conclude that at least some *Sarcocystis* species can be transmitted vertically from naturally-infected mothers to their fetuses. This is certainly an area that deserves further exploration.

SARCOCYSTIS SPP. OF WESEMEIER, ODENING, WALTER, AND BOCKHARDT, 1995

Definitive host: Unknown.
Intermediate host: Canis mesomelas Schreber, 1775, Black-backed Jackal.
Remarks: Wesemeier et al. (1995) examined fixed tissue sections of pieces of tongue from 25 black-backed jackals from Namibia in 1993.

In one tongue (4%), using LM and TEM, they found two structurally different sarcocysts. Type 1 sarcocysts had a thick wall and were textured, palisade-like, and villar protrusions had a finger-shaped outline that arose from the cyst wall. These protrusions were interwoven with microtubules in the core and showed small invaginations on their surface; the microtubules did not penetrate into the ground substance. Type 2 sarcocysts had a relatively thin wall and showed minute, naplike elevations on the surface; villar protrusions arose from the cyst walls that were flat and mushroom-like with granules in their core. Apparently, finding sarcocysts in top carnivores is not uncommon, but no other information on these, apparently different, *Sarcocystis* species has not been forthcoming, to our knowledge, so they must remain *species inquirendae*.

GENUS *CHRYSOCYON* C.E.H. SMITH, 1839 (MONOTYPIC)

CRYPTOSPORIDIUM SP. OF GILIOLI AND SILVA, 2000

Definitive host: *Chrysocyon brachyurus* (Illiger, 1815), Maned Wolf.
Remarks: Gilioli and Silva (2000) looked at fecal samples of captive maned wolves from 11 zoos in the state of São Paulo, Brazil; they found 6/31 (19%) wolves had oocysts in their feces that they identified only as *Cryptosporidium* sp.

EIMERIA SP. OF GILIOLI AND SILVA, 2000

Definitive host: *Chrysocyon brachyurus* (Illiger, 1815), Maned Wolf.
Remarks: Gilioli and Silva (2000) looked in fecal samples of captive maned wolves from 11 zoos in the state of São Paulo, Brazil; they found

3/31 (10%) wolves had oocysts in their feces that they identified only as *Eimeria* sp.

ISOSPORA SP. OF GILIOLI AND SILVA, 2000

Definitive host: *Chrysocyon brachyurus* (Illiger, 1815), Maned Wolf.
Remarks: Gilioli and Silva (2000) looked in fecal samples of captive maned wolves from 11 zoos in the state of São Paulo, and found that 1/31 (3%) wolves had oocysts in their feces that they determined only as *Isospora* sp.

SARCOCYSTIS SP. OF GILIOLI AND SILVA, 2000

Definitive host: *Chrysocyon brachyurus* (Illiger, 1815), Maned Wolf.
Intermediate host: Unknown.
Remarks: Gilioli and Silva (2000) looked in fecal samples of captive maned wolves from 11 zoos in the state of São Paulo, and found that 9/31 (29%) wolves had oocysts/sporocysts in their feces that they determined only as *Sarcocystis* sp.

GENUS *CUON* HODGSON, 1838 (MONOTYPIC)

SARCOCYSTIS SP. OF JOG, MARATHE, GOEL, RANADE, KUNTE, AND WATVE, 2003; SARCOCYSTIS AXICUONIS (?) OF JOG, MARATHE, GOEL, RANADE, KUNTE, AND WATVE, 2005

Definitive host: *Cuon alpinus* (Pallas, 1811), Dhole.
Intermediate host: *Axis axis* (Erxleben, 1777), Chital.
Remarks: Jog et al. (2003) surveyed both *C. alpinus* and *A. axis* in two protected areas near Maharashtra, India, the Mudumalai National

Park and Wildlife Sanctuary in Tamil Nadu and Tadoba National Park, in both areas chital is the most predominant ungulate species. They reported that chital is the *intermediate host* for *Sarcocystis* species in dhole. Dhole scats were sampled from 1998 to 2001, and 184/239 (77%) scats from Tadoba and 161/209 (77%) scats from Mudumalai were positive for sporocysts of a *Sarcocystis* species. Sporocysts measured L×W: 16×10, L/W ratio: 1.6, and it was common for densities of 5,000–10,000, up to 26,000, sporocysts/g of feces. Skeletal and heart muscles of chital killed by dhole, or found dead due to other causes, were collected for histopathological examination, but Jog et al. (2003) never definitively stated the number of tissue samples of chital they examined for sarcocysts. They only said that sarcocysts were small, usually <1 mm long, they were not compartmentalized, and "there was no distinct cyst wall" (?). They also said the sarcocysts were found in large numbers in the heart (prevalence 50%) and skeletal muscles (19.5%) collected from Tadoba, whereas in samples collected from Mudumalai, the prevalences were 45% and 48%, respectively. Because neither chital nor dhole are available for experimentation in India, they were unable to demonstrate the life cycle directly; however, Jog et al. (2003) were convinced of the chital–dhole life cycle because of: (1) the consistent occurrence of sarcocysts in chital and sporocysts in dhole; (2) the high proportions of chital among dhole kills; (3) the absence or very low prevalence of sporocysts in other carnivores in the region; and (4) the failure to infect domestic dogs via feeding them chital sarcocysts. Jog et al. (2005) used the same data from their 2003 paper to investigate ecological and coevolutionary aspects of this relationship. Importantly, with no more information than they provided in their 2003 paper, or addressing the guidelines for naming new species, they named the coccidian, *Sarcocystis axicuonis*. Results of their analyses indicated that sarcocyst density in heart muscles of dhole kills was greater than in chital that died of other causes, and density of sarcocysts in skeletal muscle did not differ between dhole kills and nondhole kills. Jog et al. (2005) further argued that, if *Sarcocystis* infection in chital does not alter the probability of death due to other causes, then the effect of infection increased the probability of death due to dhole predation. Large numbers of cysts in heart muscle may negatively affect chital stamina making infected chital more susceptible to pack predators (dhole), than stalkers (tigers and leopards), which reinforces the parasite–prey and parasite–host relationships in this system. Jog et al. (2005) argued that if dhole kill more infected than uninfected chital, they are "benefited" by the parasite but, is there a cost to dhole to effectively disseminate the parasite? Dhole scat with large numbers of sporocysts was not diarrheic or otherwise abnormal, which suggested to them that infection in dhole is not pathogenic but no quantitative assessment was conducted. They noted that parasites were overdispersed in the dhole pack (i.e., only a few pack members were passing large numbers of sporocysts at any time). From these observations, they made the interesting suggestion that if carrying the parasite negatively impacts hunting efficiency, then uninfected dhole may do most of the hunting, and if consistent, the "cost" would be negligible to the dhole pack. Maintaining this division of labor between infected and uninfected dhole would be maintained if infected dhole preferentially ate heart tissue with high densities of cysts, and uninfected dhole ate other tissues with no/low densities. Unfortunately, they noted there are no parasite-free dhole–chital populations to serve as a control to estimate actual costs of infection in the two hosts, thus precluding demonstration of cost-benefit analysis of *Sarcocystis* infection to dhole. If readers are interested, Jog and Watve (2005) further developed their theoretical examination and modeling of parasite–host coevolution and development of mutualistic interactions using the dhole–chital *Sarcocystis* model. Unfortunately, Jog et al. (2003, 2005) never completed the basic process of properly naming the *Sarcocystis* they studied, so it must remain a *species inquirenda*.

GENUS *LYCALOPEX* BURMEISTER, 1854 (6 SPECIES)

ISOSPORA SP. OF JIMÉNEZ, BRICEÑO, ALCAÍO, VÁSQUEZ, FUNK, AND GONZÁLEZ-ACUÑA, 2012

Original host: *Lycalopex* (syn. *Pseudalopex*) *fulvipes* (Martin, 1837), Darwin's Fox.

Remarks: Jiménez et al. (2012) did a fecal survey of Darwin's foxes from seven areas of Chiloé Island, Chile; they found 4/189 (2%) foxes to shed *Isospora* sp. oocysts in three of these areas (Huillinco, Lliuco, Quilán). No other information was given.

GENUS *LYCAON* BROOKES, 1827 (MONOTYPIC)

ISOSPORA SP. OF BERENTSEN, BECKER, STOCKDALE-WALDEN, MATANDIKO, MCROBB, AND DUNBAR, 2012

Original host: *Lycaon pictus* (Temminck, 1820), African Wild Dog.

Remarks: Berentsen et al. (2012) surveyed *L. pictus* and other African carnivore species from the Luangwa Valley, Zambia, for gastrointestinal parasites; they reported *Isospora* species in 1/13 (8%) wild dogs but gave no other information about this parasite.

ISOSPORA SP. OF FLACKE, SPIERING, COOPER, GUNTHER, ROBERTSON, PALMER, AND WARREN, 2010

Original host: *Lycaon pictus* (Temminck, 1820), African Wild Dog.

Remarks: Flacke et al. (2010) surveyed fecal samples of *L. pictus* from the KwaZulu-Natal province, South Africa, for internal parasites; they reported *Isospora* species in 2/12 (17%) wild dogs but gave no other information about this parasite.

SARCOCYSTIS SP. OF BERENTSEN, BECKER, STOCKDALE-WALDEN, MATANDIKO, MCROBB, AND DUNBAR, 2012

Definitive host: *Lycaon pictus* (Temminck, 1820), African Wild Dog.

Intermediate host: Unknown.

Remarks: Berentsen et al. (2012) surveyed wild dogs and other African carnivore species from the Luangwa Valley, Zambia, for gastrointestinal parasites; they reported a *Sarcocystis* species in 12/13 (92%) *L. pictus* but gave no other information about this parasite.

SARCOCYSTIS SP. OF FLACKE, SPIERING, COOPER, GUNTHER, ROBERTSON, PALMER, AND WARREN, 2010

Definitive host: *Lycaon pictus* (Temminck, 1820), African Wild Dog.

Intermediate host: Unknown.

Remarks: Flacke et al. (2010) surveyed *L. pictus* in the KwaZulu-Natal province, South Africa, for parasites; they found sporocysts of a *Sarcocystis* sp. in 12/12 (100%) fecal samples from *L. pictus* but gave no other information. Knowledge on the parasites of this dog could prove important to its future survival because *L. pictus* is currently the most endangered carnivore in South Africa, with its total population estimated to be only 300–400 individuals.

SARCOCYSTIS SP. OF PENZHORN, DURAND, LANE, IDE, AND HOFMEYR, 1998

Definitive host: *Lycaon pictus* (Temminck, 1820), African Wild Dog.

Intermediate host: Unknown.

Remarks: Penzhorn et al. (1998) euthanized and necropsied a terminally ill, subadult female *L. pictus*, and isolated scrapings of the intestinal mucosa; thin-walled sporulated oocysts and many free sporocysts were found, consistent with *Sarcocystis* species. Two oocysts measured 21 × 15 and 19 × 16. Sporocysts were L × W (n = 12): 15.7 × 10.2 (14–17 × 9–11), L/W ratio: 1.5; and SZ (n = 4) measured 9–11 × 2 (10.3 × 2). On histological examination, they saw large numbers of thin-walled, sporulated oocysts, each with two sporocysts and four crescent-shaped SZ with prominent N in their caudal third. Oocysts were present in the lamina propria at the tips of almost all small intestinal villi but there was no evidence of inflammatory reaction or tissue necrosis.

GENUS NYCTEREUTES TEMMINCK, 1838 (MONOTYPIC)

CRYPTOSPORIDIUM SP. OF MATSUBAYASHI, TAKAMI, KIMATA, NAKANISHI, TANI, SASAI, AND BABA, 2005

Original host: *Nyctereutes procyonoides* (Gray, 1834), Raccoon Dog.

Remarks: Matsubayashi et al. (2005) surveyed fecal samples of one captive raccoon dog, at the Osaka Municipal Tennoji Zoological Gardens in Osaka City, Japan and reported ovoidal oocysts of a *Cryptosporidium* sp. measuring 4–5 wide. The animal was asymptomatic.

CRYPTOSPORIDIUM SP. OF OSTEN-SACKEN, SŁODKOWICZ-KOWALSKA, PACOŃ, SKRZYPCZAK, AND WERNER, 2017

Original host: *Nyctereutes procyonoides* (Gray, 1834), Raccoon Dog.

Remarks: Osten-Sacken et al. (2017) surveyed endoparasites from the latrines of *N. procyonoides*

in two areas of western Poland. They collected 38 samples in Ujście Warty National Park, and 13 in the Bogdaniec Forestry District. Numerous oocysts of a *Cryptosporidium* sp. measuring 3–6 × 4–6, were detected in 17/51 (33%) samples.

SARCOCYSTIS SP. OF BRITOV, 1970

Definitive host: Unknown.

Intermediate host: *Nyctereutes procyonoides* (Gray, 1834), Raccoon Dog.

Remarks: Levine and Ivens (1981) listed this form and said that sarcocysts were found in the muscles of the raccoon dog in Primorye (former USSR). However, neither Pellérdy (1974) nor Levine and Ivens (1981), nor Levine (1986), nor Dubey et al. (2015a,b) listed the original reference (Britov, 1970), nor does it come up in Google Scholar.

SARCOCYSTIS SP. OF KUBO, OKANO, ITO, TSUBOTA, SAKAI, AND YANAI, 2009

Definitive host: Unknown.

Intermediate host: *Nyctereutes procyonoides viverrinus* Temminck, 1838, Japanese Raccoon Dog.

Remarks: Kubo et al. (2009) examined 65 free-living carnivores on Honshu Island for muscle sarcocysts of *Sarcocystis*; 12 Japanese raccoon dogs had sarcocysts in their muscles, but no inflammatory host response was associated with them. Ultrastructurally, the sarcocyst wall was thin and showed minute undulations. Kubo et al. (2009) said these sarcocysts were similar to sarcocysts seen in the Japanese red fox (*V. v. japonica*) and Japanese martens (*M. m. melampus*) during the same survey. This was the first published report of muscular sarcocystosis in Japanese carnivores. There was no attempt to identify to species so this form is a *species inquirenda*.

SARCOCYSTIS SP. OF KUBO, KAWACHI, MURAKAMI, KUBO, TOKUHIRO, AGATSUMA, ITO, OKANO, ASANO, FUKUSHI, NAGATAKI, SAKAI, AND YANAI, 2010b

Definitive host: Unknown.

Intermediate host: *Nyctereutes procyonoides viverrinus* Temminck, 1838, Japanese Raccoon Dog.

Remarks: Kubo et al. (2010b) found a free-living, adult male, Japanese raccoon dog in Gifu, Japan; the dog was weak, emaciated, and had neurological signs including head tilt, tremor, and tic. At necropsy, microscopic examination showed severe meningoencephalitis associated with asexual developmental stages consistent with *Sarcocystis* spp. Immunohistochemical tests were negative for *T. gondii* and *N. caninum* but weakly positive with antiserum specific for *S. cruzi*. Analysis of the partial 18S rRNA gene sequence indicated to Kubo et al. (2010b) that this form was most closely related to an unidentified *Sarcocystis* species isolated from the white-fronted goose (*Anser albifrons*). For the moment, this can only be considered a *species inquirenda*.

GENUS *VULPES* FRISCH, 1775 (12 SPECIES)

COCCIDIA OF CRIADO-FORNELIO, GUTIERREZ-GARCIA, RODRIGUEZ-CAABEIRO, REUS-GARCIA, ROLDAN-SORIANO, AND DIAZ-SANCHEZ, 2000

Original host: *Vulpes vulpes* (L., 1758) (syn. *V. vulgaris* Oken, 1816), Red or Silver Fox.

Remarks: Criado-Fornelio et al. (2000) did a fecal survey of wild red foxes in three valleys of Tajo basin (Jarama, Henares, and Sorbe) in Guadalajara province, central Spain. "Coccidia oocysts (*Isospora* spp.)" were detected in 2/67 (3%) foxes (1 each from Jarama, Henares).

COCCIDIA OF WILLINGHAM, OCKENS, KAPEL, AND MONRAD, 1996

Original host: *Vulpes vulpes* (L., 1758) (syn. *V. vulgaris* Oken, 1816), Red or Silver Fox.

Remarks: Willingham et al. (1996) surveyed the feces of road-killed red foxes in metropolitan Copenhagen, Denmark; "coccidia oocysts" were detected in 2/68 (3%) foxes, mostly juveniles, but no other information was given.

CRYPTOSPORIDIUM SP. OF ELMORE, LALONDE, SAMELIUS, ALISAUSKAS, GAJADHAR, AND JENKINS, 2013

Original host: *Vulpes* (syn. *Alopex*) *lagopus* (L., 1758), Arctic or Blue Fox.

Remarks: Elmore et al. (2013) examined fecal samples of Arctic foxes collected from the central Canadian Arctic (Karrak Lake ecosystem, central Nunavut, Canada). *Cryptosporidium* sp. oocysts were detected in 9/95 (9%) samples. The species was not identified.

CRYPTOSPORIDIUM SP. OF HAMNES, GJERDE, FORBERG, AND ROBERTSON, 2007a

Original host: *Vulpes vulpes* (L., 1758) (syn. *V. vulgaris* Oken, 1816), Red or Silver Fox.

Remarks: Hamnes et al. (2007a) collected feces from wild Norwegian red foxes and examined them for Giardia and *Cryptosporidium* spp. Only 6/269 (2%) foxes had *Cryptosporidium* oocysts in their feces. Hamnes et al. (2007a) did PCR of the *Cryptosporidium* 18S rRNA gene but it did not yield positive results, so they could not identify the *Cryptosporidium* species or genotype. They said that the size, morphology, and morphometry of all the oocysts seen were consistent with those described for *C. parvum* and other *C. parvum*-like species, including *C. canis*.

CRYPTOSPORIDIUM SP. OF RAVASZOVA, HALANOVA, GOLDOVA, VALENCAKOVA, MALCEKOVA, HURNÍKOVÁ, AND HALAN, 2012

Original host: *Vulpes vulpes* (L., 1758) (syn. *V. vulgaris* Oken, 1816), Red or Silver Fox.

Remarks: Ravaszova et al. (2012) examined feces of *V. vulpes* from central and eastern Slovakia from June 2010–March 2011, using *in vitro* immunoassay for the quantitative detection of the *Cryptosporidium* antigen by the sandwich ELISA method. They said 24/62 (39%) samples were positive. They said that stained fecal smears using LM was a less sensitive method, with only 13/62 (21%) positive samples.

CRYPTOSPORIDIUM SP. OF STURDEE, CHALMERS, AND NULL, 1999

Original host: *Vulpes vulpes* (L., 1758) (syn. *V. vulgaris* Oken, 1816), Red or Silver Fox.

Remarks: Sturdee et al. (1999) detected what they said was *C. parvum* in 22/184 (12%) red fox fecal samples tested with a <u>genus</u>-specific monoclonal antibody for *C. parvum*. Their results purportedly emphasized the widespread distribution of *Cryptosporidium* among wild mammals in Britain and allowed them to suggest the potential for transmission between wild mammals, via direct exposure, to those using the countryside for professional or recreational purposes (e.g., farmers and ramblers).

CRYPTOSPORIDIUM SPP. OF ZHOU, FAYER, TROUT, RYAN, SCHAEFER III, AND XIAO, 2004

Original host: *Vulpes vulpes* (L., 1758) (syn. *V. vulgaris* Oken, 1816), Red or Silver Fox.

Remarks: Zhou et al. (2004) collected the feces of 471 wild mammals from four counties in the Chesapeake Bay area of Maryland, USA, and found 6/76 foxes (8%), presumably *V. vulpes* (?) (the host binomial was not stated), to be infected with the *C. canis* fox genotype (4), the *C. canis* dog genotype (1), and a *Cryptosporidium* muskrat genotype (1). The species and genotypic nature of *Cryptosporidium* in each fecal sample was determined by a PCR-restriction fragment length polymorphism (RFLP) method based on the small-subunit rRNA gene.

EIMERIA IMANTAUICA OF NUKERBAEVA AND SVANBAEV, 1973

Original host: *Vulpes* (syn. *Alopex*) *lagopus* (L., 1758), Arctic or Blue Fox.

Remarks: Nukerbaeva and Svanbaev (1973) said they found this form in 30/1,089 (3%) Arctic foxes in Kazakhstan of the former USSR. Their oocysts were ellipsoidal, 14×10 ($13–15 \times 8–11$), L/W ratio: 1.4, with a 2-layered wall, ~1 thick; OR: present; M, PG: both absent. Sporocysts were ellipsoidal, $6–7 \times 3–4$, SB, SSB, PSB, SR: all absent. Nukerbaeva and Svanbaev (1973) presented a modest line drawing, but little structural data and this species has not been seen since its original description.

EIMERIA MESNILI OF RASTÉGAÏEFF, 1929c

Original host: *Vulpes* (syn. *Alopex*) *lagopus* (L., 1758), Arctic or Blue Fox.

Remarks: Rastégaïeff (1929c) published a note préliminaire naming this "species" from oocysts in the feces of an Arctic fox collected in Murmansk Oblast, northern Russia, on the south side of the Barents Sea. Oocysts were spheroidal to ovoidal, $18 \times 11–14$, with a 1-layered wall and a M occupying the entire small end of the oocyst, which lacked an OR. Sporocysts were ellipsoidal. Pellérdy (1974a) questioned whether this was a real species (?) of the fox, and Levine and Ivens (1981) thought it looked like a rabbit coccidium. Rastégaïeff (1930) said she found it in the same fox on both October 10 and November 19, 1928. Levine and Ivens (1981) indicated they had seen a very poor line drawing, but we have a copy of her (1929) preliminary note, which does not have a line drawing. Unfortunately, she named the species in honor of Professor F. Mesnil, Laboratory of the Parasitology School, Leningrad, but this can only be considered a *species inquirenda*.

EIMERIA SP. OF GOLEMANSKY AND RIDZHAKOV, 1975

Original host: *Vulpes vulpes* (L., 1758), (syn. *V. vulgaris* Oken, 1816), Red or Silver Fox.

Remarks: Golemansky and Ridzhakov (1975) said they found oocysts of an unnamed *Eimeria* sp. in 6/146 (4%) red foxes in Bulgaria with oocysts that were L×W: 33×20 (28–38×17–23) and had sporocysts that measured 13–15×8–10, without a SB. They said these likely were a pseudoparasite of the fox, probably oocysts of a rabbit species just passing through the gut of the fox. We agree.

EIMERIA SPP. OF MAGI, MACCHIONI, DELL'OMODARME, PRATI, CALDERINI, GABRIELLI, IORI, AND CANCRINI, 2009

Original host: *Vulpes vulpes* (L., 1758) (syn. *V. vulgaris* Oken, 1816), Red or Silver Fox.

Remarks: Magi et al. (2009) examined fecal samples of red foxes in Tuscany (Cecina, Grosseto, Pisa, Siena), central Italy. Samples were examined by "coprological methods and microscopy," and "oocysts of *Eimeria* spp." were detected in 10/110 (9%) samples.

EIMERIA VULPIS OF GALLI-VALERIO, 1929b

Original host: *Vulpes vulpes* (L., 1758), (syn. *V. vulgaris* Oken, 1816), Red or Silver Fox.

Remarks: Galli-Valerio (1929a) found this form in *V. vulgaris* collected at 1,650 m, in the Val de Bagnes, Switzerland; oocysts were ovoidal, with one end "barely flattened" as a nearly invisible M, measured 17×14, with ovoidal sporocysts, each 6×4.5, and contained two SZ, ~4×2.4. A year later he found this species in another *V. vulgaris* collected on Fignards Mountain near Torgon, Switzerland (Galli-Valerio, 1930). Watkins and Harvey (1942) reported this species in 11/52 (21%) silver fox cubs dying in England and reportedly found it in ~10% of the adults and perhaps 25% of the fox cubs from 15 fox farms in England. Svanbaev (1960) reported it in 4/18 (22%) silver foxes in the Alma Atinsk Oblast, Kazakhstan and said the oocysts sporulated in 3–4 days at 25°C in 2% $K_2Cr_2O_7$ solution. Golemansky and Ridzhakov (1975) said they found oocysts of this species in the feces of 15/146 (10%) foxes in Bulgaria. Combining descriptive features from these other authors, the sporulated oocysts are ovoidal; number of walls, 1 (?); wall characteristics: smooth, colorless, 0.8–1.5 thick; L×W: 17×14 (16–26×12–24), L/W ratio: 1.2; M; barely visible or absent; OR, PG: both absent. Likewise, sporocysts may be ovoidal to ellipsoidal; L×W: 6×4.5 (5–6×3–6); L/W ratio: 1.3; SB, SSB, PSB: all absent; SR: present; SZ: comma-shaped, 4–5×2. Frank (1978) said she found this species in *V. vulpes* trapped near Lake Neusiedl, Austria, on the border with Hungary. Nonetheless, no published description to date has provided either a line drawing or a photomicrograph of a sporulated oocyst. Thus, this form must be relegated as a *species inquirenda*.

HAMMONDIA SP. OF DAHLGREN AND GJERDE, 2010b

Original hosts: *Vulpes vulpes* (L., 1758) (syn. *V. vulgaris* Oken, 1816), Silver or Red Fox; *Vulpes* (syn. *Alopex*) *lagopus* (L., 1758), Arctic or Blue Fox.

Remarks: Dahlgren and Gjerde (2010b) infected six of each fox species with fresh portions of esophagus, diaphragm, and abdominal muscles from moose, *Alces alces*, from Norway. They reported unsporulated, subspheroidal *Hammondia* oocysts were found in the mucus along the entire posterior half of the small intestine in one of each species of fox killed on the 7th DPI and a few *Hammondia* oocysts also found in the ileum of one silver fox killed on 14 DPI. Oocysts were shed in large numbers during the first 1–5 days of patency, then in small numbers or intermittently thereafter; patency began ~13–14 DPI after foxes ingested moose meat. *Hammondia* oocysts were detected microscopically in 11/12 foxes that ingested moose flesh (their Table 2, p. 1552), and samples from 7 foxes, 4 *V. vulpes* and 3 *V. lagopus*, were positive on agarose gels after PCR using *Hammondia*-specific primers. Moose previously were reported to be an intermediate host of *H. heydorni* infecting dogs (Dubey and Williams, 1980), but this was the first report of moose as intermediate host of a *Hammondia* species infecting foxes. Citing recent molecular comparisons of *Hammondia* isolates from dogs and foxes, Dahlgren and Gjerde (2010b) suggested that the *Hammondia* oocysts they found in red and arctic foxes in Norway might be different from *H. heydorni* known from dogs.

ISOSPORA CANIVELOCIS-LIKE OOCYSTS OF DAHLGREN AND GJERDE, 2010b

Original host: *Vulpes vulpes* (L., 1758) (syn. *V. vulgaris* Oken, 1816), Red or Silver Fox.

Remarks: Dahlgren and Gjerde (2010b) found oocysts in the feces of one fox, on the 8th DPI, which measured ~35 × 25, and "resembled those of *Isospora canivelocis*." No other information was given.

ISOSPORA-LIKE OF STUART, GOLDEN, ZINTL, DE WAAL, MULCAHY, MCCARTHY, AND LAWTON, 2013

Original host: *Vulpes vulpes* (L., 1758), (syn. *V. vulgaris* Oken, 1816), Red or Silver Fox.

Remarks: Stuart et al. (2013) surveyed fecal samples of red foxes killed throughout Ireland, and "*Isospora*-like oocysts" were seen in 8/91 (9%) samples, but no other information was given.

ISOSPORA VULPIS OF GALLI-VALERIO, 1931

Synonym: *Eimeria vulpes* Patnaik and Acharjyo, *lapsus*.

Original host: *Vulpes vulpes* (L., 1758) (syn. *V. vulgaris* Oken, 1816), Silver or Red Fox.

Remarks: Galli-Valerio (1931) measured oocysts that were 25 × 24, with a visible M, and two sporocysts each with four SZ, but gave no other measurements or qualitative descriptive information and then named this "species" as new! His description was less than marginal and he did not provide a line drawing or photomicrograph as a type. Nonetheless, Svanbaev and Rachmatullina (1971) said they found it in 6/85 (7%) common foxes (*V. vulpes*). The oocysts they studied were ovoidal (25–28 × 20–22) or spheroidal (25–28 wide), light gray, with a bilayered smooth wall, ~2 thick, and M, OR, and PG all absent. Sporocysts were ovoidal (14–17 × 11–14), without SB, SSB, and PSB. Golemansky and Ridzhakov (1975) measured oocysts that were 20–23 × 18–21. The measurements by Galli-Valerio (1931) suggest that many of the oocysts measured were end-on views resulting in the mean of the measurements to be erroneously more spheroidal. It is possible that this is *Isospora ohioensis*, *Isospora neorivolta*, or *Isospora burrowsi*, but the oocyst sizes are somewhat larger suggesting *Isospora vulpis* Galli-Valerio, 1931 may represent a separate species. The exception is Golemansky and Ridzhakov (1975), who may indeed have seen a member of the *Isospora ohioensis*-complex. It is likely that Bledsoe (1976a,b) actually was working with *I.* (=C.) *vulpis* rather than *I.* (=C.) *vulpina*. However, Galli-Valerio (1931) stated that the oocysts had a micropyle and his measurements suggest subspheroidal rather than ellipsoidal oocysts. It is likely that he was in error on both accounts and that the description by Svanbaev and Rachmatullina (1971) is the most accurate. Unfortunately, however, no published description to date has provided either a line drawing or a photomicrograph of a sporulated oocyst. Thus, this form must be relegated to a *species inquirenda*.

ISOSPORA SP. (ASHFORD, 1977) OF LEVINE AND IVENS, 1981

Synonym: Hammondia sp. Ashford, 1977.

Original host: *Vulpes vulpes* (L., 1758) (syn. *V. vulgaris* Oken, 1816), Silver or Red Fox.

Remarks: Levine and Ivens (1981) placed this form in the genus *Isospora*, but it is probably best left a *species inquirenda*. Ashford (1977) found some oocysts, 14 × 12 in the feces of 1/22 (4.5%) red foxes in England. He (Ashford, 1977) said the oocysts resembled those of "*Hammondia*" *hammondi*, but they were not infective for mice so he suggested they might belong to another species of *Hammondia*. Levine and Ivens (1981) thought it could just as well be an *Isospora* or a *Besnoitia* species. It is probably best relegated to a *species inquirenda*.

KLOSSIA SP. OF GOLEMANSKY AND RIDZHAKOV, 1975

Original host: *Vulpes vulpes* (L., 1758) (syn. *V. vulgaris* Oken, 1816), Silver or Red Fox.

Remarks: Golemansky and Ridzhakov (1975) found oocysts in 2/146 (1%) red foxes in Bulgaria and measured a few; oocysts were L × W: 38 × 33 (30–52 × 25–35) and contained 5–16 spheroidal sporocysts that were about 11–12 wide, without a SB, but with a SR consisting of many residual granules. They likely had found oocysts of an *Adelina* sp. from an arthropod or annelid and this was a spurious finding.

SARCOCYSTIS CORSACI PAK, 1979

Definitive host: Unknown.

Intermediate host: *Vulpes corsac* (L., 1758), Corsac Fox.

Remarks: Levine (1986) listed this species as a valid, named *Sarcocystis* species, but gave no other information. Odening (1998) said that Pak (1979) named this species from sarcocysts found in the corsac fox, but specimens were not preserved so follow-up molecular examination of the specimens cannot be done. Gjerde and Schulze (2014) suggested that because the specimen described is unrecognizable today, it should be considered a *species inquirenda* and its name should become a nomina dubia. Neither Levine (1986) nor the three of us were able to secure a copy of the original paper, so we must concur with the opinion of Gjerde and Schulze (2014). We do, however, list its complete citation in our References.

SARCOCYSTIS GRACILIS-LIKE OF GIANNETTO, POGLAYEN, BRIANTI, GAGLIO, AND SCALA, 2005

Definitive hosts: *Vulpes* (syn. *Alopex*) *lagopus* (L., 1758), Arctic or Blue Fox; *Vulpes vulpes* (L., 1758) (syn. *V. vulgaris* Oken, 1816), Silver or Red Fox.

Intermediate host: *Ovis aries* L., 1758, Red Sheep.

Remarks: Giannetto et al. (2005) used Dubey et al.'s (1989b) classification of 24 sarcocyst-types to identify a few sarcocysts of this form (type 10 villar protrusions) in one semi-thin tissue section of diaphragm from a sheep in Sicily, Italy. Sarcocysts were 800 × 300 and divided into compartments by septa. The cyst wall was ~5 thick, with radial striations. Villar protrusions had microtubules that extended from the apex to the base of the villi, all characteristics of *S. gracilis* from roe deer. However, this identification is only circumstantial, and this form should be regarded as a *species inquirenda*. We mention this form here because we know from recent work (Gjerde, 2012) that *S. gracilis* sarcocysts in roe deer muscle can be transmitted to both *V. vulpes* and *V. lagopus*, which then shed sporocysts in their feces 9 DPI with infected deer flesh.

SARCOCYSTIS GRACILIS OF ODENING, STOLTE, AND BOCKHARDT, 1996a

Definitive hosts: *Vulpes* (syn. *Alopex*) *lagopus* (L., 1758), Arctic or Blue Fox; *Vulpes vulpes* (L., 1758) (syn. *V. vulgaris* Oken, 1816), Silver or Red Fox.

Intermediate host: *Bos taurus* L., 1758, Aurochs.

Remarks: Odening et al. (1996a) found sarcocysts in the musculature of a dwarf zebu born in a German zoo. One of the four forms they found, "mostly resembles *Sarcocystis gracilis* Rátz, 1909 from roe deer." We mention this form here because we know from recent work (Gjerde, 2012) that *S. gracilis* sarcocysts in roe deer muscle can be transmitted to both *V. vulpes* and *V. lagopus*, which then shed sporocysts in their feces 9 DPI with infected deer flesh. Obviously, this form must remain a *species inquirenda* because no other data were given to confirm its identification as *S. gracilis* in the dwarf zebu.

SARCOCYSTIS RHOMBOMYS PAK, PERMINOVA, DYMKOVA, KIM, AND PINAYEVA, 1984

Definitive host: *Vulpes vulpes* (L., 1758) (syn. *V. vulgaris* Oken, 1816), Silver or Red Fox.

Intermediate host: *Rhombomys opimus* (Lichtenstein, 1823), Great Gerbil.

Remarks: Odening (1998) mentioned this species as valid in his compilation of 189 *Sarcocystis* names and noted that it had a TEM type 1 sarcocyst wall (Dubey et al., 1989b). However, the authors were cited only in a Russian reference book (Anon, 1984) that is unavailable to us. Odening (1998) gave such little detail in his citation that we think it is best, at this time, to relegate this form to a *species inquirenda*. To our knowledge, there have been no other references to this species since 1984, other than by Odening (1998).

SARCOCYSTIS UNDULATI PAK, YESHTOKINA, PERMINOVA, AND KIM, 1984

Definitive hosts: *Vulpes* (syn. *Alopex*) *corsac* (L., 1758), Corsac Fox; *Vulpes vulpes* (L., 1758) (syn. *V. vulgaris* Oken, 1816), Silver or Red Fox; *Mustela eversmanni* Lesson, 1827, Steppe Polecat.

Intermediate host: *Urocitellus* (syn. *Citellus*) *undulatus* (Pallas, 1778), Long-tailed Ground Squirrel.

Remarks: Odening (1998) mentioned this species as valid in his compilation of 189 *Sarcocystis* names and said it was similar to *S. citellivulpes*. However, the authors are cited only in a Russian reference book (Anon, 1984) that is unavailable to us. Odening (1998) gave such little detail in his citation, that we think it is best, at this time, to relegate this form to a *species inquirenda*. To our knowledge, there have been no other references to this species since 1984, other than by Odening (1998).

SARCOCYSTIS VULPIS PAK, SKLYAROVA, AND DYMKOVA, 1991

Definitive host: Unknown.

Intermediate host: *Vulpes vulpes* (L., 1758) (syn. *V. vulgaris* Oken, 1816), Silver or Red Fox.

Remarks: Odening (1998), who listed this as a valid *Sarcocystis* species name, said that Pak et al. (1991) named it from sarcocysts found in the red fox, but specimens were not preserved so follow-up molecular examination of specimens cannot be done. Dubey et al. (2015a) listed the form by Pak (1991) from the red fox as *Sarcocystis* sp. Gjerde and Schulze (2014) suggested that because the specimen described is unrecognizable today, it should be considered a *species inquirenda* and its name should be a nomina dubia. We were not able to secure a copy of the original paper, so we must concur with the opinion of Gjerde and Schulze (2014).

SARCOCYSTIS SP. OF ASHFORD, 1977

Definitive host: *Vulpes vulpes* (L., 1758) (syn. *V. vulgaris* Oken, 1816), Silver or Red Fox.
Intermediate host: Unknown.
Remarks: Ashford (1977) said that fecal samples of 12/22 (55%) *V. vulpes* collected near Wales and Exmoor contained *Sarcocystis*-like sporocysts in their feces. The sporocysts (n = 25) measured L × W: 13.4–14.2 × 9.2–9.5. No attempt was made to identify the species nor to transmit these sporocysts to any other host. Thus, a *species inquirenda*.

SARCOCYSTIS SPP. OF BIOCCA, BALBO, GUARDA, AND COSTANTINI, 1975 AND PROBABLY OF CORNAGLIA, GIACCHERINO, AND PERACINO, 1998

Definitive hosts: *Vulpes vulpes* (L., 1758) (syn. *V. vulgaris* Oken, 1816), Silver or Red Fox; *Canis lupus* L., 1758, Wolf; *Canis lupus familiaris* (syn. *C. familiaris*) L., 1758, Domestic Dog.
Intermediate host: *Capra ibex* L., 1758, Alpine Ibex.
Remarks: Biocca et al. (1975) found sporocysts in the feces of "some" of 12 red foxes in the Gran Parasiso National Park (GPNP) in Italy; these sporocysts measured 13–15 × 8–10, with a large SR, but no SB. They also found an ibex with sarcocysts in its muscles. Levine and Ivens (1981) reported that Biocca et al. (1975) infected both the timber wolf and domestic dog by feeding them sarcocyst-infected esophageal, heart, diaphragm, intercostal, and abdominal muscles from the infected ibex. The prepatent period in the fox was 11 days, in the wolf it was 12 days, and in the domestic dog it was 20 days; the patent period in these hosts was 62, 67, and 66 days, respectively. They also tried, unsuccessfully, to infect a domestic cat, a lion, a ferret, and a kestrel (*Falco tinnunculus*) with sarcocysts from the ibex, but none of them passed sporocysts. However, there is no evidence or correlation that the sporocysts in the foxes were the same species as the sarcocysts in the ibex. Later, Cornaglia et al. (1998) described the ultrastructural morphology of the sarcocyst wall in the muscles from an ibex found dead in the same national park in Italy. They also took samples of the diaphragm from 52 ibexes of different age and sex, from the GPNP. The morphology of the cyst wall led to the identification of three types of sarcocysts in the ibex of the GPNP and a further type in one Hispanic ibex was also collected. Cornaglia et al. (1998) concluded, "the morphology of the sarcocysts' walls was similar to the wall of the species described in the domestic ruminants from several authors."

SARCOCYSTIS SPP. OF DUBEY, 1982b

Definitive host: *Vulpes vulpes* (L., 1758) (syn. *V. vulgaris* Oken, 1816), Red or Silver Fox.
Intermediate host: Unknown.
Remarks: Dubey (1982b) surveyed the feces for coccidians from a variety of wild carnivores from Montana, USA. He reported sporocysts of *Sarcocystis* in the feces of 20/198 (10%) red foxes. He measured from 3 to 14 sporocysts

from each of eight different foxes and found size differences that varied from 16.3 × 11 (largest) to 11.6 × 6.7 (smallest). No attempt was made to identify the species beyond genus; thus, a *species inquirenda*.

SARCOCYSTIS SP. OF KUBO, OKANO, ITO, TSUBOTA, SAKAI, AND YANAI, 2009

Definitive host: Unknown.

Intermediate host: *Vulpes vulpes japonica* J.E. Gray, 1868, Japanese Red Fox.

Remarks: Kubo et al. (2009) examined 65 free-living carnivores on Honshu Island for muscular sarcocysts of *Sarcocystis*. Only one Japanese red fox had sarcocysts in its muscles and no inflammatory host response was associated with the sarcocysts. Ultrastructurally, the sarcocyst wall was thin and showed minute undulations. Kubo et al. (2009) said that these sarcocysts were similar to sarcocysts they found in the Japanese raccoon dog (*N. procyonoides viverrinus*) and Japanese martens (*M. m. melampus*) during the same survey. This is the first published report of muscular sarcocystosis in Japanese carnivores. There was no attempt to identify this species so this form must remain a *species inquirenda*.

SARCOCYSTIS SPP. (?) OF GOLEMANSKY, 1975b

Definitive host: *Vulpes vulpes* (L., 1758) (syn. *V. vulgaris* Oken, 1816), Silver or Red Fox.

Intermediate host: Unknown.

Remarks: Golemansky (1975b) found free oocysts and sporocysts in the feces of 14/146 (10%) *V. vulpes* in Soria, Bulgaria. Oocysts measured L × W: 18.6 × 14.0 (17–20 × 10–18) and sporocysts were 15.3 × 10.2 (13–18 × 9.5–11). He thought these oocysts/sporocysts resembled those of *S. fusiformis* and *S. tenella*, but the only

conclusion he drew was "the European common red fox is one of the vectors in the maintenance and distribution of sarcosporidiosis in nature." This can only be considered *species inquirenda*.

FAMILY MEPHITIDAE BONAPARTE, 1845

GENUS *MEPHITIS* É. GEOFFROY SAINT-HILAIRE AND F.G. CUVIER, 1795 (2 SPECIES)

CRYPTOSPORIDIUM SP. OF ZIEGLER, WADE, SCHAAF, STERN, NADARESKI, AND MOHAMMED, 2007

Original host: *Mephitis mephitis* (Schreber, 1776), Striped Skunk.

Remarks: Ziegler et al. (2007) collected fecal samples of *M. mephitis* live-trapped in the New York City Watershed, southeastern New York state, USA. Feces were examined by LM, and by polyclonal *Cryptosporidium* antigen-capture ELISA (considered positive based on an optical density ≥0.050). They found *Cryptosporidium* in 12/86 (14%) samples.

GENUS *SPILOGALE* GRAY, 1865 (4 SPECIES)

SARCOCYSTIS SPP. OF LESMEISTER, MILLSPAUGH, WADE, AND GOMPPER, 2008

Definitive host: *Spilogale putorius* (L., 1758), Eastern Spotted Skunk.

Intermediate host: Unknown.

Remarks: Lesmeister et al. (2008) did a fecal survey of *S. putorius* in western Arkansas, USA and found 5/17 (29%) had sporocysts of (one or more) *Sarcocystis* species in their feces, but no other information was given on these structures, so this identification remains a *species inquirenda*.

FAMILY MUSTELIDAE FISCHER, 1817

SUBFAMILY LUTRINAE BONAPARTE, 1838

GENUS *ENHYDRA* FLEMMING, 1822 (MONOTYPIC)

SARCOCYSTIS SP. OF DUBEY, ROSYPAL, ROSENTHAL, THOMAS, LINDSAY, STANEK, REED, AND SAVILLE, 2001c

Definitive host: Unknown.

Intermediate host: *Enhydra lutris* (L., 1758), Sea Otter.

Remarks: Dubey et al. (2001c) found two adult female sea otters at Olympic National Park, Washington USA, naturally-infected with *Sarcocystis* sarcocysts. Their otter No. 1 had *S. neurona*, but otter No. 2 had mature sarcocysts in skeletal muscles and the tongue, which were distinctly different than those of *S. neurona*. Later, Dubey et al. (2003a) characterized this second *Sarcocystis* (otter No. 2) using TEM and saw it had thin-walled sarcocysts that were 0.5–0.7 thick, lacking protrusions, and exhibiting minute type 1 (Dubey et al., 1989b) undulations on the wall. Two of these sarcocysts measured 95×60 and 110×65. Under TEM the sarcocyst wall had minute, electron-dense undulations located at irregular intervals. Only bradyzoites were seen and three of them, in longitudinal section, were 5.0–5.7×1.6–1.9. Rhoptries were prominent, their bulbous blind end was sometimes turned toward the conoidal end, and their micronemes were in the anterior half of the bradyzoite; all these features making this species ultrastructurally distinct from *S. neurona*.

However, to our knowledge it has never formally been named.

GENUS *LONTRA* GRAY, 1843 (4 SPECIES)

CRYPTOSPORIDIUM SPP. OF GAYDOS, MILLER, GILARDI, MELLI, SCHWANT, ENGELSTOFT, FRITZ, AND CONRAD, 2007b

Original host: *Lontra canadensis* (Schreber, 1777), North American River Otter.

Remarks: Gaydos et al. (2007b) collected feces from *L. canadensis* living along the Puget Sound Georgia Basin (PSGB) marine ecosystem between Washington state, USA, and the southern tip of Vancouver Island, British Columbia, Canada, to look for the presence of *Cryptosporidium* and *Giardia* oocysts and cysts, respectively. In Washington state, they collected fecal samples from 13 locations in PSGB, and off Vancouver Island, from 30 locations; they found 4/57 (7%) samples from 4 locations in Washington state, and 5/36 (14%) fecal samples from 2 locations on Vancouver to have *Cryptosporidium* oocysts in their fecal material. Overall, they found *Cryptosporidium* oocysts in 9/93 (10%) fecal samples from river otters in the PSGB. Even when some parasites, such as *Cryptosporidium*, are only identified to genus in wildlife surveys, we can see that there are so many examples of the potential for these and other parasites to be transmitted between wildlife and humans.

GENUS *LUTRA* BRISSON, 1762 (3 SPECIES)

CRYPTOSPORIDIUM SPP. OF MÉNDEZ-HERMIDA, GÓMEZ-COUSO, ROMERO-SUANCES, AND ARES-MAZÁS, 2007

Original host: *Lutra lutra* (L., 1758), European Otter.

Remarks: Méndez-Hermida et al. (2007) did a fecal survey of 437 European otters from 161 sites in Galicia, Spain, using a direct immuno-fluorescence antibody test (IFAT). They found *Cryptosporidium* oocysts in 17/437 (4%) samples.

SARCOCYSTIS SP. OF WAHLSTRÖM, NIKKILÄ, AND UGGLA, 1999

Definitive host: Unknown.

Intermediate host: *Lutra lutra* (L., 1758), European Otter.

Remarks: Wahlström et al. (1999) found sarcocysts in the skeletal muscle of one *L. lutra* raised in Norway but had died in captivity in Sweden. The sarcocysts were 0.3–2.3 mm long and 0.05–0.25 mm wide. Under LM, sarcocyst walls were thin, <3 μm, and had a serrated surface, but did not have visible projections. By TEM, the sarcocyst wall was 0.6–1.8 thick and had minute undulations covering its entire surface, giving the wall a wavy appearance. Septa were indistinct and the sarcocysts had few metrocytes, but many bradyzoites. These sarcocysts were found in only 1/70 (1%) otters subjected to necropsy in Sweden.

SUBFAMILY MUSTELINAE FISCHER, 1817

GENUS MARTES PINEL, 1792 (8 SPECIES)

COCCIDIA SP. OF MATSCHOULSKY, 1947a,b

Original host: *Martes zibellina* (L., 1758), Sable.

Remarks: Matschoulsky (1947a,b) reported three species of coccidia in 32/144 (22%) sables, "two already known and one is new." In one sable he found oocysts that were round/ovoidal and surrounded by a 2-layered wall, ~1 thick, without a M. Ovoidal oocysts were L×W: 13.1×11.3 (12–14×10–12), L/W ratio, 1.2. Although he

could not get oocysts of this "species" to sporulate, he said the defining feature of this species is its small size, which "differs drastically from coccidia that were found in sables before. That is why we name this species as new." Fortunately, he did not give it a name, and because he never saw sporulated oocysts, it cannot be placed into a genus.

CRYPTOSPORIDIUM SP. OF RADEMACHER, JAKOB, AND BOCKHARDT, 1999

Original host: *Martes foina* (Erxleben, 1777), Beech Marten.

Remarks: Rademacher et al. (1999) reported temporary episodes of diarrhea in four captive beech martens that were not related to each other, and they found numerous oocysts of a *Cryptosporidium* sp. in the feces of all of them. The oocysts measured, L×W (n=30): 3.6×3.1 (3–4×3–4); L/W ratio: 1.2, but no other information was given.

EIMERIA SP. OF YAKIMOFF AND GOUSSEFF, 1934

Original host: *Martes martes* (L., 1758), European Pine Marten.

Remarks: Yakimoff and Gousseff (1934) described oocysts from the marten as L×W (n=101): 21.6×18.0 (20–31×16–20), L/W ratio: 1.2; M, OR, PG: all absent with elongate-ovoidal sporocysts (line drawing), 7.2 wide, SB, SSB, PSB: all absent, and SR: present (line drawing). Yakimoff and Gousseff (1934) described oocysts from the feces of one marten and one sable from the same zoo, and oocysts from the sable were L×W (n=50): 21.6×18.0 (18–25×16–20), L/W ratio: 1.2. They concluded, "The coccidia from this sable with those previously described as *E. sibirica* reveals no differences." Their (unstated) implication was that the oocysts from both the marten and the sable represented the same *Eimeria* species.

No attempt was made to identify the species beyond genus; thus, a *species inquirenda*.

HEPATOZOON SP. OF YANAI, TOMITA, MASEGI, ISHIKAWA, IWASAKI, YAMAZOE, AND UEDA, 1995

Original host: *Martes melampus* (Wagner, 1840), Japanese Marten.

Remarks: Yanai et al. (1995) studied Japanese martens in Gifu prefecture, Japan and found nodular lesions containing meronts and merozoite-gametocytes of a *Hepatozoon* species in 67/70 (96%) wild martens. The heart was the most commonly parasitized organ (67/70, 96%) followed by perirenal adipose tissue (25/70, 36%), diaphragm (9/58, 16%), mesentery (10/68, 14%), tongue (1/7, 14%), omentum (8/57, 14%), and perisplenic adipose tissues (7/70, 10%). Two types of nodular lesions were seen, each based on different developmental stages: nodules containing meronts, and nodules that consisted of an accumulation of phagocytes containing merozoites or gamonts. Nodules containing meronts were 50–400 wide. Yanai et al. (1995) studied mature meronts and membrane-bound merozoites with LM and TEM but chose not to name the parasite.

SARCOCYSTIS SP. OF DUBEY, 1982b

Definitive host: *Martes pennanti* (Erxleben, 1777), Fisher.

Intermediate host: Unknown.

Remarks: Dubey (1982b) surveyed feces for coccidians from a variety of wild carnivores in Montana, USA and reported sporocysts of *Sarcocystis* in the feces of 1/6 (17%) fishers. Sporocysts from this host varied from 12.5–13.0 × 8.5–9.0 (n = 3).

SARCOCYSTIS SP. OF GERHOLD, HOWERTH, AND LINDSAY, 2005

Definitive host: Unknown.

Intermediate host: *Martes pennanti* (Erxleben, 1777), Fisher.

Remarks: Gerhold et al. (2005 described **meningoencephalitis** due to *S. neurona* in a fisher from Maryland, USA; they also found intramuscular sarcocysts "of a possibly unrecognized *Sarcocystis* species." Although the structure and ultrastructure of the muscle sarcocysts from the fisher were similar to those of *S. neurona*, they were unable to amplify *S. neurona* DNA from these muscle forms; they said this may be related to technical difficulties, or this organism may be an unrecognized species that has sarcocysts morphologically similar to those of *S. neurona*.

SARCOCYSTIS SPP. OF KUBO, OKANO, ITO, TSUBOTA, SAKAI, AND YANAI, 2009

Definitive host: Unknown.

Intermediate host: *Martes melampus melampus* Gray, 1865, Japanese Marten.

Remarks: Kubo et al. (2009) examined 65 wild carnivores on Honshu, Japan for sarcocysts and found three Japanese red martens had sarcocysts in their muscles, and no inflammatory host response was associated with the sarcocysts. Ultrastructurally, the sarcocyst wall was thin and showed minute undulations. Kubo et al. (2009) said these sarcocysts were similar to sarcocysts they found in the Japanese raccoon dog (*N. procyonoides viverrinus*) and the Japanese red fox (*V. v. japonica*) during the same survey. This was the first published report of muscular sarcocystosis in Japanese carnivores. There was no attempt to identify the species; thus, a *species inquirenda*.

SARCOCYSTIS SPP. OF LARKIN, GABRIEL, GERHOLD, YABSLEY, WESTER, HUMPHREYS, BECKSTEAD, AND DUBEY, 2011

Definitive host: Unknown.

Intermediate host: *Martes pennanti* (Erxleben, 1777), Fisher.

Remarks: Larkin et al. (2011) examined road- or trapper-killed fishers in Pennsylvania, USA for *Sarcocystis* spp. and *Toxoplasma gondii*. DNA samples were extracted from thoracic and pelvic limb skeletal muscles using 18S rRNA PCR primers and analysis showed 38/46 (83%) fishers were positive for *Sarcocystis* species, but no specific identification was given.

GENUS *MELES* BRISSON, 1762 (3 SPECIES)

COCCIDIA SP. OF KAMIYA AND SUZUKI, 1975

Original host: *Meles anakuma* Temminck, 1844, Japanese Badger.

Remarks: Kamiya and Suzuki (1975) examined the preserved intestine of one badger, mostly for trematodes, but when they looked at tissue sections of the jejunum mucosa they saw endogenous stages of a coccidium represented by macro- and microgametocytes and oocysts. Microgametocytes with many microgametes were ~20 wide, macrogametocytes with many basophilic granules were $15-22 \times 13-20$, and unsporulated oocysts were $20-21 \times 14-17$.

Although they concluded these stages represented an *Eimeria* species there is no way to know that from the few tissue stages measured and unsporulated oocysts.

ISOSPORA-LIKE OF STUART, GOLDEN, ZINTL, DE WAAL, MULCAHY, MCCARTHY, AND LAWTON, 2013

Original host: *Meles meles* (L., 1758), European Badger.

Remarks: Stuart et al. (2013) surveyed fecal samples of *M. meles* and found "*Isospora*-like oocysts" in 8/50 (16%) samples, but no additional information was provided.

SARCOCYSTIS SP. OF KUBO, OKANO, ITO, TSUBOTA, SAKAI, AND YANAI, 2009

Definitive host: Unknown.

Intermediate host: *Meles anakuma* Temminck, 1844, Japanese Badger.

Remarks: Kubo et al. (2009) examined 65 free-living carnivores on Honshu, Japan for muscular *Sarcocystis* and two Japanese badgers had sarcocysts in their muscles, but no inflammatory host response was associated with them. Ultrastructurally, the sarcocyst wall was thick with numerous finger-like protrusions that contained microtubules. Kubo et al. (2009) said these sarcocysts were **not** similar to sarcocysts they found in the Japanese raccoon dog (*N. p. viverrinus*), the Japanese red fox (*V. v. japonica*), and the Japanese marten (*M. m. melampus*) during the same survey. This was the first published report of muscular sarcocystosis in Japanese carnivores, but there was no attempt to identify it to species, so this form must remain a *species inquirenda*.

SARCOCYSTIS SP. OF ODENING, STOLTE, WALTER, BOCKHART, AND JAKOB, 1994a

Definitive host: Unknown.
Intermediate host: *Meles meles* (L., 1758), European Badger.
Remarks: Odening et al. (1994a) found a dead female *M. meles* on the road, ~50 km northeast of Berlin, Germany. Macroscopic sarcocysts were found in the tongue and, after fixation and sectioning, they were examined through TEM. Sarcocysts were up to 1.4 mm long, with a maximum width of 185 μm, and had compartments of various sizes, with bradyzoites that measured L × W (n = 30): 12.3 × 3.1 (11–13 × 2.8–3.5). Odening et al. (1994a) said, "No sarcocysts from mustelids have been described by electron microscopy so far," but they obviously missed the paper by Cawthorn et al. (1983), who used TEM to look at sarcocysts in experimentally-infected Richardson's ground squirrels after they had fed on *Sarcocystis* sporocysts recovered from the American badger, *Taxidea taxus* (Schreber, 1777). Odening et al. (1994a) compared their form to similar sarcocysts studied from roe deer by Entzeroth (1982a,b), and Sugár et al. (1990), and said, "the similarity of the…forms from roe deer with each other and with the form from the European badger is so great, that we can regard all these forms as most likely being identical." Without more substantive data, this form must remain a *species inquirenda*.

SARCOCYSTIS SP. OF ODENING, STOLTE, WALTER, AND BOCKHART, 1994b

Synonym: cf. *Sarcocystis sebeki* of Tadros and Laarman, 1976.
Definitive host: Unknown.
Intermediate host: *Meles meles* (L., 1758), European Badger.

Remarks: Odening et al. (1994b) found four dead *M. meles* (Nos. 3, 2, 6, 9; 1 male and 3 females, respectively) on various roads, 45–75 km from Berlin, Germany. Sarcocysts were found in the tongue, thigh, loin, and thorax and, after fixation and sectioning, they were examined via LM and TEM. Sarcocysts were 6.5–9.0 mm long, and 172–200 μm wide in the fresh state, and their bradyzoites were squat and fusiform, 6.9 × 1.9 (6.1–7.2 × 1.6–2.2). In semi-thin sections bradyzoites were 5.9 × 2.0 (5.7–6.3 × 1.7–2.2). TEM showed a cyst wall 0.9–1.4 thick with no protrusions. Small elevations of the primary cyst wall were 0.08–0.09 long, the fossule-like invaginations in-between had a maximum diameter of 0.05. These small elevations and invaginations were underlayed with an osmiophilic layer. The authors (1994b) "assigned" this form to be near *S. sebeki* (cf. Tadros and Laarman, 1976, 1978, 1979, 1980a,b, 1982) "because it is morphologically very similar" to it.

GENUS *MELLIVORA* STORR, 1780 (MONOTYPIC)

SARCOCYSTIS SP. OF VILJOEN, 1921

Definitive host: Unknown.
Intermediate host: *Millivora capensis* (Schreber, 1776), Honey Badger.
Remarks: According to Levine and Ivens (1981), Viljoen (1921) found sarcocysts in the striated muscles of a honey badger, but they did not see his actual paper and got the citation from Nietz (1965). Levine (1986) did not list this species, and Dubey et al. (2015a) list neither the Viljoen nor Nietz references and make no mention of a *Sarcocystis* species in the honey badger. Viljoen (1921) does not retrieve in Google Scholar and we were unable to obtain a copy of the Nietz paper.

GENUS *MELOGALE* I. GEOFFROY SAINT-HILAIRE, 1831 (4 SPECIES)

SARCOCYSTIS SP. OF CHIOU, YEH, JENG, CHANG, CHANG, WU, CHAN, AND PANG, 2015

Definitive host: Unknown.

Intermediate host: *Melogale moschata subaurantiaca* (Swinhoe, 1862), Taiwan Ferret Badger.

Remarks: Chiou et al. (2015) examined Taiwan ferret badgers in Taiwan and found 1/31 (3%) had *Sarcocystis* sarcocysts. No other information was presented; thus, a *species inquirenda*.

GENUS *MUSTELA* L., 1758 (17 SPECIES)

COCCIDIA SP. OF BLANKENSHIP-PARIS, CHANG, AND BAGNELL, 1993

Original host: *Mustela* (syn. *Putorius*) *putorius furo* (L., 1758), Domestic Ferret.

Remarks: Blankenship-Paris et al. (1993) examined a 4-month-old ferret that was ill, dehydrated, and had pasty, dark feces. The ferret was housed with another sibling and its dam, but neither showed similar signs, and repeated fecal exams of both were negative for coccidial oocysts. Also, fecal exams of other members of the colony and necropsy of eight other ferrets in the colony did not demonstrate any coccidia. However, when the 4-month-old ferret was necropsied, Blankenship-Paris et al. (1993) reported that "enteric coccidiosis" was the cause of its illness, based on histological findings of some endogenous stages. No other identification was made.

COCCIDIA SP. OF BRONSON, BUSH, VINER, MURRAY, WISELY, AND DEEM, 2007

Original host: *Mustela* (syn. *Putorius*) *putorius furo* (L., 1758), Domestic Ferret.

Remarks: Bronson et al. (2007) examined mortality, retrospectively, based on the pathology records of 107 captive animals held at the Smithsonian's National Zoological Park, Washington, D.C., USA from 1989 to 2004. They said that "the most common cause of death among juvenile ferrets was gastrointestinal disease, found in 11/21 (52%)," with seven of those cases caused by coccidiosis. No identity of the coccidian nor other information was given.

COCCIDIA SP. OF DAVIS, CHOW, AND GORHAM, 1953

Original host: *Neovison vison* (Schreber, 1777) (syn. *Mustela vison* L., 1766), American Mink.

Remarks: Davis et al. (1953) were among the first to notice liver coccidiosis in a mink, and they described characteristic pathological and anatomical changes caused by this parasite, but because they examined only visceral organs, they did not identify the coccidian.

COCCIDIA SP. 1 OF JOLLEY, KINGSTON, WILLIAMS, AND LYNN, 1994

Original host: *Mustela nigripes* (Audubon and Bachman, 1851), Black-footed Ferret.

Remarks: Jolley et al. (1994) reported seeing meronts and oocysts of a small coccidian in the cells lining the trachea, a bronchus, and in associated bronchial glands in one black-footed ferret, which also had canine distemper. Because no sporulated oocysts could be found they could not name or characterize it further. No lesions in tracheal tissue could be attributed to the presence of this parasite.

COCCIDIA SP. 2 OF JOLLEY, KINGSTON, WILLIAMS, AND LYNN, 1994

Original host: *Mustela nigripes* (Audubon and Bachman, 1851), Black-footed Ferret.

Remarks: Jolley et al. (1994) reported seeing merozoites of another unidentified coccidian in an impression smear of the epithelium of the urinary bladder of the same ferret in which they saw the respiratory coccidian stages (above). No lesions in bladder tissue could be attributed to the presence of this parasite, but they cautioned that this form would need differentiation from *Toxoplasma*, *Neospora*, and *Hepatozoan* species, which it resembles in size, ability to invade a variety of tissue types, and merogonic development.

COCCIDIA SP. OF LI, PANG, AND FOX, 1996

Original host: *Mustela* (syn. *Putorius*) *putorius furo* (L., 1758), Domestic Ferret.

Remarks: Li et al., 1996 described proliferative bowel disease in 4/19 (21%) ferrets they found to be coinfected with a *Desulfovibrio* sp. (gram negative, comma- to spiral-shaped bacteria, often associated with proliferative bowel disease) and coccidia. Thick, rigid colons, and enlarged mesenteric lymph nodes were palpable in all four, which had a history of lethargy, anorexia, weight loss, and diarrhea. These ferrets were dehydrated and emaciated, and one had occult blood in its feces whereas another had a prolapsed rectum. Tissue sections showed proliferative changes that included a marked increase in mucosal thickness, and glandular or crypt length and irregularity with pseudovillus

formation. Epithelial cells were markedly hyperplastic, hyperchromatic, and piled on each other with numerous mitotic figures. Inflammatory cells consisted predominantly of neutrophils (two ferrets) or lymphocytes and macrophages (two ferrets), and some eosinophils in all four. They described the coccidial organisms to consist predominantly of meronts and merozoite stages. Many coccidial stages were seen within the apical cytoplasm of hyperplastic epithelial cells, but feces were not examined and no attempt was made to identify the organism other than to call them coccidia. They mentioned that the mechanism by which *Desulfovibrio* sp. and its relatives induce proliferative bowel disease is unknown, but "the presence of a second organism may in some instances be required for ICOs to cause intestinal lesions."

CRYPTOSPORIDIUM SP. OF GÓMEZ-VILLAMANDOS, CARRASCO, MOZOS, AND HERVÁS, 1995

Original host: *Mustela* (syn. *Putorius*) *putorius furo* L., 1758, Domestic Ferret.

Remarks: Gómez-Villamandos et al. (1995) reported that four of five ferrets shipped to their department in Córdoba, Spain became ill several days after arrival showing anorexia, depression, and yellow diarrhea; they died 48–72 hours after onset of the illness began. The ferrets were nonpregnant females weighing 500–550 g and originated on a goat farm. Tissue samples were fixed and prepared for LM and TEM. Microscopic examinations of the intestinal tract of all ferrets showed numerous spheroidal to ovoidal bodies, in various stages of development, attached to the brush border of enterocytes and cryptal epithelial cells of the distal large intestine. Villous atrophy was severe and a cellular infiltrate composed of neutrophils, eosinophils, and macrophages was seen in the submucosa, whereas desquamated epithelial cells with parasitic stages were seen in the intestinal lumen. All stages of the life cycle were observed including trophozoites, two types of meronts with their merozoites, macro- and microgametes, and unsporulated and sporulated oocysts. No attempt was made to name the parasite.

CRYPTOSPORIDIUM SPP. OF REHG, GIGLIOTTI, AND STOKES, 1988

Original host: *Mustela* (syn. *Putorius*) *putorius furo* L., 1758, Domestic Ferret.

Remarks: Rehg et al. (1988) identified the first case of *Cryptosporidium* in ferrets. Two unrelated young ferrets, 4- and 8-months-old, died from unknown causes on the same day. They made stained fecal smears, and then took sections of both gastrointestinal (GI) tracts and stained paraffin-embedded sections with hematoxylin-eosin for the histopathology; they also fixed, cut, and stained the GI with uranyl acetate and lead citrate for TEM. Fecal smears showed *Cryptosporidium* oocysts that were ~3–5. Histological sections demonstrated cryptosporidial stages, 2–5 wide, associated with the brush border of the epithelial cells at the tips and lateral margins, but not in the crypts, only in the small intestine (predominantly ileum); no such stages were seen in the gall bladder, trachea, or lungs. Trophozoites, meronts, macrogametes, and oocysts were detected by TEM in the small intestine. Subsequently, examination of fresh fecal samples of the ferret population at the research facility, and of the new arrivals, revealed the presence of *Cryptosporidium* as a subclinical disease in a high percentage of ferrets. The infection persisted for several weeks both in immunocompetent and immunocompromised (treated with dexamethasone) animals. Fecal smears showed *Cryptosporidium* oocysts in 9/22 (41%) ferrets at the facility, and in 31/44 (70%) new arrivals. Neither species nor genotypes of

the isolates were identified because only LM, TEM, and histopathological methods were used.

CRYPTOSPORIDIUM SP. OF SKÍRNISSON AND PÁLMADÓTTIR, 1993

Original host: *Neovison* (syn. *Mustela*) *vison* (Schreber, 1777), American Mink.

Remarks: Very small oocysts, 4–5 long, identified as *Cryptosporidium* sp. were found in the feces of 11/40 (27.5%) mink pups on 5/13 (38%) fur farms in Iceland, but no further account of this species was ever published (SkírNisson and Pálmadóttir, 1993).

CRYPTOSPORIDIUM SP. OF ZIEGLER, WADE, SCHAAF, STERN, NADARESKI, AND MOHAMMED, 2007

Original host: *Mustela erminea* L., 1758, Ermine.

Remarks: Ziegler et al. (2007) collected fecal samples of three wild *M. erminea* and one *Mustela frenata* Lichtenstein, 1831, in the New York City Watershed, southeastern New York state, USA. Their samples were examined both by LM, and by polyclonal *Cryptosporidium* antigen-capture ELISA (considered positive based on an optical density ≥ 0.050). They found *Cryptosporidium* in 1/3 (33%) *M. erminea*, but not in the sample of *M. frenata*, the long-tailed weasel.

EIMERIA BASKANICA OF NUKERBAEVA AND SVANBAEV, 1972 OR 1973 (?)

Original host: *Mustela erminea* L., 1758, Ermine or Stoat.

Remarks: The paper of Nukerbaeva and Svanbaev (1972) is unavailable to us or it may not even exist. In their survey of fur animals in Kazakhstan, Nukerbaeva and Svanbaev (1977) said they found 1/7 (14%) stoats infected with *E. baskanica* Nukerbaeva and Svanbaev, 1972; however, Global Names Index (gni.globalnames.org/) listed the authority as Nukerbaeva and Svanbaev, 1973. In their 1977 paper they briefly mentioned the oocysts of this form to be ovoidal with tapered poles, dimensions of 11.2–12.6 × 8.4–9.8, lacking both M and PG, but having an OR; the sporocysts were described only as ovoidal, with two bean-shaped SZ and an SR, but no mention was made about presence/absence of a SB.

EIMERIA MEPHITIDIS OF YAKIMOFF AND GOUSSEFF, 1936

Original host: *Mustela* (syn. *Putorius*) *putorius furo* (L., 1758), Domestic Ferret.

Remarks: Yakimoff and Gousseff (1936) reported finding oocysts in two polecats taken from the Polotsk District, in the Republic of Belarus on the Dvina River. They found only small numbers of perfectly round oocysts with a smooth, double-layered wall, that measured 21.6–23.4 wide; these oocysts lacked M, OR, and PG. The elongate-ovoidal sporocysts were 12.6 × 5.2, and apparently lacked SB, SSB, PSB. They said the oocysts they observed were somewhat similar to those of *E. furonis*, which they are not (21.6–23.4 vs.12.8 × 12.0). Ultimately, they identified their oocysts as *E. mephitidis*, a species described from the striped skunk (*M. mephitis*) from Ohio, USA, by Andrews (1928); the oocysts are similar in size, but those of *E. mephitidis* have a circular M, which was not seen in those described by Yakimoff and Gousseff (1936). The line drawing provided by Yakimoff and Gousseff (1936) is strikingly similar to the line drawing of *E. hiepei*, which was described from the European mink by Gräfner et al. (1967), but *E. hiepei* has smaller oocysts (13.5–16.6 wide).

EIMERIA SP. OF JOLLEY, KINGSTON, WILLIAMS, AND LYNN, 1994

Original host: *Mustela nigripes* (Audubon and Bachman, 1851), Black-footed Ferret.

Remarks: Jolley et al. (1994) reported finding oocysts representing three *Eimeria* species in 6/6 (100%) *M. nigripes* in Wyoming, USA. Two of the species were identified as *E. furonis* and *E. ictidea*. The third form, which they said was seen only rarely, had oocysts that were larger than those of the first two, but they made no attempt to identify or characterize it in any way other than to say it was oval and five oocysts they measured were L × W: 37.0 × 22.3 (35–39 × 21–23), L/W: 1.7. Confirming that this was likely an eimerian they said, "sporulated oocysts of the large oval form were rarely seen," and "attempts to sporulate this species were variably successful under the conditions described, often with little or no development seen after a 10-day incubation period in the potassium dichromate solution. Oocysts taken from the intestinal lumen failed to sporulate, whereas some of those passed in the feces successfully did so." They also pointed out that neither Levine and Ivens (1981), from mustelids and other carnivores, nor Levine and Ivens (1990) and Thomas and Stanton (1994) from prairie dogs, rock squirrels, or ground squirrels had reported *Eimerian* oocysts with these measurements.

EIMERIA SP. OF MUSAEV AND VEISOV, 1983

Original host: *Mustela nivalis* L., 1766, Least Weasel.

Remarks: Musaev and Veisov (1983) found oocysts of an *Eimeria* sp. in 1/43 (2%) weasels they examined; they thought these oocysts were slightly different from those of *E. mustelae*, but they declined to name their form even though they provided a line drawing. The oocyst wall was smooth, colorless, 1.5–2.0 thick. Sporulated oocysts were L×W (n=49): 20.3×14.8 (17–22×12–17), L/W ratio 1.4 (1.2–1.6); M, OR, PG: all absent. Sporocysts were described as ovoidal to pear-shaped although this is not evident in their line drawing. Sporocysts were L×W: 8.5×6.5 (6–10×4–8); SB, SSB, PSB: all absent (line drawing); SR: present, as a group of fine granules. Sporozoites measured were 5–9×3–7 and each had a RB at their broader end. Sporulation time was 48–72 hours in 2.5% potassium dichromate ($K_2Cr_2O_7$) solution at 25–30°C. They said the oocysts measured were obtained from the contents of the large intestine and the host was collected in the Batabag Shahbusk region of the Nakhitschevansk, Azerbaijan.

ISOSPORA OHIOENSIS OF PATTERSON AND FOX, 2007

Original host: *Mustela* (syn. *Putorius*) *putorius furo* (L., 1758), Domestic Ferret.

Remarks: Patterson and Fox (2007) reported oocysts they identified as *I. ohioensis* in fecal samples of healthy domestic ferret kits in a large ferret breeding operation on the same premise as juvenile domestic dogs; they neglected to mention how they arrived at this identification. It is likely their identification was either a spurious finding of a dog oocyst passing through the gut of the ferrets or is a new/different species morphologically indistinguishable from the oocysts of *I.* (=C.) *ohioensis*.

ISOSPORA SP. OF BELL, 1994

Original host: *Mustela* (syn. *Putorius*) *putorius furo* (L., 1758), Domestic Ferret.

Remarks: Bell (1994) reported that *Isospora* sp. oocysts are commonly shed by ferrets 6–16 weeks of age and is the same species that commonly affects puppies and kittens, but the "species" was not identified.

ISOSPORA SP. OF PANTCHEV, GASSMANN, AND GLOBOKAR-VRHOVEC, 2011

Original host: *Mustela* (syn. *Putorius*) *putorius furo* (L., 1758), Domestic Ferret.

Remarks: Pantchev et al. (2011) reported the results of fecal samples from domestic ferrets they examined between 2002 and 2004 and identified the species found, based on the structure of their sporulated oocysts as *E. furonis*, *E. ictidea*, *I.* (=C.) *laidlawi*, and an unidentified *Isospora* species. No other information was given about this unidentified isosporan.

SARCOCYSTIS SP. OF TADROS AND LAARMAN, 1979

Definitive host: Unknown.

Intermediate host: *Mustela nivalis* L., 1766, Least Weasel.

Remarks: Tadros and Laarman (1979) reported muscular sarcosporidiosis for the first time from the common European weasel in the Netherlands. They examined the morphology of sarcocysts both in fresh and stained histological preparations. The sarcocysts were several mm long by 0.15 mm wide and had a smooth wall without cytophaneres; the cysts were compartmentalized and had metrocytes 3.5 wide and bradyzoites about 9×2.5. Levine and Ivens (1981) speculated that these were very similar to the sarcocysts of *S. sebeki* found in *Apodemus sylvaticus* (L., 1758). In addition to its muscle sarcocysts, the weasel also had sporocysts of *S. putorii* in its feces. They attempted to complete the sexual cycle by feeding muscle sarcocysts to the tawny owl, *Strix aluco* L., 1758 and obtained a few oocysts for a short time from its feces. However, they believed that this was an abnormal host and that another genus of strigid bird might be a better definitive host. They never attempted to name the species of the weasel sarcocysts.

GENUS NEOVISON BARYSHNIKOV AND ABRAMOV, 1997 (2 SPECIES)

CRYPTOSPORIDIUM SP. OF ZIEGLER, WADE, SCHAAF, STERN, NADARESKI, AND MOHAMMED, 2007

Original host: *Neovison* (syn. *Mustela*) *vison* (Schreiber, 1777), American Mink.

Remarks: Ziegler et al. (2007) collected feces from wild *N. vison*, trapped in the New York City Watershed, southeastern New York state, USA. Samples were examined by flotation/centrifugation with sugar and/or zinc sulfate solution followed by LM and by polyclonal *Cryptosporidium* antigen-capture ELISA (considered positive based on an optical density ≥0.050). They reported finding *Cryptosporidium* in 10/58 (17%) samples.

EIMERIA SP. OF FOREYT AND TODD, 1976

Original host: *Neovison* (syn. *Mustela*) *vison* (Schreiber, 1777), American Mink.

Remarks: Foreyt and Todd (1976) collected fecal samples on 29 mink ranches (22 counties) in Wisconsin, USA, from June–December, 1975. They found that 45/79 (57%) mink feces collected from ranches that fed dry pelleted rations contained coccidian oocysts, whereas 128/244 (52%) samples from ranches that fed a wet meat mixture contained oocysts. They mentioned finding oocysts resembling an undescribed *Eimeria* species in mink on 19/29 (66%) of the ranches, but the number of mink with this species was not mentioned, stating only "the coccidia of domestic mink in Wisconsin are prevalent and widespread." They said the oocysts were 12.5 × 11.8 but gave no additional descriptive information. To our knowledge, this species has never been mentioned again in the literature.

HAMMONDIA SP. OF RYAN, WYAND, AND NIELSEN, 1982

Original host: *Neovison* (syn. *Mustela*) *vison* (Schreiber, 1777), American Mink.

Remarks: Ryan et al. (1982) studied skinned muskrat (*Ondatra zibethica*) carcasses from Connecticut and New Jersey, USA and found coccidia-like zoites in their muscles using a pepsin digestion technique. They then fed seven pairs of coccidia-free mink half of an infected muskrat carcass each. Four pairs of mink fed muskrats shed unsporulated coccidian oocysts in their feces 6–8 DPI and patency lasted 4–6 days. Sporulated oocysts were L × W (n = 80): 11.6 × 10.7 (11.5–12 × 10–11), L/W ratio: 1.1. They reported that the oocysts had a M, but we did not see one in a photomicrograph presented (their Fig. 4), and the oocysts lacked a PG and OR. Sporocysts were L × W (n = 160): 8.8 × 6.5 (8–9 × 6–7), L/W ratio: 1.4 and had a granular SR, but lacked SB and SSB. They also fed another seven pairs of coccidia-free mink ~200,000 sporulated oocysts each that were derived from the previous four pairs that shed the oocysts, but none of the second seven pairs shed oocysts during the course of the experiment. After 30 DPI, all 14 pairs of mink (those fed tissue cysts and those fed only oocysts) were killed and sections of gastrointestinal tract, pancreas, ileocecal lymph node, liver, kidney, lung, heart, brain, diaphragm, tongue, esophagus, and masseter muscles were examined for coccidian cysts and skeletal muscles were examined via pepsin digestion. All were negative. The authors concluded that their work was insufficient to establish whether this *Hammondia*-like parasite was identical to an already known species or was a new species. This interesting study certainly deserves more attention, especially now that we have molecular tools with which to work.

HEPATOZOON SP. OF PRESIDENTE AND KARSTAD, 1975

Original host: *Neovison* (syn. *Mustela*) *vison* (Schreiber, 1777), American Mink.

Remarks: Presidente and Karstad (1975) found meronts of a *Hepatozoon* in the lungs of 10/18 (56%) American minks they examined in southwestern Ontario, Canada. Meronts were found in the pulmonary parenchyma, and focal aggregations of lymphocytes, macrophages, plasma cells, and eosinophils were associated with small groups of meronts. Two kinds of meronts were seen: subspheroidal forms, 22–29 × 19–24, with a single row of 18–24 macromerozoites around the perimeter; and larger, oblong to spheroidal meronts, 29–38 × 19–24, with 34–38 micromerozoites located throughout the meront. They made no attempt to further identify or name the parasite.

ISOSPORA BIGEMINA OF SEALANDER, 1943

Original host: *Neovison* (syn. *Mustela*) *vison* (Schreiber, 1777), American Mink.

Remarks: Sealander (1943) examined 158 mink carcasses that he obtained from southern Michigan fur-buyers in the winters of 1940 and 1941. He was looking specifically to catalog helminth parasites, but briefly mentioned that "coccidia, *Isospora bigemina*, were frequently noted in fecal samples." In all likelihood, he was seeing sporocysts of an unknown *Sarcocystis* species.

SARCOCYSTIS SP. OF RAMOS-VERA, DUBEY, WATSON, WINN-ELLIOT, PATTERSON, AND YAMINI, 1997

Definitive host: Unknown.

Intermediate host: *Neovison* (syn. *Mustela*) *vison* (Schreiber, 1777), American Mink.

Remarks: Ramos-Vera et al. (1997) had three 2–3-month-old minks with signs of progressive neurological disease. One mink had variable numbers of sarcocysts, which measured up to 300 × 20, in multiple skeletal muscles. The sarcocyst wall had numerous elongated villar protrusions that measured 1.7 μm × 250 nm. These protrusions had microtubules and irregularly distanced minute undulations. The most important lesions were seen in the brains of all three minks. The authors said this was the first time *Sarcocystis* sarcocysts were described in mink muscles. The parasite was not identified to species and is considered a *species inquirenda*.

FAMILY OTARIIDAE GRAY, 1825

GENUS *CALLORHINUS* J.E. GRAY, 1859 (MONOTYPIC)

SARCOCYSTIS SP. OF BROWN, SMITH, AND KEYES, 1974

Definitive host: Unknown.

Intermediate host: *Callorhinus ursinus* (L., 1758), Northern Fur Seal.

Remarks: Brown et al. (1974) found sarcocysts in the masseter muscle of one adolescent northern fur seal among a group of 30 pups and two adults on St. Paul Island, Pribiloff Islands, Alaska, USA. Although this was the first report of an apparent *Sarcocystis* species in marine mammals, the life cycle of this species is still unknown. No other information was provided. This species has not been identified since 1974 and must remain a *species inquirenda*.

GENUS *OTARIA* PÉRON, 1816 (MONOTYPIC)

CRYPTOSPORIDIUM SPP. OF HERMOSILLA, SILVA, NAVARRO, AND TAUBERT, 2016

Original host: *Otaria flavescens* (Shaw, 1800), South American Sea Lion.

Remarks: Hermosilla et al. (2016) examined 40 fecal samples of South American sea lions, *O. flavescens*, along the shores of the river Calle-Calle and in the local fish market in Valdivia, Chile, for the presence of *Cryptosporidium*. All feces were screened by LM of stained fecal smears and also by ELISA. They determined that 4/40 (10%) samples were infected with *Cryptosporidium* species, but the authors did not identify the organism to species. This was the first report of *Cryptosporidium* in *O. flavescens*, but without more information it must remain a *species inquirenda*.

GENUS *ZALOPHUS* GILL, 1866 (3 SPECIES)

COCCIDIAN PARASITES "A," "B," "C" OF COLEGROVE, GRIGG, CARLSON-BREMER, MILLER, GULLAND, FERGUSON, REJMANEK, BARR, NORDHAUSEN, MELLI, AND CONRAD, 2011

Original host: *Zalophus californianus* (Lesson, 1828), California Sea Lion.

Remarks: Colegrove et al. (2011) discovered coccidian endogenous stages in the small intestine of five free-ranging California sea lions during routine postmortem examinations. In each case, multiple stages of both asexual (meronts, merozoites) and sexual (micro- and macrogamonts) stages were seen in the apical cytoplasm of distal jejunal enterocytes. Using standard histological techniques, IHC, TEM, DNA extraction, and PCR amplification of ITS-1 and 18S rRNA genes they were able to conclude that they identified previously undescribed intestinal protozoan species representing three previously uncharacterized gene sequences representing three new coccidian species that are most closely related to, but not identical with *Neospora caninum*.

COCCIDIA A, B, C, CSL AÑO 11 OF GIRARD, JOHNSON, FRITZ, SHAPIRO, PACKHAM, MELLI, CARLSON-BREMER, GULLAND, REJMANEK, AND CONRAD, 2016

Original host: *Zalophus californianus* (Lesson, 1828), California Sea Lion.

Remarks: Girard et al. (2016) found 16/139 (11.5%) sea lions, stranded in California, USA in 2010 and 2012, shedding oocysts in their feces. In 2011–12, they collected more fecal samples at sea lion haul-out sites at three locations in central California and 13/212 (6%) had oocysts present. Amplified ITS-1 from the samples strongly supported the presence of Coccidia A and B of Colegrove et al. (2011). One sample produced a novel sequence that had 97%–98% pairwise similarity to previously published coccidian DNA isolates in Guadalupe fur seal tissues (Gibson et al., 2011). Coccidia A and B were sporulated and inoculated into mice to investigate infectivity and pathogenicity, but no remarkable clinical signs or histologic changes were observed except ~40% of the mice had slight nephritis, pneumonia, and inflammation in lung, spleen, and lymph nodes. Brain, heart, and tongue all tested negative using pan-coccidian primers that included the ITS-1 region. Results of phylogenetic analyses using ITS-1 indicated the Coccidia A, B, C, CSL Año 11, and isolates from harbor seals and Guadalupe fur seals all shared a common ancestor with *N. caninum*. Girard et al. (2016) concluded that additional genetic and morphologic studies are required to resolve the taxonomy of these novel marine mammal coccidia, and they believe it is likely these organisms are either a new *Neospora* species or a new genus in the Sarcocystidae.

Girard et al. (2016) also inoculated excysted SZ of Coccidia A and B into tissue flasks of Green Monkey–derived MA104 cells. At 14, 21, and 35 DPI, 3/4 (75%) cultures had intra- and extracellular propagating organisms morphologically similar to *Sarcocystis* spp. Extracellular zoites were 8–11 × 1–2. As the cultures aged, the number of zoites increased suggesting they were merozoites produced via merogony, and they described active zoites to exhibit movement typical of *S. neurona*. Antigen slides, prepared from zoites, tested positive to *S. neurona* antisera from a horse and a sea lion by IFAT. PCR amplification of zoite DNA confirmed that zoites were similar to *S. neurona*, which allowed Girard et al. (2016) to conclude that in addition to the observed Coccidia A and B, a *S. neurona*-like organism is excreted by sea lions in low concentrations and sea lions are mechanical vectors.

CRYPTOSPORIDIUM SPP. OF ADELL, SMITH, SHAPIRO, MELLI, AND CONRAD, 2014

Original host: *Zalophus californianus* (Lesson, 1828), California Sea Lion.

Remarks: Adell et al. (2014) collected fecal samples from 303 *Z. californianus* at three sites in Central California, USA: White Rock near Cambria, Point Lobos State Reserve near Monterey, and Año Nuevo Island near Pescadero. Using the direct fluorescent antibody (DFA) method they detected *Cryptosporidium* oocysts in 30/303 (10%) samples including, 11/133 (8%) from White Rock, 17/113 (15%) from Point Lobos, and 2/57 (3.5%) from Año Nuevo Island. They were unable to PCR amplify the 18S rRNA and COWP gene sequences of their *Cryptosporidium* isolates, probably because of the small number of oocysts in their samples, and, thus could not confirm their specific identification by genotype analysis.

SARCOCYSTIS SP. OF MENSE, DUBEY, AND HOMER, 1992

Definitive host: Unknown.

Intermediate host: *Zalophus californianus* (Lesson, 1777), California Sea Lion.

Remarks: Mense et al. (1992) did not proof the galley of their manuscript before it went to press, so their published title reads, "Acute hepatic necrosis associated with a Savmcystis-like…," instead of *Sarcocystis*-like. We mention this only to aid those doing a search online, who may have trouble bringing up this title. In addition, the first line of their report says, "A 10-year-old (sic) male California sea lion…" so it is not clear if the affected sea lion from an aquarium in Florida, USA was 1- or 10-years-old. This animal died after 3 days of exhibiting lethargy and anorexia. Tissues were fixed and preserved for both LM and TEM and later stained with anti-*T. gondii*, anti-*N. caninum*, and anti-*S. cruzi* serum; parasite stages in the liver reacted only with the anti-*Sarcocystis* serum. Sections of infected liver demonstrated coagulative and lytic **necrosis** with associated nuclear **pyknosis**, **karyorrhexis**, and hepatocyte loss in areas adjacent to parasite stages. Sarcocysts in **myocytes**, however, were unassociated with inflammation. Parasites in the liver divided by **endopolygeny** and both meronts and merozoites were seen there. Meronts were up to 32 long and contained 6–35 merozoites, each ~5 × 1. Their TEM sections demonstrated the meronts to be located free in the hepatocyte cytoplasm, without a PV, and merozoites contained numerous micronemes, a conoid, but no rhoptries. The parasite they identified as a *Sarcocystis* species, likely was *S. neurona*, but there is no way to state that unequivocally, so their form must be relegated to a *species inquirenda*.

FAMILY PHOCIDAE GRAY, 1821

GENUS CYSTOPHORA NILSSON, 1820 (MONOTYPIC)

CRYPTOSPORIDIUM SP. OF BASS, WALLACE, YUND, AND FORD, 2012

Original host: *Cystophora cristata* (Erxleben, 1777), Hooded Seal.

Remarks: Bass et al. (2012) examined one fecal sample from a hooded seal, *C. cristata*, in the Gulf of Maine, USA, using a nested PCR amplification and subsequent sequencing of the 18S rRNA gene they determined the presence of *Cryptosporidium* sp. and found it most closely related to the genotype *Cryptosporidium* sp. seal 1 and seal 2 described by Santín et al. (2005) from ringed seals.

GENUS *ERIGNATHUS* GILL, 1866 (MONOTYPIC)

SARCOCYSTIS SP. OF BISHOP, 1979

Definitive host: Unknown.

Intermediate host: *Erignathus barbatus* (Erxleben, 1777), Bearded Seal.

Remarks: Bishop (1979) found a small number of sarcocysts in the skeletal muscle of the tongue of a bearded seal that had been killed by polar bears in the Arctic. Obviously, the life cycle of this species is unknown. No other information was provided. This species has not been identified since 1979 and must remain a *species inquirenda*.

GENUS *LEPTONYCHOTES* GILL, 1872 (MONOTYPIC)

CRYPTOSPORIDIUM SP. OF RENGIFO-HERRERA, ORTEGA-MORA, GÓMEZ-BAUTISTA, GARCÍA-PENA, GARCÍA-PÁRRAGA, AND PEDRAZA-DÍAZ, 2013

Original host: *Leptonychotes weddellii* (Lesson, 1826), Weddell Seal.

Remarks: Rengifo-Herrera et al. (2013) examined fecal samples of 14 *L. weddellii* from Deception Island in South Shetland Islands. Using PCR amplification of 18S rRNA, HSP70,

and COWP genes, they found two individuals (14%) positive for a *Cryptosporidium* sp. that represented a novel genotype they called the Weddell seal genotype.

EIMERIA SP. 2 OF DRÓŻDŻ, 1987

Original host: *Leptonychotes weddellii* (Lesson, 1826), Weddell Seal.

Remarks: Dróżdż (1987) reported cherry-orange, ellipsoidal oocysts with a thin, wrinkled, bilayered wall, M: absent, that measured L × W: 25.7 × 18.8 (22–31 × 14–22), L/W ratio: 1.4, in 5/65 (8%) Weddell seals from King George Island, South Shetlands from April, 1981 to January, 1982. No other information was provided, and this species has not been identified since 1987; thus, it must be relegated to a *species inquirenda*.

EIMERIA SP. 3 OF DRÓŻDŻ, 1987

Original host: *Leptonychotes weddellii* (Lesson, 1826), Weddell Seal.

Remarks: Dróżdż (1987) found gray, spheroidal oocysts with a thin, smooth wall without a M, that were 25–33 wide, L/W ratio: 1.0, in 3/65 (5%) Weddell seals from King George Island, South Shetlands from April, 1981 to January, 1982. No other information was provided, and this species has not been identified since 1987; thus, it must be relegated to a *species inquirenda*.

SARCOCYSTIS SP. OF IPPEN AND HENNE, 1989

Definitive host: Unknown.

Intermediate host: *Leptonychotes weddellii* (Lesson, 1826), Weddell Seal.

Remarks: Ippen and Henne (1989) examined chest, back, tongue, esophagus, diaphragm, and heart muscle tissue from a Weddell seal collected in the Antarctic. Large numbers of cysts were observed in the chest, back, tongue, and esophagus. Cross-sections of cysts were 40–70 × 50–110, and cystozoites were 4–5 × 1. Longitudinal slices of cysts were "serpentine" and measured 30–100 × 100–180. No other information was provided, and this species has not been identified since 1989; thus, it must be regarded a *species inquirenda*.

GENUS *LOBODON* GRAY, 1844 (MONOTYPIC)

EIMERIA SP. 1 OF DRÓŻDŻ, 1987

Original host: *Lobodon carcinophaga* (Hombron and Jacquinot, 1842), Crabeater Seal.

Remarks: Dróżdż (1987) said he found yellow-gray, ovoidal oocysts with a smooth, bilayered wall without a M, that measured L × W: 30.0 (sic) × 24.3 (38–40 × 24–25), L/W ratio: 1.2, in 6/43 (14%) crabeater seals from King George Island, South Shetlands from April, 1981 to January, 1982. No other information was provided, and this species has not been identified since 1987; thus, it must be regarded as a *species inquirenda*.

SARCOCYSTIS SP. OF IPPEN AND HENNE, 1989

Definitive host: Unknown.

Intermediate host: *Lobodon carcinophaga* (Hombron and Jacquinot, 1842), Crabeater Seal.

Remarks: Ippen and Henne (1989) examined chest, back, tongue, esophagus, diaphragm, and heart muscles from two crabeater seals, a male and a female, collected in the Antarctic. Male tissues were negative, but the female had a "moderate" infection with sarcocysts in her back, tongue, and esophagus. Cysts in cross-section were 40–80 × 60–110. Cysts in the esophagus measured 30–90 × 70–340. No other information was provided, and this species has not been seen

again since 1989; thus, it must be relegated to a *species inquirenda*.

GENUS *MIROUNGA* GRAY, 1827 (2 SPECIES)

CRYPTOSPORIDIUM SP. OF RENGIFO-HERRERA, ORTEGA-MORA, GÓMEZ-BAUTISTA, GARCÍA-MORENO, GARCÍA-PÁRRAGA, CASTRO-URDA, AND PEDRAZA-DÍAZ, 2011

Original host: *Mirounga leonina* (L., 1758), Southern Elephant Seal.

Remarks: Rengifo-Herrera et al. (2011) collected fecal samples from southern elephant seals, on the Antarctic Peninsula. Using immunofluorescence microscopy, and PCR amplification of 18S rRNA and HSP70 genes, they found 1/53 (2%) seals from Avian Island, Marguerite Bay, to be positive for a *Cryptosporidium* sp. they said was most closely related to a skunk genotype.

CRYPTOSPORIDIUM SP. OF RENGIFO-HERRERA, ORTEGA-MORA, GÓMEZ-BAUTISTA, GARCÍA-PENA, GARCÍA-PÁRRAGA, AND PEDRAZA-DÍAZ, 2013

Original host: *Mirounga leonina* (L., 1758), Southern Elephant Seal.

Remarks: Rengifo-Herrera et al. (2013) examined fecal samples from *M. leonina* in the South Shetland Islands and Antarctic Peninsula. Using PCR amplification of the 18S rRNA, HSP70, and COWP genes, they found 3/111 (3%) seals positive for a *Cryptosporidium* sp. they said was most closely related to the southern elephant seal genotype. One positive seal was from Avian Island, Marguerite Bay, Antarctic Peninsula, one from

Biscoe Point, and one from Byers Peninsula, Livingston Island, South Shetland Island.

SARCOCYSTIS SP. OF IPPEN AND HENNE, 1989

Definitive host: Unknown.

Intermediate host: Mirounga leonina (L., 1758), Southern Elephant Seal.

Remarks: Ippen and Henne (1989) examined chest, back, tongue, esophagus, diaphragm, and heart muscles from two male elephant seals, one adult and one juvenile, collected in the Antarctic. Adult tissues were negative, but the juvenile had cysts present in the chest, tongue, and diaphragm. Cysts were smaller than those observed in Weddell and crabeater seals reported in the same paper, measuring 20–40×30–80 in cross-section. Ippen and Henne (1989) suggested that in the juvenile the cysts might be the result of a recent infection and had not reached their full size. No other information was given by the authors, and this species has not been reported again since 1989: thus, it must be relegated to a *species inquirenda*.

GENUS PAGOPHILUS GRAY, 1844 (MONOTYPIC)

CRYPTOSPORIDIUM SP. OF BASS, WALLACE, YUND, AND FORD, 2012

Original host: *Pagophilus groenlandicus* (Erxleben, 1777), Harp Seal.

Remarks: Bass et al. (2012) examined 24 fecal samples from harp seals in the Gulf of Maine, USA using a nested PCR amplification, and subsequent sequencing of the 18S rRNA and HSP70 genes, and found one harp seal (4%) with a *Cryptosporidium* sp. genotype most closely related to the seal 1 and seal 2 genotypes described by Santín et al. (2005) from ringed seals.

GENUS PHOCA L., 1758 (2 SPECIES)

CRYPTOSPORIDIUM SP. OF BASS, WALLACE, YUND, AND FORD, 2012

Original host: *Phoca vitulina* (L., 1758), Harbor Seal.

Remarks: Bass et al. (2012) collected fecal samples from *P. vitulina* in two localities in Maine, USA, and using nested PCR amplification, with subsequent sequencing of the 18S rRNA and HSP70 genes, they reported detecting *Cryptosporidium* in 11/176 (6%) samples that were most closely related to the genotype *Cryptosporidium* sp. seal 1 and seal 2 described by Santín et al. (2005) from ringed seals.

CRYPTOSPORIDIUM SP. OF GREIG, GULLAND, SMITH, CONRAD, FIELD, FLEETWOOD, HARVEY, IP, JANG, PACKHAM, WHEELER, AND HALL, 2014

Original host: *Phoca vitulina* (L., 1758), Harbor Seal.

Remarks: Greig et al. (2014) collected fecal samples from *P. vitulina* (40 stranded, 13 wild-caught) from San Francisco, and seven wild-caught from Tomales Bay, California USA, and examined them using a direct immunofluorescent antibody test (DFA). *Cryptosporidium* was detected in only one sample of a weaned pup. Its genotype was not successfully determined.

SARCOCYSTIS SP. OF HADWEN, 1922

Definitive host: Unknown.

Intermediate host: *Phoca vitulina* L., 1758, Harbor Seal.

Remarks: While examining reindeer and caribou muscle for sarcocysts in Alaska, Hadwen (1922) also found sarcocysts in the heart and esophagus of a seal. In the heart, the sarcocysts were numerous and averaged 0.43 mm × 0.17 mm. Sarcocysts in the esophagus and other muscles were larger, 0.87 mm × 0.14 mm, with the longest cyst 2.5 mm. Hadwen (1922) said these sarcocysts looked similar to those of *Sarcocystis tenella* of sheep. Nothing more is known about this form.

SARCOCYSTIS SP. OF LAPOINTE, DUIGNAN, MARSH, GULLAND, BARR, NAYDAN, KING, FARMAN, BUREK-HUNTINGDON, AND LOWENSTINE, 1998

Definitive host: Unknown.

Intermediate host: *Phoca vitulina richardii* (Gray, 1864), Pacific Harbor Seal.

Remarks: Lapointe et al. (1998) reported seven Pacific harbor seals that, upon examination, had meningoencephalitis associated with *S. neurona*-like parasites. One seal was reported to have "rare" sarcocysts of an undetermined species in its **cardiomyocytes**.

GENUS *PUSA* SCOPOLI, 1771 (3 SPECIES)

CRYPTOSPORIDIUM SP. OF DIXON, PARRINGTON, PARENTEAU, LECLAIR, SANTÍN, AND FAYER, 2008

Original host: *Pusa hispida* (Schreber, 1775), Ringed Seal.

Remarks: Dixon et al. (2008) examined the intestinal contents of *P. hispida* in the Nunavik region, northern Québec, Canada. Using flow cytometric analyses combining fluorescence and morphological parameters, they detected *Cryptosporidium* in 5/55 (9%) of the samples. Coinfection with *Giardia duodenalis* was detected in 4/5 samples.

CRYPTOSPORIDIUM SP. OF HUGHES-HANKS, RICKARD, PANUSKA, SAUCIER, O'HARA, DEHN, AND ROLLAND, 2005

Original host: *Pusa hispida* (Schreber, 1775), Ringed Seal.

Remarks: Hughes-Hanks et al. (2005) examined fecal samples of *P. hispida* from northern Alaska, near Barrow, using the immunofluorescent assay. *Cryptosporidium* was detected in 7/31 (23%) samples (5 males, 2 females). No specific identification was attempted.

EIMERIA SP. OF KUIKEN, KENNEDY, BARRETT, VAN DE BILDT, BORGSTEEDE, BREW, CODD, DUCK, DEAVILLE, EYBATOV, FORSYTH, FOSTER, JEPSON, KYDYRMANOV, MITROFANOV, WARD, WILSON, AND OSTERHAUS, 2006

Original host: *Pusa caspica* (Gmelin, 1788) (syn. *Phoca caspica*), Caspian Seal.

Remarks: Kuiken et al. (2006) reported a large die-off of Caspian seals in the spring and summer, 2000, which they attributed to a canine distemper epidemic, and they mentioned finding *Eimeria*-like oocysts in the cytoplasm of jejunal enterocytes in 1 of the of the 18 seals they necropsied. They said the oocysts "consisted of 4–8 banana-shaped zoites (2 μm × 8 μm) with a central blue nucleus and surrounded by a narrow, birefringent wall." They did not try to identify the oocysts they saw more specifically but said they were similar to those of *E. phocae* from harbor seals. This species has not been identified since 2006 and must remain a *species inquirenda*.

SARCOCYSTIS SP. OF KUIKEN, KENNEDY, BARRETT, VAN DE BILDT, BORGSTEEDE, BREW, CODD, DUCK, DEAVILLE, EYBATOV, FORSYTH, FOSTER, JEPSON, KYDYRMANOV, MITROFANOV, WARD, WILSON, AND OSTERHAUS, 2006

Definitive host: Unknown.

Intermediate host: *Pusa caspica* (Gmelin, 1788) (syn. *Phoca caspica*), Caspian Seal.

Remarks: Kuiken et al. (2006), reported on a die-off of Caspian seals in the spring and summer, 2000, which they attributed to canine distemper, and mentioned finding *Sarcocystis*-like cysts containing many banana-shaped bradyzoites, ~6 μm × 2 μm, with a distinct N, in myocytes of the esophageal muscularis and skeletal muscle of 1/18 (5.5%) seals. The cysts distended the infected myocyte but did not induce an inflammatory response in adjacent tissue (their Fig. 12, p. 328). No other information was provided. This species has not been identified since 2006 and must remain a *species inquirenda*.

SARCOCYSTIS SP. OF MIGAKI AND ALBERT, 1980

Definitive host: Unknown.

Intermediate host: *Pusa hispida* (Schreber, 1775), Ringed Seal.

Remarks: Migaki and Albert (1980) found sarcocysts in the skeletal muscles, but not in the heart, of 12/18 (67%) apparently healthy *P. hispida* from the Arctic Ocean near Barrow, Alaska, USA. The cysts were compartment, elongate, 60–550 wide and had moderately thick, well-defined cell walls, 0.8–1.0 thick. Bradyzoites were 10–12 × 2–3. Obviously, the life cycle of this species is unknown. No other information was provided. This species has not been identified since 1980 and must remain a *species inquirenda*.

FAMILY PROCYONIDAE GRAY, 1825

GENUS POTOS É. GEOFFROY SAINT-HILAIRE AND F.G. CUVIER, 1795 (MONOTYPIC)

SARCOCYSTIS SP. OF TAKOS, 1957

Definitive host: Unknown.

Intermediate host: *Potos* sp., Kinkajou.

Remarks: Takos (1957) found a sarcosporidian infection in an old male kinkajou shot near the Rio Mandinga Bridge, Panama Canal Zone, Panama. Sarcocysts were found in striated muscle, but not in the myocardium or other organs. Sarcocysts were broadly ovoidal and measured 123–216 × 85–100. Each sarcocyst was bounded by a dense, well-defined, unstriated wall, ~1 thick. Sarcocysts were divided into compartments by thin septa and the chambers they formed were densely packed with banana-shaped zoites that measured 7.5–9 × 2. Takos (1957) said there was no evidence of tissue reaction to the parasite and that this was the first report of a *Sarcocystis* species in the muscles of a kinkajou. No other information was given.

GENUS PROCYON STORR, 1780 (3 SPECIES)

COCCIDIUM OF CARLSON AND NIELSEN, 1982

Original host: *Procyon lotor* (L., 1758), Raccoon.

Remarks: Carlson and Nielsen (1982) reported the presence of "macrogametocytes containing multiple substructures identified as macrogametes and red-staining residual bodies, as well as oocysts" in the villi and intestinal lumen of the small intestine of a young raccoon in which they also described a *Cryptosporidium* sp. (below). No other information was given.

CRYPTOSPORIDIUM SP. OF CARLSON AND NIELSEN, 1982

Original host: *Procyon lotor* (L., 1758), Raccoon.
Remarks: Carlson and Nielsen (1982) first reported the presence of *Cryptosporidium* in a young male raccoon from Waterford, Connecticut, USA. The raccoon did not show any clinical signs of infection. Histology revealed endogenous stages of a *Cryptosporidium* sp. at the tips of the small intestinal villi, but not in the crypts. The villi were reduced in length, blunted, and increased in width; lamina propria was infiltrated with eosinophils and mononuclear cells.

CRYPTOSPORIDIUM SPP. OF FENG, ALDERISIO, YANG, BLANCERO, KUHNE, NADARESKI, REID, AND XIAO, 2007

Original host: *Procyon lotor* (L., 1758), Raccoon.
Remarks: Feng et al. (2007) surveyed fecal samples of wild *P. lotor* from the watershed of the New York City drinking water supply, USA, for *Cryptosporidium* spp. Using 18S rDNA and RFLP gene sequencing and analysis they reported 4/21(19%) positive samples, 1 for a cervine genotype (syn. genotype W4) and 3 for a skunk genotype (syn. genotype W13).

CRYPTOSPORIDIUM SPP. OF LEŚNIAŃSKA, PEREC-MATYSIAK, HILDEBRAND, BUŃKOWSKA-GAWLIK, PIRÓG, AND POPIOŁEK, 2016

Original host: *Procyon lotor* (L., 1758), Raccoon.
Remarks: Leśniańska et al. (2016) collected feces from *P. lotor* that were introduced and

are now invasive, to Europe; 32 samples were from two areas in Poland (Kostrzyn on the Oder, and Warta Mouth National Park), and 17 samples from Germany (Müritz National Park, Mecklenburg-Vorpommern). *Cryptosporidium* was detected in 17/49 (35%) samples (14 from Poland, 3 from Germany). Amplification of 18S rRNA, COWP, and actin genes demonstrated that 9/17 (53%) infected raccoons had *Cryptosporidium* skunk genotype. This study was the first evidence of *Cryptosporidium* in raccoons from Poland and Germany.

CRYPTOSPORIDIUM SP. OF MARTIN AND ZEIDNER, 1992

Original host: *Procyon lotor* (L., 1758), Raccoon.
Remarks: Martin and Zeidner (1992) described a case of cryptosporidiosis in a juvenile *P. lotor* found moribund in Fort Collins, Colorado, USA. The animal was emaciated, dehydrated, and had diarrhea. Microscopically, *Cryptosporidium* endogenous stages, spheroidal to ovoidal, 2–7 wide, were seen on intact intestinal villi. The raccoon also was infected with coronavirus and parvovirus.

CRYPTOSPORIDIUM SP. OF ZHOU, FAYER, TROUT, RYAN, SCHAEFER III, AND XIAO, 2004

Original host: *Procyon lotor* (L., 1758), Raccoon.
Remarks: Zhou et al. (2004) collected the feces of 471 mammals from four counties in the Chesapeake Bay area of Maryland, USA; they found 2/51 (4%) raccoons (presumably *P. lotor*) to be infected with a *Cryptosporidium* skunk genotype. The species and genotype of *Cryptosporidium* in each fecal sample was determined by a PCR-RFLP method based on the 18S rRNA gene.

CRYPTOSPORIDIUM SPP. OF ZIEGLER, WADE, SCHAAF, STERN, NADARESKI, AND MOHAMMED, 2007

Original host: *Procyon lotor* (L., 1758), Raccoon.
Remarks: Ziegler et al. (2007) collected fecal samples of wild *P. lotor* in the New York City Watershed, southeastern New York state, USA. Samples were examined by LM and by poly-clonal *Cryptosporidium* antigen-capture ELISA (considered positive based on an optical density ≥0.050). They found *Cryptosporidium* in 49/173 (28%) samples.

EIMERIA (?) SPP. OF ROBEL, BARNES, AND UPTON, 1989

Original host: *Procyon lotor* (L., 1758), Raccoon.
Remarks: Robel et al. (1989) collected rac-coons from two locations in Kansas, USA and reported that 8/36 (22%) raccoons from Ft. Riley and 25/92 (27%) from rural Manhattan had eimerian oocysts in their rectal contents. However, because all intestinal tracts had been frozen for 1–3 months at −5°C, which should have prevented sporulation, it is not clear to us how they were able to state these were eimerian oocysts.

EIMERIA SPP. OF SNYDER, 1984, 1988

Original host: *Procyon lotor* (L., 1758), Raccoon.
Remarks: Snyder (1984, 1988) reported oocysts of *Eimeria* spp. in 67/100 (67%) fecal samples from *P. lotor* in Illinois, USA. He examined the samples for *C. parvum*, using sucrose flotation (1984) or an indirect immunofluorescent detec-tion procedure (1988) and reported that "*Eimeria* spp. oocysts were routinely seen in samples but never exhibited any fluorescence."

EIMERIA SP. OF FOSTER, MCCLEERY, AND FORRESTER, 2004

Original host: *Procyon lotor* (L., 1758), Raccoon.
Remarks: Foster et al. (2004) recovered oocysts of three *Eimeria* spp. from raccoons collected in Key Largo, Monroe county, Florida, USA; two were previously described (*E. procyonis*, *E. nuttalli*), but the third form, found in 2/61 (3%) samples, was unknown. Oocysts were ellipsoidal, L×W (n=22): 29.2×15.7 (28–31×14–17), L/W ratio: 1.9; with a smooth, 2-layered wall; M, OR, PG: all absent. Sporocysts were ellipsoidal, 10.1×7.7 (10–11×6–8); SB, SSB, PSB, SR: all absent. Foster et al. (2004) speculated this was likely a spurious coccidium originating from a food item passing through the raccoon's gastrointestinal tract.

SARCOCYSTIS SP. OF ADAMS, LEVINE, AND TODD, JR., 1981

Definitive host: *Procyon lotor* (L., 1758), Raccoon.
Intermediate host: Unknown.
Remarks: Adams et al. (1981) mentioned finding two naturally-infected raccoons in Illinois, USA that were discharging *Sarcocystis*-like sporocysts in their feces, but they did not attempt to determine the species. Sporocysts were ellipsoidal or had one side flattened, L×W (n=17): 13.0×9.3 (11–13×8–10), with a smooth wall; SB, SSB, PSB: all absent; SR: present, and SZ were "elongate" lying length-wise in SP. An attempt to infect four pigs resulted in no sarcocysts in pig muscles or other tissues at necropsy and no oocysts in the pig's feces.

SARCOCYSTIS SP. OF DUBEY, HAMIR, HANLON, TOPPER, AND RUPPRECHT, 1990b

Definitive host: Unknown.
Intermediate host: *Procyon lotor* (L., 1758), Raccoon.

Remarks: Dubey et al. (1990b) received 45 raccoons from Ohio, USA for experiments to develop an oral rabies recombinant vaccine for wildlife. One juvenile female was unsteady on its feet, had difficulty with balance, and its head was constantly turned to the left. Seven days after arrival, it was anorectic, had mucopurulent nasal and serous ocular discharge, and was moribund. On necropsy they observed the carcass was dehydrated, mucous membranes were pale, and lungs were consolidated. Numerous developmental stages of a *Sarcocystis* species were found in the cytoplasm of macrophages, neurons, and multinucleated giant cells. In mature meronts, merozoites were arranged in a rosette around a residual body; individual merozoites measured $4-5 \times 1$ and were seen in mononuclear cells located within meningeal blood vessels. Organisms were located in host cell cytoplasm without a PV, and merozoites had no rhoptries. Moderate numbers of sarcocysts were found in striated muscles of the heart, tongue, diaphragm, esophagus, masseter, and extraorbital muscles. In all likelihood, this species is *S. neurona* but must be considered a *species inquirenda* at this time.

SARCOCYSTIS SP. OF FOSTER, MCCLEERY, AND FORRESTER, 2004

Definitive host: *Procyon lotor* (L., 1758), Raccoon.
Intermediate host: Unknown.
Remarks: Foster et al. (2004) collected sporocysts from the feces of 2/61 (3%) raccoons on Key Largo, Monroe county, Florida, USA. Sporocysts were ellipsoidal, L×W (n=10): 13.3×8.5 ($12-14 \times 7-10$). There was no attempt to identify the species.

SARCOCYSTIS (?) SP. OF ROBEL, BARNES, AND UPTON, 1989

Definitive host: *Procyon lotor* (L., 1758), Raccoon.
Intermediate host: Unknown.

Remarks: Robel et al. (1989) collected raccoons from two locations in Kansas, USA and reported that 5/92 (5%) from rural Manhattan, but 0/36 from Ft. Riley, had sporocysts of a *Sarcocystis* sp. in their rectal contents. However, these numbers only were present in their Table I, and they never mentioned the presence of *Sarcocystis* in the body of their paper. It also should be noted that all intestinal tracts had been frozen, for 1–3 months at $-5°C$, before they were examined, so it is not clear to us if the sporocysts they saw had SZ in them or not.

SARCOCYSTIS SP. OF SENEVIRATNA, EDWARD, AND DEGIUSTI, 1975

Definitive host: Unknown.
Intermediate host: *Procyon lotor* (L., 1758), Raccoon.
Remarks: Seneviratna et al. (1975) examined the muscles of domestic animals and a few wild animals killed in Detroit, Michigan, USA from April to September, 1973. They found 2/6 (33%) raccoons, both female, with sarcocysts in their muscles. They were unable to make a species identification; thus, another *species inquirenda*.

SARCOCYSTIS SPP. OF THULIN, GRANSTROM, GELBERG, MORTON, FRENCH, AND GILES, 1992

Definitive host: *Procyon lotor* (L., 1758), Raccoon.
Intermediate host: *Procyon lotor* (L., 1758), Raccoon.
Remarks: Thulin et al. (1992) reported an adult male raccoon with protozoal encephalitis associated with a *Sarcocystis*-like organism and concurrently infected with canine distemper. The *Sarcocystis* species was intracellular in the cytoplasm, without a PV. Histologically, sarcocysts were present in skeletal muscle and occasionally

in the heart; these cysts were 19 × 25 to 40 × 506 and had striated walls that were 1.5–2.0 thick. Individual merozoites were 2.0 × 1.5. A second raccoon had numerous *Sarcocystis*-type oocysts in the lamina propria of its small intestine. It is possible that the form in the first raccoon was *S. neurona* because of its intracellular location without a PV, with the raccoon serving as an intermediate host; similarly, the isosporoid oocysts in the gut of the second raccoon may represent another species of *Sarcocystis*, with the raccoon serving as the definitive host. Both forms can only be considered *species inquirendae* at this time.

FAMILY *URSIDAE* FISCHER DE WALDHEIM, 1817

GENUS *AILUROPODA* MILNE-EDWARDS, 1870 (MONOTYPIC)

CRYPTOSPORIDIUM SP. OF LIU, HE, ZHONG, ZHANG, WANG, DONG, WANG, LI, DENG, PENG, AND ZHANG, 2013

Original host: *Ailuropoda melanoleuca* (David, 1869), Giant Panda.

Remarks: Liu et al. (2013) examined fecal samples of 57 giant pandas from the China Conservation and Research Centre for the Giant Panda in Ya'an City, Sichuan, China. No clinical signs were observed in the pandas at the time of feces collections. One 18-year-old panda was positive for *Cryptosporidium* oocysts that were L × W (n = 50): 4.6 × 4.0 (4–6 × 3–5). Using the sequences of 18S rRNA, HSP70, COWP, and actin genes, Liu et al. (2013) discovered that this parasite represented a new genotype of *Cryptosporidium*, which was most closely related to the *Cryptosporidium* bear genotype, and they designated this new genotype, *Cryptosporidium* giant panda genotype, but did not give it a binomial.

GENUS *HELARCTOS* HORSFIELD, 1825 (MONOTYPIC)

CRYPTOSPORIDIUM SP. OF SIAM, SALEM, GHONEIM, MICHAEL, AND EL-REFAY, 1994

Original host: *Helarctos malayanus* (Raffles, 1821), Sun Bear.

Remarks: Siam et al. (1994) examined 81 captive carnivores in the Giza Zoological Gardens Zoo, Egypt, including two sun bears; they found 1/2 (50%) sun bears to be passing oocysts of a *Cryptosporidium* sp. No other information was provided.

CRYPTOSPORIDIUM SP. OF WANG AND LIEW, 1990

Original host: *Helarctos malayanus* (Raffles, 1821), Sun Bear.

Remarks: Wang and Liew (1990) first reported the presence of oocysts of *Cryptosporidium* in both captive sun bears in a bird park in Taiwan. Parasites were detected in fecal smears stained with modified Ziehl-Neelsen karbolfuchsin staining method. No other information was provided.

SARCOCYSTIS SP. OF LATIF, VELLAYAN, OMAR, ABDULLAH, AND DESA, 2010

Definitive host: Unknown.

Intermediate host: *Helarctos malayanus* (Raffles, 1821), Sun Bear.

Remarks: Latif et al. (2010) examined one Malayan sun bear in a zoo in Korea and found that it had sarcocysts of *Sarcocystis* only in the diaphragm, but they did not find sarcocysts in the tongue, esophagus, heart, or skeletal muscles. There was no attempt to identify the species beyond genus so their finding can only be considered a *species inquirenda*.

GENUS *URSUS* L., 1758
(4 SPECIES)

COCCIDIA SPP. OF GAU, KUTZ, AND ELKIN, 1999

Original host: *Ursus arctos* L., 1758 (syn. *Ursus horribilis* Ord, 1815), Brown Bear.

Remarks: Gau et al. (1999) reported the presence of "gastrointestinal coccidia" in 8/56 (14%) fecal samples of *U. arctos* from the Central Canadian Arctic (Northwest Territories, Canada), but they neither measured oocysts nor identified the genus of the coccidia they observed (probably because fecal samples all had been frozen in the field and stored at −20°C until analyzed, which would have prevented sporulation). They suggested that the coccidians may be enzootic in *U. arctos* in the central Arctic, rather than incidentally occurring through the ingestion of infected prey species. This species, or these species, can only be considered *species inquirendae*.

COCCIDIUM OF BEMRICK AND O'LEARY, 1979

Original host: *Ursus arctos* L., 1758 (syn. *Ursus horribilis* Ord, 1815), Brown Bear.

Remarks: Bemrick and O'Leary (1979) reported that a 1-week-old female grizzly (brown) bear cub, from the Como Park Zoo, St. Paul, Minnesota, USA had severe diarrhea. The cub weighed only 454 g and died. Routine histological examination of the lamina propria of the small intestine showed exceptionally large asexual stages (meronts) present, but these were not measured and, although four photomicrographs of tissue sections were published, no structural measurements were given. Bemrick

and O'Leary (1979) mentioned that fecal samples of other grizzly bears in the zoo had been examined periodically in previous years, but no coccidian oocysts were found. They could not say with certainty that these endogenous stages were the etiological agent of the diarrhea seen in the bear cub or not. Their coccidium must be considered a *species inquirenda*.

CRYPTOSPORIDIUM SP. OF FAGIOLINI, LIA, LARICCHIUTA, CAVICCHIO, MANNELLA, CAFARCHIA, OTRANTO, FINOTELLO, AND PERRUCCI, 2010

Original host: *Ursus thibetanus* G. [Baron] Cuvier, 1823, Asian Black Bear.

Remarks: Fagiolini et al. (2010) reported finding oocysts of a *Cryptosporidium* species in an Asian black bear at the Fasano Zoo Safari in Italy. No other information was given.

CRYPTOSPORIDIUM SPP. OF RAVASZOVA, HALANOVA, GOLDOVA, VALENCAKOVA, MALCEKOVA, HURNÍKOVÁ, AND HALAN, 2012

Original host: *Ursus arctos* L., 1758 (syn. *Ursus horribilis* Ord, 1815), Brown Bear.

Remarks: Ravaszova et al. (2012) studied the feces of brown bears from central and eastern Slovakia (Europe) from June 2010–March 2011, using *in vitro* immunoassay for the quantitative detection of *Cryptosporidium* antigen by the sandwich ELISA method and found 35/63 (56%) samples to be positive. They also examined the fecal smears stained by a modified Kinyoun's acid-fast stain using LM; this method was less sensitive and only 17/63 (27%) of the samples were positive. No attempt to identify the species was made.

CRYPTOSPORIDIUM SP. OF SIAM, SALEM, GHONEIM, MICHAEL, AND EL-REFAY, 1994

Original host: *Ursus arctos* L., 1758 (syn. *Ursus horribilis* Ord, 1815), Brown Bear.

Remarks: Siam et al. (1994) examined 81 captive carnivores in the Giza Zoological Gardens Zoo, Egypt, including brown bears; they found 2/7 (29%) brown bears passing oocysts of a *Cryptosporidium* sp. No other information was provided.

CRYPTOSPORIDIUM SP. OF SIAM, SALEM, GHONEIM, MICHAEL, AND EL-REFAY, 1994

Original host: *Ursus maritimus* Phipps, 1774, Polar Bear.

Remarks: Siam et al. (1994) examined 81 captive carnivores in the Giza Zoological Gardens Zoo, Egypt, including polar bears; they found 1/7 (14%) polar bears passing oocysts of a *Cryptosporidium* sp. No other information was provided.

EIMERIA SP. OF AGHAZADEH, ELSON-RIGGINS, RELJIC, AMBROGI, HUBER, MAJNARIC, AND HERMOSILLA, 2015

Original host: *Ursus arctos* L., 1758 (syn. *Ursus horribilis* Ord, 1815), Brown Bear.

Remarks: Aghazadeh et al. (2015) examined fecal samples from European brown bears collected in Croatia and found 1/94 (1%) positive for *Eimeria* oocysts. The authors provided no description except that oocysts were unsporulated and had a thin, white-gray double oocyst wall, but no M. They noted that the oocysts could have occurred incidentally via infected prey.

ISOSPORA SP. OF YAKIMOFF AND MATSCHOULSKY, 1935

Original host: *Ursus arctos* L., 1758 (syn. *Ursus horribilis* Ord, 1815), Brown Bear.

Remarks: *Isospora* oocysts were found in 2/7 (29%) brown bears in the Leningrad Zoo, former USSR. The animals were imported from north of the former USSR, which likely is the natural habitat for both the host and these oocysts. Oocysts sporulated in 4 days in 2% $K_2Cr_2O_7$ solution at 24°C. The oocysts had two forms, with a wall ~1.5 thick. Spheroidal oocysts were 24.6 (19–32), whereas ovoidal oocysts were L × W: 26.4 × 24.0 (23–33 × 21–29), L/W ratio: 1.1; M: absent; OR: present (line drawing); PG: present. Ovoidal to piriform sporocysts were L × W: 16.9 × 11.6 (15–19 × 11–13), L/W ratio, 1.5; SB, SSB: both present; PSB: absent; SR: present; SR characteristics: a clump of granules or granules spread among SZ; SZ: crescent-shaped. Yakimoff and Matschoulsky (1935) thought this was not a parasite of bears, but may be a bird isosporan because its morphological features were similar to sporulated oocysts described as *Isospora lacazei* (Labbé, 1893). Its occurrence in this bear's feces may be explained by the fact that bears lick their paws contaminated by the soil where the sparrows defecate. No one knows for sure.

SARCOCYSTIS SP. OF CRUM, NETTLES, AND DAVIDSON, 1978

Definitive host: Unknown.

Intermediate host: *Ursus americanus* Pallas, 1780, American Black Bear.

Remarks: Crum et al. (1978) found 6/53 (11%) *U. americanus* collected from six states in the southeastern United States to have sarcocysts, which they found histologically in the cardiac and skeletal muscles. No other information was given.

SARCOCYSTIS SP. OF DUBEY, HUMPHREYS, AND FRITZ, 2008a

Definitive host: Unknown.

Intermediate host: *Ursus americanus* Pallas, 1780, American Black Bear.

Remarks: Sarcocysts were found in 1/374 (~0.3%) black bears legally shot in Pennsylvania, USA, but only one cyst was found in this bear. The sarcocyst from this bear was structurally different from the sarcocysts found in two bears, during the same collection, which allowed Dubey et al. (2008a) to name a new species at that time, *S. ursusi*. The wall of these sarcocysts was ~2 thick and had finger-like villi on the cyst wall giving the sarcocyst wall a striated appearance that the sarcocysts of *S. ursusi* lacked. Nothing else is yet known about the identity of the *Sarcocystis* species in bears with these kinds of sarcocysts.

SARCOCYSTIS SP. OF DUBEY, TOPPER, AND NUTTER, 1998b

Definitive host: Unknown.

Intermediate host: *Ursus americanus* Pallas, 1780, American Black Bear.

Remarks: Dubey et al. (1998b) were able to examine diaphragm, abdominal muscles, and carcass muscles from 92 hunter-killed bears in North Carolina, USA. They found two sarcocysts in cross-sections of muscle from one bear (1%). The sarcocysts were 45 × 37.5 and 67.5 × 50. Under TEM they saw that the bradyzoites butted against the ground substance of the cyst wall; five longitudinally-cut bradyzoites were 6.0–6.6 × 2.5–3.3 and contained organelles typically found in *Sarcocystis* bradyzoites. Dubey et al. (1998b) reiterated a previous (perhaps questionable) argument that the structure of the sarcocyst wall is a reliable taxonomic criterion to distinguish *Sarcocystis* species within a given host. They concluded their reasoning as to why they did not call this the same species as the one seen by Zeman et al. (1993), below, by saying, "A *Sarcocystis*-like parasite has been reported as causing fatal hepatitis in a black bear from South Dakota (Zeman et al., 1993) and in two polar bears from Alaska (Garner et al., 1997). Only schizonts and merozoites were found in bears that died of hepatitis; sarcocysts were not seen." Thus, the observational data between this report and those of Zeman et al. (1993) and Garner et al. (1997) is not comparable, and all of these can only be considered as *species inquirendae*.

SARCOCYSTIS SP. OF GARNER, BARR, PACKHAM, MARSH, BUREK-HUNTINGTON, WILSON, AND DUBEY, 1997

Definitive host: Unknown.

Intermediate host: *Ursus maritimus* Phipps, 1774, Polar Bear.

Remarks: Garner et al. (1997) diagnosed fatal hepatic sarcocystosis in two zoo polar bears in Anchorage, Alaska, USA. Gross lesions were icterus and systemic petechiae, whereas microscopic lesions were detected only in the liver and included severe random necrotizing hepatitis with hemorrhage. They observed only asexual stages of the parasite within hepatocytes along with rare extracellular zoites. This parasite divided by endopolygeny, and occasionally merozoites formed rosettes around a central residual body. TEM of merozoites showed a conoid and a small number of micronemes at their apical pole, a central N, but rhoptries were absent. These parasites failed to react with anti-*Neurospora* sp., anti-*T. gondii*, and anti-*S. neurona* sera. Nothing more about this parasite is known, including the life cycle. Thus, it must be considered a *species inquirenda*.

SARCOCYSTIS SP. OF ZEMAN, DUBEY, AND ROBISON, 1993

Definitive host: Unknown.

Intermediate host: *Ursus americanus* Pallas, 1780, American Black Bear.

Remarks: Zeman et al. (1993) reported a case of fatal sarcocystosis in an American black bear from a wild-animal park, Black Hills, South Dakota, USA; initially, they found different developmental stages of a protozoan parasite in the cytoplasm of several hepatocytes. There was no inflammation associated with parasitized hepatocytes, but they saw both inflammation and necrosis associated with maturation and rupture of mature meronts. Zeman et al. (1993) reported that mature meronts occupied 50%–80% of hepatocyte cytoplasm and moved the HCN to the periphery of the cell. They also noted that the meronts divided by **endopolygeny**, characteristic of *Sarcocystis* species. Mature meronts were 30×20 and contained up to 36 merozoites. When liver tissue sections were deparaffinized, they reacted with antiserum to *T. gondii*, *N. caninum*, and *S. cruzi*, but the parasite tissue only reacted with *S. cruzi*, not with *T. gondii* or *N. caninum* antisera. Zeman et al. (1993) compared the hepatic lesions seen in the bear to those reported from a sea lion (Mense et al., 1992) and said these lesions also were identical to those described in a 2-day-old dog with congenital sarcocystosis (Dubey et al., 1992a). The canine parasite was morphologically and antigenically identical to *Sarcocystis canis*, but unlike in the bear, the *S. canis* infection was found in many of the dog's tissues including skin, brain, liver, and lungs. This was the first report of a fatal hepatic sarcocystosis in a bear, but its true identity is still unknown.

SUBORDER FELIFORMIA KRETZOI, 1945

FAMILY FELIDAE FISCHER DE WALDHEIM, 1817

SUBFAMILY FELINAE FISCHER DE WALDHEIM, 1817

GENUS ACINONYX BROOKES, 1828 (MONOTYPIC)

CRYPTOSPORIDIUM SP. OF SIAM, SALEM, GHONEIM, MICHAEL, AND EL-REFAY, 1994

Original host: *Acinonyx jubatus* (Schreber, 1775), Cheetah.

Remarks: Siam et al. (1994) examined 81 captive carnivores in the Giza Zoological Gardens Zoo, Egypt including four cheetahs; they found 2/4 (50%) to be passing oocysts of a *Cryptosporidium* sp. No other information was provided.

GENUS *FELIS* L., 1758 (7 SPECIES)

BESNOITIA SP. OF MCKENNA AND CHARLESTON, 1980c

Original host: *Felis catus* L., 1758, Domestic Cat.

Remarks: McKenna and Charleston (1980c) infected rats with isosporan oocysts recovered from the feces of a feral cat. Later, they found macroscopically visible, spheroidal cysts up to 260 wide, which resembled a *Besnoitia* cyst. Kittens were fed infected rats and, at 11–12 DPI, they shed similar oocysts that measured 16.9×14.6 in their feces. These sporulated oocysts were fed to mice, rats, rabbits, and guinea pigs, all of which developed *Besnoitia*-type cysts, except the guinea pigs. Unfortunately, they did not attempt to name their organism.

COCCIDIA SPP. OF BALLWEBER, PANUSKA, HUSTON, VASILOPULOS, PHARR, AND MACKIN, 2009

Original host: *Felis catus* L., 1758, Domestic Cat.
Remarks: Ballweber et al. (2009) surveyed fecal samples of domestic cats both indoor and outdoor, with and without diarrhea, from 159 households in northeastern Mississippi, and northwestern Alabama, USA. "Coccidial oocysts" were found in 19/250 (8%) cats, but the authors did not differentiate them.

COCCIDIA SPP. OF DE SANTIS-KERR, RAGHAVAN, GLICKMAN, CALDANARO, MOORE, LEWIS, SCHANTZ, AND GLICKMAN, 2006

Original host: *Felis catus* L., 1758, Domestic Cat.
Remarks: De Santis-Kerr et al. (2006) surveyed the feces of 211,105 pet cats for feline *Giardia* and coccidia by visiting pet hospitals in 40 US states, 2003–04. Coccidia were detected in 14/1,000 fecal tests (1%), mostly in cats under 4 years of age, and in summer months; most infections were in the Southeast Central region, with the fewest in the North Pacific. Patient medical records did not distinguish between *T. gondii*, *Cryptosporidium* species, *Isospora* species, and other coccidial intestinal parasites.

COCCIDIA SPP. OF FARIAS, CHRISTOVÃO, AND STOBBE, 1995

Original host: *Felis catus* L., 1758, Domestic Cat.
Remarks: Farias et al. (1995) examined fecal samples of cats in the Araçatuba Region, São Paulo, Brazil. Oocysts of "coccidia" were seen in 3/32 (9%) samples, but no identifications were determined.

COCCIDIA SPP. OF JOFFE, VAN NIEKERK, GAGNÉ, GILLEARD, KUTZ, AND LOBINGIER, 2011

Original host: *Felis catus* L., 1758, Domestic Cat.
Remarks: Joffe et al. (2011) examined fecal samples of 68 household and 85 sheltered cats in the Calgary, Alberta, Canada; "Coccidian oocysts" were detected in 1 (<1%) sheltered cat.

COCCIDIA SPP. OF KRECEK, MOURA, LUCAS, AND KELLY, 2010

Original host: *Felis catus* L., 1758, Domestic Cat.
Remarks: Krecek et al. (2010) examined feces of trapped stray cats in Basseterre, St. Kitts, West Indies. "Coccidian oocysts" were detected in 12/100 (12%) samples; identifications were not attempted.

COCCIDIA OF NASH, MTAMBO, AND GIBBS, 1993

Original host: *Felis catus* L., 1758, Domestic Cat.
Remarks: Nash et al. (1993) surveyed fecal samples of cats from eight farms in Glasgow, Scotland, United Kingdom. "Coccidial oocysts measuring 11×8 to $13 \mu m \times 12 \mu m$ in diameter" were detected in 2/57 (3.5%) cats. The authors stated that based on oocyst size, these may represent *T. gondii*, *Sarcocystis* sp., or *Hammondia* sp.

COCCIDIA OF VISCO, CORWIN, AND SELBY, 1978

Original host: *Felis catus* L., 1758, Domestic Cat.
Remarks: Visco et al. (1978) examined pet cats in Missouri, USA, from 1974 to 1976. "Coccidia"

were detected in 87/1,294 (7%) cats of all age categories but mostly in those <6-months-old. Oocysts found were not determined to genus or species, and the authors admit that everything was reported as *Isospora* sp. or as "coccidia."

CRYPTOSPORIDIUM BAILEYI (?) OF MCGLADE, ROBERTSON, ELLIOT, READ, AND THOMPSON, 2003

Original host: *Felis catus* L., 1758, Domestic Cat.

Remarks: McGlade et al. (2003) examined 418 fecal samples of 125 domestic cats, from various sources in Perth, Western Australia; 40 randomly-selected samples were screened by nested PCR of the 18S rRNA gene. None of the 418 samples was positive by microscopy, but 4/40 (10%) PCR-sequenced samples were positive for *Cryptosporidium* spp. and one successfully-sequenced PCR product, "most closely resembled" *C. baileyi* (commonly found in chickens).

CRYPTOSPORIDIUM SPP. OF NASH, MTAMBO, AND GIBBS, 1993

Original host: *Felis catus* L., 1758, Domestic Cat.

Remarks: Nash et al. (1993) studied fecal samples of cats from 8 farms in Glasgow, Scotland, by several tests including a specific monoclonal antibody against *Cryptosporidium* (Northumbria Biologicals); *Cryptosporidium* was detected in 7/57 (12%) cats (3 kittens, 4 adults) on three farms. They euthanized 32 cats, all without diarrhea, and processed them for histology. Histology revealed the presence of endogenous developmental stages and oocysts in the epithelium of the ileum, and two types of oocysts were recorded, smaller, 5.0 × 4.5, and larger, 6.0 × 5.0, which were detected in one farm, whereas in the other two farms only smaller oocysts were found.

CRYPTOSPORIDIUM CURYI (?) CITED BY OGASSAWARA, BENASSI, LARSSON, AND HAGIWARA, 1986

Original host: *Felis catus* L., 1758, Domestic Cat.

Remarks: Ogassawara et al. (1986) surveyed the feces of domestic cats from different areas in São Paulo, Brazil, and reported finding oocysts of a "species" they called *C. curyi* in 8/215 (4%) cats. However, the citation they gave for this species (Ogassawara, S., Benassi, S., Larsson, C.E., Hagiwara, M.K. 1986. *Cryptosporidium curyi* n. sp. in the feces of *Felis catus domesticus* in the city of São Paulo, Brazil. Rev. Microbiol., São Paulo.) apparently was never published. They refer to *C. curyi*, and the paper in which it was presumably published as follows: "This agent has recently been described by us and is still being studied for its true identity." This species and citation do not appear in Wikipedia, Google Scholar, or in more recent reviews of *Cryptosporidium* species names by Plutzer and Karanis (2009) and by Fayer (2010).

CRYPTOSPORIDIUM SP. OF ASAHI, KOYAMA, ARAI, FUNAKOSHI, YAMAURA, SHIRASAKA, AND OKUTOMI, 1991

Original host: *Felis catus* L., 1758, Domestic Cat.

Remarks: Asahi et al. (1991) reported a cat in Japan, naturally-infected with "a small type of *Cryptosporidium* sp. oocysts," measuring 4.5 wide. Necropsy showed endogenous stages in the villous epithelia of the small intestine and cecum, but not in the stomach. Oocysts from this cat were inoculated per os into six cats (weight < 1 kg), and all six discharged oocysts; the prepatent period was 8–10 days and peak oocyst shedding was 14–19 DPI, followed by 7–14 more peaks during patency (i.e., 69–203 DPI). All the cats were asymptomatic. After patency ended, the cats were injected s.c. with prednisolone, 10 mg/kg daily for 4–9 days, which caused the recurrence of oocyst shedding. Experimental infections with oocysts in specific pathogen-free (SPF) mice, BALB/c mice, BALB/c mice injected with hydrocortisone acetate, SPF Wistar rats, SPF guinea pigs, and dogs, all failed.

CRYPTOSPORIDIUM SP. OF BARR, GUILFORD, JAMROSZ, HORNBUCKLE, AND BOWMAN, 1994a

Original host: *Felis catus* L., 1758, Domestic Cat.
Remarks: Barr et al. (1994a) diagnosed cryptosporidiosis in three cats suffering from diarrhea, based on the presence of *Cryptosporidium* oocysts in their feces. The cats were administered paromomycin for 5 days, and the diarrhea resolved 5 days after the last dose in two cats, and within 30 days in the third cat. No other information is given.

CRYPTOSPORIDIUM SP. OF BARR, JAMROSZ, HORNBUCKLE, BOWMAN, AND FAYER, 1994b

Original host: *Felis catus* L., 1758, Domestic Cat.
Remarks: Barr et al. (1994b) diagnosed *Cryptosporidium* oocysts and *Toxocara cati* eggs in the feces of a 6-month-old spayed domestic cat that had diarrhea for 2 months. The cat was properly vaccinated and was both FeLV and FIV negative. It was administered pyrantel pamoate (against *Toxocara*), metronidazole (against protozoans), and a special diet (Hill's c/d), but after 14 days the cat still had diarrhea and still shed *Cryptosporidium* oocysts in its feces. It was then given paromomycin, 165 mg/kg, p.o., twice daily for 5 days, and *Cryptosporidium* was not detected in its feces 1, 8, or 34 days after treatment. On days 1 and 8, the diarrhea persisted, but by day 34 the cat was nondiarrheic ~80% of the time. Thus, paromomycin successfully treated the *Cryptosporidium* infection, although it was not identified to species.

CRYPTOSPORIDIUM SP. OF BORKATAKI, KATOCH, GOSWAMI, GODARA, KHAJURIA, YADAV, AND KAUR, 2013

Original host: *Felis catus* L., 1758, Domestic Cat.
Remarks: Borkataki et al. (2013) surveyed fecal samples of stray cats in Jammu, a humid subtropical zone in northwestern India. Oocysts of *Cryptosporidium* were detected in 4/100 (4%) samples, but not identified to species.

CRYPTOSPORIDIUM SPP. OF CIRAK AND BAUER, 2004

Original hosts: *Felis catus* L., 1758, Domestic Cat; *Canis lupus familiaris* (syn. *C. familiaris*) L., 1758, Domestic Dog.
Remarks: Cirak and Bauer (2004) examined fecal samples of cats in Germany to compare conventional fecal exam methods versus a commercial coproantigen ELISA kit (ProSpecT *Cryptosporidium* Microplate Assay) to detect *Cryptosporidium*. No cats examined had diarrhea. Direct fecal smears, fast-stained with carbol fuchsin, found only 1/100 (1%) cats infected with *Cryptosporidium*, whereas ELISA detected infection in 30/100 (30%) cats. Thus, the ELISA kit used can better determine the presence of *Cryptosporidium* but cannot distinguish between the species.

CRYPTOSPORIDIUM SP. OF COELHO, DO AMARANTE, DE SOUTELLO, MEIRELES, AND BRESCIANI, 2009

Original host: *Felis catus* L., 1758, Domestic Cat.
Remarks: Coelho et al. (2009) examined fecal samples of cats in Andradina, São Paulo, Brazil. Samples were collected from the rectum,

and *Cryptosporidium* oocysts were detected in 2/51 (4%) cats using a malachite green negative stain, and in 3/51 (6%) cats with ELISA. Positive samples mostly originated from young animals and did not depend on the sex or breed.

CRYPTOSPORIDIUM SP. OF COX, GRIFFITH, ANGLES, DEERE, AND FERGUSON, 2005

Original host: *Felis catus* L., 1758, Domestic Cat.

Remarks: Cox et al. (2005) examined fecal samples of various domestic, native, and feral animals during a survey of protozoal, bacterial, and viral pathogens, in four drinking-water watersheds in Sydney, Australia. Fecal samples were fluorescence-stained and examined with an epifluorescence microscope. Oocysts of *Cryptosporidium* were detected in 3/7 (43%) domestic cats, but not in the only feral cat examined.

CRYPTOSPORIDIUM SP. OF DADO, IZQUIERDO, VERA, MONTOYA, MATEO, FENOY, GALVÁN, GARCÍA, GARCÍA, ARÁNGUEZ, LÓPEZ, DEL ÁGUILA, AND MIRÓ, 2012

Original host: *Felis catus* L., 1758, Domestic Cat.

Remarks: Dado et al. (2012) examined 625 soil samples and 79 fecal samples ("presumably from dogs and cats") from 67 playgrounds and public parks in southeastern Madrid, Spain. Soil samples were examined using the modified Telemann and MIF methods and fecal samples by a modified Ziehl-Neelsen staining, followed by a rapid immunochromatographic assay. *Cryptosporidium* oocysts were only found in 7/79 (9%) fecal samples found in four parks.

CRYPTOSPORIDIUM SP. OF DE OLIVEIRA LEMOS, ALMOSNY, SOARES, AND ALENCAR, 2012

Original host: *Felis catus* L., 1758, Domestic Cat.

Remarks: de Oliveira Lemos et al. (2012) examined fecal samples of diarrheic (acute or chronic) domestic cats from Rio de Janeiro, Niterói, and Praia de Mauá, Brazil. *Cryptosporidium* oocysts were detected in 5/60 (8%) samples, and 4 of the positive samples also were FeLV-positive. They noted that animals infected with retroviruses were more prone to the *Cryptosporidium* infection and may exhibit more severe clinical signs.

CRYPTOSPORIDIUM SP. OF DUBEY AND PANDE, 1963b

Original host: *Felis chaus* Schreber, 1777, Jungle Cat.

Remarks: Dubey and Pande (1963b) found a "sporulated stage" that measured 11×7 (10–12×7–8), L/W ratio: 1.2–1.5; this "stage" had 4 SZ that were 7–9×1–2, each with a large RB at their broader end. They called these stages "Cryptosporodial/Coccidial bodies," in their discussion and labeled their drawing (Fig. 16) a *Cryptosporidium*. It's likely they were looking at a sporocyst of a *Sarcocystis* sp. because we think the cyst was too large to be a *Cryptosporidium*.

CRYPTOSPORIDIUM SP. OF EGGER, NGUYEN, SCHAAD, AND KRECH, 1990

Original host: *Felis catus* L., 1758, Domestic Cat.

Remarks: Egger et al. (1990) described intestinal cryptosporidiosis in an 8-year-old boy who suffered from coughing and bronchitis prior to having watery, nonbloody diarrhea, vomiting, and **colics**. The boy became ill during a visit to a dairy farm, where some kittens suffered from diarrhea and showed failure to thrive. The boy's stool was negative for rotaviruses and pathogenic bacteria, but using auramine fluorescence staining, oocysts of *Cryptosporidium* were found both in the stool of the boy and in feces of a skinny kitten he had contact with. This indicated that the infection "was acquired from a cat that had probably been infected by feces from calves."

CRYPTOSPORIDIUM SPP. OF FUNADA, PENA, SOARES, AMAKU, AND GENNARI, 2007

Original host: *Felis catus* L., 1758, Domestic Cat.
Remarks: Funada et al. (2007) examined fecal samples of domestic cats in São Paulo, Brazil. *Cryptosporidium* oocysts were detected in 37/327 (11%) samples, mostly in cats younger than 1-year-old.

CRYPTOSPORIDIUM SP. OF HOOPES, POLLEY, WAGNER, AND JENKINS, 2013

Original host: *Felis catus* L., 1758, Domestic Cat.
Remarks: Hoopes et al. (2013) surveyed fecal samples of cats in Saskatchewan and Alberta, western Canada; 3/635 (0.4%) samples were positive when examined by sucrose flotation, and 6/635 (1%) were positive when examined by a commercial immunofluorescence assay.

CRYPTOSPORIDIUM SP. OF HOOPES, HILL, POLLEY, FERNANDO, WAGNER, SCHURER, AND JENKINS, 2015

Original host: *Felis catus* L., 1758, Domestic Cat.
Remarks: Hoopes et al. (2015) examined fecal samples of rural, free-roaming, and pet cats

from urban areas of Saskatchewan and from a rural region in southwestern Alberta, Canada. *Cryptosporidium* was detected in 11/161 (7%) free-ranging cats, only in Saskatchewan, but not in 31 cats from pet shops in Saskatchewan nor in 27 cats tested from rural Alberta.

CRYPTOSPORIDIUM SP. OF HUBER, BOMFIM, AND GOMES, 2002

Original host: *Felis catus* L., 1758, Domestic Cat.
Remarks: Huber et al. (2002) examined fecal samples of 28 shelter, and 20 household adult cats in Rio de Janeiro, Brazil; all cats were apparently healthy. Oocysts of *Cryptosporidium* were detected in 6/48 (12.5%) samples, 5/20 (25%) household cats, and 1/28 (4%) shelter cats. The authors said that household cats were more parasitized with protozoa, whereas more shelter cats harbored worms.

CRYPTOSPORIDIUM SP. OF KORKMAZ, GOKPINAR, AND YILDIZ, 2016

Original host: *Felis catus* L., 1758, Domestic Cat.
Remarks: Korkmaz et al. (2016) examined fecal samples of pet and stray cats in Kirikkale province, Turkey. Oocysts of *Cryptosporidium* were detected in 1/100 (1%) samples.

CRYPTOSPORIDIUM SP. OF LIM, NGUI, SHUKRI, ROHELA, AND NAIM, 2008

Original host: *Felis chaus* Schreber, 1777, Jungle Cat.
Remarks: Lim et al. (2008) found *Cryptosporidium* oocysts in the feces of 1/3 (33%) jungle cats examined at Zoo Negra, Kuala Lumpur, Malaysia. No other information was given.

CRYPTOSPORIDIUM SPP. OF LUCIO-FORSTER AND BOWMAN, 2011

Original host: *Felis catus* L., 1758, Domestic Cat.

Remarks: Lucio-Forster and Bowman (2011) examined 1,272 fecal samples from two shelters and 50 from foster homes in upstate New York, USA. *Cryptosporidium* oocysts were detected in 50/1,322 (4%) samples.

CRYPTOSPORIDIUM SPP. OF MARKS, HANSON, AND MELLI, 2004

Original host: *Felis catus* L., 1758, Domestic Cat.

Remarks: Marks et al. (2004) examined 416 feces of 104 domestic shorthair kittens, 8–16-weeks-old, in Davis, California, USA, which were naturally-exposed to *Cryptosporidium* spp. The kittens were housed individually, and their fecal samples were collected once daily for four consecutive days. Samples were examined by five diagnostic tests to evaluate and compare their sensitivity: (1) a modified Ziehl-Neelsen acid-fast staining technique (mZN); (2) direct immunofluorescence (DIC) by a commercial kit (Merifluor *Cryptosporidium*/Giardia direct immunofluorescent kit) that used a monoclonal antibody against antigen of *C. parvum*; (3) enzyme immunoassay-1 (EIA-1) that used a monoclonal antibody (Premier *Cryptosporidium* EIA); (4) EIA-2 that used a polyclonal antibody (ProSpecT *Cryptosporidium* microplate assay) and (5) EIA-3 that used a polyclonal antibody (ProSpecT *Cryptosporidium* rapid assay) to detect *Cryptosporidium* antigen in feces. *Cryptosporidium* was detected in at least one test in 101/104 (92%) kittens. Regarding positive cats, 96 (92%) were positive by EIA-2, 91 (88%) by EIA-1, 89 (86%) by mZN, 80 (77%) by DIC, but only 46 (44%) by EIA-3. Similarly, regarding the number of positive samples, 344/416 (83%) were positive by EIA-2, 304/416 (73%) by EIA-1, 259/416 (62%) by mZN, 195/416 (47%) by DIC, and only 77/416 (19%) by EIA-3. Marks et al. (2004) suggested higher sensitivity of mZN over DIC due to the preparation procedure in the manufacturer's guidelines (loss of oocysts during the rinsing procedure), and because oocyst fluorescence intensity was variable. A markedly low sensitivity of EIA-3 was likely caused by its high detection limit compared with that of EIA-1 and EIA-2. To summarize: EIA-2 and EIA-1 had the highest sensitivities when only a single fecal sample was examined, and mZN and EIA-1 had similar sensitivities when two consecutive samples were examined.

CRYPTOSPORIDIUM SPP. OF MEKARU, MARKS, FELLEY, CHOUICHA, AND KASS, 2007

Original host: *Felis catus* L., 1758, Domestic Cat.

Remarks: Mekaru et al. (2007), in northern California, USA, examined feces of 344 diarrheic and nondiarrheic cats from four animal shelters. Samples were examined by three methods to evaluate/compare their specificity and sensitivity: flotation, commercial available enzyme (ProSpecT *Cryptosporidium* Microplate Assay), and nonenzymatic (ImmunoCard STAT! *Cryptosporidium*/*Giardia* Rapid Assay, Xpect *Giardia*/*Cryptosporidium*) immunoassay; these were compared with a reference standard, the MeriFluor direct immunofluorescence assay. They wanted to test the credibility of using human-based immunoassays for the diagnosis of *Cryptosporidium* spp. infections in cats and other animals. *Cryptosporidium* spp. was detected in 14/344 (5%) cats (9/177 diarrheic, 5/177 nondiarrheic). Two diarrheic cats were coinfected with *Giardia*. Flotation only detected 3/14 positive samples; the best specificity and sensitivity was found using the enzyme immunoassay ProSpecT *Cryptosporidium* Microplate Assay.

CRYPTOSPORIDIUM SP. OF MIRZAGHAVAMI, SADRAEI, AND FOROUZANDEH, 2016

Original host: *Felis catus* L., 1758, Domestic Cat.

Remarks: Mirzaghavami et al. (2016) surveyed fecal samples of stray cats in Tehran, Iran. *Cryptosporidium* oocysts, measuring 6.9×4.6, were detected in 5/50 (10%) samples.

CRYPTOSPORIDIUM SPP. OF NUTTER, DUBEY, LEVINE, BREITSCHWERDT, FORD, AND STOSKOPF, 2004

Original host: *Felis catus* L., 1758, Domestic Cat.

Remarks: Nutter et al. (2004) surveyed the blood and fecal samples of feral cats and healthy pet cats (mostly strays or in shelters) in rural Randolph county, North Carolina, USA. Fecal samples were concentrated by sedimentation, and then tested by a commercially-available indirect fluorescent antibody test (Merifluor, Meridian Diagnostics, Cincinnati, Ohio). *Cryptosporidium* was detected in 6/87 (7%) feral and in 4/66 (6%) pet cats. The antibody test reacted with both *C. parvum* and *C. felis* and, thus, was not able to distinguish between these *Cryptosporidium* species.

CRYPTOSPORIDIUM SPP. OF NYAMBURA NJUGUNA, KAGIRA, MUTURI KARANJA, NGOTHO, MUTHARIA, AND WANGARI MAINA, 2017

Original host: *Felis catus* L., 1758, Domestic Cat.

Remarks: Nyambura Njuguna et al. (2017) examined fecal samples of household cats (indoors and outdoors) in Thika, Kiambu county, Kenya. *Cryptosporidium* oocysts were seen in 42/103 (41%) cats.

CRYPTOSPORIDIUM SP. OF OVERGAAUW, VAN ZUTPHEN, HOEK, YAYA, ROELFSEMA, PINELLI, VAN KNAPEN, AND KORTBEEK, 2009

Original host: *Felis catus* L., 1758, Domestic Cat.

Remarks: Overgaauw et al. (2009) surveyed fecal samples of 22 clinically healthy household cats from different provinces in the Netherlands. *Cryptosporidium* sp. was detected in 1 (5%) sample. Genotyping based on PCR of 18S rDNA failed, therefore the species/genotype remained unknown.

CRYPTOSPORIDIUM SPP. OF PALMER, THOMPSON, TRAUB, REES, AND ROBERTSON, 2008a

Original host: *Felis catus* L., 1758, Domestic Cat.

Remarks: Palmer et al. (2008a) surveyed fecal samples of cats from both urban and rural areas across Australia, which were collected from 59 veterinary clinics (572 samples) and 26 refuges (491 samples). *Cryptosporidium* was detected in 23/1,063 (2%) cats, mostly from refuges.

CRYPTOSPORIDIUM SPP. OF PARIS, WILLS, BALZER, SHAW, AND GUNN-MOORE, 2014

Original host: *Felis catus* L., 1758, Domestic Cat.

Remarks: Paris et al. (2014) examined fecal samples of diarrheic cats in the United Kingdom. Samples were examined by the real-time PCR assay for the 18S rRNA gene. *Cryptosporidium* was detected in 265/1,088 (24%) cats, mostly in young animals.

CRYPTOSPORIDIUM SP. OF PAVLÁSEK, 1983

Original hosts: *Bos taurus* L., 1758, Aurochs; *Felis catus* L., 1758, Domestic Cat.

Remarks: Pavlásek (1983) isolated oocysts of *Cryptosporidium* from a 12-day-old calf in the Czech Republic, purified them on a sugar gradient, and inoculated 5×10^5 sporulated oocysts *per os* into a 21-day-old coccidia-free cat and two chickens, and examined their feces for 45 DPI. The cat started to discharge cryptosporidial oocysts 5–12 DPI and diarrhea was observed 5–9 DPI. Chickens discharged oocysts within several hours after the inoculation until 2 DPI, so the author supposed it was just a passage through the gut and that their transmission was not successful.

CRYPTOSPORIDIUM SP. OF POONACHA AND PIPPIN, 1982

Original host: *Felis catus* L., 1758, Domestic Cat.

Remarks: Poonacha and Pippin (1982) reported a case of a 5-year-old male domestic longhair cat suffering from anorexia, weight loss, and persistent diarrhea for 2.5 months. The cat was FeLV negative, and did not respond to treatment with Azithromycin, B-12, B-plex, fluids, and lincocin. Both fecal flotation and direct microscopic examination of feces also were negative. Exploratory surgery followed by necropsy revealed dilatation and thickening of the small intestine and cecum, enlarged mesenteric lymph nodes, fusion of small intestinal villi, increased number of goblet cells, and hyperplastic crypt epithelium with a few dilated cystic crypts containing necrotic cell debris. Changes were apparent only in the small intestine and cecum, where numerous round or ovoidal organisms, 1–3 wide, were found located more in crypts and the lower half of the villi, and only rarely on the villous tips. TEM showed meronts and trophozoites in the lumen and attached to the microvillous border of intestinal epithelial cells. Morphology of the organisms and lesions corresponded to those caused by *Cryptosporidium*.

CRYPTOSPORIDIUM SPP. OF QUEEN, MARKS, AND FARVER, 2012

Original host: *Felis catus* L., 1758, Domestic Cat.

Remarks: Queen et al. (2012) examined feces of 22 different breeds of diarrheic and nondiarrheic cats from northern California, USA, and *Cryptosporidium* was detected in 6/190 (3%) diarrheic and in 0/54 nondiarrheic cats. Younger cats were significantly more likely to be infected.

CRYPTOSPORIDIUM SPP. OF RAMBOZZI, MENZANO, MANNELLI, ROMANO, AND ISAIA, 2007

Original host: *Felis catus* L., 1758, Domestic Cat.

Remarks: Rambozzi et al. (2007) surveyed fecal samples of domestic cats in Turin, Italy. *Cryptosporidium* oocysts were seen in 49/200 (24.5%) samples, mostly in cats <1-year-old, with diarrhea, and concurrently infected with other enteric parasites (*Cystoisospora, Toxocara, Toxascaris*). Oocysts found were spheroidal, 4.5 wide.

CRYPTOSPORIDIUM SPP. OF SABSHIN, LEVY, TUPLER, TUCKER, GREINER, AND LEUTENEGGER, 2012

Original host: *Felis catus* L., 1758, Domestic Cat.

Remarks: Sabshin et al. (2012) surveyed fecal samples of cats in Alachua county, Florida, USA; 50 cats had diarrhea and 50 cats had normal feces. Fecal samples were examined using fecal flotation and RT-PCR assay for *Cryptosporidium* 18S rDNA. *Cryptosporidium* was detected in 5/50 (10%) cats with diarrhea and in 10/50 (20%) cats with normal feces.

CRYPTOSPORIDIUM SP. OF SHUKLA, GIRALDO, KRALIZ, FINNIGAN, AND SANCHEZ, 2006

Original host: *Felis catus* L., 1758, Domestic Cat.

Remarks: Shukla et al. (2006) collected fecal samples from domestic cats in the Niagara Region, Ontario, Canada. Samples were examined by three different methods to test and compare their sensitivity: a concentration method, acid-fast staining, and *Cryptosporidium* EIA (ProSpecT *Cryptosporidum* Microplate Assay). *Cryptosporidium* was detected only by EIA in 3/41 (7%) cats.

CRYPTOSPORIDIUM SPP. OF SPAIN, SCARLETT, WADE, AND MCDONOUGH, 2001

Original host: *Felis catus* L., 1758, Domestic Cat.

Remarks: Spain et al. (2001) surveyed cats, 1–12-month-old, in central New York state, USA. Fecal samples were examined by sugar and zinc-sulfate flotation, and by ELISA kit (ProSpecT *Cryptosporidium* Microplate Assay), with 90% sensitivity, originally developed for use in humans. *Cryptosporidium* oocysts were found in 10/263 (4%) cats, but the number of ELISA-positive cats was not given.

CRYPTOSPORIDIUM SP. OF TYSNES, GJERDE, NØDTVEDT, AND SKANCKE, 2011

Original host: *Felis catus* L., 1758, Domestic Cat.

Remarks: Tysnes et al. (2011) examined feces of clinically healthy cats participating in cat

shows in Norway. *Cryptosporidium* was detected in only 1/52 (2%) samples.

CRYPTOSPORIDIUM SPP. OF TZANNES, BATCHELOR, GRAHAM, PINCHBECK, WASTLING, AND GERMAN, 2008

Original host: *Felis catus* L., 1758, Domestic Cat.

Remarks: Tzannes et al. (2008) examined cat fecal samples from mainland Great Britain, Northern Ireland, the Isle of Man, and the Channel Islands. Three populations of cats were surveyed: (1) 1,355 domestic cats displaying signs of gastrointestinal disease; (2) 48 domestic cats with signs of gastrointestinal disease; and (3) 45 pet cats with no gastrointestinal signs. *Cryptosporidium* was detected only in population No. 1, where 13/1,355 (1%) cats had oocysts of a *Cryptosporidium* in their feces.

CRYPTOSPORIDIUM SP. OF TZIPORI AND CAMPBELL, 1981

Original host: *Felis catus* L., 1758, Domestic Cat.

Remarks: Tzipori and Campbell (1981) did a serosurvey for antibodies to *Cryptosporidium* by an indirect immunofluorescence test of the sera of cats, probably all from the Glasgow area, United Kingdom; they found 20/23 (87%) sera were positive. This was the first serological procedure for the detection of antibodies against *Cryptosporidium*, but there was no attempt to identify the species.

CRYPTOSPORIDIUM SPP. OF UGA, MATSUMURA, ISHIBASHI, YODA, YATOMI, AND KATAOKA, 1989

Original host: *Felis catus* L., 1758, Domestic Cat.

Remarks: Uga et al. (1989) examined rectal contents of cats captured in Hyogo prefecture, Japan. Oocysts of *Cryptosporidium* were detected in 20/507 (4%) cats, mostly in those with diarrhea. Cats suffering from diarrhea shed significantly more oocysts than cats without diarrhea.

CRYPTOSPORIDIUM SPP. OF YANG, YING, MONIS, AND RYAN, 2015

Original host: *Felis catus* L., 1758, Domestic Cat.

Remarks: Yang et al. (2015) examined fecal samples of both kittens and adult cats of different breeds from Perth, Western Australia. Cats originated from a cat refuge center (179), three pet shops (29), a breeding establishment (10), and private homes (127); none of the cats showed any clinical symptoms. Samples were examined by nested PCR amplification and sequencing of the 18S rRNA gene. *Cryptosporidium* was detected in 34/345 (10%) samples; five were identified as *Cryptosporidium* rat genotype III, and one as *Cryptosporidium* related to *C*. rat genotype III. This was the first report of *Cryptosporidium* rat genotype III in cats.

CYSTOISOSPORA RIVOLTA-LIKE OF GATES AND NOLAN, 2009

Definitive host: *Felis catus* L., 1758, Domestic Cat.

Intermediate host: Unknown.

Remarks: Between 1997 and 2007, Gates and Nolan (2009) surveyed fecal samples of cats at the University of Pennsylvania, USA; "*Cystoisospora rivolta*-like" oocysts were detected in 19/1,566 (1%) samples, mostly in cats less than 3-years-old but increased when the cats were >13-years-old.

CYSTOISOSPORA SPP. OF BARUTZKI AND SCHAPER, 2003

Definitive host: *Felis catus* L., 1758, Domestic Cat.
Intermediate host: Unknown.

Remarks: During a survey on endoparasites, Barutzki and Schaper (2003) examined fecal samples of cats in Freiburg, Germany. *Cystoisospora* oocysts were detected in 693/3,167 (22%) samples, and the infection was higher in cats up to 1-year-old.

CYSTOISOSPORA SPP. OF COELHO, DO AMARANTE, DE SOUTELLO, MEIRELES, AND BRESCIANI, 2009

Definitive host: *Felis catus* L., 1758, Domestic Cat.
Intermediate host: Unknown.

Remarks: Coelho et al. (2009) examined fecal samples of cats in Andradina, São Paulo, Brazil. *Cystoisospora* oocysts were reported in 22/51 (43%) samples, but they did not attempt to determine the species.

CYSTOISOSPORA SPP. OF FUNADA, PENA, SOARES, AMAKU, AND GENNARI, 2007

Definitive host: *Felis catus* L., 1758, Domestic Cat.

Intermediate host: Unknown.

Remarks: Funada et al. (2007) examined fecal samples of domestic cats in São Paulo, Brazil. *Cystoisospora* oocysts were detected in 27/327 (8%) samples but no identifications were made.

CYSTOISOSPORA SPP. OF GENNARI, KASAI, PENA, AND CORTEZ, 1999

Definitive host: *Felis catus* L., 1758, Domestic Cat.
Intermediate host: Unknown.

Remarks: Gennari et al. (1999) examined fecal samples of domestic cats from different areas of the city of São Paulo, Brazil. *Cystoisospora* oocysts were detected in 72/187 (38.5%) samples, but no attempt was made to identify the oocysts to species.

CYSTOISOSPORA SP. OF HUBER, BOMFIM, AND GOMEZ, 2002

Definitive host: *Felis catus* L., 1758, Domestic Cat.

Intermediate host: Unknown.

Remarks: Huber et al. (2002) examined fecal samples of healthy adult cats (28 in a shelter, 20 pet cats from six different owners) in Rio de Janeiro, Brazil. Oocysts of a *Cystoisospora* species were detected in 4/48 (8%) samples, all shelter cats, but the species was not identified.

CYSTOISOSPORA SP. OF HUBER, DA SILVA, BOMFIM, TEIXEIRA, AND BELLO, 2007

Definitive host: *Felis catus* L., 1758, Domestic Cat.

Intermediate host: Unknown.

Remarks: Huber et al. (2007) surveyed fecal samples of stray cats in an animal shelter in Nova Iguaçu, Rio de Janeiro State, Brazil; 4/30 (13%) samples were positive for a *Cystoisospora* species. No attempt was made to identify the oocysts.

CYSTOISOSPORA SPP. OF LUCIO-FORSTER AND BOWMAN, 2011

Definitive host: *Felis catus* L., 1758, Domestic Cat.

Intermediate host: Unknown.

Remarks: Lucio-Forster and Bowman (2011) surveyed fecal samples of cats from two shelters (1,272 cats) and affiliated foster homes (50 cats) in upstate New York, USA. *Cystoisospora* oocysts were detected in 278/1,322 (21%) samples, but there was no attempt to identify to species.

CYSTOISOSPORA SPP. OF RAMBOZZI, MENZANO, MANNELLI, ROMANO, AND ISAIA, 2007

Definitive host: *Felis catus* L., 1758, Domestic Cat.

Intermediate host: Unknown.

Remarks: Rambozzi et al. (2007) surveyed fecal samples of domestic cats in Turin, Italy. Oocysts of *Cystoisospora*, not identified to species, were detected in 15/200 (7.5%) samples and 5/200 (2.5%) positive samples were concurrently infected with *Cryptosporidium* oocysts.

CYSTOISOSPORA SPP. OF SABSHIN, LEVY, TUPLER, TUCKER, GREINER, AND LEUTENEGGER, 2012

Definitive host: *Felis catus* L., 1758, Domestic Cat.

Intermediate host: Unknown.

Remarks: Sabshin et al. (2012) surveyed fecal samples of cats in Alachua county, Florida, USA; 50 cats had diarrhea and 50 cats had normal feces. *Cystoisospora* oocysts were detected in 7/50 (14%) cats with diarrhea, and in 5/50 (10%) cats with normal feces.

CYSTOISOSPORA SPP. OF SERRA, UCHÔA, AND COIMBRA, 2003

Definitive host: *Felis catus* L., 1758, Domestic Cat.

Intermediate host: Unknown.

Remarks: Serra et al. (2003) examined fecal samples of domestic and stray cats in Rio de Janeiro, Brazil. *Cystoisospora* oocysts were detected in 57/131 (43.5%) samples, with 8/65 (12%) domestic cats and 49/66 (74%) stray cats demonstrating oocysts in their feces.

EIMERIA SP. OF CHRISTIE, DUBEY, AND PAPPAS, 1976

Original host: *Felis catus* L., 1758, Domestic Cat.

Remarks: Christie et al. (1976) surveyed feces from cats, all >3-months-old, from a humane shelter in Ohio, USA; they found 4/1,000 (0.4%) samples to have oocysts of an *Eimeria* species. After sporulation in 2.5% $K_2Cr_2O_7$ solution, they inoculated ~1,000 oocysts into 16 mice and 2 cats. After 1 month, the mice were fed to 4 SPF cats. None of the 6 cats shed oocysts within the next 30 days. Thus, this must be considered a *species inquirenda*.

EIMERIA SP. OF MILSTEIN AND GOLDSMID, 1997

Original host: *Felis catus* L., 1758, Domestic Cat.

Remarks: Milstein and Goldsmid (1997) surveyed feral cats in southern Tasmania. Rectal fecal samples and intestinal contents at necropsy demonstrated oocysts of an *Eimeria* species in 2/39 (5%) samples.

EIMERIA SP. OF OGASSAWARA, BENASSI, LARSSON, AND HAGIWARA, 1986

Original host: *Felis catus* L., 1758, Domestic Cat.

Remarks: Ogassawara et al. (1986) examined fecal samples of domestic cats from different areas of São Paulo, Brazil. "Coccidia" were found in 73/215 (34%) samples, along with ascarid and hookworm eggs. Oocysts of an *Eimeria* were reported in 1/215 (<0.5%) samples, in an animal 4–6-months-old, but no attempt was made to identify the eimerian.

EIMERIA SP. OF YAMAMOTO, KON, SAITO, MAENO, KOYAMA, SUNAOSHI, YAMAGUCHI, MORISHIMA, AND KAWANAKA, 2009

Original host: *Felis catus* L., 1758, Domestic Cat.

Remarks: Yamamoto et al. (2009) surveyed fecal samples of cats in animal shelters in the Saitama prefecture, Japan. LM examination revealed the presence of *Eimeria* oocysts in 3/1,079 (0.3%) of the samples, but the species identification was not attempted.

HAMMONDIA–TOXOPLASMA OF BARUTZKI AND SCHAPER, 2003

Original host: *Felis catus* L., 1758, Domestic Cat.

Remarks: During a survey of endoparasites, Barutzki and Schaper (2003) examined fecal samples of cats in Freiburg, Germany. They reported *Hammondia–Toxoplasma*-like oocysts in 142/3,167 (4.5%) samples.

HAMMONDIA–TOXOPLASMA OF FUNADA, PENA, SOARES, AMAKU, AND GENNARI, 2007

Original host: *Felis catus* L., 1758, Domestic Cat.

Remarks: Funada et al. (2007) examined fecal samples of domestic cats in São Paulo, Brazil. *Hammondia–Toxoplasma*-like oocysts were detected in 2/327 (<1%) samples.

HAMMONDIA–TOXOPLASMA OF GENNARI, KASAI, PENA, AND CORTEZ, 1999

Original host: *Felis catus* L., 1758, Domestic Cat.

Remarks: Gennari et al. (1999) examined fecal samples of domestic cats from São Paulo,

Brazil. *Hammondia–Toxoplasma*-like oocysts were reported in 3/187 (<2%) samples.

HAMMONDIA–TOXOPLASMA OF PALMER, THOMPSON, TRAUB, REES, AND ROBERTSON, 2008a

Original host: *Felis catus* L., 1758, Domestic Cat.

Remarks: Palmer et al. (2008a) surveyed fecal samples of cats from 59 veterinary clinics (572 samples) and 26 refuges (491 samples), from both urban and rural areas across Australia. *Hammondia–Toxoplasma*-like oocysts (not identified to genus) were detected in only 1/1,063 cats, the one from a refuge.

HAMMONDIA–TOXOPLASMA–BESNOITIA OF SPAIN, SCARLETT, WADE, AND MCDONOUGH, 2001

Original host: *Felis catus* L., 1758, Domestic Cat.

Remarks: Spain et al. (2001) surveyed 1–12-month-old cats in central New York state, USA. Fecal samples from 149 cats in three county shelters and from 144 cats with their primary-care veterinarians were examined and *Toxoplasma*/*Hammondia*/*Besnoitia*-like oocysts were detected incidentally in the fecal flotations of 3/263 (1%) cats, all from the shelters. A serological test confirming the identity of the oocysts was not performed.

HEPATOZOON SP. OF PEREZ, RUBINI, AND O'DWYER, 2004

Original host: *Felis catus* L., 1758, Domestic Cat.

Remarks: Perez et al. (2004) were the first to diagnose *Hepatozoon* sp. in three naturally-infected domestic cats from São Paulo State, Brazil. During a hematological exam, *Hepatozoon* gamonts were identified within polymorphonuclear cells of a cat with renal failure. Two other cats, which lived in the same house, also were positive for this hemoparasite.

ISOSPORA RIVOLTA OF TRIFFITT, 1927

Original host: *Felis catus* L., 1758, Domestic Cat or *Felis silvestris* Schreber, 1777, Wildcat (?).

Remarks: Triffitt (1927) described oocysts from an Eyot cat in the Zoological Gardens, London. Yakimoff et al. (1933b) said that Triffitt found the oocysts in an ocelot, but an Eyot cat is not an ocelot. Aston's Eyot is a 12 ha "island" owned by Christ Church and bordered by the Thames, Cherwell New Cut, and Shire Lake Ditch. It can be approached from Meadow Lane via the Kidneys and across a footbridge, or from Jackdaw Lane off Iffley Road (http://friendsofastonseyot.org.uk/history/). Levine and Ivens (1981) speculated that the cat examined by Triffitt (1927) was either *F. catus* or *F. silvestris*, but although domestic cats sometimes penetrate deep into the Eyot from nearby housing, there is no evidence of feral cats doing so (http://friendsofastonseyot.org.uk/wildlife/197-2/). Oocysts found by Triffitt (1927) were described by her to be L×W: 20–26×14–18, with a M that was distinct, ~3 wide, but oocysts of *I. rivolta* do not have a M, so there is no way to determine what species Triffitt (1927) examined.

ISOSPORA SP. OF BORKATAKI, KATOCH, GOSWAMI, GODARA, KHAJURIA, YADAV, AND KAUR, 2013

Original host: *Felis catus* L., 1758, Domestic Cat.

Remarks: Borkataki et al. (2013) surveyed fecal samples of stray cats in Jammu, a humid subtropical zone in northwestern India. Oocysts of *Isospora* were detected in 80/100 (80%) samples. There was no attempt to identify these oocysts to species, thus a *species inquirenda*.

ISOSPORA SPP. OF COLLINS, EMSLIE, FARROW, AND WATSON, 1983

Original host: *Felis catus* L., 1758, Domestic Cat.
Remarks: Collins et al. (1983) reported *Isospora* spp. in 3/71 (4%) fecal samples from cats in Sydney, Australia, which were examined for "sporozoa." No other information was given.

ISOSPORA SPP. OF EPE, COATI, AND SCHNIEDER, 2004

Original host: *Felis catus* L., 1758, Domestic Cat.
Remarks: Epe et al. (2004), in northern Germany, surveyed fecal samples of cats between 1998 and 2002 and found 47/441 (11%) to pass *Isospora* spp. oocysts, which were not identified further.

ISOSPORA SPP. OF EPE, ISING-VOLMER, AND STOYE, 1993

Original host: *Felis catus* L., 1758, Domestic Cat.
Remarks: Epe et al. (1993), in Germany, surveyed fecal samples from cats between 1984 and 1991 and found 53/1,147 (5%) to pass *Isospora* spp. oocysts, which were not identified to species.

ISOSPORA SPP. OF HOOPES, HILL, POLLEY, FERNANDO, WAGNER, SCHURER, AND JENKINS, 2015

Original host: *Felis catus* L., 1758, Domestic Cat.
Remarks: Hoopes et al. (2015) examined fecal samples of rural, free-roaming, and pet cats

from urban areas of Saskatchewan, and from a rural region in southwestern Alberta, Canada. *Isospora* spp. were detected in 19% rural cats from Alberta, 6% free-ranging cats in Saskatchewan, and in 3% pet cats in Saskatchewan. Moreover, blood was observed in two samples to be positive for *Isospora*.

ISOSPORA SPP. OF KORKMAZ, GOKPINAR, AND YILDIZ, 2016

Original host: *Felis catus* L., 1758, Domestic Cat.
Remarks: Korkmaz et al. (2016) examined fecal samples of owned and stray cats in Kirikkale province, Turkey; oocysts of *Isospora* spp., which were not identified to species, were detected in 31/100 (31%) samples.

ISOSPORA SPP. OF MALLOY AND EMBIL, 1978

Original host: *Felis catus* L., 1758, Domestic Cat.
Remarks: Malloy and Embil (1978) examined fecal samples of stray cats in Halifax, Nova Scotia, Canada. Oocysts of *Isospora* spp. were detected in 19/299 (6%) cats, mostly in young animals 0.5–2-years-old, but no attempt was made to identify the species of these isosporans.

ISOSPORA SP. OF MILSTEIN AND GOLDSMID, 1997

Original host: *Felis catus* L., 1758, Domestic Cat.
Remarks: Milstein and Goldsmid (1997) surveyed feral cats in southern Tasmania. Rectal fecal samples and intestinal contents from necropsy were examined, and oocysts of an *Isospora* sp. were recorded, but not identified, in 3/39 (8%) cats.

ISOSPORA SPP. OF NYAMBURA NJUGUNA, KAGIRA, MUTURI KARANJA, NGOTHO, MUTHARIA, AND WANGARI MAINA, 2017

Original host: *Felis catus* L., 1758, Domestic Cat.
Remarks: Nyambura Njuguna et al. (2017) examined fecal samples of household cats (both indoors and outdoors) in Thika, Kiambu county, central Kenya. Oocysts of *Isospora* spp. were detected in 45/103 (44%) cats but no attempt was made to identify them to species.

ISOSPORA SP. OF SPADA, PROVERBIO, DELLA PEPA, DOMENICHINI, BAGNAGATTI DE GIORGI, TRAIDI, AND FERRO, 2013

Original host: *Felis catus* L., 1758, Domestic Cat.
Remarks: Spada et al. (2013) examined fecal samples of stray colony cats in Milan, Italy. They reported the presence of *Isospora* sp. oocysts in 6/139 (4%) samples. There was no attempt to identify to species.

ISOSPORA SPP. OF LORENZINI, TASCA, AND CARLI, 2007

Original host: *Felis catus* L., 1758, Domestic Cat.
Remarks: Lorenzini et al. (2007) examined fecal samples of 288 cats from different neighborhoods in Porto Alegre, Rio Grande do Sul, Brazil, and they detected the presence of oocysts of *Isospora* spp.

SARCOCYSTIS SP. OF ARBABI AND HOOSHYAR, 2009

Definitive host: *Felis catus* L., 1758, Domestic Cat.
Intermediate host: Unknown.

Remarks: Arbabi and Hooshyar (2009) examined fecal samples of stray cats trapped and necropsied in urban and rural areas of the Kashan region, central Iran. Sporocysts of *Sarcocystis* were detected in 9/113 (8%) samples, in 5 males and 4 females.

SARCOCYSTIS SPP. OF BARUTZKI AND SCHAPER, 2003

Definitive host: *Felis catus* L., 1758, Domestic Cat.
Intermediate host: Unknown.
Remarks: Barutzki and Schaper (2003) examined fecal samples of 3,167 cats in Freiburg, Germany. Sporocysts of *Sarcocystis* were detected in 70/3,167 (2%) samples.

SARCOCYSTIS SP. OF BÖTTNER, CHARLESTON, POMROY, AND ROMMEL, 1987

Definitive host: *Felis catus* L., 1758, Domestic Cat.
Intermediate host: *Bos taurus* L., 1758, Aurochs.
Remarks: Böttner et al. (1987) surveyed muscle samples by LM, TEM, and SEM of 500 beef cattle slaughtered in New Zealand and found 100% to be infected; of these, 399/500 (80%) were infected with thick-walled sarcocysts, but they were not able to distinguish whether these sarcocysts were *S. hirsuta* or *S. hominis*. They took 305 cysts from 31 samples of diaphragm and esophagus, measured them, and examined them via LM, TEM, and SEM; cyst wall thickness was ~5 (2–7) and was normally distributed throughout the cyst. Protrusion widths were ~1.0 (0.6–2.2) and they formed a continuous, though skewed, distribution. They fed these thick-walled cysts to 3 cats and one human volunteer; the human did not pass sporocysts, but 1/3 (33%) cats shed a few sporocysts in its feces on 11–17 DPI. Nonetheless, they chose not to name this form so it must remain a *species inquirenda*, until further study.

SARCOCYSTIS SP. OF CHRISTIE, DUBEY, AND PAPPAS, 1976

Definitive host: *Felis catus* L., 1758, Domestic Cat.

Intermediate host: Unknown.

Remarks: Christie et al. (1976) surveyed feces from cats, all >3-months-old, from a shelter in Ohio, USA, but found only 2/1,000 (0.2%) samples had sporocysts of a *Sarcocystis* species. These sporocysts were orally inoculated into mice on the same day they were collected from cats. The mice were killed 1–6 months PI, and unstained squashes of skeletal muscles and brain were examined for cysts of *Sarcocystis* species and *Toxoplasma*. The remainder of mouse carcasses were homogenized in a blender and force-fed to 29 SPF cats. Neither of the two mice that had sarcocysts were infectious for either mice or cats. This indicated the species was not *S. muris*.

SARCOCYSTIS SP. (DUBEY AND PANDE, 1963b) OF LEVINE AND IVENS, 1981

Synonym: *Cryptosporodial/Coccidial* (sic) bodies of Dubey and Pande, 1963b.

Definitive host: *Felis chaus* Schreber, 1777, Jungle Cat.

Intermediate host: Unknown.

Remarks: Dubey and Pande (1963b) looked at the feces of three *F. chaus* and found coccidian oocysts in two. They said these oocysts represented six species. Three of the forms they identified were already named, *E. cati* Yakimoff, 1933, *E. felina* Nieschulz, 1924b, and *I. rivolta* (Grassi, 1879) Wenyon, 1923, and two of the forms they named as new species, *E. hammondi* and *E. mathurai*. The sixth form they found was thought to represent a species of *Cryptosporidium*, but these "oocysts," of course were sporocysts of a *Sarcocystis* species, and Levine and Ivens (1981) corrected the name. The sporocysts were ellipsoidal and measured L×W: 11×7 (10–12×7–8), L/W ratio, 1.6; the sausage-shaped SZ measured 7–9×1–2 and had

a clear RB at their rounded ends. The presence of an SR was not mentioned but their drawing (their Fig. 16) indicated it consisted of large globules congregated at one end of the SP.

SARCOCYSTIS SP. DUBEY AND STREITEL, 1976c

Definitive host: *Felis catus* L., 1758, Domestic Cat.

Intermediate host: *Bos taurus* L., 1758, Aurochs.

Remarks: Dubey and Streitel (1976c) did cross-infections between dogs, cats, sheep, pigs, and cattle from Iowa or Ohio, USA. Cats fed bovine tissues shed sporocysts in small numbers; two cats had patent periods that lasted for 2 and 12 days after ingesting bovine tissue; sporocysts (n=72) were 12.4×8.5 (11–14×8–11). The sporocysts they measured in cat feces were smaller than those in canine feces after ingesting infected bovine flesh. Fayer et al. (1976) earlier the same year fed 16 cats *Sarcocystis*-infected musculature from bovines, but none of them became infected. Dubey and Streitel (1976c) suggested that separate species of *Sarcocystis* parasitize cattle in different areas of the United States, but they did not suggest a name for any of their *Sarcocystis* species.

SARCOCYSTIS SP. OF EDWARDS, FICKEN, LUTGEN, AND FREY, 1988

Definitive host: Unknown.

Intermediate host: *Felis catus* L., 1758, Domestic Cat.

Remarks: Edwards et al. (1988) reported numerous cysts in a 1.5-year-old cat from College Station, Texas, USA. Sarcocysts were found in muscles of the heart, forelimbs, hind limbs, diaphragm, eyes, and intercostal spaces. Sarcocysts were (n=50): 48 (30–60) wide × 1.5–2.2 long, had a thick wall, and septa subdivided the cyst into compartments, all with banana-shaped bradyzoites that were 7–10 long. TEM showed the primary cyst wall differed slightly from those of sarcocysts found in cats by Kirkpatrick et al. (1986), and now thought to be identical with *S. felis* (Dubey et al., 1992b). Primary cyst walls seen by Edwards et al. (1988) had a Pvm with regularly-spaced, villus projections, which were round in cross-section and all about 1 long, whereas the villus projections of Kirkpatrick et al. (1986) and Dubey et al. (1992b) had shorter, irregularly-spaced projections. This led Edwards et al. (1988) to conclude that the form they saw may be a different species. No inflammatory response was associated with the sarcocysts in any of the muscles examined. This form must also be relegated to a *species inquirenda*.

SARCOCYSTIS SP. OF EINSTEIN AND INNES, 1956

Definitive host: Unknown.
Intermediate host: *Felis catus* L., 1758, Domestic Cat.
Remarks: Levine and Ivens (1981) say that Einstein and Innes (1956) found sarcocysts in the striated muscles of a cat. We do not have, nor can we find a copy of, this reference.

SARCOCYSTIS SPP. OF EPE, ISING-VOLMER, AND STOYE, 1993

Definitive host: *Felis catus* L., 1758, Domestic Cat.
Intermediate host: Unknown.
Remarks: Epe et al. (1993), in Germany, surveyed fecal samples from cats between 1984 and 1991 and found 3/1,147 (0.3%) to have sporocysts of *Sarcocystis*, which were not identified to species.

SARCOCYSTIS SP. OF FUNADA, PENA, SOARES, AMAKU, AND GENNARI, 2007

Definitive host: *Felis catus* L., 1758, Domestic Cat.
Intermediate host: Unknown.

Remarks: Funada et al. (2007) examined fecal samples of domestic cats in São Paulo, Brazil. *Sarcocystis* sporocysts were detected in 6/327 (2%) samples, but no other information was given.

SARCOCYSTIS SPP. OF GENNARI, KASAI, PENA, AND CORTEZ, 1999

Definitive host: *Felis catus* L., 1758, Domestic Cat.
Intermediate host: Unknown.
Remarks: Gennari et al. (1999) examined fecal samples of domestic cats from São Paulo, Brazil. Sporocysts of *Sarcocystis* were found in 16/187 (9%) samples.

SARCOCYSTIS SP. OF HUBER, DA SILVA, BOMFIM, TEIXEIRA, AND BELLO, 2007

Definitive host: *Felis catus* L., 1758, Domestic Cat.
Intermediate host: Unknown.
Remarks: Huber et al. (2007) surveyed fecal samples of cats (originally stray) from an animal shelter in Nova Iguaçu, Rio de Janeiro State, Brazil. Cat fecal samples were collected from the floor of the cat shelter; only 1/30 (3%) was positive for *Sarcocystis* sporocysts.

SARCOCYSTIS SPP. OF JANITSCHKE, PROTZ, AND WERNER, 1976

Definitive host: *Felis catus* L., 1758, Domestic Cat.
Intermediate host: *Nanger granti* (Brooke, 1872) (syn. *Gazella granti*), Grant's Gazelle.
Remarks: Janitschke et al. (1976) found sarcocysts in Grant's gazelle in Tanzania, fed infected flesh to both cats and dogs, and reported finding sporocysts and sporulated oocysts in the feces of both. Sporocysts shed by the cat were L×W: 13×9 (11–16×8–12), L/W ratio, 1.4; the prepatent period

in cats was 20 days and patency lasted 44–48 days. Janitschke et al. (1976) thought they were dealing with two *Sarcocystis* species, but without further infection and/or molecular studies, it is not possible to tell which one was which. Therefore, these must remain *species inquirendae* until they can be differentiated and named. There are at least three *Sarcocystis* species that have been named from gazelles, but only from sarcocysts in their muscle tissues. All three, *S. gazellae* Balfour, 1913, *S. mongolica* Matschoulsky, 1947a,b, and *S. woodhousei* Dogel, 1916, are mentioned in Levine (1986) and in Dubey et al. (2015a), but the carnivore definitive host is not known for any of them. Clearly a lot of work still needs to be done just sorting out the various *Sarcocystis* species in gazelles.

SARCOCYSTIS SP. OF LUCIO-FORSTER AND BOWMAN, 2011

Definitive host: *Felis catus* L., 1758, Domestic Cat.

Intermediate host: Unknown.

Remarks: Lucio-Forster and Bowman (2011) surveyed fecal samples of cats from two shelters (1,272 samples) and their affiliated foster homes (50 samples) in upstate New York, USA. *Sarcocystis* sporocysts were detected in 11/1,322 (<1%) samples. Determination was based on microscopy and morphology, and there was no attempt to identify to species.

SARCOCYSTIS SPP. OF MCKENNA AND CHARLESTON, 1980a

Definitive host: *Felis catus* L., 1758, Domestic Cat.

Intermediate host: Unknown.

Remarks: McKenna and Charleston (1980a) working on the North Island, New Zealand, examined fecal samples from domestic cats and identified sporocysts of *Sarcocystis* in 86/508 (17%) samples. There was no attempt to identify to species.

SARCOCYSTIS SP. MUNDAY, MASON, HARTLEY, PRESIDENTE, AND OBENDORF, 1978

Definitive host: *Felis catus* L., 1758, Domestic Cat.

Intermediate host: Unknown.

Remarks: Munday et al. (1978) examined muscle samples from 1,497 Australian mammals including 3 red foxes (*Vulpes vulpes*) and 27 brown fur seals (*Arctocephalus pusillus* (syn. *S. doriferus*)), but all 30 were negative. They also examined intestinal mucosal scrapings or feces from 55 feral cats and found small numbers of sporocysts in 1, and these measured 13–14 × 8.5. They (1978) concluded the sporocysts were "typical of *Sarcocystis* or Frenkelia."

SARCOCYSTIS SP. OF OGASSAWARA, BENASSI, LARSSON, AND HAGIWARA, 1986

Definitive host: *Felis catus* L., 1758, Domestic Cat.

Intermediate host: Unknown.

Remarks: Ogassawara et al. (1986) examined fecal samples of domestic cats from different areas of São Paulo, Brazil and reported finding sporocysts of *Sarcocystis* in 18/215 (8%) fecal samples, mostly in animals 4–6-months-old (their Table 2).

SARCOCYSTIS SP. OF SERRA, UCHÔA, AND COIMBRA, 2003

Definitive host: *Felis catus* L., 1758, Domestic Cat.

Intermediate host: Unknown.

Remarks: Serra et al. (2003) examined fecal samples of 65 household and 66 stray cats in Rio de Janeiro, Brazil. *Sarcocystis* sporocysts were seen in 1/131 (<1%) cats, from one household.

SARCOCYSTIS SP. OF WALLACE, 1975

Definitive host: *Felis catus* L., 1758, Domestic Cat (?).

Intermediate host: *Mus musculus* L., 1758, House Mouse.

Remarks: Wallace (1975) looked at two morphologically different cysts in mouse skeletal muscles, which resulted when he inoculated them "with fecal material from a stray cat containing *Isospora*-type oocysts." The most common cyst type turned out to belong to *T. gondii*, which he confirmed by feeding the cysts to lab cats that produced oocysts that were 13 × 11 and resembled those of *T. gondii*. The second type of cyst found in mouse skeletal muscles was "observed in only a few mice, contained bradyzoites resembling those of *Sarcocystis*, but the oocyst or sporocyst that gave rise to it was overlooked and apparently lost."

TOXOPLASMA-LIKE OF EPE, COATI, AND SCHNIEDER, 2004

Original host: *Felis catus* L., 1758, Domestic Cat.

Remarks: Epe et al. (2004), in northern Germany, surveyed fecal samples of cats from 1998 to 2002 and found 3/441 (<1%) to pass *Toxoplasma*-like oocysts, which did not "fit" in any particular genus.

TOXOPLASMA-LIKE OF LUCIO-FORSTER AND BOWMAN, 2011

Original host: *Felis catus* L., 1758, Domestic Cat.

Remarks: Lucio-Forster and Bowman (2011) surveyed fecal samples of cats from two shelters (1,272 samples) and their affiliated foster homes (50 samples) in upstate New York, USA. "*Toxoplasma*-like" oocysts were detected in 11/1,322 (<1%) samples. Determination was based only on general morphology.

TOXOPLASMA-LIKE OF NYAMBURA NJUGUNA, KAGIRA, MUTURI KARANJA, NGOTHO, MUTHARIA, AND WANGARI MAINA, 2017

Original host: *Felis catus* L., 1758, Domestic Cat.

Remarks: Nyambura Njuguna et al. (2017) examined fecal samples of household cats in the Thika region, Kiambu county, central Kenya. *Toxoplasma*-like oocysts of uncertain etiology were detected in 5/103 (5%) cats. However, these samples were *Toxoplasma*-negative by both mouse bioassay and PCR. Thus, it could have been *Hammondia* species.

HAMMONDIA–TOXOPLASMA OF BORKATAKI, KATOCH, GOSWAMI, GODARA, KHAJURIA, YADAV, AND KAUR 2013

Original host: *Felis catus* L., 1758, Domestic Cat.

Remarks: Borkataki et al. (2013) studied fecal samples from stray cats in Jammu, a humid subtropical zone in northwestern India. Oocysts of *Toxoplasma*/*Hammondia* (not distinguished) were detected in 88/100 (88%) samples.

HAMMONDIA–TOXOPLASMA OF CHRISTIE, DUBEY, AND PAPPAS, 1976

Original host: *Felis catus* L., 1758, Domestic Cat.

Remarks: Christie et al. (1976) surveyed intestinal parasites of cats, all >3-months-old, from a shelter in Columbus, Ohio, USA. "*Toxoplasma*-like" oocysts, 12 × 11, were detected in 9/1,000 (0.9%) cats. The oocysts were orally inoculated into mice, then the inoculated mice were fed to SPF cats; 1 SPF cat began to shed similar oocysts in its feces.

GENUS *LEOPARDUS* GRAY, 1842 (9 SPECIES)

CRYPTOSPORIDIUM SP. OF HOLSBACK, CARDOSO, FAGNANI, AND PATELLI, 2013

Original host: *Leopardus tigrinus* (Schreber, 1775), Oncilla.

Remarks: Holsback et al. (2013) found oocysts of *Cryptosporidium* in fecal samples of two oncillas at the wild animal rehabilitation center in the state of São Paulo, Brazil, using flotation–centrifugation. No other information was given.

HEPATOZOON SP. OF MERCER, JONES, RAPPOLE, TWEDT, LAACK, AND CRAIG, 1988

Original host: *Leopardus pardalis* (L., 1758), Ocelot.

Remarks: Mercer et al. (1988) collected blood samples from ocelots trapped in Cameron and Willacy counties, Texas, USA; the authors found 6/13 (46%) samples infected with a *Hepatozoon* species. They made no attempt to name or identify the species.

HEPATOZOON SP. OF METZGER, DOS SANTOS PADUAN, RUBINI, DE OLIVEIRA, PEREIRA, AND O'DWYER, 2008

Original hosts: *Leopardus pardalis* (L., 1758), Ocelot; *Leopardus tigrinus* (Schreber, 1775), Oncilla or Little Spotted Cat; *Leopardus wiedii* (Schinz, 1821) Margay.

Remarks: Metzger et al. (2008) collected blood samples from 29 non-domestic neotropical felids in northeastern Brazil and found an ocelot, a little spotted cat, and a margay

infected with an *Hepatozoon* species. They confirmed each infection by light microscopy and molecular analysis of partial sequences of the 18S rRNA gene of *Hepatozoon*, but no specific identification was attempted.

ISOSPORA SP. OF PATTON, RABINOWITZ, RANDOLPH, AND JOHNSON, 1986

Original host: *Leopardus pardalis* (L., 1758), Ocelot.

Remarks: Patton et al. (1986) did a coprological survey of parasites of wild neotropical Felidae from the Cockscomb Basin, Belize, Central America and said they found oocysts of an *Isospora* species in 3/8 (37.5%) fecal samples from ocelots. No other information was given.

GENUS *LEPTAILURUS* SEVERTZOV, 1858 (MONOTYPIC)

ISOSPORA FELIS OF MACKINNON AND DIBB, 1938

Original host: *Leptailurus serval* (Schreber, 1776) (syn. *Felis serval* Schreber, 1776), Serval.

Remarks: Mackinnon and Dibb (1938) looked at the feces of several serval at the London Zoo and reported oocysts they identified as those of *I. felis*. However, the oocysts they measured were 26–33 × 22–27, with sporocysts only 13 in mean length. They indicated the oocysts were partially sporulated when passed by their hosts. However, both the oocysts, and especially the sporocysts, are too small to be those of *I. felis* (now *C. felis*) and they are larger than those of *I. rivolta* (now *C. rivolta*). Levine and Ivens (1981) suggested these oocysts belong to a separate (unknown) species. We agree. It can only be relegated to a *species inquirenda*.

GENUS *LYNX* KERR, 1752 (4 SPECIES)

CRYPTOSPORIDIUM SPP. OF CARVER, SCORZA, BEVINS, RILEY, CROOKS, VANDEWOUDE, AND LAPPIN, 2012

Original host: *Lynx rufus* (Schreber, 1777), Bobcat.

Remarks: Carver et al. (2012) collected fecal samples from 141 bobcats in California (Ventura county) and Colorado (Front Range and Western Slope), USA. Samples were examined by flotation and direct immunofluorescence followed by PCR assays, but the authors did not specify what genes were amplified (!) and the PCR amplification failed. The authors said they detected *Cryptosporidium* across all studied sites but did not provide the number of positive animals nor the prevalence.

CRYPTOSPORIDIUM SP. OF ZIEGLER, WADE, SCHAAF, STERN, NADARESKI, AND MOHAMMED, 2007

Original host: *Lynx rufus* (Schreber, 1777), Bobcat.

Remarks: Ziegler et al. (2007) examined fecal samples from bobcats in southeastern New York state, USA, by flotation and LM, and by polyclonal *Cryptosporidium* antigen-capture ELISA (considered positive based on an optical density ≥0.050). *Cryptosporidium* was found in 1/14 (7%) samples, but not identified to species.

EIMERIA LYNCIS OF ANPILOGOVA AND SOKOV, 1973

Original host: *Lynx lynx isabellinus* (Blyth, 1847), Central Asian Lynx.

Remarks: Levine and Ivens (1981) listed this eimerian as having been described by Anpilogova and Sokov (1973) from Tadzhikistan (former USSR). They said the ellipsoidal oocysts measured 33×23 (30–38×19–27) and had a bilayered wall with a M in the inner wall. However, neither pair of authors provided a line drawing or photomicrograph; thus, it can only be a *species inquirenda*.

EIMERIA SP. OF ANPILOGOVA AND SOKOV, 1973

Original host: *Lynx lynx isabellinus* (Blyth, 1847), Central Asian Lynx.

Remarks: Levine and Ivens (1981) listed this eimerian as having been described by Anpilogova and Sokov (1973) from Tadzhikistan (former USSR). They said the elongate-ovoidal oocysts were truncated at the M and measured 40.5×27, with sporocysts that were 13.5×11, with no other information. Neither pair of authors provided a line drawing or a photomicrograph; thus, it can only be considered a *species inquirenda*.

EIMERIA TADZHIKISTANICA OF ANPILOGOVA AND SOKOV, 1973

Original host: *Lynx lynx isabellinus* (Blyth, 1847), Central Asian Lynx.

Remarks: Levine and Ivens (1981) listed this *eimerian* as having been described by Anpilogova and Sokov (1973) from Tadzhikistan (former USSR). They said the ovoidal oocysts measured L × W: 31.0×23.5 (24–32×19–27), with a 2-layered wall and without a M, OR, PG. Neither pair of authors provided a line drawing or photomicrograph; thus, a *species inquirenda*.

HEPATOZOON SP. OF LANE AND KOCAN, 1983

Original host: *Lynx rufus* (Schreber, 1777), Bobcat.

Remarks: Lane and Kocan (1983) reported a *Hepatozoon* species infection in bobcats. No other information was given.

HEPATOZOON SP. OF MERCER, JONES, RAPPOLE, TWEDT, LAACK, AND CRAIG, 1988

Original host: *Lynx rufus* (Schreber, 1777), Bobcat.

Remarks: Mercer et al. (1988) collected blood samples from bobcats trapped in Aransa, LaSalle, Cameron, Starr, and Willacy counties, Texas, USA. They found that 3/20 (15%) were infected with a *Hepatozoon* species but made no attempt to name or identify the species.

ISOSPORA BIGEMINA LARGE FORM OF DUSZYNSKI AND SPEER, 1976

Original host: *Lynx rufus* (Schreber, 1777), Bobcat.

Remarks: In 1972, Dr. David Worley, Montana State University, Bozeman, Montana, USA collected feces from a bobcat and sent it to Duszynski, the University of New Mexico, Albuquerque, USA. Duszynski and Speer (1976) found oocysts they called *I. bigemina* large form and were among the first to use them to look at *in vitro* excystation of sporocysts that lack Stieda bodies. The oocysts and sporocysts were, of course, an unknown species of *Sarcocystis*. Although the species from the bobcat remains a *species inquirenda*, the interesting observation was that during excystation, the walls of the sporocyst collapsed, apparently along predetermined lines, allowing sporozoites to escape. As the sporocyst collapsed, the wall separated into two halves, each with two pieces attached together at a point corresponding to one pole of the original sporocyst.

ISOSPORA LYNCIS LEVINE AND IVENS, 1981

Synonym: *Isospora felis* (Wasielewski, 1904) Wenyon, 1923.

Original host: *Lynx* sp., Bobcat.

Remarks: Triffitt (1927) said she found oocysts of an *Isospora* in the rectal contents of a lynx that died in the Zoological Gardens, London, but did not specify the host species (*L. lynx* or *L. canadensis*). She did state that its oocysts were identical to those of *I. felis*, but that they had a M, which those of *I. felis* lack. Based on that difference, Levine and Ivens (1981) named the form partially described by Triffitt (1927) as *I. lyncis* because she also gave some mensural data. Triffitt (1927) said the oocysts were ovoidal, 40–47 × 28–37, and had an oocyst wall with 3-layers, ~0.75 thick, and a M, ~4–5 wide; ovoidal SP were 20–33 × 14–18, with a SR, and SZ measured 15 long, with a large RB at their more rounded end and a smaller one at their more pointed end. Triffitt (1927) said that sporulation was completed in 7–9 days at room temperature. However, neither Triffitt (1927) nor Levine and Ivens (1981) provided a line drawing or a photomicrograph. Thus, there is no evidence that this species actually exists, so the name only can be a *species inquirenda*.

SARCOCYSTIS SP. OF DUBEY, 1982b

Definitive host: *Lynx rufus* (Schreber, 1777), Bobcat.

Intermediate host: Unknown.

Remarks: Dubey (1982b) surveyed the feces for coccidians from a variety of wild carnivores from Montana, USA. He reported sporocysts of *Sarcocystis* in the feces of 2/61 (3%) bobcats. No attempt was made to identify the species beyond genus; thus, a *species inquirenda*.

GENUS *PRIONAILURUS* SEVERTZOV, 1858 (5 SPECIES)

SARCOCYSTIS SP. OF KUBO AND KUNIYOSHI, 2014

Definitive host: Unknown.

Intermediate host: *Prionailurus bengalensis*, Tsushima Leopard Cat.

Remarks: Kubo and Kuniyoshi (2014) examined tissues from wild Tsushima leopard cats in Japan; 5/36 (14%) had cysts presumed to be *Sarcocystis* in their muscles. Cysts were 33–745 × 17–65, cyst walls were 1.4–1.7 thick, and there were numerous finger-like protrusions. No attempt was made to identify the species beyond genus; thus, it must be considered a *species inquirenda*.

GENUS *PUMA* JARDINE, 1834 (2 SPECIES)

HEPATOZOON SP. OF METZGER, DOS SANTOS PADUAN, RUBINI, DE OLIVEIRA, PEREIRA, AND O'DWYER, 2008

Original host: *Puma yagouaroundi* (É. Geoffroy Saint-Hilaire, 1803), Jaguarundi.

Remarks: Metzger et al. (2008) collected blood samples from 29 non-domestic neotropical felids in northeastern Brazil and found a jaguarundi infected with an *Hepatozoon* species. They confirmed this infection by light microscopy and molecular analysis of partial sequences of the 18S rRNA gene of *Hepatozoon*, but no specific identification was attempted.

SARCOCYSTIS SP. OF DUBEY, 1982b

Definitive host: *Puma* (syn. *Felis*) *concolor* (L., 1771), Puma, Cougar.

Intermediate host: Unknown.

Remarks: Dubey (1982b) surveyed feces for coccidians from a variety of wild carnivores in Montana, USA and reported sporocysts of *Sarcocystis* in 2/12 (17%) pumas. Sporocysts were 11.5–13.0 × 7.5–8.8. No attempt was made to identify the species beyond genus; thus, a *species inquirenda*.

SARCOCYSTIS SP. OF KLUGE, 1967

Definitive host: Unknown.

Intermediate host: *Puma* (syn. *Felis*) *concolor* (L., 1771), Puma, Cougar.

Remarks: Kluge (1967) found sarcocysts in the skeletal muscles of a 13-year-old puma that died in the National Zoological Park, Washington, D.C., USA. Sarcocysts, examined with LM, had a thin wall, composed of a single layer without septa projecting from the internal surface. The cyst contained numerous banana-shaped structures (bradyzoites?), "each of which had a round to oval subterminal nucleus and small basophilic granules within the cytoplasm." Kluge (1967) said these cysts "replaced approximately two-thirds of the sarcoplasm in the slightly swollen affected muscle bundles," but that no inflammatory reaction was seen. No other information and no measurements were given, but because he reported "no septa" to be present, it is unlikely that this form can be attributed to *S. felis*, so it must be considered a *species inquirenda*.

SUBFAMILY PANTHERINAE POCOCK, 1917

GENUS *PANTHERA* (L., 1758) (4 SPECIES)

APICOMPLEXAN PROTOZOA OF BJORK, AVERBECK, AND STROMBERG, 2000

Original host: *Panthera leo* (L., 1758) (syn. *Leo leo* Frisch, 1775), Lion.

Remarks: Bjork et al. (2000) published, "the first documentation of enteric parasites in a wild population of African lions in the Serengeti region" of northern Tanzania, Africa. They collected 33 freshly deposited fecal samples from wild lions, preserved them in 10% formalin, and examined both direct smears and fecal flotations for transmission stages. They said they found the following apicomplexans: *Eimeria* sp. in 1 lion, *Isospora felis* in 16, *I. rivolta* in 2, *Isospora* sp. in 1, *Sarcocystis* sp. in 15, and *Toxoplasma*-like oocysts in 4 samples. Unfortunately, they made these spurious identifications by measuring only one or a few oocysts, and all oocysts (except the oocysts/sporocysts of *Sarcocystis*) were unsporulated, which, of course, makes their identifications to genus completely unreliable, if not impossible.

APICOMPLEXAN PROTOZOA OF PATTON AND RABINOWITZ, 1994

Original hosts: *Panthera pardus* (L., 1758), Leopard; *Panthera tigris* (L., 1758), Tiger; *Panthera tigris bengalensis* (L., 1758), Bengal Tiger.

Remarks: Patton and Rabinowitz (1994) did a coprological survey of wild felids in Thailand and preserved the feces in 10% formalin, but made no mention that they took time to sporulate potential oocysts that may have been in their samples. Nonetheless, they reported finding *Isospora*-like oocysts that measured 40 × 32 in 2/54 (4%) *P. pardus* and in 1/3 (33%) *P. t. bengalensis*; *Isospora*-like oocysts that were 20 × 20 in 4/54 (7%) *P. pardus*; *Toxoplasma*-like oocysts in 1/54 (2%) *P. pardus*; *Sarcocystis* spp. oocysts/sporocysts in 11/54 (20%) *P. pardus* and 7/19 (37%) *P. tigris*. These generalist determinations to genus seem completely unreliable to us.

COCCIDIA SP. OF MÜLLER-GRAF, 1995

Original host: *Panthera leo* (L., 1758) (syn. *Leo leo* Frisch, 1775), Lion.

Remarks: Müller-Graf (1995) conducted a coprological survey of intestinal parasites of wild *P. leo* in the Serengeti and the Ngorongoro Crater, Tanzania, East Africa. She examined feces from lions and found "Coccidia" in 59/112 (53%) samples. No other information was given on the oocysts she saw.

COCCIDIA SP. OF DUBEY AND JARDINE, 2008

Original host: *Panthera leo* (L., 1758) (syn. *Leo leo* Frisch, 1775), Lion.

Remarks: Dubey and Jardine (2008) examined formalin-fixed tissues of a <2-day-old captive-born lion cub, *P. leo*, from Pretoria, South Africa. Meronts, merozoites, gamonts, and unsporulated oocysts were found in epithelial cells of the cub's ileum and examined by LM and TEM. Endogenous stages did not stain with antibodies to *T. gondii* and/or *N. caninum* and the morphology and size of various tissue stages eliminated *I.* (syn. *C.*) *felis* and *I.* (syn. *C.*) *rivolta* as suspects. Stages also differed from those of *H. hammondi*, and *H. hammondi* is not known to be transmitted transplacentally, nor are felids suspected to be definitive hosts of *N. caninum*. The age of the cub and the advanced development of the parasite supported the assumption that it was acquired in utero but no identification was/could be made. This seems a great opportunity for a future research project but, until then, it must be considered a *species inquirenda*.

CRYPTOSPORIDIUM SP. OF KARANIS, PLUTZER, HALIM, IGORI, NAGASAWA, ONGERTH, AND LIQING, 2007

Original host: *Panthera pardus* (L., 1758), Leopard.

Remarks: Karanis et al. (2007) examined feces of *P. pardus* in the Xining Zoo, Qinghai province, China, using an immunofluorescence test, nested PCR, and sequencing of a partial 18S rRNA gene; they reported *Cryptosporidium* oocysts in *P. pardus* and said they were *C. parvum* mouse genotype. Neither the number of examined leopards nor their origin was given.

CRYPTOSPORIDIUM SP. OF LIM, NGUI, SHUKRI, ROHELA, AND NAIM, 2008

Original host: *Panthera tigris corbetti*, Indochinese Tiger.

Remarks: Lim et al. (2008) said they found oocysts of a *Cryptosporidium* sp. in the feces of 1/3 (33%) Indochinese tigers examined at Zoo Negra, Kuala Lumpur, Malaysia. No other information was given.

CRYPTOSPORIDIUM SP. OF LIM, NGUI, SHUKRI, ROHELA, AND NAIM, 2008

Original host: *Panthera tigris jacksoni*, Malayan Tiger.

Remarks: Lim et al. (2008) said they found oocysts of a *Cryptosporidium* sp. in the feces of 1/3 (33%) Malayan tigers examined at Zoo Negra, Kuala Lumpur, Malaysia. No other information was given.

CRYPTOSPORIDIUM SP. OF LIM, NGUI, SHUKRI, ROHELA, AND NAIM, 2008

Original host: *Panthera tigris sumatrae*, Sumatran Tiger.

Remarks: Lim et al. (2008) said they found oocysts of a *Cryptosporidium* sp. in the feces of 1/3 (33%) Sumatran tigers examined at Zoo Negra, Kuala Lumpur, Malaysia. No other information was given.

CRYPTOSPORIDIUM SP. OF WANG AND LIEW, 1990

Original host: *Panthera* (?), identified only as "leopard."

Remarks: Wang and Liew (1990) reported oocysts of *Cryptosporidium* in a "leopard" from a bird park in Taiwan; the oocysts were detected in a fecal smear stained with modified Ziehl-Neelsen karbolfuchsin. No other information was given.

EIMERIA NOVOWENYONI OF RASTÉGAÏEFF, 1929a

Original host: *Panthera tigris* (L., 1758), Tiger (?).

Remarks: Rastégaïeff (1929a) in a "note preliminaire" reported finding oocysts of this form in the feces of a tiger (species name not given) of the Zoological Gardens of Leningrad. She described the oocysts as spheroidal, 14–15 wide, without a M. She gave no other structural information other than it had four sporocysts. Rajasekariah et al. (1971) reported that they found this same "species" in a captured "panther" cub kept at the Dharmaram College, Bangalore, India and that it had spheroidal oocysts, 18–20 wide, with a 2-layered wall, ~2.0 thick, and without a M, OR, PG, SB, SR but that it had ellipsoidal SP, 10×6, with SZ that measured 8×4. They also reported another eimerian, *E. anekalensis*, which they described as new, also from this panther (see Chapter 10, Felidae). It is questionable whether this poorly described form can be a parasite of both the tiger and the leopard. It is likely not a parasite of either, in our opinion.

HEPATOZOON SP. OF BROCKLESBY, 1971

Original host: *Panthera leo* (L., 1758), Lion.

Remarks: Brocklesby (1971) illustrated only a gamont/gametocyte in a granulocyte (PMN) of an east African lion; its size was given as 8.5 (8–10).

HEPATOZOON SP. OF KEYMER AND BROCKLESBY, 1971

Original host: *Panthera pardus* (L., 1758), Leopard.

Remarks: Keymer and Brocklesby (1971) described intraleukocytic gametocytes and extracellular forms of a *Hepatozoon* species in the blood, and two forms of meronts of a *Hepatozoon* in *P. pardus* from central Africa. Meronts were found, both in cardiac muscle and lungs. They said that the gametocytes were indistinguishable from *H. canis* of the dog, but unlike the *Hepatozoon* of the dog, no meronts were found in liver, bone marrow, spleen, or lymph nodes. This was the first description of *Hepatozoon* meronts from a leopard, but its actual identity remains a mystery.

HEPATOZOON SP. OF KRAMPITZ, SACHS, SCHALLER, AND SCHINDLER, 1968

Original host: *Panthera leo massaica* (Neumann, 1900), Massai Lion.

Remarks: Krampitz et al. (1968) said that about 28/56 (50%) Massai lions had "gametocytes in its monocytes, which differed from all other species described so far."

ISOSPORA RIVOLTA-LIKE OF MANDAL AND CHOUDHURY, 1983

Original host: *Panthera pardus* (L., 1758), Leopard.

Remarks: Mandal and Choudhury (1983) collected feces from one *P. pardus*, in the Betla Forest Palamau Tiger Reserve, Bihar, India. They incubated the sample in 2%–2.5% potassium dichromate solution and concentrated oocysts via centrifugation. They found ovoidal isosporan oocysts with a 2-layered wall, ~0.9 thick,

that measured, L × W: 29.2 × 23.4 (26–31 × 22–24), L/W ratio: 1.2; M, OR, PG: all absent. Sporocysts were spheroidal, 15.3 (12–17); L/W ratio: 1.0; SB, SSB, PSB: all absent, but SR was present as a large, granular, spheroidal mass, 5.8 (5–7) wide; SZ were banana-shaped, 10.3 × 2.6 (7.5–10 × 2–3), with a prominent RB at the broad end. They chose only to identify the oocysts measured as *I. rivolta*-like. Its true identity is anyone's guess.

ISOSPORA SP. OF CHAUHAN, BHATIA, ARORA, AGRAWAL, AND AHLUWALIA, 1973

Original hosts: *Panthera leo* (L., 1758), Lion; *Panthera tigris* (L., 1758), Tiger.

Remarks: Chauhan et al. (1973) did a "preliminary survey" of parasitic infections among mammals and birds at the Lucknow Zoological Garden, India and reported finding *Isospora* sp. oocysts in the feces of *P. leo* and *P. tigris*, but the number of lions and tigers examined was not stated.

ISOSPORA SP. OF HOU, HUA, LIU, ZENG, CHAI, SUN, LIU, AND XIA, 2008

Original host: *Panthera tigris altaica* Temminck, 1844, Tiger.

Remarks: Hou et al. (2008) found coccidian oocysts in a naturally-infected tiger in China; based on morphology, sporulation, and phylogenetic analysis, they concluded the coccidian from their tiger was *Isospora*. No other information was given.

ISOSPORA SP. OF PANDE, BHATIA, CHAUHAN, AND GARG, 1970

Original host: *Panthera leo* (L., 1758), Lion.

Remarks: Pande et al. (1970) examined feces of 23 mammal species in the Zoological Gardens, Lucknow, India for coccidian oocysts, including four samples from zoo lions, two of which had isosporan oocysts in them. Ovoidal oocysts were L×W (n=30): 26×22 (23–33×20–28), L/W ratio: 1.2 (1.1–1.4); the oocyst wall was 2-layered, ~1.3 thick, and lacked M, OR, PG. Sporocysts were ellipsoidal, 17×12 (16–18×11–13), L/W ratio: 1.4; SB, SSB, PSB: all absent, but SR was present and SZ were banana-shaped, 13×4 (12–15×3–9), with a central N and a prominent RB at the broad end. Pande et al. (1970) compared their sporulated oocysts to those of *I. felis*, *I. laidlawi*, and *I. leonine* and thought theirs was sufficiently different. Nonetheless, they wrote, "It is not possible to assign present material categorically to any of these" and, "pending the availability of more material, these oocysts are, therefore described under an unnamed species, *Isospora* sp." Levine and Ivens (1981) questioned whether or not this is a true parasite of the lion, and so do we. This morphotype has not been seen or described since its original discovery, but if it is found again and, indeed, is a true parasite of the lion, it must be placed in the *Cystoisospora*.

ISOSPORA SP. OF PATTON, RABINOWITZ, RANDOLPH, AND JOHNSON, 1986

Original host: *Panthera pardus* (L., 1758), Leopard.
Remarks: Patton et al. (1986) did a coprological survey of neotropical felids in Belize; they found oocysts of an *Isospora* species in the feces of 2/25 (8%) jaguars from the Cockscomb Basin of Belize, Central America. No other information was presented.

ISOSPORA SP. OF RAVINDRAN, KUMAR, AND GAFOOR, 2011

Original host: *Panthera pardus* (L., 1758), Leopard.
Remarks: Ravindran et al. (2011) said they found oocysts of an *Isospora* sp. in the fecal sample from 1/1 *P. pardus*. No other information was given.

ISOSPORA SPP. OF SINGH, GUPTA, SINGLA, SINGH, AND SHARMA, 2006

Original host: *Panthera leo* (L., 1758) (syn. *Leo leo* Frisch, 1775), Lion.
Remarks: Singh et al. (2006) said they found *Isospora* spp. in 4/50 (9%) fecal samples from lions in Mahendra Choudhury Zoological Park, Punjab, India. No other information was given.

ISOSPORA SPP. OF SINGH, GUPTA, SINGLA, SINGH, AND SHARMA, 2006

Original host: *Panthera tigris* (L., 1758), Tiger.
Remarks: Singh et al. (2006) said they found *Isospora* spp. in 5/50 (11%) fecal samples from tigers, Mahendra Choudhury Zoological Park, Punjab, India. No other information was given.

SARCOCYSTIS SP. OF BERENTSEN, BECKER, STOCKDALE-WALDEN, MATANDIKO, MCROBB, AND DUNBAR, 2012

Definitive host: *Panthera leo* (L., 1758) (syn. *Leo leo* Frisch, 1775), Lion.
Intermediate host: Unknown.
Remarks: Berentsen et al. (2012) surveyed African lions and other carnivore species from the Luangwa Valley, Zambia, and reported sporocysts of a *Sarcocystis* species in 1/15 (7%) *P. leo* but gave no other information about this parasite.

SARCOCYSTIS SP. OF BHATAVDEKAR AND PUROHIT, 1963

Definitive host: Unknown.
Intermediate host: *Panthera leo* (L., 1758) (syn. *Leo leo* Frisch, 1775), Lion.
Remarks: Bhatavdekar and Purohit (1963) may have been the first to document sarcocysts in the muscles of felids. They said they found, "a very thin hyaline capsule and the cavity was filled

with numerous crescentic bodies" in sections of heart muscle from two zoo lions (presumably *P. leo*) that had died in India. The sarcocysts, examined only under LM, were, 12.3 × 2.4, did not have "discernable" septa, and they were found in both striated and cardiac muscle fibers and in the cells of Purkinje fibers. Because of the small size and lack of septa (?), it is unlikely that this form can be attributed to *S. felis*, so it must be considered a *species inquirenda*. Bhatvdekar and Purohit (1963) said they fed sarcocysts in muscle tissue to mice and injected "the spores" (bradyzoites?) intramuscularly into mice and that "typical sarcocysts developed within four to seven weeks after feeding the infective stages." This remains to be confirmed.

SARCOCYSTIS SP. OF BWANGAMOI, ROTTCHER, AND WEKESA, 1990

Definitive host: Unknown.
Intermediate host: *Panthera leo* (L., 1758) (syn. *Leo leo* Frisch, 1775), Lion.
Remarks: Bwangamoi et al. (1990) found numerous sarcocysts measuring 730–760 × 113–114 in the skeletal muscles of a 7-year-old lioness from Nairobi National Park, Africa. No other information was given, thus, a *species inquirenda*.

SARCOCYSTIS SP. OF JOG, MARATHE, GOEL, RANADE, KUNTE, AND WATVE, 2003

Definitive host: *Panthera tigris* (L., 1758), Tiger.
Intermediate host: Unknown.
Remarks: Jog et al. (2003) surveyed the feces of 69 tigers from Tadoba National Park, Maharashtra, India, and found 3/69 (4%) passed sporocysts of a *Sarcocystis* species, and 2/36 (5.5%) tigers from Mudumalai National Park and Wildlife Sanctuary passed similar sporocysts in their feces. No attempt was made to further characterize the species, but Jog et al. (2003) also mentioned that 0/28 leopards, presumably *Panthera pardus* (L., 1758), were never found to have sporocysts in their feces when examined.

SARCOCYSTIS SP. OF MÜLLER-GRAF, 1995

Definitive host: *Panthera leo* (L., 1758) (syn. *Leo leo* Frisch, 1775), Lion.
Intermediate host: Unknown.
Remarks: Müller-Graf (1995) did a coprological survey of wild *P. leo* in the Serengeti and the Ngorongoro Crater, Tanzania, East Africa. She examined feces from lions and found "Coccidia" in 59/112 (53%) samples. She also reported finding sporocysts representing a *Sarcocystis* species in 16/112 (28%) samples. No other information was given on these samples.

SARCOCYSTIS SP. OF PATTON AND RABINOWITZ, 1994

Definitive host: *Panthera pardus* (L., 1758), Leopard.
Intermediate host: Unknown.
Remarks: Patton and Rabinowitz (1994) did a coprological survey of wild felids in Thailand and found *Sarcocystis* sporocysts in the feces of 11/54 (20%) samples examined. No other information was presented; thus, another *species inquirenda*.

SARCOCYSTIS SP. OF PATTON AND RABINOWITZ, 1994

Definitive host: *Panthera tigris* (L., 1758), Tiger.
Intermediate host: Unknown.
Remarks: Patton and Rabinowitz (1994) did a coprological survey of wild felids in Thailand and found *Sarcocystis* sporocysts in the feces of 7/19 (37%) samples examined. No other information was presented, thus another *species inquirenda*.

SARCOCYSTIS SP. OF SOMVANSHI, KOUL, AND BISWAS, 1987

Definitive host: Unknown.
Intermediate host: *Panthera pardus* (L., 1758), Leopard.

Remarks: Somvanshi et al. (1987) examined the carcass of a young leopard that was shot in Ramgarh, Uttarakhand, India, in the foothills of the Himalayas. Numerous elongated sarcocysts were found in the myocardium; the sarcocyst wall was thin, with numerous trophozoites. In spite of the large number of sarcocysts seen, the authors reported no inflammatory reaction. No other information was presented; thus, another *species inquirenda*.

FAMILY HERPESTIDAE BONAPARTE, 1845

GENUS CYNICITIS OGILBY, 1833 (MONOTYPIC)

ISOSPORA SP. OF MARKUS, 1972

Original host: *Cynictis penicillata* (G. [Baron] Cuvier, 1829), Yellow Mongoose.
Remarks: Markus (1972) reported isosporan-like oocysts from the yellow mongoose in South Africa, but no measurements were given.

GENUS HELOGALE GRAY, 1862 (2 SPECIES)

SARCOCYSTIS SP. OF VILJOEN, 1921

Definitive host: Unknown.
Intermediate host: *Helogale parvula* (Sundevall, 1847), Common Dwarf Mongoose.
Remarks: According to Levine and Ivens (1981), Viljoen (1921) found sarcocysts in the striated muscles of *H. parvula* in South Africa, but they did not see that actual paper, and got the citation from Nietz (1965). Levine (1986) did not list this species, and Dubey et al. (2015a) listed neither the Viljoen nor Nietz references and made no mention of a *Sarcocystis* species in *H. parvula*. Viljoen (1921) does not come up in Google Scholar and we were unable to obtain a copy of the Nietz paper.

GENUS HERPESTES ILLIGER, 1811 (10 SPECIES)

ISOSPORA ICHNEUMONIS OF LEVINE, IVENS, AND HEALY, 1975

Original host: *Herpestes ichneumon* (L., 1758), Egyptian Mongoose.
Remarks: Balozet (1933) found oocysts in fecal matter of two *H. ichneumon* from the Zaghousan region, Tunisia. He measured 100 sporulated oocysts and offered a very superficial description saying the subspheroidal oocysts were L×W: 22×19 (19–26×16–20), with a transparent, 2-layered wall and a poorly visible M. He said oocysts sporulated in 4 days when fecal material was placed on filter paper impregnated with potassium dichromate. Balozet (1933) fed sporulated oocysts in fecal material to a 4-day-old puppy and 9 days later, reinfected it with more oocysts. Four days after the second inoculation, oocysts were "extremely numerous" in the dog's feces, and the pup was described as having dysentery; after the fourth day of patency, oocysts became rare in the feces and the pup was sacrificed 30 days after the first inoculation. Balozet (1933) found no visible intestinal lesions and concluded that he had found *Isospora rivolta* (Grassi, 1879) Wenyon, 1923, saying, "…which appears to be a rather ubiquitous species capable of parasitizing several species of carnivorous species." In spite of this very modest description, and the lack of line drawing or photomicrograph, Levine et al. (1975) named the form seen by Balozet (1933) a new species, *I. ichneumonis*, when they should have relegated it, as we are here, to a *species inquirenda*.

GENUS MUNGOS É. GEOFFROY SAINT-HILAIRE, AND F.G. CUVIER, 1795 (2 SPECIES)

SARCOCYSTIS SP. OF VILJOEN, 1921

Definitive host: Unknown.

Intermediate host: *Mungos mungo* (Gmelin, 1788), Banded Mongoose.

Remarks: According to Levine and Ivens (1981), Viljoen (1921) found sarcocysts in the striated muscles of *M. mungo* in South Africa, but they did not see Viljoen's paper and got the citation from Nietz (1965). Levine (1986) did not list this species, and Dubey et al. (2015a) listed neither the Viljoen nor Nietz references and made no mention of a *Sarcocystis* species in *M. mungo*. Viljoen (1921) does not come up in Google Scholar and we were unable to obtain a copy of the Nietz paper.

GENUS *SURICATA* DESMAREST, 1804 (MONOTYPIC)

ISOSPORA SP. OF USHIGOME, YOSHINO, SUZUKI, KAWAJIRI, MASAKI, ENDO, AND ASAKAWA, 2011

Original host: *Suricata suricatta* (Schreber, 1776), Meerkat.

Remarks: Ushigome et al. (2011) examined fecal materials of 53 species of captive animals in Kawasaki Yumemigasaki Zoological Park, Japan, and found some *Isospora* sp. oocysts in meerkats. Not much to go on, but certainly an area that could bear fruitful research.

FAMILY HYAENIDAE GRAY, 1821

GENUS *CROCUTA* KAUP, 1828 (MONOTYPIC)

CYSTOISOSPORA SP. OF FERREIRA, 2015

Original host: *Crocuta crocuta* (Erxleben, 1777), Spotted Hyaena.

Intermediate host: Unknown.

Remarks: Ferreira (2015) collected 164 fecal samples from 104 known spotted hyaena juveniles (*C. crocuta*), ages 36- to 726-days-old, from March, 2010 to August, 2011 and examined them for parasite eggs and oocysts. She also extracted parasite DNA from the feces of two spotted hyaenas to obtain 18S rRNA gene fragments of 556 and 803 bp (minus primers), using the template *Cystoisospora felis* (of Carreno et al., 1998, GenBank accession #L76471.1). Her fecal samples showed two *Cystoisospora* forms, type 1 (small form, ~14 µm) in 33/104 (32%) hyaenas and *Cystoisospora* type 2 (large form, 31 µm) in 44/104 (42%) hyaenas. Her type 1 isolate (hyaena #I550) was closely related to *B. besnoiti*, *H. triffittae*, *T. gondii*, and *N. caninum*, indicating that it does not belong to *Cystoisospora*, whereas her type 2 isolate (hyaena #M661) aligned with the *Isospora/Cystoisospora* clade.

HEPATOZOON SP. OF KRAMPITZ, SACHS, SCHALLER, AND SCHINDLER, 1968

Original host: *Crocuta crocuta* (Erxleben, 1777), Spotted Hyaena.

Remarks: Krampitz et al. (1968) said that about 4/9 (44%) spotted hyaenas in the Serengeti National Park, Tanzania had gametocytes of a *Hepatozoon* species in their monocytes and neutrophiles.

ISOSPORA SP. OF BERENTSEN, BECKER, STOCKDALE-WALDEN, MATANDIKO, MCROBB, AND DUNBAR, 2012

Original host: *Crocuta crocuta* (Erxleben, 1777), Spotted Hyaena.

Remarks: Berentsen et al. (2012) surveyed hyaenas and other African carnivore species from the Luangwa Valley, Zambia for gastrointestinal parasites; they reported *Isospora* species in 3/9 (33%) *C. crocuta* but gave no other information about this parasite.

ISOSPORA SP. OF ENGH, NELSON, PEEBLES, HERNANDEZ, HUBBARD, AND HOLEKAMP, 2003

Original host: *Crocuta crocuta* (Erxleben, 1777), Spotted Hyaena.

Remarks: Engh et al. (2003) collected fecal samples from *C. crocuta* in the Masai Mara National Reserve, Kenya, and found oocysts of an *Isospora* sp. in 18/70 (26%) hyaenas. The size of the oocysts, ~35.3 μm, was intermediate between that of *I.* (=C.) *felis* and *I.* (=C.) *leonina*, two species recorded in African lions, but not in hyaenas.

FAMILY VIVERRIDAE GRAY, 1821

SUBFAMILY PARADOXURINAE GRAY, 1865

GENUS *PARADOXURUS* F.G. CUVIER, 1821 (3 SPECIES)

COCCIDIA, CYCLOSPORA, EIMERIA SPP. OF CHAKRABORTY, TIWARI, REDDY, AND UMAPATHY, 2016

Original hosts: *Paradoxurus hermaphroditus* (Pallas, 1777), Asian Palm Civet; *Paradoxurus jerdoni* Blanford, 1885, Jerdon's Palm Civet.

Remarks: Chakraborty et al. (2016) did a field survey of civets in the Anamalai Tiger Reserve (10° 12–35′N, 76° 49′–77° 24′E) and adjoining Valparai plateau, southern Western Ghats, India. They collected fecal samples of 108 civets from December, 2014 to March, 2015; samples were taken from 10 "forest fragments" that ranged from 8–2,000 ha. All samples were collected in 10% formalin, and they (2016) could not identify to which of the three endemic civets each fecal sample belonged. Samples thought to be infected with a *Cyclospora* sp. were found in two forest fragments, those infected with *Eimeria* species were found in four forest fragments and those identified only as Coccidia species were found in seven forest fragments. It is not clear how they defined "Coccidia" species nor how they were able to distinguish oocysts of *Cyclospora* and *Eimeria* species, given that feces were collected in 10% formalin and, apparently, not placed into thin layers in Petri dishes to allow sporulation.

EIMERIA SP. OF COLÓN AND PATTON, 2012

Original host: *Paradoxurus hermaphroditus* (Pallas, 1777), Asian Palm Civet.

Remarks: Colón and Patton (2012) did a coprological survey of civets in Sabah, Borneo, and feces from a road-killed *P. hermaphroditus* was reported to have oocysts of an *Eimeria* species in its feces. No other information was given.

SUBFAMILY VIVERRINAE GRAY, 1821

GENUS *GENETTA* F.G. COUVIER, 1816 (14 SPECIES)

CRYPTOSPORIDIUM SP. OF MATEO, DE MINGO, DE LUCIO, MORALES, BALSEIRO, ESPÍ, BARRAL, LIMA-BARBERO, HABELA, FERNÁNDEZ-GARCÍA, BERNAL, KÖSTER, CARDONA, AND CARMENA, 2017

Original host: *Genetta genetta* (L., 1758), Common Genet.

Remarks: Mateo et al. (2017) examined fecal samples of genets, from three autonomous regions of Spain (Basque Country, Castile-La Mancha, Extremadura) and examined them by nested PCR targeting the 18S rRNA gene, followed by genotyping based on the gp60 gene. *Cryptosporidium* was detected in 1/6 (17%) samples, the one from Extremadura.

EIMERIA GENETTAE OF AGOSTINUCCI AND BRONZINI, 1953

Original host: *Genetta dongolana* (L., 1758) (syn. *Genetta dongolana* Hemprich and Ehrenberg, 1832), Common Genet.

Remarks: Agostinucci and Bronzini (1953) examined the intestinal contents of one *G. dongolana* that died in the Zoological Garden of Rome, Italy, a few days after it arrived from Somalia (East coast of Africa) and found unsporulated oocysts. They kept the fecal material in 3% potassium dichromate solution at ~18°C and said, "the oocysts reached full maturity in ~7–8 days." Sporulated oocysts were slightly ellipsoidal and "featured a micropyle in each of the poles, with rather thin-walled, smooth, and seemingly double outline." The oocysts were L×W: 25.4×19.9 (20–30×12.5–25), L/W ratio: 1.3; OR, PG: both absent. Sporocysts were reported to be "pear-shaped pods," 8.4×6.0 (6–12.5×5–7.5); SR: absent. There was no mention of presence or absence of SB, SSB, PSB, and there was no line drawing or photomicrograph, presented as a type, to support this inadequate description. No one in the literature has referred to this species since its original description. Therefore, it must be relegated to a *species inquirenda*.

HEPATOZOON SP. OF KEYMER AND BROCKLESBY, 1971

Original hosts: *Genetta genet* (L., 1758), Common Genet; *Genetta thierryi* Matschie, 1902 (syn. *Genetta rubiginosa* Pucheran, 1855), Haussa Genet; *Genetta tigrine* (Schreber, 1776), Cape Genet.

Remarks: Keymer and Brocklesby (1971) studied and described intraleukocytic and extracellular stages of a *Hepatozoon* sp. they found in the blood of *G. rubiginosa* and *G. tigrina*, and meronts in the liver and cardiac muscle of *G. rubiginosa*. They found two forms of meronts in the heart, and both differed from meronts found in the liver. This was the first time *Hepatozoon* meronts have been described in *Genetta* spp.

GENUS VIVERRA L., 1758 (4 SPECIES)

EIMERIA, ISOSPORA, AND SARCOCYSTIS SPP. OF COLÓN AND PATTON, 2012

Original host: *Viverra tangalunga* (Gray, 1832), Malayan Civet.

Remarks: Colón and Patton (2012) did a coprological survey of civets in Sabah, Borneo, and a female *V. tangalunga* was reported to have *Eimeria* and *Isospora* oocysts and sporocysts of a *Sarcocystis* sp. in her feces. But no other information was given.

NOMENA NUDA (2)

Some authors, especially in some of the very old literature, gave new names to organisms they saw, but for which they presented no other substantive information. Such a name is called a "nude name" or *nomen nudum* (pl. *nomena nuda*). These names become preoccupied and unavailable names; however, the same name may be made available at a later time for the same or a different concept, but in such case, it would take authorship and date from the act of establishment, not from the earlier publication as a *nomen nudum*.

GENUS FELIS L., 1758

ISOSPORA NOVOCATI OF PELLÉRDY, 1974b

Original host: *Felis catus* L., 1758, Domestic Cat.

Remarks: Pellérdy (1974b) proposed this name for *I. rivolta* from the cat because he believed *I. rivolta* was first discovered and named from the dog. However, Wenyon (1923) reviewed all of the literature on the coccidia known to that date from dogs and cats and convinced most colleagues that *I. rivolta* was first discovered in the cat. Thus, as concluded by Dubey (1975c), and we agree, this renders *I. novocati* to be rendered a nomen nudum.

GENUS *MARTES* PINEL, 1792

ISOSPORA MUSTELAE OF GALLI-VALERIO, 1932

Original host: *Martes martes* (L., 1758), European Pine Marten.

Remarks: Galli-Valerio (1932) said he saw an ovoidal coccidium that was, 7 × 2.25 with a flattened micropyle in the feces of the European pine marten and that it developed two sporocysts each with four sporozoites. We know of no oocysts in any apicomplexan family that has oocysts this small. No other structural data were given nor did he include a line drawing. Therefore, this name must be considered a nomen nudum.

DISCUSSION

In the <u>Caniformia</u>, there are no casual, common-name-only, or genus-name-only references in these family and genera: **Canidae**: *Atelocynus* Cabrera, 1940 (monotypic); *Cerdocyon* C.E.H. Smith, 1839 (monotypic); *Dusicyon* C.E.H. Smith, 1839 (monotypic); *Otocyon* Müller, 1836 (monotypic); *Speothos* Lund, 1836 (monotypic); *Urocyon* Baird, 1857 (2 species); **Mephitidae**: *Conepatus* Gray, 1837 (4 species); *Mydaus* F.G. Cuvier, 1821 (2 species); **Mustelidae**: *Aonyx* Lesson 1827 (2 species); *Hydrictis* Pocock, 1921 (monotypic); *Lutrogale* Gray, 1865 (monotypic); *Pteronura* Gray, 1837 (monotypic); *Arctonyx* F.G.

Cuvier, 1825 (monotypic); *Eira* C.E.H. Smith, 1842 (monotypic); *Galictis* Bell, 1826 (2 species); *Gulo* Pallas, 1780 (monotypic); *Ictonyx* Kaup, 1835 (2 species); *Lycodon* Gervais, 1845 (monotypic); *Poecilogale* Thomas, 1883 (monotypic); *Taxidea* Waterhouse, 1839 (monotypic); *Vormela* Blasius, 1884 (monotypic); **Odobenidae**: *Odobenus* Brisson, 1762 (monotypic); **Otariidae**: *Arctocephalus* É. Geoffroy Saint-Hilaire, and F.G. Cuvier, 1826 (8 species); *Eumetopias* Gill, 1866 (monotypic); *Neophoca* Gray, 1866 (monotypic); *Phocarctos* Peters, 1866 (monotypic); **Phocidae**: *Halichoerus* Nilsson, 1820 (monotypic); *Histriophoca* Gill, 1873 (monotypic); *Hydrurga* Gistel, 1848 (monotypic); *Monachus* Fleming, 1822 (3 species); *Ommatophoca* Gray, 1844 (monotypic); **Procyonidae**: *Bassaricyon* J.A. Allen, 1876 (5 species); *Bassariscus* Coues, 1887 (2 species); *Nasua* Storr, 1780 (2 species); *Nasuella* Hollister, 1915 (monotypic); and **Ursidae**: *Melursus* Meyer, 1793 (monotypic); and *Tremarctos* Gervais, 1855 (monotypic). In total, there is no record that 37/72 (51%) Caniformia genera, and their 60 species (above), have any abbreviated coccidian identifications associated to them. And, in the 35 genera that have been surveyed, only 52/105 (49.5%) species in those genera have been looked at sufficiently to have various coccidian forms known from them.

In the <u>Feliformia</u>, we found no casual, common-name-only, or genus-name-only references in these family and genera: **Eupleridae**: *Cryptoprocta* Bennett, 1833 (monotypic); *Eupleres* Doyère, 1835 (monotypic); *Fossa* Gray, 1865 (monotypic); *Galidia* I. Geoffroy Saint-Hilaire, 1837 (monotypic); *Galidictis* I. Geoffroy Saint-Hilaire, 1839 (2 species); *Mungotictis* Pocock, 1915 (monotypic); *Salanoia* Gray, 1865 (monotypic); **Felidae**: *Caracal* Gray, 1843 (monotypic); *Catopuma* Severtzov, 1858 (2 species); *Pardofelis* Severtzov, 1858 (monotypic); *Profelis* Severtzov, 1858 (monotypic); *Neofelis* Gray, 1867 (monotypic); *Uncia* Gray, 1854 (monotypic); **Herpestidae**: *Atilax* F.G. Cuvier, 1826 (monotypic); *Bdeogale* Peters, 1850 (3 species); *Crossarchus* F.G. Cuvier, 1825 (4 species); *Dologale*

Thomas, 1926 (monotypic); *Galerella* Gray, 1865 (4 species); *Ichneumia* I. Geoffroy Saint-Hilaire, 1837 (monotypic); *Liberiictis* Hayman, 1958 (monotypic); *Paracynictis* Pocock, 1916 (monotypic); *Rhynchogale* Thomas, 1894 (monotypic); **Hyaenidae**: *Hyaena* Brisson, 1762 (2 species); *Proteles* I. Geoffroy Saint-Hilaire, 1824 (monotypic); **Nandiniidae**: *Nandinia* Gray, 1843 (monotypic); **Viverridae**: *Arctictis* Temminck, 1824 (monotypic); *Arctogalidia* Merriam, 1897 (monotypic); *Macrogalidia* Schwarz, 1910 (monotypic); *Paguma* Gray, 1831 (monotypic); *Chrotogale* Thomas, 1912 (monotypic); *Cynogale* Gray, 1837 (monotypic); *Diplogale* Thomas, 1912 (monotypic); *Hemigalus* Jourdan, 1837 (monotypic); *Prionodon* Horsfield, 1822 (2 species); *Civettictis* Pocock, 1915 (monotypic); *Poiana* Gray, 1865 (2 species); and *Viverricula* Hodgson, 1838 (monotypic). In total, there is no record that 37/54 (68.5%) Feliformia genera, and their 50 species (above), have any abbreviated coccidian identifications associated to them. And, in the 17 genera that have been surveyed, only 27/71 (38%) species in those genera have been looked at sufficiently to have various coccidian forms known from them.

In total, we found 483 apicomplexans that have been mentioned in the literature and placed into 17 genera or generic categories, but that either have not been described sufficiently or there was so little information provided by the author(s), that their validity, and sometimes even their identity was in question. These include: 2 "Apicomplexa protozoa," 1 *Besnoitia* sp., 34 Coccidia-like or Coccidia spp., 135 *Cryptosporidium* spp., 2 Cyclospora spp., 26 *Cystoisospora* spp., 36 *Eimeria* spp., 3 *Hammondia*-like forms; 7 *Hammondia–Neospora*-like forms; 7 *Hammondia–Toxoplasma*-like forms; 14 *Hepatozoon* spp., 1 *Hoareosporidium* sp., 72 *Isospora* spp., 1 *Klossia* sp., 1 "oocysts," 135 *Sarcocystis* spp., and 3 *Toxoplasma*-like forms. All are considered *species inquirendae*. In addition, two names, *Isospora novocati* of Pellérdy, 1974b, and *Isospora mustelae*

of Galli-Valerio, 1932, are considered nomena nuda, by definition.

If one takes time to look into any of the individual entries cited above in this chapter, you might imagine each as the beginning of a short story that may wet your appetite for more information, but the story ends and leaves you wanting to know more. Even though many of these citations may seem trivial on first examination, they all present some modest baseline data, and virtually any one of these efforts could be expanded on by the right person(s). From the above numbers, two things may be obvious; (1) most carnivore populations have been poorly surveyed for apicomplexan parasites; and (2) there are a plethora of apicomplexan genera and species to be discovered, studied in much more detail, and be defined in many different ways.

We are just now beginning to have a basic understanding of most of the apicomplexan genera mentioned in this chapter and we now know where and how to look for them. For example, *Besnoitia* species are often overlooked or misidentified as sarcocysts of *Sarcocystis* when carcasses are examined. It is still worthwhile and useful to study the oocysts of *Eimeria*, *Isospora*, *Caryospora*, and *Cystoisospora* species, but they must be carefully defined by measurements, photomicrographs, and line drawings. Sporocysts of *Isospora* species must be examined carefully to determine the presence or absence of a Stieda body. If a Stieda body is present, cross-transmission and feeding experiments will be needed to determine if sporulated oocysts can infect the host species in which they were discovered, or their nearest relatives, or the original oocysts may belong to a prey item and simply be passing through the gut of the original host from environmental contamination. If the sporocysts of larger isosporan-like oocysts do not have a Stieda body, it is most likely they are a species of *Cystoisospora* and lab mice should be infected to determine if they can act as intermediate/transport hosts for some asexual stage(s).

Lots of surveys look at certain muscles of potential host species for the presence of sarcocysts and if there are none present (or none are "seen") in the specific muscles examined, the animal necropsied is considered negative for *Sarcocystis*. However, those doing surveys should understand that some sarcocysts are not visible to the naked eye, especially if they are very young, some are very small even when mature and can best be found by pepsin digestion versus gross inspection, and many species have their highest densities in different tissues; to some, this may seem reminiscent of how *Eimeria* species seem to divide up the intestinal tract, each destined to live in its own site-specific location. To illustrate the point we are making, Mohammed (2000) and Mohammed et al. (2000) looked for *Sarcocystis* infections in different gazelle species at the King Khalid Wildlife Research Centre in Saudi Arabia. They detected no macroscopic sarcocysts by fibre optic examination, a 40% infection rate was detected by histological examination, and an overall prevalence of infection of 67% was reached when they used pepsin digestion of muscle. In addition, the esophagus, diaphragm, heart, tongue, and skeletal muscles had different rates of infection dependent on the host gazelle species that was examined. They also reported that *Sarcocystis* infection was significantly higher in free-ranging gazelles kept in a main enclosure than in gazelles kept in breeding pens and higher in adult versus juvenile gazelles. Thus, there are lots of ways to examine every problem and, with the plethora of inquiries presented in this chapter, there are lots of problems awaiting future study.

Discussion, Summary and Conclusions

Within the mammalian order Carnivora there are four families of protist parasites (Apicomplexa: Conoidasida) common in carnivores. These include Adeleidae Mesnil, 1903, Cryptosporidiidae Léger, 1911, Eimeriidae Minchin, 1903, and Sarcocystidae Poche, 1913, which we will refer to as the coccidia. In this book we recognized about 217 valid coccidian species in the order Carnivora, including 5 *Besnoitia*, 1 *Caryospora*, 10 *Cryptosporidium*, 1 *Cyclospora*, 53 *Cystoisospora*, 39 *Eimeria*, 3 *Hammondia*, 6 *Hepatozoon*, 9 *Isospora*, 1 *Neospora*, 78 *Sarcocystis*, and 1 *Toxoplasma* species. In addition, there are about 483 incompletely named species recorded from carnivores that fit taxonomically into these taxa only as genus names, or less. Below we provide brief discussions and summaries of what we know, and do not know, about these parasites in carnivores in the Eimeriorina and Adeleorina from each carnivore family and three sarcocystid subfamilies: Cystoisosporinae Frenkel et al., 1987, Sarcocystinae Poche, 1913, and Toxoplasmatinae Biocca, 1957; therapy and treatment; improperly reported coccidia (or *Species inquirendae*); and final concluding thoughts.

APICOMPLEXA: EIMERIIDAE

Ailuridae. We know very little about eimeriid coccidia infecting the red (or lesser) panda, *Ailurus fulgens*, the single species in this monotypic family. *Eimeria ailuri* was reported and described from a red panda (or pandas?) in a zoo in India by Agrawal et al. (1981). This is all we know. There are no additional reports of coccidia from red pandas in the literature. Given the endangered status of the red panda and the pressures on its remaining wild relatives, any opportunities we may have to learn more about them and their parasites and biology are rapidly decreasing. In addition, efforts at maintaining and rearing red pandas in captivity run the risk of exposure to coccidia from other hosts if zoo keepers are not careful to maintain animals in clean, sanitary, low-stress conditions to avoid cross-contamination from other hosts.

Canidae. Relative to other carnivore families, we know quite a bit about Eimeriidae found in members of this family. This is not surprising as the family includes domestic dogs (*Canis lupus familiaris*) and other popular and widely distributed members including coyotes (*C. latrans*), foxes (*Vulpes* spp.), and wolves (*C. lupus*). All the attention paid to protist parasites in this family has helped illuminate some important taxonomic issues that have contributed to our understanding of the phylogenetic relationships and life histories of these parasites. Three issues in particular require our future and immediate attention to be able to better understand the intestinal and tissue apicomplexan parasites in these hosts. First, research on *Caryospora* species requires much more study. Caryosporans were

575

© 2018 Donald W. Duszynski published by Elsevier Inc. All rights reserved.

initially and traditionally thought to be primarily parasites of snakes and birds, but there is a growing body of evidence now that they can infect canids in nonintestinal locations and cause serious disease and death in our companion animals. Second, it is our opinion, and one shared with many parasitologists, that the *Eimeria* species reported from canids are not really their parasites, but represent oocysts from prey hosts just passing through the canid gut after their normal host was ingested by the canid in which they were reported. Third, based on analysis of molecular data, *Isospora*-type oocysts without Stieda bodies (SB) on their sporocysts, which once were assigned to the genus *Isospora* (family Eimeriidae), all now need to be reassigned to the genus *Cystoisospora* (family Sarcocystidae). Of the 14 species of *Isospora* we found described from canids in the literature, all but one lacks a SB and, thus we reassigned them to their appropriate taxonomic position. The one species we believe that does possess a SB complex, *I. fennechi*, is a spurious finding of oocysts from a prey item of the fennec fox. And one last and important point about the Canidae is that, realistically, we know very little about what eimeriid and sarcocystid species are and may continue to be found in species comprising this family. Only 3/13 genera (13%) and 9/35 species (26%) in the family have been examined for such coccidian parasites, and these are found only in small numbers and in limited localities within their various ranges. Thus, we hope we may have cleaned up some taxonomic confusion within this host–parasite assemblage, but we still have a lot to learn.

Mephitidae. Our knowledge of eimeriids in skunks, like so many carnivore host lineages, is limited. In this case it could be due to the unpleasant smell of the host constraining interest, but this is not certain. Only two species of *Eimeria* have been described and both are from the striped skunk, *Mephitis mephitis* and two species from the Eastern spotted skunk, *Spilogale putorius*, originally placed in the *Isospora*, are now reassigned to the *Cystoisospora*. For the entire family, only 2/4 (50%) of the genera and only 2/12 (17%) of extant skunk species have been examined for eimeriid parasites.

Mustelidae. This is the most species-rich carnivore family with 22 genera and 59 species. Some of the more commonly-recognized animals include the badger (*Taxidea taxus*), fishers and martens (*Martes* spp.), mink (*Neovison vison*), otters (*Lutra* spp.), polecats and weasels (*Ictonyx* spp., *Mustela* spp., *Vormela* spp.), sable (*M. zibellina*), sea otter (*Enhydra lutris*), and wolverine (*Gulo gulo*). Possibly because of the mink pelt trade and the efforts to save the endangered black-footed ferret, mustelids have been studied more for internal parasites than other carnivore families except for the Canidae and Felidae. Overall, only 9/59 (15%) extant species in 7/22 (32%) genera have been looked at for coccidia, and from these 9 host species, 10 *Eimeria*, 12 *Cystoisospora*, 1 *Isospora*, and 1 *Hammondia* are known. This leaves 68% of the mustelid genera and 85% of the species yet to be examined. We clearly have much to discover about eimeriids from this host family. What an excellent opportunity this presents.

Odobenidae, Otariidae, Phocidae. These three families include most marine carnivores such as fur seals, sea lions, walruses, and true (earless) seals. Only five intestinal coccidians (3 *Eimeria*, 2 *Cystoisospora*) have been named and described, three of these are not well-described, and all are reported from different species in the Phocidae. There are no eimeriid coccidians known from the only extant species of Odobenidae, the walrus. Only a single species of *Isospora* has been reported in the Otariidae, that in a sea lion that died in the Giza Zoological Garden (Egypt), and we reassigned it to *Cystoisospora*. Three of the coccidian species that we think are valid species are not very well-described and only one, *E. phocae*, from harbor and gray seals, has been studied in enough detail that includes its endogenous development and associated pathology. This lack of knowledge is concerning because 8/36 (22%) species in these families are on IUCN lists of species endangered or at risk. Many marine mammals spend part of the year in high-density breeding colonies, and this presents an ideal opportunity to collect fecal samples for study. Because these breeding colonies concentrate hundreds to thousands of individuals, coccidian prevalence should be at its highest, and fecal–oral transmission of multiple coccidia species should be facilitated; what a wonderful and opportune time to do collecting of feces.

Procyonidae. This is a small carnivore family that includes several well-known animals including coatis (*Nasua* spp.), the kinkajou (*Potos flavus*), and raccoons (*Procyon* spp.). Four *Eimeria* species have been described from 3/14 (14%) species in this family, 1 from the raccoon (*Procyon lotor*), 1 from the pygmy raccoon (*P. pygmaeus*), 1 from the white-nosed coati (*N. narica*), and 1 from the kinkajou. Of these four described species, only *E. procyonis* has received extensive study that includes information on both oocyst and sporocyst exogenous stages and their ultrastructure, endogenous development, and histopathology. The South American coati (*N. nasua*) and kinkajou both have been infected experimentally with *Cystoisospora arctopitheci*, a species originally described from a marmoset, a New World monkey. Given what we think we know about host-specificity for *Eimeria* and *Cystoisospora* species, this is a curious report that should be repeated! For the Procyonidae 11/14 (79%) of the species have not been examined for coccidia. The IUCN also notes that 11 species in this family are decreasing in numbers, except the raccoon, which seems to be increasing its populations worldwide because it adapts so easily to human habitations. Nothing is known at this time about the population trends of the cacomistle (*Bassariscus sumichrasti*) and ringtail (*Bassariscus astutus*), the remaining two species in this family. Thus, the opportunity to explore eimeriid presence, biology, and biodiversity in this tractable carnivore host group is

disappearing. This is unfortunate as this is an entire mammalian family in which every host species population could be surveyed with good sample sizes and a lot of knowledge could be gained on how many coccidia species actually exist in an entire family population.

Ursidae. The bears comprise another small carnivore family from which only three species of *Eimeria* have been described, two from black bears (*Ursus americanus*) in North America and one from the brown bear (*U. arctos*) in Russia. One species of *Isospora* has been described from brown bears (presumably) in Zoos in Russia, Uzbekistan, and Ukraine, and one species of *Cystoisospora* is now known from a sloth bear in India. In this family, 5/8 (62.5%) species have not been examined for coccidia and of the 4 named coccidian species, none have a type specimen deposited in an accredited museum. The IUCN lists 6/8 (75%) bears as vulnerable so, once again, the opportunity to learn more about their coccidia is rapidly diminishing with time. However, as primarily solitary animals, the prevalence of coccidia in them likely will be low, but one never knows when you study the coccidia what surprises such efforts will bring. And, like the bear populations themselves, their coccidians will continue to decline and, ultimately, go extinct with them.

Felidae. Much like the canids, we know a lot more about Eimeriidae and Sarcocystidae found in cats than in other carnivores, *relatively speaking*. Like the canids, this is due in large part to attention paid to domestic cats (*Felis catus*) as lab and companion animals, as well as our interest in the variety of felids kept in zoos and zoological parks, and especially those that are of concern to our conservation efforts including cheetahs (*Acinonyx jubatus*), leopards, lions, and tigers (*Panthera* spp.). And also like in the Canidae, the biology and life history of eimeriid coccidia in felids are confusing. First, although a number of *Eimeria* species have been found in felid feces, all described and named *Eimeria* infections in felids are thought by most/many parasitologists to be spurious findings; that is, the oocysts found and named are likely those of prey species passing through the cat's gut at the time its feces were examined. Thus, members of the Felidae and Canidae may be unique among mammal lineages in that they have no *Eimeria* species that parasitize them. This "observation" certainly bears further exploration. Second, the known *Isospora* species from felids, almost all of which have sporocysts without SB, now belong in the *Cystoisospora* because of their unusual heteroxenous life histories, and their molecular affinities with the Sarcocystidae. And those *Isospora*-like oocysts having sporocysts with a SB complex are likely spurious objects in passage through the felid gut after ingesting a prey item.

Herpestidae. This family includes the meerkat (*Suricata suricatta*), mongooses (e.g., *Atilax, Bdeogale, Dologale, Helogale, Herpestes, Mungos* spp.), and kusimanses (*Crossarchus* spp.). Only 2/14 (14%) genera and 5/33 (15%) species in this family have been examined for intestinal coccidia and only 3 *Eimeria* species have been described, all from the Indian gray mongoose. However, it must be recognized that, as for the Canidae and Felidae, one or all three might be oocysts of the *Eimeria* species of prey items just passing through the intestine, and present in the feces of these herpestids, at the time fecal samples were collected. Six of the seven *Isospora* species discovered from herpestid hosts belong within the *Cystoisospora* because their sporocysts lack a SB, along with *C. timoni*, which was discovered and named by El-Gayar et al. (2008) from the slender-tailed meerkat from South Africa. Here once again, we have a small number of very interesting animals in the Herpestidae, which makes it a tractable group in which virtually every species could be sampled throughout its range.

Eupleridae, Hyaenidae, Nandiniidae, Viverridae. These four families comprise an assortment of carnivores including fossas, Malagasy civets, and Malagasy mongooses in the Eupleridae;

hyaenas and aardwolf in the Hyaenidae; African palm civets in the Nandiniidae; and binturongs, civets, and genets in the Viverridae. Only a few animals from these four lineages have been examined for apicomplexan parasites. Two *Isospora* species have been described, one from the African civet (*Civettictis civetta*) and the other from the brown or Indian hyaena (*Hyaena brunnea*). Both, given our current knowledge on *Isospora*-type oocysts that have sporocysts without SB, have been placed into the *Cystoisospora*. These four families clearly need more study.

ADELEIDAE

The Adeleorina are a poorly studied group of coccidian species that parasitize the blood and tissues of many vertebrate and invertebrate species with a defining characteristic being a form of gamete formation termed syzygy, a process during which microgametes and macrogamonts are pressed together during their development. There are seven families in the Adeleorina including members that have both homoxenous and heteroxenous life cycles. All known species that infect carnivores are in one family, Hepatozoidae, within the genus *Hepatozoon*, which includes more than 300 species. *Hepatozoon* species infect various vertebrates as their *intermediate host*, including species in the Carnivora. The *definitive* hosts for these species are invertebrates that include mites, ticks, and various insects, and infection of the vertebrate host occurs when it ingests the infected invertebrate (that is, not by its bite). There are six named species of *Hepatozoon* described from six carnivore families (Canidae, Felidae, Hyaenidae, Mustelidae, Procyonidae, and Ursidae), and a goodly number of "*Hepatozoon* species" have been reported from individual species in these and at least one other family, Viverridae. At one time, when gamonts were observed in the WBCs of a vertebrate the observation was sufficient to name a new species whenever a new vertebrate host species was infected. We now know that certain *Hepatozoon* species are not host-specific and can infect a variety of reasonably unrelated host lineages (e.g., *H. canis*); that is, *Hepatozoon* species found in many vertebrate groups have low host-specificity for both their definitive and intermediate hosts. With the increasing use of molecular technologies for identifying and differentiating species, we believe there is now a great deal of knowledge yet to be discovered by any interested parasitologist about the taxonomy and systematics of the Adeleorina.

SARCOCYSTIDAE: CYSTOISOSPORINAE

This subgroup of sarcocystid coccidia is defined by the production of monozoic cysts that can occur in intermediate or paratenic hosts. Almost all the species in this group were originally named as species of *Isospora*. However, following the initial direction of Frenkel (1977), and later following the molecular evidence, we reassigned all *Isospora* species with oocysts lacking a SB complex to the *Cystoisospora*. As a result of our 38 new name assignments, the total number of *Cystoisospora* spp. now known to infect carnivores is about 50. Clearly, much of what we know now of the biology of these parasites resulted from studies of domestic and laboratory dogs and cats. A limited number of wild and zoo carnivore species have had their feces examined for coccidian oocysts in 11/15 (73%) families, which include only 30/126 (24%) genera and 48/286 (17%) species. From these studies, 50 named *Cystoisospora* species have been described, or about one per each carnivore species that has been examined. We believe it likely that all true carnivores can serve as definitive hosts for at least one *Cystoisospora* species unique to it. If our assumption is reasonable, then there may be another 250 *Cystoisospora* species yet to be discovered just from carnivores.

SARCOCYSTIDAE: SARCOCYSTINAE

This subfamily was comprised of two genera, *Sarcocystis* and *Frenkelia*, both with heteroxenous life cycles involving predator–prey hosts; the intermediate stage is encysted in tissues (typically muscle for *Sarcocystis* and nervous tissue for *Frenkelia*) of the prey while the predator/definitive hosts shed infective sporocysts in their feces. However, no *Frenkelia* have ever been recorded from carnivorous mammals and recent molecular evidence indicates the genus is likely a synonym of *Sarcocystis*. For the Carnivora, with few exceptions (domestic and lab dogs and cats), only a few wild or zoo carnivores, usually 1–2 specimens per species, have been examined in 9/15 (60%) families, 44/126 (23%) genera, and 63/286 (22%) species. From these reports, 78 named *Sarcocystis* species, and a lot of partially-named forms, have been described. Also, because tissue stages can be and are involved, 58 of the named *Sarcocystis* species parasitize carnivores that serve as definitive hosts and discharge sporocysts into the environment, whereas 16 *Sarcocystis* species are in carnivores that serve as intermediate hosts in which sarcocysts occur in their muscles. There are also four *Sarcocystis* species in which either the same carnivore or two different carnivores serve both as definitive and intermediate hosts in the cycle. Only a few studies have used molecular methods to discriminate sarcocysts found in carnivore muscles from other known sarcocyst species via sequence comparisons and phylogenetic analyses, so there is great opportunity for much more research using this approach to fill in the gaps in our knowledge about these *Sarcocystis* species.

Also, there is a long history of taxonomic issues involving *Sarcocystis*-like organisms that include proposals to erect new genera based on questionable characters, invalid names based on insufficient descriptions, and existing names that need to be validated and cryptic species identified. Assessing biodiversity within the *Sarcocystis* species will require systematic sampling of the 78% of carnivore hosts and geographic regions not yet studied. For 58/78 (74%) named species we have a modest start and know something about their biology and life histories and we know at least one or more definitive and intermediate hosts, but for the remaining 20 *Sarcocystis* species, we know virtually nothing about their life cycles, and there are large numbers of reports of sarcocysts that have been found in many animal species without any attempts to name the species or determine the definitive host(s). Finally, we know very little about endogenous development in both intermediate and definitive hosts.

SARCOCYSTIDAE: TOXOPLASMATINAE

This subfamily is composed of four genera, *Besnoitia*, *Hammondia*, *Neospora*, and *Toxoplasma*. *Besnoitia* species are obligatorily heteroxenous coccidia, but they differ from *Sarcocystis* species in three unique ways: (1) oocysts are shed unsporulated by their definitive hosts and have relatively thick walls; (2) the completion of the sexual cycle in the definitive host is dependent on ingestion of tissue cysts from a suitable intermediate host—that is, the ability of oocysts to initiate gametogenesis in the definitive host has been lost; and (3) these species can be successfully propagated asexually by mechanical transmission from intermediate host to intermediate host by blood-sucking arthropods. There are only four *Besnoitia* species with known life cycles and all utilize cats as their definitive host. Whether there are other hosts for these four is not known. The genus *Hammondia* has an interesting history that encapsulates many of the taxonomic issues that have confused and complicated the taxonomy of many other coccidia; interested readers are encouraged to review Chapter 16. There are three valid species of *Hammondia* recorded only from canids, felids, mustelids, and a single sea lion; these likely reflect the close association of these host groups with humans. There is one species of *Neospora* recorded from carnivores, *N. caninum*, and it has only been since the early 1970s that it was recognized as the cause of meningoencephalitis, polymyositis, polyradiculoneuritis, and dermatological diseases in dogs (definitive host), whereas cats and a variety of hoof-stock animals are natural intermediate hosts. The story of the discovery and naming of *N. caninum* (Chapter 16) is another tale illustrating the confusing twists and turns the taxonomy and nomenclature of a coccidian species can take when investigators do not pay attention to how to correctly name and describe new genera and species such that they are in agreement with the International Code of Zoological Nomenclature. Using a variety of diagnostic techniques, *N. caninum* exposure has been demonstrated in canids in 21 countries, in noncanid carnivores in 8 countries, and in domestic cats in 7 and wild felids in 87 countries. It is interesting to us that there is no evidence for clinical neosporosis in felids. *Toxoplasma gondii* has an indirect life cycle with only cats and other felids serving as definitive hosts in which the parasite goes through both asexual and sexual endogenous development in intestinal epithelial cells, while virtually any vertebrate species may serve as the intermediate host in which *T. gondii* stages encyst in a variety of tissues. It has a global distribution, it is likely the most ubiquitous parasite on Earth, and it can be transmitted directly, transplacentally, and by carnivorism/cannibalism. Clinical toxoplasmosis has been reported in virtually all species of warm-blooded animals, including humans, domestic and wild animals. The wide host and geographic range of *T. gondii* is based on tens of thousands of surveys around the world looking at cat feces for oocysts, testing blood for antibodies from various animals and examining tissues for cysts. *Toxoplasma gondii* is a significant public health concern, especially for women in their first trimester of pregnancy and for individuals who are immunocompromised.

CRYPTOSPORIDIIDAE

The single genus *Cryptosporidium* has about 10 species and genotypes described, named, and/or genetically characterized from carnivores and there is not a great deal of information known about the general biology, life history, and morphology of these species/genotypes. *Cryptosporidium* species lack strict host-specificity and can be transmitted between carnivores and other wild, feral, domestic, zoo, and food animals, and humans. *Cryptosporidium* species are obligate, monoxenous, intracellular, but extracytoplasmic parasites. In Caniformia, we have knowledge that about 9 distinct species of *Cryptosporidium* are known to be present in 8/9 (89%) families, 15/72 (21%) genera with 17/165 (10%) species. In addition, there are 22 genera and 29 species in the Caniformia from which *Cryptosporidium* sp. have been reported, most based only on oocysts in the feces. For the Feliformia, 5 *Cryptosporidium* species are known in 2/6 (33%) families, 6/54 (11%) genera, and in 3/121 (2%) species, and *Cryptosporidium* sp. has been found in an additional 5 genera and species. In carnivores, most surveys worldwide have involved dogs and cats, both stray and domestic, although most of these identifications are made as *Cryptosporidium* sp. *Cryptosporidium canis* and *C. felis* are the most frequently identified species in our pets, although small numbers of zoonotic *C. parvum* and *C. muris* also have been reported. Both *C. canis* and *C. felis* are considered potentially zoonotic, particularly in children, those who are immunocompromised, and/or elderly people, and because so many mammalian species can be infected with *C. parvum*, a large potential zoonotic reservoir exists in wild, domestic, and companion animals. Each of these species deserves special concern.

TREATMENT AND DRUG THERAPIES

Treatment and therapy of coccidiosis in Carnivora is difficult because most anticoccidials have not been tested and/or registered for the majority of the carnivore genera making their use often only experimental and off-label. In addition, most infections are self-limiting in immunocompetent hosts and resolve without intervention, and following exposure hosts may develop partial or total immunity to reinfection. These factors, in addition to the longevity of coccidian oocysts in the external environment, complicate further the transmission scenarios, and in most cases make prevention more important than therapy. Prevention measures include maintenance of sanitary rearing/holding facilities and proper use of household and clinical disinfectants. We listed chemotherapeutics (Chapter 18 and Table 3) used for treatment of coccidiosis in carnivores, but it is important to note that many of the antiprotozoal drugs are effective against a restricted range of coccidian genera and for many infections, treatment may not result in a complete cure. Therapy of coccidiosis is complicated in carnivores and is becoming more so as resistance of coccidian parasites to antiprotozoal drugs is an emerging problem.

SPECIES INQUIRENDAE IN THE CARNIVORA

Finally, we found 483 apicomplexans mentioned in the literature and placed into 17 genera or generic categories, but they were not described sufficiently, or there was so little information provided by the author(s), that their validity and sometimes even their identity was in question. We believe it is important to think of each *species inquirenda* as representing a baseline of information that can be developed further into research leading to a valid species description, a contribution to documenting the biodiversity of this important parasitic group, and additional contributions to the growing knowledge base about life histories and biology of this amazingly diverse and important parasitic group.

CONCLUSIONS

The Carnivora comprises a diverse group of mammals that are hosts to a fascinating diversity of apicomplexan parasites (Williams and Thorne, 1996). According to Wozencraft (2005), the order is composed of two major lineages, Feliformia Kretzoi, 1945 and Caniformia Kretzoi, 1938. Feliformia has 121 extant species consisting of 6 families, and the Caniformia lineage is somewhat larger with 165 species identified in 9 family lineages. Here we have attempted to provide a comprehensive, if not the most comprehensive, treatise describing the structural and biological knowledge of all known, named, and some unnamed, species within the coccidia that infect Carnivora species. In compiling the literature, and from our own research studying coccidia in many wild and domestic hosts, several issues relating to research on, and our current understanding of, these ubiquitous protozoan parasites require emphasis.

Historically, the taxonomy and identification of coccidian parasites was based primarily on studying the morphology of oocysts found in the feces, because this was the most readily available stage of these parasites, they were easy to collect by noninvasive methods, and they could be stored in a refrigerator for sometimes lengthy periods of time. Morphology is still a useful taxonomic tool, as evidenced by the large number of species descriptions in the literature for these apicomplexan parasites from carnivores and other animals. However, morphology alone is no longer sufficient by itself to identify many coccidian species, especially those in genera that have species with very small oocysts and sporocysts, because they have only a limited number of mensural characters for comparisons. Thus,

identifications ideally should be supplemented by multiple data sets with information collected from, but not limited to, location of sporulation (endogenous vs. exogenous), length of time needed for exogenous sporulation at a constant temperature, morphology and timing of some or all of the developmental stages in their endogenous life cycle (e.g., merogony, gamogony), length of prepatent and patent periods in experimentally-infected definitive hosts, host specificity as determined via carefully-controlled cross-transmission experiments, observations on histological changes, and pathology due to asexual and sexual endogenous development, and others, to clarify and compliment the complex taxonomy of these parasites. And now, with all the advances in DNA/RNA technologies, sequence data should be employed as a component of contemporary species descriptions, and used to conduct phylogenetic analyses to more robustly assign a parasite to a group, genus, or even species (e.g., see Merino et al., 2008, 2009, 2010). Thus, molecular tools to ensure accurate species identifications are becoming part of one's common taxonomic practice to better understand the host–parasite associations of these species and genera. The combination of as many of the above data sets as possible will enable more robust phylogenetic inferences to be made and will result in a more stable taxonomy for the coccidia. Numerous examples in this book may begin to affirm we are moving in the right direction, albeit slowly.

The taxonomic state of affairs for the majority of protist parasites of carnivores is sometimes confusing because many previous investigators either have not provided adequate morphological descriptions and/or have not adhered to accepted practices for identifying and naming new species (or higher taxa) of coccidia. For investigators planning to engage in taxonomic research on the coccidia in Carnivora, or any host taxon, we encourage them to evaluate both the formal requirements of the International Rules of Zoological Nomenclature (Ride et al., 1999), and the specific scientific reasons why they believe the description of new taxa (genera, species) is needed. When creating a new coccidian genus, the criteria should be established as to how and why this suite of characters differs from already existing genera within the familial lineage, and a formal, detailed definition of the new genus should be presented that convincingly differentiates it from existing, presumably closely related genera. We further encourage reviewers and editors to embrace and understand the use of the internationally accepted rules of properly naming new genera and species. Every competent journal editor and peer reviewer should understand *and* appreciate that taxonomy and nomenclature are instruments to prevent confusion, not to produce confusion, and the complete scientific name acts as the anchor for that species being described in perpetuity, whether parasite or host. As we move forward chronologically, we can expect that the application of new technologies/methods/tools will result in new knowledge that may demonstrate unknown differences in organisms that were previously thought to be well-known (e.g., sporocysts with SB vs. those without). The question then becomes which differences are essential or useful for strain, species, genus, or family discrimination? It only creates confusion when investigators discriminate species or genera and give them new names before they are investigated and compared with already existing ones.

Carnivora species, especially domestics, are important because they engage humans in so many different ways. Both domestic and, increasingly, nondomestic carnivore species are kept captive for educational and recreational purposes including, but not limited to: household pets, fur production, scientific research (e.g., chemotherapeutics, food additives, parasite immunity, and cross-transmission), and as research models in captive breeding programs for endangered species recovery programs (e.g., black-footed ferret). However, we should not ignore the magnitude of domesticated carnivore

populations directly attributable to human needs for companionship, migrations, and population growth on Earth. For example, the American Veterinary Medical Association estimated that there are now about 70 million dogs and 74 million cats in the continental United States (US Pet Ownership Statistics); China has >27 million dogs and 53 million cats; and almost all other countries have similar burgeoning dog and cat populations relative to their landmass and the numbers of people inhabiting each country (https://www.petsecure.com.au/pet-care/a-guide-to-worldwide-pet-ownership/). Despite all of the physical, social, and emotional benefits that close contact with dogs and cats provide for humans, they also can pose threats to public health, they are reservoirs of infectious apicomplexans with propagules transmissible to people and other animals, and they can contaminate pristine environments with these transmission stages (oocysts, sporocysts) capable of infecting and causing morbidity and mortality in previously unexposed wild carnivores (e.g., sea otters, polar bears) (Awadallah and Salem, 2015). Thus, domestic animals may transmit pathogens to endemic wildlife through direct contact or environmental contamination.

To expand and reiterate, domestic and wild carnivores are facing increasing perturbation because human population growth and expansive development leads to enhanced contact, disease transmission, parasite exchange, and increased disease susceptibility. That is, introduced animals impact endemic populations through predation, competition, and disease transmission. For example, some free-ranging carnivores, such as red foxes (*V. vulpes*), coyotes (*C. latrans*), and raccoons (*P. lotor*), often approach human settlements, which may enhance the possibility of their direct contact with domestic pets and humans, again with zoonotic potential for disease transmission. This has been termed "pathogen spillover;" it is a particular threat to endangered species and may lead to local extinctions (Woodroffe, 1999;

Daszak et al., 2000). For example, rabies and canine distemper viruses, from dogs, have decimated populations of African wild dogs (*Lycaon pictus*), Ethiopian wolves (*Canis simensis*), and African lions (*Panthera leo*) (Gascoyne et al., 1993a,b; Laurenson et al., 1998). A sound knowledge base of all the parasites that are out there (including the many coccidian lineages), who are their hosts, where are they found, and if they cause pathology and/or mortality can address many of the concerns regarding preventing and managing coccidiosis and other outbreaks to the good of all carnivores and other vertebrates in any particular ecosystem.

Appendix A

TABLE A1   Alphabetical List of All Apicomplexan Parasites Covered in This Book and the Carnivore Hosts From Which They Have Been Reported

APICOMPLEXAN PROTOZOA OF BJORK ET AL., 2000 (*SPECIES INQUIRENDA*)
Panthera leo (syn. *Leo leo*), Lion

APICOMPLEXAN PROTOZOA OF PATTON AND RABINOWITZ, 1994 (*SPECIES INQUIRENDA*)
Panthera pardus, Leopard
Panthera tigris, Tiger
Panthera tigris bengalensis, Bengal Tiger

BESNOITIA BESNOITI OF (MAROTEL, 1912) HENRY, 1913
Felis catus, Domestic Cat

BESNOITIA DARLINGI (BRUMPT, 1913) MANDOUR, 1965
Felis catus, Domestic Cat

BESNOITIA NEOTOMOFELIS DUBEY AND YABSLEY, 2010
Felis catus, Domestic Cat

BESNOITIA ORYCTOFELISI DUBEY ET AL., 2003c
Felis catus, Domestic Cat

BESNOITIA SP. OF MCKENNA AND CHARLESTON, 1980c (*SPECIES INQUIRENDA*)
Felis catus, Domestic Cat

BESNOITIA WALLACEI (WALLACE AND FRENKEL, 1975) FRENKEL, 1977 N. COMB.
Felis catus, Domestic Cat

CARYOSPORA BIGENETICA WACHA AND CHRISTIANSEN, 1982
Canis lupus familiaris (syn. *C. familiaris*), Domestic Dog

COCCIDIA, *CYCLOSPORA, EIMERIA* SPP. OF CHAKRABORTY ET AL., 2016 (*SPECIES INQUIRENDAE*)
Paradoxurus hermaphroditus, Asian Palm Civet
Paradoxurus jerdoni, Jerdon's Palm Civet

COCCIDIA/COCCIDIAN/COCCIDIA-LIKE/COCCIDIUM SPP. (*SPECIES INQUIRENDAE*) OF MANY AUTHORS (SEE CHAPTER 19)
Canis lupus, Wolf
Canis lupus familiaris (syn. *C. familiaris*), Domestic Dog
Felis catus, Domestic Cat
Martes foina, Beech Marten
Martes zibellina, Sable
Meles anakuma, Japanese Badger
Mustela nigripes, Black-footed Ferret
Mustela (syn. *Putorius*) *putorius furo*, Domestic Ferret
Neovison vison (syn. *Mustela vison*), American Mink
Panthera leo (syn. *Leo leo*), Lion
Procyon lotor, Raccoon
Ursus arctos (syn. *U. horribilis*), Brown Bear
Vulpes vulpes (syn. *V. vulgaris* Oken, 1816), Red or Silver Fox
Zalophus californianus, California Sea Lion

CRYPTOSPORIDIUM ANDERSONI LINDSAY ET AL., 2000
Ailuropoda melanoleuca, Giant Panda
Ailurus fulgens, Red Panda
Neovison vison, American Mink

CRYPTOSPORIDIUM BAILEYI (?) OF MCGLADE ET AL., 2003 (*SPECIES INQUIRENDA*)
Felis catus, Domestic Cat

CRYPTOSPORIDIUM CANIS FAYER ET AL., 2001
Canis latrans, Coyote
Canis lupus familiaris (syn. *C. familiaris*), Domestic Dog
Herpestes ichneumon, Egyptian Mongoose
Neovison vison, American Mink
Nyctereutes procyonoides, Raccoon Dog
Vulpes (syn. *Alopex*) *lagopus*, Arctic Fox or Blue Fox
Vulpes vulpes, Red Fox or Silver Fox
Vulpes spp.

CRYPTOSPORIDIUM CURYI (?) CITED BY OGASSAWARA ET AL., 1986 (*SPECIES INQUIRENDA*)
Felis catus, Domestic Cat

CRYPTOSPORIDIUM FELIS ISEKI, 1979
Felis catus, Domestic Cat
Vulpes vulpes, Red Fox or Silver Fox

CRYPTOSPORIDIUM HOMINIS MORGAN-RYAN ET AL., 2002
Meles meles, European Badger

CRYPTOSPORIDIUM MELEAGRIDIS SLAVIN, 1955
Canis lupus familiaris (syn. *C. familiaris*), Domestic Dog
Neovison vison (syn. *Mustela vison*), American Mink

CRYPTOSPORIDIUM MURIS (TYZZER, 1907) TYZZER, 1910
Canis lupus familiaris (syn. *C. familiaris*), Domestic Dog
Felis catus, Domestic Cat
Pusa hispida, Ringed Seal

CRYPTOSPORIDIUM PARVUM TYZZER, 1912
Ailurus fulgens, Red Panda
Canis lupus familiaris (syn. *C. familiaris*), Domestic Dog
Felis catus, Domestic Cat
Lontra canadensis, North American River Otter
Martes foina, Beech Marten
Meles meles, European Badger
Mephitis mephitis, Striped Skunk
Mungos mungo, Banded Mongoose
Mustela erminea, Ermine
Mustela putorius furo, Domestic Ferret
Neovison vison, American Mink
Nyctereutes procyonoides viverrinus, Korean Raccoon Dog
Procyon lotor, Raccoon
Ursus americanus, American Black Bear
Vulpes vulpes, Red or Silver Fox
Zalophus californianus, California Sea Lion

CRYPTOSPORIDIUM RYANAE **FAYER ET AL., 2008**
 Felis catus, Domestic Cat

CRYPTOSPORIDIUM SCROFARUM **KVÁČ ET AL., 2013**
 Canis lupus familiaris (syn. *C. familiaris*), Domestic Dog

CRYPTOSPORIDIUM **SPP. (***SPECIES INQUIRENDAE***) OF MANY AUTHORS (SEE CHAPTER 19)**
 Acinonyx jubatus, Cheetah
 Ailuropoda melanoleuca, Giant Panda
 Canis latrans, Coyote
 Canis lupus, Wolf
 Canis lupus dingo, Dingo
 Canis lupus familiaris (syn. *C. familiaris*), Domestic Dog
 Chrysocyon brachyurus, Maned Wolf
 Cystophora cristata, Hooded Seal
 Felis catus, Domestic Cat
 Felis chaus, Jungle Cat
 Genetta genetta, Common Genet
 Helarctos malayanus, Sun Bear
 Leopardus pardalis, Ocelot
 Leopardus tigrinus, Oncilla
 Lontra canadensis, North American River Otter
 Leptonychotes weddellii, Weddell Seal
 Lutra lutra, European Otter
 Lynx (syn. *Felis*) *rufus*, Bobcat
 Martes foina, Beech Marten
 Mephitis mephitis, Striped Skunk
 Mirounga leonina, Southern Elephant Seal
 Mustela erminea, Ermine
 Mustela (syn. *Putorius*) *putorius furo*, Domestic Ferret
 Neovison (*Mustela*) *vison*, American Mink
 Nyctereutes procyonoides, Raccoon Dog
 Otaria flavescens (syn. *O. byronia*), South American Sea Lion
 Pagophilus groenlandicus, Harp Seal
 Panthera pardus, Leopard
 Panthera tigris, Tiger
 Panthera tigris corbetti, Indochinese Tiger
 Panthera tigris jacksoni, Malayan Tiger
 Panthera tigris sumatrae, Sumatran Tiger
 Panthera sp., Leopard
 Phoca vitulina (syn. *P. richardii*), Harbor Seal
 Procyon lotor, Raccoon
 Pusa hispida, Ringed Seal
 Ursus arctos, Brown Bear
 Ursus maritimus, Polar Bear
 Ursus thibetanus, Asian Black Bear
 Vulpes (syn. *Alopex*) *lagopus*, Arctic or Blue Fox
 Vulpes vulpes (syns. *V. fulvus, V. vulgaris*), Red or Silver Fox
 Zalophus californianus, California Sea Lion

CRYPTOSPORIDIUM UBIQUITUM **FAYER ET AL., 2010**
 Neovison vison, American Mink
 Vulpes vulpes (syns. *V. fulvus, V. vulgaris*), Red or Silver Fox

CYCLOSPORA CAYETANENSIS OF AWADALLAH AND SALEM, 2015 (*SPECIES INQUIRENDA*)

Canis lupus familiaris (syn. *C. familiaris*), Domestic Dog

CYSTOISOSPORA AFRICANA (SYN. *ISOSPORA AFRICANA* PRASAD, 1961b) N. COMB.

Ictonyx (syn. *Poecilictis*) *libyca alexandrae*, Saharan Striped Polecat

CYSTOISOSPORA ALTAICA (SYN. *ISOSPORA ALTAICA* SVANBAEV AND RACHMATULLINA, 1971) N. COMB.

Mustela altaica, Mountain Weasel

CYSTOISOSPORA ARCTOPITHECI (SYN. *ISOSPORA ARCTOPITHECI* RODHAIN, 1933) N. COMB.

Canis lupus familiaris (syn. *C. familiaris*), Domestic Dog
Eira barbara, Tayra
Felis catus, Domestic Cat
Nasua nasua, South American Coati
Potos flavus, Kinkajou

CYSTOISOSPORA BENGALENSIS (SYN. *ISOSPORA BENGALENSIS* PATNAIK AND ACHARJYO, 1971) N. COMB.

Panthera tigris tigris, Bengal Tiger

CYSTOISOSPORA BURIATICA (SYN. *ISOSPORA BURIATICA* YAKIMOFF AND MATSCHOULSKY, 1940) N. COMB.

Vulpes bengalensis, Bengal Fox
Vulpes corsac, Corsac Fox
Vulpes vulpes (syns. *V. fulvus*, *V. vulgaris*), Red or Silver Fox

CYSTOISOSPORA BURROWSI (SYN. *ISOSPORA BURROWSI* TRAYSER AND TODD, 1978) N. COMB.

Canis lupus familiaris (syn. *C. familiaris*), Domestic Dog

CYSTOISOSPORA CANIS (SYN. *ISOSPORA CANIS* NEMESÉRI, 1959) N. COMB.

Canis aureus, Golden Jackal
Canis latrans, Coyote
Canis lupus familiaris (syn. *C. familiaris*), Domestic Dog
Felis catus, Domestic Cat (experimental intermediate host as newborn kittens)
Vulpes vulpes (syns. *V. fulvus*, *V. vulgaris*), Red or Silver Fox

CYSTOISOSPORA CANIVELOCIS (SYN. *ISOSPORA CANIVELOCIS* WEIDMAN, 1915 EMEND. WENYON, 1923) N. COMB.

Vulpes (syn. *Alopex*) *lagopus*, Arctic or Blue Fox (experimental)
Vulpes velox, Swift Fox
Vulpes vulpes (syns. *V. fulvus*, *V. vulgaris*), Red or Silver Fox

CYSTOISOSPORA CHOBOTARI (SYN. *ISOSPORA CHOBOTARI* LEVINE AND IVENS, 1981) N. COMB.

Procyon lotor, Raccoon

CYSTOISOSPORA DASGUPTAI (SYN. *ISOSPORA DASGUPTAI* LEVINE ET AL., 1975) N. COMB.

Herpestes edwardsi (syn. *Her. mungo*), Indian Gray Mongoose
Herpestes javanicus (syn. *Her. auropunctatus*), Small Asian Mongoose

CYSTOISOSPORA DUTOITI (YAKIMOFF ET AL., 1933a) N. COMB.

Canis aureus, Golden Jackal

CYSTOISOSPORA EVERSMANNI (SVANBAEV, 1956) EMEND. YI-FAN ET AL., 2012

Mustela eversmanii, Steppe polecat
Mustela putorius (syn. *Mustela vison*), European Polecat

CYSTOISOSPORA FELINA (SYN. *ISOSPORA FELINA* PATNAIK AND ACHARJYO, 1971) N. COMB.

Panthera tigris tigris (L., 1758), Bengal Tiger

CYSTOISOSPORA FELIS (WENYON, 1923) FRENKEL, 1977
Canis lupus familiaris (syn. *C. familiaris*), Domestic Dog (experimental intermediate host)
Felis catus, Domestic Cat (definitive host, experimental intermediate host)
Felis chaus, Jungle Cat
Felis silvestris, Wildcat
Leopardus pardalis, Ocelot
Leptailurus serval, Serval
Lynx lynx, Eurasian Lynx
Lynx pardinus, Iberian Lynx
Panthera leo, Lion
Panthera onca, Jaguar
Panthera tigris, Tiger

CYSTOISOSPORA FONSECAI (SYN. *ISOSPORA FONSECAI* YAKIMOFF AND MATSCHOULSKY, 1940) N. COMB.
Ursus arctos isabellinus (syn. *Ursus pamirensis*), Brown or Red Bear

CYSTOISOSPORA FRENKELI ARCAY, 1981
Felis catus, Domestic Cat

CYSTOISOSPORA GARNHAMI (SYN. *ISOSPORA GARNHAMI* BRAY, 1954) N. COMB.
Crossarchus obscurus, Common Kusimanse
Helogale parvula (syn. *Hel. undulatus*), Common Dwarf Mongoose
Herpestes edwardsi (syn. *Her. mungo*), Indian Gray Mongoose

CYSTOISOSPORA GOTTSCHALKI (SYN. *ISOSPORA LUTRAE* VON CORD GOTTSCHALK, 2000) N. COMB., N. SP.
Lutra lutra, European Otter

CYSTOISOSPORA GOUSSEVI (SYN. *ISOSPORA GOUSSEVI* MUSAEV AND VEISOV, 1983) N. COMB.
Mustela nivalis, Least Weasel

CYSTOISOSPORA HERPESTEI (SYN. *ISOSPORA HERPESTEI* LEVINE ET AL., 1975) N. COMB.
Herpestes edwardsi (syn. *Her. mungo*), Indian Gray Mongoose
Herpestes javanicus (syn. *Her. auropunctatus*), Small Asian Mongoose

CYSTOISOSPORA HOAREI (SYN. *ISOSPORA HOAREI* BRAY, 1954) N. COMB.
Herpestes edwardsi (syn. *Her. mungo*), Indian Gray Mongoose
Helogale parvula (syn. *Hel. undulatus*), Common Dwarf Mongoose

CYSTOISOSPORA HOOGSTRAALI (SYN. *ISOSPORA HOOGSTRAALI* PRASAD, 1961b) N. COMB.
Ictonyx (syn. *Poecilictis*) *libyca alexandrae*, Saharan Striped Polecat

CYSTOISOSPORA ISRAELI KUTTIN AND KALLER, 1992
Arctocephalus pusillus, Brown (South African) Fur Seal

CYSTOISOSPORA LAIDLAWI (SYN. *ISOSPORA LAIDLAWI* HOARE, 1927) N. COMB.
Mustela (syn. *Putorius*) *putorius furo*, European Polecat (Domestic Ferret)
Neovison vison (syns. *Mustela vison*, *Lutreola vison*), American Mink
Vulpes vulpes (syns. *V. fulvus*, *V. vulgaris*), Red or Silver Fox

CYSTOISOSPORA LEONINA (SYN. *ISOSPORA LEONINA* MANDAL AND RAY, 1960) N. COMB.
Panthera leo, Lion

CYSTOISOSPORA LEOPARDI (SYN. *ISOSPORA LEOPARDI* AGRAWAL ET AL., 1981) N. COMB.
Neofelis nebulosa, Clouded Leopard

CYSTOISOSPORA LEVINEI (SYN. *ISOSPORA LEVINEI* DUBEY, 1963a) N. COMB.
Hyaena hyaena (syn. *H. striata*), Brown, Indian, or Striped Hyaena

CYSTOISOSPORA LUTRAE **(SYN.** *ISOSPORA LUTRAE* **TORRES ET AL., 2000) N. COMB.**
  Lutra lutra, European Otter

CYSTOISOSPORA MARTESSII **(SYN.** *ISOSPORA MARTESSII* **NUKERBAEVA, 1981a) N. COMB.**
  Martes zibellina, Sable

CYSTOISOSPORA MELIS **(PELLÉRDY, 1955) N. COMB.**
  Meles meles (syn. *Meles taxus*), European Badger

CYSTOISOSPORA MIRUNGAE **(SYN.** *ISOSPORA MIRUNGAE* **DRÓŻDŻ, 1987) N. COMB.**
  Mirounga leonina, Southern Elephant Seal

CYSTOISOSPORA MOHINI **(SYN.** *ISOSPORA MOHINI* **AGRAWAL ET AL., 1981) N. COMB.**
  Panthera leo, Lion

CYSTOISOSPORA MUNGOI **(SYN.** *ISOSPORA MUNGOI* **LEVINE ET AL., 1975) N. COMB.**
  Herpestes edwardsi (syn. *Her. mungo*), Indian Gray Mongoose

CYSTOISOSPORA NEORIVOLTA **(SYN.** *ISOSPORA NEORIVOLTA* **DUBEY AND MAHRT, 1978) N. COMB.**
  Canis latrans, Coyote
  Canis lupus familiaris (syn. *C. familiaris*), Domestic Dog

CYSTOISOSPORA **(?)** *NEOTOMAFELIS* **(GALAVÍZ-SILVA ET AL., 1991) N. COMB.**
  Felis catus, Domestic Cat

CYSTOISOSPORA NIVALIS **(SYN.** *ISOSPORA NIVALIS* **MUSAEV AND VEISOV, 1983) N. COMB.**
  Mustela nivalis, Least Weasel

CYSTOISOSPORA OHIOENSIS **(SYN.** *ISOSPORA OHIOENSIS* **DUBEY, 1975c) FRENKEL, 1977**
  Canis latrans, Coyote
  Canis lupus dingo, Dingo (?)
  Canis lupus familiaris (syn. *C. familiaris*), Domestic Dog
  Nyctereutes procyonoides ussuriensis, Raccoon Dog
  Vulpes vulpes (syns. *V. fulvus*, *V. vulgaris*), Red or Silver Fox (?)

CYSTOISOSPORA OHIOENSIS **COMPLEX OF PALMER ET AL., 2008a (***SPECIES INQUIRENDA***)**
  Canis lupus familiaris (syn. *C. familiaris*), Domestic Dog

CYSTOISOSPORA OHIOENSIS-**LIKE OF GATES AND NOLAN, 2009 (***SPECIES INQUIRENDA***)**
  Canis lupus familiaris (syn. *C. familiaris*), Domestic Dog

CYSTOISOSPORA PANTHERI **(***ISOSPORA PANTHERI* **AGRAWAL ET AL., 1981) N. COMB.**
  Panthera leo (syn. *Leo leo*), Lion

CYSTOISOSPORA PARDUSI **(***ISOSPORA PARDUSI* **PATNAIK AND ACHARJYO, 1971) N. COMB.**
  Panthera pardus, Leopard

CYSTOISOSPORA PAVLODARICA **(NUKERBAEVA AND SVANBAEV, 1973) N. COMB.**
  Vulpes (syn. *Alopex*) *lagopus*, Blue or Arctic Fox
  Vulpes vulpes (syns. *V. fulvus*, *V. vulgaris*), Red or Silver Fox

CYSTOISOSPORA PAVLOVSKYI **(SVANBAEV, 1956) EMEND. YI-FAN ET AL., 2012**
  Mustela eversmanii, Steppe Polecat

CYSTOISOSPORA PELLERDYI **(SYN.** *ISOSPORA PELLERDYI* **DUBEY AND PANDE, 1964) N. COMB.**
  Herpestes edwardsi (syn. *Her. mungo*), Indian Gray Mongoose

***CYSTOISOSPORA RIVOLTA* (GRASSI, 1879) FRENKEL, 1977**

Acinonyx jubatus, Cheetah
Canis lupus dingo, Dingo
Canis lupus familiaris (syn. *C. familiaris*), Domestic Dog
Felis catus, Domestic Cat (definitive host, experimental intermediate host)
Felis chaus, Jungle Cat
Felis silvestris, Wildcat
Leptailurus serval, Serval
Leopardus pardalis, Ocelot
Lynx lynx, Eurasian Lynx
Panthera leo, Lion
Panthera onca, Jaguar
Panthera pardus, Leopard
Panthera tigris, Tiger

***CYSTOISOSPORA RIVOLTA*-LIKE OF GATES AND NOLAN, 2009 (*SPECIES INQUIRENDA*)**

Felis catus, Domestic Cat

***CYSTOISOSPORA SENGERI* (SYN. *ISOSPORA SENGERI* LEVINE AND IVENS, 1964) N. COMB.**

Spilogale putorius ambarvalis, Eastern Spotted Skunk

***CYSTOISOSPORA SPILOGALES* (SYN. *ISOSPORA SPILOGALES* LEVINE AND IVENS, 1964) N. COMB.**

Spilogale putorius ambarvalis, Eastern Spotted Skunk

***CYSTOISOSPORA* SPP. (*SPECIES INQUIRENDAE*) OF MANY AUTHORS (SEE CHAPTER 19)**

Canis lupus familiaris (syn. *C. familiaris*), Domestic Dog
Crocuta crocuta, Spotted Hyaena
Felis catus, Domestic Cat

***CYSTOISOSPORA THEILERI* (SYN. *ISOSPORA THEILERI* YAKIMOFF AND LEWKOWITSCH, 1932) N. COMB.**

Canis aureus, Golden Jackal

***CYSTOISOSPORA TIMONI* EL-GAYAR ET AL., 2008**

Suricata suricatta, Meerkat, Suricate, Slender-tailed Meerkat

***CYSTOISOSPORA TRIFFITTI* (NUKERBAEVA AND SVANBAEV, 1973) N. COMB.**

Vulpes (syn. *Alopex*) *lagopus*, Blue or Arctic Fox
Vulpes vulpes (syns. *V. fulvus*, *V. vulgaris*), Red or Silver Fox

***CYSTOISOSPORA URSI* (SYN. *ISOSPORA URSI*) AGRAWAL ET AL., 1981**

Melursus ursinus, Sloth Bear

***CYSTOISOSPORA VIVERRAE* (SYN. *ISOSPORA VIVERRAE* ADLER, 1924) N. COMB.**

Civettictis civetta (syn. *Viverra civetta*), African Civet

***CYSTOISOSPORA VIVERRINA* (SYN. *ISOSPORA VIVERRINA* AGRAWAL AND CHAUHAN, 1993) N. COMB.**

Prionailurus (syn. *Felis*) *viverrinus*, Fishing Cat

***CYSTOISOSPORA VULPINA* (NIESCHULZ AND BOS, 1933) FRENKEL, 1977**

Canis lupus familiaris (syn. *C. familiaris*), Domestic Dog (experimental)
Vulpes bengalensis, Bengal Fox
Vulpes (syn. *Alopex*) *lagopus*, Blue or Arctic Fox
Vulpes vulpes (syns. *V. fulvus*, *V. vulgaris*), Red or Silver Fox

***CYSTOISOSPORA ZORILLAE* (SYN. *ISOSPORA ZORILLAE* (PRASAD, 1961b) EMEND. PELLÉRDY, 1963) N. COMB.**

Ictonyx (syn. *Poecilictis*) *libyca alexandrae*, Saharan Striped Polecat

EIMERIA ADLERI YAKIMOFF AND GOUSSEFF, 1936
Vulpes vulpes (syns. *V. fulvus, V. vulgaris*), Red or Silver Fox

EIMERIA AILURI AGRAWAL ET AL., 1981
Ailurus fulgens, Red Panda

EIMERIA ALBERTENSIS HAIR AND MAHRT, 1970
Ursus americanus, American Black Bear

EIMERIA ANEKALENSIS RAJASEKARIAH ET AL., 1971
Panthera pardus, Leopard

EIMERIA ARCTOWSKI DRÓŻDŻ, 1987
Leptonychotes weddellii, Weddell Seal

EIMERIA AUREI BHATIA ET AL., 1979
Canis aureus naria Wroughton, 1916, Golden Jackal

EIMERIA BAKANENSIS SVANBAEV AND RACHMATULLINA, 1971
Vulpes vulpes (syns. *V. fulvus, V. vulgaris*), Red or Silver Fox

EIMERIA BASKANICA OF NUKERBAEVA AND SVANBAEV, 1972 OR 1973 (?) (*SPECIES INQUIRENDA*)
Mustela erminea, Ermine or Stoat

EIMERIA BOREALIS HAIR AND MAHRT, 1970
Ursus americanus, American Black Bear

EIMERIA CANIS WENYON, 1923
Canis latrans, Coyote
Canis lupus dingo, Dingo
Canis lupus familiaris (syn. *C. familiaris*), Domestic Dog
Felis catus, Domestic Cat (?)

EIMERIA CATI YAKIMOFF, (1932) 1933
Felis catus, Domestic Cat
Felis chaus, Jungle Cat

EIMERIA CHAUS RYŠAVÝ, 1954
Felis chaus, Jungle Cat

EIMERIA FELINA NIESCHULZ, 1924b
Felis catus, Domestic Cat
Felis chaus, Jungle Cat
Felis silvestris, Wildcat
Panthera leo, Lion

EIMERIA FURONIS HOARE, 1927
Mustela ermine, Ermine (Stoat)
Mustela nigripes, Black-footed Ferret
Mustela (syn. *Putorius*) *putorius furo*, European Polecat (Domestic Ferret)
Neovison vison (syns. *Mustela vison, Lutreola vison*), American Mink

EIMERIA GENETTAE OF AGOSTINUCCI AND BRONZINI, 1955 (*SPECIES INQUIRENDA*)
Genetta gemetta (syn. *G. dongolana*), Common Genet

EIMERIA HAMMONDI DUBEY AND PANDE, 1963b
Felis chaus, Jungle Cat

EIMERIA HARTMANNI **RASTEGAÏEFF, 1930**
Panthera pardus, Leopard (?)
Panthera tigris, Tiger

EIMERIA HEISSINI **SVANBAEV, 1956**
Vulpes corsac, Corsac Fox

EIMERIA HIEPEI **GRÄFNER ET AL., 1967**
Mustela lutreola, European mink
Neovison vison (syns. *Mustela vison, Lutreola vison*), American Mink

EIMERIA ICTIDEA **HOARE, 1927**
Mustela eversmanii, Steppe Polecat (?)
Mustela nigripes, Black-footed Ferret
Mustela (syn. *Putorius*) *putorius furo*, European Polecat (Domestic Ferret)
Neovison vison (syns. *Mustela vison, Lutreola vison*), American Mink

EIMERIA IMANTAUICA **OF NUKERBAEVA AND SVANBAEV, 1973**
Vulpes (syn. *Alopex*) *lagopus*, Arctic or Blue Fox

EIMERIA IRARA **CARINI AND FONSECA, 1938**
Eira barbara, Tayra

EIMERIA JALPAIGURIENSIS **BANDYOPADHYAY, 1982**
Herpestes edwardsi (syn. *Her. mungo*), Indian Gray Mongoose

EIMERIA LI **OF GOLEMANSKI, 1975a**
Vulpes vulpes (syns. *V. fulvus, V. vulgaris*), Red or Silver Fox

EIMERIA LOMARII **DUBEY, 1963a**
Vulpes bengalensis, Bengal Fox

EIMERIA, ISOSPORA, **AND** *SARCOCYSTIS* **SPP. OF COLÓN AND PATTON, 2012 (***SPECIES INQUIRENDAE***)**
Viverra tangalunga, Malayan Civet

EIMERIA MATHURAI **DUBEY AND PANDE, 1963b**
Felis chaus, Jungle Cat

EIMERIA MELIS **KOTLÁN AND POSPESCH, 1933**
Meles meles (syn. *Meles taxus*), European Badger
Neovison vison (syns. *Mustela vison, Lutreola vison*), American Mink

EIMERIA MEPHITIDIS **ANDREWS, 1928**
Mephitis mephitis (syn. *M. hudsonica*), Striped Skunk
Spilogale putorius, Eastern Spotted Skunk

EIMERIA MEPHITIDIS **OF YAKIMOFF AND GOUSSEFF, 1936 (***SPECIES INQUIRENDA***)**
Mephitis mephitis (syn. *M. hudsonica*), Striped Skunk
Mustela (syn. *Putorius*) *putorius furo*, Domestic Ferret
Spilogale putorius, Eastern Spotted Skunk

EIMERIA MESNILI **OF RASTEGAÏEFF, 1929c (***SPECIES INQUIRENDA***)**
Vulpes (syn. *Alopex*) *lagopus*, Arctic or Blue Fox

EIMERIA MUSTELAE **IWANOFF-GOBZEM, 1934**
Mustela nivalis, Least Weasel
Neovison vison (syns. *Mustela vison, Lutreola vison*), American Mink

***EIMERIA NASUAE* CARINI AND GRECHI, 1938**
  Nasua narica, Coati

***EIMERIA NEWALAI* DUBEY AND PANDE, 1963a**
  Herpestes edwardsi (syn. *Her. mungo*), Indian Gray Mongoose

***EIMERIA NOVOWENYONI* OF RASTEGAÏEFF, 1929a (*SPECIES INQUIRENDA*)**
  Panthera pardus, Leopard (?)
  Panthera tigris, Tiger (?)

***EIMERIA NUTTALLI* YAKIMOFF AND MATIKASCHWILI, 1933**
  Procyon lotor, Raccoon
  Procyon pygmaeus, Pygmy Raccoon

***EIMERIA PANDEI* (PATNAIK AND RAY, 1965) PATNAIK AND RAY, 1966**
  Herpestes edwardsi (syn. *Her. mungo*), Indian Gray Mongoose

***EIMERIA PHOCAE* HSU ET AL., 1974a**
  Halichoerus grypus (?), Grey Seal
  Phoca vitulina concolor, Harbor Seal

***EIMERIA POTI* LAINSON, 1968**
  Potos flavus (Schreber, 1774), Kinkajou

***EIMERIA PROCYONIS* INABNIT ET AL., 1972**
  Procyon lotor, Raccoon

***EIMERIA RAYII* OF RAO AND BHATAVDEKAR, 1957 (*SPECIES INQUIRENDA*)**
  Canis lupus familiaris (syn. *C. familiaris*), Domestic Dog

***EIMERIA SABLII* NUKERBAEVA, 1981a**
  Martes zibellina, Sable

***EIMERIA SIBIRICA* YAKIMOFF AND TERWINSKY, 1931**
  Martes martes, European Pine Marten
  Martes zibellina, Sable

***EIMERIA STIEDAE* OF GUILLEBEAU, 1916 (*SPECIES INQUIRENDA*)**
  Canis lupus familiaris (syn. *C. familiaris*), Domestic Dog

***EIMERIA* SPP. (*SPECIES INQUIRENDAE*) OF MANY AUTHORS (SEE CHAPTER 19)**
  Canis lupus familiaris (syn. *C. familiaris*), Domestic Dog
  Chrysocyon brachyurus, Maned Wolf
  Felis catus, Domestic Cat
  Leptonychotes weddellii, Weddell Seal
  Lobodon carcinophaga, Crabtree Seal
  Lynx lynx isabellinus, Central Asian Lynx
  Martes martes, European Pine Marten
  Mustela nigripes, Black-footed Ferret
  Mustela nivalis, Least Weasel
  Neovison (syn. *Mustela*) *vison,* American Mink
  Otaria flavescens (syn. *O. byronia* (de Blainville, 1820)), South American Sea Lion
  Paradoxurus hermaphroditus, Asian Palm Civet
  Procyon lotor, Raccoon
  Pusa caspica (syn. *Phoca caspica*), Caspian Seal
  Ursus arctos (syn. *U. horribilis*), Brown Bear
  Vulpes vulpes (syn. *V. vulgaris*), Red or Silver Fox

EIMERIA TADZHIKISTANICA OF ANPILOGOVA AND SOKOV, 1973 (*SPECIES INQUIRENDA*)

Lynx lynx isabellinus, Central Asian Lynx

EIMERIA URSI YAKIMOFF AND MATSCHOULSKY, 1935

Ursus arctos, Brown Bear

EIMERIA VISON (KINGSCOTE, 1934a,b) KINGSCOTE, 1935

Mustela (syn. *Putorius*) *putorius furo*, European Polecat, Domestic Ferret
Neovison vison (syns. *Mustela vison*, *Lutreola vison*), American Mink

EIMERIA VISONLEVINEI (LEVINE, 1948) N. COMB., N. SP.

Neovison vison (syns. *Mustela vison*, *Lutreola vison*), American Mink

EIMERIA VORONEZBENSIS LEVINE AND IVENS, 1981

Mephitis mephitis (syn. *M. hudsonica*), Striped Skunk

EIMERIA VULPIS OF GALLI-VALERIO, 1929b (*SPECIES INQUIRENDA*)

Vulpes vulpes (syn. *V. vulgaris*), Red or Silver Fox

EIMERIA WEDDELLI DRÓŻDŻ, 1987

Leptonychotes weddellii, Weddell Seal

HAMMONDIA HAMMONDI FRENKEL, 1974

Felis catus, Domestic Cat

HAMMONDIA HEYDORNI (TADROS AND LAARMAN, 1976) DUBEY, 1977c

Canis latrans, Coyote
Canis lupus dingo, Dingo
Canis lupus familiaris (syn. *C. familiaris*), Domestic Dog
Cerdocyon thous, Crab-eating Fox
Neovison vison (syn. *Mustela vison*), American mink
Otaria flavescens (syn. *Otaria byronia*), South American Sea Lion
Vulpes (syn. *Alopex*) *lagopus*, Arctic or Blue Fox
Vulpes vulpes (syns. *V. fulvus*, *V. vulgaris*), Red or Silver Fox

HAMMONIDA SPP./*HAMMONDIA–NEOSPORA*-LIKE/*HAMMONDIA–TOXOPLASMA*-LIKE (*SPECIES INQUIRENDAE*) OF ONE OR MORE AUTHORS (SEE CHAPTER 19)

Canis lupus, Wolf
Canis lupus familiaris (syn. *C. familiaris*), Domestic Dog
Felis catus, Domestic Cat
Neovison (syn. *Mustela*) *vison*, American Mink
Vulpes (syn. *Alopex*) *lagopus*, Arctic or Blue Fox
Vulpes vulpes (syn. *V. vulgaris*), Silver or Red Fox

HAMMONDIA PARDALIS HENDRICKS ET AL., 1979

Panthera (syn. *Puma*) *onca*, Jaguar
Puma concolor, Cougar

HEPATOZOON AMERICANUM VINCENT-JOHNSON ET AL., 1997

Canis latrans, Coyote (intermediate host)
Canis lupus familiaris (syn. *C. familiaris*), Domestic Dog (intermediate host)

HEPATOZOON CANIS (JAMES, 1905) WENYON, 1926b

Acinonyx jubatus, Cheetah (intermediate host)
Canis latrans, Coyote (intermediate host)
Canis lupus familiaris (syn. *C. familiaris*), Domestic Dog (intermediate host)

Canis mesomelas, Black-backed Jackal (intermediate host)
Cerdocyon thous, Crab-eating Fox (intermediate host)
Crocuta crocuta, Spotted Hyaena (intermediate host)
Felis catus, Domestic Cat (intermediate host)
Vulpes vulpes silacea, Red or Silver Fox (intermediate host)
Panthera leo, Lion (intermediate host)
Panthera pardus, Leopard (intermediate host)

HEPATOZOON FELIS PATTON, 1908
Felis catus, Domestic Cat (intermediate host)
Lycalopex gymnocercus, Pampas Fox (?) (intermediate host)
Prionailurus bengalensis, Leopard Cat (intermediate host)
Prionailurus bengalensis euptilurus, Tsushima Leopard Cat (intermediate host)
Panthera onca, Jaguar (intermediate host)
Prionailurus iriomotensis (syn. *P. bengalensis iriomotensis*), Iriomote Wild Cat (intermediate host)

HEPATOZOON MUSTELIS NOVILLA ET AL., 1980
Mustela eversmanni satunini, Siberian Polecat (intermediate host)

HEPATOZOON PROCYONIS RICHARDS, 1961
Nasua nasua, South American Coati (intermediate host)
Procyon cancrivorus, Crab-eating Raccoon (intermediate host)
Procyon cancrivorus panamensis, Panamanian Crab-eating Raccoon (intermediate host)
Procyon lotor, Raccoon (intermediate host)

HEPATOZOON SPP. (*SPECIES INQUIRENDAE*) OF ONE OR MORE AUTHORS (SEE CHAPTER 19)
Canis adustus, Side-striped Jackal; and lions, cheetahs, hyaenas, and leopards
Canis latrans, Coyote
Canis lupus (syn. *C. familiaris*), Domestic Dog
Crocuta crocuta, Spotted Hyaena
Felis catus, Domestic Cat
Genetta genetta (syn. *G. dongolana*), Common Genet
Genetta thierryi (syn. *Genetta rubiginosa*), Haussa Genet
Genetta tigrine, Cape Genet
Leopardus pardalis, Ocelot
Lynx (syn. *Felis*) *rufus*, Bobcat
Martes melampus, Japanese Marten
Neovison (syn. *Mustela*) *vison*, American Mink
Panthera leo, Lion
Panthera leo massaica, Massai Lion
Panthera pardus, Leopard

HEPATOZOON URSI KUBO ET AL., 2008
Ursus thibetanus japonicus, Japanese Black Bear (intermediate host)

HOAREOSPORIDIUM PELLERDYI OF PANDE ET AL., 1972 (*SPECIES INQUIRENDA*)
Canis lupus familiaris (syn. *C. familiaris*), Domestic Dog

ISOSPORA ARCTOPITHECI RODHAIN, 1933
Callithrix penicillata, Black Tufted-ear Marmoset

ISOSPORA BIGEMINA (STILES, 1891) OF LÜHE, 1906 (*SPECIES INQUIRENDA*)
Canis lupus familiaris (syn. *C. familiaris*), Domestic Dog

ISOSPORA BIGEMINA FREE SPOROCYSTS OF GASSNER, 1940 (*SPECIES INQUIRENDA*)
Canis lupus familiaris (syn. *C. familiaris*), Domestic Dog

ISOSPORA BIGEMINA **LARGE FORM OF DUSZYNSKI AND SPEER, 1976 (*SPECIES INQUIRENDA*)**
Lynx (syn. *Felis*) *rufus*, Bobcat

ISOSPORA BIGEMINA **OF SEALANDER, 1943 (*SPECIES INQUIRENDA*)**
Neovison (syn. *Mustela*) *vison*, American Mink

ISOSPORA BURROWSI/ISOSPORA OHIOENSIS-**LIKE OF CIRAK AND BAUER, 2004 (*SPECIES INQUIRENDA*)**
Canis lupus familiaris (syn. *C. familiaris*), Domestic Dog

ISOSPORA CANIVELOCIS-**LIKE OOCYSTS. OF DAHLGREN AND GJERDE, 2010b**
Vulpes vulpes (syn. *V. vulgaris*), Silver or Red Fox

ISOSPORA DUTOITI **OF YAKIMOFF ET AL., 1933a (*SPECIES INQUIRENDA*)**
Canis aureus, Golden Jackal

ISOSPORA FELIS **OF MACKINNON AND DIBB, 1938**
Leptailurus serval (syn. *Felis serval*), Serval

ISOSPORA FENNECHI **PRASAD, 1961a (?)**
Vulpes (syn. *Fennecus*) *zerda*, Fennec Fox

ISOSPORA ICHNEUMONIS **OF LEVINE ET AL., 1975 (*SPECIES INQUIRENDA*)**
Herpestes ichneumon, Egyptian Mongoose

ISOSPORA LYNCIS **LEVINE AND IVENS, 1981 (*SPECIES INQUIRENDA*)**
Lynx sp., Bobcat

ISOSPORA MUSTELAE **OF GALLI-VALERIO, 1932 (NOMEN NUDUM)**
Martes martes, European Pine Marten

ISOSPORA NOVOCATI **OF PELLÉRDY, 1974b (NOMEN NUDUM)**
Felis catus, Domestic Cat

ISOSPORA OHIOENSIS **DUBEY, 1975c**
Canis lupus familiaris (syn. *C. familiaris*), Domestic Dog
Procyon lotor, Raccoon (?)

ISOSPORA OHIOENSIS **COMPLEX OF FONTANARROSA ET AL., 2006 (*SPECIES INQUIRENDA*)**
Canis lupus familiaris (syn. *C. familiaris*), Domestic Dog

ISOSPORA OHIOENSIS **OF PATTERSON AND FOX, 2007 (*SPECIES INQUIRENDA*)**
Mustela (syn. *Putorius*) *putorius furo*, Domestic Ferret

ISOSPORA-**LIKE/*ISOSPORA* SPP. (*SPECIES INQUIRENDAE*) OF ONE OR MORE AUTHORS (SEE CHAPTER 19)**
Canis lupus, Wolf
Canis lupus familiaris (syn. *C. familiaris*), Domestic Dog
Chrysocyon brachyurus, Maned Wolf
Crocuta crocuta, Spotted Hyaena
Cynictis penicillata, Yellow Mongoose
Felis catus, Domestic Cat
Leopardus pardalis, Ocelot
Lycalopex (syn. *Pseudalopex*) *fulvipes*, Darwin's Fox
Lycaon pictus, African Wild Dog
Meles meles, European Badger
Mustela (syn. *Putorius*) *putorius furo*, Domestic Ferret
Panthera leo, Lion

Panthera pardus, Leopard
Panthera tigris, Tiger
Procyon lotor, Raccoon
Suricata suricatta, Meerkat
Ursus arctos, Brown Bear
Vulpes vulpes (syn. *V. vulgaris*), Silver or Red Fox

ISOSPORA RIVOLTA-LIKE OF MANDAL AND CHOUDHURY, 1983
Panthera pardus, Leopard

ISOSPORA RIVOLTA OF TRIFFITT, 1927
Felis catus, Domestic Cat
Felis silvestris, Wildcat (?)

ISOSPORA THEILERI OF YAKIMOFF AND LEWKOWITSCH, 1932
Canis aureus, Golden Jackal

ISOSPORA VULPIS OF GALLI-VALERIO, 1931
Vulpes vulpes (syn. *V. vulgaris*), Silver or Red Fox

KLOSSIA SP. OF GOLEMANSKY AND RIDZHAKOV, 1975
Vulpes vulpes (syn. *V. vulgaris*), Silver or Red Fox

NEOSPORA CANINUM DUBEY ET AL., 1988a
Acinonyx jubatus, Cheetah
Ailurus fulgens, Red Panda
Canis aureus, Golden Jackal
Canis latrans, Coyote
Canis lupus, Wolf
Canis lupus dingo, Australian Dingo
Canis lupus familiaris (syn. *C. familiaris*), Domestic Dog
Caracal caraacal, Caracal
Cerdocyon thous, Crab-eating Fox
Chrysocyon brachyurus, Maned Wolf
Crocuta crocuta, Spotted Hyaena
Enhydra lutris, Sea Otter
Erignathus barbatus, Bearded Seal
Felis catus, Domestic Cat
Felis silvestris, Wildcat
Genetta genetta (syn. *G. dongolana*), Common Genet
Herpestes ichneumon, Egyptian Mongoose
Leopardus (syn. *Oncifelis*) *colocolo*, Colocolo or Pampas Cat
Leopardus (syn. *Oncifelis*) *geoffroyi*, Geoffroy's Cat
Leopardus pardalis, Ocelot
Leopardus tigrinus, Oncilla or Little Spotted Cat
Leptailurus serval, Serval
Lutra lutra, European Otter
Lycalopex (syn. *Dusicyon*) *culpaeus*, Culpeo
Lycalopex (syn. *Pseudalopex*) *fulvipes*, Darwin's or Chiloé Fox
Lycalopex (syn. *Dusicyon*) *griseus*, South American Gray Fox
Lycalopex gymnocercus, Pampas or Azara's Fox
Lycalopex (syn. *Pseudalopex*) *vetulus*, Hoary Fox
Lynx lynx, Eurasian Lynx
Lynx pardinus, Iberian Lynx
Martes foina, Beech Marten
Martes martes, European Pine Marten

Martes pennanti, Fisher
Meles meles, European Badger
Mustela putorius, European Polecat
Mustela (syn. *Putorius*) *putorius furo*, Domestic Ferret
Neofelis nebulosa, Clouded Leopard
Neovison vison (syn. *Mustela vison*), American Mink
Nyctereutes procyonoides koreensis, Korean Raccoon Dog
Odobenus rosmarus, Walrus
Otaria flavescens (syn. *Otaria byronia*), South American Sea Lion
Panthera leo, Lion
Panthera (syn. *Puma*) *onca*, Jaguar
Panthera pardus, Leopard
Panthera tigris, Tiger
Phoca largha, Spotted Seal
Phoca vitulina, Harbor Seal
Phoca vitulina stejnegeri, Kuril Harbor Seal
Prionailurus viverrinus, Fishing Cat
Procyon lotor, Raccoon
Puma concolor, Cougar
Puma yagouaroundi, Jaguarundi
Pusa (syn. *Phoca*) *hispida*, Ringed Seal
Speothos venaticus, Bush Dog
Uncia uncia, Snow Leopard
Urocyon cinereoargenteus, Gray Fox
Ursus arctos, Brown or Grizzly Bear
Vulpes (syn. *Alopex*) *lagopus*, Arctic or Blue Fox
Vulpes vulpes, Red or Silver Fox
Vulpes zerda, Fennec Fox
Zalophus californianus, California Sea Lion

OOCYSTS OF CARLSLAKE ET AL., 2017
Canis lupus familiaris (syn. *Canis dingo*), Domestic Dog

SARCOCYSTIS ALBIFRONSI KUTKIENĖ ET AL., 2012
Vulpes (syn. *Alopex*) *lagopus*, Arctic or Blue Fox (definitive host)

SARCOCYSTIS ALCES DAHLGREN AND GJERDE, 2008
Vulpes (syn. *Alopex*) *lagopus*, Arctic or Blue Fox (definitive host)
Vulpes vulpes, Red or Silver Fox (definitive host)

SARCOCYSTIS ALCESLATRANS DUBEY, 1980b
Canis latrans, Coyote (definitive host)
Canis lupus familiaris (syn. *Canis dingo*), Domestic Dog (definitive host)

SARCOCYSTIS ALECTORIVULPES PAK ET AL., 1989
Vulpes (syn. *Alopex*) *corsac*, Corsac Fox (definitive host)
Vulpes vulpes (syns. *V. fulvus*, *V. vulgaris*), Red or Silver Fox (definitive host)

SARCOCYSTIS ARCTICA GJERDE AND SCHULZE, 2014
Vulpes (syn. *Alopex*) *lagopus*, Arctic or Blue Fox (intermediate host)

SARCOCYSTIS ARIETICANIS HEYDORN, 1985
Canis lupus familiaris (syn. *Canis dingo*), Domestic Dog (definitive host)

SARCOCYSTIS AUCHENIAE BRUMPT, 1913
Canis lupus familiaris (syn. *Canis dingo*), Domestic Dog (definitive host)

SARCOCYSTIS BAIBACINACANIS **UMBETALIEV, 1979**
    Canis lupus, Wolf (definitive host)
    Canis lupus familiaris (syn. *Canis dingo*), Domestic Dog (definitive host)
    Vulpes vulpes, Red or Silver Fox (definitive host)

SARCOCYSTIS BERTRAMI **DOFLEIN, 1901**
    Canis lupus familiaris (syn. *Canis dingo*), Domestic Dog (definitive host)

SARCOCYSTIS BOVIFELIS **HEYDORN ET AL., 1975b**
    Felis catus, Domestic Cat (definitive host)

SARCOCYSTIS BUFFALONIS **HUONG ET AL., 1997a**
    Felis catus, Domestic Cat (definitive host)

SARCOCYSTIS CAMELI **(MASON, 1910) BABUDIERI, 1932**
    Canis lupus familiaris (syn. *Canis dingo*), Domestic Dog (definitive host)

SARCOCYSTIS CAMPESTRIS **CAWTHORN ET AL., 1983**
    Taxidea taxus, American Badger (definitive host)

SARCOCYSTIS CANINUM **DUBEY ET AL., 2015b**
    Canis lupus familiaris (syn. *Canis dingo*), Domestic Dog (intermediate host)

SARCOCYSTIS CANIS **DUBEY AND SPEER, 1991**
    Canis lupus familiaris (syn. *Canis dingo*), Domestic Dog (intermediate host)
    Monachus schauinslandi, Hawaiian Monk Seal (intermediate host—natural)
    Eumetopias jubatus, Steller Sea Lion (intermediate host—natural)
    Ursus americanus, American Black Bear (intermediate host)
    Ursus maritimus, Polar Bear (intermediate host)
    Zalophus californianus, California Sea Lion (intermediate host—natural)

SARCOCYSTIS CAPRACANIS **FISCHER, 1979**
    Canis latrans, Coyote (definitive host)
    Canis lupus familiaris (syn. *Canis dingo*), Domestic Dog (definitive host)
    Cerdocyon thous, Crab-eating Dog (definitive host)
    Vulpes (syn. *Alopex*) *corsac*, Corsac Fox (definitive host)
    Vulpes vulpes, Red or Silver Fox (definitive host)

SARCOCYSTIS CAPREOLI **OF LEVCHENKO, 1963 (*SPECIES INQUIRENDA*)**
    Canis lupus familiaris (syn. *C. familiaris*), Domestic Dog (definitive host)
    Vulpes vulpes, Red Fox (definitive host)

SARCOCYSTIS CAPREOLICANIS **ERBER ET AL., 1978**
    Canis lupus familiaris (syn. *Canis dingo*), Domestic Dog (definitive host)
    Vulpes velox, Swift Fox (definitive host)
    Vulpes vulpes, Red or Silver Fox (definitive host)

SARCOCYSTIS CAPRIFELIS **EL-RAFAII ET AL., 1980**
    Felis catus, Domestic Cat (definitive host)

SARCOCYSTIS CERVICANIS **HERNANDEZ ET AL., 1981**
    Canis lupus familiaris (syn. *Canis dingo*), Domestic Dog (definitive host)

SARCOCYSTIS CITELLIVULPES **PAK ET AL., 1979**
    Mustela eversmanii, Steppe Polecat (definitive host)
    Vulpes (syn. *Alopex*) *corsac*, Corsac Fox (definitive host)
    Vulpes vulpes, Red or Silver Fox (definitive host)

SARCOCYSTIS CORSACI PAK, 1979 (*SPECIES INQUIRENDA*)

Vulpes (syn. *Alopex*) *corsac*, Corsac Fox (definitive host, intermediate host)

SARCOCYSTIS CRUZI (HASSELMANN, 1926) WENYON, 1926c

Canis latrans, Coyote (definitive host)
Canis lupus, Wolf (definitive host)
Canis lupus familiaris (syn. *Canis dingo*), Domestic Dog (definitive host)
Cerdocyon thous, Crab-eating Dog (definitive host)
Nyctereutes procyonoides, Raccoon Dog (definitive host)
Procyon lotor, Raccoon (definitive host)
Vulpes vulpes, Red or Silver Fox (definitive host)

SARCOCYSTIS CUNICULORUM (BRUMPT, 1913) ODENING ET AL., 1996b

Felis catus, Domestic Cat (definitive host—experimental)

SARCOCYSTIS CYMRUENSIS ASHFORD, 1978

Felis catus, Domestic Cat (definitive host)

SARCOCYSTIS DASYPI HOWELLS ET AL., 1975

Ailurus fulgens, Red Panda (?) (intermediate host)

SARCOCYSTIS ERDMANAE ODENING, 1997

Canis lupus familiaris (syn. *Canis dingo*), Domestic Dog (definitive host)
Mephitis mephitis, Striped Skunk (intermediate host)

SARCOCYSTIS EVERSMANNI PAK ET AL., 1991

Mustela eversmanni, Steppe Polecat (intermediate host)

SARCOCYSTIS FAYERI DUBEY ET AL., 1977b

Canis lupus familiaris (syn. *Canis dingo*), Domestic Dog (definitive host)

SARCOCYSTIS FELIS DUBEY ET AL., 1992b

Acinonyx jubatus, Cheetah (intermediate host)
Felis catus, Domestic Cat (intermediate host)
Leopardus colocolo, Colocolo (intermediate host)
Leopardus geoffroyi, Geoffroy's Cat (intermediate host)
Leopardus tigrinus (syn. *Leopardus guttulus*), Oncilla (intermediate host)
Leopardus wiedii, Margay (intermediate host)
Lynx (syn. *Felis*) *rufus*, Bobcat (intermediate host)
Panthera leo, Lion (intermediate host)
Puma (syn. *Felis*) *concolor coryi*, Florida Panther (intermediate host)
Puma (syn. *Felis*) *concolor stanleyana*, Cougar (intermediate host)
Puma yagouaroundi, Jaguarundi (intermediate host)

SARCOCYSTIS FEROVIS DUBEY, 1983b

Canis latrans, Coyote (definitive host)

SARCOCYSTIS FUSIFORMIS (RAILLIET, 1897) BERNARD AND BAUCHE, 1912

Felis catus, Domestic Cat (definitive host)

SARCOCYSTIS FUSIFORMIS OF MEHLHORN ET AL., 1975a (*SPECIES INQUIRENDA*)

Canis lupus familiaris (syn. *C. familiaris*), Domestic Dog (definitive host)
Felis catus, Domestic Cat (definitive host)

SARCOCYSTIS GIGANTEA (RAILLIET, 1886a) ASHFORD, 1977

Felis catus, Domestic Cat (definitive host)
Vulpes vulpes, Red or Silver Fox (definitive host—experimental)

SARCOCYSTIS GRACILIS RÁTZ, 1909
Vulpes (syn. *Alopex*) *lagopus*, Arctic or Blue Fox (definitive host)
Vulpes vulpes, Red or Silver Fox (definitive host)

SARCOCYSTIS GRACILIS-LIKE OF GIANNETTO ET AL., 2005 (*SPECIES INQUIRENDA*)
Vulpes (syn. *Alopex*) *lagopus*, Arctic or Blue Fox (? See Chapter 19)
Vulpes vulpes (syn. *V. vulgaris*), Silver or Red Fox (? See Chapter 19)

SARCOCYSTIS GRACILIS OF ODENING ET AL., 1996a (*SPECIES INQUIRENDA*)
Vulpes (syn. *Alopex*) *lagopus*, Arctic or Blue Fox (? See Chapter 19)
Vulpes vulpes (syn. *V. vulgaris*), Silver or Red Fox (? See Chapter 19)

SARCOCYSTIS GRUENERI YAKIMOFF AND SOKOLOFF, 1934
Canis lupus familiaris (syn. *Canis dingo*), Domestic Dog (definitive host?)
Nyctereutes procyonoides, Raccoon Dog (definitive host)
Vulpes (syn. *Alopex*) *lagopus*, Arctic or Blue Fox (definitive host?)
Vulpes vulpes, Red or Silver Fox (definitive host) (?)

SARCOCYSTIS HEMIONILATRANTIS HUDKINS AND KISTNER, 1977
Canis latrans, Coyote (definitive host)
Canis lupus familiaris (syn. *Canis dingo*), Domestic Dog (definitive host)

SARCOCYSTIS HIRCICANIS HEYDORN AND UNTERHOLZNER, 1983
Canis lupus familiaris (syn. *Canis dingo*), Domestic Dog (definitive host)

SARCOCYSTIS HIRSUTA MOULÉ, 1888
Felis catus, Domestic Cat (definitive host)
Felis silvestris, Wildcat (definitive host)

SARCOCYSTIS HJORTI DAHLGREN AND GJERDE, 2010a
Vulpes (syn. *Alopex*) *lagopus*, Arctic or Blue Fox (definitive host)
Vulpes vulpes, Red or Silver Fox (definitive host)

SARCOCYSTIS HOFMANNI ODENING ET AL., 1994b
Meles meles, European Badger (intermediate host)
Procyon lotor, Raccoon (intermediate host) (?)

SARCOCYSTIS HORVATHI RÁTZ, 1908
Canis lupus familiaris (syn. *Canis dingo*), Domestic Dog (definitive host?)
Felis catus, Domestic Cat (definitive host?)

SARCOCYSTIS HUETI (MOULÉ, 1888) LABBÉ, 1899
Zalophus (syn. *Otaria*) *californicus*, California Sea Lion (intermediate host)

SARCOCYSTIS HYDRURGAE ODENING AND ZIPPER, 1986
Hydrurga leptonyx, Leopard Seal (intermediate host, definitive host—unlikely)

SARCOCYSTIS KALVIKUS DUBEY ET AL., 2010b
Gulo gulo, Wolverine (intermediate host)

SARCOCYSTIS KIRKPATRICKI SNYDER ET AL., 1990
Procyon lotor, Raccoon (intermediate host)

SARCOCYSTIS KITIKMEOTENSIS DUBEY ET AL., 2010b
Gulo gulo, Wolverine (intermediate host)

SARCOCYSTIS LEPORUM CRAWLEY, 1914
Felis catus, Domestic Cat (definitive host)
Procyon lotor, Raccoon (definitive host)

SARCOCYSTIS LEVINEI DISSANAIKE AND KAN, 1978
Canis lupus familiaris (syn. *Canis dingo*), Domestic Dog (definitive host)

SARCOCYSTIS LUTRAE GJERDE AND JOSEFSEN, 2015
Lutra lutra, European Otter (intermediate host)
Vulpes (syn. *Alopex*) *lagopus*, Arctic or Blue Fox (intermediate host)

SARCOCYSTIS MEDUSIFORMIS COLLINS ET AL., 1979
Felis catus, Domestic Cat (definitive host)

SARCOCYSTIS MELIS ODENING ET AL., 1994b
Meles meles, European Badger (intermediate host)
Mustela nivalis, Least Weasel (intermediate host) (?)
Procyon lotor, Raccoon (intermediate host) (?)

SARCOCYSTIS MEPHITISI DUBEY ET AL., 2002c
Mephitis mephitis, Striped Skunk (intermediate host)

SARCOCYSTIS MICROS WANG ET AL., 1988
Canis lupus familiaris (syn. *Canis dingo*), Domestic Dog (definitive host)

SARCOCYSTIS MIESCHERIANA (KÜHN, 1865) LABBÉ, 1899
Canis aureus, Golden Jackal (definitive host)
Canis lupus, Wolf (definitive host)
Canis lupus familiaris (syn. *Canis dingo*), Domestic Dog (definitive host)
Procyon lotor, Raccoon (definitive host)
Vulpes vulpes, Red or Silver Fox (definitive host)

SARCOCYSTIS MIESCHERIANA OF FARMER ET AL., 1978 (*SPECIES INQUIRENDA*)
Canis lupus familiaris (syn. *C. familiaris*), Domestic Dog (definitive host)

SARCOCYSTIS MIHOENSIS SAITO ET AL., 1997
Canis lupus famialiaris (syn. *Canis dingo*), Domestic Dog (definitive host)

SARCOCYSTIS MOULEI NEVEU-LEMAIRE, 1912
Felis catus, Domestic Cat (definitive host)

SARCOCYSTIS MURIS (RAILLIET, 1886a,b) LABBÉ, 1899
Felis catus, Domestic Cat (definitive host)
Felis chaus, Jungle Cat (definitive host)
Mustela (syn. *Putorius*) *putorius furo*, European Polecat/Domestic Ferret (definitive host)

SARCOCYSTIS NEOTOMAFELIS GALAVÍZ-SILVA ET AL., 1991 (?)
Felis catus, Domestic Cat (definitive host)

SARCOCYSTIS NEURONA DUBEY ET AL., 1991b
Arctocephalus townsendi, Guadalupe Fur Seal (intermediate host—natural)
Ailurus fulgens, Red Panda (intermediate host)
Callorhinus ursinus, Northern Fur Seal (intermediate host—natural).
Canis lupus familiaris (syn. *Canis dingo*), Domestic Dog (intermediate host—natural)
Enhydra lutris neris, Sea Otter (intermediate host—natural)
Eumetopias jubatus, Steller Sea Lion (intermediate host—natural)
Felis catus, Domestic Cat (intermediate host—natural and experimental)
Lynx canadensis, Canadian Lynx (intermediate host)
Martes pennanti, Fisher (intermediate host)
Mephitis mephitis, Striped Skunk (intermediate host—natural and experimental)
Mirounga angustirostris, Northern Elephant Seal (intermediate host—natural)

Mustela (syn. *Putorius*) *putorius furo*, European Polecat/Domestic Ferret (intermediate host)
Nasua narica molaris, White-nosed Coati (intermediate host—natural)
Neovison (syn. *Mustela*) *vison*, American Mink (intermediate host)
Phoca vitulina richardii, Harbor Seal (intermediate host)
Procyon lotor, Raccoon (intermediate host)
Zalophus (syn. *Otaria*) *californicus*, California Sea Lion (intermediate host—natural)

SARCOCYSTIS NEURONA/SARCOCYSTIS DASYPI OF ZOLL ET AL., 2015 (SPECIES INQUIRENDA)
Ailurus fulgens, Red Panda (intermediate host)

SARCOCYSTIS ODOCOILEOCANIS CRUM ET AL., 1981
Canis latrans, Coyote (definitive host)
Canis lupus familiaris (syn. *Canis dingo*), Domestic Dog (definitive host)
Urocyon cinereoargenteus, Gray Fox (definitive host)
Vulpes vulpes, Red or Silver Fox (definitive host)

SARCOCYSTIS ODOI DUBEY AND LOZIER, 1983
Felis catus, Domestic Cat (definitive host)

SARCOCYSTIS PECKAI ODENING, 1997
Canis lupus familiaris (syn. *Canis dingo*), Domestic Dog (definitive host)
Felis catus, Domestic Cat (definitive host) (?)

SARCOCYSTIS POEPHAGI WEI ET AL., 1985
Felis catus, Domestic Cat (definitive host)

SARCOCYSTIS POEPHAGICANIS WEI ET AL., 1985
Canis lupus familiaris (syn. *Canis dingo*), Domestic Dog (definitive host)

SARCOCYSTIS PORCIFELIS DUBEY, 1976
Felis catus, Domestic Cat (definitive host)

SARCOCYSTIS PUTORII (RAILLIET AND LUCET, 1891), TADROS AND LAARMAN, 1978a
Mustela erminea, Ermine (definitive host)
Mustela nivalis, Least Weasel (definitive host)
Mustela (syn. *Putorius*) *putorius furo*, European Polecat, Domestic Ferret (definitive host)
Neovison (syn. *Mustela*) *vison*, American Mink (definitive host)

SARCOCYSTIS RANGI GJERDE, 1984b
Vulpes (syn. *Alopex*) *lagopus*, Arctic or Blue Fox (definitive host)
Vulpes vulpes, Red or Silver Fox (definitive host)

SARCOCYSTIS RHOMBOMYS PAK ET AL., 1984 (SPECIES INQUIRENDA)
Vulpes vulpes (syn. *V. vulgaris*), Silver or Red Fox (definitive host)

SARCOCYSTIS RICHARDII HADWEN, 1922
Phoca vitulina (syn. *Phoca richardii*), Harbor Seal (intermediate host)

SARCOCYSTIS RILEYI (STILES, 1893) LABBÉ, 1899
Mephitis mephitis, Striped Skunk (definitive host)
Nyctereutes procyonoides, Raccoon Dog (definitive host)
Vulpes vulpes, Red or Silver Fox (definitive host)

SARCOCYSTIS ROMMELI DUBEY ET AL., 2016b
Felis catus, Domestic Cat (definitive host)

SARCOCYSTIS SPP. (*SPECIES INQUIRENDAE*) OF ONE OR MORE AUTHORS (SEE CHAPTER 19)

Ailurus fulgens, Red Panda (intermediate host)
Callorhinus ursinus, Northern Fur Seal (intermediate host)
Canis latrans, Coyote (definitive host)
Canis lupus, Wolf (definitive and intermediate host)
Canis lupus familiaris (syn. *C. familiaris*), Domestic Dog (definitive and intermediate host)
Canis mesomelas, Black-backed Jackal (intermediate host)
Chrysocyon brachyurus, Maned Wolf (definitive host)
Cuon alpinus, Dhole (definitive host)
Enhydra lutris, Sea Otter (intermediate host)
Erignathus barbatus, Bearded Seal (intermediate host)
Felis catus, Domestic Cat (definitive and intermediate host)
Felis chaus, Jungle Cat (definitive host)
Helarctos malayanus, Sun Bear (intermediate host)
Helogale parvula, Common Dwarf Mongoose (intermediate host)
Leptonychotes weddellii, Weddell Seal (intermediate host)
Lobodon carcinophaga, Crabeater Seal (intermediate host)
Lutra lutra, European Otter (intermediate host)
Lycaon pictus, African Wild Dog (definitive host)
Lynx rufus, Bobcat (definitive host)
Martes melampus melampus, Japanese Marten (intermediate host)
Martes pennanti, Fisher (definitive and intermediate host)
Meles anakuma, Japanese Badger (intermediate host)
Meles meles, European Badger (intermediate host)
Melogale moschata subaurantiaca, Taiwan Ferret Badger (intermediate host)
Mellivora capensis, Honey Badger (intermediate host)
Mirounga leonina, Southern Elephant Seal (intermediate host)
Mungos mungo, Banded Mongoose (intermediate host)
Mustela nivalis, Least Weasel (intermediate host)
Neovison (syn. *Mustela*) *vison*, American Mink (intermediate host)
Nyctereutes procyonoides, Raccoon Dog (intermediate host)
Nyctereutes procyonoides viverrinus, Japanese Raccoon Dog (intermediate host)
Panthera leo (syn. *Leo leo*), Lion (definitive and intermediate host)
Panthera pardus, Leopard (definitive and intermediate host)
Panthera tigris, Tiger (definitive host)
Phoca vitulina (syn. *P. richardii*), Pacific Harbor Seal (intermediate host)
Phoca vitulina richardii, Pacific Harbor Seal (intermediate host)
Potos sp., Kinkajou (intermediate host)
Prionailurus bengalensis, Tsushima Leopard Cat
Procyon lotor, Raccoon (definitive and intermediate host)
Puma (syn. *Felis*) *concolor*, Puma or Cougar (definitive and intermediate host)
Pusa caspica (syn. *Phoca caspica*), Caspian Seal (intermediate host)
Pusa hispida (syn. *Phoca hispida*), Ringed Seal (intermediate host)
Spilogale putorius, Eastern Spotted Skunk (definitive host)
Ursus americanus, American Black Bear (intermediate host)
Ursus maritimus, Polar Bear (intermediate host)
Vulpes vulpes (syn. *V. vulgaris*), Silver or Red Fox (definitive host)
Vulpes vulpes japonica, Japanese Red Fox (intermediate host)
Zalophus californianus, California Sea Lion (intermediate host)

SARCOCYSTIS SVANAI DUBEY ET AL., 2015c

Canis lupus familiaris (syn. *Canis dingo*), Domestic Dog (intermediate host)
Lycalopex gymnocercus, Pampas Fox (intermediate host)

SARCOCYSTIS SYBILLENSIS **DUBEY ET AL., 1983**
   Canis lupus familiaris (syn. *Canis dingo*), Domestic Dog (definitive host)

SARCOCYSTIS TARANDIVULPES **GJERDE, 1984d**
   Canis lupus familiaris (syn. *Canis dingo*), Domestic Dog (definitive host) (?)
   Lycalopex gymnocercus, Pampas Fox (definitive host)
   Nyctereutes procyonoides (Gray, 1834), Raccoon Dog (definitive host)
   Vulpes (syn. *Alopex*) *lagopus*, Arctic or Blue Fox (definitive host)
   Vulpes vulpes, Red or Silver Fox (definitive host) (?)

SARCOCYSTIS TENELLA **(RAILLIET, 1886a,b) MOULÉ, 1886**
   Canis latrans, Coyote (definitive host)
   Canis lupus, Wolf (definitive host)
   Canis lupus familiaris (syn. *Canis dingo*), Domestic Dog (definitive host)
   Vulpes vulpes, Red or Silver Fox (definitive host)

SARCOCYSTIS TILOPODI **QUIROGA ET AL., 1969**
   Canis lupus familiaris (syn. *Canis dingo*), Domestic Dog (definitive host)

SARCOCYSTIS TROPICALIS **(MUKHERJEE AND KRASSNER, 1965) LEVINE AND TADROS, 1980**
   Canis aureus, Golden Jackal (definitive host)

SARCOCYSTIS UNDULATI **PAK ET AL., 1984 (*SPECIES INQUIRENDA*)**
   Mustela eversmanni, Steppe Polecat (definitive host)
   Vulpes (syn. *Alopex*) *corsac*, Corsac Fox (definitive host)
   Vulpes vulpes (syn. *V. vulgaris*), Silver or Red Fox (definitive host)

SARCOCYSTIS URSUSI **DUBEY ET AL., 2008a**
   Ursus americanus, American Black Bear (intermediate host)

SARCOCYSTIS VULPIS **PAK ET AL., 1991 (*SPECIES INQUIRENDA*)**
   Vulpes vulpes (syn. *V. vulgaris*), Silver or Red Fox (intermediate host)

SARCOCYSTIS WAPITI **SPEER AND DUBEY, 1982**
   Canis latrans, Coyote (definitive host)
   Canis lupus familiaris (syn. *Canis dingo*), Domestic Dog (definitive host)

SARCOCYSTIS WENZELI **ODENING, 1997**
   Canis lupus familiaris (syn. *Canis dingo*), Domestic Dog (definitive host)
   Felis catus, Domestic Cat (definitive host) (?)

SARCOCYSTIS WETZELI **(SUGÁR, 1980) N. COMB.**
   Vulpes vulpes, Red or Silver Fox (definitive host)

TOXOPLASMA GONDII **(NICOLLE AND MANCEAUX, 1908) NICOLLE AND MANCEAUX, 1909**
   Acinonyx jubatus, Cheetah
   Ailurus fulgens, Red Panda
   Ailuropoda melanoleuca, Giant Panda
   Arctictis binturong, Binturong
   Arctocephalus australis, South American Fur Seal
   Arctocephalus forsteri, Australian Fur Seal
   Arctocephalus gazella, Antarctic Fur Seal
   Bassariscus astutus, Civet or Ringtail Cat
   Callorhinus ursinus, Northern Fur Seal
   Canis aureus, Golden Jackal
   Canis latrans, Coyote
   Canis lupus, Wolf

Canis lupus dingo, Australian Dingo
Canis lupus familiaris (syn. *C. familiaris*), Domestic Dog
Caracal caraacal, Caracal
Catopuma temminckii, Asian Golden Cat
Cerdocyon thous, Crab-eating Fox
Chrysocyon brachyurus, Maned Wolf
Crocuta crocuta, Spotted Hyaena
Cryptoprocta ferox, Fossa
Cystophora cristata, Hooded Seal
Eira barbara, Tayra
Enhydra lutris, Sea Otter
Erignathus barbatus, Bearded Seal
Felis catus, Domestic Cat
Felis manul, Pallas's Cat
Felis margarita, Sand Cat
Felis silvestris, Wildcat
Genetta genetta, Common Genet
Halichoerua grypus, Gray Seal
Herpestes edwardsi, Indian Gray Mongoose
Herpestes ichneumon, Egyptian Mongoose
Hyaena brunnea (syn. *Parahyaena brunnea*), Brown Hyaena
Hyaena hyaena, Striped Hyaena
Ichneumia albicauda, White-tailed Mongoose
Leopardus (syn. *Oncifelis*) *colocolo*, Colocolo or Pampas Cat
Leopardus (syn. *Oncifelis*) *geoffroyi*, Geoffroy's Cat
Leopardus pardalis, Ocelot
Leopardus tigrinus, Oncilla or Little Spotted Cat
Leopardus wiedii, Margay
Leptailurus serval, Serval
Leptonychotes weddellii, Weddell Seal
Lobodon carcinophaga, Crabeater Seal
Lontra canadensis, North American River Otter
Lutra lutra, European Otter
Lycalopex (syn. *Dusicyon*) *culpaeus*, Culpeo
Lycalopex (syn. *Dusicyon*) *griseus*, South American Gray Fox
Lycalopex (syn. *Pseudalopex*) *vetulus*, Hoary Fox
Lycaon pictus, African Wild Dog
Lynx lynx, Eurasian Lynx
Lynx pardinus, Iberian Lynx
Lynx rufus, Bobcat
Martes foina, Beech Marten
Martes martes, European Pine Marten
Martes pennanti, Fisher
Meles meles, European Badger
Mephitis mephitis, Striped Skunk
Mirounga angustirostris, Northern Elephant Seal
Mirounga leonina, Southern Elephant Seal
Monachus schauinslandi, Hawaiian Monk Seal
Mungotictis decemlineata, Narrow-striped Mongoose
Mustela erminea, Ermine or Stoat
Mustela nigripes, Black-footed Ferret
Mustela putorius, European Polecat
Mustela (syn. *Putorius*) *putorius furo*, Domestic Ferret
Nasua nasua, South American Coati

Neofelis nebulosa, Clouded Leopard
Neovison vison (syn. *Mustela vison*), American mink
Nyctereutes procyonoides viverrinus, Korean Raccoon Dog
Odobenus rosmarus, Walrus
Otaria flavescens (syn. *Otaria byronia*), South American Sea Lion
Paguma larvata, Masked Palm Civet
Panthera leo, Lion
Panthera (syn. *Puma*) *onca*, Jaguar
Panthera pardus, Leopard
Panthera tigris, Tiger
Paradoxurus hermaphroditus, Asian Palm Civet
Phoca largha, Spotted Seal
Phoca vitulina, Harbor Seal
Phoca vitulina richardsi, Pacific Harbor Seal
Phocarctos hookeri, New Zealand Sea Lion
Potos flavus, Kinkajou
Prionailurus bengalensis, Leopard Cat
Prionailurus iriomotensis, Iriomote Cat
Prionailurus viverrinus, Fishing Cat
Procyon cancrivorus, Crab-eating Raccoon
Procyon lotor, Raccoon
Procyon pygmaeus, Pygmy Raccoon
Puma concolor, Cougar
Puma yagouaroundi, Jaguarundi
Pusa (syn. *Phoca*) *hispida*, Ringed Seal
Speothos venaticus, Bush Dog
Spilogale gracilis, Western Spotted Skunk
Suricata suricatta, Meerkat
Uncia uncia, Snow Leopard
Urocyon littoralis, Island Fox
Urocyon cinereoargenteus, Gray Fox
Ursus americanus, American Black Bear
Ursus arctos, Brown or Grizzly Bear
Ursus maritimus, Polar Bear
Viverra tangalunga, Malayan Civet
Vulpes cana, Blanford's Fox
Vulpes (syn. *Alopex*) *lagopus*, Arctic or Blue Fox
Vulpes rueppellii, Rüppell's Fox
Vulpes vulpes, Red or Silver Fox
Vulpes zerda, Fennec Fox
Zalophus californianus, California Sea Lion

TOXOPLASMA-LIKE OF EPE ET AL., 2004 (*SPECIES INQUIRENDA*)
Felis catus, Domestic Cat (definitive host)

TOXOPLASMA-LIKE OF LUCIO-FORSTER AND BOWMAN, 2011 (*SPECIES INQUIRENDA*)
Felis catus, Domestic Cat (definitive host)

TOXOPLASMA-LIKE OF NYAMBURA NJUGUNA ET AL., 2017 (*SPECIES INQUIRENDA*)
Felis catus, Domestic Cat (definitive host)

Appendix B

Alphabetical List of All Carnivora Suborders, Families, Genera, and Species Covered in This Book and the Apicomplexa Parasites Which Have Been Reported From Them

Suborder: Caniformia

FAMILY AILURIDAE

Ailurus fulgens, Red Panda

Cryptosporidium andersoni Lindsay et al., 2000
Cryptosporidium parvum Tyzzer, 1912
Eimeria ailuri Agrawal et al., 1981
Neospora caninum Dubey et al., 1988a
Sarcocystis dasypi Howells et al., 1975 (intermediate host) (?)
Sarcocystis neurona Dubey et al., 1991b (intermediate host)
Sarcocystis neurona / Sarcocystis dasypi of Zoll et al., 2015 (*species inquirenda*) (intermediate host)
Sarcocystis spp. (*species inquirendae*) of one or more authors (see Chapter 19) (intermediate host)
Toxoplasma gondii (Nicolle and Manceaux, 1908) Nicolle and Manceaux, 1909

FAMILY CANIDAE

Canis adustus, Side-striped Jackal

Hepatozoon sp. (*species inquirendae*) of one or more authors (see Chapter 19)

Canis aureus, Golden Jackal

Cystoisospora canis (syn. *Isospora canis* Neméséri, 1959) Frenkel, 1977
Cystoisospora dutoiti (Yakimoff et al., 1933a) N. Comb.
Cystoisospora theileri (syn. *Isospora theileri* Yakimoff and Lewkowitsch, 1932) N. Comb.
Isospora dutoiti of Yakimoff et al., 1933a (*species inquirenda*)
Isospora theileri of Yakimoff and Lewkowitsch, 1932
Neospora caninum Dubey et al., 1988a
Sarcocystis miescheriana (Kühn, 1865) Labbé, 1899 (definitive host)
Sarcocystis tropicalis (Mukherjee and Krassner, 1965) Levine and Tadros, 1980 (definitive host)
Toxoplasma gondii (Nicolle and Manceaux, 1908) Nicolle and Manceaux, 1909

Canis aureus naria, Golden Jackal

Eimeria aurei Bhatia et al., 1979

Canis latrans, Coyote

Cryptosporidium canis Fayer et al., 2001
Cryptosporidium sp. (*species inquirendae*)
Cystoisospora canis (syn. *Isospora canis* Neméséri, 1959) Frenkel, 1977
Cystoisospora neorivolta (Dubey and Mahrt, 1978), N. Comb.
Cystoisospora ohioensis (syn. *Isospora ohioensis* Dubey, 1975c) Frenkel, 1977
Hammondia heydorni (Tadros and Laarman, 1976) Dubey, 1977c
Hepatozoon americanum Vincent-Johnson et al., 1997 (intermediate host)
Hepatozoon sp. (*species inquirendae*) of one or more authors (see Chapter 19)
Eimeria canis Wenyon, 1923
Hepatozoon canis (James, 1905) Wenyon, 1926b (intermediate host)
Neospora caninum Dubey et al., 1988a
Sarcocystis alceslatrans Dubey, 1980b (definitive host)
Sarcocystis capracanis Fischer, 1979 (definitive host)
Sarcocystis cruzi (Hasselmann, 1923) Wenyon, 1926b (definitive host)

Sarcocystis ferovis Dubey, 1983b (definitive host)
Sarcocystis hemionilatrantis Hudkins and Kistner, 1977 (definitive host)
Sarcocystis odocoileocanis Crum et al., 1981 (definitive host)
Sarcocystis sp. (*species inquirendae*) of one or more authors (see Chapter 19) (definitive host)
Sarcocystis tenella (Railliet, 1886a) Moulé, 1886 (definitive host)
Sarcocystis wapiti Speer and Dubey, 1982 (definitive host)
Toxoplasma gondii (Nicolle and Manceaux, 1908) Nicolle and Manceaux, 1909

Canis lupus, Wolf

Coccidia/Coccidian/Coccidia-like/Coccidium spp. (*species inquirendae*) of many authors (see Chapter 19)
Cryptosporidium sp. (*species inquirendae*)
Hammonida spp./*Hammondia–Neospora*-like/*Hammondia–Toxoplasma*-like (*species inquirendae*) of one or more authors (see Chapter 19)
Isospora-like/*Isospora* spp. (*species inquirendae*) of one or more authors (see Chapter 19)
Neospora caninum Dubey et al., 1988a
Sarcocystis baibacinacanis Umbetaliev, 1979 (definitive host)
Sarcocystis cruzi (Hasselmann, 1923) Wenyon, 1926 (definitive host)
Sarcocystis miescheriana (Kühn, 1865) Labbé, 1899 (definitive host)
Sarcocystis sp. (*species inquirendae*) of one or more authors (see Chapter 19) (definitive and intermediate host)
Sarcocystis tenella (Railliet, 1886a) Moulé, 1886 (definitive host)
Toxoplasma gondii (Nicolle and Manceaux, 1908) Nicolle and Manceaux, 1909

Canis lupus dingo, Dingo

Cryptosporidium sp. (*species inquirendae*)
Cystoisospora ohioensis (syn. *Isospora ohioensis* Dubey, 1975c) Frenkel, 1977 (?)
Eimeria canis Wenyon, 1923
Cystoisospora rivolta (Grassi, 1879) Frenkel, 1977
Hammondia heydorni (Tadros and Laarman, 1976) Dubey, 1977c
Neospora caninum Dubey et al., 1988a
Toxoplasma gondii (Nicolle and Manceaux, 1908) Nicolle and Manceaux, 1909

Canis lupus familiaris (syn. *C. familiaris*), Domestic Dog

Caryospora bigenetica Wacha and Christiansen, 1982
Coccidia/Coccidian/Coccidia-like/Coccidium spp. (*species inquirendae*) of many authors (see Chapter 19)
Cryptosporidium canis Fayer et al., 2001
Cryptosporidium meleagridis Slavin, 1955
Cryptosporidium muris (Tyzzer, 1907) Tyzzer, 1910
Cryptosporidium parvum Tyzzer, 1912
Cryptosporidium scrofarum Kváč et al., 2013
Cryptosporidium sp. (*species inquirendae*)
Cyclospora cayetanensis of Awadallah and Salem, 2015 (*species inquirenda*)
Cystoisospora arctopitheci (syn. *Isospora arctopitheci* Rodhain, 1933) N. Comb.
Cystoisospora burrowsi (syn. *Isospora burrowsi* Trayser and Todd, 1978) Rommel and Zielasko, 1981
Cystoisospora canis (syn. *Isospora canis* Neméséri, 1959) Frenkel, 1977
Cystoisospora felis (Wenyon, 1923) Frenkel, 1977
Cystoisospora neorivolta (syn. *Isospora neorivolta* Dubey and Mahrt, 1978) N. Comb.
Cystoisospora ohioensis (syn. *Isospora ohioensis* Dubey, 1975c) Frenkel, 1977
Cystoisospora ohioensis complex of Palmer et al., 2008a (*species inquirenda*)
Cystoisospora ohioensis-like of Gates and Nolan, 2009 (*species inquirenda*)
Cystoisospora rivolta (Grassi, 1879) Frenkel, 1977
Cystoisospora sp. *species inquirendae* of many authors (see Chapter 19)
Cystoisospora vulpina (Nieschulz and Bos, 1933) Frenkel, 1977
Eimeria canis Wenyon, 1923
Eimeria rayii of Rao and Bhatavdekar, 1957 (*species inquirenda*)
Eimeria stiedae of Guillebeau, 1916 (*species inquirenda*)

Eimeria sp. (*species inquirendae*) of many authors (see Chapter 19)

Hammondia heydorni (Tadros and Laarman, 1976) Dubey, 1977c

Hammonida spp./*Hammondia–Neospora*-like/*Hammondia–Toxoplasma*-like (*species inquirendae*) of one or more authors (see Chapter 19)

Hepatozoon americanum Vincent-Johnson et al., 1997 (intermediate host)

Hepatozoon canis (James, 1905) Wenyon, 1926b (intermediate host)

Hepatozoon sp. (*species inquirendae*) of one or more authors (see Chapter 19)

Hoareosporidium pellerdyi of Pande et al., 1972 (*species inquirenda*)

Isospora bigemina (Stiles, 1891) of Lühe, 1906 (*species inquirenda*)

Isospora bigemina free sporocysts of Gassner, 1940 (*species inquirenda*)

Isospora burrowsi/*Isospora ohioensis*-like of Cirak and Bauer, 2004 (*species inquirenda*)

Isospora ohioensis Dubey, 1975c

Isospora ohioensis complex of Fontanarrosa et al., 2006 (*species inquirenda*)

Isospora-like/*Isospora* spp. (*species inquirendae*) of one or more authors (see Chapter 19)

Neospora caninum Dubey et al., 1988a

Oocysts of Carlslake et al., 2017

Sarcocystis alceslatrans Dubey, 1980b (definitive host)

Sarcocystis arieticanis Heydorn, 1985 (definitive host)

Sarcocystis aucheniae Brumpt, 1913 (definitive host)

Sarcocystis baibacinacanis Umbetaliev, 1979 (definitive host)

Sarcocystis bertrami Doflein, 1901 (definitive host)

Sarcocystis cameli (Mason, 1910) Babudieri, 1932 (definitive host)

Sarcocystis caninum Dubey et al., 2015c (intermediate host)

Sarcocystis canis Dubey and Speer, 1991 (intermediate host)

Sarcocystis capreoli of Levchenko, 1963 (*species inquirenda*) (definitive host)

Sarcocystis capracanis Fischer, 1979 (definitive host)

Sarcocystis capreolicanis Erber et al., 1978 (definitive host)

Sarcocystis cervicanis Hernandez et al., 1981 (definitive host)

Sarcocystis cruzi (Hasselmann, 1923) Wenyon, 1926b (definitive host)

Sarcocystis erdmanae Odening, 1997 (definitive host)

Sarcocystis fayeri Dubey et al., 1977b (definitive host)

Sarcocystis fusiformis of Mehlhorn et al., 1975a (*species inquirenda*) (definitive host)

Sarcocystis grueneri Yakimoff and Sokoloff, 1934 (definitive host) (?)

Sarcocystis hemionilatrantis Hudkins and Kistner, 1977 (definitive host)

Sarcocystis hircicanis Heydorn and Unterholzner, 1983 (definitive host)

Sarcocystis horvathi Rátz, 1908 (definitive host) (?)

Sarcocystis levinei Dissanaike and Kan, 1978 (definitive host)

Sarcocystis micros Wang et al., 1988 (definitive host)

Sarcocystis miescheriana (Kühn, 1865) Labbé, 1899 (definitive host)

Sarcocystis miescheriana of Farmer et al., 1978 (*species inquirenda*)

Sarcocystis mihoensis Saito et al., 1997 (definitive host)

Sarcocystis neurona Dubey et al., 1991b (intermediate host—natural)

Sarcocystis odocoileocanis Crum et al., 1981 (definitive host)

Sarcocystis peckai Odening, 1997 (definitive host)

Sarcocystis poephagicanis Wei et al., 1985 (definitive host)

Sarcocystis sp. (*species inquirendae*) of one or more authors (see Chapter 19) (definitive and intermediate host)

Sarcocystis svanai Dubey et al., 2015c (intermediate host)

Sarcocystis sybillensis Dubey et al., 1983 (definitive host)

Sarcocystis tarandivulpes Gjerde, 1984d (definitive host)

Sarcocystis tenella (Railliet, 1886a) Moulé, 1886 (definitive host)

Sarcocystis tilopodi Quiroga et al., 1969 (definitive host)

Sarcocystis wapiti Speer and Dubey, 1982 (definitive host)

Sarcocystis wenzeli Odening, 1997 (definitive host)

Toxoplasma gondii (Nicolle and Manceaux, 1908) Nicolle and Manceaux, 1909

Canis mesomelas, **Black-backed Jackal**

Hepatozoon canis (James, 1905) Wenyon, 1926b (intermediate host)
Sarcocystis sp. (*species inquirendae*) of one or more authors (see Chapter 19) (intermediate host)

Caracal caracal, **Caracal**

Neospora caninum Dubey et al., 1988a
Toxoplasma gondii (Nicolle and Manceaux, 1908) Nicolle and Manceaux, 1909

Cerdocyon thous, **Crab-eating Dog**

Hammondia heydorni (Tadros and Laarman, 1976) Dubey, 1977
Hepatozoon canis (James, 1905) Wenyon, 1926b (intermediate host)
Neospora caninum Dubey et al., 1988a
Sarcocystis capracanis Fischer, 1979 (definitive host)
Sarcocystis cruzi (Hasselmann, 1923) Wenyon, 1926 (definitive host)
Toxoplasma gondii (Nicolle and Manceaux, 1908) Nicolle and Manceaux, 1909

Chrysocyon brachyurus, **Maned Wolf**

Cryptosporidium sp. (*species inquirendae*)
Eimeria sp. (*species inquirendae*) of one or more authors (see Chapter 19)
Isospora-like/*Isospora* spp. (*species inquirendae*) of one or more authors (see Chapter 19)
Neospora caninum Dubey et al., 1988a
Sarcocystis sp. (*species inquirendae*) of one or more authors (see Chapter 19) (definitive host)
Toxoplasma gondii (Nicolle and Manceaux, 1908) Nicolle and Manceaux, 1909

Cuon alpinus, **Dhole**

Sarcocystis sp. (*species inquirendae*) of one or more authors (see Chapter 19) (definitive host)

Lycalopex (syn. *Dusicyon*) *culpaeus*, **Culpeo**

Neospora caninum Dubey et al., 1988a
Toxoplasma gondii (Nicolle and Manceaux, 1908) Nicolle and Manceaux, 1909

Lycalopex (syn. *Pseudalopex*) *fulvipes*, **Darwin's or Chiloé Fox**

Isospora-like/*Isospora* spp. (*species inquirendae*) of one or more authors (see Chapter 19)
Neospora caninum Dubey et al., 1988a

Lycalopex (syn. *Dusicyon*) *griseus*, **South American Gray Fox**

Neospora caninum Dubey et al., 1988a
Toxoplasma gondii (Nicolle and Manceaux, 1908) Nicolle and Manceaux, 1909

Lycalopex gymnocercus, **Pampas Fox**

Hepatozoon felis Patton, 1908 (intermediate host)
Neospora caninum Dubey et al., 1988a
Sarcocystis svanai Dubey et al., 2015c (intermediate host)
Sarcocystis tarandivulpes Gjerde, 1984d (definitive host)

Lycalopex (syn. *Pseudalopex*) *fulvipes*, **Darwin's Fox**

Isospora-like/*Isospora* spp. (*species inquirendae*) of one or more authors (see Chapter 19)

Lycalopex (syn. *Pseudalopex*) *vetulus*, **Hoary Fox**

Neospora caninum Dubey et al., 1988a
Toxoplasma gondii (Nicolle and Manceaux, 1908) Nicolle and Manceaux, 1909

Lycaon pictus, **African Wild Dog**

Isospora-like/*Isospora* spp. (*species inquirendae*) of one or more authors (see Chapter 19)
Sarcocystis sp. (*species inquirendae*) of one or more authors (see Chapter 19) (definitive host)
Toxoplasma gondii (Nicolle and Manceaux, 1908) Nicolle and Manceaux, 1909

Nyctereutes procyonoides, **Raccoon Dog**
  Cryptosporidium canis Fayer et al., 2001
  Cryptosporidium parvum Tyzzer, 1912
  Cryptosporidium sp. (*species inquirendae*)
  Sarcocystis cruzi (Hasselmann, 1923) Wenyon, 1926 (definitive host)
  Sarcocystis grueneri Yakimoff and Sokoloff, 1934 (definitive host)
  Sarcocystis rileyi (Stiles, 1893) Labbé, 1899 (definitive host)
  Sarcocystis tarandivulpes Gjerde, 1984d (definitive host)
  Sarcocystis sp. (*species inquirendae*) of one or more authors (see Chapter 19) (intermediate host)

Nyctereutes procyonoides koreensis, **Korean Raccoon Dog**
  Neospora caninum Dubey et al., 1988a

Nyctereutes procyonoides ussuriensis, **Raccoon Dog**
  Cystoisospora ohioensis (syn. *Isospora ohioensis* Dubey, 1975c) Frenkel, 1977 (?)

Nyctereutes procyonoides viverrinus, **Korean Raccoon Dog**
  Cryptosporidium parvum Tyzzer, 1912
  Sarcocystis sp. (*species inquirendae*) of one or more authors (see Chapter 19) (intermediate host)
  Toxoplasma gondii (Nicolle and Manceaux, 1908) Nicolle and Manceaux, 1909

Speothos venaticus, **Bush Dog**
  Neospora caninum Dubey et al., 1988a
  Toxoplasma gondii (Nicolle and Manceaux, 1908) Nicolle and Manceaux, 1909

Urocyon cinereoargenteus, **Gray Fox**
  Neospora caninum Dubey et al., 1988a
  Sarcocystis odocoileocanis Crum et al., 1981 (definitive host)
  Toxoplasma gondii (Nicolle and Manceaux, 1908) Nicolle and Manceaux, 1909

Urocyon littoralis, **Island Fox**
  Toxoplasma gondii (Nicolle and Manceaux, 1908) Nicolle and Manceaux, 1909

Vulpes bengalensis, **Bengal Fox**
  Cystoisospora buriatica (syn. *Isospora buriatica* Yakimoff and Matschoulsky, 1940) N. Comb.
  Cystoisospora vulpina (Nieschulz and Bos, 1933) Frenkel, 1977
  Eimeria lomarii Dubey, 1963a

Vulpes cana, **Blanford's Fox**
  Toxoplasma gondii (Nicolle and Manceaux, 1908) Nicolle and Manceaux, 1909

Vulpes (syn. *Alopex*) *corsac*, **Corsac Fox**
  Cystoisospora buriatica (syn. *Isospora buriatica* Yakimoff and Matschoulsky, 1940) N. Comb.
  Eimeria heissini Svanbaev, 1956
  Sarcocystis alectorivulpes Pak et al., 1989 (definitive host)
  Sarcocystis capracanis Fischer, 1979 (definitive host)
  Sarcocystis citellivulpes Pak et al., 1979 (definitive host)
  Sarcocystis corsaci Pak, 1979 (definitive host)
  Sarcocystis undulati Pak et al., 1984 (*species inquirenda*) (definitive host)

Vulpes (syn. *Alopex*) *lagopus*, **Arctic or Blue Fox**
  Cryptosporidium canis Fayer et al., 2001
  Cryptosporidium sp. (*species inquirendae*)
  Cystoisospora canivelocis (syn. *Isospora canivelocis* Weidman, 1915 emend. Wenyon, 1923) N. Comb. (experimental)
  Cystoisospora pavlodarica (Nukerbaeva and Svanbaev, 1973) N. Comb.
  Cystoisospora triffitti (Nukerbaeva and Svanbaev, 1973) N. Comb.

Cystoisospora vulpina (Nieschulz and Bos, 1933) Frenkel, 1977
Eimeria imantauica of Nukerbaeva and Svanbaev, 1973
Eimeria mesnili of Rastegaïeff, 1929c (*species inquirenda*)
Hammondia heydorni (Tadros and Laarman, 1976) Dubey, 1977c
Hammonida spp./*Hammondia–Neospora*-like/*Hammondia–Toxoplasma*-like (*species inquirendae*) of one or more authors (see Chapter 19)
Neospora caninum Dubey et al., 1988a
Sarcocystis albifronsi Kutkienė et al., 2012 (definitive host)
Sarcocystis alces Dahlgren and Gjerde, 2008 (definitive host)
Sarcocystis arctica Gjerde and Schulze, 2014 (intermediate host)
Sarcocystis gracilis Rátz, 1909 (definitive host)
Sarcocystis gracilis of Odening et al., 1996a (*species inquirenda*) (?)
Sarcocystis gracilis-like of Giannetto et al., 2005 (*species inquirenda*) (?)
Sarcocystis grueneri Yakimoff and Sokoloff, 1934 (definitive host)
Sarcocystis hjorti Dahlgren and Gjerde, 2010a (definitive host)
Sarcocystis lutrae Gjerde and Josefsen, 2015 (intermediate host)
Sarcocystis rangi Gjerde, 1984b (definitive host)
Sarcocystis tarandivulpes Gjerde, 1984d (definitive host)
Sarcocystis undulati Pak et al., 1984 (*species inquirenda*) (definitive host)
Toxoplasma gondii (Nicolle and Manceaux, 1908) Nicolle and Manceaux, 1909

Vulpes rueppellii, **Rüppell's Fox**
Toxoplasma gondii (Nicolle and Manceaux, 1908) Nicolle and Manceaux, 1909

Vulpes **spp.**
Cryptosporidium canis Fayer et al., 2001

Vulpes velox, **Swift Fox**
Cystoisospora canivelocis (syn. *Isospora canivelocis* Weidman, 1915 emend. Wenyon, 1923) N. Comb.
Sarcocystis capreolicanis Erber et al., 1978 (definitive host)

Vulpes vulpes (syns. *V. fulvus*, *V. vulgaris*), **Red or Silver Fox**
Coccidia/Coccidian/Coccidia-like/Coccidium spp. (*species inquirendae*) of many authors (see Chapter 19)
Cryptosporidium canis Fayer et al., 2001
Cryptosporidium felis Iseki, 1979
Cryptosporidium parvum Tyzzer, 1912
Cryptosporidium sp. (*species inquirendae*)
Cryptosporidium ubiquitum Fayer et al., 2010
Cystoisospora buriatica (syn. *Isospora buriatica* Yakimoff and Matschoulsky, 1940) N. Comb.
Cystoisospora canis (syn. *Isospora canis* Nemeséri, 1959) Frenkel, 1977
Cystoisospora canivelocis (syn. *Isospora canivelocis* Weidman, 1915 emend. Wenyon, 1923) N. Comb.
Cystoisospora laidlawi (syn. *Isospora laidlawi* Hoare, 1927) N. Comb.
Cystoisospora ohioensis (syn. *Isospora ohioensis* Dubey, 1975c) Frenkel, 1977 (?)
Cystoisospora pavlodarica (Nukerbaeva and Svanbaev, 1973) N. Comb.
Cystoisospora triffitti (Nukerbaeva and Svanbaev, 1973) N. Comb.
Cystoisospora vulpina (Nieschulz and Bos, 1933) Frenkel, 1977
Eimeria adleri Yakimoff and Gousseff, 1936
Eimeria bakanensis Svanbaev and Rachmatullina, 1971
Eimeria li of Golemanski, 1975
Eimeria sp. (*species inquirendae*) of one or more authors (see Chapter 19)
Eimeria vulpis of Galli-Valerio, 1929b (*species inquirenda*)
Hammondia heydorni (Tadros and Laarman, 1976) Dubey, 1977c
Hammonida spp./*Hammondia–Neospora*-like/*Hammondia–Toxoplasma*-like (*species inquirendae*) of one or more authors (see Chapter 19)
Isospora canivelocis-like oocysts. of Dahlgren and Gjerde, 2010b

Isospora-like/*Isospora* spp. (*species inquirendae*) of one or more authors (see Chapter 19)
Isospora vulpis of Galli-Valerio, 1931
Klossia sp. of Golemansky and Ridzhakov, 1975
Neospora caninum Dubey et al., 1988a
Sarcocystis alces Dahlgren and Gjerde, 2008 (definitive host)
Sarcocystis alectorivulpes Pak et al., 1989 (definitive host)
Sarcocystis arctica Gjerde and Schulze, 2014
Sarcocystis baibacinacanis Umbetaliev, 1979 (definitive host)
Sarcocystis capracanis Fischer, 1979 (definitive host)
Sarcocystis capreoli of Levchenko, 1963 (*species inquirenda*) (definitive host)
Sarcocystis capreolicanis Erber et al., 1978 (definitive host)
Sarcocystis citellivulpes Pak et al., 1979 (definitive host)
Sarcocystis cruzi (Hasselmann, 1923) Wenyon, 1926 (definitive host)
Sarcocystis gigantea (Railliet, 1886a,b) Ashford, 1977 (definitive host)
Sarcocystis gracilis Rátz, 1909 (definitive host)
Sarcocystis gracilis of Odening et al., 1996a (*species inquirenda*) (?)
Sarcocystis gracilis-like of Giannetto et al., 2005 (*species inquirenda*) (?)
Sarcocystis grueneri Yakimoff and Sokoloff, 1934 (definitive host)
Sarcocystis hjorti Dahlgren and Gjerde, 2010a (definitive host)
Sarcocystis miescheriana (Kühn, 1865) Labbé, 1899 (definitive host)
Sarcocystis odocoileocanis Crum et al., 1981 (definitive host)
Sarcocystis rangi Gjerde, 1984b (definitive host)
Sarcocystis rhombomys Pak et al., 1984 (*species inquirenda*) (definitive host)
Sarcocystis rileyi (Stiles, 1893) Labbé, 1899 (definitive host)
Sarcocystis sp. (*species inquirendae*) of one or more authors (see Chapter 19) (definitive host)
Sarcocystis tarandivulpes Gjerde, 1984c (definitive host)
Sarcocystis tenella (Railliet, 1886a) Moulé, 1886 (definitive host)
Sarcocystis vulpis Pak et al., 1991 (*species inquirenda*) (intermediate host)
Sarcocystis wetzeli (Sugár, 1980) N. Comb. (definitive host)
Toxoplasma gondii (Nicolle and Manceaux, 1908) Nicolle and Manceaux, 1909

Vulpes vulpes japonica, **Japanese Red Fox**
Sarcocystis sp. (*species inquirendae*) of one or more authors (see Chapter 19) (intermediate host)

Vulpes vulpes silacea, **Red or Silver Fox**
Hepatozoon canis (James, 1905) Wenyon, 1926b (intermediate host)

Vulpes (syn. *Fennecus*) *zerda*, **Fennec Fox**
Cystoisospora fennechi (syn. *Isospora fennechi* Prasad, 1961a) N. Comb.
Isospora fennechi Prasad, 1961a,b (?)
Neospora caninum Dubey et al., 1988a
Toxoplasma gondii (Nicolle and Manceaux, 1908) Nicolle and Manceaux, 1909

FAMILY MEPHITIDAE
Mephitis mephitis (syn. *M. hudsonica*), **Striped Skunk**
Cryptosporidium parvum Tyzzer, 1912
Cryptosporidium sp. (*species inquirendae*)
Eimeria mephitidis Andrews, 1928
Eimeria mephitidis of Yakimoff and Gousseff, 1936 (*species inquirenda*)
Eimeria voronezbensis Levine and Ivens, 1981
Sarcocystis erdmanae Odening, 1997 (intermediate host)
Sarcocystis mephitisi Dubey et al., 2002c (intermediate host)
Sarcocystis neurona Dubey et al., 1991b (intermediate host—natural and experimental)
Sarcocystis rileyi (Stiles, 1893) Labbé, 1899 (definitive host)
Toxoplasma gondii (Nicolle and Manceaux, 1908) Nicolle and Manceaux, 1909

Spilogale gracilis, **Western Spotted Skunk**
  Toxoplasma gondii (Nicolle and Manceaux, 1908) Nicolle and Manceaux, 1909

Spilogale putorius, **Eastern Spotted Skunk**
  Eimeria mephitidis Andrews, 1928
  Eimeria mephitidis of Yakimoff and Gousseff, 1936 (*species inquirenda*)
  Sarcocystis sp. (*species inquirendae*) of one or more authors (see Chapter 19) (definitive host)

Spilogale putorius ambarvalis, **Eastern Spotted Skunk**
  Cystoisospora sengeri (syn. *Isospora sengeri* Levine and Ivens, 1964) N. Comb.
  Cystoisospora spilogales (syn. *Isospora spilogales* Levine and Ivens, 1964) N. Comb.

FAMILY MUSTELIDAE
Eira barbara, **Tayra**
  Cystoisospora arctopitheci (syn. *Isospora arctopitheci* Rodhain, 1933) N. Comb.
  Eimeria irara Carini and Fonseca, 1938
  Toxoplasma gondii (Nicolle and Manceaux, 1908) Nicolle and Manceaux, 1909

Enhydra lutris, **Sea Otter**
  Neospora caninum Dubey et al., 1988a,b
  Sarcocystis neurona Dubey et al., 1991b (intermediate host—natural)
  Sarcocystis sp. (*species inquirendae*) of one or more authors (see Chapter 19) (intermediate host)
  Toxoplasma gondii (Nicolle and Manceaux, 1908) Nicolle and Manceaux, 1909

Gulo gulo, **Wolverine**
  Sarcocystis kalvikus Dubey et al., 2010b (intermediate host)
  Sarcocystis kitikmeotensis Dubey et al., 2010b (intermediate host)

Ictonyx **(Poecilictis)** *libyca alexandrae,* **Saharan Striped Polecat**
  Cystoisospora africana (syn. *Isospora africana* Prasad, 1961b) N. Comb.
  Cystoisospora hoogstraali (syn. *Isospora hoogstraali* Prasad, 1961b) N. Comb.
  Cystoisospora zorillae (syn. *Isospora zorillae* (Prasad, 1961b) emend. Pellérdy, 1963) N. Comb.

Lontra canadensis, **North American River Otter**
  Cryptosporidium parvum Tyzzer, 1912
  Cryptosporidium sp. (*species inquirendae*)
  Toxoplasma gondii (Nicolle and Manceaux, 1908) Nicolle and Manceaux, 1909

Lutra lutra, **European Otter**
  Cryptosporidium sp. (*species inquirendae*)
  Cystoisospora lutrae (syn. *Isospora lutrae* Torres et al., 2000) N. Comb.
  Cystoisospora gottschalki (syn. *Isospora lutrae* von Cord Gottschalk, 2000) N. Comb., N. Sp.
  Neospora caninum Dubey et al., 1988a
  Sarcocystis lutrae Gjerde and Josefsen, 2015 (intermediate host)
  Sarcocystis sp. (*species inquirendae*) of one or more authors (see Chapter 19) (intermediate host)
  Toxoplasma gondii (Nicolle and Manceaux, 1908) Nicolle and Manceaux, 1909

Martes foina, **Beech Marten**
  Coccidia/Coccidian/Coccidia-like/Coccidium spp. (*species inquirendae*) of many authors (see Chapter 19)
  Cryptosporidium parvum Tyzzer, 1912
  Cryptosporidium sp. (*species inquirendae*)
  Neospora caninum Dubey et al., 1988a
  Toxoplasma gondii (Nicolle and Manceaux, 1908) Nicolle and Manceaux, 1909

Martes martes, **European Pine Marten**
  Eimeria sibirica Yakimoff and Terwinsky, 1931
  Eimeria sp. (*species inquirendae*) of one or more authors (see Chapter 19)

Isospora mustelae of Galli-Valerio, 1932 (nomen nudum)
Neospora caninum Dubey et al., 1988a
Toxoplasma gondii (Nicolle and Manceaux, 1908) Nicolle and Manceaux, 1909

Martes melampus, Japanese Marten

Hepatozoon sp. (*species inquirendae*) of one or more authors (see Chapter 19)
Sarcocystis sp. (*species inquirendae*) of one or more authors (see Chapter 19) (intermediate host)

Martes pennanti, Fisher

Neospora caninum Dubey et al., 1988a
Sarcocystis neurona Dubey et al., 1991b (intermediate host)
Sarcocystis sp. (*species inquirendae*) of one or more authors (see Chapter 19) (definitive and intermediate host)
Toxoplasma gondii (Nicolle and Manceaux, 1908) Nicolle and Manceaux, 1909

Martes zibellina, Sable

Coccidia/Coccidian/Coccidia-like/Coccidium spp. (*species inquirendae*) of many authors (see Chapter 19)
Cystoisospora martessii (syn. *Isospora martessii* Nukerbaeva, 1981a) N. Comb.
Eimeria sablii Nukerbaeva, 1981a
Eimeria sibirica Yakimoff and Terwinsky, 1931

Meles anakuma, Japanese Badger

Coccidia/Coccidian/Coccidia-like/Coccidium spp. (*species inquirendae*) of many authors (see Chapter 19)
Sarcocystis sp. (*species inquirendae*) of one or more authors (see Chapter 19) (intermediate host)

Meles meles, European Badger

Cryptosporidium hominis Morgan-Ryan et al., 2002
Cryptosporidium parvum Tyzzer, 1912
Cystoisospora melis (Pellérdy, 1955) N. Comb.
Eimeria melis Kotlán and Pospesch, 1933
Isospora-like/*Isospora* spp. (*species inquirendae*) of one or more authors (see Chapter 19)
Neospora caninum Dubey et al., 1988a
Sarcocystis hofmanni Odening et al., 1994b (intermediate host)
Sarcocystis melis Odening et al., 1994b (intermediate host)
Sarcocystis sp. (*species inquirendae*) of one or more authors (see Chapter 19) (intermediate host)
Toxoplasma gondii (Nicolle and Manceaux, 1908) Nicolle and Manceaux, 1909

Mellivora capensis, Honey Badger

Sarcocystis sp. (*species inquirendae*) of one or more authors (see Chapter 19) (intermediate host)

Melogale moschata subaurantiaca, Taiwan Ferret Badger

Sarcocystis sp. (*species inquirendae*) of one or more authors (see Chapter 19) (intermediate host)

Mustela altaica, Mountain Weasel

Cystoisospora altaica (syn. *Isospora altaica* Svanbaev and Rachmatullina, 1971) N. Comb.

Mustela erminea, Ermine (Stoat)

Cryptosporidium parvum Tyzzer, 1912
Cryptosporidium sp. (*species inquirendae*)
Eimeria baskanica of Nukerbaeva and Svanbaev, 1972 or 1973 (?) (*species inquirenda*)
Eimeria furonis Hoare, 1927
Sarcocystis putorii (Railliet and Lucet, 1891), Tadros and Laarman, 1978a (definitive host)
Toxoplasma gondii (Nicolle and Manceaux, 1908) Nicolle and Manceaux, 1909

Mustela eversmanii, Steppe Polecat

Cystoisospora eversmanni (Svanbaev, 1956) emend. Yi-Fan et al., 2012
Cystoisospora pavlovskyi (Svanbaev, 1956) emend. Yi-Fan et al., 2012
Eimeria ictidea Hoare, 1927
Sarcocystis citellivulpes Pak et al., 1979 (definitive host)

Sarcocystis eversmanni Pak et al., 1991 (intermediate host)
Sarcocystis undulati Pak et al., 1984 (*species inquirenda*) (definitive host)

***Mustela eversmanni saturnini*, Siberian Polecat**
Hepatozoon mustelis Novilla et al., 1980 (intermediate host)

***Mustela lutreola*, European Mink**
Eimeria hiepei Gräfner et al., 1967

***Mustela nigripes*, Black-footed Ferret**
Coccidia/Coccidian/Coccidia-like/Coccidium spp. (*species inquirendae*) of many authors (see Chapter 19)
Eimeria furonis Hoare, 1927
Eimeria ictidea Hoare, 1927
Eimeria sp. (*species inquirendae*) of one or more authors (see Chapter 19)
Toxoplasma gondii (Nicolle and Manceaux, 1908) Nicolle and Manceaux, 1909

***Mustela nivalis*, Least Weasel**
Cystoisospora goussevi (syn. *Isospora goussevi* Musaev and Veisov, 1983) N. Comb.
Cystoisospora nivalis (syn. *Isospora nivalis* Musaev and Veisov, 1983) N. Comb.
Cystoisospora nivalis (syn. *Isospora goussevi* Musaev and Veisov, 1983) N. Comb.
Eimeria mustelae Iwanoff-Gobzem, 1934
Eimeria sp. (*species inquirendae*) of one or more authors (see Chapter 19)
Sarcocystis melis Odening et al., 1994b (intermediate host) (?)
Sarcocystis putorii (Railliet and Lucet, 1891), Tadros and Laarman, 1978a (definitive host)
Sarcocystis sp. (*species inquirendae*) of one or more authors (see Chapter 19) (intermediate host)

***Mustela putorius*, European Polecat**
Coccidia/Coccidian/Coccidia-like/Coccidium spp. (*species inquirendae*) of many authors (see Chapter 19)
Cystoisospora eversmanni (Svanbaev, 1956) emend. Yi-Fan et al., 2012
Neospora caninum Dubey et al., 1988a
Toxoplasma gondii (Nicolle and Manceaux, 1908) Nicolle and Manceaux, 1909

***Mustela* (syn. *Putorius*) *putorius furo*, European Polecat/Domestic Ferret**
Cryptosporidium parvum Tyzzer, 1912
Cryptosporidium sp. (*species inquirendae*)
Cystoisospora laidlawi (syn. *Isospora laidlawi* Hoare, 1927) N. Comb.
Eimeria furonis Hoare, 1927
Eimeria ictidea Hoare, 1927
Eimeria mephitidis of Yakimoff and Gousseff, 1936 (*species inquirenda*)
Eimeria vison (syn. *Eimeria mustelae* Kingscote, 1934a,b) Kingscote, 1935
Isospora ohioensis of Patterson and Fox, 2007 (*species inquirenda*)
Isospora-like/*Isospora* spp. (*species inquirendae*) of one or more authors (see Chapter 19)
Neospora caninum Dubey et al., 1988a
Sarcocystis muris (Railliet, 1885) Labbé, 1899 (definitive host)
Sarcocystis neurona Dubey et al., 1991b (intermediate host)
Sarcocystis putorii (Railliet and Lucet, 1891), Tadros and Laarman, 1978a (definitive host)
Toxoplasma gondii (Nicolle and Manceaux, 1908) Nicolle and Manceaux, 1909

***Neovison* (syn. *Mustela*) *vison*, American Mink**
Coccidia/Coccidian/Coccidia-like/Coccidium spp. (*species inquirendae*) of many authors (see Chapter 19)
Cryptosporidium andersoni Lindsay et al., 2000
Cryptosporidium canis Fayer et al., 2001
Cryptosporidium meleagridis Slavin, 1955
Cryptosporidium parvum Tyzzer, 1912
Cryptosporidium sp. (*species inquirendae*)
Cryptosporidium ubiquitum Fayer et al., 2010
Cystoisospora laidlawi (syn. *Isospora laidlawi* Hoare, 1927) N. Comb.
Eimeria furonis Hoare, 1927

Eimeria hiepei Gräfner et al., 1967
Eimeria ictidea Hoare, 1927
Eimeria melis Kotlán and Pospesch, 1933
Eimeria mustelae Iwanoff-Gobzem, 1934
Eimeria sp. (*species inquirendae*) of one or more authors (see Chapter 19)
Eimeria vison (syn. *Eimeria mustelae* Kingscote, 1934a,b) Kingscote, 1935
Eimeria visonlevinei (Levine, 1948) N. Comb., N. Sp.
Hammondia heydorni (Tadros and Laarman, 1976) Dubey, 1977c
Hammonida spp./*Hammondia–Neospora*-like/*Hammondia–Toxoplasma*-like (*species inquirendae*) of one or more authors (see Chapter 19)
Hepatozoon sp. (*species inquirendae*) of one or more authors (see Chapter 19)
Isospora bigemina of Sealander, 1943 (*species inquirenda*)
Neospora caninum Dubey et al., 1988a
Sarcocystis neurona Dubey et al., 1991b (intermediate host)
Sarcocystis putorii (Railliet and Lucet, 1891), Tadros and Laarman, 1978a (definitive host)
Sarcocystis sp. (*species inquirendae*) of one or more authors (see Chapter 19) (intermediate host)
Toxoplasma gondii (Nicolle and Manceaux, 1908) Nicolle and Manceaux, 1909

Taxidea taxus, American Badger
Sarcocystis campestris Cawthorn et al., 1983 (definitive host)

FAMILY ODOBENIDAE
Odobenus rosmarus, Walrus
Neospora caninum Dubey et al., 1988a
Toxoplasma gondii (Nicolle and Manceaux, 1908) Nicolle and Manceaux, 1909

FAMILY OTARIIDAE
Eumetopias jubatus, Steller Sea Lion
Sarcocystis canis Dubey and Speer, 1991 (intermediate host—natural)
Sarcocystis neurona Dubey et al., 1991b (intermediate host—natural)

Zalophus californianus (syn. *Otaria californiana*), California Sea Lion
Coccidia/Coccidian/Coccidia-like/Coccidium spp. (*species inquirendae*) of many authors (see Chapter 19)
Cryptosporidium parvum Tyzzer, 1912
Cryptosporidium sp. (*species inquirendae*)
Neospora caninum Dubey et al., 1988a
Sarcocystis canis Dubey and Speer, 1991 (intermediate host—natural)
Sarcocystis hueti (Moulé, 1888) Labbé, 1899 (intermediate host)
Sarcocystis neurona Dubey et al., 1991b (intermediate host—natural)
Sarcocystis sp. (*species inquirendae*) of one or more authors (see Chapter 19) (intermediate host)
Toxoplasma gondii (Nicolle and Manceaux, 1908) Nicolle and Manceaux, 1909

FAMILY PHOCIDAE

Arctocephalus australis, South American Fur Seal
Toxoplasma gondii (Nicolle and Manceaux, 1908) Nicolle and Manceaux, 1909

Arctocephalus forsteri, Australian Fur Seal
Toxoplasma gondii (Nicolle and Manceaux, 1908) Nicolle and Manceaux, 1909

Arctocephalus gazella, Antarctic Fur Seal
Toxoplasma gondii (Nicolle and Manceaux, 1908) Nicolle and Manceaux, 1909

Arctocephalus pusillus, Brown (South African) Fur Seal
Cystoisospora israeli Kuttin and Kaller, 1992

Arctocephalus townsendi, Guadalupe Fur Seal
Sarcocystis neurona Dubey et al., 1991b (intermediate host—natural)

Callorhinus ursinus, Northern Fur Seal
  Sarcocystis neurona Dubey et al., 1991b (intermediate host—natural)
  Sarcocystis spp. (*species inquirendae*) of one or more authors (see Chapter 19) (intermediate host)
  Toxoplasma gondii (Nicolle and Manceaux, 1908) Nicolle and Manceaux, 1909

Cystophora cristata, Hooded Seal
  Cryptosporidium sp. (*species inquirendae*)
  Toxoplasma gondii (Nicolle and Manceaux, 1908) Nicolle and Manceaux, 1909

Erignathus barbatus, Bearded Seal
  Neospora caninum Dubey et al., 1988a
  Sarcocystis sp. (*species inquirendae*) of one or more authors (see Chapter 19) (intermediate host)
  Toxoplasma gondii (Nicolle and Manceaux, 1908) Nicolle and Manceaux, 1909

Halichoerus grypus, Gray Seal
  Eimeria phocae Hsu et al., 1974a (?)
  Toxoplasma gondii (Nicolle and Manceaux, 1908) Nicolle and Manceaux, 1909

Hydrurga leptonyx, Leopard Seal
  Sarcocystis hydrurgae Odening and Zipper, 1986 (intermediate host, definitive host—unlikely)

Leptonychotes weddellii, Weddell Seal
  Cryptosporidium sp. (*species inquirendae*)
  Eimeria arctowski Dróżdż, 1987
  Eimeria weddelli Dróżdż, 1987
  Eimeria sp. (*species inquirendae*) of one or more authors (see Chapter 19)
  Sarcocystis sp. (*species inquirendae*) of one or more authors (see Chapter 19) (intermediate host)
  Toxoplasma gondii (Nicolle and Manceaux, 1908) Nicolle and Manceaux, 1909

Lobodon carcinophaga, Crabeater Seal
  Eimeria sp. (*species inquirendae*) of one or more authors (see Chapter 19)
  Sarcocystis sp. (*species inquirendae*) of one or more authors (see Chapter 19) (intermediate host)
  Toxoplasma gondii (Nicolle and Manceaux, 1908) Nicolle and Manceaux, 1909

Mirounga angustirostris, Northern Elephant Seal
  Sarcocystis neurona Dubey et al., 1991b (intermediate host—natural)
  Toxoplasma gondii (Nicolle and Manceaux, 1908) Nicolle and Manceaux, 1909

Mirounga leonina, Southern Elephant Seal
  Cryptosporidium sp. (*species inquirendae*)
  Cystoisospora mirungae (syn. *Isospora mirungae* Dróżdż, 1987) N. Comb.
  Sarcocystis sp. (*species inquirendae*) of one or more authors (see Chapter 19) (intermediate host)
  Toxoplasma gondii (Nicolle and Manceaux, 1908) Nicolle and Manceaux, 1909

Monachus schauinslandi, Hawaiian Monk Seal
  Sarcocystis canis Dubey and Speer, 1991 (intermediate host—natural)
  Toxoplasma gondii (Nicolle and Manceaux, 1908) Nicolle and Manceaux, 1909

Otaria flavescens (syn. Otaria byronia), South American Sea Lion
  Cryptosporidium sp. (*species inquirendae*)
  Eimeria sp. (*species inquirendae*) of one or more authors (see Chapter 19)
  Hammondia heydorni (Tadros and Laarman, 1976) Dubey, 1977c
  Neospora caninum Dubey et al., 1988a
  Toxoplasma gondii (Nicolle and Manceaux, 1908) Nicolle and Manceaux, 1909

Pagophilus groenlandicus, Harp Seal
  Cryptosporidium sp. (*species inquirendae*)

Phoca largha, **Spotted Seal**
    Neospora caninum Dubey et al., 1988a
    Toxoplasma gondii (Nicolle and Manceaux, 1908) Nicolle and Manceaux, 1909

Phoca vitulina **(syn.** *P. richardii***), Harbor Seal**
    Cryptosporidium sp. (*species inquirendae*)
    Neospora caninum Dubey et al., 1988a
    Sarcocystis neurona Dubey et al., 1991b (intermediate host)
    Sarcocystis richardii Hadwen, 1922 (intermediate host)
    Sarcocystis sp. (*species inquirendae*) of one or more authors (see Chapter 19) (intermediate host)
    Toxoplasma gondii (Nicolle and Manceaux, 1908) Nicolle and Manceaux, 1909

Phoca vitulina concolor, **Harbor Seal**
    Eimeria phocae Hsu et al., 1974a

Phoca vitulina richardsi, **Pacific Harbor Seal**
    Sarcocystis neurona Dubey et al., 1991b (intermediate host)
    Sarcocystis sp. (*species inquirendae*) of one or more authors (see Chapter 19) (intermediate host)
    Toxoplasma gondii (Nicolle and Manceaux, 1908) Nicolle and Manceaux, 1909

Phoca vitulina stejnegeri, **Kuril Harbor Seal**
    Neospora caninum Dubey et al., 1988a

Phocarctos hookeri, **New Zealand Sea Lion**
    Toxoplasma gondii (Nicolle and Manceaux, 1908) Nicolle and Manceaux, 1909

Pusa capsica **(syn.** *Phoca capsica***), Caspian Seal**
    Sarcocystis sp. (*species inquirendae*) of one or more authors (see Chapter 19) (intermediate host)

Pusa hispida **(syn.** *Phoca hispida***), Ringed Seal**
    Cryptosporidium muris (Tyzzer, 1907) Tyzzer, 1910
    Cryptosporidium sp. (*species inquirendae*)
    Eimeria sp. (*species inquirendae*) of one or more authors (see Chapter 19)
    Neospora caninum Dubey et al., 1988a
    Sarcocystis sp. (*species inquirendae*) of one or more authors (see Chapter 19) (intermediate host)
    Toxoplasma gondii (Nicolle and Manceaux, 1908) Nicolle and Manceaux, 1909

FAMILY PROCYONIDAE

Bassariscus astutus, **Civet or Ringtail Cat**
    Toxoplasma gondii (Nicolle and Manceaux, 1908) Nicolle and Manceaux, 1909

Nasua narica **(syn.** *Nasua nasica***), White-nosed Coati or Coatimundi**
    Eimeria nasuae Carini and Grechi, 1938

Nasua narica molaris, **White-nosed Coati**
    Sarcocystis neurona Dubey et al., 1991b (intermediate host—natural)

Nasua nasua, **South American Coati**
    Cystoisospora arctopitheci (syn. *Isospora arctopitheci* Rodhain, 1933) N. Comb.
    Hepatozoon procyonis Richards, 1961 (intermediate host)
    Toxoplasma gondii (Nicolle and Manceaux, 1908) Nicolle and Manceaux, 1909

Potos flavus, **Kinkajou**
    Cystoisospora arctopitheci (syn. *Isospora arctopitheci* Rodhain, 1933) N. Comb.
    Eimeria poti Lainson, 1968
    Sarcocystis sp. (*species inquirendae*) of one or more authors (see Chapter 19) (intermediate host)
    Toxoplasma gondii (Nicolle and Manceaux, 1908) Nicolle and Manceaux, 1909

Procyon cancrivorus, **Crab-eating Raccoon**
  Hepatozoon procyonis Richards, 1961 (intermediate host)
  Toxoplasma gondii (Nicolle and Manceaux, 1908) Nicolle and Manceaux, 1909

Procyon cancrivorus panamensis, **Panamanian Crab-eating Raccoon**
  Hepatozoon procyonis Richards, 1961 (intermediate host)

Procyon lotor, **Raccoon**
  Coccidia/Coccidian/Coccidia-like/Coccidium spp. (*species inquirendae*) of many authors (see Chapter 19)
  Cryptosporidium parvum Tyzzer, 1912
  Cryptosporidium sp. (*species inquirendae*)
  Cystoisospora chobotari (syn. *Isospora chobotari* Levine and Ivens, 1981) N. Comb.
  Cystoisospora ohioensis (syn. *Isospora ohioensis* Dubey, 1975c) N. Comb. (?)
  Eimeria nuttalli Yakimoff and Matikaschwili, 1933
  Eimeria procyonis Inabnit et al., 1972
  Eimeria sp. (*species inquirendae*) of one or more authors (see Chapter 19)
  Hepatozoon procyonis Richards, 1961 (intermediate host)
  Isospora ohioensis Dubey, 1975c
  Isospora-like/*Isospora* spp. (*species inquirendae*) of one or more authors (see Chapter 19)
  Neospora caninum Dubey et al., 1988a
  Sarcocystis cruzi (Hasselmann, 1923) Wenyon, 1926 (definitive host)
  Sarcocystis hofmanni Odening et al., 1994b (intermediate host) (?)
  Sarcocystis kirkpatricki Snyder et al., 1990 (intermediate host)
  Sarcocystis leporum Crawley, 1914 (definitive host)
  Sarcocystis melis Odening et al., 1994b (intermediate host)
  Sarcocystis miescheriana (Kühn, 1865) Labbé, 1899 (definitive host)
  Sarcocystis neurona Dubey et al., 1991b (intermediate host)
  Sarcocystis sp. (*species inquirendae*) of one or more authors (see Chapter 19) (definitive and intermediate host)
  Toxoplasma gondii (Nicolle and Manceaux, 1908) Nicolle and Manceaux, 1909

Procyon pygmaeus, **Pygmy Raccoon**
  Eimeria nuttalli Yakimoff and Matikaschwili, 1933
  Toxoplasma gondii (Nicolle and Manceaux, 1908) Nicolle and Manceaux, 1909

FAMILY URSIDAE

Ailuropoda melanoleuca, **Giant panda**
  Cryptosporidium andersoni Lindsay et al., 2000
  Cryptosporidium sp. (*species inquirendae*)
  Toxoplasma gondii (Nicolle and Manceaux, 1908) Nicolle and Manceaux, 1909

Helarctos malayanus, **Sun Bear**
  Cryptosporidium sp. (*species inquirendae*)
  Sarcocystis sp. (*species inquirendae*) of one or more authors (see Chapter 19) (intermediate host)

Melursus ursinus, **Sloth Bear**
  Cystoisospora ursi (syn. *Isospora ursi* Agrawal et al., 1981) N. Comb.

Ursus americanus, **American Black Bear**
  Cryptosporidium parvum Tyzzer, 1912
  Eimeria albertensis Hair and Mahrt, 1970
  Eimeria borealis Hair and Mahrt, 1970
  Sarcocystis canis Dubey and Speer, 1991 (intermediate host)
  Sarcocystis ursusi Dubey et al., 2008a (intermediate host)
  Sarcocystis sp. (*species inquirendae*) of one or more authors (see Chapter 19) (intermediate host)
  Toxoplasma gondii (Nicolle and Manceaux, 1908) Nicolle and Manceaux, 1909

Ursus arctos, **Brown or Grizzly Bear**

Coccidia/Coccidian/Coccidia-like/Coccidium spp. (*species inquirendae*) of many authors (see Chapter 19)
Cryptosporidium sp. (*species inquirendae*)
Eimeria sp. (*species inquirendae*) of one or more authors (see Chapter 19)
Eimeria ursi Yakimoff and Matschoulsky, 1935
Isospora-like/*Isospora* spp. (*species inquirendae*) of one or more authors (see Chapter 19)
Neospora caninum Dubey et al., 1988a
Toxoplasma gondii (Nicolle and Manceaux, 1908) Nicolle and Manceaux, 1909

Ursus arctos isabellinus (syn. *Ursus pamirensis*), **Brown or Red Bear**

Cystoisospora fonsecai (syn. *Isospora fonsecai* Yakimoff and Matschoulsky, 1940) N. Comb.

Ursus maritimus, **Polar Bear**

Cryptosporidium sp. (*species inquirendae*)
Sarcocystis canis Dubey and Speer, 1991 (intermediate host)
Sarcocystis sp. (*species inquirendae*) of one or more authors (see Chapter 19) (intermediate host)
Toxoplasma gondii (Nicolle and Manceaux, 1908) Nicolle and Manceaux, 1909

Ursus thibetanus japonicus, **Japanese Black Bear**

Cryptosporidium sp. (*species inquirendae*)
Hepatozoon ursi Kubo et al., 2008 (intermediate host)

Suborder: Feliformia

FAMILY EUPLERIDAE
Cryptoprocta ferox, **Fossa**

Toxoplasma gondii (Nicolle and Manceaux, 1908) Nicolle and Manceaux, 1909

Mungotictis decemlineata, **Narrow-striped Mongoose**

Toxoplasma gondii (Nicolle and Manceaux, 1908) Nicolle and Manceaux, 1909

FAMILY FELIDAE
Acinonyx jubatus, **Cheetah**

Cryptosporidium sp. (*species inquirendae*)
Cystoisospora rivolta (Grassi, 1879) Frenkel, 1977
Hepatozoon canis (James, 1905) Wenyon, 1926b (intermediate host)
Neospora caninum Dubey et al., 1988a
Sarcocystis felis Dubey et al., 1992b (intermediate host)
Toxoplasma gondii (Nicolle and Manceaux, 1908) Nicolle and Manceaux, 1909

Catopuma temminckii, **Asian Golden Cat**

Toxoplasma gondii (Nicolle and Manceaux, 1908) Nicolle and Manceaux, 1909

Felis catus, **Domestic Cat**

Besnoitia besnoiti of (Marotel, 1912) Henry, 1913
Besnoitia darlingi (Brumpt, 1913) Mandour, 1965
Besnoitia neotomofelis Dubey and Yabsley, 2010
Besnoitia oryctofelisi Dubey et al., 2003c
Besnoitia sp. of McKenna and Charleston, 1980c (*species inquirenda*)
Besnoitia wallacei (Wallace and Frenkel, 1975) Frenkel, 1977 N. Comb.
Cryptosporidium baileyi (?) of McGlade et al., 2003 (*species inquirenda*)
Cryptosporidium curyi (?) cited by Ogassawara et al., 1986 (*species inquirenda*)
Cryptosporidium felis Iseki, 1979
Cryptosporidium muris (Tyzzer, 1907) Tyzzer, 1910
Cryptosporidium parvum Tyzzer, 1912
Cryptosporidium ryanae Fayer et al., 2008

Cryptosporidium sp. (*species inquirendae*)
Cystoisospora arctopitheci (syn. *Isospora arctopitheci* Rodhain, 1933) N. Comb.
Cystoisospora canis (syn. *Isospora canis* Nemeséri, 1959) N. Comb.
Cystoisospora felis (Wenyon, 1923) Frenkel, 1977
Cystoisospora frenkeli Arcay, 1981
Cystoisospora (?) *neotomafelis* (Galavíz-Silva et al., 1991) N. Comb.
Cystoisospora rivolta (Grassi, 1879) Frenkel, 1977
Cystoisospora rivolta-like of Gates and Nolan, 2009 (*species inquirenda*)
Cystoisospora spp. *species inquirendae* of many authors (see Chapter 19)
Eimeria canis (?) Wenyon, 1923
Eimeria cati Yakimoff, (1932) 1933
Eimeria felina Nieschulz, 1924b
Eimeria sp. (*species inquirendae*) of one or more authors (see Chapter 19)
Hammondia hammondi Frenkel, 1974
Hammonida spp./*Hammondia–Neospora*-like/*Hammondia–Toxoplasma*-like (*species inquirendae*) of one or more authors (see Chapter 19)
Hepatozoon canis (James, 1905) Wenyon, 1926b (intermediate host)
Hepatozoon felis Patton, 1908 (intermediate host)
Hepatozoon sp. (*species inquirendae*) of one or more authors (see Chapter 19)
Isospora novocati of Pellérdy, 1974b (nomen nudum)
Isospora-like/*Isospora* spp. (*species inquirendae*) of one or more authors (see Chapter 19)
Isospora rivolta of Triffitt, 1927
Neospora caninum Dubey et al., 1988a
Sarcocystis bovifelis Heydorn et al., 1975b (definitive host)
Sarcocystis buffalonis Huong et al., 1997 (definitive host)
Sarcocystis caprifelis El-Rafaii et al., 1980 (definitive host)
Sarcocystis cuniculorum (Brumpt, 1913) Odening et al., 1996b (definitive host—experimental)
Sarcocystis cymruensis Ashford, 1978 (definitive host)
Sarcocystis felis Dubey et al., 1992b (intermediate host)
Sarcocystis fusiformis (Railliet, 1897) Bernard and Bauche, 1912 (definitive host)
Sarcocystis fusiformis of Mehlhorn et al., 1975a (*species inquirenda*) (definitive host)
Sarcocystis gigantea (Railliet, 1886b) Ashford, 1977 (definitive host)
Sarcocystis hirsuta Moulé, 1888 (definitive host)
Sarcocystis horvathi Rátz, 1908 (definitive host) (?)
Sarcocystis leporum Crawley, 1914 (definitive host)
Sarcocystis medusiformis Collins et al., 1979 (definitive host)
Sarcocystis moulei Neveu-Lemaire, 1912 (definitive host)
Sarcocystis muris (Railliet, 1885) Labbé, 1899 (definitive host)
Sarcocystis neotomafelis Galavíz-Silva et al., 1991 (definitive host) (?)
Sarcocystis neurona Dubey et al., 1991b (intermediate host—natural and experimental)
Sarcocystis odoi Dubey and Lozier, 1983 (definitive host)
Sarcocystis peckai Odening, 1997 (definitive host) (?)
Sarcocystis poephagi Wei et al., 1985 (definitive host)
Sarcocystis porcifelis Dubey, 1976 (definitive host)
Sarcocystis rommeli Dubey et al., 2016b (definitive host)
Sarcocystis sp. (*species inquirendae*) of one or more authors (see Chapter 19) (definitive and intermediate host)
Sarcocystis wenzeli Odening, 1997 (definitive host) (?)
Toxoplasma gondii (Nicolle and Manceaux, 1908) Nicolle and Manceaux, 1909
Toxoplasma-like of Epe et al., 2004 (*species inquirenda*)
Toxoplasma-like of Lucio-Forster and Bowman, 2011 (*species inquirenda*)
Toxoplasma-like of Nyambura Njuguna et al., 2017 (*species inquirenda*)

Felis chaus, Jungle Cat

Cryptosporidium sp. (*species inquirendae*)
Cystoisospora felis (Wenyon, 1923) Frenkel, 1977

Cystoisospora rivolta (Grassi, 1879) Frenkel, 1977
Eimeria cati Yakimoff, (1932) 1933
Eimeria chaus Ryšavý, 1954
Eimeria felina Nieschulz, 1924b
Eimeria hammondi Dubey and Pande, 1963b
Eimeria mathurai Dubey and Pande, 1963b
Sarcocystis muris (Railliet, 1885) Labbé, 1899 (definitive host)
Sarcocystis sp. (*species inquirendae*) of one or more authors (see Chapter 19) (definitive host)

Felis manul, **Pallas's Cat**
Toxoplasma gondii (Nicolle and Manceaux, 1908) Nicolle and Manceaux, 1909

Felis margarita, **Sand Cat**
Toxoplasma gondii (Nicolle and Manceaux, 1908) Nicolle and Manceaux, 1909

Felis silvestris, **Wildcat**
Cystoisospora felis (Wenyon, 1923) Frenkel, 1977
Cystoisospora rivolta (Grassi, 1879) Frenkel, 1977
Eimeria felina Nieschulz, 1924b
Isospora rivolta of Triffitt, 1927
Neospora caninum Dubey et al., 1988a
Sarcocystis hirsuta Moulé, 1888 (definitive host)
Toxoplasma gondii (Nicolle and Manceaux, 1908) Nicolle and Manceaux, 1909

Leopardus (syn. *Oncifelis*) *colocolo*, **Colocolo**
Neospora caninum Dubey et al., 1988a
Sarcocystis felis Dubey et al., 1992b (intermediate host)
Toxoplasma gondii (Nicolle and Manceaux, 1908) Nicolle and Manceaux, 1909

Leopardus (syn. *Oncifelis*) *geoffroyi*, **Geoffroy's Cat**
Neospora caninum Dubey et al., 1988a
Sarcocystis felis Dubey et al., 1992b (intermediate host)
Toxoplasma gondii (Nicolle and Manceaux, 1908) Nicolle and Manceaux, 1909

Leopardus pardalis, **Ocelot**
Cryptosporidium sp. (*species inquirendae*)
Cystoisospora felis (Wenyon, 1923) Frenkel, 1977
Cystoisospora rivolta (Grassi, 1879) Frenkel, 1977
Hepatozoon sp. (*species inquirendae*) of one or more authors (see Chapter 19)
Isospora-like/*Isospora* spp. (*species inquirendae*) of one or more authors (see Chapter 19)
Neospora caninum Dubey et al., 1988a
Toxoplasma gondii (Nicolle and Manceaux, 1908) Nicolle and Manceaux, 1909

Leopardus tigrinus (syn. *Leopardus guttulus*), **Oncilla**
Cryptosporidium sp. (*species inquirendae*)
Neospora caninum Dubey et al., 1988a
Sarcocystis felis Dubey et al., 1992b (intermediate host)
Toxoplasma gondii (Nicolle and Manceaux, 1908) Nicolle and Manceaux, 1909

Leopardus wiedii, **Margay**
Sarcocystis felis Dubey et al., 1992b (intermediate host)
Toxoplasma gondii (Nicolle and Manceaux, 1908) Nicolle and Manceaux, 1909

Leptailurus serval, **Serval**
Cystoisospora felis (Wenyon, 1923) Frenkel, 1977
Cystoisospora rivolta (Grassi, 1879) Frenkel, 1977
Isospora felis of Mackinnon and Dibb, 1938
Neospora caninum Dubey et al., 1988a
Toxoplasma gondii (Nicolle and Manceaux, 1908) Nicolle and Manceaux, 1909

Lynx canadensis, **Canadian Lynx**
    Sarcocystis neurona Dubey et al., 1991b (intermediate host)

Lynx lynx, **Eurasian Lynx**
    Cystoisospora felis (Wenyon, 1923) Frenkel, 1977
    Cystoisospora rivolta (Grassi, 1879) Frenkel, 1977
    Neospora caninum Dubey et al., 1988a
    Toxoplasma gondii (Nicolle and Manceaux, 1908) Nicolle and Manceaux, 1909

Lynx lynx isabellinus, **Central Asian Lynx**
    Eimeria sp. (*species inquirendae*) of one or more authors (see Chapter 19)
    Eimeria tadzhikistanica of Anpilogova and Sokov, 1973 (*species inquirenda*)

Lynx pardinus, **Iberian Lynx**
    Cystoisospora felis (Wenyon, 1923) Frenkel, 1977
    Neospora caninum Dubey et al., 1988a
    Toxoplasma gondii (Nicolle and Manceaux, 1908) Nicolle and Manceaux, 1909

Lynx (**syn.** *Felis*) *rufus*, **Bobcat**
    Cryptosporidium sp. (*species inquirendae*)
    Hepatozoon sp. (*species inquirendae*) of one or more authors (see Chapter 19)
    Isospora bigemina large form of Duszynski and Speer, 1976 (*species inquirenda*)
    Sarcocystis felis Dubey et al., 1992b (intermediate host)
    Sarcocystis sp. (*species inquirendae*) of one or more authors (see Chapter 19) (definitive host)
    Toxoplasma gondii (Nicolle and Manceaux, 1908) Nicolle and Manceaux, 1909

Lynx **sp., Bobcat**
    Cystoisospora felis (Wenyon, 1923) Frenkel, 1977
    Isospora lyncis Levine and Ivens, 1981 (*species inquirenda*)

Neofelis nebulosa, **Clouded Leopard**
    Cystoisospora leopardi (syn. *Isospora leopardi* Agrawal et al., 1981) N. Comb.
    Neospora caninum Dubey et al., 1988a
    Toxoplasma gondii (Nicolle and Manceaux, 1908) Nicolle and Manceaux, 1909

Panthera leo, **Lion**
    Apicomplexan Protozoa of Bjork et al., 2000 (*species inquirenda*)
    Coccidia/Coccidian/Coccidia-like/Coccidium spp. (*species inquirendae*) of many authors (see Chapter 19)
    Cystoisospora felis (Wenyon, 1923) Frenkel, 1977
    Cystoisospora leonina (syn. *Isospora leonina* Mandal and Ray, 1960) N. Comb.
    Cystoisospora mohini (syn. *Isospora mohini* Agrawal et al., 1981) N. Comb.
    Cystoisospora pantheri (syn. *Isospora pantheri* Agrawal et al., 1981) N. Comb.
    Cystoisospora rivolta (Grassi, 1879) Frenkel, 1977
    Eimeria felina Nieschulz, 1924b
    Hepatozoon canis (James, 1905) Wenyon, 1926b (intermediate host)
    Hepatozoon sp. (*species inquirendae*) of one or more authors (see Chapter 19)
    Isospora-like/*Isospora* spp. (*species inquirendae*) of one or more authors (see Chapter 19)
    Neospora caninum Dubey et al., 1988a
    Sarcocystis felis Dubey et al., 1992b (intermediate host)
    Sarcocystis sp. (*species inquirendae*) of one or more authors (see Chapter 19) (definitive and intermediate host)
    Toxoplasma gondii (Nicolle and Manceaux, 1908) Nicolle and Manceaux, 1909

Panthera leo massaica, **Massai Lion**
    Hepatozoon sp. (*species inquirendae*) of one or more authors (see Chapter 19)

Panthera (**syn.** *Puma*) *onca*, **Jaguar**
    Cystoisospora felis (Wenyon, 1923) Frenkel, 1977
    Cystoisospora rivolta (Grassi, 1879) Frenkel, 1977

Hammondia pardalis Hendricks et al., 1979
Hepatozoon felis Patton, 1908 (intermediate host)
Neospora caninum Dubey et al., 1988a
Toxoplasma gondii (Nicolle and Manceaux, 1908) Nicolle and Manceaux, 1909

Panthera pardus, Leopard

Apicomplexan Protozoa of Patton and Rabinowitz, 1994 (*species inquirenda*)
Cryptosporidium sp. (*species inquirendae*)
Cystoisospora pardusi (syn. *Isospora pardusi* et al., 1971) N. Comb.
Cystoisospora rivolta (Grassi, 1879) Frenkel, 1977
Eimeria anekalensis Rajasekariah et al., 1971
Eimeria hartmanni Rastegaïeff, 1930 (?)
Eimeria novowenyoni Rastegaïeff, 1930 (?)
Hepatozoon canis (James, 1905) Wenyon, 1926b (intermediate host)
Hepatozoon sp. (*species inquirendae*) of one or more authors (see Chapter 19)
Isospora-like/*Isospora* spp. (*species inquirendae*) of one or more authors (see Chapter 19)
Isospora-rivolta-like of Mandal and Choudhury, 1983
Neospora caninum Dubey et al., 1988a
Sarcocystis sp. (*species inquirendae*) of one or more authors (see Chapter 19) (definitive and intermediate host)
Toxoplasma gondii (Nicolle and Manceaux, 1908) Nicolle and Manceaux, 1909

Panthera tigris, Tiger

Apicomplexan Protozoa of Patton and Rabinowitz, 1994 (*species inquirenda*)
Cryptosporidium sp. (*species inquirendae*)
Cystoisospora felis (Wenyon, 1923) Frenkel, 1977
Cystoisospora rivolta (Grassi, 1879) Frenkel, 1977
Eimeria hartmanni Rastegaïeff, 1930
Eimeria novowenyoni Rastegaïeff, 1930
Isospora-like/*Isospora* spp. (*species inquirendae*) of one or more authors (see Chapter 19)
Neospora caninum Dubey et al., 1988a
Sarcocystis sp. (*species inquirendae*) of one or more authors (see Chapter 19) (definitive host)
Toxoplasma gondii (Nicolle and Manceaux, 1908) Nicolle and Manceaux, 1909

Panthera tigris corbetti, Indochinese Tiger

Cryptosporidium sp. (*species inquirendae*)

Panthera tigris jacksoni, Malayan Tiger

Cryptosporidium sp. (*species inquirendae*)

Panthera tigris sumatrae, Sumatran Tiger

Cryptosporidium sp. (*species inquirendae*)

Panthera sp., Leopard

Cryptosporidium sp. (*species inquirendae*)

Panthera tigris tigris, Bengal Tiger

Apicomplexan Protozoa of Patton and Rabinowitz, 1994 (*species inquirenda*)
Cystoisospora bengalensis (syn. *Isospora bengalensis* Patnaik and Acharjyo, 1971) N. Comb.
Cystoisospora felina (syn. *Isospora felina* Patnaik and Acharjyo, 1971) N. Comb.

Prionailurus bengalensis, Leopard Cat

Hepatozoon felis Patton, 1908 (intermediate host)
Sarcocystis sp. (*species inquirendae*) of one or more authors (see Chapter 19) (definitive host)
Toxoplasma gondii (Nicolle and Manceaux, 1908) Nicolle and Manceaux, 1909

Prionailurus bengalensis euptilurus, Tsushima Leopard Cat

Hepatozoon felis Patton, 1908 (intermediate host)

Prionailurus iriomotensis (syn. *P. bengalensis iriomotensis*), **Iriomote Wild Cat**
  Hepatozoon felis Patton, 1908 (intermediate host)
  Toxoplasma gondii (Nicolle and Manceaux, 1908) Nicolle and Manceaux, 1909

Prionailurus (syn. *Felis*) *viverrinus*, **Fishing Cat**
  Cystoisospora viverrina (syn. *Isospora viverrina* Agrawal and Chauhan, 1993) N. Comb.
  Neospora caninum Dubey et al., 1988a
  Toxoplasma gondii (Nicolle and Manceaux, 1908) Nicolle and Manceaux, 1909

Puma (syn. *Felis*) *concolor*, **Cougar**
  Hammondia pardalis Hendricks et al., 1979
  Neospora caninum Dubey et al., 1988a
  Sarcocystis sp. (*species inquirendae*) of one or more authors (see Chapter 19) (definitive and intermediate host)
  Toxoplasma gondii (Nicolle and Manceaux, 1908) Nicolle and Manceaux, 1909

Puma (syn. *Felis*) *concolor coryi*, **Florida Panther**
  Sarcocystis felis Dubey et al., 1992b (intermediate host)

Puma (syn. *Felis*) *concolor stanleyana*, **Cougar**
  Sarcocystis felis Dubey et al., 1992b (intermediate host)

Puma yagouaroundi, **Jaguarundi**
  Neospora caninum Dubey et al., 1988a
  Sarcocystis felis Dubey et al., 1992b (intermediate host)
  Toxoplasma gondii (Nicolle and Manceaux, 1908) Nicolle and Manceaux, 1909

Uncia uncia, **Snow Leopard**
  Neospora caninum Dubey et al., 1988a
  Toxoplasma gondii (Nicolle and Manceaux, 1908) Nicolle and Manceaux, 1909

FAMILY HERPESTIDAE

Crossarchus obscurus, **Common Kusimanse**
  Cystoisospora garnhami (syn. *Isospora garnhami* Bray, 1954) N. Comb.

Cynictis penicillate, **Yellow Mongoose**
  Isospora-like/*Isospora* spp. (*species inquirendae*) of one or more authors (see Chapter 19)

Helogale parvula (syn. *Hel. undulatus*), **Common Dwarf Mongoose**
  Cystoisospora garnhami (syn. *Isospora garnhami* Bray, 1954) N. Comb.
  Cystoisospora hoarei (syn. *Isospora hoarei* Bray, 1954) N. Comb.
  Sarcocystis sp. (*species inquirendae*) of one or more authors (see Chapter 19) (intermediate host)

Herpestes edwardsi (syn. *Her. mungo*), **Indian Gray Mongoose**
  Cystoisospora dasguptai (syn. *Isospora dasguptai* Levine et al., 1975) N. Comb.
  Cystoisospora garnhami (syn. *Isospora garnhami* Bray, 1954) N. Comb.
  Cystoisospora herpestei (syn. *Isospora herpestei* Levine et al., 1975) N. Comb.
  Cystoisospora hoarei (syn. *Isospora hoarei* Bray, 1954) N. Comb.
  Cystoisospora mungoi (syn. *Isospora mungoi* Levine et al., 1975) N. Comb.
  Cystoisospora pellerdyi (syn. *Isospora pellerdyi* Dubey and Pande, 1964) N. Comb.
  Eimeria jalpaiguriensis Bandyopadhyay, 1982
  Eimeria newalai Dubey and Pande, 1963a
  Eimeria pandei (Patnaik and Ray, 1965) Patnaik and Ray (sic), 1966
  Toxoplasma gondii (Nicolle and Manceaux, 1908) Nicolle and Manceaux, 1909

Herpestes ichneumon, **Egyptian Mongoose**
  Cryptosporidium canis Fayer et al., 2001
  Isospora ichneumonis of Levine et al., 1975 (*species inquirenda*)

Neospora caninum Dubey et al., 1988a
Toxoplasma gondii (Nicolle and Manceaux, 1908) Nicolle and Manceaux, 1909

Herpestes javanicus (syn. *Her. auropunctatus*), Small Asian Mongoose
Cystoisospora dasguptai (syn. *Isospora dasguptai* Levine et al., 1975) N. Comb.
Cystoisospora herpestei (syn. *Isospora herpestei* Levine et al., 1975) N. Comb.

Ichneumia albicauda, White-tailed Mongoose
Toxoplasma gondii (Nicolle and Manceaux, 1908) Nicolle and Manceaux, 1909

Mungos mungo, Banded Mongoose
Cryptosporidium parvum Tyzzer, 1912
Sarcocystis sp. (*species inquirendae*) of one or more authors (see Chapter 19) (intermediate host)

Suricata suricatta, Meerkat or Suricate or Slender-tailed Meerkat
Cystoisospora timoni El-Gayar et al., 2008
Isospora-like/*Isospora* spp. (*species inquirendae*) of one or more authors (see Chapter 19)
Toxoplasma gondii (Nicolle and Manceaux, 1908) Nicolle and Manceaux, 1909

FAMILY HYAENIDAE

Crocuta crocuta, Spotted Hyaena
Cystoisospora spp. *species inquirendae* of many authors (see Chapter 19)
Hepatozoon canis (James, 1905) Wenyon, 1926b (intermediate host)
Hepatozoon sp. (*species inquirendae*) of one or more authors (see Chapter 19)
Isospora-like/*Isospora* spp. (*species inquirendae*) of one or more authors (see Chapter 19)
Neospora caninum Dubey et al., 1988a
Toxoplasma gondii (Nicolle and Manceaux, 1908) Nicolle and Manceaux, 1909

Hyaena hyaena (syn. *H. striata*), Brown, Indian, or Striped Hyaena
Cystoisospora levinei (syn. *Isospora levinei* Dubey, 1963a) N. Comb.
Toxoplasma gondii (Nicolle and Manceaux, 1908) Nicolle and Manceaux, 1909

FAMILY VIVERIIDAE

Arctictis binturong, Binturong
Toxoplasma gondii (Nicolle and Manceaux, 1908) Nicolle and Manceaux, 1909

Civettictis civetta (syn. *Viverra civetta*), African Civet
Cystoisospora viverrae (syn. *Isospora viverrae* Adler, 1924) N. Comb., N. Sp.

Genetta genetta (syn. *G. dongolana*), Common Genet
Cryptosporidium sp. (*species inquirendae*)
Eimeria genettae of Agostinucci and Bronzini, 1955 (*species inquirenda*)
Hepatozoon sp. (*species inquirendae*) of one or more authors (see Chapter 19)
Neospora caninum Dubey et al., 1988a
Toxoplasma gondii (Nicolle and Manceaux, 1908) Nicolle and Manceaux, 1909

Genetta thierryi (syn. *Genetta rubiginosa*), Haussa Genet
Hepatozoon sp. (*species inquirendae*) of one or more authors (see Chapter 19)

Genetta tigrine, Cape Genet
Hepatozoon sp. (*species inquirendae*) of one or more authors (see Chapter 19)

Paguma larvata, Masked Palm Civet
Toxoplasma gondii (Nicolle and Manceaux, 1908) Nicolle and Manceaux, 1909

Paradoxurus hermaphroditus, Asian Palm Civet
Coccidia, *Cyclospora*, *Eimeria* spp. of Chakraborty et al., 2016 (*species inquirendae*)
Eimeria sp. (*species inquirendae*) of one or more authors (see Chapter 19)
Toxoplasma gondii (Nicolle and Manceaux, 1908) Nicolle and Manceaux, 1909

Paradoxurus jerdoni, Jerdon's Palm Civet
Coccidia, *Cyclospora, Eimeria* spp. of Chakraborty et al., 2016 (*species inquirendae*)

Viverra tangalunga, Malayan Civet
Eimeria, Isospora, and *Sarcocystis* spp. of Colón and Patton, 2012 (*species inquirendae*)
Toxoplasma gondii (Nicolle and Manceaux, 1908) Nicolle and Manceaux, 1909

Appendix C

TABLE A3   Overview of Some Recommended Therapies for Carnivore Coccidioses

Drug (Efficacy Against)	Treatment Regime	References
Amprolium (*Cystoisospora*, *Eimeria*)	300–400 mg total for 5 days (dogs)	CAPC, 2013
	110–200 mg/day for 7–12 days (dogs)	CAPC, 2013
	60–100 mg/kg/day for 7 days (cats)	CAPC, 2013
	19 mg/kg/day PO for 2 wk or longer (domestic ferrets)	CAPC, 2013
Amprolium + sulfadimethoxine (*Cystoisospora*)	150 mg/kg/day + 25 mg/kg/day for 14 days (dogs)	CAPC, 2013
Azithromycin (*T. gondii*, *Cryptosporidium*)	5.3 mg/kg PO b.i.d. for 2 wk (dogs, cats)	Fitzgerald et al., 2011
Clindamycin (*Neospora*, *T. gondii*)	5.5–11 mg/kg PO s.i.d. or b.i.d. for at least 3 wk (adult dogs and cats)	Šimůnek and Smola, 1998; Poli et al., 1998
	12 mg/kg PO each 8 h for 18 wk	Crookshanks et al., 2007
	75 mg/puppy PO b.i.d. (puppies at 9 wk old) for 6 months	Lyon, 2010
	150 mg/puppy PO b.i.d. (puppies at 13 wk old) for 6 months	Lyon, 2010
	11 mg/kg IM s.i.d. or b.i.d. (dogs)	Šimůnek and Smola, 1998
Clindamycin + trimethoprim sulfadiazine (*Neospora*)	10 mg/kg PO each 8 h + 15 mg/kg PO b.i.d. for 4 wk or longer (dogs)	Lyon, 2010
Decoquinate (*Eimeria*, *Hepatozoon*, *Sarcocystis*)	10–20 mg/kg PO s.i.d. or b.i.d. (dogs)	CAPC, 2013; Sykes and Papich, 2014
	0.5 mg/kg/day PO for 2 wk or longer (domestic ferrets)	Bell, 1994; Patterson and Fox, 2007; Patterson et al., 2014
Diclazuril (*Cystoisospora*, *Eimeria*)	25 mg/kg PO one dose (cats)	CAPC, 2013
Furazolidone (*Cystoisospora*, *Eimeria*)	8–20 mg/kg s.i.d. or b.i.d. for 5 days (dogs, cats)	CAPC, 2013
Imidocarb dipropionate (*Hepatozoon*)	5–6 mg/kg SC or IM twice a month at least for 8 wk (dogs)	Sasanelli et al., 2010; de Tommasi et al., 2014
Imidocarb dipropionate (*Hepatozoon*)	(the above recommended dose) + 10 mg/kg PO doxycycline monohydrate for 21 days (dogs)	Sasanelli et al., 2010; Pasa et al., 2011

TABLE A3   Overview of Some Recommended Therapies for Carnivore Coccidioses—cont'd

Drug (Efficacy Against)	Treatment Regime	References
Nitazoxanide (*Cryptosporidium, Sarcocystis neurona*)	25 mg/kg/day for days 1–5, then	http://www.vin.com
	50/mg/kg/day for days 6–28 (horses)	Li et al., 2003
	500 mg b.i.d. for 14 days, or 300 mg t.i.d. for 7 days, or 1 g b.i.d. for 7 days (humans)	https://reference.medscape.com
	50, 100 or 200 mg/kg/day for 7 days (rats)	Li et al., 2003
Quinacrine (Eimeriidae, Cystoisosporinae)	10 mg/kg/day for 5 days (cats)	CAPC, 2013
Paromomycin (*Cryptosporidium*)	125–165 mg/kg PO b.i.d. for 5 days (dogs, cats)	Barr et al., 1994a,b
Ponazuril (Eimeriidae, Cystoisosporinae, Sarcocystinae)	20–50 mg/kg/day PO for 1–18 days (dogs, cats)	http://www.vin.com; CAPC, 2013; Litster et al., 2014; Sykes and Papich, 2014
	50 mg/kg/day PO for 3 days (domestic ferrets)	Litster et al., 2014
	30 mg/kg/day PO once or twice (black-footed ferrets)	
Pyrimethamine (*Neospora, T. gondii, Sarcocystis*)	1 mg/kg PO s.i.d. or b.i.d. for 4 wk or longer (dogs, cats)	Löschenberger et al., 2000; Parzefall et al., 2014
Pyrimethamine + trimethoprim sulfadiazine (*Neospora*)	1 mg/kg/day PO + 15 mg/kg PO b.i.d. for 4 wk or longer (dogs)	Lyon, 2010
Spiramycin (*T. gondii*)	10–12 mg/kg/day IM (dogs, cats)	Šimůnek and Smola, 1998
	75,000 int. units/kg/day PO (dogs, cats)	www.uskvbl.cz
Sulfonamides in general (Eimeriidae, Sarcocystidae)	1.2–1.5 g/10 kg/day PO (dogs, cats)	Šimůnek and Smola, 1998
	0.6–0.75 g/10 kg parenterally (dogs, cats)	Šimůnek and Smola, 1998
Sulfadiazine + trimethoprim (coccidia)	30 mg/kg/day PO for 2 wk or longer (domestic ferrets)	Bell, 1994; Patterson and Fox, 2007; Patterson et al., 2014
Sulfadimethoxine (*Cystoisospora*)	50–60 mg/kg/day for 5–20 days (dogs, cats)	CAPC, 2013
	20–40 mg/kg/day PO for 5–7 days (dogs, cats)	https://imedikament.de/kokzidiol-sd
	300 mg/kg PO in drinking water for 2 wk or longer (domestic ferrets)	Bell, 1994; Patterson and Fox, 2007; Patterson et al., 2014
Sulfadimethoxine + ormetoprim (*Cystoisospora*)	55 mg/kg/day + 11 mg/kg/day for 7–23 days (dogs)	CAPC, 2013
Sulfaguanidine (*Cystoisospora*)	150–200 mg/kg/day for 6 days (dogs, cats)	CAPC, 2013
	100–200 mg/kg every 8 h for 5 days (dogs, cats)	CAPC, 2013
Sulfamethoxypyridazine (Eimeriidae, Cystoisosporinae)	25–50 mg/kg/day **IM** for 7 days (dogs, cats)	Šimůnek and Smola, 1998; Rademacher et al., 1999

TABLE A3   Overview of Some Recommended Therapies for Carnivore Coccidioses—cont'd

Drug (Efficacy Against)	Treatment Regime	References
Toltrazuril (Eimeriidae, Cystoisosporinae, Sarcocystinae)	10–30 mg/kg/day PO for 1–7 days (dogs) 20 mg/kg PO (domestic ferrets)	Daugschies et al., 2000; CAPC, 2013
(Hepatozoon)	14 mg/kg PO s.i.d. for 5 days (dogs) 10 mg/kg/day PO for 5 days in combination with trimethoprim sulfamethoxazole (dogs)	Perez Tort et al., 2007 Voyvoda et al., 2004
Tylosin (Cryptosporidium)	10 mg/kg IM b.i.d. (dogs, cats)	Šimůnek and Smola, 1998
	5–15 mg/kg PO each 6–8 h (dogs, cats)	Šimůnek and Smola, 1998

References

Abal-Fabeiro, J.L., Maside, X., Llovo, J., Bello, X., Torres, M., Treviño, M., Moldes, L., Muñoz, A., Carracedo, A., Bartolomé, C., 2014. High-throughput genotyping assay for the large-scale genetic characterization of *Cryptosporidium* parasites from human and bovine samples. Parasitology 141 (4), 491–500.

Abarca, V.K., López del, P.J., Peña, D.A., López, G.J.C., 2011. Pet ownerships and health status of pets from immunocompromised children, with emphasis in zoonotic diseases. Revista Chilena de Infectología 28 (3), 205–210 (in Spanish).

Abbitt, B., Craig, T.M., Jones, L.P., Huey, R.L., Eugster, A.K., 1993. Protozoal abortion in a herd of cattle concurrently infected with *Hammondia pardalis*. Journal of the American Veterinary Medical Association 303 (3), 444–448.

Abe, N., Iseki, M., 2003. Identification of genotypes of *Cryptosporidium parvum* isolates from ferrets in Japan. Parasitology Research 89 (5), 422–424.

Abe, N., Takami, K., Kimata, I., Iseki, M., 2004. Molecular characterization of a *Cryptosporidium* isolate from a banded mongoose *Mungos mungo*. Journal of Parasitology 90 (1), 167–171.

Abel, J., Schares, G., Orzeszko, K., Gasser, R.B., Ellis, J.T., 2006. *Hammondia* isolated from dogs and foxes are genetically distinct. Parasitology 132 (2), 187–192.

Adams, J.H., Levine, N.D., Todd, K.S., 1981. *Eimeria* and *Sarcocystis* in raccoons in Illinois. Journal of Protozoology 28 (2), 221–222.

Adamu, H., Petros, B., Zhang, G., Kassa, H., Amer, S., Ye, J., Feng, Y., Xiao, L., 2014. Distribution and clinical manifestations of *Cryptosporidium* species and subtypes in HIV/AIDS patients in Ethiopia. PLoS Neglected Tropical Diseases 8 (4), e2831.

Adell, A.D., Smith, W.A., Shapiro, K., Melli, A., Conrad, P.A., 2014. Molecular epidemiology of *Cryptosporidium* spp. and *Giardia* spp. in mussels (*Mytilus californianus*) and California sea lions (*Zalophus californianus*) from Central California. Applied and Environmental Microbiology 80 (24), 7732–7740.

Adl, S.M., Simpson, A.G.B., Lane, C.E., Lukeš, J., Bass, D., Bowser, S.S., Brown, M.W., Burki, F., Dunthorn, M., Hampl, V., Heiss, A., Hoppenrath, M., Lara, E., le Gall, L., Lynn, D.H., McManus, H., Mitchell, E.A.D., Mozley-Stanridge, S.E., Parfrey, L.W., Pawlowski, J., Rueckert, S., Shadwick, L., Schoch, C.L., Smirnov, A., Spiegel, F.W., 2012. The revised classification of Eukaryotes. Journal of Eukaryotic Microbiology 59 (5), 429–493.

Adler, S., 1924. An *Isospora* of civet cats. Annals of Tropical Medicine and Parasitology 18 (1), 87–94.

Aghazadeh, M., Elson-Riggins, J., Reljic, S., de Ambrogi, M., Huber, D., Majnaric, D., Hermosilla, C., 2015. Gastrointestinal parasites and the first report of *Giardia* spp. in a wild population of European brown bears (*Ursus arctos*) in Croatia. Veterinarski Arhiv 82 (2), 201–210.

Agostinucci, G., Bronzini, E., 1953. *Eimeria genettae* n. sp. parasita della *Genetta dongolana*. In: Proceedings of the 6th International Congress of Microbiology, vol. 5, pp. 284–285.

Agrawal, R.D., Chauhan, P.P.S., 1993. On a new coccidium *Isospora viverrina* from fishing cat (*Felis viverrina*). Indian Journal of Animal Sciences 63, 628–629.

Agrawal, R.D., Ahluwalia, S.S., Bhatia, B.B., Chauhan, P.P.S., 1981. Note on mammalian coccidia at Lucknow zoo. Indian Journal of Animal Sciences 51 (1–6), 125–128.

Ajjampur, S.S., Gladstone, B.P., Selvapandian, D., Muliyil, J.P., Ward, H., Kang, G., 2007. Molecular and spatial epidemiology of cryptosporidiosis in children in a semi-urban community in South India. Journal of Clinical Microbiology 45 (3), 915–920.

Akinbo, F.O., Okaka, C.E., Omoregie, R., Adamu, H., Xiao, L., 2013. Unusual *Enterocytozoon bieneusi* genotypes and *Cryptosporidium hominis* subtypes in HIV-infected patients on highly active antiretroviral therapy. The American Journal of Tropical Medicine and Hygiene 89 (1), 157–161.

Akuzawam, M., Mochizukmi, M., Yasudan, N., 1987. Hematological and parasitological study of the Iriomate cat (*Prionailurus iriomotensis*). Canadian Journal of Zoology 65 (4), 946–949.

Alcaino, H., Tagle, I., 1970. Estudio sobre enteroparasitosis del perro en Santiago. Boletin Chileno de Parasitologia 25 (1), 5–8 (in Spanish).

Al-Kappany, Y.M., Abu-Elwafa, S.A., Hilali, M., Rosenthal, B.M., Dunams, D.B., Dubey, J.P., 2013. Experimental transmission of *Sarcocystis muris* (Apicomplexa: Sarcocystidae) sporocysts from a naturally infected cat (*Felis catus*) to immunocompetent and immunocompromised mice. Journal of Parasitology 99 (6), 997–1001.

Almería, S., 2013. *Neospora caninum* and wildlife. ISRN Parasitology 2013, 23 947347. https://doi.org/10.5402/2013/947347.

Almería, S., Ferrer, D., Pabón, M., Castellà, J., Mañas, S., 2002. Red foxes (*Vulpes vulpes*) are a natural intermediate host of *Neospora caninum*. Veterinary Parasitology 107 (4), 287–294.

Almería, S., Vidal, D., Ferrer, D., Pabón, M., Fernández-de-Mera, M.I.G., Ruiz-Fons, F., Alzaga, V., Marco, I., Calvete, C., Lavin, S., Gortazar, C., 2007. Seroprevalence of Neospora caninum in non-carnivorous wildlife from Spain. Veterinary Parasitology 143 (1), 21–28.

Altreuther, G., Gasda, N., Schroeder, I., Joachim, A., Settje, T., Schimmel, A., Hutchens, D., Krieger, K.J., 2011a. Efficacy of emodepside plus toltrazuril suspension (Procox® oral suspension for dogs) against prepatent and patent infection with Isospora canis and Isospora ohioensis-complex in dogs. Parasitology Research 109 (Suppl. 1), S9–S20.

Altreuther, G., Gasda, N., Adler, K., Hellmann, K., Thurieau, H., Schimmel, A., Hutchens, D., Krieger, K.J., 2011b. Field evaluations of the efficacy and safety of emodepside plus toltrazuril (Procox® oral suspension for dogs) against naturally acquired nematode and Isospora spp. infections in dogs. Parasitology Research 109 (Suppl. 1), S21–S28.

Alvarado-Esquivel, C., Liesenfeld, O., Herrera-Flores, R.G., Ramírez-Sánchez, B.E., González-Herrera, A., Martínez-García, S.A., Dubey, J.P., 2007. Seroprevalence of Toxoplasma gondii antibodies in cats from Durango city, Mexico. Journal of Parasitology 93 (5), 1214–1216.

Alves, M., Matos, O., Pereira Da Fonseca, I., Delgado, E., Lourenço, A.M., Antunes, F., 2001. Multilocus genotyping of Cryptosporidium isolates from human HIV-infected and animal hosts. Journal of Eukaryotic Microbiology (Suppl.), 17S–18S.

Alwar, V.S., Lalitha, C.M., 1958. Parasites of domestic cats (Felis catus) in Madras. Indian Veterinary Journal 35 (6), 292–295.

Amaral, V.D., Amaro, R.G., Birgel, E.H., 1964. Sobre a presença de Isospora felis Wenyon, 1923 (Protozoa: Eimeriidae Poche, 1913) em Canis familiaris em São Paulo (On the presence of Isospora felis Wenyon, 1923 (Protozoa: Eimeriidae Poche, 1913) in Canis familiaris, in São Paulo). Arquivos do Instituto Biológico 31 (3), 101–102 (in Portuguese, English summary).

Anderson, M.L., Barr, B., Conrad, P., Thurmond, M., Picanso, J., Dubey, J.P., 1991. Bovine protozoal abortions in California. Bovine Practitioner 26, 102–104.

Anderson, A.J., Greiner, E.C., Atkinson, C.T., Roelke, M.E., 1992. Sarcocysts in the Florida bobcat (Felis rufus floridanus). Journal of Wildlife Diseases 28 (1), 116–120.

André, M.R., Adania, C.H., Teixeira, R.H.F., Silva, K.F., Jusi, M.M.G., Machado, S.T.Z., de Bortolli, C.P., Falcade, M., Sousa, L., Alegretti, S.M., Felippe, P.A.N., Machado, R.Z., 2010. Antibodies to Toxoplasma gondii and Neospora caninum in captive neotropical and exotic wild canids and felids. Journal of Parasitology 96 (5), 1007–1009.

Andrews, J., 1926a. Coccidiosis in mammals. American Journal of Hygiene 6 (6), 784–798.

Andrews, J., 1926b. The specificity of the Isospora of cats and dogs with respect to host. Journal of Parasitology 13 (1), 89.

Andrews, J., 1928. New species of coccidia from the skunk and prairie dog. Journal of Parasitology 14 (1), 143–145.

Angus, K.W., 1987. Cryptosporidiosis in domestic animals and humans. In Practice 9, 47–49.

Anon, 1984. Sarcosporidians of Animals in Kazakhstan. Institute of Zoology, Kazakh Academy of Sciences, Nauka, Alma-Ata, Kazakhstan. 258 p. (in Russian). (nos non videbo illum).

ANOPHEL, 2010. Cryptosporidium National Network. https://www.ncbi.nlm.nih.gov/pubmed/20739000.

Anpilogova, N.V., Sokov, A.I., 1973. Novye vidy koktsidis iz blendnoy ili srednoaziatska, rysi v Tadzhikistane (New types of coccidia from Blend or Middle Asian, lynx in Tajikistan). Izvestia Akademii Nauk Tadzhikskoi SSR, Otdelenie Biologicheskich Nauk 4 (53), 89–90 (in Russian, no English summary).

Anwar, M.A., Newman, C., MacDonald, D.W., Woolhouse, M.E., Kelly, D.W., 2000. Coccidiosis in the European badger (Meles meles) from England, an epidemiological study. Parasitology 120 (3), 255–260.

Appelbee, A.J., Thompson, R.C., Measures, L.M., Olson, M.E., 2010. Giardia and Cryptosporidium in harp and hooded seals from the Gulf of St. Lawrence, Canada. Veterinary Parasitology 173 (1–2), 19–23.

Aramini, J.J., Stephen, C., Dubey, J.P., 1998. Toxoplasma gondii in Vancouver Island cougars (Felis concolor vancouverensis): serology and oocyst shedding. Journal of Parasitology 84 (2), 438–440.

Araujo, F.G., Remington, J.S., 1974. Effect of clindamycin on acute and chronic toxoplasmosis in mice. Antimicrobial Agents and Chemotherapy 5 (6), 647–651.

Araujo, F.G., Shepard, R.M., Remington, J.S., 1991. In vivo activity of the macrolide antibiotics azithromycin, roxithromycin and spiramycin against Toxoplasma gondii. European Journal of Clinical Microbiology and Infectious Diseases 10 (6), 519–524.

Arbabi, M., Hooshyar, H., 2009. Gastrointestinal parasites of stray cats in Kashan, Iran. Tropical Biomedicine 26 (1), 16–22.

Arcay, L., 1981. Nuevo coccidia de gato: Cystoisospora frenkeli sp. nova (Toxoplasmatinae) y su desarrollo en la membrana corio-alantoidea de embrion de pollo (A new coccidian of the cat: Cystoisospora frenkeli sp. nov (Toxoplasmatinae) and its development in chick allantoic membrane of chick embryo). Acta Cientifica Venezolana 32, 401–410 (in Spanish, English abstract).

Arcay, L., 1987. Cultivo de Cystoisospora felis Frenkel, 1977 (Isospora felis Wasielewski, 1904, Wenyon, 1923) en la membrana chorioalantoidea de embrion de pollo (Cultivation of Cystoisospora felis Frenkel, 1977 (Isospora felis Wasielewski, 1904, Wenyon, 1923) in chorioalantoic membrane of chicken embryo). Acta Cientifica Venezolana 38, 474–483.

Arcay-de-Peraza, L., 1967. Coccidiosis en monos y su comparacion con la isosporosis humana, con descripcion de una nueva especie de Isospora en Cacajoa rubicundus

(Uakari monkey o mono chucuto) (Coccidiosis in monkeys and their comparison with human isosporosis, with a description of a new species of *Isospora* in *Cacajoa rubicundus* (Uakari monkey or chucuto monkey)). Acta Biologia Venezuelica 5, 203–222 (in Spanish).

Arcay-de-Peraza, L., 1976. Desarrollo en la membrana corio-alantoidea de embrión de pollo (MCA) de un nuevo coccidia de gato: *Isospora frenkeli* sp. nov. In: Resumenes de Trabajos de Parasitologia, San Jose, Costa Rica, 7–11 December, p. 26 (in Spanish, abstract).

Armitage, K., Flanigan, T., Carey, J., Frank, I., MacGregor, R.R., Ross, P., Goodgame, R., Turner, J., 1992. Treatment of cryptosporidiosis with paromomycin. A report of five cases. Archives of Internal Medicine 152 (12), 2497–2499.

Armson, A., Reynoldson, J.A., Thompson, R.C.A., 2003. A review of chemotherapeutic approaches to the treatment of *Cryptosporidium*. In: Thompson, R.C.A., Armson, A., Morgan-Ryan, U.M. (Eds.), *Cryptosporidium* from Molecules to Disease. Elsevier, Amsterdam, The Netherlands, pp. 395–403.

Arnastauskienė, T., 1989. Sarcosporidia of wild boars in the Lithuanian SSR. Acta Parasitologica Lituanica 23, 51–58.

Arnastauskienė, T., Grikienienė, J., 1989. Possibility of the development of *Sarcocystis* sp. taken from the bank vole in the organism of laboratory rats without the definitive host's participation. Lietuvos TSR Mokslų Akademijos Darbai 4, 51–60.

Arther, R.G., Post, G., 1977. Coccidia of coyotes in eastern Colorado. Journal of Wildlife Diseases 13 (1), 97–100.

Aryeetey, M.E., Piekarski, G., 1976. Serologische *Sarcocystis*-Studien am Menschen und Ratten. Zeitschrift für Parasitenkunde 50 (2), 109–124.

Aryeetey, M., Mehlhorn, H., Heydorn, A.O., 1980. Electron microscopic studies on development of *Sarcocystis capracanis* in experimentally infected goats. Zentralblatt für Bakteriologie. I. Abteilung Originale Reihe A: Medizinische Mikrobiologie, Infektionskrankheiten und Parasitologie 247 (4), 543–556.

Asahi, H., Koyama, T., Arai, H., Funakoshi, Y., Yamaura, H., Shirasaka, R., Okutomi, K., 1991. Biological nature of *Cryptosporidium* sp. isolated from a cat. Parasitology Research 77 (3), 237–240.

Ashford, R.W., 1977. The fox, *Vulpes vulpes*, as a final host for *Sarcocystis* of sheep. Annals of Tropical Medicine and Parasitology 71 (1), 29–34.

Ashford, R.W., 1978. *Sarcocystis cymruensis* n. sp., a parasite of rats *Rattus norvegicus* and cats *Felis catus*. Annals of Tropical Medicine and Parasitology 72 (1), 37–43.

Asma, I., Sim, B.L., Brent, R.D., Johari, S., Yvonne Lim, A.L., 2015. Molecular epidemiology of *Cryptosporidium* in HIV/AIDS patients in Malaysia. Tropical Biomedicine 32 (2), 310–322.

Atkinson, E.M., 1978. A *Sarcocystis* species in rats. Journal of Protozoology 25, 13B (Abstract).

Atkinson, C.T., Wright, S.D., Telford Jr., S.R., McLaughlin, G.S., Forrester, D.J., Roelke, M.E., McCown, J.W., 1993. Morphology, prevalence, and distribution of *Sarcocystis* spp. in white-tailed deer (*Odocoileus virginianus*) from Florida. Journal of Wildlife Diseases 29 (1), 73–84.

Awadallah, M.A.I., Salem, L.M.A., 2015. Zoonotic enteric parasites transmitted from dogs in Egypt with special concern to *Toxocara canis* infection. Veterinary World 8 (8), 946–957.

Babudieri, B., 1932. I sarcosporidi e le sarcosporidiosi (Studio monografico) (Sarcosporidia and sarcosporidiosis (monographic study)). Archiv für Protistenkunde 76 (421), 421–580 (in Italian).

Bacchi, C.J., Nathan, H.C., Hutner, S.H., Duch, D.S., Nichol, C.A., 1981. Prevention by polyamines of the curative effect of amicarbalide and imidocarb for *Trypanosoma brucei* infections in mice. Biochemical Pharmacology 30 (8), 883–886.

Baek, B.K., Kim, C.S., Kim, J.H., Han, K.S., Kim, Y.G., 1993. Studies on isosporsis in dogs I: isolation and sporulation of *Isospora ohioensis*. The Korean Journal of Parasitology 31 (3), 201–206.

Ballweber, L.R., Panuska, C., Huston, C.L., Vasilopulos, R., Pharr, G.T., Mackin, A., 2009. Prevalence and risk factors associated with shedding of *Cryptosporidium felis* in domestic cats of Mississippi and Alabama. Veterinary Parasitology 160 (3–4), 306–310.

Balozet, L., 1933. Sur une coccidie de la mangouste (On a mongoose coccidia). Bulletin de la Société de Pathologie Exotique 26, 913–914 (in French).

Bandoni, S.M., Duszynski, D.W., 1988. A plea for improved presentation of type material for coccidia. Invited Critical Comment Journal of Parasitology 74 (4), 519–523.

Bandyopadhyay, S., 1982. A new coccidium, *Eimeria jalpaiguriensis* n. sp. from a mongoose, *Herpestes edwardsi* (Geoffroy). Journal of the Bengal Natural History Society 1, 23–27.

Baneth, G., 2006. Hepatozoonosis. In: Greene, E. (Ed.), Infectious Diseases of the Dog and Cat. Elsevier, Philadelphia, USA, pp. 698–705.

Baneth, G., Shkap, V., 2003. Monozoic cysts of *Hepatozoon canis*. Journal of Parasitology 89 (2), 379–381.

Baneth, G., Harmelin, A., Presentez, B.Z., 1995. *Hepatozoon canis* in two dogs. Journal of the American Veterinary Medical Association 206 (12), 1891–1894.

Baneth, G., Aroch, I., Tal, N., Harrus, S., 1998. *Hepatozoon* species infection in domestic cats: a retrospective study. Veterinary Parasitology 79 (2), 123–133.

Baneth, G., Samish, M., Alekseev, E., Aroch, I., Shkap, V., 2001. Transmission of *Hepatozoon canis* to dogs by naturally-fed or percutaneously-injected *Rhipicephalus sanguineus* ticks. Journal of Parasitology 87 (3), 606–611.

Baneth, G., Samish, M., Shkap, V., 2007. Life cycle of *Hepatozoon canis* (Apicomplexa: Adeleorina: Hepatozoidae) in the tick *Rhipicephalus sanguineus* and domestic dog (*Canis familiaris*). Journal of Parasitology 93 (2), 283–299.

Baneth, G., Sheiner, A., Eyal, O., Hahn, S., Beaufils, J.-P., Anug, Y., Talmi-Frank, D., 2013. Redescription of *Hepatozoon felis* (Apicomplexa: Hepatozoidae) based on phylogenetic analysis, tissue and blood form morphology, and possible transplacental transmission. Parasites and Vectors 6, 102.

Barber, J.S., Trees, A.J., 1996. Clinical aspects of 27 cases of neosprosis in dogs. Veterinary Record 139 (18), 439–443.

Barber, J.S., Gasser, R.B., Ellis, J., Reichel, M.P., McMillan, D., Trees, A.J., 1997. Prevalence of antibodies to *Neospora caninum* in different canid populations. Journal of Parasitology 83 (6), 1056–1058.

Barbosa, L., Johnson, C.K., Lambourn, D.M., Gibson, A.K., Haman, K.H., Huggins, J.L., Sweeny, A.R., Sundar, N., Raverty, S.A., Grigg, M.E., 2015. A novel *Sarcocystis neurona* genotype XIII is associated with severe encephalitis in an unexpectedly broad range of marine mammals from the northeastern Pacific Ocean. International Journal for Parasitology 45 (9–10), 595–603.

Barham, M., Stützer, H., Karanis, P., Latif, B.M., Neiss, W.F., 2005. Seasonal variation in *Sarcocystis* species infections in goats in northern Iraq. Parasitology 130 (2), 151–156.

Barling, K.S., Sherman, M., Peterson, M.J., Thompson, J.A., McNeill, J.W., Craig, T.M., Adams, L.G., 2000. Spatial associations among density of cattle, abundance of wild canids, and seroprevalence to *Neospora caninum* in a population of beef calves. Journal of the American Veterinary Medical Association 217 (9), 1361–1365.

Barna, F., Debache, K., Vock, C.A., Kuster, T., Hemphill, A., 2013. In vitro effects of novel ruthenium complexes in *Neospora caninum* and *Toxoplasma gondii* tachyzoites. Antimicrobial Agents and Chemotherapy 57 (11), 5747–5754.

Barr, F., 1997. Cryptosporidiosis. Journal of Small Animal Practice 38 (7), 319–320.

Barr, S.C., Bowman, D.D., 2006. Cryptosporidiosis. In: Barr, S.C., Bowman, D.D. (Eds.), The 5-Minute Veterinary Consult Clinical Companion: Canine and Feline Infectious Diseases and Parasitology. Blackwell Publishing, pp. 157–161.

Barr, B.C., Anderson, M.L., Dubey, J.P., Conrad, P.A., 1991. *Neospora*-like protozoal infections associated with bovine abortions. Veterinary Pathology 28, 110–116.

Barr, S.C., Guilford, W.G., Jamrosz, G.F., Hornbuckle, W.E., Bowman, D.E., 1994a. Paromomycin for the treatment of *Cryptosporidium* in dogs and cats. Journal of Veterinary Internal Medicine 8, 177.

Barr, S.C., Jamrosz, G.F., Hornbuckle, W.E., Bowman, D.E., Fayer, R., 1994b. Use of paromomycin for treatment of cryptosporidiosis in a cat. Journal of the American Veterinary Medical Association 205 (12), 1742–1743.

Barreto, J.F., de Almeida, J.L., 1937. Primeiras observacões sobre a presenca de *Isospora felis* Wenyon, 1923 (Protozoa-Eimeridia) em felideos no Brasil (First observation on the presence of *Isospora felis* Wenyon 1923 (Protozoa-Eimeridia) in felids in Brazil). Boletim da Sociedade Brasileira de Medicina Veterinária 7, 356–360.

Barrows, P.L., Smith Jr., H.M., Prestwood, A.K., Brown, J., 1981. Prevalence and distribution of *Sarcocystis* sp. among wild swine of southeastern United States. Journal of the American Veterinary Medical Association 179 (11), 1117–1118.

Barta, J.R., 1989. Phylogenetic analysis of the class Sporozoea (Phylum Apicomplexa Levine, 1970): evidence for the independent evolution of heteroxenous life cycles. Journal of Parasitology 75 (2), 195–206.

Barta, J.R., 2000. Suborder Adeleorina Léger, 1911. In: Lee, J.J., Leedale, G.F., Bradbury, P. (Eds.), An Illustrated Guide to the Protozoa, vol. 1. second ed. Society of Protozoologists, Lawrence, KS, USA, pp. 305–318.

Barta, J.R., Thompson, R.A., 2006. What is *Cryptosporidium*? Reappraising its biology and phylogenetic affinities. Trends in Parasitology 22 (10), 463–468.

Barta, J.R., Schrenzel, M.D., Carreno, R., Rideout, B.A., 2005. Critical Comment: the genus *Atoxoplasma* (Garnham 1950) as a junior objective synonym of the genus *Isospora* (Schneider 1881) species infecting birds and resurrection of *Cystoisospora* (Frenkel 1977) as the correct genus for *Isospora* species infecting mammals. Journal of Parasitology 91 (3), 726–727.

Bartley, P.M., Wright, S.E., Zimmer, I.A., Roy, S., Kitchener, A.C., Meredith, A., Innes, E.A., Katzer, F., 2013. Detection of *Neospora caninum* in wild carnivores in Great Britain. Veterinary Parasitology 192 (1–3), 279–283.

Barton, C.L., Russon, E.A., Craig, T.M., Green, R.W., 1985. Canine hepatozoonosis: a retrospective study of 15 naturally occurring cases. Journal of the American Animal Hospital Association 21, 125–134.

Barutzki, D., Schaper, R., 2003. Endoparasites in dogs and cats in Germany 1999–2002. Parasitology Research 90, S148–S150.

Bass, A.L., Wallace, C.C., Yund, P.O., Ford, T.E., 2012. Detection of *Cryptosporidium* sp. in two new seal species, *Phoca vitulina* and *Cystophora cristata*, and a novel *Cryptosporidium* genotype in a third seal species, *Pagophilus groenlandicus*, from the Gulf of Maine. Journal of Parasitology 98 (2), 316–322.

Basso, W., Venturini, L., Venturini, M.C., Hill, D.E., Kwok, O.C.H., Shen, S.K., Dubey, J.P., 2001. First isolate of *Neospora caninum* from the feces of a naturally infected dog. Journal of Parasitology 87 (3), 612–618.

Basso, W., More, G., Quiroga, M.Z., Pardini, L., Bacigalupe, D., Venturini, L., Valenzuela, M.C., Balducchi, D., Maksimov, P., Schares, G., Venturini, M.C., 2009. Isolation and molecular characterization of *Toxoplasma gondii* from captive slender-tailed meerkats (*Suricata suricatta*) with fatal toxoplasmosis in Argentina. Veterinary Parasitology 161 (3–4), 201–206.

Basso, W., Schares, G., Gollnick, N.S., Rütten, M., Deplazers, P., 2011. Exploring the life cycle of *Besnoitia besnoiti*—experimental infection of putative definitive and intermediate host species. Veterinary Parasitology 178 (3–4), 223–234.

Batchelor, D.J., Tzannes, S., Graham, P.A., Wastling, J.M., Pinchbeck, G.L., German, A.J., 2007. Detection of endoparasites with zoonotic potential in dogs with gastrointestinal disease in the UK. Transboundary and Emerging Diseases 55 (2), 99–104.

Batzias, G.C., Delis, G.A., Athanasiou, L.V., 2005. Clindamycin bioavailability and pharmacokinetics following oral administration of clindamycin hydrochloride capsules in dogs. The Veterinary Journal 170 (3), 339–345.

Bearup, A.J., 1954. The coccidia of carnivores in Sydney. Australian Veterinary Journal 30, 185–186.

Beaufils, J.P., Martin-Granel, J., Jumelle, P., 1996. Hepatozoonosis in dogs and foxes: epidemiology, clinical findings and treatment. Pratique Médicale et Chirurgicale de l'Animal de Compagnie 31, 243–253.

Becker, E.R., 1934. A check-list of the coccidia of the genus *Isospora*. Journal of Parasitology 20, 195–196.

Becker, B., Mehlhorn, H., Heydorn, A.-O., 1979. Light and electron microscope studies on gamogony and sporogony of 5 *Sarcocystis* species in vivo and in tissue cultures. Zentralblatt für Bakteriologie, Mikrobiologie und Hygiene. I. Abteilung Originale Reihe A: Medizinische Mikrobiologie, Infektionskrankheiten und Parasitologie 244 (2–3), 394–404.

Bell, J.A., 1994. Parasites of domesticated pet ferrets. Compendium on Continuing Education for the Practicing Veterinarian 16 (5), 617–620.

Bell, W.B., Trelkeld, W.Z., 1948. *Isospora laidlawi* in mink. The Cornell Veterinarian 38, 3–6.

Bemrick, W.J., O'Leary, T.P., 1979. A coccidian from a grizzly bear. Veterinary Medicine, Small Animal Clinician 74, 389–390.

Bennett, M., Baxby, D., Blundell, N., Gaskell, C.J., Hart, C.A., Kelly, D.F., 1985. Cryptosporidiosis in the domestic cat. The Veterinary Record 116 (3), 73–74.

Bentley, C.A., 1905. Preliminary note upon a leucocytozoan of the dog. British Medical Journal 1 (2314), 988.

Berdoy, M., Webster, J.P., Macdonald, D.W., 2000. Fatal attraction in rats infected with *Toxoplasma gondii*. In: Proceedings of the Royal Society of London. B, vol. 267, pp. 1591–1594.

Berentsen, A.R., Becker, M.S., Stockdale-Walden, H., Matandiko, W., McRobb, R., Dunbar, M.R., 2012. Survey of gastrointestinal parasite infection in African lion (*Panthera leo*), African wild dog (*Lycaon pictus*) and spotted hyaena (*Crocuta crocuta*) in the Luangwa Valley, Zambia. African Zoology 47 (2), 363–368.

Bergman, A.M., 1913. Beitrag zur Kenntnis des Vorkommens der Sarkosporidien bei den Haustieren (Occurrence of Sarcosporidia in domestic animals). Zeitschrift für Fleisch – und Milch Hygiene 23, 169–180.

Bergmann, V., Kinder, E., 1976. Elektronenmikroskopische Untersuchungen zur Wandstruktur von Sarkozysten in der Skelettmuskulatur von Wildschwein und Reh. Monatshefte für Veterinärmedizin 31, 785–788.

Bern, C., Kjos, S., Yabsley, M.J., Montgomery, S.P., 2011. *Trypanosoma cruzi* and Chagas' disease in the United States. Clinical Microbiology Reviews 24 (2), 655–681.

Berrocal, A., López, A., 2003. Pulmonary sarcocystosis in a puppy with canine distemper in Costa Rica. Journal of Veterinary Diagnostic Investigation 15 (3), 292–294.

Bertelsen, M.F., Meyland-Smith, F., Willesen, J.L., Jefferies, R., Morgan, E.R., Monrad, J., 2010. Diversity and prevalence of metastrongyloid nematodes infecting the red panda (*Ailurus fulgens*) in European zoos. Veterinary Parasitology 172 (3–4), 299–304.

Beser, J., Toresson, L., Eltrem, R., Troell, K., Winiecka-Krusnell, J., Lebbad, M., 2015. Possible zoonotic transmission of *Cryptosporidium felis* in a household. Infection Ecology and Epidemiology 6 (5), 28463.

Besnoit, C., Robin, V., 1912. Sarcosporidiose cutanée chez une vache (Cutaneous sarcosporidiosis in a cow). Revue Vétérinaire 37 (11), 649–663.

Bhatavdekar, M.Y., Purohit, B.L., 1963. A record of sarcosporidiosis in a lion. Indian Veterinary Journal 40, 44–45.

Bhatia, B.B., 1996. On the species of *Sarcocystis* of the pig from Uttar Pradesh, India with a description of a sarcocyst of hitherto unrecognised species. Journal of Veterinary Parasitology 10 (1), 57–61.

Bhatia, B.B., Chauhan, P.P.S., Agrawal, R.D., Ahluwalia, S.S., 1979. *Eimeria aurei* n. sp. from jackal. Indian Journal of Parasitology 3 (1), 49–50.

Binninger, C.E., Beecham, J.J., Thomas, L.A., Winward, L.D., 1980. A serologic survey for selected infectious diseases of black bears in Idaho. Journal of Wildlife Diseases 16, 423–430.

Biocca, E., 1968. Class Toxoplasmatea: critical review and proposal of the new name *Frenkelia* gen. n. for M-organism. Parasitologia 10 (1), 89–98.

Biocca, E., Balbo, T., Guarda, E., Costantini, R., 1975. L'importanza della volpe (*Vulpes vulpes*) nella trasmissione della sarcosporidiosi dello stambecco (*Capra ibex*) nel Parco Nazionale dei Gran Paradiso. Parassitologia 17, 17–24.

Birhane, M.G., Cleaton, J.M., Monroe, B.P., Wadhwa, A., Orciari, L.A., Yager, P., Blanton, J., Velasco-Villa, A., Petersen, B.W., Wallace, R.M., 2017. Rabies surveillance in the United States during 2015. Journal of the American Veterinary Medical Association 250 (10), 1117–1130.

Bishop, L., 1979. Parasite-related lesions in a bearded seal *Erignathus barbatus*. Journal of Wildlife Diseases 15 (2), 285–293.

Bjerkås, I., Dubey, J.P., 1991. Evidence that *Neospora caninum* is identical to the *Toxoplasma*-like parasite of Norwegian dogs. Acta Veterinaria Scandinavica 32 (3), 407–410.

Bjerkås, I., Mohn, S.F., Presthus, J., 1984. Unidentified cyst-forming sporozoon causing encephalomyelitis and myositis in dogs. Zeitschrift für Parasitenkdunde 70, 271–274.

Bjork, K.E., Averbeck, G.A., Stromberg, B.E., 2000. Parasites and parasite stages of free-ranging wild lions (*Panthera leo*) of northern Tanzania. Journal of Zoo and Wildlife Medicine 31 (1), 56–61.

Björkman, C., Lundén, A., Holmdahl, J., Barber, J., Trees, A.J., Uggla, A., 1994. *Neospora caninum* in dogs: detection of antibodies by ELISA using an iscom antigen. Parasite Immunology 16 (12), 643–648.

Björkman, C., Jakubek, E.-B., Arnemo, J.M., Malmsten, J., 2010. Seroprevalence of *Neospora caninum* in gray wolves in Scandinavia. Veterinary Parasitology 173 (1–2), 139–142.

Blagburn, B.L., Lindsay, D.S., Swango, L.J., Pidgeon, G.L., Braund, K.G., 1988. Further characterization of the biology of *Hammondia heydorni*. Veterinary Parasitology 27 (3–4), 193–198.

Blagburn, B.L., Braund, K.G., Amling, K.A., Toivo-Kinnucan, M., 1989. Muscular *Sarcocystis* in a dog. Proceedings of the Helminthological Society of Washington 56 (2), 207–210.

Blais, J., Garneau, V., Chamberland, S., 1993. Inhibition of *Toxoplasma gondii* protein synthesis by azithromycin. Antimicrobial Agents and Chemotherapy 37 (8), 1701–1703.

Blanchard, R., 1885. Note sur les Sarcosporidies et sur un Essai de Classification de ces Sporozoaires (Note on the Sarcosporidia and on a classification test of these Sporozoa). Bulletin de la Societe Zoologique de France (Paris) 10, 244–276 (in French).

Blankenship-Paris, T.L., Chang, J., Bagnell, C.R., 1993. Enteric coccidiosis in a ferret. Laboratory Animal Science 43 (4), 361–363.

Blazius, R.D., Emerick, S., Prophiro, J.S., Romão, P.R.T., da Silva, O.S., 2005. Occurrence of protozoa and helminthes in faecal samples of stray dogs from Itapema City, Santa Catarina. Revista da Sociedade Brasileira de Medicina Tropical 38 (1), 73–74 (in Portuguese).

Bledsoe, B., 1976a. Transmission of *Isospora vulpina* from the silver fox to the dog; establishment of the mouse as an intermediate host of *I. vulpina*. In: Proceedings of the 40th Annual Meeting of the American Society of Parasitologists, 12–17 April 1965, Atlanta, Georgia. Allen Press, Lawrence, KS, USA. 51 (Abstract 96):46.

Bledsoe, B., 1976b. *Isospora vulpina* Nieschulz and Bos, 1933: description, and transmission from the fox (*Vulpes vulpes*) to the dog. Journal of Protozoology 23 (3), 365–367.

Boch, V.J., Walter, D., 1979. Vier verschiedene Kokzidienarten bei Katzen in Süddeutschland (Four different coccidia species in cats in southern Germany). Tierärztliche Umschau 11 (1), 749–752 (in German, English summary).

Boch, V.J., Mannewitz, U., Erber, M., 1978. Sarkosporidien bein Schlachtschweinen in Süddeutschland (Sarcosporidia in slaughter pigs in southern Germany). Berliner und Münchener Tierärztliche Wochenschrift 91, 106–111 (in German, English summary).

Böhm, L.K., 1923. Morphologische und experimentelle Beiträge zur Kenntnis der Hunde und Katzenkokzidiose (Morphological and experimental contributions to dog knowledge and cat coccidiosis). Wiener Tierärztliche Monatschrift 10137–10140 (*nos non videbo illum*, from Andrews, 1926b).

Bohrmann, R., 1991. Treatment with toltrazuril in a natural outbreak of coccidiosis in calves. Deutsche Tierärztliche Wochenschrift 98, 343–345.

Boothe, D.M., 1990. Anaerobic infections in small animals. Problems in Veterinary Medicine 2 (2), 330–347.

Borkataki, S., Katoch, R., Goswami, P., Godara, R., Khajuria, J.K., Yadav, A., Kaur, R., 2013. Prevalence of parasitic infections of stray cats in Jammu, India. Sokoto Journal of Veterinary Sciences 11 (1), 1–6.

Bornay-Llinares, F.J., da Silva, A.J., Moura, L.N.S., Myjak, P., Pietkiewicz, H., Kruminis-Lozowska, W., Graczyk, T.K., Pieniazek, N.J., 1999. Identification of *Cryptosporidium felis* in a cow by morphologic and molecular methods. Applied and Environmental Microbiology 65 (4), 1455–1458.

de Bortoli, C.P., André, M.R., Braga Mdo, S., Machado, R.Z., 2011. Molecular characterization of *Hepatozoon* sp. in cats from São Luis Island, Maranhão, northeastern Brazil. Parasitology Research 109 (4), 1189–1192.

Böttner, A., Charleston, W.A.G., Pomroy, W.E., Rommel, M., 1987. The prevalence and identity of *Sarcocystis* in beef cattle in New Zealand. Veterinary Parasitology 24 (1), 157–168.

Box, E.D., Duszynski, D.W., 1978. Experimental transmission of *Sarcocystis* from icterid birds to sparrows and canaries by sporocysts from opossums. Journal of Parasitology 64 (4), 682–688.

Box, E.D., Meier, J.L., Smith, J.H., 1984. Description of *Sarcocystis falcatula* Stiles, 1893, a parasite of birds and opossums. Journal of Protozoology 31 (4), 521–524.

Braun, J.L., Thayer, C.B., 1962. A survey for intestinal parasites in Iowa dogs. Journal of the American Veterinary Medical Association 141 (9), 1049–1050.

Bray, R.S., 1954. On the coccidia of the mongoose. Annals of Tropical Medicine and Parasitology 48 (4), 405–415.

Bray, R.S., 1959. On the parasitic protozoa of Liberia. VI. A further note on the coccidia of the mongoose. Acta Veterinaria (Budapest) 9, 233–234.

Briggs, M.B., Leathers, C.W., Foreyt, W.J., 1993. *Sarcocystis felis* in captive cheetahs (*Acinonyx jubatus*). Journal of the Helminthological Society of Washington 60 (2), 277–279.

Britton, A.P., Dubey, J.P., Rosenthal, B.M., 2010. Rhinitis and disseminated disease in a ferret (*Mustela putorius furo*) naturally infected with *Sarcocystis neurona*. Veterinary Parasitology 169 (1), 226–231.

Brocklesby, D.W., 1971. Illustration of a *Hepatozoon* species in the heart of a lion. Journal of Zoology (London) 164 (4), 525–528.

Bronson, E., Bush, M., Viner, T., Murray, S., Wisely, S.M., Deem, S.L., 2007. Mortality of captive black-footed ferrets (*Mustela nigripes*) at Smithsonian's National Zoological Park, 1989–2004. Journal of Zoo and Wildlife Medicine 38 (2), 169–176.

Brooks, D.R., Hoberg, E.P., 2007. How will global climate change affect parasite-host assemblages? Trends in Parasitology 23 (12), 571–574.

Brösigke, S., Heine, J., Boch, J., 1982. Der Nachweis extraintestinaler Entwicklungsstadien (Dormozoiten) in experimentell mit *Cystoisospora rivolta* oozysten infizierten Mäusen (The detection of extracellular developmental stages (dormozoites) in mice experimentally infected with *Cystoisospora rivolta* oocysts). Kleintier Praxis 27, 25–34 (in German, English summary).

Brown, H.C., Stammers, G.E.F., 1922. Observations on canine faeces on London pavements: bacteriological, helminthological, and protozoological. Lancet 200 (5179), 1165–1167.

Brown, R.J., Smith, A.W., Keyes, M.C., 1974. *Sarcocystis* in the northern fur seal. Journal of Wildlife Diseases 10 (1), 53.

Brown, S.A., Dieringer, T.M., Hunter, R.P., Zaya, M.J., 1989. Oral clindamycin disposition after single and multiple doses in normal cats. Journal of Veterinary Pharmacology and Therapeutics 12 (2), 209–216.

Brown, S.A., Zaya, M.J., Dieringer, T.M., Hunter, R.P., Nappier, G.A., Hoffman, G.A., Hornish, R.E., Yein, F.S., 1990. Tissue concentrations of clindamycin after multiple oral doses in normal cats. Journal of Veterinary Pharmacology and Therapeutics 13 (3), 270–277.

Bru, P., 1913. Seance du 17 Novembre 1912. Sarcosporidiose cutanée chez une vache, par M.M. Besnoit et Robin. Revue Vétérinaire 70, 165–167 (in French).

Brumpt, E., 1913. Précis de Parasitologie, second ed. Masson et Cie Editeurs, Paris. 1011 p. (in French).

Bryant, H.N., Russell, A.P., Fitch, W.D., 1993. Phylogenetic relationships within the extant Mustelidae (Carnivora): appraisal of the cladistic status of the Simpsonian subfamilies. Zoological Journal of the Linnean Society 108, 301–334.

Budsberg, S.C., Kemp, D.T., Wolski, N., 1992. Pharmacokinetics of clindamycin phosphate in dogs after single intravenous and intramuscular administrations. American Journal of Veterinary Research 53 (12), 2333–2336.

Bugg, R.J., Robertson, I.D., Elliott, A.D., Thompson, R.C.A., 1999. Gastrointestinal parasites in urban dogs in Perth, Western Australia. The Veterinary Journal 157 (3), 295–301.

Bugmyrin, S., Tirronen, K., Panchenko, D., Kopatz, A., Hagen, S., Eiken, H., Kuznetsova, A., 2017. Helminths of brown bears (*Ursus arctos*) in the Kola Peninsula. Parasitology Research 116 (6), 1755–1760.

Burney, D.A., Flannery, T.F., 2005. Fifty millennia of catastrophic extinctions after human contact. Trends in Ecology and Evolution 20 (7), 395–401.

Burns, R., Williams, E.S., O'Toole, D., Dubey, J.P., 1993. Toxoplasmosis in black-footed ferrets (*Mustela nigripes*) at the Louisville zoo. In: Junge, R.E. (Ed.), Proceedings of the American Association of Zoo Veterinarians [AAZV], 10–15 October, Philadelphia, PA. St. Louis, Montana, USA, p. 48.

Burrells, A., Bartley, P.M., Zimmer, I.A., Roy, S., Kitchener, A.C., Meredith, A., Wright, S.E., Innes, E.A., Katzer, F., 2013. Evidence of the three main clonal *Toxoplasma gondii* lineages from wild mammalian carnivores in the UK. Parasitology 140 (14), 1768–1776.

Burrows, R.B., 1968. Internal parasites of dogs and cats from central New Jersey. Bulletin of the New Jersey Academy of Sciences 13 (2), 3–8.

Burrows, R.B., Hunt, G.R., 1970. Intestinal protozoan infections in cats. Journal of the American Veterinary Medical Association 157 (12), 2065–2067.

Buxton, D., Maley, S.W., Pastoret, P.P., Brocher, B., Innes, E.A., 1997. Examination of red foxes (*Vulpes vulpes*) from Belgium for antibody to *Neospora caninum* and *Toxoplasma gondii*. Veterinary Research 141 (12), 308–309.

Bwangamoi, O., Rottcher, D., Wekesa, C., 1990. Rabies, microbesnoitiosis and sarcocystosis in a lion. The Veterinary Record 127 (16), 411.

Bwangamoi, O., Ngatia, T.A., Richardson, J.D., 1993. *Sarcocystis*-like organisms in musculature of a domestic dog (*Canis familiaris*) and wild dogs (*Lycaon pictus*) in Kenya. Veterinary Parasitology 49 (2–4), 201–205.

Cabezón, O., Hall, A.J., Vincent, C., Pabón, M., García-Bocanegra, L., Dubey, J.P., Almería, S., 2011. Seroprevalence of *Toxoplasma gondii* in North-eastern Atlantic harbor seal (*Phoca vitulina vitulina*) and grey seal (*Halichoerus grypus*). Veterinary Parasitology 179 (1), 253–256.

Calvopina, M., Armijos, R.X., Hashiguchi, Y., 2004. Epidemiology of leishmaniasis in Ecuador: current status of knowledge – a review. Memorias do Instituto Oswaldo Cruz 69 (7), 663–672.

Cama, V.A., Bern, C., Sulaiman, I.M., Gilman, R.H., Ticona, E., Vivar, A., Kawai, V., Vargas, D., Zhou, L., Xiao, L., 2003. *Cryptosporidium* species and genotypes in HIV-positive patients in Lima, Peru. Journal of Eukaryotic Microbiology 50 (Suppl.), 531–533.

Cama, V.A., Gilman, R.H., Vivar, A., Ticona, E., Ortega, Y., Bern, C., Xiao, L., 2006. Mixed *Cryptosporidium* infections and HIV. Emerging Infectious Diseases 12 (6), 1025–1028.

Cama, V.A., Ross, J.M., Crawford, S., Kawai, V., Chavez-Valdez, R., Vargas, D., Vivar, A., Ticona, E., Navincopa, M., Williamson, J., Ortega, Y., Gilman, R.H., Bern, C., Xiao, L., 2007. Differences in clinical manifestations among *Cryptosporidium* species and subtypes in HIV-infected persons. The Journal of Infectious Diseases 196 (5), 684–691.

Cama, V.A., Bern, C., Roberts, J., Cabrera, L., Sterling, C.R., Ortega, Y., Gilman, R.H., Xiao, L., 2008. *Cryptosporidium* species and subtypes and clinical manifestations in children, Peru. Emerging Infectious Diseases 14 (10), 1567–1574.

de Camps, S., Dubey, J.P., Saville, W.J.A., 2008. Seroepidemiology of *Toxoplasma gondii* in zoo animals in selected zoos in the midwestern United States. Journal of Parasitology 94 (3), 648–653.

Cañón-Franco, W.A., Yai, L.E.D., Souza, L.P., Santos, L.C., Farias, N.A.R., Ruas, J., Rossi, F.W., Gomes, A.A.B., Dubey, J.P., Gennari, S.M., 2004. Detection of antibodies to *Neospora caninum* in two species of wild canids, *Lycalopex gymnocercus* and *Cerdocyon thous* from Brazil. Veterinary Parasitology 123 (3), 275–277.

Cañón-Franco, W.A., Araújo, F.A.P., López-Orozco, N., Jardim, M.M.A., Keid, L.B., Dalla-Rosa, C., Cabral, A.D., Pena, H.F.J., Gennari, S.M., 2013. *Toxoplasma gondii* in free-ranging wild small felids from Brazil: molecular detection and genotypic characterization. Veterinary Parasitology 197 (3–4), 461–469.

Cañón-Franco, W.A., López-Orozco, N., Christoff, A.U., de Castilho, C.S., de Araújo, F.A., Verma, S.K., Dubey, J.P., Soares, R.M., Gennari, S.M., 2016. Molecular and morphologic characterization of *Sarcocystis felis* (Apicomplexa: Sarcocystidae) in South American wild felids from Brazil. Veterinary Parasitology 217 (1), 15–20.

CAPC, 2013. Current Advice on Parasite Control: Intestinal Parasites – Coccidia. http://www.capcvet.org/capc-recommendations/coccidia.

Cardona, G.A., de Lucio, A., Bailo, B., Cano, L., de Fuentes, I., Carmena, D., 2015. Unexpected finding of feline-specific *Giardia duodenalis* assemblage F and *Cryptosporidium felis* in asymptomatic adult cattle in Northern Spain. Veterinary Parasitology 209 (3–4), 258–263.

Cardoso, L., Cortes, H.C.E., Eyal, O., Reis, A., Lopes, A.P., Vila-Viçosa, M.J., Rodrigues, P.A., Baneth, G., 2014. Molecular and histopathological detection of *Hepatozoon canis* in red foxes (*Vulpes vulpes*) from Portugal. Parasites and Vectors 7 (1), 113.

Carini, A., Fonseca, F., 1938. Sobre uma nova *Eimeria* (*E. irara* n. sp.) parasita da *Tayra barbara*. Archivos de Biologia 22, 36 (in Portuguese).

Carini, A., Grechi, D., 1938. Sobre uma nova *Eimeria*, parasita do *Nasua narica*. Archivos de Biologia 22, 104–105 (in Portuguese).

Carletti, T., Martin, M., Romero, S., Morrison, D.A., Marcoppido, G., Florin-Christensen, M., Schnittger, L., 2013. Molecular identification of *Sarcocystis aucheniae* as the macrocyst-forming parasite of llamas. Veterinary Parasitology 198 (3–4), 396–400.

Carlslake, R.J., Hill, K.E., Sjölander, K., Hii, S.F., Prattley, D., Acke, E., 2017. Cross-sectional survey of health management and prevalence of vector-borne diseases, endoparasites and ectoparasites in Samoan dogs. Australian Veterinary Journal 95 (12), 462–468.

Carlson, B.L., Nielsen, S.W., 1982. Cryptosporidiosis in a raccoon. Journal of the American Veterinary Medical Association 181 (11), 1405–1406.

Carlson, C.J., Burgio, K.R., Dougherty, E.R., Phillips, A.J., Bueno, V.M., Clements, C.F., Castaldo, G., Dallas, T.A., Cizauskas, C.A., Cumming, G.S., Dona, J., Harris, N.C., Jovani, R., Mironov, S., Muellerklein, O.C., Proctor, H.C., Getz, W.M., 2017. Parasite biodiversity faces extinction and redistribution in a changing climate. Science Advances 3 (8), e1602422.

Carlson-Bremer, D.P., Gulland, F.M., Johnson, C.K., Colegrove, K.M., 2012. Diagnosis and treatment of *Sarcocystis neurona*-induced myositis in a free-ranging California sea lion. Journal of the American Veterinary Medical Association 240 (3), 324–328.

Carreno, R.A., Barta, J.R., 1999. An eimeriid origin of isosporid coccidia with Stieda bodies as shown by phylogenetic analysis of small subunit ribosomal RNA gene sequences. Journal of Parasitology 85 (1), 77–83.

Carreno, R.A., Schnitzler, B.E., Jeffries, A.C., Tenter, A.M., Johnson, A.M., Barta, J.R., 1998. Phylogenetic analysis of coccidia based on 18S rDNA sequence comparison indicates that *Isospora* is most closely related to *Toxoplasma* and *Neospora*. Journal of Eukaryotic Microbiology 45 (2), 184–188.

Carreno, R.A., Martin, D.S., Barta, J.R., 1999. *Cryptosporidium* is more closely related to the gregarines than to coccidia as shown by phylogenetic analysis of apicomplexan parasites inferred using small-subunit ribosomal RNA gene sequences. Parasitology Research 85 (11), 899–904.

Carreno, R.A., Pokorny, N.J., Lee, H., Trevors, J.T., De Grandis, S.A., 2001. Phenotypic and genotypic characterization of *Cryptosporidium* species and isolates. Journal of Industrial Microbiology and Biotechnology 26 (3), 95–106.

Carver, S., Scorza, A.V., Bevins, S.N., Riley, S.P., Crooks, K.R., Vandewoude, S., Lappin, M.R., 2012. Zoonotic parasites of bobcats around human landscapes. Journal of Clinical Microbiology 50 (9), 3080–3083.

Catalano, S., Lejeune, M., Tizzani, P., Verocai, G., Schwantje, H., Nelson, C., Duignan, P., 2015. Helminths of grizzly bears (*Ursus arctos*) and American black bears (*Ursus americanus*) in Alberta and British Columbia, Canada. Canadian Journal of Zoology 93 (10), 765–772.

Catcott, E.J., 1946. The incidence of intestinal protozoa in the dog. Journal of the American Veterinary Medical Association 108, 34–36.

Causapé, A.C., Quílez, J., Sánchez-Acedo, C., del Cacho, E., 1996. Prevalence of intestinal parasites, including *Cryptosporidium parvum*, in dogs in Zaragoza city, Spain. Veterinary Parasitology 67 (3–4), 161–167.

Cavalcante, G.T., Monteiro, R.M., Soares, R.M., Nishi, S.M., Alves Neto, A.F., Esmerini, P.O., Sercundes, M.K., Martins, J., Gennari, S.M., 2011. Shedding of *Neospora caninum* oocysts by dogs fed different tissues from naturally infected cattle. Veterinary Parasitology 179 (1–3), 220–223.

Cawthorn, R.J., Rainnie, D., 1981. Experimental transmission of *Sarcocystis* sp. (Protozoa: Sarcocystidae) between the shoveler (*Anas clypeata*) duck and the striped skunk (*Mephitis mephitis*). Journal of Wildlife Diseases 17 (3), 389–394.

Cawthorn, R.J., Wobeser, G.A., Gajadhar, A.A., 1983. Description of *Sarcocystis campestris* sp. n. (Protozoa: Sarcocystidae): a parasite of the badger *Taxidea taxus* with experimental transmission to the Richardson's ground squirrel, *Spermophilus richardsonii*. Canadian Journal of Zoology 61 (2), 370–377.

Cawthorn, R.J., Reduker, D.W., Speer, C.A., Dubey, J.P., 1986. *In vitro* excystation of *Sarcocystis capracanis, Sarcocystis cruzi* and *Sarcocystis tenella* (Apicomplexa). Journal of Parasitology 72 (6), 880–884.

Center for Disease Control, 2012. Parasites: Trichinellosis (Also Known as Trichinosis). https://www.cdc.gov/parasites/trichinellosis/epi.html.

Černá, Z., Loučková, A.M., Nedvědová, A.H., Vávra, J., 1981. Spontaneous and experimental infection of domestic rabbits by *Sarcocystis cuniculi* Brumpt, 1913. Folia Parasitologica (Praha) 28 (4), 313–318.

Chabreck, R.H., 1965. Sarcosporidiosis in ducks in Louisiana. Transactions of the North American Wildlife Conference 30, 174–184.

Chakraborty, D., Tiwari, S., Reddy, D.M., Umapathy, G., 2016. Prevalence of gastrointestinal parasites in civets of fragmented rainforest patches in Anamalai Hills, Western Ghats, India. Journal of Parasitology 102 (4), 463–467.

Chalmers, R.M., Elwin, K., Thomas, A.L., Guy, E.C., Mason, B., 2009. Long-term *Cryptosporidium* typing reveals the aetiology and species-specific epidemiology of human cryptosporidiosis in England and Wales, 2000 to 2003. Euro Surveillance: Bulletin European sur les Maladies Transmissibles 14 (2), 19086.

Chalmers, R.M., Smith, R., Elwin, K., Clifton-Hadley, F.A., Giles, M., 2011. Epidemiology of anthroponotic and zoonotic human cryptosporidiosis in England and Wales, 2004–2006. Epidemiology and Infection 139 (5), 700–712.

Chambers, D., Ulrey, W., Guthrie, J., Kwok, O., Cox, J., Maehr, D., Dubey, J., 2012. Seroprevalence of *Toxoplasma gondii* from free-ranging black bears (*Ursus americanus*) from Florida. Journal of Parasitology 98 (3), 674–675.

Chapman, J., Mense, M., Dubey, J.P., 2005. Clinical muscular sarcocystosis in a dog. Journal of Parasitology 91 (1), 187–190.

Charles, R.A., Ellis, A.E., Dubey, J.P., Barnes, J.C., Yabsley, M.J., 2011. Besnoitiosis in a southern plains woodrat (*Neotoma*

micropus) from Uvalde, Texas. Journal of Parasitology 97 (5), 838–841.

Chaudhuri, S.K., Choudhury, A., 1982. Relationship between sporulation and effects of temperature and chemical exposures of isosporid coccidium in a white tiger (*Panthera tigris tigris* Linn.) in Zoological Garden of Calcutta. In: Negotiation Report of the XXIV International Symposium on the Diseases of the Zootiere, 19–21 May, 1982, in Veszprém. Akademia-Verlag, Berlin, pp. 331–336.

Chaudhuri, S.K., Das, S.K., 1992. Studies on host-specificity of coccidian parasites in captive and wild mammals of India. Verhandlungen bericht Erkrankungen der Zootiere 34, 317–327.

Chauhan, P.P.S., Bhatia, B.B., Arora, G.S., Agrawal, R.D., Ahluwalia, S.S., 1973. A preliminary survey of parasitic infections among mammals and birds at Lucknow and Delhi zoos. Indian Journal of Animal Science 43, 163–168.

Chavez, D.J., LeVan, I.K., Miller, M.W., Ballweber, L.R., 2012. *Baylisascaris procyonis* in raccoons (*Procyon lotor*) from eastern Colorado, an area of undefined prevalence. Veterinary Parasitology 185 (2–4), 330–334.

Cheadle, M.A., Spencer, J.A., Blagburn, B.L., 1999. Seroprevalences of *Neospora caninum* and *Toxoplasma gondii* in nondomestic felids from southern Africa. Journal of Zoo and Wildlife Medicine 30 (2), 248–251.

Cheadle, M., Yowell, C., Selton, D., Hines, M., Ginn, P., Marsh, A., Dame, J., Greiner, E., 2001. The striped skunk (*Mephitis mephitis*) is an intermediate host for *Sarcocystis neurona*. International Journal for Parasitology 31 (8), 843–849.

Chen, X., He, Y., Liu, Y., Olias, P., Rosenthal, B.M., Cui, L., Zuo, Y., Yang, Z., 2012. Infections with *Sarcocystis wenzeli* are prevalent in the chickens of Yunnan Province, China, but not in the flocks of domesticated pigeons or ducks. Experimental Parasitology 131 (1), 31–34.

Chessum, B.S., 1972. Reactivation of *Toxoplasma* oocyst production in the cat by infection with *Isospora felis*. British Veterinary Journal 128 (7), 33–36.

Chhabra, M.B., Mahajan, S.K., Gupta, S.L., Gautam, O.P., 1984. Sporozoa and helminthes encountered in faeces of cats from North India. Indian Journal of Parasitology 2, 211–213.

Chinchilla, M., Ruiz, A., 1976. Cockroaches as possible transport hosts of *Toxoplasma gondii* in Costa Rica. Journal of Parasitology 62 (1), 140–142.

Chiou, H.-Y., Yeh, K.-S., Jeng, C.-R., Chang, H.W., Chang, L.-J., Wu, Y.-H., Chan, F.-T., Pang, V.F., 2015. Disease surveillance in rescued and road-killed wild-ranging carnivores in Taiwan. Taiwan Veterinary Journal 41 (2), 73–84.

Chomel, B.B., Zarnke, R.L., Kasten, R.W., Kass, P.H., Mendes, E., 1995. Serologic survey of *Toxoplasma gondii* in grizzly bears (*Ursus arctos*) and black bears (*Ursus americanus*) from Alaska, 1988–1991. Journal of Wildlife Diseases 31 (4), 472–479.

Choquette, L.P.E., Gelinas, L.G., 1950. The incidence of intestinal nematodes and protozoa of dogs in the Montreal district. Canadian Journal of Comparative Medicine and Veterinary Science 14 (2), 33–38.

Christie, E., Dubey, J.P., Pappas, P.W., 1976. Prevalence of *Sarcocystis* infection and other intestinal parasitisms in cats from a humane shelter in Ohio. Journal of the American Veterinary Medical Association 168 (5), 421–422.

Christie, E., Dubey, J.P., Pappas, P.W., 1977. Prevalence of *Hammondia hammondi* in the feces of cats in Ohio. Journal of Parasitology 63 (5), 929–931.

Christophers, S.R. (Ed.), 1906. *Leucocytozoon canis*. Scientific Memoirs by Officers of the Medical and Sanitary Departments of the Government of India. New Series, vol. 26 16 pp.

Cieloszyk, J., Goñi, P., García, A., Remacha, M.A., Sánchez, E., Clavel, A., 2012. Two cases of zoonotic cryptosporidiosis in Spain by the unusual species *Cryptosporidium ubiquitum* and *Cryptosporidium felis*. Enfermedades Infecciosas y Microbiologia Clinica 30 (9), 549–551.

Cirak, V.Y., Bauer, C., 2004. Comparison of conventional coproscopical methods and commercial coproantigen ELISA kits for the detection of *Giardia* and *Cryptosporidium* infections in dogs and cats. Berliner und Münchener Tierärztliche Wochenschrift 117 (9–10), 410–413.

Clark, K.A., Robinson, R.M., Weishuhn, L.L., Horvath, K., 1973. *Hepatozoon procyonis* infections in Texas. Journal of Wildlife Diseases 9 (2), 182–192.

Clarke, L., Fodey, T.L., Crooks, S.R.H., Moloney, M., O'Mahony, J., Delahaut, P., O'Kennedy, R., Danaher, M., 2014. A review of coccidiostats and the analysis of their residues in meat and other food. Meat Science 97 (3), 358–374.

Clifford, D.L., Mazet, J.A.K., Dubovi, E.J., Garcelon, D.K., Coonan, T.J., Conrad, P.A., Munson, L., 2006. Pathogen exposure in endangered island fox (*Urocyon littoralis*) populations: implications for conservation management. Biological Conservation 131, 230–243.

Čobádiová, A., Víchová, B., Majláthová, V., Reiterová, K., 2013. First molecular detection of *Neospora caninum* in European brown bears (*Ursus arctos*). Veterinary Parasitology 197 (1–2), 346–349.

Coelho, W.M., do Amarante, A.F., de Soutello, R.V., Meireles, M.V., Bresciani, K.D., 2009. Occurrence of gastrointestinal parasites in fecal samples of cats in Andradina City, São Paulo. Revista Brasileira de Parasitologia Veterinaria 18 (2), 46–49 (in Portuguese).

Cole, R.A., Lindsay, D.S., Blagburn, G.L., Sorjonen, D.C., Dubey, J.P., 1995. Vertical transmission of *Neospora caninum* in dogs. Journal of Parasitology 81 (2), 208–211.

Colegrove, K.M., Grigg, M.E., Carlson-Bremer, D., Miller, R.H., Gulland, F.M.D., Ferguson, D.J.P., Rejmanek, D., Rarr, B.C., Nordhausen, R., Melli, A.C., Conrad, P.A., 2011. Discovery of three novel coccidian parasites infecting California sea lions (*Zalophus californianus*), with evidence of sexual replication and interspecies pathogenicity. Journal of Parasitology 97 (5), 868–877.

Collins, G.H., Emslie, D.R., Farrow, B.R.H., Watson, A.D.J., 1983. Sporozoa in dogs and cats. Australian Veterinary Journal 60 (10), 289–290.

Colón, C.P., Patton, S., 2012. Parasites of civets (Mammalia, Viverridae) in Sabah, Borneo: a coprological survey. Malayan Nature Journal 64 (2), 87–94.

Colwell, D.D., Mahrt, J.L., 1981. Ultrastructure of the cyst wall and merozoites of *Sarcocystis* from moose (*Alces alces*) in Alberta, Canada. Zeitschrift für Parasitenkunde 65 (3), 317–329.

Coman, B.J., Jones, E.H., Westbury, H.A., 1981. Protozoan and viral infections of feral cats. Australian Veterinary Journal 57 (7), 319–323.

Conceição-Silva, F.M., Abranches, P., Silva-Pereira, M.C.D., Janz, J.G., 1988. Hepatozoonosis in foxes from Portugal. Journal of Wildlife Diseases 24 (2), 344–347.

Conrad, P.A., Miller, M.A., Kreuder, C., James, E.R., Mazet, J., Dabritz, H., Jessup, D.A., Gulland, F., Grigg, M.E., 2005. Transmission of *Toxoplasma*: clues from the study of sea otters as sentinels of *Toxoplasma gondii* flow into marine environments. International Journal for Parasitology 35 (11), 1155–1168.

Constantin, E.M., Schares, G., Großmann, E., Sauter, K., Romig, T., Hartmann, S., 2011. Untersuchungen zur Rolle des Rotfuchses (*Vulpes vulpes*) als möglicher Endwirt von *Neospora caninum* (Studies on the role of the red fox (*Vulpes vulpes*) as a potential definitive host of *Neospora caninum*). Berliner und Münchener Tierärztliche Wochenschrift 124, 148–153 (in German, English summary).

Cooley, A.J., Barr, B., Rejmanek, D., 2007. *Saracocystis neurona* encephalitis in a dog. Veterinary Pathology 44 (6), 956–961.

Cornaglia, E., Giaccherino, A.R., Peracino, V., 1998. Ultrastructural morphology of sarcosporidiosis in alpine ibex (*Capra ibex*). Veterinary Parasitology 75 (1), 21–32.

Cornwell, G., 1963. New waterfowl host records for *Sarcocystis rileyi* and a review of sarcosporidiosis in birds. Avian Diseases 7 (2), 212–216.

Corpa, J.M., Garcia-Quirós, A., Casares, M., Gerique, A.C., Carbonell, M.D., Gómez-Muñoz, M.T., Uzal, F.A., Ortega, J., 2013. Encephalomyelitis by *Toxoplasma gondii* in a captive fossa (*Cryptoprocta ferox*). Veterinary Parasitology 193 (1–3), 281–283.

Costa, H.M.A., Freitas, M.G., 1959. *Isospora felis* Wenyon, 1923 e *Isospora rivolta* Grassi, 1879, em cães de Belo Horizonte (*Isospora felis* Wenyon, 1923 and *Isospora rivolta* Grassi, 1879, in dogs from Belo Horizonte). Arquivos de Escola Superior de Veterinâaria de Universidad Rural do Estado de Minas Gerais 12, 127–130 (in Portuguese, English summary).

Costa, D.G.C., Marvulo, M.F.V., Silva, J.S.A., Santana, S.C., Magalhães, F.J.R., Lima Filho, C.D.F., Ribeiro, V.O., Alves, L.C., Mota, R.A., Dubey, J.P., Silva, J.C.R., 2012. Seroprevalence of *Toxoplasma gondii* in domestic and wild animals from the Fernando de Noronha, Brazil. Journal of Parasitology 98 (3), 679–680.

Coupe, S., Sarfati, C., Hamane, S., Derouin, F., 2005. Detection of *Cryptosporidium* and identification to the species level by nested PCR and restriction fragment length polymorphism. Journal of Clinical Microbiology 43 (3), 1017–1023.

Cox, P., Griffith, M., Angles, M., Deere, D., Ferguson, C., 2005. Concentrations of pathogens and indicators in animal feces in the Sydney watershed. Applied and Environmental Microbiology 71 (10), 5929–5934.

Cox, J., Murphy, S., Augustine, B., Guthrie, J., Hast, J., Maehr, S., McDermott, J., 2017. Seroprevalence of *Toxoplasma gondii* in American black bears (*Ursus americanus*) of the central Appalachians, USA. Journal of Wildlife Diseases 53 (3), 671–673.

de Craeye, S., Speybroeck, N., Ajzenberg, D., Dardé, M.L., Collinet, F., Tavernier, P., Van Gucht, S., Dorny, P., Dierick, K., 2011. *Toxoplasma gondii* and *Neospora caninum* in wildlife: common parasites in Belgian foxes and Cervidae? Veterinary Parasitology 178 (1–2), 64–69.

Craig, T.M., 1990. Hepatozoonosis. In: Greene, C.E. (Ed.), Clinical Microbiology and Infectious Diseases of the Dog and Cat. W.B. Saunders, Philadelphia, PA, USA, pp. 778–785.

Craig, T.M., 2001. *Hepatozoon* spp. and hepatozoonosis. In: Samuel, W.M., Pybus, M.J., Kocan, A.A. (Eds.), Parasitic Diseases of Wild Mammals. Iowa State University Press, Ames, Iowa, pp. 462–468.

Crawley, H., 1914. Two new sarcosporidia. Proceedings of the Academy of Natural Sciences of Philadelphia 66 (1), 214–218.

Criado-Fornelio, A., Gutiéerrez-Garcia, L., Rodriguez-Caabeiro, F., Reus-Garcia, E., Roldan-Soriano, M.A., Diaz-Sanchez, M.A., 2000. A parasitological survey of wild red foxes (*Vulpes vulpes*) from the province of Guadalajara, Spain. Veterinary Parasitology 92 (4), 245–251.

Crookshanks, J.L., Taylor, S.M., Haines, D.M., Shelton, G.D., 2007. Treatment of canine pediatric *Neospora caninum* myositis following immunohistochemical identification of tachyzoites in muscle biopsies. The Canadian Veterinary Journal 48 (5), 506–508.

Crum, J.M., Prestwood, A.K., 1977. Transmission of *Sarcocystis leporum* from a cottontail rabbit to domestic cats. Journal of Wildlife Diseases 13 (2), 174–175.

Crum, J.M., Nettles, V.F., Davidson, W.B., 1978. Studies on endoparasites of the black bear (*Ursus americanus*) in the southeastern United States. Journal of Wildlife Diseases 14 (2), 178–186.

Crum, J.M., Fayer, R., Prestwood, A.K., 1981. *Sarcocystis* spp. in white-tailed deer. I. Definitive and intermediate host spectrum with a description of *Sarcocystis odocoileocanis* n. sp. Journal of Wildlife Diseases 17 (4), 567–579.

Cuvier, F.G., 1825. Éléphant d'Afrique. In: Saint-Hilaire, G., Cuvier, F.G. (Eds.), Histoire Naturelle des Mammifères. Chez A. Belin, Paris, France 3.52:2, p. VI (in French).

Dado, D., Izquierdo, F., Vera, O., Montoya, A., Mateo, M., Fenoy, S., Galván, A.L., García, S., García, A., Aránguez, E., López, L., del Águila, C., Miró, G., 2012. Detection of zoonotic intestinal parasites in public parks of Spain. Potential epidemiologic role of microsporidia. Zoonoses and Public Health 59 (1), 23–28.

Dahlgren, S.S., Gjerde, B., 2007. Genetic characterization of six *Sarcocystis* species from reindeer (*Rangifer tarandus tarandus*) in Norway based on the small subunit rRNA gene. Veterinary Parasitology 146 (3), 204–213.

Dahlgren, S.S., Gjerde, B., 2008. *Sarcocystis* in moose (*Alces alces*): molecular identification and phylogeny of six *Sarcocystis* species in moose, and a morphological description of three new species. Parasitology Research 103 (1), 93–110.

Dahlgren, S.S., Gjerde, B., 2009. *Sarcocystis* in Norwegian roe deer (*Capreolus capreolus*): molecular and morphological identification of *Sarcocystis gracilis* and their phylogenetic relationship with other *Sarcocystis* species. Parasitology Research 104 (5), 993–1003.

Dahlgren, S.S., Gjerde, B., 2010a. Molecular characterization of five *Sarcocystis* species in red deer (*Cervus elaphus*), including *Sarcocystis hjoerti* n. sp., reveals that these species are not intermediate host specific. Parasitology 137 (5), 815–840.

Dahlgren, S.S., Gjerde, B., 2010b. The red fox (*Vulpes vulpes*) and the arctic fox (*Vulpes lagopus*) are definitive hosts of *Sarcocystis alces* and *Sarcocystis hjorti* from moose (*Alces alces*). Parasitology 137 (10), 1547–1557.

Daly, T.J.M., Markus, M.G., 1981. Enteric multiplication of *Isospora felis* by endodyogeny. In: Proceedings of the Electron Microscopy Society of Southern Africa, vol. 11. Elektronmikroskopievereniging van Suidelike Afrika, pp. 99–100.

Dannemann, B., McCutchan, J.A., Israelski, D., Antoniskis, D., Leport, C., Luft, B., Nussbaum, J., Clumeck, N., Morlat, P., Chiu, J., Vilde, J.-L., Orellana, M., Feigal, D., Bartok, A., Heseltine, P., Leedom, J., Remington, J., 1992. Treatment of toxoplasmic encephalitis in patients with AIDS (a randomized trial comparing pyrimethamine plus clindamycin to pyrimethamine plus sulfadiazine). Annals of Internal Medicine 116 (1), 33–43.

Darius, A.K., Mehlhorn, H., Heydorn, A.O., 2004. Effects of toltrazuril and ponazuril on the fine structure and multiplication of tachyzoites of the NC-1 strain of *Neospora caninum* (a synonym of *Hammondia heydorni*) in cell cultures. Parasitology Research 92 (6), 453–458.

Darling, S.T., 1910. Sarcosporidiosis in an opossum and its experimental production in the guinea pig by the intramuscular injection of sporozoites. Bulletin de la Societe de Pathologie Exotique 3, 513–518.

Das, P., Roy, S.S., MitraDhar, K., Dutta, P., Bhattacharya, M.K., Sen, A., Ganguly, S., Bhattacharya, S.K., Lal, A.A., Xiao, L., 2006. Molecular characterization of *Cryptosporidium* spp. from children in Kolkata, India. Journal of Clinical Microbiology 44 (11), 4246–4249.

Daszak, P., Cunningham, A.A., Hyatt, A.D., 2000. Wildlife ecology - emerging infectious diseases of wildlife—threats to biodiversity and human health. Science 287 (5452), 443–449.

Daugschies, A., Mundt, H.C., Letkova, V., 2000. Toltrazuril treatment of cystoisosporosis in dogs under experimental and field conditions. Parasitology Research 86 (10), 797–799.

Davis, C.L., Chow, T.L., Gorham, J.R., 1953. Hepatic coccidiosis in mink. Small Animal Practice 48 (9), 371–375.

Davis, D.S., Robinson, R.M., Craig, T.M., 1978. Naturally occurring hepatozoonosis in a coyote. Journal of Wildlife Diseases 14 (2), 244–246.

Debache, K., Hemphill, A., 2012. Effects of miltefosine treatment in fibroblast cell cultures and in mice experimentally infected with *Neospora caninum* tachyzoites. Parasitology 139 (7), 934–944.

Debache, K., Guionaud, C., Kropf, C., Boykin, D., Stephens, C.E., Hemphill, A., 2011. Experimental treatment of *Neospora caninum*-infected mice with the arylimidamide DB750 and the thiazolide nitazoxanide. Experimental Parasitology 129 (2), 95–100.

Deem, S.L., Spelman, L.H., Yates, R.A., Montali, R.J., 2000. Canine distemper in terrestrial carnivores: a review. Journal of Zoo and Wildlife Medicine 31 (4), 441–451.

de Graaf, D.C., Spano, F., Petry, F., Sagodira, S., Bonnin, A., 1999. Speculation on whether a vaccine against cryptosporidiosis is a reality or fantasy. International Journal for Parasitology 29 (8), 1289–1306.

Delport, T.C., Asher, A.J., Beaumont, L.J., Webster, K.N., Harcourt, R.G., Power, M.L., 2014. *Giardia duodenalis* and *Cryptosporidium* occurrence in Australian sea lions (*Neophoca cinerea*) exposed to varied levels of human interaction. International Journal for Parasitology. Parasites and Wildlife 3 (3), 269–275.

Deng, M.Q., Peterson, R.P., Cliver, D.O., 2000. First findings of *Cryptosporidium* and *Giardia* in California sea lions (*Zalophus californianus*). Journal of Parasitology 86 (3), 490–494.

Denholm, K.M., Haitjema, H., Gwynne, B.J., Morgan, U.M., Irwin, P.J., 2001. Concurrent *Cryptosporidium* and parvovirus infections in a puppy. Australian Veterinary Journal 79 (2), 98–101.

Dewey, T., Myers, P., 2005. Ursidae. (On-line), Animal Diversity Web http://animaldiversity.ummz.umich.edu/site/accounts/information/Ursidae.html.

Diesing, L., Heydorn, A.O., Matuschka, F.R., Bauer, C., Pipano, E., De Waal, D.T., Potgieter, F.T., 1988. *Besnoitia besnoiti*: studies on the definitive host and experimental infetions in cattle. Parasitology Research 75, 114–117.

Dijkstra, T., Eysker, M., Schares, G., Conraths, F.J., Wouda, W., Barkema, H.W., 2001. Dogs shed *Neospora caninum* oocysts after ingestion of naturally infected bovine placenta but not after ingestion of colostrum spiked with *Neospora caninum* tachyzoites. International Journal for Parasitology 31 (8), 747–752.

Dissanaike, A.S., Kan, S.O., Retnasabapathy, A., Baskavar, G., 1977. Developmental stages of *Sarcocystis fusiformis* (Railliet, 1897) and *Sarcocystis* sp. of the water buffalo, in the small intestines of cats and dogs, respectively. Southeast Asian Journal of Tropical Medicine and Public Health 8 (3), 417.

Dixon, B.R., Parrington, L.J., Parenteau, M., Leclair, D., Santín, M., Fayer, R., 2008. *Giardia duodenalis* and *Cryptosporidium* spp. in the intestinal contents of ringed seals (*Phoca hispida*) and bearded seals (*Erignathus barbatus*) in Nunavik, Quebec, Canada. Journal of Parasitology 94 (5), 1161–1163.

Dobell, C.C., 1919. A revision of the coccidia parasitic in man. Parasitology 11 (2), 147–197.

Doflein, F.J.T., 1901. Die Protozoen als Parasiten und Krankheitserreger: nach biologischen Gesichtspunkten dargestellt (The Protozoans are Represented as Parasites and Pathogens from a Biological Point of View). Fischer, Jena, Germany. xiii + 274 p. (in German).

Donahoe, S.L., Rose, K., Šlapeta, J., 2014. Multisystemic toxoplasmosis associated with a type II-like *Toxoplasma gondii* strain in a New Zealand fur seal (*Arctocephalus forsteri*) from New South Wales, Australia. Veterinary Parasitology 205 (1–2), 347–353.

Donley, D.W., Olson, A.R., Raisbeck, M.F., Fox, J.H., Gigley, J.P., 2016. Huntington's disease mice infected with *Toxoplasma gondii* demonstrate early kynurenine pathway activation, altered CD8+ T-cell responses, and premature mortality. PLoS One 11 (9), e0162404.

Dorny, P., Fransen, J., 1989. Toxoplasmosis in a Siberian tiger (*Panthera tigris altaica*). The Veterinary Record 125 (26–27), 647.

Dow, S.W., 1988. Management of anaerobic infections. The Veterinary Clinics of North America. Small Animal Practice 18 (6), 1167–1182.

Dreesen, D.W., 1990. *Toxoplasma gondii* infections in wildlife. Journal of the American Veterinary Medical Association 196 (2), 274–276.

Dróżdż, J., 1987. Oocysts of six new Coccidiomorpha species from pinnipeds of King George Island (South Shetlands Antarctic). Acta Protozoologica 26, 263–266.

Dryburgh, E.L., Marsh, A.E., Dubey, J.P., Howe, D.K., Reed, S.M., Bolten, K.E., Pei, W., Saville, J.A., 2015. Sarcocyst development in raccoons (*Procyon lotor*) inoculated with different strains of *Sarcocystis neurona* culture-derived merozoites. Journal of Parasitology 101 (4), 462–467.

Dubey, J.P., 1963a. Observations on coccidian oocysts from Indian hyaena (*Hyaena striata*). Indian Journal of Microbiology 3 (1), 121–122.

Dubey, J.P., 1963b. Observations on the coccidian oocysts from the Indian fox (*Vulpes bengalensis*). Indian Journal of Microbiology 3 (1), 143–146.

Dubey, J.P., 1973. Feline toxoplasmosis and coccidiosis: a survey of domiciled and stray cats. Journal of the American Veterinary Medical Association 162 (10), 873–877.

Dubey, J.P., 1975a. Experimental *Hammondia hammondi* infection in dogs. British Veterinary Journal 131 (6), 741–743.

Dubey, J.P., 1975b. Experimental *Isospora canis* and *Isospora felis* infection in mice, cats, and dogs. Journal of Protozoology 22 (3), 416–417.

Dubey, J.P., 1975c. *Isospora ohioensis* sp. n. proposed for *I. rivolta* of the dog. Journal of Parasitology 61 (3), 462–465.

Dubey, J.P., 1976. A review of *Sarcocystis* of domestic animals and of other coccidia of cats and dogs. Journal of the American Veterinary Medical Association 169 (10), 1061–1078.

Dubey, J.P., 1977a. Attempted transmission of feline coccidia from chronically infected queens to their kittens. Journal of the American Veterinary Medical Association 170 (5), 541–543.

Dubey, J.P., 1977b. Letters: taxonomy of *Sarcocystis* and other coccidia of cats and dogs. Journal of the American Veterinary Medical Association 170 (8), 778–779.

Dubey, J.P., 1977c. *Toxoplasma, Hammondia, Besnoitia, Sarcocystis*, and other tissue cyst-forming coccidia of man and animals. In: Kreier, J.P. (Ed.), Parasitic Protozoa, vol. III. Academic Press, Inc., New York, NY, USA, pp. 102–237.

Dubey, J.P., 1978a. Life cycle of *Isospora ohioensis* in dogs. Parasitology 77 (1), 1–11.

Dubey, J.P., 1978b. Pathogenicity of *Isospora ohioensis* infection in dogs. Journal of the American Veterinary Medical Association 173 (2), 192–197.

Dubey, J.P., 1979a. Frequency of *Sarcocystis* in pigs in Ohio and attempted transmission to cats and dogs. American Journal of Veterinary Research 40 (6), 867–868.

Dubey, J.P., 1979b. Life cycle of *Isospora rivolta* (Grassi 1879) in cats and mice. Journal of Protozoology 26 (3), 433–443.

Dubey, J.P., 1980a. Coyote as a final host for *Sarcocystis* species of goats, sheep, cattle, elk, bison, and moose in Montana. American Journal of Veterinary Research 41 (8), 1227–1229.

Dubey, J.P., 1980b. *Sarcocystis* species in moose (*Alces alces*), bison (*Bison bison*), and pronghorn (*Antilocapra americana*) in Montana. American Journal of Veterinary Research 41 (12), 2063–2065.

Dubey, J.P., 1982a. *Baylisascaris procyonis* and eimerian infections in raccoons. Journal of the American Veterinary Medical Association 181 (11), 1292–1294.

Dubey, J.P., 1982b. *Sarcocystis* and other coccidia in foxes and other wild carnivores from Montana. American Veterinary Medical Association 181 (11), 1270–1271.

Dubey, J.P., 1983a. Experimental infections of *Sarcocystis cruzi, Sarcocystis tenella, Sarcocystis capracanis* and *Toxoplasma gondii* in red foxes (*Vulpes vulpes*). Journal of Wildlife Diseases 19 (3), 200–203.

Dubey, J.P., 1983b. *Sarcocystis ferovis* sp. n. from the bighorn sheep (*Ovis canadensis*) and coyote (*Canis latrans*). Proceedings of the Helminthological Society of Washington 50 (1), 153–158.

Dubey, J.P., 1993. Intestinal protozoa. Veterinary Clinics of North America: Small Animal Practice 23 (1), 37–55.

Dubey, J.P., 1998. *Toxoplasma gondii* oocyst survival under defined temperatures. Journal of Parasitology 84 (4), 862–865.

Dubey, J.P., 1999. Recent advances in *Neospora* and neosporosis. Veterinary Parasitology 84 (3), 349–367.

Dubey, J.P., 2003. Review of *Neospora caninum* and neosporosis in animals. Korean Journal of Parasitology 41 (1), 1–16.

Dubey, J.P., 2007. The history and life cycle of *Toxoplasma gondii*. In: Weiss, L.M., Kim, K. (Eds.), *Toxoplasma gondii*. The Model Apicomplexan: Perspectives and Methods. Elsevier/Academic Press, London, United Kingdom, pp. 1–17.

Dubey, J.P., 2009. The evolution of the knowledge of cat and dog coccidia. Parasitology 136 (12), 1469–1475.

Dubey, J.P., 2010. *Toxoplasma gondii* infections in chickens (*Gallus domesticus*): prevalence, clinical disease, diagnosis, and public health significance. Zoonoses and Public Health 57 (1), 60–73.

Dubey, J.P., 2013. Neosporosis in dogs. Commonwealth Agricultural Bureau Reviews 8, 055.

Dubey, J.P., Beattie, C.P., 1988. Toxoplasmosis of Animals and Man. CRC Press, Boca Raton, Florida, USA. 220 p.

Dubey, J.P., Blagburn, B.L., 1983. Failure to transmit *Sarcocystis* species from ox, sheep, goats, moose, elk, and mule deer to raccoons. American Journal of Veterinary Research 44 (6), 1079–1080.

Dubey, J.P., Carpenter, J.L., 1991. *Toxoplasma gondii*-like schizonts in the tracheal epithelium of a cat. Journal of Parasitology 77 (5), 792–796.

Dubey, J.P., Desmonts, G., 1987. Serological responses of equids fed *Toxoplasma gondii* oocysts. Equine Veterinary Journal 19 (4), 337–339.

Dubey, J.P., Fayer, R., 1976. Development of *Isospora bigemina* in dogs and other mammals. Parasitology 73 (3), 371–380.

Dubey, J.P., Frenkel, J.K., 1972a. Cyst-induced toxoplasmosis in cats. Journal of Protozoology 19 (1), 155–177.

Dubey, J.P., Frenkel, J.K., 1972b. Extra-intestinal stages of *Isospora felis* and *I. rivolta* (Protozoa: Eimeriidae) in cats. Journal of Protozoology 19 (1), 89–92.

Dubey, J.P., Hamir, A.N., 2000. Immunohistochemical confirmation of *Sarcocystis neurona* infections in raccoons, mink, cat, skunk and pony. Journal of Parasitology 86 (5), 1150–1152.

Dubey, J.P., Hedstrom, O.R., 1993. Meningoencephalitis in mink associated with a *Sarcocystis neurona*-like organism. Journal of Veterinary Diagnostic Investigation 5 (3), 467–471.

Dubey, J.P., Jardine, J.E., 2008. Severe intestinal coccidiosis in a newborn lion (*Panthera leo*). Acta Protozoologica 47 (1), 63–68.

Dubey, J.P., Lappin, M.R., 2006. Toxoplasmosis and neosporosis. In: Greene, C.E. (Ed.), Infectious Diseases of the Dog and Cat, third ed. W.B. Saunders, Philadelphia, USA, pp. 768–775.

Dubey, J.P., Lindsay, D.S., 1989a. Transplacental *Neospora caninum* infection in cats. Journal of Parasitology 75 (5), 765–771.

Dubey, J.P., Lindsay, D.S., 1989b. Transplacental *Neospora caninum* infection in dogs. American Journal of Veterinary Research 50 (9), 1578–1579.

Dubey, J.P., Lindsay, D.S., 1990. *Neospora caninum* induced abortion in sheep. Journal of Veterinary Diagnostic Investigation 2 (3), 230–233.

Dubey, J.P., Lindsay, D.S., 1996. A review of *Neospora caninum* and neosporosis. Veterinary Parasitology 67 (1), 1–59.

Dubey, J.P., Lozier, S.M., 1983. *Sarcocystis* infection in the white-tailed deer (*Odocoileus virginianus*) in Montana: intensity and description of *Sarcocystis odoi* n. sp. American Journal of Veterinary Research 44 (9), 1738–1743.

Dubey, J.P., Mehlhorn, H., 1978. Extraintestinal stages of *Isospora ohioensis* from dogs in mice. Journal of Parasitology 64 (4), 689–695.

Dubey, J.P., Odening, K., 2001. Toxoplasmosis and related infections. In: Samuel, W.M., Pybus, M.J., Kocan, A.A. (Eds.), Parasitic Diseases of Wild Mammals. Iowa State University Press, Ames, Iowa, USA, pp. 478–519.

Dubey, J.P., Pande, B.P., 1963a. Observations on the coccidian oocysts from Indian mongoose (*Herpestes mungo*). Indian Journal of Microbiology 3, 49–54.

Dubey, J.P., Pande, B.P., 1963b. Observations on the coccidian oocysts from the Indian jungle cat (*Felis chaus*). Indian Journal of Microbiology 3, 103–108.

Dubey, J.P., Pande, B.P., 1964. Letter to the editor. Indian Journal of Microbiology 4, 29.

Dubey, J.P., Pas, A., 2008. *Toxoplasma gondii* infection in Blanford's fox (*Vulpes cana*). Veterinary Parasitology 153 (1), 147–151.

Dubey, J.P., Slife, L.N., 1990. Fatal encephalitis in a dog associated with an unidentified coccidian parasite. Journal of Veterinary Diagnostic Investigation 2 (3), 233–236.

Dubey, J.P., Speer, C.A., 1985. Prevalence and ultrastructure of three types of *Sarcocystis* in mule deer, *Odocoileus hemionus* (Rafinesque), in Montana. Journal of Wildlife Diseases 21 (3), 219–228.

Dubey, J.P., Speer, C.A., 1991. *Sarcocystis canis* n. sp. (Apicomplexa: Sarcocystidae), the etiologic agent of generalized coccidiosis in dogs. Journal of Parasitology 77 (4), 522–527.

Dubey, J.P., Streitel, R.H., 1976a. Further studies on the transmission of *Hammondia hammondi* in cats. Journal of Parasitology 62 (4), 548–551.

Dubey, J.P., Streitel, R.H., 1976b. *Isospora felis* and *I. rivolta* infections in cats induced by mouse tissue or oocysts. British Veterinary Journal 132 (6), 649–651.

Dubey, J.P., Streitel, R.H., 1976c. Shedding of *Sarcocystis* in feces of dogs and cats fed muscles of naturally infected food animals in the Midwestern United States. Journal of Parasitology 62 (5), 628–630.

Dubey, J.P., Thayer, D.W., 1994. Killing of different strains of *Toxoplasma gondii* tissue cysts by irradiation under defined conditions. Journal of Parasitology 80 (5), 764–767.

Dubey, J.P., Thulliez, P., 2005. Prevalence of antibodies to *Neospora caninum* in wild animals. Journal of Parasitology 91 (5), 1217–1218.

Dubey, J.P., Williams, C.S.F., 1980. *Hammondia heydorni* infection in sheep, goats, moose, dogs and coyotes. Parasitology 81 (1), 123–127.

Dubey, J.P., Yabsley, M.J., 2010. *Besnoitia neotomofelis* n. sp. (Protozoa: Apicomplexa) from the southern plains woodrat (*Neotoma micropus*). Parasitology 137 (12), 1731–1747.

Dubey, J.P., Miller, N.L., Frenkel, J.P., 1970. Characterization of the new fecal form of *Toxoplasma gondii*. Journal of Parasitology 56 (3), 447–456.

Dubey, J.P., Christie, E., Pappas, P.W., 1977a. Characterization of *Toxoplasma gondii* from the feces of naturally infected cats. Journal of Infectious Diseases 136 (3), 432–435.

Dubey, J.P., Streitel, R.H., Stromberg, P.C., Toussant, M.J., 1977b. *Sarcocystis fayeri* n. sp. from the horse. Journal of Parasitology 63 (3), 443–447.

Dubey, J.P., Fayer, R., Seesee, F.M., 1978a. *Sarcocystis* in feces of coyotes from Montana: prevalence and experimental transmission to sheep and cattle. Journal of the American Veterinary Medical Association 173 (9), 1167–1170.

Dubey, J.P., Weisbrode, S.E., Rogers, W.A., 1978b. Canine coccidiosis attributed to an *Isospora ohioensis*-like organism: a case report. Journal of the American Veterinary Medical Association 173 (1), 185–192.

Dubey, J.P., Speer, C.A., Callis, G., Blixt, J.A., 1982. Development of the sheep-canid cycle of *Sarcocystis tenella*. Canadian Journal of Zoology 60 (10), 2464–2477.

Dubey, J.P., Jolley, W.R., Thorne, E.T., 1983. *Sarcocystis sybillensis* sp. nov. from the North American elk (*Cervus elaphus*). Canadian Journal of Zoology 61 (4), 737–742.

Dubey, J.P., Quinn, W.J., Weinandy, D., 1987. Fatal neonatal toxoplasmosis in a bobcat. Journal of Wildlife Diseases 23 (2), 324–327.

Dubey, J.P., Carpenter, J.L., Speer, C.A., Topper, M.J., Uggla, A., 1988a. Newly recognized fatal protozoan disease of dogs. Journal of the American Veterinary Medical Association 192 (9), 1269–1285.

Dubey, J.P., Gendron-Fitzpatrick, A.P., Lenhard, A.L., Bowman, D., 1988b. Fatal toxoplasmosis and entero-epithelial stages of *Toxoplasma gondii* in a Pallas cat (*Felis manul*). Journal of Protozoology 35 (4), 528–530.

Dubey, J.P., Hattel, A.L., Lindsay, D.S., Topper, M.J., 1988c. Neonatal *Neospora caninum* infection in dogs: isolation of the causative agent and experimental transmission. Journal of the American Veterinary Medical Association 193 (10), 1259–1263.

Dubey, J.P., Lindsay, D.S., Speer, C.A., Fayer, R., Livingston Jr., C.W., 1988d. *Sarcocystis arieticanis* and other *Sarcocystis* species in sheep in the United States. Journal of Parasitology 74 (6), 1033–1038.

Dubey, J.P., Hartely, W.J., Badman, R.T., 1989a. Fatal perinatal sarcocystosis in a lamb. Journal of Parasitology 75 (6), 980–982.

Dubey, J.P., Speer, C.A., Fayer, R., 1989b. Sarcocystosis of Animals and Man. CRC Press, Boca Raton, Florida, USA. 215 p.

Dubey, J.P., Black, S.S., Sangster, L.T., Lindsay, D.S., Sundermann, C.A., Topper, M.J., 1990a. *Caryospora*-associated dermatitis in dogs. Journal of Parasitology 76 (4), 552–556.

Dubey, J.P., Hamir, A.N., Hanlon, C.A., Topper, M.J., Rupprecht, C.E., 1990b. Fatal necrotizing encephalitis in a raccoon associated with a *Sarcocystis*-like protozoan. Journal of Veterinary Diagnostic Investigation 2 (4), 345–347.

Dubey, J.P., Koestner, A., Piper, R.C., 1990c. Repeated transplacental transmission of *Neospora caninum* in dogs. Journal of the American Veterinary Medical Association 197 (7), 857–860.

Dubey, J.P., Cosenza, S.F., Lipscomb, T.P., Topper, M.J., Hoban, L.D., Davis, S.W., Kincaid, A.L., Seely, J.C., Marrs Jr., G.E., 1991a. Acute sarcocystosis-like disease in a dog. Journal of the American Veterinary Medical Association 198 (3), 439–444.

Dubey, J.P., Davis, S.W., Speer, C.A., Bowman, D.D., de Lahunta, A., Granstrom, D.E., Topper, M.J., Hamir, A.N., Cummings, J.E., Suter, M.M., 1991b. *Sarcocystis neurona* n. sp. (Protozoa: Apicomplexa), the etiologic agent of equine protozoal myeloencephalitis. Journal of Parasitology 77 (2), 212–218.

Dubey, J.P., Slife, L.N., Lipscomb, T.P., Speer, C.A., Topper, M.T., 1991c. Fatal cutaneous and visceral infection in a Rottweiler dog due to a *Sarcocystis*-like organism. Journal of Veterinary Diagnostic Investigation 3 (1), 72–75.

Dubey, J.P., Speer, C.A., Hamir, A.N., Topper, M.J., Brown, C., Rupprecht, C.E., 1991d. Development of a *Sarcocystis*-like Apicomplexan protozoan in the brain of a raccoon (*Procyon lotor*). Journal of the Helminthological Society of Washington 58, 250–255.

Dubey, J.P., Duncan, D.E., Speer, C.A., Brown, C., 1992a. Congenital sarcocystosis in a two-day-old dog. Journal of Veterinary Diagnostic Investigation 4 (1), 89–93.

Dubey, J.P., Hamir, A.N., Kirkpatrick, C.E., Todd Jr., K.S., Rupprecht, C.E., 1992b. Sarcocystis felis sp. n. (Protozoa: Sarcocystidae) from the bobcat (*Felis rufus*). Journal of the Helminthological Society of Washington 59 (2), 227–229.

Dubey, J.P., Lindsay, D.S., Anderson, M.L., Davis, S.W., Shen, S.K., 1992c. Induced transplacental transmission of *Neospora caninum* in cattle. Journal of the American Veterinary Medical Association 201 (5), 709–713.

Dubey, J.P., Higgins, R.J., Barr, B.C., Spangler, W.L., Kollin, B., Jorgensen, L.S., 1994. *Sarcocystis*-associated meningoencephalomyelitis in a cat. Journal of Veterinary Diagnostic Investigation 6 (1), 118–120.

Dubey, J.P., Humphreys, J.G., Thulliez, P., 1995a. Prevalence of viable *Toxoplasma gondii* tissue cysts and antibodies to *T. gondii* by various serologic tests in black bears (*Ursus americanus*) from Pennsylvania. Journal of Parasitology 81 (1), 109–112.

Dubey, J.P., Metzger, F.L., Hattel, A.L., Lindsay, D.S., Fritz, D.L., 1995b. Canine cutaneous neosporosis: clinical improvement with clindamycin. Veterinary Dermatology 6, 37–43.

Dubey, J.P., Jenkins, M.C., Thayer, D.W., 1996a. Irradiation killing of *Toxoplasma gondii* oocysts. Journal of Eukaryotic Microbiology 43 (5), 123S.

Dubey, J.P., Jenkins, M.C., Thayer, D.W., Kwok, O.C.H., Shen, S.K., 1996b. Killing of *Toxoplasma gondii* oocysts by irradiation and protective immunity induced by vaccination with irradiated oocysts. Journal of Parasitology 82 (5), 724–727.

Dubey, J.P., Hamir, A.N., Niezgoda, M., Rupprecht, C.E., 1996c. A *Sarcocystis neurona*-like organism associated with encephalitis in a striped skunk (*Mephitis mephitis*). Journal of Parasitology 82 (1), 172–174.

Dubey, J.P., Jenkins, M.C., Adams, D.S., McAllister, M.M., Anderson-Sprecher, R., Baszler, T.V., Kwok, O.C.H., Lally, N.C., Björkman, C., Uggla, A., 1997. Antibody responses of cows during an outbreak of neosporosis evaluated by indirect fluorescent antibody test and different enzyme-linked immunosorbent assays. Journal of Parasitology 83 (6), 1063–1069.

Dubey, J.P., Thayer, D.W., Speer, C.A., Shen, S.K., 1998a. Effect of gamma irradiation on unsporulated and sporulated *Toxoplasma gondii* oocysts. International Journal for Parasitology 28 (3), 369–375.

Dubey, J.P., Topper, M.J., Nutter, F.B., 1998b. Muscular *Sarcocystis* infection in a bear (*Ursus americanus*). Journal of Parasitology 84 (2), 452–454.

Dubey, J.P., Garner, M.M., Rosenthal, B.M., DeGhetto, D., 2000a. Clinical coccidiosis in raccoons (*Procyon lotor*). Journal of Parasitology 86 (6), 1299–1303.

Dubey, J.P., Saville, W.J.A., Lindsay, D.S., Sitch, R.W., Stanek, J.F., Speer, C.A., Rosenthal, B.M., Njoku, C.J., Kwok, O.C.H., Shen, S.K., Reed, S.M., 2000b. Completion of the life cycle of *Sarcocystis neurona*. Journal of Parasitology 86 (6), 1276–1280.

Dubey, J.P., Lindsay, D.S., Kerber, C.E., Kasai, N., Pena, H.F.J., Gennari, S.M., Kwok, O.C.H., Shen, S.K., Rosenthal, B.M., 2001a. First isolation of *Sarcocystis neurona* from the South American opossum, *Didelphis albiventris*, from Brazil. Veterinary Parasitology 95 (2–4), 295–304.

Dubey, J.P., Lindsay, D.S., Saville, W.J.A., Reed, S.M., Granstrom, D.E., Speer, C.A., 2001b. A review of *Sarcocystis neurona* and equine protozoal myeloencephalitis (EPM). Veterinary Parasitology 95 (1), 89–131.

Dubey, J.P., Rosypal, A.C., Rosenthal, B.M., Thomas, N.J., Lindsay, D.S., Stanek, J.F., Reed, S.M., Saville, W.J.A., 2001c. *Sarcocystis neurona* infection in sea otter (*Enhydra lutris*): evidence for natural infections with sarcocysts and transmission of infection to opossums (*Didelphis virginiana*). Journal of Parasitology 87 (6), 1387–1393.

Dubey, J.P., Saville, W.J.A., Stanek, J.F., Lindsay, D.S., Rosenthal, B.M., Oglesbee, M.J., Rosypal, A.C., Njoku, C.J., Stich, R.W., Kwok, O.C.H., Shen, S.K., Hamir, A.N., Reed, S.M., 2001d. *Sarcocystis neurona* infections in raccoons (*Procyon lotor*): evidence for natural infection with sarcocysts, transmission of infection to opossums (*Didelphis virginiana*), and experimental induction of neurologic disease in raccoons. Veterinary Parasitology 100 (3–4), 117–129.

Dubey, J.P., Barr, B.C., Barta, J.R., Bjerkås, I., Björkman, C., Blagburn, B.L., Bowman, D.D., Buxton, D., Ellis, J.T., Gottstein, B., Hemphill, A., Hill, D.E., Howe, D.K., Jenkens, M.C., Kobayashi, Y., Koudela, B., Marsh, A.E., Mattsson, J.G., McAllister, M.M., Modrý, D., Omata, Y., Sibley, L.D., Speer, C.A., Trees, A.J., Uggla, A., Upton, S.J., Williams, D.J.L., Lidsay, D.S., 2002a. Redescription of *Neospora caninum* and its differentiation from related coccidia. International Journal for Parasitology 32 (8), 929–946.

Dubey, J.P., Carpenter, J.L., Topper, M.J., Uggla, A., 2002b. Fatal toxoplasmosis in dogs. Journal of the American Animal Hospital Association 25, 659–664.

Dubey, J.P., Hamir, A.N., Topper, M.J., 2002c. *Sarcocystis mephitisi* n. sp. (Protozoa: Sarcocystidae), *Sarcocystis neurona*-like and *Toxoplasma*-like infections in striped skunks (*Mephitis mephitis*). Journal of Protozoology 88 (1), 113–117.

Dubey, J.P., Lindsay, D.S., Hill, D., Romand, S., Thulliez, P., Kwok, O.C.H., Silva, J.C.R., Oliveira-Camargo, M.C., Gennari, S.M., 2002d. Prevalence of antibodies to *Neospora caninum* and *Sarcocystis neurona* in sera of domestic cats from Brazil. Journal of Parasitology 88 (6), 1251–1252.

Dubey, J.P., Cawthorn, R.J., Speer, C.A., Wobeser, G.A., 2003a. Redescription of the sarcocysts of *Sarcocystis rileyi* (Apicomplexa: Sarcocystidae). Journal of Eukaryotic Microbiology 50 (6), 476–482.

Dubey, J.P., Lindsay, D.S., Rosenthal, B.M., Thomas, N.J., 2003b. Sarcocysts of an unidentified species of *Sarcocystis* in the sea otter (*Enhydra lutris*). Journal of Parasitology 89 (2), 397–399.

Dubey, J.P., Sreekumar, C., Lindsay, D.S., Hill, D., Rosenthal, B.M., Venturini, L., Venturini, M.C., Greiner, E.C., 2003c. *Besnoitia oryctofelis* n. sp. (Protozoa: Apicomplexa) from domestic rabbits. Parasitology 126 (6), 521–539.

Dubey, J.P., Zamke, R., Thomas, N.J., Wong, S.K., van Bonn, W., Briggs, M., Davis, J.W., Weing, R., Mense, M., Kwok, O.C.H., Romand, S., Thulliez, P., 2003d. *Toxoplasma gondii, Neospora caninum, Sarcocystis neurona,* and *Sarcocystis canis*-like infections in marine mammals. Veterinary Parasitology 116 (4), 275–296.

Dubey, J.P., Lipscomb, T.P., Mense, M., 2004a. Toxoplasmosis in an elephant seal (*Mirounga angustirostris*). Journal of Parasitology 90 (2), 410–411.

Dubey, J.P., Sreekumar, C., Rosenthal, B.M., Vianna, M.C.B., Nylund, M., Nikander, S., Oksanen, A., 2004b. Redescription of *Besnoitia tarandi* (Protozoa: Apicomplexa) from the reindeer (*Rangifer tarandus*). International Journal for Parasitology 34 (11), 1273–1287.

Dubey, J.P., Hill, D.E., Jones, J.L., Hightower, A.W., Kirkland, E., Roberts, J.M., Marcet, P.L., Lehmann, T., Vianna, M.C.B., Miska, K., Sreekumar, C., Kwok, O.C.H., Shen, S.K., Gamble, H.R., 2005. Prevalence of viable *Toxoplasma gondii* in beef, chicken, and pork from retail meat stores in the United States: risk assessment to consumers. Journal of Parasitology 91 (5), 1082–1093.

Dubey, J.P., Chapman, J.L., Rosenthal, B.M., Mense, M., Schueler, R.L., 2006. Clinical *Sarcocystis neurona, Sarcocystis canis, Toxoplasma gondii,* and *Neospora caninum* infections in dogs. Veterinary Parasitology 137 (1), 36–49.

Dubey, J.P., Schares, G., Ortega-Mora, L.M., 2007. Epidemiology and control of neosporosis and *Neospora caninum*. Clinical Microbiology Reviews 20 (2), 323–367.

Dubey, J.P., Humphreys, J.G., Fritz, D., 2008a. A new species of *Sarcocystis* (Apicomplexa: Sarcocystidae) from the black bear (*Ursus americanus*). Journal of Parasitology 94 (2), 496–499.

Dubey, J.P., Stone, D., Kwok, O.C.H., Sharma, R.N., 2008b. *Toxoplasma gondii* and *Neospora caninum* antibodies in dogs from Grenada, West Indes. Journal of Parasitology 94 (3), 750–751.

Dubey, J.P., Mergl, J., Gehring, E., Sundar, N., Velmurugan, G.V., Kwok, O.C.H., Grigg, M.E., Su, C., Martineau, D., 2009. Toxoplasmosis in captive dolphins (*Tursiops truncatus*) and walrus (*Odobenus rosmarus*). Journal of Parasitology 96 (1), 82–85.

Dubey, J.P., Pas, A., Rajendran, C., Kwok, O.C.H., Ferreira, L.R., Martin, J., Hebel, C., Hammer, S., Su, C., 2010a. Toxoplasmosis in sand cats (*Felis margarita*) and other animals in the breeding centre for endangered Arabian wildlife in the United Arab Emirates and Al Wabra wildlife preservation, the State of Qatar. Veterinary Parasitology 172 (3), 195–203.

Dubey, J.P., Reichard, M.V., Torretti, L., Garvon, J.M., Sundar, N., Grigg, M.E., 2010b. Two new species of *Sarcocystine* (Apicomplexa: Sarcocystidae) infecting the wolverine (*Gulo gulo*) from Nunavut, Canada. Journal of Parasitology 96 (5), 972–976.

Dubey, J.P., Rosenthal, B.M., Felix, T.A., 2010c. Morphologic and molecular characterization of the sarcocysts of *Sarcocystis rileyi* (Apicomplexa: Sarcocystidae) from the mallard duck (*Anas platyrhynchos*). Journal of Parasitology 96 (4), 765–770.

Dubey, J.P., Jenkins, M.C., Rajendran, C., Miska, K., Ferreira, L.R., Martins, J., Kwok, O.C.H., Choudhary, S., 2011. Gray wolf (*Canis lupus*) is a natural definitive host for *Neospora caninum*. Veterinary Parasitology 181 (2–4), 382–387.

Dubey, J.P., Tilahun, G., Boyle, J.P., Schares, G., Verma, S.K., Ferreira, L.R., Oliveira, S., Tiao, N., Darrington, C., Gebreyes, A., 2013. Molecular and biological characterization of first isolates of *Hammondia hammondi* from cats from Ethiopia. Journal of Parasitology 99 (4), 614–618.

Dubey, J.P., Black, S.S., Verma, S.K., Calero-Bernal, R.C., Morris, E., Hanson, M.A., Cooley, A.J., 2014. *Sarcocystis neurona* schizonts-associated encephalitis, chorioretinitis, and myositis in a two-month-old dog simulating toxoplasmosis, and presence of mature sarcocysts in the muscles. Veterinary Parasitology 202 (3), 194–200.

Dubey, J.P., Calero-Bernal, R., Rosenthal, B.M., Speer, C.A., Fayer, R., 2015a. Sarcocystis of Animals and Humans, second ed. CRC Press, Inc., Boca Raton, Florida, USA. 501 p.

Dubey, J.P., Howe, D.K., Furr, M., Saville, W.J., Marsh, A.E., Reed, S.M., Grigg, M.E., 2015b. An update on *Sarcocystis neurona* infections in animals and equine protozoal myeloencephalitis (EPM). Veterinary Parasitology 209 (1–2), 1–42.

Dubey, J.P., Sykes, J.E., Shelton, G.D., Sharp, N., Verma, S.K., Calero-Bernal, R., Viviano, J., Sundar, N., Khan, A., Grigg, M.E., 2015c. *Sarcocystis caninum* and *Sarcocystis svanai* n. spp. (Apicomplexa: Sarcocystidae) associated with severe myositis and hepatitis in the domestic dog (*Canis familiaris*). Journal of Eukaryotic Microbiology 62 (3), 307–317.

Dubey, J., Brown, J., Ternent, M., Vermaa, S., Hill, D., Cerqueira-Cézar, C., Kwoka, O., Calero-Bernal, R., Humphreys, J., 2016a. Seroepidemiologic study on the prevalence of *Toxoplasma gondii* and *Trichinella* spp. infections in black bears (*Ursus americanus*) in Pennsylvania, USA. Veterinary Parasitology 229, 76–80.

Dubey, J.P., Moré, G., van Wilpe, E., Calero-Bernal, R., Verma, S.K., Schares, G., 2016b. *Sarcocystis rommeli* n. sp. (Apicomplexa: Sarcocystidae) from cattle (*Bos taurus*) and its differentiation from *Sarcocystis hominis*. Journal of Eukaryotic Microbiology 63 (1), 62–68.

Dubey, J.P., A'aji, N.N., Mowery, J.D., Verma, S.K., Calero-Bernal, R., 2017a. Identification of macroscopic sarcocysts of *Sarcocystis cameli* from one-humped camel (*Camelus dromidarius*) in Iraq. Journal of Parasitology 103 (2), 168–169.

Dubey, J.P., Hemphill, A., Calero-Bernal, R., Schares, G., 2017b. Neosporosis in Animals. CRC Press, Inc., Boca Raton, Florida, USA. 448 p.

Dubey, J.P., Trupkiewicz, J.G., Verma, S.K., Mowery, J.D., Adedoyin, G., Georoff, T., Grigg, M.E., 2017c. Atypical fatal sarcocystosis associated with *Sarcocystis neurona* in a white-nosed coati (*Nasua narica molaris*). Veterinary Parasitology 247, 80–84.

Dubná, S., Langrová, I., Nápravník, J., Jankovská, I., Vadlejch, J., Pekár, S., Fechtner, J., 2007. The prevalence of intestinal parasites in dogs from Prague, rural areas, and shelters of the Czech Republic. Veterinary Parasitology 145 (1–2), 120–128.

Duncan, R.B., Caudell, D., Lindsay, D.S., Moll, H.D., 1999. Cryptosporidiosis in a black bear in Virginia. Journal of Wildlife Diseases 35 (2), 381–383.

Dunlap, J.S., 1956. Experimental coccidial infection in the fox. Western Veterinarian 56, 64–67.

Dupouy-Camet, J., Bourée, P., Year, H., 2017. *Trichinella* and polar bears: a limited risk for humans. Journal of Helminthology 91 (4), 440–446.

Duszynski, D.W., 1999. Revisiting the code: clarifying name-bearing types for photomicrographs of protozoa. Invited Critical Comment Journal of Parasitology 85 (4), 769–770.

Duszynski, D.W., 2002. Coccidia (Apicomplexa: Eimeriidae) of the Mammalian Order Chiroptera. Special Publication of the Museum of Southwestern Biology, No. 5. First Impressions, Inc., Albuquerque, NM. 42 p.

Duszynski, D.W., 2016. The Biology and Identification of the Coccidia (Apicomplexa) of Marsupials of the World. Elsevier/Academic Press Inc. ISBN: 978-0-12-802709-7. 241 p.

Duszynski, D.W., Box, E.D., 1978. The opossum (*Didelphis virginiana*) as a host for *Sarcocystis debonei* from cowbirds (*Molothrus ater*) and grackles (*Cassidix mexicanus, Quiscalus quiscula*). Journal of Parasitology 64 (2), 326–329.

Duszynski, D.W., Couch, L., 2013. The Biology and Identification of the Coccidia (Apicomplexa) of Rabbits of the World. Elsevier/Academic Press Inc. ISBN: 978-0-12-397899-8. 340 p.

Duszynski, D.W., Morrow, J.J., 2014. The Biology and Identification of the Coccidia (Apicomplexa) of Turtles of the World. Elsevier/Academic Press Inc. ISBN: 978-0-12-801367-0. 210 p.

Duszynski, D.W., Speer, C.A., 1976. Excystation of *Isospora arctopitheci* Rodhain, 1933 with notes on a similar process in *Isospora bigemina* (Stiles, 1891) Lühe, 1906. Zeitschrift für Parasitenkunde 48 (3–4), 191–197.

Duszynski, D.W., Upton, S.J., 2000. Coccidia (Apicomplexa: Eimeriidae) of the Mammalian Order Insectivora. Special Publication of the Museum of Southwestern Biology, No. 4. University of New Mexico Printing Services, Albuquerque, NM. 67 p.

Duszynski, D.W., Upton, S.J., 2001. *Cyclospora, Eimeria, Isospora,* and *Cryptosporidium* spp. In: Samuel, W.M., Pybus, M.J., Kocan, A.A. (Eds.), Parasitic Diseases of Wild Mammals, second ed. Iowa State University Press, Ames, Iowa, pp. 416–459.

Duszynski, D.W., Upton, S.J., 2010. The Biology of the Coccidia (Apicomplexa) of Snakes of the World. A Scholarly Handbook for Identification and Treatment. CreateSpace Independent Publishing Platform, USA. ISBN: 1448617995. 422 p.

Duszynski, D.W., Speer, C.A., Chobotar, B., Marchiondo, A.A., 1981. Fine structure of the oocyst wall and excystation of *Eimeria procyonis* from the American raccoon (*Procyon lotor*). Zeitschrift für Parasitenkunde 65 (2), 131–136.

Duszynski, D.W., Wilson, W.D., Upton, S.J., Levine, N.D., 1999. Coccidia (Apicomplexa: Eimeriidae) in the Primates and Scandentia. International Journal of Primatology 20, 761–797.

Duszynski, D.W., Upton, S.J., Bolek, M., 2007. Coccidia (Apicomplexa: Eimeriidae) of the Amphibians of the world. Zootaxa (Magnolia Press) 1667, 1–77.

Ebner, J., Koehler, A.V., Robertson, G., Bradbury, R.S., Jex, A.R., Haydon, S.R., Stevens, M.A., Norton, R., Joachim, A., Gasser, R.B., 2015. Genetic analysis of *Giardia* and *Cryptosporidium* from people in Northern Australia using PCR-based tools. Infection, Genetics and Evolution: Journal of Molecular Epidemiology and Evolutionary Genetics in Infectious Diseases 36, 389–395.

Edwards, J.F., Ficken, M.D., Luttgen, P.J., 1988. Disseminated sarcocystosis in a cat with lymphosarcoma. Journal of the American Veterinary Medical Association 193 (7), 831–832.

Egger, M., Nguyen, X.M., Schaad, U.B., Krech, T., 1990. Intestinal cryptosporidiosis acquired from a cat. Infection 18 (3), 177–178.

Egyed, Z., Sréter, T., Széll, Z., Varga, I., 2003. Characterization of *Cryptosporidium* spp. – recent developments and future needs. Veterinary Parasitology 111 (2–3), 103–114.

Ehrensperger, F., Pospischil, A., 1989. Spontaneous mixed infections with distemper virus and *Toxoplasma* in dogs. Deutsche Tierärztliche Wochenschrift 96 (4), 184–186.

Einstein, R., Innes, J.R.M., 1956. Sarcosporidiosis in man and animals. Veterinary Reviews and Annotations 2 (2), 61–78.

el Wakeel, E.S., Homeida, M.M., Ali, H.M., Geary, T.G., Jensen, J.B., 1985. Clindamycin in the treatment of falciparum malaria in Sudan. The American Journal of Tropical Medicine and Hygiene 34 (6), 1065–1068.

Elias, E., Homans, P.A., 1988. *Hepatozoon canis* infection in dogs: clinical and hematological findings; treatment. Journal of Small Animal Practice 29, 55–62.

El-Ahraf, A., Tacal, J.V., Sobih, M., Amin, M., Lawrence, W., Wilcke, B.W., 1991. Prevalence of cryptosporidiosis in dogs and human beings in San Bernardino County, California. Journal of the American Veterinary Medical Association 198 (4), 631–634.

El-Gayar, A.K., Holman, P.J., Craig, T.M., Demaar, T.W., Wilson, S.C., Chung, P., Woods, K.M., Norris, C., Upton, S.J., 2008. A new species of coccidia (Apicomplexa: Sarcocystidae) from the slender-tailed meerkat *Suricata suricatta* (Schreber, 1776) from South Africa. Acta Protozoologica 47 (1), 69–76.

Elias, E., Homans, P.A., 1988. Hepatozoon canis infection in dogs: clinical and hematological findings; treatment. Journal of Small Animal Practice 29 (1), 55–62.

Ellis, J.T., Morrison, D.A., Liddell, S., Jenkins, M.C., Mohammed, O.B., Ryce, D., Dubey, J.P., 1999. The genus *Hammondia* is paraphyletic. Parasitology 118 (Pt4), 357–362.

Elmore, S.A., Lalonde, L.F., Samelius, G., Alisauskas, R.T., Gajadhar, A.A., Jenkins, E.J., 2013. Endoparasites in the feces of arctic foxes in a terrestrial ecosystem in Canada. International Journal for Parasitology. Parasites and Wildlife 2, 90–96.

El-Rafaii, A.H., Abdel-Baki, G., Selim, M.K., 1980. Sarcosporidia in goats of Egypt. Journal of the Egyptian Society of Parasitology 10 (2), 471–472.

Elsheikha, H.M., Mansfield, L.S., 2007. Molecular typing of *Sarcocystis neurona*: current status and future trends. Veterinary Parasitology 149 (1), 43–55.

Elsheikha, H.M., Mansfield, L.S., Fitzgerald, S.D., Saeed, M.A., 2003. Prevalence and tissue distribution of *Besnoitia darlingi* cysts in the Virginia opossum (*Didelphis virginiana*) in Michigan. Veterinary Parasitology 115 (4), 321–327.

Elwasila, M., Entzeroth, R., Chobotar, B., Scholtyseck, E., 1984. Comparison of the structure of *Sarcocystis cuniculi* of the European rabbit (*Oryctolagus cuniculus*) and *Sarcocystis leporum* of the cottontail rabbit (*Sylvilagus floridanus*) by light and electron microscopy. Acta Veterinaria Hungarica 32 (1), 71–78.

Elwin, K., Hadfield, S.J., Robinson, G., Chalmers, R.M., 2012. The epidemiology of sporadic human infections with unusual cryptosporidia detected during routine typing in England and Wales, 2000–2008. Epidemiology and Infection 140 (4), 673–683.

Engh, A.L., Nelson, K.G., Peebles, R., Hernandez, A.D., Hubbard, K.K., Holekamp, K.E., 2003. Coprologic survey of parasites of spotted hyenas (*Crocuta crocuta*) in the Masai Mara National Reserve, Kenya. Journal of Wildlife Diseases 39 (1), 224–227.

Entzeroth, R., 1982a. A comparative light and electron microscope study of the cysts of *Sarcocystis* species of roe deer (*Capreolus capreolus*). Zeitschrift für Parasitenkunde 66 (3), 281–292.

Entzeroth, R., 1982b. Ultrastructure of gamonts and gametes and fertilization of *Sarcocystis* sp. from the roe deer (*Capreolus capreolus*) in dogs. Zeitschrift für Parasitenkunde 67 (1), 147–153.

Entzeroth, R., 1983. Electron microscope study of merogony preceding cyst formation of *Sarcocystis* sp. in roe deer (*Capreolus capreolus*). Zeitschrift für Parasitenkunde 69 (4), 447–456.

Entzeroth, R., 1984. Electron microscope study of host-parasite interactions of *Sarcocystis muris* (Protozoa, Coccidia) in tissue culture and in vivo. Zeitschrift für Parasitenkunde 70 (1), 131–134.

Entzeroth, R., 1985. Light-, scanning-, and transmission electron microscope study of the cyst wall of *Sarcocystis gracilis* Rátz, 1909 (Sporozoa, Coccidia) from the roe deer (*Capreolus capreolus* L.). Archiv für Protistenkunde 129 (1–4), 183–186.

Entzeroth, R., Scholtyseck, E., Greuel, E., 1978. The roe deer intermediate host of different coccidia. Naturwissenschaften 65 (7), 395.

Entzeroth, R., Chobotar, B., Scholtyseck, E., 1982a. Ultrastructure of *Sarcocystis* sp. from the muscle of a white-tailed deer (*Odocoileus virginianus*). Zeitschrift für Parasitenkunde 68 (1), 33–38.

Entzeroth, R., Stuht, N., Chobotar, B., Scholtyseck, E., 1982b. *Sarcocystis* of white-tailed deer (*Odocoileus virginianus*) and its transmission to the dog (*Canis familiaris*). Tropenmedizin und Parasitologie 33 (2), 111–112.

Entzeroth, R., Chobotar, B., Scholtyseck, E., 1985. Electron microscope study of gamogony of *Sarcocystis muris* (Protozoa, Apicomplexa) in the small intestine of cats (*Felis catus*). Protistologica 21 (3), 399–408.

Epe, C., Ising-Volmer, S., Stoye, M., 1993. Ergebnisse parasitologischer Kotuntersuchungen von Equiden, Hunden, Katzen und Igeln der Jahre 1984–1991 (Results of parasitological examinations of faecal samples from horses, donkeys, dogs, cats and hedgehogs between 1984 and 1991). Deutsche Tierärztliche Wochenschrift 100 (11), 426–428 (in German, English summary).

Epe, C., Coati, N., Schnieder, T., 2004. Results of parasitological examinations of faecal samples from horses, ruminants, pigs, dogs, cats, hedgehogs and rabbits between 1998 and 2002. Deutsche Tierärztliche Wochenschrift 111 (6), 243–247 (in German).

Erber, M., 1978. *Sarcocystis* spp. of wild boar and roe deer. In: Short Communication, Fourth International Congress of Parasitology (ICOPA IV), Warsaw, Poland, 1976. B, p. 79.

Erber, M., Boch, J., Barth, D., 1978. Drei Sarkosporidienarten des Rehwildes (Three *Sarcocystis* species in roe deer (*Capreolus capreolus*)). Berliner und Münchener Tierärztliche Wochenschrift 91 (24), 482–486 (in German, English summary).

Ercolani, G.B., 1859. Nuovi elementi teorico-pratici di medicina veterinaria (New Theoretical-Practical Elements of Veterinary Medicine). Giacomo Monti Tipografo Editore, Bologna, Italy. 550 p. (in Italian, no English translation). (*nos non videbo illum*, as cited by Wenyon, 1923).

Erdman, L.F., 1978. *Sarcocystis* in striped skunks. Iowa State University Veterinarian 40 (3), 112.

Eriksson, P., Zidar, J., White, D., Westander, J., Andersson, M., 2010. Current husbandry of red pandas (*Ailurus fulgens*) in zoos. Zoo Biology 29 (6), 732–740.

Esposito, M., Stettler, R., Moores, S.L., Pidathala, C., Müller, N., Stachulski, A., Berry, N.G., Rossignol, J.F., Hemphill, A., 2005. In vitro efficacies of nitazoxanide and other thiazolides against *Neospora caninum* tachyzoites reveal antiparasitic activity independent of the nitro group. Antimicrobial Agents and Chemotherapy 49 (9), 3715–3723.

Esposito, M., Moores, S., Naguleswaran, A., Muller, J., Hemphill, A., 2007. Induction of tachyzoite egress from cells infected with the protozoan *Neospora caninum* by nitro- and bromo-thiazolides, a class of broad-spectrum anti-parasitic drugs. International Journal for Parasitology 37 (10), 1143–1152.

Everitt, J.I., Basgall, E.J., Hooser, S.B., 1987. *Sarcocystis* sp. in the striated muscle of domestic cats, *Felis catus*. Proceedings of the Helminthological Society of Washington 54 (2), 279–281.

Eydelloth, M., 1977. Experimentelle Untersuchungen über das Wirtsspektrum von *Hammondia hammondi* (Investigations into the Host Range of *Hammondia hammondi*). (Inaugural dissertation). Universität München, München, Germany. 47 p. (in German, English summary).

Fagiolini, M., Lia, R.P., Laricchiuta, P., Cavicchio, P., Mannella, R., Cafarchia, C., Otranto, D., Finotello, R., Perrucci, S., 2010. Gastrointestinal parasites in mammals of two Italian zoological gardens. Journal of Zoo and Wildlife Medicine 41 (4), 662–670.

Fameree, L., Cotteleer, C., 1976. Toxoplasmose et hygiène. Prévalence de la coccidiose féline en Belgique (Toxoplasmosis and hygiene. Prevalence of feline coccidiosis in Belgium). Journal of Protozoology 23 (4), A10 (in French, abstract).

Farias, N.A., Christovão, M.L., Stobbe, N.S., 1995. Frequência de parasitas intestinais em cães (*Canis familiaris*) e gatos (*Felis catus* domesticus) em Araçatuba, São Paulo. Revista Brasileira de Parasitologia Veterinaria 4 (1), 57–60 (in Portuguese).

Farmer, J.N., Herbert, I.V., Partridge, M., Edwads, G.T., 1978. The prevalence of *Sarcocystis* spp. in dogs and red foxes. The Veterinary Record 102 (1), 78–80.

Fayer, R., 1970. Sarcocystis: development in cultured avian and mammalian cells. Science 168 (3935), 1104–1105.

Fayer, R., 1972a. Cultivation of feline *Isospora rivolta* in mammalian cells. Journal of Parasitology 58 (6), 1207–1208.

Fayer, R., 1972b. Gametogony of *Sarcocystis* sp. in cell culture. Science 175 (4017), 65–67.

Fayer, R., 1974. Development of *Sarcocystis fusiformis* in the small intestine of the dog. Journal of Parasitology 60 (4), 660–665.

Fayer, R., 1977a. Production of *Sarcocystis cruzi* sporocysts by dogs fed experimentally infected and naturally infected beef. Journal of Parasitology 63 (6), 1072–1075.

Fayer, R., 1977b. The first asexual generation in the life cycle of *Sarcocystis bovicanis*. Proceedings of the Helminthological Society of Washington 44 (2), 206–209.

Fayer, R., 1979. Multiplication of *Sarcocystis bovicanis* in the bovine bloodstream. Journal of Parasitology 65 (6), 980–982.

Fayer, R., 2010. Taxonomy and species delimitation in *Cryptosporidium*. Experimental Parasitology 124 (1), 90–97.

Fayer, R., Dubey, J.P., 1987. Comparative epidemiology of coccidia: clues to the etiology of equine protozoal myelo-encephalitis. International Journal for Parasitology 17 (2), 615–620.

Fayer, R., Ellis, W., 1993a. Glycoside antibiotics alone and combined with tetracyclines for prophylaxis of experimental cryptosporidiosis in neonatal BALB/c mice. Journal of Parasitology 79 (4), 553–558.

Fayer, R., Ellis, W., 1993b. Paromomycin is effective as prophylaxis for cryptosporidiosis in dairy calves. Journal of Parasitology 79 (5), 771–774.

Fayer, R., Frenkel, J.K., 1979. Comparative infectivity for calves of oocysts of feline coccidia: *Besnoitia*, *Hammondia*, *Cystoisospora*, *Sarcocystis*, and *Toxoplasma*. Journal of Parasitology 65 (5), 756–762.

Fayer, R., Johnson, A.J., 1973. Development of *Sarcocystis fusiformis* in calves infected with sporocysts from dogs. Journal of Parasitology 59 (6), 1135–1137.

Fayer, R., Johnson, A.J., 1974. *Sarcocystis fusiformis*: development of cysts in calves infected with sporocysts from dogs. Proceedings of the Helminthological Society of Washington 41 (1), 105–108.

Fayer, R., Kradel, D., 1977. *Sarcocystis leporum* in cottontail rabbits and its transmission to carnivores. Journal of Wildlife Diseases 13 (2), 170–173.

Fayer, R., Leek, R.G., 1973. Excystation of *Sarcocystis fusiformis* sporocysts from dogs. Proceedings of the Helminthological Society of Washington 40 (2), 294–296.

Fayer, R., Leek, R.G., 1979. *Sarcocystis* transmitted by blood transfusion. Journal of Parasitology 65 (6), 890–893.

Fayer, R., Mahrt, J.L., 1972. Development of *Isospora canis* (Protozoa: Sporozoa) in cell culture. Zeitschrift für Parasitenkunde 38 (4), 313–318.

Fayer, R., Thompson, D.E., 1974. *Isospora felis*: development in cultured cells with some cytological observations. Journal of Parasitology 60 (1), 160–168.

Fayer, R., Johnson, A.J., Hildebrandt, P.K., 1976. Oral infection of mammals with *Sarcocystis fusiformis* bradyzoites from cattle and sporocysts from dogs and coyotes. Journal of Parasitology 62 (1), 10–14.

Fayer, R., Dubey, J.P., Leek, R.G., 1982. Infectivity of *Sarcocystis* spp. from bison, elk, moose, and cattle for cattle via sporocysts from coyotes. Journal of Parasitology 68 (4), 681–685.

Fayer, R., Morgan, U., Upton, S.J., 2000. Epidemiology of *Cryptosporidium*: transmission, detection and identification. International Journal for Parasitology 30 (12–13), 1305–1322.

Fayer, R., Trout, J.M., Xiao, L., Morgan, U.M., Lal, A.A., Dubey, J.P., 2001. *Cryptosporidium canis* n. sp. from domestic dogs. Journal of Parasitology 87 (6), 1415–1422.

Fayer, R., Santín, M., Trout, J.M., Dubey, J.P., 2006. Detection of *Cryptosporidium felis* and *Giardia duodenalis* Assemblage F in a cat colony. Veterinary Parasitology 140 (1–2), 44–53.

Fayer, R., Santín, M., Trout, J.M., 2008. *Cryptosporidium ryanae* n. sp. (Apicomplexa: Cryptosporidiidae) in cattle (*Bos taurus*). Veterinary Parasitology 156 (3–4), 191–198.

Fayer, R., Santín, M., Macarisin, D., 2010. *Cryptosporidium ubiquitum* n. sp. in animals and humans. Veterinary Parasitology 172 (1), 23–32.

Feng, Y., Alderisio, K.A., Yang, W., Blancero, L.A., Kuhne, W.G., Nadareski, C.A., Reid, M., Xiao, L., 2007. *Cryptosporidium* genotypes in wildlife from a New York watershed. Applied and Environmental Microbiology 73 (20), 6475–6483.

Feng, Y., Dearen, T., Cama, V., Xiao, L., 2009. 90-kilodalton heat shock protein, Hsp90, as a target for genotyping *Cryptosporidium* spp. known to infect humans. Eukaryotic Cell 8 (4), 478–482.

Fenger, C.K., Granstrom, D.E., Langemeier, J.L., Stamper, S., Donahue, J.M., Patterson, J.S., Gajadhar, A.A., Marteniuk, J.V., Xiaomin, Z., Dubey, J.P., 1995. Identification of opossums (*Didelphis virginiana*) as the putative definitive host of *Sarcocystis neurona*. Journal of Parasitology 81 (6), 916–919.

Ferguson, D.J.P., Birch-Andersen, A., Hutchison, W.M., Siim, J.C., 1980a. Ultrastructural observations on macrogametogenesis and the structure of the macrogamete of *Isospora felis*. Acta Pathologica et Microbiologica Scandinavica. Section B 88, 161–168.

Ferguson, D.J.P., Birch-Andersen, A., Hutchison, W.M., Siim, J.C., 1980b. Ultrastructural observations on microgametogenesis and the structure of the microgamete of *Isospora felis*. Acta Pathologica et Microbiologica Scandinavica. Section B 88, 151–159.

Ferguson, D.J.P., Birch-Andersen, A., Hutchison, W.M., Siim, J.C., 1980c. Ultrastructural observations showing enteric multiplication of *Cystoisospora* (*Isospora*) *felis* by endodyogeny. Zeitschrift für Parasitenkunde 63 (3), 289–291.

Ferreira, S.C.M., 2015. Parasite Ecology in Spotted Hyena in Serengeti National Park in Tanzania (M.S. thesis). Universidade de Lisboa, Faculdade de Medicina Vetereinária, Lisboa, Lisbon, Portugal. 58 p.

Ferreira, J.I., Pena, H.F., Azevedo, S.S., Labruna, M.B., Gennari, S.M., 2016. Occurrences of gastrointestinal parasites in fecal samples from domestic dogs in São Paulo, SP, Brazil. Revista Brasileira de Parasitologia Veterinaria 25 (4), 435–440.

Ferroglio, E., Wambwa, E., Castiello, M., Trisciuoglio, A., Prouteau, A., Pradere, E., Ndungu, S., De Meneghi, D., 2003. Antibodies to *Neospora caninum* in wild animals from Kenya, East Africa. Veterinary Parasitology 118 (1–2), 43–49.

Fichtenbaum, C.J., Ritchia, D.J., Powderly, W.G., 1993. Use of paromomycin for treatment of cryptosporidiosis in patients with AIDS. Clinical Infectious Diseases: An Official Publication of the Infectious Diseases Society of America 16 (2), 298–300.

Finch, H., 1854. Sur la physiologie de l'épithélium intestinal (On the Physiology of the Intestinal Epithelium). (Doctoral dissertation). Faculté de médecine de Strasbourg (in French). (*nos non videbo illum*, as cited in Wenyon, 1923).

Findley, J.S., 1987. The Natural History of New Mexico Mammals. University of New Mexico press, Albuquerque, NM. 164 p.

Fiori, M.G., Lowndes, H.E., 1988. Histochemical study of *Sarcocystis* sp. intramuscular cysts in gastrocnemius and soleus of the cat. Parasitology Research 75 (2), 123–131.

Fischer, G., 1979. Die Entwicklung von *Sarcocystis capracanis* n. spec. in der Ziege (The Development of *Sarcocystis capracanis* n. Spec., in the Goat). (D.V.M. thesis). Freien University, Berlin, Germany. 45 p.

Fischer, S., Odening, K., 1998. Characterization of bovine *Sarcocystis* species by analysis of their 18S ribosomal DNA sequences. Journal of Parasitology 84 (1), 50–54.

Fitzgerald, L., Bennett, M., Ng, J., Nicholls, P., James, F., Elliot, A., Slaven, M., Ryan, U., 2011. Morphological and molecular characterisation of a mixed *Cryptosporidium muris/Cryptosporidium felis* infection in a cat. Veterinary Parasitology 175 (1–2), 160–164.

Flacke, G., Spiering, P., Cooper, D., Gunther, M.S., Robertson, I., Palmer, C., Warren, K., 2010. A survey of internal parasites in free-ranging African wild dogs (*Lycaon pictus*) from KwaZulu-Natal, South Africa. South African Journal of Wildlife Research 40 (2), 176–180.

Flegr, J., 2013. Influence of latent *Toxoplasma* infection on human personality, physiology and morphology: pros and cons of the *Toxoplasma*-human model in studying the manipulation hypothesis. Journal of Experimental Biology 216, 127–133.

Fok, É., Szatmári, V., Busák, K., Rozgonyi, F., 2001. Prevalence of intestinal parasites in dogs in some urban and rural areas of Hungary. The Veterinary Quarterly 23 (2), 96–98.

Fontanarrosa, M.F., Vezzani, D., Basabe, J., Eiras, D.F., 2006. An epidemiological study of gastrointestinal parasites of dogs from Southern Greater Buenos Aires (Argentina): age, gender, breed, mixed infections, and seasonal and spatial patterns. Veterinary Parasitology 136 (3–4), 283–295.

Forest, T.W., Abou-Madi, N., Summers, B.A., Tornquist, S.J., Cooper, B.J., 2001. *Sarcocystis neurona*-like encephalitis in a Canada lynx (*Felis lynx canadensis*). Journal of Zoo and Wildlife Medicine 31 (3), 383–387.

Foreyt, W.J., Todd, A.C., 1976. Prevalence of coccidia in domestic mink in Wisconsin. Journal of Parasitology 62 (3), 496.

Forlano, M., Scofield, A., Elisei, C., Fernandes, K.R., Ewing, S.A., Massard, C.L., 2005. Diagnosis of *Hepatozoon* spp. in *Amblyomma ovale* and its experimental transmission in domestic dogs in Brazil. Veterinary Parasitology 134 (1), 1–7.

Forrester, D., 1992. Parasites and Diseases of Wild Mammals in Florida, first ed. University Press of Florida, USA. 480 p.

Foster, G.W., McCleery, R.A., Forrester, D.J., 2004. Intestinal coccidia of raccoons (*Procyon lotor*) from Key Largo, Florida, USA. Comparative Parasitology 71, 175–177.

Frank, C., 1978. Kleinsaugerprotozoen im Neusiedlerseegebiet (Small suction protozoa in Lake Neusiedl area). Anoewandte Parasitologie 19, 137–154 (in German).

Franti, C.E., Riemann, H.P., Behymer, D.E., Suther, D., Ruppanner, R., 1976. Prevalence of *Toxoplasma gondii* antibodies in wild and domestic animals in northern California. Journal of the American Veterinary Medical Association 169 (9), 901–906.

Franzen, C., Miller, A., Bailek, R., Diehl, V., Salzberger, R., Fätkenheuer, G., 2000. Taxonomic position of the human intestinal protozoan parasite *Isospora belli* as based on ribosomal RNA sequences. Parasitology Research 86 (8), 669–676.

Freitas-Girau, L.S., 2002. Estudo anátomo-patológico da toxoplasmose canina em Belo Horizonte (Anatomopathological study of canine toxoplasmosis in Belo Horizonte). Arquivos da Escola de Veterinaria da Universidade Federal de Minas Geraus 3, 482–483 (in Portuguese).

Frenkel, J.K., 1953. Infections with organisms resembling *Toxoplasma*, together with the description of a new organism *Besnoitia jellisoni*. In: Atti del VI Congresso Internazionale di Microbiologia, vol. 5, pp. 426–434.

Frenkel, J.K., 1956. Pathogenesis of toxoplasmosis and of infections with organisms resembling *Toxoplasma*. Annals of the New York Academy of Sciences 64, 215–251.

Frenkel, J.K., 1973. Toxoplasmosis: parasite life cycle, pathology, and immunology. In: Hammond, D.M., Long, P.L. (Eds.), The Coccidia. *Eimeria*, *Isospora*, *Toxoplasma*, and Related Genera. University Park Press, Baltimore, MD, USA, pp. 344–410.

Frenkel, J.K., 1974. Advances in the biology of Sporozoa. Zeitschrift für Parasitenkunde 45 (2), 125–162.

Frenkel, J.K., 1977. *Besnoitia wallacei* of cats and rodents: with a reclassification of other cyst-forming isosporoid coccidia. Journal of Parasitology 63 (4), 611–628.

Frenkel, J.K., Dubey, J.P., 1972a. Rodents as vectors for feline coccidia, *Isospora felis* and *Isospora rivolta*. The Journal of Infectious Diseases 125 (1), 69–72.

Frenkel, J.K., Dubey, J.P., 1972b. Toxoplasmosis and its prevention in cats and man. The Journal of Infectious Diseases 126 (6), 664–673.

Frenkel, J.K., Dubey, J.P., 1973. Effects of freezing on the viability of *Toxoplasma* oocysts. Journal of Parasitology 59 (3), 587–588.

Frenkel, J.K., Dubey, J.P., 1975a. *Hammondia hammondi*: a new coccidium of cats producing cysts in muscle of other mammals. Science 189 (4198), 222–224.

Frenkel, J.K., Dubey, J.P., 1975b. *Hammondia hammondi* gen. nov., sp. nov., from domestic cats, a new coccidian related to *Toxoplasma* and *Sarcocystis*. Zeitschrift für Parasitenkunde 46 (1), 3–12.

Frenkel, J.K., Smith, D.D., 2003. Determination of the genera of cyst-forming coccidia. Parasitology Research 91 (5), 384–389.

Frenkel, J.K., Sousa, O.E., 1983. Antibodies to *Toxoplasma* in panamanian mammals. Journal of Parasitology 69 (1), 244–245.

Frenkel, J.K., Dubey, J.P., Miller, N.L., 1970. *Toxoplasma gondii* in cats: fecal stages identified as coccidian oocysts. Science 167 (3919), 892–896.

Frenkel, J.K., Ruiz, A., Chinchilla, M., 1975. Soil survival of *Toxoplasma* oocysts in Kansas and Costa Rica. American Journal of Tropical Medicine and Hygiene 24 (3), 439–443.

Frenkel, J.K., Mehlhorn, H., Heydorn, A.O., 1987. Beyond the oocyst: over the molehills and mountains of coccidialand. Parasitology Today 3 (8), 250–252.

Frey, J.K., Yates, T.L., Duszynski, D.W., Gannon, W.L., Gardner, S.L., 1992. Designation and curatorial management of type host specimens (symbiotypes) for new parasite species. Journal of Parasitology 78 (5), 930–932.

Fry, M., Williams, R.B., 1984. Effects of decoquinate and clopidol on electron transport in mitochondria of *Eimeria tenella* (Apicomplexa: Coccidia). Biochemical Pharmacology 33 (2), 229–240.

Fry, D.R., McSporran, K.D., Ellis, J.T., Harvey, C., 2009. Protozoal hepatitis associated with immunosuppressive therapy in a dog. Journal of Veterinary Internal Medicine 23 (2), 366–368.

Fujii, K., Kakumoto, C., Kobayashi, M., Saito, S., Kariya, T., Watanabe, Y., Xuan, X., Igarashi, I., Suzuki, M., 2007. Seroepidemiology of *Toxoplasma gondii* and *Neospora caninum* in seals around Hokkaido, Japan. Journal of Veterinary Medical Science 69 (4), 393–398.

Fukushima, K., Helman, R.G., 1984. Cryptosporidiosis in a pup with distemper. Veterinary Pathology 21, 247–248.

Funada, M.R., Pena, H.F.J., Soares, R.M., Amaku, M., Gennari, S.M., 2007. Freqüência de parasitos gastrintestinais em cães e gatos atendidos em hospital-escola veterinário da cidade de São Paulo (Frequency of gastrointestinal parasites in dogs and cats treated at a veterinary school hospital in the city of São Paulo). Arquivo Brasileiro de Medicina Veterinária e Zootecnia 59 (5), 1338–1340 (in Portuguese, English abstract).

Furr, M., Kennedy, T., MacKay, R., Reed, S., Andrews, F., Bernard, B., Bain, F., Byars, D., 2001. Efficacy of ponazuril 15% oral paste as a treatment for equine protozoal myeloencephalitis. Veterinary Therapeutics: Research in Applied Veterinary Medicine 2 (3), 215–222.

Furr, M., McKenzie, H., Saville, W.J., Dubey, J.P., Reed, S.M., Davis, W., 2006. Prophylactic administration of ponazuril reduces clinical signs and delays seroconversion in horses challenged with *Sarcocystis neurona*. Journal of Parasitology 92 (3), 637–643.

Furtado, M.M., Metzger, B., de Almeida Jácomo, A.T., Labruna, M.B., Martins, T.F., O'Dwyer, L.H., dos Santos-Paduan, K., Porfirio, G.E.O., Silveira, L., Sollmann, R., Taniwaki, S.A., Tôrres, N.M., Neto, J.S.F., 2017. *Hepatozon* spp. infect free-ranging jaguars (*Panthera onca*) in Brazil. Journal of Parasitology 103 (3), 243–250.

Gabor, M., Gabor, L.J., Srivastava, M., Booth, M., Reece, R., 2010. Chronic myositis in an Australian alpaca (*Llama pacos*) associated with *Sarcocystis* spp. Journal of Veterinary Diagnostic Investigation 22 (6), 966–969.

Gajadhar, A.A., Marquardt, W.C., 1992. Ultrastructural and transmission evidence of *Sarcocystis cruzi* associated with eosinophilic myositis in cattle. Canadian Journal of Veterinary Research 56 (1), 41–46.

Gajadhar, A.A., Measures, L., Forbes, L.B., Kapel, C., Dubey, J.P., 2004. Experimental *Toxoplasma gondii* infection in grey seals (*Halichoerus grypus*). Journal of Parasitology 90 (2), 255–259.

Galavíz-Silva, L., Mercardo-Hernández, R., Ramírez-Bon, E., Arredondo-Cantú, J.M., Lazcano-Villarreal, D., 1991. *Sarcocystis neotomafelis* n. sp. (Protozoa: Apicomplexa) from the woodrat *Neotoma micropus* in Mexico. Revista Latinoamericana de Microbiologia 33 (4), 313–322.

Galli-Valerio, B., 1929a. Notes de parasitologie. Zentralblatt für Bakteriologie, Parasitenkunde und Infektionskrankheiten. I. Abteilung Originale 112, 54–59 (in French).

Galli-Valerio, B., 1929b. Observations et recherches sur les parasites et les maladies parasitaires des animaux sauvages (Observations and research on parasites and parasitic diseases of wildlife). Bulletin de la Murithienne 47, 50–89 (in French).

Galli-Valerio, B., 1930. Notes de parasitologie. Zentralblatt für Bakteriologie, Parasitenkunde und Infektionskrankheiten. I. Abteilung Originale 115, 212–219 (in French).

Galli-Valerio, B., 1931. Notes de parasitologie. Zentralblatt für Bakteriologie, Parasitenkunde und Infektionskrankheiten. I. Abteilung Originale 120, 98–106 (in French).

Galli-Valerio, B., 1932. Notes de parasitologie et de technique parasitologique. Zentralblatt für Bakteriologie, Parasitenkunde und Infektionskrankheiten. I. Abteilung Originale 125, 129–142 (in French).

Galli-Valerio, B., 1935. Parasitologische Untersuchungen und parasitologische Technik (Parasitological examinations and parasitological technique). Zentralblatt für Bakteriologie. I. Abteilung Originale 135, 318–327 (pn German).

Gao, S.S., Wu, S.Q., Luo, J., Wang, C.M., Zhang, M., Zhao, B.H., He, H.X., 2013. Development of an IMS-qPCR method for detection of *Cryptosporidium parvum* in water. Zhongguo Ji Sheng Chong Xue Yu Ji Sheng Chong Bing Za Zhi (Chinese Journal of Parasitology and Parasitic Diseases) 31 (3), 180–184 (in Chinese).

Garner, M.M., Barr, B.C., Packham, A.E., Marsh, A.E., Burek-Huntington, K.A., Wilson, R.K., Dubey, J.P., 1997. Fatal hepatic sarcocystosis in two polar bears (*Ursus maritimus*). Journal of Protozoology 83 (3), 523–526.

Garner, M.M., Gardiner, C.H., Wellehan, J.F.X., Johnson, A.J., McNamara, T., Linn, M., Terrell, S.P., Childress, A., Jacobson, E.R., 2006. Intranuclear coccidiosis in tortoises: nine cases. Veterinary Pathology 43, 311–320.

Gascoyne, S.C., Laurenson, M.K., Lelo, Borner, M., 1993a. Rabies in African wild dogs (*Lycaon pictus*) in the Serengeti region, Tanzania. Journal of Wildlife Diseases 29 (3), 396–402.

Gascoyne, S.C., King, A.A., Laurenson, M.K., Borner, M., Schildger, B., Barrat, J., 1993b. Aspects of rabies infection and control in the conservation of the African wild dog (Lycaon pictus) in the Serengeti Region, Tanzania. Onderstepoort Journal of Veterinary Research 60 (4), 415–420.

Gasser, R.B., Zhu, X., Caccio, S., Chalmers, R., Widmer, G., Morgan, U.M., Thompson, R.C., Pozio, E., Browning, G.F., 2001. Genotyping *Cryptosporidium parvum* by single-strand conformation polymorphism analysis of ribosomal and heat shock gene regions. Electrophoresis 22 (3), 433–437.

Gassner, F.X., 1940. Studies in canine coccidiosis. Journal of the American Veterinary Medical Association 96, 225–229.

Gatei, W., Suputtamongkol, Y., Waywa, D., Ashford, R.W., Bailey, J.W., Greensill, J., Beeching, N.J., Hart, C.A., 2002. Zoonotic species of *Cryptosporidium* are as prevalent as the anthroponotic in HIV-infected patients in Thailand. Annals of Tropical Medicine and Parasitology 96 (8), 797–802.

Gatei, W., Wamae, C.N., Mbae, C., Waruru, A., Mulinge, E., Waithera, T., Gatika, S.M., Kamwati, S.K., Revathi, G., Hart, C.A., 2006. Cryptosporidiosis: prevalence, genotype analysis, and symptoms associated with infections in children in Kenya. The American Journal of Tropical Medicine and Hygiene 75 (1), 78–82.

Gatei, W., Das, P., Dutta, P., Sen, A., Cama, V., Lal, A.A., Xiao, L., 2007. Multilocus sequence typing and genetic structure of *Cryptosporidium hominis* from children in Kolkata, India. Infection, Genetics and Evolution: Journal of Molecular Epidemiology and Evolutionary Genetics in Infectious Diseases 7 (2), 197–205.

Gatei, W., Barrett, D., Lindo, J.F., Eldemire-Shearer, D., Cama, V., Xiao, L., 2008. Unique *Cryptosporidium* population in HIV-infected persons, Jamaica. Emerging Infectious Diseases 14 (5), 841–843.

Gates, M.C., Nolan, T.J., 2009. Endoparasite prevalence and recurrence across different age groups of dogs and cats. Veterinary Parasitology 166 (1–2), 153–158.

Gatesy, J., Meredith, R.W., Janecka, J.E., Simmons, M.P., Murphy, W.J., Springer, M.S., 2016. Resolution of a concatenation/coalescence kerfuffle: partitioned coalescence support and a robust family-level tree for Mammalia. Cladistics 33, 295–332.

Gau, R.J., Kutz, S., Elkin, B.T., 1999. Parasites in grizzly bears from the Central Canadian Arctic. Journal of Wildlife Diseases 35 (3), 618–621.

Gaydos, J.K., Conrad, P.A., Gilardi, K.V.K., Blundell, G.M., Ben-David, M., 2007a. Does human proximity affect antibody prevalence in marine-foraging river otters (*Lontra canadensis*)? Journal of Wildlife Diseases 43 (1), 116–123.

Gaydos, J.K., Miller, W.A., Gilardi, K.V.K., Melli, A., Schwant, H., Engelstoft, C., Fritz, H., Conrad, P.A., 2007b. *Cryptosporidium* and *Giardia* in marine-foraging river otters (*Lotra canadensis*) from the Puget Sound Georgia basin ecosystem. Journal of Parasitology 93 (1), 198–202.

Gaydos, J.K., Miller, W.A., Johnson, C., Zornetzer, H., Melli, A., Packham, A., Jeffries, S.J., Lance, M.M., Conrad, P.A., 2008. Novel and canine genotypes of *Giardia duodenalis* in harbor seals (*Phoca vitulina richardsi*). Journal of Parasitology 94 (6), 1264–1268.

Gennari, S.M., Kasai, N., Pena, H.F.J., Cortez, A., 1999. Ocorrência de protozoários e helmintos em amostras de fezes de cães e gatos da cidade de São Paulo. Brazilian Journal of Veterinary Research and Animal Science 36 (2), 87–91 (in Portuguese).

Gerhold, R.W., Howerth, E.W., Lindsay, D.S., 2005. *Sarcocystis neurona*-associated meningoencephalitis and description of intramuscular sarcocysts in a fisher (*Martes pennanti*). Journal of Wildlife Diseases 41 (1), 224–230.

Gerhold, R.W., Newman, S.J., Grunenwald, G.M., Crews, A., Hodshon, A., Su, C., 2014. Acute onset of encephalomyelitis with atypical lesions associated with dual infection of *Sarcocystis neurona* and *Toxoplasma gondii* in a dog. Veterinary Parasitology 205 (3), 697–701.

Gestrich, R., Heydorn, A.O., Baysu, N., 1975. Beitrage zum Lebenszyklus der Sarkosporidien. VI. Berliner und Münchener Tierärztliche Wochenschrift 88, 191–197 (in German).

Ghaffar, F.A., Entzeroth, R., Chobotar, B., Scholtyseck, E., 1979. Ultrastructural studies of *Sarcocystis* sp. from the camel (*Camelus dromedarius*) in Egypt. Tropenmedicin und Parasitologie 30, 434–438.

Gharekhani, J., 2014. Study on gastrointestinal zoonotic parasites in pet dogs in western Iran. Turkiye Parazitolojii Dergisi 38 (3), 172–176.

Gherasim, A., Lebbad, M., Insulander, M., Decraene, V., Kling, A., Hjertqvist, M., Wallensten, A., 2012. Two geographically separated food-borne outbreaks in Sweden linked by an unusual *Cryptosporidium parvum* subtype, October 2010. Euro Surveillance: Bulletin Europeen sur les Maladies Transmissibles 17 (46), 20318.

Gherman, M., Mihalca, A.D., 2017. A synoptic overview of golden jackal parasites reveals high diversity of species. Parasites and Vectors 10, 419.

Giangaspero, A., Iorio, R., Paoletti, B., Traversa, D., Capelli, G., 2006. Molecular evidence for *Cryptosporidium* infection in dogs in Central Italy. Parasitology Research 99 (3), 297–299.

Giannetto, S., Poglayen, G., Brianti, E., Gaglio, G., Scala, A., 2005. *Sarcocystis gracilis*-like sarcocysts in a sheep. The Veterinary Record 156 (10), 322–323.

Giannitti, F., Diab, S.S., Uzal, F.A., Fresneda, K., Rossi, D., Talmi-Frank, D., Baneth, G., 2012. Infection with a *Hepatozoon* sp. closely related to *Hepatozoon felis* in a wild Pampas gray fox (*Lycalopex – Pseudalopex – gymnocercus*) co-infected with canine distemper virus. Veterinary Parasitology 186 (3), 497–502.

Gibson, A.K., Raverty, S., Lambourn, D.M., Huggins, J., Margagal, S.L., Grigg, M.E., 2011. Polyparasitism is associated with increased disease severity in *Toxoplasma gondii*-infected marine sentinel species. PLoS Neglected Tropical Diseases 5 (5), e1142.

Gil, H., Cano, L., de Lucio, A., Bailo, B., de Mingo, M.H., Cardona, G.A., Fernández-Basterra, J.A., Aramburu-Aguirre, J., López-Molina, N., Carmena, D., 2017. Detection and molecular diversity of *Giardia duodenalis* and *Cryptosporidium* spp. in sheltered dogs and cats in Northern Spain. Infection, Genetics and Evolution 50, 62–69.

Gilioli, R., Silva, F.A., 2000. Freqüência de parasitas e infecção por *Salmonella* em lobos uará, *Chrysocyon brachyurus*, mantidos em zoológicos no Estado de São Paulo (Frequency of parasites and *Salmonella* infection in captive maned-wolf, *Chrysocyon brachyurus*, kept in zoos at the State of São Paulo, Brazil). Arquivo Brasileiro de Medicina Veterinária e Zootecnia 52 (4), 337–341 (in Portuguese).

Gill, H.S., Singh, A., Vadehra, V., Sethi, S.K., 1978. Shedding of unsporulated isosporan oocysts in feces by dogs fed diaphragm muscles from water buffalo (*Bubalus bubalis*) naturally infected with Sarcocystis. Journal of Parasitology 64 (3), 549–551.

Gillis, K.D., MacKay, R.J., Yowell, C.A., Levy, J.K., Greiner, E.C., Dame, J.B., Cheadle, M.A., Hernandez, J., Massey, E.T., 2003. Naturally occurring *Sarcocystis* infection in domestic cats (*Felis catus*). International Journal for Parasitology 33 (8), 877–883.

Gingrich, E.N., Scorza, A.V., Clifford, E.L., Olea-Popelka, F.J., Lappin, M.R., 2010. Intestinal parasites of dogs on the Galápagos Islands. Veterinary Parasitology 169 (3–4), 404–407.

Girard, Y.A., Johnson, C.K., Fritz, H.M., Shapiro, K., Packham, A.E., Melli, A.C., Carlson-Bremer, D., Gulland, F.M., Rejmanek, D., Conrad, P.A., 2016. Detection and characterization of diverse coccidian protozoa shed by California sea lions. International Journal for Parasitology. Parasites and Wildlife 5 (1), 5–16.

Gjerde, B., 1984a. A light microscopic comparison of the cysts of four species of *Sarcocystis* infecting domestic reindeer (*Rangifer tarandus*) in northern Norway. Acta Veterinaria Scandinavica 25 (3), 195–204.

Gjerde, B., 1984b. *Sarcocystis hardangeri* and *Sarcocystis rangi* n. sp. from the domestic reindeer (*Rangifer tarandus*) in northern Norway. Acta Veterinaria Scandinavica 25 (3), 411–418.

Gjerde, B., 1984c. *Sarcocystis* infection in wild reindeer (*Rangifer tarandus*) from Hardangervidda in southern Norway: with description of the cysts of *Sarcocystis hardangeri* n. sp. Acta Veterinaria Scandinavica 25 (3), 205–212.

Gjerde, B., 1984d. The fox as a definitive host for *Sarcocystis* sp. Gjerde, 1984 from skeletal muscle of reindeer (*Rangifer tarandus*) with a proposal for *Sarcocystis tarandivulpes* n. sp. as replacement name. Acta Veterinaria Scandinavica 25, 403–410.

Gjerde, B., 1984e. The raccoon dog (*Nyctereutes procyonoides*) as definitive host for *Sarcocystis* spp. of reindeer (*Rangifer tarandus*). Acta Veterinaria Scandinavica 25 (3), 419–424.

Gjerde, B., 1985a. The fox as a definitive host for *Sarcocystis rangi* from reindeer (*Rangifer tarandus tarandus*). Acta Veterinaria Scandinavica 26 (1), 140–142.

Gjerde, B., 1985b. Ultrastructure of the cysts of *Sarcocystis grueneri* from cardiac muscle of reindeer (*Rangifer tarandus tarandus*). Zeitschrift für Parasitenkunde 71 (1), 189–198.

Gjerde, B., 1985c. Ultrastructure of the cysts of *Sarcocystis hardangeri* from skeletal muscle of reindeer (*Rangifer tarandus tarandus*). Canadian Journal of Zoology 63 (11), 2676–2683.

Gjerde, B., 1986. Scanning electron microscopy of the sarcocysts of six species of *Sarcocystis* from reindeer (*Rangifer tarandus tarandus*). Acta Pathologica, Microbiologica, et Immunologica 94 (1–6), 309–317.

Gjerde, B., 2012. Morphological and molecular characterization and phylogenetic placement of *Sarcocystis capreolicanis* and *Sarcocystis silva* n. sp. from roe deer (*Capreolus capreolus*) in Norway. Parasitology Research 110 (3), 1225–1237.

Gjerde, B., 2013. Phylogenetic relationships among *Sarcocystis* species in cervids, cattle and sheep inferred from the mitochondrial cytochrome c oxidase subunit I gene. International Journal for Parasitology 43 (7), 579–591.

Gjerde, B., 2014a. Molecular characterisation of *Sarcocystis rileyi* from a common eider (*Somateria mollissima*) in Norway. Parasitology Research 113 (9), 3501–3509.

Gjerde, B., 2014b. Morphological and molecular characteristics of four *Sarcocystis* spp. in Canadian moose (*Alces alces*), including *Sarcocystis taeniata* n. sp. Parasitology Research 113 (4), 1591–1604.

Gjerde, B., 2014c. *Sarcocystis* species in the red deer revisited: with a redescription of two known species as *Sarcocystis elongata* n. sp. and *Sarcocystis truncata* n. sp. based on mitochondrial cox1 sequences. Parasitology 141 (3), 441–452.

Gjerde, B., 2016a. The resurrection of a species: *Sarcocystis bovifelis* Heydorn et al., 1975 is distinct from the current *Sarcocystis hirsuta* in cattle and morphologically indistinguishable from *Sarcocystis sinensis* in water buffaloes. Parasitology Research 115 (1), 1–21.

Gjerde, B., 2016b. Molecular characteristics of *Sarcocystis bovifelis*, *Sarcocystis bovini* n. sp., *Sarcocystis hirsuta* and *Sarcocystis cruzi* from cattle (*Bos taurus*) and *Sarcocystis sinensis* from water buffaloes (*Bubalus bubalis*). Parasitology Research 115 (4), 1473–1492.

Gjerde, B., Bratberg, B., 1984. The domestic reindeer (*Rangifer tarandus*) from northern Norway as interemediate host for three species of *Sarcocystis*. Acta Veterinaria Scandinavica 25 (1), 187–194.

Gjerde, G., Dahlgren, S.S., 2011. *Hammondia triffittae* n. comb. of foxes (*Vulpes* spp.): biological and molecular characteristics and differentiation from *Hammondia heydorni* of dogs. Parasitology 138 (3), 303–321.

Gjerde, B., Josefsen, T.D., 2015. Molecular characterisation of *Sarcocystis lutrae* n. sp. and *Toxoplasma gondii* from the musculature of two Eurasian otters (*Lutra lutra*) in Norway. Parasitology Research 114 (3), 873–886.

Gjerde, B., Schulze, J., 2014. Muscular sarcocystosis in two arctic foxes (*Vulpes lagopus*) due to *Sarcocystis arctica* n. sp.: sarcocyst morphology, molecular characteristics and phylogeny. Parasitology Research 113 (3), 811–821.

Gjerde, B., Giacomelli, S., Bianchi, A., Bertoletti, I., Mondani, H., Gibelli, L.R., 2017. Morphological and molecular characteriztion of four *Sarcocystis* spp. including *Sarcocystis linearis* n. sp., from roe deer (*Capreolus capreolus*) in Italy. Parasitology Research 116 (4), 1317–1338.

Glebezdin, V.S., 1978. About coccidia fauna of wild mammals of south-western Turkmenistan. Izvestia Akademii Nauk Turkmenskoi SSR, Seria Biologicheskich Nauk (Academy of Sciences of Turkmenistan, SSR, Biology Series) 3, 71–78 (in Russian).

Göbel, E., 1976. Elektronenmikroskopische Untersuchungen zur Feinstrukter der Zystenstadien von Pferdesarkosporidien (*Sarcocystis equicanis*). Zeitschrift für Parasitenkunde 50, 201.

Goh, S., Reacher, M., Casemore, D.P., Verlander, N.Q., Chalmers, R., Knowles, M., Williams, J., Osborn, K., Richards, S., 2004. Sporadic cryptosporidiosis, North Cumbria, England, 1996–2000. Emerging Infectious Diseases 10 (6), 1007–1015.

Golemansky, V., 1975a. *Eimeria li* nov. sp. et *Klossia* sp. (Protozoa: Coccidia) trouvés dans le gros intestin du renard cummun (*Vulpes vulpes* L.) en Bulgarie. Zoologischer Anzeiger, Jena 194 (1–2), 133–139 (in French, English summary).

Golemansky, V., 1975b. Observations des oocystes et des spores libres de *Sarcocystis* sp. (Protozoa: coccidia) dans le gros intestin du renard commun (*Vulpes vulpes* L.) en Bulgarie (Observation of the oocysts and free spores of *Sarcocystis* sp. (Protozoa: Coccidia) in the large intestine of the fox (*Vulpes vulpes* L.) in Bulgaria). Acta Protozoologica (Warszawa) 14 (3–4), 291–296 (in French, English summary).

Golemansky, V.G., 1986. Coccidia of game animals in Bulgaria. Symposium Biologica Hungarica 33, 357–361.

Golemansky, V., Ridzhakov, N., 1975. V'rkho koktsidite (Protozoa, Coccidia) na lisitsite v B'lgariya (On coccidia (Protozoa, Coccidia) in the foxes in Bulgaria). Acta Zoologica Bulgarica 3 (1), 3–18 (in Russian, English summary).

Golubkov, I.A., 1979. Zarazhenie sobak i koshek sarcotsistami ot kur i vtok (Infection of dogs and cats with sarcocysts from chickens and ducks). Veterinariya Moscow 1979 (1), 35–36 (in Russian).

Golubkov, V.I., Rybaltovskii, O.V., Kislyakova, Z.I., 1974. Plotoyadnye-istochnik zarasheniya svinei sarkotsistami (Carnivores – source of infection of swine with sarcocysts). Veterinariya 11, 85–86 (in Russian).

Gómez-Couso, H., Méndez-Hermida, F., Ares-Mazás, E., 2007. First report of *Cryptosporidium parvum* 'ferret' genotype in American mink (*Mustela vison* Schreber 1777). Parasitology Research 100 (4), 877–879.

Gómez-Villamandos, J.C., Carrasco, L., Mozos, E., Hervás, J., 1995. Fatal cryptosporidiosis in ferrets (*Mustela putorius furo*): a morphopathologic study. Journal of Zoo and Wildlife Medicine 26 (4), 539–544.

Gompper, M.E., Goodman, R.M., Kays, R.W., Ray, J.C., Fiorello, C.V., 2003. A survey of the parasites of coyotes (*Canis latrans*) in New York based on fecal analysis. Journal of Wildlife Diseases 39 (3), 712–717.

Gondim, L.F.P., 2006. *Neospora caninum* in wildlife. Trends in Parasitology 22 (6), 247–251.

Gondim, L.F.P., McAllister, M.M., Mateus-Pinilla, N.E., Pitt, W.C., Mech, L.D., Nelson, M.E., 2004a. Transmission of *Neospora caninum* between wild and domestic animals. Journal of Parasitology 90 (6), 1361–1365.

Gondim, L.F.P., McAllister, M.M., Pitt, W.C., Zemlicka, D.E., 2004b. Coyotes (*Canis latrans*) are definitive hosts of *Neospora caninum*. International Journal for Parasitology 34 (2), 159–161.

González-Díaz, M., Urrea-Quezada, A., Villegas-Gómez, I., Durazo, M., Garibay-Escobar, A., Hernández, J., Xiao, L., Valenzuela, O., 2016. *Cryptosporidium canis* in two Mexican toddlers. The Pediatric Infectious Disease Journal 35 (11), 1265–1266.

Goodrich, H.P., 1944. Coccidian oocysts. Parasitology 36 (1–2), 72–79.

Goodwin, M.A., Barsanti, J.A., 1990. Intractable diarrhea associated with intestinal cryptosporidiosis in a domestic cat also infected with feline leukemia virus. Journal of the American Animal Hospital Association 26, 365–368.

Gookin, J.L., Riviere, J.E., Gilger, B.C., Papich, M.G., 1999. Acute renal failure in four cats treated with paromomycin. Journal of the American Veterinary Medical Association 215 (12), 1821–1823.

Gookin, J.L., Levy, M.G., Law, J.M., Papich, M.G., Poore, M.F., Breitschwerdt, E.B., 2001. Experimental infection of cats with *Tritrichomonas foetus*. American Journal of Veterinary Research 62 (11), 1690–1697.

Gorman, T.R., Alcaíno, H.A., Muñoz, H., Cunazza, C., 1984. *Sarcocystis* sp. in guanaco (*Lama guanicoe*) and effect of temperature on its viability. Veterinary Parasitology 15 (2), 95–101.

Gothe, R., Reichler, I., 1990. Spectrum of species and infection frequency of endoparasites in bitches and their puppies in south Germany. Tierärztliche Praxis 18 (1), 61–64.

Gottstein, B., Eperon, S., Dai, W.J., Cannas, A., Hemphill, A., Greif, G., 2001. Efficacy of toltrazuril and ponazuril against experimental *Neospora caninum* infection in mice. Parasitology Research 87 (1), 43–48.

Gottstein, B., Razmi, G.R., Ammann, P., Sager, H., Müller, N., 2005. Toltrazuril treatment to control diaplacental *Neospora caninum* transmission in experimentally infected pregnant mice. Parasitology 130 (Pt1), 41–48.

Gousseff, W.F., 1933. Zur Frage der Coccidien der Füchse in Transkaukasien (On the question of coccidia of foxes in Transcaucasia). Archiv für Wissenschaftliche und Praktische Tierheilkunde 66, 424–428 (in German).

Gräfner, G., Graubmann, H.-D., Dobbriner, W., 1967. Leberkokzidiose beim Nerz (*Lutreola vison* Schreb.), hervorgrufen durch eine neue Kokzidienart, *Eimeria hiepei* n. sp. Monatshefte für Veterinärmedizin 22, 696–700 (in German).

Grassi, B., 1879. Dei protozoi parassiti e specialmente di quelli che sono nell'uomo (Protozoan parasites and especially those that are in humans). Gazzetta Medica Italiana 39, 445–448 (in Italian).

Greig, D.J., Gulland, F.M.D., Smith, W.A., Conrad, P.A., Field, C.L., Fleetwood, M., Harvey, J.T., Ip, H.S., Jang, S., Packham, A., Wheeler, E., Hall, A.J., 2014. Surveillance for zoonotic and selected pathogens in harbor seals *Phoca vitulina* from central California. Diseases of Aquatic Organisms 111 (2), 93–106.

Greiner, E.C., Roelke, M.E., Atkinson, C.T., Dubey, J.P., Wright, S.D., 1989. *Sarcocystis* sp. in muscles of free-ranging Florida panthers and cougars (*Felis concolor*). Journal of Wildlife Diseases 25 (4), 623–628.

Grikienienė, J., 1993. New experimental data on development cycle of sarcosporidians (Sarcosporidia) of rodents. Ekologija 1, 33–46.

Grikienienė, J., Arnastauskienė, T., 1992. On the possibility of the development of bank vole parasite *Sarcocystis* sp. in the organism of other intermediate hosts, avoiding the definitive host. Ekologija 1, 48–58.

Grikienienė, J., Kutkienė, L., 1998. New experimental data on the laboratory rat as a definitive host of *Sarcocystis rodentifelis*. Acta Zoologica Lituanica Parasitologia 8 (1), 121–124.

Grikienienė, J., Arnastauskienė, T., Kutkienė, L., 1993. On some disregarded ways of sarcosporidians' circulation and remarks about systematics of the genus *Sarcocystis* Lankester, 1882 with the description of the new species from rodents. Ekologija 1, 16–24.

Grüner, S.A., 1927. Sarcosporidiosis in reindeer. Veterinarnyi Truzhenik 3 (9), 27–30 (in Russian).

Gu, Y.F., Wang, K., Liu, D.Y., Mei, N., Chen, C., Chen, T., Han, M.M., Zhou, L., Cao, J.T., Zhang, H., Zhang, X.L., Fan, Z.L., Li, W.C., 2015. Molecular detection of *Giardia lamblia* and *Cryptosporidium* species in pet dogs. Chinese Journal of Parasitology and Parasitic Diseases 33 (5), 362–367.

Guillebeau, A., 1916. Parasitisches Vorkommen von *Eimeria stiedae* in der Leber des Hundes (Parasitic occurrence of *Eimeria stiedae* in the liver of a dog). Archiv für Tierheilkunde Bd 58, 596 (in German).

Guo, P.F., Chen, T.T., Tsaihong, J.C., Ho, G.D., Cheng, P.C., Tseng, Y.C., Peng, S.Y., 2014. Prevalence and species identification of *Cryptosporidium* from fecal samples of horses in Taiwan. The Southeast Asian Journal of Tropical Medicine and Public Health 45 (1), 6–12.

Guterbock, W.M., Levine, N.D., 1977. Coccidia and intestinal nematodes of east central Illinois cats. Journal of the American Veterinary Medical Association 170 (12), 1411–1413.

Gutiérrez, F., Arcay, L., 1987. Cultivo de *Cystoisospora felis* Frenkel, 1977 (*Isospora felis* Wasielewski, 1904, Wenyon, 1923) in la membrana corioalantoidea de embrion de pollo. Acta Cientifica Venezolana 38, 474–483 (in Spanish, English summary).

Guyot, K., Follet-Dumoulin, A., Lelièvre, E., Sarfati, C., Rabodonirina, M., Nevez, G., Cailliez, J.C., Camus, D., Dei-Cas, E., 2001. Molecular characterization of *Cryptosporidium* isolates obtained from humans in France. Journal of Clinical Microbiology 39 (10), 3472–3480.

Guyot, K., Follet-Dumoulin, A., Recourt, C., Lelièvre, E., Cailliez, J.C., Dei-Cas, E., 2002. PCR-restriction fragment length polymorphism analysis of a diagnostic 452-base-pair DNA fragment discriminates between *Cryptosporidium parvum* and *C. meleagridis* and between *C. parvum* isolates of human and animal origin. Applied and Environmental Microbiology 68 (4), 2071–2076.

Haberkorn, A., Stoltefuss, J., 1987. Studies on the activity spectrum of toltrazuril, a new anti-coccidial agent. Veterinary Medicine Review 1, 22–32.

Hackett, T., Lappin, M.R., 2003. Prevalence of enteric pathogens in dogs of north-central Colorado. Journal of the American Animal Hospital Association 39 (1), 52–56.

Hadwen, S., 1922. Cyst-forming protozoa in reindeer and caribou and a sarcosporidean parasite of the seal (*Phoca richardi*). Journal of the American Veterinary Medical Association 61, 282–374.

Haerdi, C., Haessig, M., Sager, H., Greif, G., Staubli, D., Gottstein, B., 2006. Humoral immune reaction of newborn calves congenitally infected with *Neospora caninum* and experimentally treated with toltrazuril. Parasitology Research 99 (5), 534–540.

Hair, J.D., Mahrt, J.L., 1970. *Eimeria albertensis* n.sp. and *E. borealis* n.sp. (Sporozoa: Eimeriidae) in black bears *Ursus americanus* from Alberta. Journal of Protozoology 17 (4), 663–664.

Hajdušek, O., Ditrich, O., Šlapeta, J., 2004. Molecular identification of *Cryptosporidium* spp. in animal and human hosts from the Czech Republic. Veterinary Parasitology 122 (3), 183–192.

Hall, M.C., Wigdor, M., 1918. Canine coccidiosis, with a note regarding other protozoan parasites from the dog. Journal of the American Veterinary Medical Association 53, 64–76.

Hamilton, C.M., Gray, R., Wright, S.E., Gangadharan, B., Laurenson, K., Innes, E.A., 2005. Prevalence of antibodies to *Toxoplasma gondii* and *Neospora caninum* in red foxes (*Vulpes vulpes*) from around the UK. Veterinary Parasitology 130 (1), 169–173.

Hamnes, I.S., Gjerde, B.K., Forberg, T., Robertson, L.J., 2007a. Occurrence of *Giardia* and *Cryptosporidium* in Norwegian red foxes (*Vulpes vulpes*). Veterinary Parasitology 143 (3), 347–353.

Hamnes, I.S., Gjerde, B.K., Robertson, L.J., 2007b. A longitudinal study on the occurrence of *Cryptosporidium* and *Giardia* in dogs during their first year of life. Acta Veterinaria Scandinavica 49, 22.

von Hänichen, T., Geyer, C., Hegel, G., 1991. Plazentitis durch *Toxoplasma gondii* als Ursache von perinatalem Tod bei einem Südamerikanischen Zwergseebären (*Arctocephalus australis*) (*Toxoplasma gondii* placentitis as a cause of perinatal death in a South American dwarf (*Arctocephalus australis*)). Erkrankungen der Zootiere: Verhandlungsbericht des Internationalen Symposiums über die Erkrankungen der Zoo-und Wildtiere 1991, 33–38 (in German, English summary).

Haralabidis, S.T., Papazachariadou, M.G., Koutinas, A.F., Rallis, T.S., 1988. A survey on the prevalence of gastrointestinal parasites of dogs in the area of Thessaloniki, Greece. Journal of Helminthology 62 (1), 45–49.

Harder, A., Haberkorn, A., 1989. Possible mode of action of toltrazuril: studies on two *Eimeria* species and mammalian and *Ascaris suum* enzymes. Parasitology Research 76 (1), 8–12.

Harp, J.A., Goff, J.G., 1998. Strategies for the control of *Cryptosporidium parvum* infection in calves. Journal of Dairy Science 81 (1), 289–294.

Harp, J.A., Woodmansee, D.B., Moon, H.W., 1989. Effect of colostral antibody on susceptibility of calves to *Cryptosporidium parvum* infection. American Journal Research 50 (12), 2117–2119.

Hawkins, C.E., Racey, P.A., 2005. Low population density of a tropical forest carnivore, *Cryptoprocta ferrox*: implications for protected area management. Oryx 39 (1), 35–43.

Head, K.W., 1959. Diseases of mink. Veterinary Record 71, 1025–1032.

Healey, M.C., Yang, S., Rasmussen, K.R., Jackson, M.K., Du, C., 1995. Therapeutic efficacy of paromomycin in immunosuppressed adult mice infected with *Cryptosporidium parvum*. Journal of Parasitology 81 (1), 114–116.

Hedges, S.B., Dudley, J., Kumar, S., 2006. TimeTree: a public knowledge-base of divergence times among organisms. Bioinformatics 22 (23), 2971–2972.

Hedges, S.B., Marin, J., Suleski, M., Paymer, M., Kumar, S., 2015. Tree of life reveals clock-like speciation and diversification. Molecular Biology and Evolution 32 (4), 835–845.

Heine, J., 1981. Die tryptische Organverdauung als Methode zum Nachweis extraintestinaler Stadien bei *Cystoisospora* spp. Infektionen (The tryptic digestion as a method for demonstration of extraintestinal stages in *Cryptosporidium* spp. infections). Berliner und Münchener Tierärztliche Wochenschrift 94, 103–104 (in German, English summary).

Hendricks, L.D., 1974. A redescription of *Isospora arctopitheci* Rodhain, 1933 (Protozoa: Eimeriidae) from primates of Panama. Proceedings of the Helminthological Society of Washington 41, 229–233.

Hendricks, L.D., 1977. Host range characteristics of the primate coccidian, *Isospora arctopitheci* Rodhain, 1933 (Protozoa: Eimeriidae). Journal of Parasitology 63 (1), 32–35.

Hendricks, L.D., Walton, B.C., 1974. Vertebrate intermediate hosts in the life cycle of an isosporan from a non-human primate. Proceedings of the International Congress of Parasitology 1, 96–97.

Hendricks, L.D., Ernst, J.V., Courtney, C.H., Speer, C.A., 1979. *Hammondia pardalis* sp. n. (Sarcocystidae) from the ocelot, *Felis pardalis*, and experimental infection of other felines. Journal of Protozoology 26 (1), 39–43.

Henry, A., 1913. Le travail de M.M. Besnoit et Robin (The work of M.M. Besnoit and Robin). Également communique a la Société des Sciences Vétérinaires de Lyon (Séance du 17 Novembre 1912). Revue Médicine Vétérinaire 90 (9), 328 (in French).

Hermosilla, C., Silva, L.M., Navarro, M., Taubert, A., 2016. Anthropozoonotic endoparasites in free-ranging "urban" South American sea lions (*Otaria flavescens*). Journal of Veterinary Medicine:7507145 7 p.

Hermosilla, C., Kleinertz, S., Silva, L.M., Hirzmann, J., Huber, D., Kusak, J., Taubert, A., 2017. Protozoan and helminth parasite fauna of free-living Croatian wild wolves (*Canis lupus*) analyzed by scat collection. Veterinary Parasitology 233, 14–19.

Hernández-Rodriguez, S., Martinez-Gómez, F., Navarrete, I., Acosta-Garcia, I., 1981. Estudio al microscopio optico y electronico del quiste de *Sarcocystis cervicanis*. Revista Ibérica de Parasitologia 41 (3), 351–361 (in Spanish, English summary).

Herrmann, D.C., Wibbelt, G., Götz, M., Conraths, F.J., Schares, G., 2013. Genetic characterization of *Toxoplasma gondii* isolates from European beavers (*Castor fiber*) and European wildcats (*Felis silvestris silvestris*). Veterinary Parasitology 191 (1–2), 108–111.

Heuer, C., Nicholson, C., Russel, D., Weston, J., 2004. Field study in dairy cattle from New Zealand. Veterinary Parasitology 125, 137–146.

Heydorn, A.O., 1973. Zum Lebenszyklus der kleinen Form von *Isospora bigemina* des Hundes I. Rind und Hund als mögliche Zwischenwirte (To the life cycle of the small form of *Isospora bigemina* of the dog I. Cattle and the dog as possible intermediate hosts). Berliner und Münchener Tierärztliche Wochenschrift 86, 323–329 (in German).

Heydorn, A.O., 1985. Zur Entwicklung von *Sarcocystis arieticanis* n. sp. (On the development of *Sarcocystis arieticanis* n. sp.). Berliner und Münchener Tierärztliche Wochenschrift 98, 231–241.

Heydorn, A.O., Haralambidis, S., 1982. Zur Entwicklung von *Sarcocystis capracanis* Fischer, 1979 (On the development of *Sarcocystis capracanis* Fisher, 1979). Berliner und Münchener Tierärztliche Wochenschrift 95 (14), 265–271 (in German, English summary).

Heydorn, A.O., Karaer, Z., 1986. Zur schizogonie von *Sarcocystis ovicanis* (On the schizogony of *Sarcocystis ovicanis*). Berliner und Münchener Tierärztliche Wochenschrift 99, 185–189 (in German, English summary).

Heydorn, A.O., Mehlhorn, H., 1987. Fine structure of *Sarcocystis arieticanis* Heydorn, 1985 in its intermediate and final hosts (sheep and dog). Zentralblatt für Bakteriologie, Mikrobiologie und Hygiene. I. Abteilung Originale Reihe A: Medizinische Mikrobiologie, Infektionskrankheiten und Parasitologie 264 (3–4), 353–362.

Heydorn, A.O., Mehlhorn, H., 2002. *Neospora caninum* is an invalid species name: an evaluation of facts and statements. Parasitology Research 88 (2), 175–184.

Heydorn, A.O., Rommel, M., 1972. Beiträge zum Lebenszyklus der Sarkosporidien. II. Hund und Katze als Überträger der Sarkosporidien des Rindes (Contributions to the life cycle of sarcosporidia II. Dog and cat as transmitters of cattle sarcosporidia). Berliner und Münchener Tierärztliche Wochenschrift 85, 121–123 (in German).

Heydorn, A.O., Unterholzner, J., 1983. Zur Entwicklung von *Sarcocystis hircicanus* sp. n. (For the development of *Sarcocystis hircicanis* sp. n.). Berliner und Münchener Tierärztliche Wochenschrift 96, 276–282 (in German).

Heydorn, A.O., Mehlhorn, G., Gestrich, R., 1975a. Licht- und elektronenmikroskopische Untersuchungen an Cysten von *Sarcocystis fusiformis* in der Muskulatur von Kälbern nach experimenteller Infektion mit Oocysten und Sporocysten der großen Form von *Isospora bigemina* des Hundes. 2. Die Feinstruktur der Cystenstadien. Zentralblatt für Bakteriologie, Parasitenkunde, Infektionskrankheiten und Hygiene, I. Abteilung Originale Reihe A: Medizinische Mikrobiologie und Parasitologie 233, 123–137 (in German).

Heydorn, A.O., Gestrich, R., Mehlhorn, H., Rommel, M., 1975b. Proposal for a new nomenclature of the Sarcosporidia. Zeitschrift für Parasitenkunde 48 (2), 73–82.

Heydorn, A.O., Gestrich, R., Ipczynski, V., 1975c. Zum Lebenszyklus der kleinen Form von *Isospora bigemina* des Hundes. II. Entwicklungsstadien im Darm des Hundes. Berliner und Münchener Tierärztliche Wochenschrift 88, 449–453 (in German).

Hijjawi, N., Ng, J., Yang, R., Atoum, M.F., Ryan, U., 2010. Identification of rare and novel *Cryptosporidium* GP60 subtypes in human isolates from Jordan. Experimental Parasitology 125 (2), 161–164.

Hilali, M., Mohamed, A., 1980. The dog (*Canis familiaris*) as the final host of *Sarcocystis cameli* (Mason, 1910). Tropenmedizin und Parasitologie 31 (2), 213–214.

Hilali, M., Nassar, A.M., El-Ghaysh, A., 1992. Camel (*Camelus dromedarius*) and sheep (*Ovis aries*) meat as a source of dog infection with some coccidian parasites. Veterinary Parasitology 43 (1), 37–43.

Hill, J.E., Chapman, W.L., Prestwood, A.K., 1988. Intramuscular *Sarcocystis* sp. in two cats and a dog. Journal of Parasitology 74 (4), 724–727.

Hill, D.E., Liddell, S., Jenkins, M.C., Dubey, J.P., 2001. Specific detection of *Neospora caninum* oocysts in fecal samples from experimentally-infected dogs using the polymerase chain reaction. Journal of Parasitology 87 (2), 395–398.

Himsworth, C.G., Skinner, S., Chaban, B., Jenkins, E., Wagner, B.A., Harms, N.J., Leighton, F.A., Thompson, R.C., Hill, J.E., 2010. Multiple zoonotic pathogens identified in canine feces collected from a remote Canadian indigenous community. The American Journal of Tropical Medicine and Hygiene 83 (2), 338–341.

Hindsbo, O., Andreassen, A., Nielsen, F., 1991. Age related prevalence of coccidia in Danish farmed foxes. Scientifur 15 (3), 245–248.

Hindsbo, O., Andreassen, J., Nielsen, F., Lodal, J., 1995. Occurrence of the coccidia *Isospora laidlawi* and *Eimeria vison* in Danish farm mink, 1987–1993; Age related resistance to infection. Scientifur 19, 231–237.

Hinney, B., Ederer, C., Stengl, C., Wilding, K., Štrkolcová, G., Harl, J., Flechl, E., Fuehrer, H.P., Joachim, A., 2015. Enteric protozoa of cats and their zoonotic potential – a field study of Austria. Parasitology Research 114 (5), 2003–2006.

Hitchcock, D.J., 1955. The life cycle of *Isospora felis* in the kitten. Journal of Parasitology 41 (4), 383–397.

Hoare, C.A., 1927. On the coccidia of the ferret. Annals of Tropical Medicine and Parasitology 21, 313–321.

Hoare, C.A., 1928. On the coccidia of the ferret. Jahresbericht Veterinär Medizin (Berlin) 47, 1066.

Hoare, C.A., 1935a. A histological reaction of a special type on the part of the intestinal villi in ferret coccidiosis. Transactions of the Royal Society of Tropical Medicine and Hygiene 29, 2–3.

Hoare, C.A., 1935b. The endogenous development of the coccidia of the ferret, and the histopathological reaction of the infected intestinal wall. Annals of Tropical Medicine and Parasitology 29, 111–123.

Hobbs, R.P., Twigg, L.E., Elliot, A.D., Wheeler, A.G., 1999. Factors influencing the faecal egg and oocyst counts of parasites of wild European rabbits *Oryctolagus cuniculus* (L.) in southern western Australia. Journal of Parasitology 85 (5), 796–802.

Holsback, L., Cardoso, M.J., Fagnani, R., Patelli, T.H., 2013. Natural infection by endoparasites among free-living wild animals. Revista Brasileira de Parasitologia Veterinaria 22 (2), 302–306.

Holshuh, H.J., Sherrod, A.E., Taylor, C.R., Andrews, B.F., Howard, E.B., 1985. Toxoplasmosis in a feral northern fur seal. Journal of the American Veterinary Medical Association 187 (11), 1229–1230.

Homem, C.G., Nakamura, A.A., Silva, D.C., Teixeira, W.F., Coelho, W.M., Meireles, M.V., 2012. Real-time PCR assay targeting the actin gene for the detection of *Cryptosporidium parvum* in calf fecal samples. Parasitology Research 110 (5), 1741–1745.

Hong, C.B., Giles Jr., R.C., Newman, L.E., Fayer, R., 1982. Sarcocystosis in an aborted bovine fetus. Journal of the American Veterinary Medical Association 181 (6), 585.

Honnold, S.P., Braun, R., Scott, D.P., Sreekumar, C., Dubey, J.P., 2005. Toxoplasmosis in a Hawaiian Monk seal (*Monachus schauinslandi*). Journal of Parasitology 91 (3), 695–697.

Hoopes, J.H., Polley, L., Wagner, B., Jenkins, E.J., 2013. A retrospective investigation of feline gastrointestinal parasites in western Canada. The Canadian Veterinary Journal 54 (4), 359–362.

Hoopes, J., Hill, J.E., Polley, L., Fernando, C., Wagner, B., Schurer, J., Jenkins, E., 2015. Enteric parasites of free-roaming, owned, and rural cats in prairie regions of Canada. The Canadian Veterinary Journal 56 (5), 495–501.

Hoskins, J., Malone, J., Smith, P., 1982. Prevalence of parasitism diagnosed by fecal examination in Louisiana dogs. American Journal of Veterinary Research 43 (6), 1106–1109.

Hou, Z., Hia, Y., Liu, J., Zeng, X., Chai, H., Sun, Y., Liu, D., Xia, X., 2008. Discovery of *Isospora* from *Panthera tigris altaica*. Acta Theriologica Sinica 28 (1), 96–100.

Houk, A.E., Rosypal, A.C., Grant, D.C., Dubey, J.P., Zajac, A.M., Yabsley, M.J., Lindsay, D.S., 2011. Serological response of cats to experimental *Besnoitia darlingi* and *Besnoitia heotomofelis* infections and prevalence of antibodies to these parasites in cats from Virginia and Pennsylvania. Journal of Parasitology 97 (2), 259–261.

Houk, A.E., O'Connor, T., Pena, H.F.J., Gennari, S.M., Zajac, A.M., Lindsay, D.S., 2013. Experimentally induced clinical *Cystoisospora canis* coccidiosis in dogs with prior natural patent *Cystoisospora ohioensis*-like or *C. canis* infections. Journal of Parasitology 99 (5), 892–895.

House, P.K., Vyas, A., Sapolsky, R., 2011. Predator cat odors activate sexual arousal pathways in brains of *Toxoplasma gondii* infected rats. PLoS One 6 (8), e23277.

Hsu, C.K., Melby, E.C., Altman, N.H., 1974a. *Eimeria phocae* n. sp. from the harbor seal (*Phoca vitulina concolor*). Journal of Parasitology 60 (3), 399–402.

Hsu, C.K., Melby, E.C., Altman, N.H., Burek, J.D., 1974b. Coccidiosis in harbor seals. Journal of the American Veterinary Medical Association 164 (7), 700–702.

Hu, J.-J., Liao, J.Y., Meng, Y., Guo, Y.M., Chen, X.W., Zuo, Y.X., 2011. Identification of *Sarcocystis cymruensis* in wild *Rattus flavipectus* and *Rattus norvegicus* from Peoples Republic of China and its transmission to rats and cats. Journal of Parasitology 97 (3), 421–424.

Hu, J.J., Huang, S., Wen, T., Esch, G.W., Liang, Y., Li, H.L., 2017. Morphology, molecular characteristics, and demonstration of a definitive host for *Sarcocystis rommeli* from cattle (*Bos taurus*) in China. Journal of Parasitology 103 (5), 471–476.

Huber, F., Bomfim, T.C.B., Gomes, R.S., 2002. Comparação entre infecção por *Cryptosporidium* sp. e por *Giardia* sp. em gatos sob dois sistemas de criação. Revista Brasileira de Parasitologia Veterinaria 11 (1), 7–12 (in Portuguese).

Huber, F., Bomfim, T.C.B., Gomes, R.S., 2005. Comparison between natural infection by *Cryptosporidium* sp., *Giardia* sp. in dogs in two living situations in the West Zone of the municipality of Rio de Janeiro. Veterinary Parasitology 130 (1–2), 69–72.

Huber, F., da Silva, S., Bomfim, T.C., Teixeira, K.R., Bello, A.R., 2007. Genotypic characterization and phylogenetic analysis of *Cryptosporidium* sp. from domestic animals in Brazil. Veterinary Parasitology 150 (1–2), 65–74.

Hudkins, G., Kistner, T.P., 1977. *Sarcocystis hemionilatrantis* (Sp. N.) life cycle in mule deer and coyotes. Journal of Wildlife Diseases 13 (1), 80–84.

Hueffer, K., Holcomb, D., Ballweber, L.R., Gende, S.M., Blundell, G., O'Hara, T.M., 2011. Serologic surveillance of pathogens in a declining harbor seal (*Phoca vitulina*) population in Glacier Bay National Park, Alaska, USA and a reference site. Journal of Wildlife Diseases 47 (4), 984–988.

Huet, L., 1882. Note sur des parasites trouves dans les poumons et dans les muscles de l'*Otaria californiana* (Note on parasite found in the lungs and muscles of *Otaria californiana*). Comptes Rendus des Memórias Seances Socété de Biologie 34, 321–322 (in French).

Hughes-Hanks, J.M., Rickard, L.G., Panuska, C., Saucier, J.R., O'Hara, T.M., Dehn, L., Rolland, R.M., 2005. Prevalence of *Cryptosporidium* spp. and *Giardia* spp. in five marine mammal species. Journal of Parasitology 91 (5), 1225–1228.

Hung, C.C., Tsaihong, J.C., Lee, Y.T., Deng, H.Y., Hsiao, W.H., Chang, S.Y., Chang, S.C., Su, K.E., 2007. Prevalence of intestinal infection due to *Cryptosporidium* species among Taiwanese patients with human immunodeficiency virus infection. Journal of the Formosan Medical Association 106 (1), 31–35.

Hunt Jr., R.M., 1996. Biogeography of the order Carnivora. In: Gittleman, J.L. (Ed.), Carnivore Behavior, Ecology and Evolution. Cornell University Press, Ithaca, New York, USA, pp. 485–541.

Huo, G.-Y., Zhao, J.-M., Zhou, H.-L., Rong, G., 2016. Seroprevalence and genetic characterization of *Toxoplasma gondii* in masked palm civet (*Paguma larvata*) in Hainan province, tropical China. Acta Tropica 162, 103–106.

Huong, L.T.T., 1999. Prevalence of *Sarcocystis* spp. in water buffaloes in Vietnam. Veterinary Parasitology 86 (1), 33–39.

Huong, L.T.T., Dubey, J.P., Nikkilä, T., Uggla, A., 1997a. *Sarcocystis buffalonis* n. sp. (Protozoa: Sarcocystidae) from the water buffalo (*Bubalus bubalis*) in Vietnam. Journal of Parasitology 83 (3), 471–474.

Huong, L.T.T., Dubey, J.P., Uggla, A., 1997b. Redescription of *Sarcocystis levinei* Dissanaike and Kan, 1978. (Protozoa: Sarcocystidae) of the water buffalo (*Bubalus bubalis*). Journal of Parasitology 83 (6), 1148–1152.

Hůrková, L., Modrý, D., 2006. PCR detection of *Neospora caninum*, *Toxoplasma gondii* and *Encephalitozoon cuniculi* in brains of wild carnivores. Veterinary Parasitology 137 (1–2), 150–154.

Hutchison, W.M., 1965. Experimental transmission of *Toxoplasma gondii*. Nature 206 (987), 961–962.

Hutchison, W.M., 1967. The nematode transmission of *Toxoplasma gondii*. Transactions of the Royal Society of Tropical Medicine and Hygiene 61 (1), 80–89.

Hutchison, W.M., Dunachie, J.F., Work, K., 1968. The faecal transmission of *Toxoplasma gondii*. Acta Pathologica et Microbiologica Scandinavica 74 (3), 462–464.

Hutchison, W.M., Pittilo, R.M., Ball, S.J., Siim, J.C., 1981. Scanning electron microscopy of the cat small intestine during *Isospora felis* infection. Annals of Tropical Medicine and Parasitology 75 (1), 15–16.

Imre, K., Sala, C., Morar, A., Ilie, M.S., Plutzer, J., Imre, M., Hora, F.Ş., Badea, C., Herbei, M.V., Dărăbuş, G., 2017. *Giardia duodenalis* and *Cryptosporidium* spp. as contaminant protozoa of the main rivers of western Romania: genetic characterization and public health potential of the isolates. Environmental Science and Pollution Research International 24 (22), 18672–18679.

Inabnit, R., Chobotar, B., Ernst, J.V., 1972. *Eimeria procyonis* sp. n., an *Isopora* sp., and a redescription of *E. nuttalli* Yakimoff and Matikaschwili, 1932 (Protozoa: Eimeriidae) from the American raccoon (*Procyon lotor*). Journal of Protozoology 19 (2), 244–247.

Inpankaew, T., Traub, R., Thompson, R.C.A., Sukthana, Y., 2007. Canine parasitic zoonoses in Bangkok temples. The Southeast Asian Journal of Tropical Medicine and Public Health 38 (2), 247–255.

Insulander, M., Silverlås, C., Lebbad, M., Karlsson, L., Mattsson, J.G., Svenungsson, B., 2013. Molecular epidemiology and clinical manifestations of human cryptosporidiosis in Sweden. Epidemiology and Infection 141 (5), 1009–1020.

International Union for Conservation of Nature (IUCN), 2017. IUCN Red List of Threatened Species. Version 2017.1. www.iucnredlist.org.

Ippen, R., Henne, D., 1989. Weitere sarcocystisbefunde bei Vögeln und Säugetieren der Antarktis. Erkrankungen der Zootiere 31, 371–376.

Irwin, P.J., 2002. Companion animal parasitology: a clinical perspective. International Journal for Parasitology 32 (5), 581–593.

Iseki, M., 1979. *Cryptosporidium felis* sp. n. (Protozoa: Eimeriorina) from the domestic cat. Japanese Journal of Parasitology 28 (5), 285–307.

Iseki, M., Tanabe, K., Uni, S., Sano, R., Takada, S., 1974. A survey on *Toxoplasma* and other protozoal and helminthic parasites of adult stray cats in Osaka Area. Japanese Journal of Parasitology 23, 317–322.

Iskander, A.R., 1984. On *Isospora bigemina* and *Heterophyes heterophyes* from the sea lion, *Otaria byronia* at Giza zoological garden. Bulletin of the Zoological Society of Egypt 34, 141–143.

Ito, S., Shimura, K., 1986. The comparison of *Isospora bigemina* large type of the cat and *Besnoitia wallacei*. Japanese Journal of Veterinary Science 48 (2), 433–435.

Ito, S., Tsunoda, K., Nishikawa, H., Matsui, T., 1974. Small type of *Isospora bigemina*: isolation from naturally infected cats and relations with *Toxoplasma* oocysts. National Institute of Animal Health Quarterly 14 (3), 137–144.

Ito, S., Tsunoda, K., Shimura, K., 1978. Life cycle of the large type of *Isospora bigemina* of the cat. National Institute of Animal Health Quarterly 18 (2), 69–82.

Ito, Y., Itoh, N., Kimura, Y., Kanai, K., 2016. Molecular detection and characterization of *Cryptosporidium* spp. among breeding cattery cats in Japan. Parasitology Research 115 (5), 2121–2123.

Ito, Y., Itoh, N., Iijima, Y., Kimura, Y., 2017. Molecular prevalence of *Cryptosporidium* species among household cats and pet shop kittens in Japan. Journal of Feline Medicine and Surgery Open Reports 3 (2). https://doi.org/10.1177/2055116917730719. 4 p.

Itoh, N., Kanai, K., Hori, Y., Hoshi, F., Higuchi, S., 2009. Prevalence of *Giardia intestinalis* and other zoonotic intestinal parasites in private household dogs of the Hachinohe area in Aomori prefecture, Japan in 1997, 2002 and 2007. Journal of Veterinary Science 10 (4), 305–308.

Ivanov, A., Kanakov, D., 2003. First case of canine hepatozoonosis in Bulgaria. Bulgarian Journal of Veterinary Medicine 6 (1), 43–46.

Ivanov, A., Tsachev, I., 2008. *Hepatozoon canis* and hepatozoonosis in the dog. Trakia Journal of Sciences 6 (2), 27–35.

Iwanoff-Gobzem, P.S., 1934. Zum Vorkommen von Coccidien bei kleinen wilden Säugetieren (On the occurrence of coccidia in small wild mammals). Deutsche Tierärztliche Wochenschrift 42, 149–151 (in German).

Iwanoff-Gobzem, P.S., 1935. K voprosy o koktsidiyakh domashnikh i dikikh zhivotnykh severnogo Kazakhstana (On the question of coccidia of domestic and wild animals of the norther Kazakhstan). In: Pavlovsky, E.N. (Ed.), Vrediteli sel'skokh. Zhivot. Bor'ba Nimi. Po materalam parasitologicheskoi ekspeditsii v Severnom Kazakhstana 1932. Izdat Akademii Nauk SSSR, pp. 243–263.

Jacobs, L., Melton, M.J., Cook, M.K., 1955. Observations on toxoplasmosis in dogs. Journal of Parasitology 41 (4), 353–362.

Jacquiet, P., Liénard, E., Franc, M., 2010. Bovine besnoitiosis: epidemiological and clinical aspects. Veterinary Parasitology 174 (1–2), 30–36.

Jäkel, T., Khoprasert, Y., Borger, I., Kliemt, D., Seehabutr, V., Suasa-ard, K., Hongnark, S., 1997. Sarcosporidiasis in rodents from Thailand. Journal of Wildlife Diseases 33 (4), 860–867.

Jakubek, E.B., Bröjer, C., Regnersen, C., Uggla, A., Schares, G., Björkman, C., 2001. Seroprevalence of *Toxoplasma gondii* and *Neospora caninum* in Swedish red foxes (*Vulpes vulpes*). Veterinary Parasitology 102 (1–2), 167–172.

Jakubek, E.B., Farkas, R., Pálfi, V., Mattsson, J.G., 2007. Prevalence of antibodies against *Toxoplasma gondii* and *Neospora caninum* in Hungarian red foxes (*Vulpes vulpes*). Veterinary Parasitology 144 (1–2), 39–44.

Janitschke, K., Werner, H., 1972. Untersuchungen über die Wirtsspezifität des geschlechtlichen Entwicklungszyklus von *Toxoplasma gondii* (Investigations about host specificity of the oocyst-forming life-cycle of *Toxoplasma gondii*). Zeitschrift für Parasitenkunde 39 (3), 247–254 (in German, short English summary).

Janitschke, K., Protz, D., Werner, H., 1976. Beitrag zum Entwicklungszyklus von Sarkosporidien der Grantgazelle (*Gazella granti*) (Contribution to life-cycle of sarcosporidia in the Grant's Gazelle (*Gazella granti*)).

Zeitschrift für Parasitenkunde 48 (3), 215–219 (in German).

Jaskoski, B.J., Barr, V., Borges, M., 1982. Intestinal parasites of well-cared-for dogs: an area revisited. American Journal of Tropical Medicine and Hygiene 31 (6), 1107–1110.

Jatusevich, A., Gerasimchik, V., 1995. Mink coccidiosis in Belorussia. Bulletin of the Scandinavian Society of Parasitology 5, 63–64.

Jellison, W.L., 1956. On the nomenclature of *Besnoitia besnoiti*, a protozoan parasite. Annals of the New York Academy of Sciences 64 (1), 268–270.

Jenkins, M.C., 2001. Advances and prospects for subunit vaccines against protozoa of veterinary importance. Veterinary Parasitology 101 (3–4), 291–310.

Jensen, S.-K., Aars, J., Lydersen, C., Kovacs, K.M., Åsbakk, K., 2010. The prevalence of *Toxoplasma gondii* in polar bears and their marine mammal prey: evidence for a marine transmission pathway? Polar Biology 33 (5), 599–606.

Jensen, S.-K., Nymo, I.H., Forcada, J., Godfroid, J., Hall, A., 2012. Prevalence of *Toxoplasma gondii* in pinnipeds from Antarctica. Microbiology 11, 562–568.

Jewell, M.L., Frenkel, J.K., Johnson, K.M., Reed, V., Ruiz, A., 1972. Development of *Toxoplasma* oocysts in neotropical Felidae. American Journal of Tropical Medicine and Hygiene 21 (5), 512–517.

Jiang, J., Xiao, L., 2003. An evaluation of molecular diagnostic tools for the detection and differentiation of human-pathogenic *Cryptosporidium* spp. Journal of Eukaryotic Microbiology 50 (Suppl.), 542–547.

Jiménez, J.E., Briceño, C., Alcaíno, H., Vávquez, P., Funk, S., González-Acuña, D., 2012. Coprologic survey of endoparasites from Darwin's fox (*Pseudalopex fulvipes*) in Chiloé, Chile. Archivos de Medicina Veterinaria 44, 93–97.

Jirků, M., Valigurová, A., Koudela, B., Křížek, J., Modrý, D., Šlapeta, J., 2008. New species of *Cryptosporidium* Tyzzer, 1907 (Apicomplexa) from amphibian host: morphology, biology and phylogeny. Folia Parasitologica (Praha) 55 (2), 81–94.

Joffe, D., Van Niekerk, D., Gagné, F., Gilleard, J., Kutz, S., Lobingier, R., 2011. The prevalence of intestinal parasites in dogs and cats in Calgary, Alberta. The Canadian Veterinary Journal 52 (12), 1323–1328.

Jog, M.M., Watve, M.G., 2005. Sarcocystosis of chital-dhole: conditions for evolutionary stability of a predator parasite mutualism. BMC Ecology 5, 3. https://doi.org/10.1186/1472-6785-5-3.

Jog, M.M., Marathe, R.R., Goel, S.S., Ranade, S.P., Kunte, K.K., Watve, M.G., 2003. *Sarcocystis* infection in chital (*Axis axis*) and dhole (*Cuon alpinus*) in two Indian protected areas. Zoos' Print Journal 18 (10), 1220–1222.

Jog, M.M., Marathe, R.R., Goel, S.S., Ranade, S.P., Kunte, K.K., Watve, M.G., 2005. Sarcocystosis of chital (*Axis axis*) and dhole (*Cuon alpinus*): ecology of a mammalian prey–predator–parasite system in Peninsular India. Journal of Tropical Ecology 21 (4), 479–482.

Johnson, A.M., 1998. Is there more than one species in the genus *Toxoplasma*?? Tokai Journal of Experimental and Clinical Medicine 23 (6), 383–389.

Johnson, E.M., Allen, K.E., Panciera, R.J., Little, S.E., Ewing, S.A., 2008. Infectivity of *Hepatozoon americanum* cystozoites for a dog. Veterinary Parasitology 154 (1–2), 148–150.

Jolley, W.R., Kingston, N., Williams, E.S., Lynn, C., 1994. Coccidia, *Giardia* sp., and a physalopteran nematode parasite from black footed ferrets (*Mustela nigripes*) in Wyoming. Journal of the Helminthological Society of Washington 61 (1), 89–94.

Jordan, H.E., Mullins, S.T., Stebbins, M.E., 1993. Endoparasitism in dogs: 1, 583 cases (1981–1990). Journal of the American Veterinary Medical Association 203 (4), 547–549.

Juan-Sallés, C., Prats, N., López, S., Domingo, M., Marco, A.J., Morán, J.F., 1997. Epizootic disseminated toxoplasmosis in captive slender-tailed meerkats (*Suricata suricatta*). Veterinary Parasitology 34 (1), 1–7.

Kalyakin, V.N., Zasukhin, D.S., 1975. Distribution of *Sarcocystis* (Protozoa: Sporozoa) in vertebrates. Folia Parasitologica (Praha) 22 (4), 289–307.

Kamga-Waladjo, A.R., Gbati, O.B., Kone, P., Lapo, R.A., Dombou, E., Chatagnon, G., Bakou, S.N., Diop, P.E.H., Pangui, L.J., Tainturier, D., Akakpo, J.A., 2009. *Neospora caninum* and *Toxoplasma gondii* in lion (*Panthera leo*) from Senegal, West Africa. Asian Journal of Animal Veterinary Advances 4 (6), 346–349.

Kamiya, H., Suzuki, Y., 1975. Parasites of the Japanese badger, *Meles meles anakuma* Temminck, especially on *Isthmiophora melis* (Schrank, 1788) Lühe, 1909. Japanese Journal of Veterinary Research 23 (4), 125–130.

Karanis, P., Plutzer, J., Halim, N.A., Igori, K., Nagasawa, H., Ongerth, J., Liqing, M., 2007. Molecular characterization of *Cryptosporidium* from animal sources in Qinghai province of China. Parasitology Research 101 (6), 1575–1580.

Katagiri, S., Oliveira-Sequeira, T.C.G., 2008. Prevalence of dog intestinal parasites and risk perception of zoonotic infection by dog owners in São Paulo State, Brazil. Zoonoses and Public Health 55 (8–10), 406–413.

Katlama, C., 1991. Evaluation of the efficacy and safety of clindamycin plus pyrimethamine for induction and maintenance therapy of toxoplasmic encephalitis in AIDS. European Journal of Clinical Microbiology and Infectious Diseases 10 (3), 189–191.

Katsumata, T., Hosea, D., Wasito, E.B., Kohno, S., Hara, K., Soeparto, P., Ranuh, I.G., 1998. Cryptosporidiosis in Indonesia: a hospital-based study and a community-based survey. American Journal of Tropical Medicine and Hygiene 59 (4), 628–632.

Kauffman, C.A., Bergman, A.G., O'Connor, R.P., 1982. Distemper virus infection in ferrets: an animal model of measles-induced immunosuppression. Clinical and Experimental Immunology 47 (3), 617–625.

Kaye, S.W., Ossiboff, R.J., Noonan, B., Stokol, T., Buckles, E., Seimon, T.A., Morrisey, J., Matos, R., 2015. Biliary coccidiosis associated with immunosuppressive treatment of pure red cell aplasia in an adult ferret (*Mustela putorius furo*). Journal of Exotic Pet Medicine 24 (2), 215–222.

Kellnerová, K., Holubová, N., Jandová, A., Vejčík, A., McEvoy, J., Sak, B., Kváč, M., 2017. First description of *Cryptosporidium ubiquitum* XIIa subtype family in farmed fur animals. European Journal of Protistology 59, 108–113.

Kemp, T.S., 2005. The Origin and Evolution of Mammals. Oxford University Press, Oxford, England. 331 pp.

Keymer, I.F., Brocklesby, D.W., 1971. Blood protozoa of wild carnivores in Central Africa. Journal of Zoology (London) 164 (4), 513–524.

Khoshnegah, J., Mohri, M., 2009. The first report of *Hepatozoon canis* infection of a dog in Iran. Comparative Clinical Pathology 18 (4), 455–458.

Kiehl, E., Heydorn, A.O., Schein, E., Al-Rasheid, K.A., Selmair, J., Abdel-Ghaffar, F., Mehlhorn, H., 2010. Molecular biological comparison of different *Besnoitia* species and stages from different countries. Parasitology Research 106 (4), 889–894.

Kim, J.T., Wee, S.H., Lee, C.G., 1998. Detection of *Cryptosporidium* oocysts in canine fecal samples by immunofluorescence assay. The Korean Journal of Parasitology 36 (2), 147–149.

Kim, J.T., Park, J.Y., Seo, H.S., Oh, H.G., Noh, J.W., Kim, J.H., Kim, D.Y., Youn, H.J., 2002. In vitro antiprotozoal effects of artemisinin on *Neospora caninum*. Veterinary Parasitology 103 (1–2), 53–63.

Kim, J.H., Kang, M.-S., Lee, B.-C., Hwang, W.-S., Lee, C.-W., So, B.-W., Dubey, J.P., Kim, D.-Y., 2003. Seroprevalence of antibodies to *Neospora caninum* in dogs and raccoon dogs in Korea. Korean Journal of Parasitology 41 (4), 243–245.

King, J.S., Šlapeta, J., Jenkins, D.J., Al-Qassab, S.E., Ellis, J.T., Windsor, P.A., 2010. Australian dingoes are definitive host of *Neospora caninum*. International Journal for Parasitology 40 (8), 945–950.

King, J.S., Jenkins, D.J., Ellis, J.T., Fleming, P., Windsor, P.A., Šlapeta, J., 2011. Implications of wild dog ecology on the sylvatic and domestic life cycle of *Neospora caninum* in Australia. Veterinary Journal 188 (1), 24–33.

King, J.S., Brown, G.K., Jenkins, D.J., Ellis, J.T., Fleming, P.J.S., Windsor, P.A., Šlapeta, J., 2012. Oocysts and high seroprevalence of *Neospora caninum* in dogs living in remote Aboriginal communities and wild dogs in Australia. Veterinary Parasitology 187 (1), 85–92.

Kingscote, A.A., 1934a. Coccidiosis in mink. In: Ontario Department of Agriculture, Report of the Ontario Veterinary College 1933, Sessional Paper No. 29. Herbert H. Ball Publisher, Toronto, Ontario, Canada, pp. 30–41.

Kingscote, A.A., 1934b. *Eimeria mustelae* n. sp. from *Mustela vison*. Journal of Parasitology 20, 252–253.

Kingscote, A.A., 1935. A note on the coccidia of minks. Journal of Parasitology 21, 126.

Kirkpatrick, C.E., Dubey, J.P., Goldschmidt, M.H., Salk, J.E., Schmitz, J.A., 1986. *Sarcocystis* sp. in muscles of domestic cats. Veterinary Parasitology 23 (1), 88–90.

Kirkpatrick, C.E., Hamir, A.N., Dubey, J.P., Rupprecht, C.E., 1987. *Sarcocystis* in muscles of raccoons (*Procyon lotor* L.). Journal of Protozoology 34 (4), 445–447.

Kiupel, H., Ritscher, D., Fricke, G., 1987. Toxoplasmose bei jungen Kodiakbären (*Ursus arctos* Middendorffi) (Toxoplasmosis in young bears (*Ursus arctos* Middendorffi)). In: Ippen, R., Schröder, H.D. (Eds.), Erkrankungen der Zootiere. Verhandlungsbericht des 29. Internationalen Symposiums über die Erkrankungen der Zootiere von 20. Mai bis 24. Mai 1987 in Cardiff. Akademie-Verlag, Berlin, pp. 335–340 (in German).

Klein, B.U., Muller, E., 2001. Seroprevalence of antibodies to *Neospora caninum* in dogs with and without clinical suspicion for neosporosis in Germany. Praktische Tierärztliche 82, 437–440.

Klopfer, U., Neumann, F., 1970. A note on coccidiosis in minks. Refuah Veterinarith 27, 122–124.

Klopfer, U., Nobel, T.A., Neumann, F., 1973. *Hepatozoon*-like parasite (schizonts) in the myocardium of the domestic cat. Veterinary Pathology 10 (3), 185–190.

Kluge, J.P., 1967. Trichinosis and sarcosporidiosis in a puma. Bulletin of the Wildlife Disease Association 3, 110–111.

Knowles, R., Gupta, B.M.D., 1931. A note on two intestinal protozoa of the Indian Mongoose. Indian Journal of Medical Research 19, 175–176.

Koepfli, K.-P., Wayne, R.K., 1998. Phylogenetic relationships of otters (Carnivora: Mustelidae) based on mitochondrial cytochrome b sequences. Journal of Zoology (London) 246, 401–416.

Koepfli, K.-P., Deere, K.A., Slater, G.J., Begg, C., Begg, K., Grassman, L., Lucherini, M., Veron, G., Wayne, R.K., 2008. Multigene phylogeny of the Mustelidae: resolving relationships, tempo and biogeographic history of a mammalian adaptive radiation. BioMed Central Biology 6 (1), 10.

Koompapong, K., Mori, H., Thammasonthijarern, N., Prasertbun, R., Pintong, A.R., Popruk, S., Rojekittikhun, W., Chaisiri, K., Sukthana, Y., Mahittikorn, A., 2014. Molecular identification of *Cryptosporidium* spp. in seagulls, pigeons, dogs, and cats in Thailand. Parasite 21, 52.

Korkmaz, U.F., Gokpinar, S., Yildiz, K., 2016. Prevalence of intestinal parasites in cats and their importance in terms of public health. Turkiye Parazitolojii Dergisi 40 (4), 194–198 (in Turkish, English summary).

Kostopoulou, D., Claerebout, E., Arvanitis, D., Ligda, P., Voutzourakis, N., Casaert, S., Sotiraki, S., 2017. Abundance, zoonotic potential and risk factors of intestinal parasitism amongst dog and cat populations: the scenario of Crete, Greece. Parasites and Vectors 10, 43.

Kotlán, A., Pospesch, L., 1933. Coccidial infections in the badger *Meles taxus* L. Parasitology 25, 102–107.

Kotschwar Logan, M., Gerber, B., Karpanty, S., Justin, S., Rabenahy, F., 2015. Assessing carnivore distribution from local knowledge across a human-dominated landscape in central-southeastern Madagascar. Animal Conservation 18 (1), 82–91.

Koudela, B., 1993. Experimental transmission of *Caryospora bigenetica* Wacha and Christiansen, 1982 (Apicomplexa: Eimeriidae) from a rattlesnake *Crotalus atrox* to rodents and pigs. Folia Parasitologica (Praha) 40 (1), 81–84.

Koudela, B., Modrý, D., 2000. *Sarcocystis muris* possesses both diheteroxenous and dihomoxenous characters of life cycle. Journal of Parasitology 86 (4), 877–879.

Kramer, A.M., Wouda, W., Kooistra, H.S., 2000. Clinical neosporosis in the dog: a review. Tijdschrift voor Diergeneeskunde 125 (20), 609–613.

Krampitz, H.E., Haberkorn, A., 1988. Experimental treatment of *Hepatozoon* infections with the anticoccidial agent toltrazuril. Journal of Veterinary Medicine. Series B 35 (2), 131–137.

Krampitz, H.E., Sachs, R., Schaller, G.B., Schindler, R., 1968. Zur Verbreitung von Parasiten der Gattung *Hepatozoon* Miller, 1908 (Protozoa, Adeleidae) in ostafrikanischen Wildsäugetieren (Distribution of *Hepatozoon* Miller, 1908 (Protozoa, Adeleidae) in East African wild mammals). Zeitschrift für Parasitenkunde 31 (3), 203–210 (in German, English summary).

Krause, C., Goranoff, S., 1933. Ueber Sarkosporidiosis bei Huhn und Wildente (About sarcosporidiosis in chicken and wild duck). Zeitschrift für Infektionskrankheiten der Haustieren 43, 261–278 (in German).

Krecek, R.C., Moura, L., Lucas, H., Kelly, P., 2010. Parasites of stray cats (*Felis domesticus* L., 1758) on St. Kitts, west Indies. Veterinary Parasitology 172 (1–2), 147–149.

Kritzner, S., Sager, H., Blum, J., Krebber, R., Greif, G., Gottstein, B., 2002. An explorative study to assess the efficacy of toltrazuril-sulfone (Ponazuril) in calves experimentally infected with *Neospora caninum*. Annals of Clinical Microbiology and Antimicrobials 1, 4.

Kruuk, H., 1978. Foraging and spatial organization of the European badger *Meles meles* L. Behavioral Ecology and Sociobiology 4, 75–89.

Kubo, M., Kuniyoshi, S., 2014. Parasitology muscular *Sarcocystis* sp. Infection in Tsushima leopard cats (*Prionailurus bengalensis euptilurus*). Japanese Journal of Zoo Wildlife Medicine 19 (3), 101–103.

Kubo, M., Miyoshi, N., Yasuda, N., 2006. Hepatozoonosis in two species of Japanese wild cats. Journal of Veterinary Medical Science 68 (8), 833–837.

Kubo, M., Uni, S., Agatsuma, T., Nagataki, M., Panciera, R.J., Tsubota, T., Nakamura, S., Sakai, H., Masegi, T., Yanai, T., 2008. *Hepatozoon ursi* n. sp. (Apicomplexa: Hepatozoidae) in Japanese black bear (*Ursus thibetanus japonicus*). Parasitology International 57 (3), 287–294.

Kubo, M., Okano, T., Ito, K., Tsubota, T., Sakai, H., Yanai, T., 2009. Muscular sarcocystosis in wild carnivores in Honshu, Japan. Parasitology Research 106 (1), 213–219.

Kubo, M., Jeong, A., Kim, S.-I., Kim, Y.-J., Lee, H., Kimura, J., Agatsuma, T., Sakai, H., Yanai, T., 2010a. The first report of *Hepatozoon* species infection in leopard cats (*Prionailurus bengalensis*) in Korea. Journal of Parasitology 96 (2), 437–439.

Kubo, M., Kawachi, T., Murakami, M., Kubo, M., Tokuhiro, S., Agatsuma, T., Ito, K., Okano, T., Asano, M., Fukushi, H., Nagataki, M., Sakai, H., Yanai, T., 2010b. Meningoencephalitis associated with *Sarcocystis* spp. in a free-living Japanese raccoon dog (*Nyctereutes procyonoides viverrinus*). Journal of Comparative Pathology 143 (2–3), 185–189.

Kuiken, T., Kennedy, S., Barrett, T., Van de Bildt, M.W.G., Borgsteede, F.H., Brew, S.D., Codd, G.A., Duck, C., Deaville, R., Eybatov, T., Forsyth, M.A., Foster, G., Jepson, P.D., Kydyrmanov, A., Mitrofanov, I., Ward, C.J., Wilson, S., Osterhaus, A.D.M.E., 2006. The 2000 canine distemper epidemic in Caspian seals (*Phoca caspica*): pathology and analysis of contributory factors. Veterinary Pathology 43 (3), 321–338.

Kumar, S., Hedges, S.B., 2011. TimeTree2: species divergence times on the iPhone. Bioinformatics 27, 2023–2024.

Kumar, S., Stecher, G., Suleski, M., Hedges, S.B., 2017. TimeTree: a resource for timelines, timetrees, and divergence times. Molecular Biology and Evolution 34 (7), 1812–1819.

Kuo, C.H., Wares, J.P., Kissinger, J.C., 2008. The Apicomplexan whole-genome phylogeny: an analysis of incongruence among gene trees. Molecular Biology and Evolution 25 (12), 2689–2698.

Kurniawan, A., Dwintasari, S.W., Connelly, L., Nichols, R.A., Yunihastuti, E., Karyadi, T., Djauzi, S., 2013. *Cryptosporidium* species from human immunodeficiency-infected patients with chronic diarrhea in Jakarta, Indonesia. Annals of Epidemiology 23 (11), 720–723.

Kutkienė, L., 2001. The species composition of European roe deer (*Capreolus Capreolus* (sic)) *Sarcocystis* in Lithuania. Acta Zoologica Lituanica 11 (1), 97–101.

Kutkienė, L., 2003. Investigations of red deer (*Cervus elaphus*) *Sarcocystis* species composition in Lithuania. Acta Zoologica Lituanica 13 (4), 390–395.

Kutkienė, L., Grikienienė, J., 1993. Transplacental transmission as one of the ways of circulation of some sarcosporidian species in rodents. Ekologija 1, 25–32.

Kutkienė, L., Grikienienė, J., 1995. New experimental data on transplacental transmission of *Sarcocystis* in laboratory rats. Acta Zoologica Lituanica Parasitologia 25 (1), 42–44.

Kutkienė, L., Grikienienė, J., 1998. Transmission of *Sarcocystis rodentifelis* from female rats (*Rattus norvegicus*) to their offspring. Acta Zoologica Lituanica Parasitologia 8 (1), 76–83.

Kutkienė, L., Grikienienė, J., 2003. The importance of coprophagy and transplacental transmission in spread of *Sarcocystis rodentifelis* in rats. Acta Zoologica Lituanica Parasitologia 13 (3), 322–326.

Kutkienė, L., Sruoga, A., 2004. *Sarcocystis* spp. in birds of the order Anseriformes. Parasitology Research 92 (1), 171–172.

Kutkienė, L., Sruoga, A., Butkauskas, D., 2006. *Sarcocystis* sp. from white-fronted goose (*Anser albifrons*): cyst morphology and life cycle studies. Parasitology Research 99 (5), 562–565.

Kutkienė, L., Prakas, P., Sruoga, A., Butkauskas, D., 2011. Identification of *Sarcocystis rileyi* from the mallard duck (*Anas platyrhynchos*) in Europe: cyst morphology and results of DNA analysis. Parasitology Research 108 (3), 709–714.

Kutkienė, L., Prakas, P., Sruoga, A., Butkauskas, D., 2012. Description of *Sarcocystis anasi* sp. nov. and *Sarcocystis albifronsi* sp. nov. in birds of the order Anseriformes. Parasitology Research 110 (2), 1043–1046.

Kuttin, E.S., Kaller, A., 1992. *Cystoisospora israeli* n. sp. causing enteritis in a South African fur seal. Aquatic Mammals 18 (3), 79–81.

Kváč, M., Kestřánová, M., Pinková, M., Květoňová, D., Kalinová, J., Wagnerová, P., Kotková, M., Vítovec, J., Ditrich, O., McEvoy, J., Stenger, B., Sak, B., 2013. *Cryptosporidium scrofarum* n. sp. (Apicomplexa: Cryptosporidiidae) in domestic pigs (*Sus scrofa*). Veterinary Parasitology 191 (3–4), 218–227.

Kvičerová, J., Hypša, V., 2013. Host-parasite incongruences in rodent *Eimeria* suggest significant role of adaptation rather than cophylogeny in maintenance of host specificity. PLoS One 8 (7), e63601.

Labbé, A., 1899. Sporozoa. In: Schulze, F.E., Butschi, O. (Eds.), Tierreich. Verlag von R. Friedlander & Sohn, Berlin, Germany, pp. 115–119.

Lainson, R., 1968. Parasitological studies in British Honduras. III. Some coccidial parasites of mammals. Annals of Tropical Medicine and Parasitology 62 (2), 252–259.

Laird, M., 1959. Malayan protozoa and *Hepatozoon* Miller (Sporozoa: Coccidia) with an unusual host record for *H. canis* (James). Journal of Protozoology 6 (4), 316–318.

Lalonde, L.F., Gajadhar, A.A., 2011. Detection and differentiation of coccidian oocysts by real-time PCR and melting curve analysis. Journal of Parasitology 97 (4), 725–730.

Lalonde, L.F., Reyes, J., Gajadhar, A.A., 2013. Application of a qPCR assay with melting curve analysis for detection and differentiation of protozoan oocysts in human fecal samples from Dominican Republic. The American Journal of Tropical Medicine and Hygiene 89 (5), 892–898.

Lambourn, D.M., Jeffries, S.J., Dubey, J.R., 2001. Seroprevalence of *Toxoplasma gondii* in harbor seals (*Phoca vitulina*) in southern Puget Sound, Washington. Journal of Parasitology 87 (5), 1196–1197.

Lan, J., Fu, Y., Yang, Z., Zhang, Z., Wang, C., Luo, L., Liu, L., Gu, X., Wang, S., Peng, X., Yang, G., 2012. Treatment and prevention of natural heartworm (*Dirofilaria immitis*) infections in red pandas (*Ailurus fulgens*) with selamectin and ivermectin. Parasitology International 61 (2), 372–374.

Landau, I., 1982. Hypothèses sur la phylogénie des Coccidiomorphes de vertébrés: Évolution des cycles et spectre d'hôtes. In: Metrick, D.F., Desser, S.S. (Eds.), Parasites – Their World and Ours. Elsevier Biomedical Press, Amsterdam, The Netherlands, pp. 169–171.

Lane, J.R., Kocan, A.A., 1983. *Hepatozoon* sp. infection in bobcats. Journal of the American Veterinary Medical Association 183 (11), 1323.

Lankester, E.R., 1882. On *Drepanidium ranarum* the cell parasite of the frog's blood and spleen (Gaule's Wurmchen). Quarterly Journal of Microscopy 22, 53–65.

Lapointe, J.M., Duignan, P.J., Marsh, A.E., Gulland, F.M., Barr, B.C., Naydan, D.K., King, D.P., Farman, C.A., Burek-Huntingdon, K.A., Lowenstine, L.J., 1998. Meningoencephalitis due to a *Sarcocystis neurona*-like protozoan in Pacific harbor seals (*Phoca vitulina richardsi*). Journal of Parasitology 84 (6), 1184–1189.

Lappin, M.R., 2000. Protozoal and miscellaneous infections. In: Ettinger, S.J., Feldman, E.C. (Eds.), Textbook of Veterinary Internal Medicine, fifth ed. W.B. Saunders, Philadelphia, USA, pp. 408–417.

Lappin, M.R., 2005. Enteric protozoal diseases. The Veterinary Clinics of North America. Small Animal Practice 35 (1), 81–88.

Lappin, M.R., 2010. Update on the diagnosis and management of *Isospora* spp. infections in dogs and cats. Topics in Companion Animal Medicine 25 (3), 133–135.

Lappin, M.R., Greene, C.E., Prestwood, A.K., Dawe, D.L., Marks, A., 1989. Prevalence of *Toxoplasma gondii* infections in cats in Georgia using enzyme-linked immunosorbent assays for IgM, IgG, and antigens. Veterinary Parasitology 33 (3–4), 225–230.

Lappin, M.R., Jacobson, E.R., Kollias, G.V., Powell, C.C., Stover, J., 1991. Comparison of serologic assays for the diagnosis of toxoplasmosis in nondomestic felids. Journal of Zoo and Wildlife Medicine 22 (2), 169–174.

Larkin, J.L., Gabriel, M., Gerhold, R.W., Yabsley, M.J., Wester, J.C., Humphreys, J.G., Beckstead, R., Dubey, J.P., 2011. Prevalence to *Toxoplasma gondii* and *Sarcocystis* spp. in a reintroduced Fisher (*Martes pennanti*) population in Pennsylvania. Journal of Parasitology 93 (3), 425–429.

Latif, B., Vellayan, S., Omar, E., Abdullah, S., Desa, N.M., 2010. Sarcocystosis among wild captive and zoo animals in Malaysia. The Korean Journal of Parasitology 48 (3), 213–217.

Lauckner, G., 1985. Diseases of mammalia: Pinnipedia. In: Kinne, O. (Ed.), Diseases of Marine Animals, Vol. IV, Pt. 2, Introduction, Reptilia, Aves, Mammalia. Biologische Anstalt Helgoland, Hamburg, Germany, pp. 1–33.

Laurenson, K., Sillero-Zubiri, C., Thompson, H., Shiferaw, F., 1998. Disease as a threat to endangered species: Ethiopian wolves, domestic dogs and canine pathogens. Animal Conservation Fourm 1 (4), 273–280.

Lavy, E., Ziv, G., Shem-Tov, M., Glickman, A., Dey, A., 1999. Pharmacokinetics of clindamycin HCl administered intravenously, intramuscularly and subcutaneously to dogs. Journal of Veterinary Pharmacology and Therapeutics 22 (4), 261–265.

Lee, C.D., 1934. The pathology of coccidiosis in the dog. Journal of the American Veterinary Medical Association 85, 760–781.

Lee, J.J., Leedale, G.F., Bradbury, P., 2000. In: An Illustrated Guide to the Protozoa, vol. 1. second ed. Society of Protozoologists, Lawrence, KS, p. 689.

Leek, R.G., Fayer, R., Johnson, A.J., 1977. Sheep experimentally infected with *Sarcocystis* from dogs. I. Disease in young lambs. Journal of Parasitology 63 (4), 642–650.

Leguía, G., 1991. The epidemiology and economic impact of llama parasites. Parasitology Today 7 (2), 54–56.

Leighton, F.A., Gajadhar, A.A., 2001. Tissue inhabiting protozoans. In: Samuel, W.M., Pybus, M.J., Kocan, A.A. (Eds.), Parasitic Diseases of Wild Mammals. Iowa State University Press, Ames, Iowa, USA, pp. 468–478.

Lemberger, K.Y., Gondim, L.F.P., Pressier, A.P., McAllister, M.M., Kinsel, M.J., 2005. *Neospora caninum* infection in a free-ranging raccoon (*Procyon lotor*) with concurrent canine distemper virus infection. Journal of Parasitology 91 (4), 960–961.

Leoni, F., Gallimore, C.I., Green, J., McLauchlin, J., 2003. Molecular epidemiological analysis of *Cryptosporidium* isolates from humans and animals by using a heteroduplex mobility assay and nucleic acid sequencing based on a small double-stranded RNA element. Journal of Clinical Microbiology 41 (3), 981–992.

Leoni, F., Gallimore, C.I., Green, J., McLauchlin, J., 2006. Characterisation of small double stranded RNA molecule in *Cryptosporidium hominis*, *Cryptosporidium felis* and *Cryptosporidium meleagridis*. Parasitology International 55 (4), 299–306.

Lepp, D.L., Todd Jr., K.S., 1974. Life cycle of *Isospora canis* Nemeséri, 1959 in the dog. Journal of Protozoology 21 (2), 199–206.

Lepp, D.L., Todd Jr., K.S., 1976. Sporogony of the oocysts of *Isospora canis*. Transactions of the American Microscopical Society 95 (1), 98–103.

Lesmeister, D.G., Millspaugh, J.J., Wade, S.E., Gompper, M.W., 2008. A survey of parasites identified in the feces of eastern spotted skunks (*Spilogale putorius*) in western Arkansas. Journal of Wildlife Diseases 44 (4), 1041–1044.

Leśniańska, K., Perec-Matysiak, A., Hildebrand, J., Buńkowska-Gawlik, K., Piróg, A., Popiołek, M., 2016. *Cryptosporidium* spp. and *Enterocytozoon bieneusi* in introduced raccoons (*Procyon lotor*) - first evidence from Poland and Germany. Parasitology Research 115 (12), 4535–4541.

Levchenko, N.G., 1963. Ein Fall von Sarkosporidiose beim Rehwild (*Capreolus capreolus*) (A case of Sarcosporidiosis in Roe Deer (*Capreolus capreolus*)). Trudy Instituta Zoologii Akademii Nauk Kazakhstan, SSR 19, pp. 244–245 (in Russian). (*nos non videbo illum*, found in Odening et al., 1994b and in Sedlaczek and Wesemeier, 1995, respectively).

Levine, N.D., 1948. *Eimeria* and *Isospora* in the mink (*Mustela vison*). Journal of Parasitology 34, 486–492.

Levine, N.D., 1973. Protozoan Parasites of Domestic Animals and of Man, second ed. Burgess Publishing, Minneapolis, Minnesota, USA. 406 p.

Levine, N.D., 1977. Nomenclature of *Sarcocystis* in the ox and sheep and of fecal coccidia of the dog and cat. Journal of Parasitology 63 (1), 36–51.

Levine, N.D., 1978. Textbook of Veterinary Parasitology. Burgess Publishing, Minneapolis, Minnesota, USA. 236 p.

Levine, N.D., 1986. Invited review. The taxonomy of *Sarcocystis* (Protozoa, Apicomplexa) species. Journal of Parasitology 72 (3), 372–382.

Levine, N.D., 1988. The Protozoan Phylum Apicomplexa. CRC Press, Boca Raton, Florida, USA. Vols. I and II. 357 p.

Levine, N.D., Ivens, V., 1964. *Isospora spilogales* and *I. sengeri* n. sp. (Protozoa: Eimeriidae) from the spotted skunk, *Spilogale putorius ambarvalis*. Journal of Protozoology 11, 505–509.

Levine, N.D., Ivens, V., 1965. *Isospora* species in the dog. Journal of Parasitology 51 (5), 859–864.

Levine, N.D., Ivens, V., 1981. The Coccidian Parasites (Protozoa, Apicomplexa) of Carnivores. Illinois Biological Monograph No. 51. University of Illinois Press, Urbana, Illinois, USA. 249 p.

Levine, N.D., Ivens, V., 1990. The Coccidian Parasites (Protozoa, Apicomplexa) of Rodents. CRC Press, Inc, Boca Raton, Florida USA. 228 p.

Levine, N.D., Tadros, W., 1980. Named species and hosts of *Sarcocystis* (Protozoa: Apicomplexa: Sarcocystidae). Systematic Parasitology 2 (1), 41–59.

Levine, N.D., Ivens, V., Healy, G.R., 1975. *Isospora herpestei* n. sp. (Protozoa, Apicomplexa) and other new species of *Isospora* from mongooses. Proceedings of the Oklahoma Academy of Sciences 55, 150–153.

Lewis, I.J., Hart, C.A., Baxby, D., 1985. Diarrhoea due to *Cryptosporidium* in acute lymphoblastic leukaemia. Archives of Disease in Childhood 60 (1), 60–62.

Lewis, R.E., Klepser, M.E., Ernst, E.J., Lund, B.C., Biedenbach, D.J., Jones, R.N., 1999. Evaluation of low-dose, extended-interval clindamycin regimens against *Staphylococcus aureus* and *Streptococcus pneumoniae* using a dynamic in vitro model of infection. Antimicrobial Agents and Chemotherapy 43 (8), 2005–2009.

Li, X., Pang, J., Fox, J.G., 1996. Coinfection with intracellular *Desulfovibrio* species and coccidia in ferrets with proliferative bowel disease. Laboratory Animal Science 46, 569–571.

Li, Q.-Q., Yang, Z.-Q., Zuo, Y.-X., Attwood, S.W., Chen, X.-W., Zhang, Y.-P., 2002. A PCR-based RFLP analysis of *Sarcocystis cruzi* (Protozoa: Sarcocystidae) in Yunnan province, PR China, reveals the water buffalo (*Bubalus bubalis*) as a natural intermediate host. Journal of Parasitology 88 (6), 1259–1261.

Li, X., Brasseur, P., Agnamey, P., Leméteil, D., Favennec, L., Ballet, J.J., Rossignol, J.F., 2003. Long-lasting anticryptosporidial activity of nitazoxanide in an immunosuppressed rat model. Folia Parasitologica (Praha) 50 (1), 19–22.

Li, W., Li, Y., Song, M., Lu, Y., Yang, J., Tao, W., Jiang, Y., Wan, Q., Zhang, S., Xiao, L., 2015. Prevalence and genetic characteristics of *Cryptosporidium*, *Enterocytozoon bieneusi* and *Giardia duodenalis* in cats and dogs in Heilongjiang province, China. Veterinary Parasitology 208 (3–4), 125–134.

Lickfeld, K.G., 1959. Untersuchungen über das Katzencoccid *Isospora felis* (Wenyon 1923) (Studies on the canine coccid *Isospora felis* [Wenyon 1923]). Archiv für Protistenkunde 103 (3–4), 427–460 (in German).

Lim, Y.A.L., Ngui, R., Shukri, J., Rohela, M., Naim, H.R.M., 2008. Intestinal parasites in various animals at a zoo in Malaysia. Veterinary Parasitology 157 (1), 154–159.

Lim, Y.A., Iqbal, A., Surin, J., Sim, B.L., Jex, A.R., Nolan, M.J., Smith, H.V., Gasser, R.B., 2011. First genetic classification of *Cryptosporidium* and *Giardia* from HIV/AIDS patients in Malaysia. Infection, Genetics and Evolution: Journal of Molecular Epidemiology and Evolutionary Genetics in Infectious Diseases 11 (5), 968–974.

Lindergard, G., Nydam, D.V., Wade, S.E., Schaaf, S.L., Mohammed, H.O., 2003. A novel multiplex polymerase chain reaction approach for detection of four human infective *Cryptosporidium* isolates: *Cryptosporidium parvum*, types H and C, *Cryptosporidium canis*, and *Cryptosporidium felis* in fecal and soil samples. Journal of Veterinary Diagnostic Investigation 15 (3), 262–267.

Lindsay, D.S., Dubey, J.P., 1989a. Evaluation of anti-coccidial drugs' inhibition of *Neospora caninum* development in cell cultures. Journal of Parasitology 75 (6), 990–992.

Lindsay, D.S., Dubey, J.P., 1989b. Immunohistochemical diagnosis of *Neospora caninum* in tissue sections. American Journal of Veterinary Research 50 (11), 1981–1983.

Lindsay, D.S., Dubey, J.P., 1989c. In vitro development of *Neospora caninum* (Protozoa: Apicomplexa) from dogs. Journal of Parasitology 75 (1), 163–165.

Lindsay, D.S., Dubey, J.P., 1990. Effects of sulfadiazine and amprolium on *Neospora caninum* (Protozoa: Apicomplexa) infections in mice. Journal of Parasitology 76 (2), 177–179.

Lindsay, D.S., Dubey, J.P., 2000. Canine neosporosis. Journal of Veterinary Parasitology 14 (1), 1–11.

Lindsay, D.S., Blagburn, B.L., Mason, W.H., Frandsen, C., 1988. Prevalence of *Sarcocystis odocoileocanis* from white-tailed deer in Alabama and its attempted transmission to goats. Journal of Wildlife Diseases 24 (1), 154–156.

Lindsay, D.S., Rippey, N.S., Cole, R.A., Parsons, L.C., Dubey, J.P., Tidwell, R.R., Blagburn, B.L., 1994. Examination of the activities of 43 chemotherapeutic agents against *Neospora caninum* tachyzoites in cultured cells. American Journal of Veterinary Research 55 (7), 976–981.

Lindsay, D.S., Dubey, J.P., Blagburn, B.L., 1997. Biology of *Isospora* spp. from humans, nonhuman primates, and domestic animals. Clinical Microbiology Reviews 10 (1), 19–34.

Lindsay, D.S., Dubey, J.P., Kennedy, T.J., 2000a. Determination of the activity of ponazuril against *Sarcocystis neurona* in cell cultures. Veterinary Parasitology 92 (2), 165–169.

Lindsay, D.S., Thomas, N.J., Dubey, J.P., 2000b. Biological characterization of *Sarcocystis neurona* isolated from a southern sea otter (*Enhydra lutris nereis*). International Journal for Parasitology 30 (5), 617–624.

Lindsay, D.S., Thomas, N.J., Rosypal, A.C., Dubey, J.P., 2001a. Dual *Sarcocystis neurona* and *Toxoplasma gondii* infection in a northern sea otter from Washington state, USA. Veterinary Parasitology 97 (4), 319–327.

Lindsay, D.S., Spencer, J., Rupprecht, C., Blagburn, B.L., 2001b. Prevalence of agglutinating antibodies to *Neospora caninum* in raccoons, *Procyon lotor*. Journal of Parasitology 87 (5), 1197–1198.

Lindsay, D.S., Weston, J.L., Little, S.E., 2001c. Prevalence of antibodies to *Neospora caninum* and *Toxoplasma gondii* in gray foxes (*Urocyon cinereoargenteus*) from South Carolina. Veterinary Parasitology 97 (2), 159–164.

Lindsay, D.S., Houk, A.E., Mitchell, S.M., Dubey, J.P., 2014. Developmental biology of *Cystoisospora* (Apicomplexa: Sarcocystidae) monozoic tissue cysts. Journal of Parasitology 100 (4), 392–398.

Lipscomb, T.P., Dubey, J.P., Pletcher, J.M., Altman, N.H., 1989. Intrahepatic biliary coccidiosis in a dog. Veterinary Pathology 26 (4), 343–345.

Little, S.E., Johnson, E.M., Lewis, D., Jaklitsch, R.P., Payton, M.E., Blagburn, B.L., Bowman, D.D., Moroff, S., Tams, T., Rich, L., Aucoin, D., 2009. Prevalence of intestinal parasites in pet dogs in the United States. Veterinary Parasitology 166 (1–2), 144–152.

Litvenkova, A.E., 1969. Coccidia of wild mammals in Byelorussia. In: Progress in Protozoology, 3rd International Congress on Protozoology (Leningrad), vol. 3, pp. 340–341.

Liu, X., He, T., Zhong, Z., Zhang, H., Wang, R., Dong, H., Wang, C., Li, D., Deng, J., Peng, G., Zhang, L., 2013. A new genotype of *Cryptosporidium* from giant panda (*Ailuropoda melanoleuca*) in China. Parasitology International 62 (5), 454–458.

Lloyd, S., Smith, J., 1997. Pattern of *Cryptosporidium parvum* oocyst excretion by experimentally infected dogs. International Journal for Parasitology 27 (7), 799–801.

Llorente, M.T., Clavel, A., Varea, M., Pilar Goñi, M., Sahagún, J., Olivera, S., 2006. *Cryptosporidium felis* infection, Spain. Emerging Infectious Diseases 12 (9), 1471–1472.

Llorente, M.T., Clavel, A., Goñi, M.P., Varea, M., Seral, C., Becerril, R., Suarez, L., Gómez-Lus, R., 2007. Genetic characterization of *Cryptosporidium* species from humans in Spain. Parasitology International 56 (3), 201–205.

Loeffler, I.K., Howard, J.G., Montali, R.J., Hayek, L.-A., Dubovi, E., Zhang, Z., Yan, Q., Guo, W., Wildt, D.E., 2007. Serosurvey of ex situ giant pandas (*Ailuropoda melanoleuca*) and red pandas (*Ailurus fulgens*) in China with implications for species conservation. Journal of Zoo and Wildlife Medicine 38 (4), 559–566.

López, C., Panadero, R., Bravo, A., Paz, A., Sánchez-Andrade, R., Díez-Baños, P., Lugo, P.M., 2003. *Sarcocystis* spp. infection in roe deer (*Capreolus capreolus*) from the north-west of Spain. Zeitschrift für Jagdwissenschaft 49 (3), 211–288.

Lorenzini, G., Tasca, T., de Carli, G.A., 2007. Prevalência de parasitas intestinais em cães e gatos sob cuidado veterinário em Porto Alegre, Rio Grande do Sul, Brasil (Prevalence of intestinal parasites in dogs and cats under veterinary care in Porto Alegre Rio Grande do Sul, Brazil). Brazilian Journal of Veterinary Research and Animal Science 44 (2), 137–145 (in Portuguese, English summary).

Loveless, R.M., Andersen, F.L., 1975. Experimental infection of coyotes with *Echinococcus granulosus*, *Isospora canis*, and *Isospora rivolta*. Journal of Parasitology 61 (3), 546–547.

Lucca, Pd., De Gaspari, E.N., Bozzoli, L.M., Funada, M.R., Silva, S.O., Iuliano, W., Soares, R.M., 2009. Molecular characterization of *Cryptosporidium* spp. from HIV infected patients from an urban area of Brazil. Revista do Instituto de Medicina Tropical de Sao Paulo 51 (6), 341–343.

de Lucio, A., Merino, F.J., Martínez-Ruiz, R., Bailo, B., Aguilera, M., Fuentes, I., Carmena, D., 2016. Molecular genotyping and sub-genotyping of *Cryptosporidium* spp. isolates from symptomatic individuals attending two major public hospitals in Madrid, Spain. Infection, Genetics and Evolution. Journal of Molecular Epidemiology and Evolutionary Genetics in Infectious Diseases 37, 49–56.

de Lucio, A., Bailo, B., Aguilera, M., Cardona, G.A., Fernández-Crespo, J.C., Carmena, D., 2017. No molecular epidemiological evidence supporting household transmission of zoonotic *Giardia duodenalis* and *Cryptosporidium* spp. from pet dogs and cats in the province of Álava, Northern Spain. Acta Tropica 170, 48–56.

Lucio-Forster, A., Bowman, D.D., 2011. Prevalence of fecal-borne parasites detected by centrifugal flotation in feline samples from two shelters in upstate New York. Journal of Feline Medicine and Surgery 13 (4), 300–303.

Lucio-Forster, A., Griffiths, J.K., Cama, V.A., Xiao, L., Bowman, D.D., 2010. Minimal zoonotic risk of cryptosporidiosis from pet dogs and cats. Trends in Parasitology 26 (4), 174–179.

Lukešová, D., Literák, I., 1998. Shedding of *Toxoplasma gondii* oocysts by Felidae in zoos in the Czech Republic. Veterinary Parasitology 74 (1), 1–7.

Lupo, P.J., Langer-Curry, R.C., Robinson, M., Okhuysen, P.C., Chappell, C.L., 2008. *Cryptosporidium muris* in a Texas canine population. The American Journal of Tropical Medicine and Hygiene 78 (6), 917–921.

Lyon, C., 2010. Update on the diagnosis and management of *Neospora caninum* infections in dogs. Topics in Companion Animal Medicine 25 (3), 170–175.

Ma, H., Wang, Z., Wang, C., Li, C., Wei, F., Liu, Q., 2015. Fatal *Toxoplasma gondii* infection in the giant panda. Parasite 22, 30.

Macintire, D.K., Vincent-Johnson, N., Dillon, A.R., Blagburn, B., Lindsay, D., Whitley, E.M., Banfield, C., 1997. Hepatozoonosis in dogs. 22 cases (1989–1994). Journal of the American Veterinary Medical Association 210 (7), 916–922.

MacKinnon, D.L., Dibb, M.J., 1938. Report on intestinal protozoa of some mammals in the zoological gardens at Regent's park. Proceedings of the Zoological Society of London 108, 323–345.

Magi, M., Macchioni, F., Dell'Omodarme, M., Prati, M.C., Calderini, P., Gabrielli, S., Iori, A., Cancrini, G., 2009. Endoparasites of red fox (*Vulpes vulpes*) in central Italy. Journal of Wildlife Diseases 45 (3), 881–885.

Mahrt, J.L., 1966. Life Cycle of *Isospora rivolta* (Grassi, 1879) Wenyon, 1923 in the Dog (Ph.D. dissertation). University of Illinois, Urbana, Illinois.

Mahrt, J.L., 1967. Endogenous stages of the life cycle of *Isospora rivolta* in the dog. Journal of Protozoology 14 (4), 754–759.

Mahrt, J.L., 1968. Sporogony of *Isospora rivolta* oocysts from the dog. Journal of Protozoology 15 (2), 308–312.

Mahrt, J.L., 1973. Cinemicrographic observations on the asexual development of *Isospora canis* in cultured cells. Progress in Protozoology 4, 267.

Malloy, W.F., Embil, J.R., 1978. Prevalence of *Toxocara* spp. and other parasites in dogs and cats in Halifax, Nova Scotia. Canadian Journal of Comparative Medicine 42 (1), 29–31.

Mancianti, F., Nardoni, S., Mugnaini, L., Zambernardi, L., Guerrini, A., Gazzola, V., Papini, R.A., 2015. A retrospective molecular study of select intestinal protozoa in healthy pet cats from Italy. Journal of Feline Medicine and Surgery 17 (2), 163–167.

Mandal, A.K., 1976. Coccidia of Indian vertebrates. Record of the Zoological Survey of India 70, 94–106.

Mandal, A.K., Chakravarty, M.M., 1964. Studies on some aspects of avian coccidia (Protozoa: Sporozoa). 2. Five new species of *Isospora* Schneider, 1881. Proceedings of the Zoological Society of Calcutta 17 (1), 35–45.

Mandal, D., Choudhury, A., 1983. Coccidian parasites of some wild mammals in Betla Forest Palaman Tiger Reserve, Bihar, India. In: Ippen, R., Schröder (Eds.), International Symposium Erkrankungen der Zootiere, Wein, Austria, 11-15 May 1983, pp. 309–313.

Mandal, A.K., Ray, H.N., 1960. A new coccidium *Isospora leonina* n. sp. from a lion cub. Bulletin Calcutta School of Tropical Medicine 8, 107–108.

Manharth, A., February 6, 2004. Meerkat (AZA Small Carnivore TAG). Veterinary Advisor Report.

Mantovani, A., 1965. Osservazioni sulla coccidiosi delle volpi in Abruzzo (Observations on the coccidiosis of foxes in Abruzzo). Parassitologia 7 (1), 9–17 (in Italian).

Mao, J.B., Zuo, Y.X., 1994. Studies on the prevalence and experimental transmission of *Sarcocystis* sp. in chickens. Acta Veterinaria et Zootechnica Sinica 25, 555–559.

Marco, I., Ferroglio, E., López-Olvera, R., Montané, J., Lavin, S., 2008. High sereoprevalence of *Neospora caninum* in the red fox (*Vulpes vulpes*) in the Pyrenees (NE Spain). Veterinary Parasitology 152 (3–4), 321–324.

Margolin, J.H., Jolley, W.R., 1979. Experimental infection of dogs with *Sarcocystis* from wapiti. Journal of Wildlife Diseases 15 (2), 259–262.

Marks, S.L., Hanson, T.E., Melli, A.C., 2004. Comparison of direct immunofluorescence, modified acid-fast staining, and enzyme immunoassay techniques for detection of *Cryptosporidium* spp. in naturally exposed kittens. Journal of the American Veterinary Medical Association 225 (10), 1549–1553.

Markus, M.B., 1972. Diagnosis of isosporosis and toxoplasmosis. Transactions of the Royal Society of Tropical Medicine and Hygiene 66 (4), 673–674.

Markus, M.B., 1979. The authorship of *Hammondia hammondi*. Annals of Tropical Medicine and Parasitology 73 (4), 393–394.

Markus, M.B., 1983. The hypnozoite of *Isospora canis*. South African Journal of Science 79 (3), 117.

Markus, M.B., Draper, C.C., Hutchinson, W.H., Killick-Kendrick, R., Garnham, P.C.C., 1974a. Attempted infection of chimpanzees and cats with *Sarcocystis* of cattle. Transactions of the Royal Society of Tropical Medicine and Hygiene 68 (1), 3.

Markus, M.B., Killick-Kendrick, R., Garnham, P.C.C., 1974b. The coccidial nature and life-cycle of *Sarcocystis*. Journal of Tropical Medicine and Hygiene 77 (11), 248–259.

Marmi, J., López-Giráldez, J.F., Domingo-Roura, X., 2004. Phylogeny, evolutionary history and taxonomy of the Mustelidae based on sequences of the cytochrome b gene and a complex repetitive flanking region. Zoological Science 33, 481–499.

Marotel, M., 1912. Discussion paper by Besnoit and Robin. Bulletin et Mémoires de la Société des Sciences Vétérinaires de Lyon et de la Société de Médecine Vétérinaire des Lyon et du Sud-Est 15, 196–217.

Marsh, A.E., Barr, B.C., Packham, A.E., Conrad, P.A., 1998. Description of a new *Neospora* species (Protozoa: Apicomplexa: Sarcocystidae). Journal of Parasitology 84 (5), 983–991.

Martin, H.D., Zeidner, N.S., 1992. Concomitant cryptosporidia, coronavirus and parvovirus infection in a raccoon (Procyon lotor). Journal of Wildlife Diseases 28 (1), 113–115.

Martino, P.E., Montenegro, J.L., Preziosi, J.A., Venturini, C., Bacigalupe, D., Stanchi, N.O., Bautista, E.L., 2004. Serological survey of selected pathogens of free-ranging foxes in southern Argentina, 1998–2001. OIE Revue Scientifique et Technique 23 (3), 801–806.

Mason, F.E., 1910. Sarcocysts in the camel in Egypt. Journal of Comparative Pathology and Therapy 23, 168–176.

Mason, R.W., 1978. The detection of Hammondia hammondi in Australia and the identification of a free-living intermediate host. Zeitschrift für Parasitenkunde 57 (2), 101–106.

Mason, R.W., 1980. The discovery of Besnoitia wallacei in Australia and the identification of a free-living intermediate host. Zeitschrift für Parasitenkunde 61 (2), 173–178.

Mason, P., Orr, M., 1993. Sarcocystosis and hydatidosis in lamoids – diseases we can do without. Surveillance 20, 14.

Mateo, M., de Mingo, M.H., de Lucio, A., Morales, L., Balseiro, A., Espí, A., Barral, M., Lima Barbero, J.F., Habela, M.Á., Fernández-García, J.L., Bernal, R.C., Köster, P.C., Cardona, G.A., Carmena, D., 2017. Occurrence and molecular genotyping of Giardia duodenalis and Cryptosporidium spp. in wild mesocarnivores in Spain. Veterinary Parasitology 235, 86–93.

Matjila, P.T., Leisewitz, A.L., Jongejan, F., Bertschinger, H.J., Penzhorn, B.L., 2008. Molecular detection of Babesia rossi and Hepatozoon sp. in African wild dogs (Lycaon pictus) in South Africa. Veterinary Parasitology 157 (1), 123–127.

Matoba, Y., Asano, M., Masubuchi, H., Asakawa, M., 2002. First record of the genera Eimeria and Isospora (Protozoa: Eimeriidae) obtained from feral raccoons (Procyon lotor) alien species in Japan and prevalence of serum antibodies to Toxoplasma gondii among the raccoons. Japanese Journal of Zoo and Wildlife Medicine 7 (1), 87–90 (in Japanese, English summary).

Matos, O., Alves, M., Xiao, L., Cama, V., Antunes, F., 2004. Cryptosporidium felis and C. meleagridis in persons with HIV, Portugal. Emerging Infectious Diseases 10 (12), 2256–2257.

Matschoulsky, S.N., 1947a. About coccidia of fur animals in Buryat-Mongol, SSR, vol. 3. Trudy Buryat-Mongol'skoi Zooveterinarnogo Instituta, Ulan-Ude, pp. 78–86.

Matschoulsky, S.N., 1947b. K voprosu o koktsidiyakh zverei Buryat-Mongol'skoi ASSR. (Sarcosporidiosis of wildlife in Buryat-Mongolia), vol. 3. Trudy Buryat-Mongol'skoi Zooveterinarnogo Instituta, Ulan-Ude, pp. 87–92 (in Russian).

Matsubayashi, M., Abe, N., Takami, K., Kimata, I., Iseki, M., Nakanishi, T., Tani, H., Sasai, K., Baba, E., 2004. First record of Cryptosporidium infection in a raccoon dog (Nyctereutes procyonoides viverrinus). Veterinary Parasitology 120 (3), 171–175.

Matsubayashi, M., Takami, K., Kimata, I., Nakanishi, T., Tani, H., Sasai, K., Baba, E., 2005. Survey of Cryptosporidium spp. and Giardia spp. infections in various animals at a zoo in Japan. Journal of Zoo and Wildlife Medicine: Official Publication of the American Associations of Zoo Veterinarians 36 (2), 331–335.

Matsui, T., Morii, T., Iijima, T., Ito, S., Tsunoda, K., Correa, W.M., Fujino, T., 1981. Cyclic transmission of the small type of Isospora bigemina of the dog. Japanese Journal of Parasitology 30 (3), 179–186.

Matsui, T., Morii, T., Iijima, T., Ito, S., Tsunoda, K., Kobayashi, F., Fujino, T., 1986. Isospora heydorni isolated in Brazil: endogenous stages in dogs. Japanese Journal of Parasitology 35 (3), 215–222.

Matsui, T., Morii, T., Iijima, T., Ohnaga, H., Tohgou, S., Ishii, T., 1987. Isospora heydorni isolated in Brazil: infectivity to cattle. Japanese Journal of Parasitology 36 (5), 343–346.

Matsui, T., Morii, T., Iijima, T., Kobayashi, F., Fujino, T., 1989. Transformation of oocysts from several coccidian species by heat treatment. Parasitology Research 75 (4), 264–267.

Matsui, T., Fujino, T., Morii, T., Ito, S., 1993a. Infectivity to mice of the merozoites and zoites of Isospora rivolta in cats. Japanese Journal of Parasitology 42 (6), 457–460.

Matsui, T., Fujino, T., Morii, T., Kobayashi, F., Tsuji, M., 1993b. Invasion of the extra-intestinal organs of cats by the merozoites and zoites of Isospora rivolta. Journal of the Kyorin Medical Society 24 (2), 201–204.

Matsui, T., Ito, S., Fujino, T., Morii, T., 1993c. Infectivity and sporogony of Caryospora-type oocysts of Isospora rivolta obtained by heating. Parasitology Research 79 (7), 599–602.

Mattos, B.C., Patrício, L.L., Plugge, N.E., Lange, R.R., Richartz, R.R., Dittrich, R.L., 2008. Seroprevalence of antibodies anti-Neospora caninum and anti-Toxoplasma gondii in captive wild canids. Revista Brasileira de Parasitologia Veterinaria 17 (1), 267–272 (in Portuguese, English summary).

Matuschka, F.-R., Bannert, B., 1987. Canibalism and autonomy as predator-prey relationship for monoxenous Sarcosporidia. Parasitology Research 74 (1), 88–93.

Mayberry, L.F., Bristol, J.R., Duszynski, D.W., Reid, W.H., 1980. Eimeria macrotis sp. n. from Vulpes macrotis neomexicanus Merriam, 1902. Zeitschrift für Parasitenkunde 61, 197–200.

Mayer, H., 1965. Investigaciones sobre toxoplasmosis (Experiments and results in toxoplasmosis). Boletin de la Oficina Sanitaria Panamericana 58, 485–497 (in Spanish, English summary).

Mayhew, I.G., Smith, K.C., Dubey, J.P., Gatwards, L.K., McGlennon, N.J., 1991. Treatment of encephalomyelitis due to Neospora caninum in a litter of puppies. Journal of Small Animal Practice 32, 609–612.

Mayr, E., 1986. Uncertainty in Science: is the giant panda a bear or a raccoon? Nature 323 (6091), 769–771.

Mazuz, M.L., Haynes, R., Shkap, V., Fish, L., Wollkomirsky, R., Leibovich, B., Molad, T., Savitsky, I., Golenser, J., 2012. *Neospora caninum*: in vivo and in vitro treatment with artemisone. Veterinary Parasitology 187 (1–2), 99–104.

Mbae, C., Mulinge, E., Waruru, A., Ngugi, B., Wainaina, J., Kariuki, S., 2015. Genetic diversity of *Cryptosporidium* in children in an urban informal settlement of Nairobi, Kenya. PLoS One 10 (12), e0142055.

McAllister, M.M., Dubey, J.P., Lindsay, D.S., Jolley, W.R., Wills, R.A., McGuire, A.M., 1998a. Dogs are definitive hosts of *Neospora caninum*. International Journal for Parasitology 28 (9), 1473–1478.

McAllister, M.M., Jolley, W.R., Wills, R.A., Lindsay, D.S., McGuire, A.M., Tranas, J.D., 1998b. Oral inoculation of cats with tissue cysts of *Neospora caninum*. American Journal of Veterinary Research 59 (4), 441–444.

McClelland, G., 1993. *Eimeria phocae* (Apicomplexa: Eimeriidae) in harbour seals *Phoca vitulina* from Sable Island, Canada. Diseases of Aquatic Organisms 17, 1–8.

McCully, R.M., Basson, P.A., Bigalke, R.D., De Vos, V., Young, E., 1975. Observations on naturally acquired hepatozoonosis of wild carnivores and dogs in the Republic of South Africa. Onderstepoort Journal of Veterinary Research 42 (4), 117–134.

McFadden, K.W., Wade, S.E., Dubovi, E.J., Gompper, M.E., 2005. A serological and fecal parasitologic survey of the critically endangered pygmy raccoon (*Procyon pygmaeus*). Journal of Wildlife Diseases 41 (3), 615–617.

McGlade, T.R., Robertson, E.D., Elliot, A.D., Read, C., Thompson, R.C.A., 2003. Gastrointestinal parasites of domestic cats in Perth, Western Australia. Veterinary Parasitology 117 (4), 251–262.

McHardy, N., Woollon, R.M., Clampitt, R.B., James, J.A., Crawley, R.J., 1986. Efficacy, toxicity and metabolism of imidocarb dipropionate in the treatment of *Babesia ovis* infection in sheep. Research in Veterinary Science 41 (1), 14–20.

McKenna, P.B., Charleston, W.A.G., 1980a. Coccidia (Protozoa: Sporozoasida) of cats and dogs. I. Identity and prevalence in cats. New Zealand Veterinary Journal 28 (5), 86–88.

McKenna, P.B., Charleston, W.A.G., 1980b. Coccidia (Protozoa: Sporozoasida) of cats and dogs. II. Experimental induction of *Sarcocystis* infections in mice. New Zealand Veterinary Journal 28 (6), 117–119.

McKenna, P.B., Charleston, W.A.G., 1980c. Coccidia (Protozoa: Sporozoasida) of cats and dogs. III. The occurrence of a species of *Besnoitia* in cats. New Zealand Veterinary Journal 28 (6), 120–122.

McKenna, P.B., Charleston, W.A.G., 1980d. Coccidia (Protozoa: Sporozoasida) of cats and dogs. IV. Identity and prevalence in dogs. New Zealand Veterinary Journal 28 (7), 128–130.

McKenna, P.B., Charleston, W.A.G., 1982. Activation and excystation of *Isospora felis* and *Isospora rivolta* sporozoites. Journal of Parasitology 68 (2), 276–286.

McReynolds, C.A., Lappin, M.R., Ungar, B., McReynolds, L.M., Bruns, C., Spilker, M.M., Thrall, M.A., Reif, J.S., 1999. Regional seroprevalence of *Cryptosporidium parvum*-specific IgG of cats in the United States. Veterinary Parasitology 80 (3), 187–195.

McTaggart, H.S., 1960. Coccidia from mink in Britain. Journal of Parasitology 46, 201–205.

Measures, L.N., Dubey, J.P., Labelle, P., Martineau, D., 2004. Seroprevalence of *Toxoplasma gondii* in Canadian Pinnipeds. Journal of Wildlife Diseases 40 (2), 294–300.

Mech, L.D., Kurtz, H.J., 1999. First record of coccidiosis in wolves, *Canis lupus*. The Canadian Field Naturalist 113, 305–306.

Meeusen, E.N., Walker, J., Peters, A., Pastoret, P.P., Jungersen, G., 2007. Current status of veterinary vaccines. Clinical Microbiology Reviews 20 (3), 489–510.

Mehlhorn, H., 1974. Light and electron microscope studies on stages of *Sarcocystis tenella* in the intestine of cats. In: Proceedings of the 3rd International Congress of Parasitology, vol. 1, pp. 105–106.

Mehlhorn, H., Aspöck, H., 2008. Coccidial drugs. In: Mehlhorn, H. (Ed.), Encyclopedia of Parasitology, third ed. Springer-Verlag Berlin Heidelberg, Germany, pp. 269–286.

Mehlhorn, H., Heydorn, A.O., 2000. *Neospora caninum*: is it really different from *Hammondia heydorni* or is it a strain of *Toxoplasma gondii*? An opinion. Parasitology Research 86 (2), 169–178.

Mehlhorn, H., Markus, M.B., 1976. Electron microscopy of stages of *Isospora felis* of the cat in the mesenteric lymph nodes of the mouse. Zeitschrift für Parasitenkunde 51 (1), 15–24.

Mehlhorn, H., Scholtyseck, E., 1973. Elektronenmikroskopische Untersuchungen an Cystenstadien von *Sarcocystis tenella* aus der Oesophagus-muskulatur des Schafes (Electron microscope studies on cyst staging of *Sarcocystis tenella* from the esophageal musculature of the sheep). Zeitschrift für Parasitenkunde 41 (4), 291–310 (in German).

Mehlhorn, H., Scholtyseck, E., 1974a. Die Parasit-Wirtsbeziehungen bei verscheidenen gattungen der Sporozoen (*Eimeria, Toxoplasma, Sarcocystis, Frenkelia, Hepatozoon, Plasmodium* und *Babesia*) unter Anwendung spezieller Verfahren. Microscopica Acta 75 (5), 429–451 (in German).

Mehlhorn, H., Scholtyseck, E., 1974b. Licht und elektronenmikroskopische Untersuchungen an Entwicklungsstadien von *Sarcocystis tenella* aus der Darmwand der Hauskatze. I. Die Oocysten und Sporocysten. Zeitschrift für Parasitenkunde 43 (4), 251–270 (in German).

Mehlhorn, H., Senaud, J., Heydorn, A.G., Gestrich, R., 1975a. Comparison des ultrastructures des kystes de *Sarcocystis fusiformis* Railliet, 1897 dans la musculature du bœuf, après infection naturelle et après infection expérimentale par des sporocystes d'*Isospora hominis* et par des sporocystes des grandes formes d'*Isospora bigemina* du chien et du chat (Comparison of ultrastructures of the cysts of *Sarcocystis fusiformis* Railliet, 1897 in the musculature of the beef, after natural infection and after experimental infection by sporocysts of *Isospora hominis* and sporocysts of the large forms of *Isospora bigemina* of the dog and the cat). Protistologica 11 (4), 445–455 (in French, English summary).

Mehlhorn, H., Heydorn, A.-O., Gestrich, R., 1975b. Licht- und elektronenmikroskopische Untersuchungen an Cysten von *Sarcocystis fusiformis* in der Muskulatur von Kälbern nach experimenteller Infektion mit Oocysten und Sporocysten der grossen Form von *Isospora bigemina* des Hundes (Light and electron microscope studies on cysts of *Sarcocystis fusiformis* in the muscles of calves infected experimentally with oocysts and sporocysts of the large form of *Isospora bigemina* from dogs. 1. The development of cyst and cyst wall). Zentralblatt für Bakteriologie, Parasitenkunde, Infektionskrankheiten und Hygiene. I. Abteilung Originale Reihe A: Medizinische Mikrobiologie und Parasitologie 232 (2–3), 392–409 (in German, English summary).

Mehlhorn, H., Hartley, W.J., Heydorn, A.-O., 1976. A comparative ultrastructural study of the cyst wall of 13 *Sarcocystis* species. Protistologica 12, 451–467.

Mehlhorn, H., Ortmann-Falkenstein, G., Haberkorn, A., 1984. The effects of the sym. trianzinons on developmental stages of *Eimeria tenella*, *E. maxima* and *E. acervulina*: a light and electron microscopical study. Zeitschrift für Parasitenkunde 70 (2), 173–182.

Meireles, M.V., 2010. *Cryptosporidium* infection in Brazil: implications for veterinary medicine and public health. Revista Brasileira de Parasitologia Veterinaria 19 (4), 197–204.

Mekaru, S.R., Marks, S.L., Felley, A.J., Chouicha, N., Kass, P.H., 2007. Comparison of direct immunofluorescence, immunoassays, and fecal flotation for detection of *Cryptosporidium* spp. and *Giardia* spp. in naturally exposed cats in 4 Northern California animal shelters. Journal of Veterinary Internal Medicine 21 (5), 959–965.

Meloni, B.P., Thompson, R.C., Hopkins, R.M., Reynolds, J.A., Gracey, M., 1993. The prevalence of *Giardia* and other intestinal parasites in children, dogs and cats from aboriginal communities in the Kimberley. The Medical Journal of Australia 158 (3), 157–159.

Memmedov, I., 2010. Nahcivan ozerk cumhuriyetinde bazi kanatlilarda *Sarcocystis* turlerinin yayginligi (The prevalence of *Sarcocystis* species in some birds in Nakhichevan republic). Kafkas Üniversitesi Veteriner Fakültesi Dergisi 16, 857–860 (in Russian).

Méndez-Hermida, F., Gómez-Couso, H., Romero-Suances, R., Ares-Mazás, E., 2007. *Cryptosporidium* and *Giardia* in wild otters (*Lutra lutra*). Veterinary Parasitology 144 (1–2), 153–156.

Mense, M.G., Dubey, J.P., Homer, B.L., 1992. Acute hepatic necrosis associated with a *Sarcocystis*-like protozoa in a sea lion (*Zalophus californianus*). Journal of Veterinary Diagnostic Investigation 4 (4), 486–490.

Mercer, S.H., Jones, L.P., Rappole, J.H., Twedt, D., Laack, L.L., Craig, T.M., 1988. *Hepatozoon* sp. in wild carnivores in Texas. Journal of Wildlife Diseases 24 (3), 574–576.

Meredith, R.W., Janečka, J.E., Gatesy, J., Ryder, O.A., Fisher, C.A., Teeling, E.C., Goodbla, A., Eizirik, E., Simão, T.L., Stadler, T., Rabosky, D.L., Honeycutt, R.L., Flynn, J.J., Ingram, C.M., Steiner, C., Williams, T.L., Robinson, T.J., Burk-Herrick, A., Westerman, M., Ayoub, N.A., Springer, M.S., Murphy, W.J., 2011. Impacts of the cretaceous terrestrial revolution and KPg extinction on mammal diversification. Science 334 (6055), 521–524.

Merino, S., Vásquez, R.A., Martínez, J., Celis-Diez, J.L., Martínez-de la Puente, J., Marín-Vial, P., Sánchez-Monsalvez, I., Peirce, M.A., 2008. A sarcocystid misidentified as *Hepatozoon didelphydis*: molecular data from a parasitic infection in the blood of the southern mouse opossum (*Thylamys elegans*) from Chile. Journal of Eukaryotic Microbiology 55, 536–540.

Merino, S., Vásquez, R.A., Martínez, J., Celis-Diez, J.L., Gutiérrez-Jiménez, L., Ippi, S., Sánchez-Monsalvez, I., Martínez-de la Puente, J., 2009. Molecular characterization of an ancient *Hepatozoon* species parasitizing the "living fossil" marsupial "monito del monte" *Dromiciops gliroides* from from Chile. Biological Journal of the Linnean Society 98, 568–576.

Merino, S., Martínez, J., Vasquez, R.A., Šlapeta, J., 2010. Monophyly of marsupial intraerythrocytic apicomplexan parasites from South America and Australia. Parasitology 137, 37–43.

Metzger, B., dos Santos Paduan, K., Rubini, A.S., de Oliveira, T.G., Pereira, C., O'Dwyer, L.H., 2008. The first report of *Hepatozoon* sp. (Apicomplexa: Hepatozoidae) in neotropical felids from Brazil. Veterinary Parasitology 152 (1–2), 28–33.

Michael, S.A., Howe, L., Chilvers, B.I., Morel, P.C.H., Roe, W.D., 2016. Seroprevalence of *Toxoplasma gondii* in mainland and sub-Antarctic New Zealand sea lion (*Phocarctos hookeri*) populations. New Zealand Veterinary Journal 64 (5), 293–297.

Miescher, F., 1843. Über eigenthümliche Schläuche in den Muskein einer Hausmaus (On peculiar tubes in the muscle of a house mouse). Bericht der Verhandlungen der Naturforschender Gesellschaft 5, 198–202 (in German).

Migaki, G., Albert, T.F., 1980. Sarcosporidiosis in the ringed seal. Journal of the American Veterinary Medical Association 177 (9), 917–918.

Migaki, G., Allen, J.F., Casey, H.W., 1977. Toxoplasmosis in a California sea lion. American Journal of Veterinary Research 38 (1), 135–136.

Millán, J., Cabezón, O., Pabón, M., Dubey, J.P., Almería, S., 2009. Seroprevalence of *Toxoplasma gondii* and *Neospora caninum* in feral cats (*Felis silvestris catus*) in Majorca, Balearic Islands, Spain. Veterinary Parasitology 165 (3–4), 323–326.

Millán, J., Sobrino, R., Rodríguez, A., Oleaga, Á., Gortazar, C., Schares, G., 2012. Large-scale serosurvey of *Besnoitia besnoiti* in free-living carnivores in Spain. Veterinary Parasitology 190 (1), 241–245.

Miller, W.W., 1908. *Hepatozoon perniciosum* (n.g., n.sp.) a haemogregarine pathogenic for white rats; with a brief description of the sexual cycle in the intermediate host, a mite (*Laelaps echidninus* Berlese). Bulletin of the Hygiene Laboratory (Washington) 46, 51–123.

Miller, N.L., Frenkel, J.K., Dubey, J.P., 1972. Oral infections with toxoplasma cysts and oocysts in felines, other mammals, and in birds. Journal of Parasitology 58 (5), 928–937.

Miller, M.A., Crosbie, P.R., Sverlow, K., Hanni, K., Barr, B.C., Kock, N., Murray, M.J., Lowenstine, L.J., Conrad, P.A., 2001a. Isolation and characterization of *Sarcocystis* from brain tissue of a free-living southern sea otter (*Enhydra lutris nereis*) with fatal meningoencephalitis. Parasitology Research 87 (3), 252–257.

Miller, M.A., Sverlow, K., Crosbie, P.R., Barr, B.C., Lowenstein, L.J., Gulland, F.M., Packham, A., Conrad, P.A., 2001b. Isolation and characterization of two parasitic protozoa from a Pacific harbor seal (*Phoca vitulina richardsi*) with meningoencephlomyelitis. Journal of Parasitology 87 (4), 816–822.

Miller, M.A., Gardner, I.A., Kreuder, C., Paradies, D.M., Worcester, K.R., Jessup, D.A., Dodd, E., Harris, M.D., Ames, J.A., Packham, A.E., Conrad, P.A., 2002. Coastal freshwater runoff is a risk factor for *Toxoplasma gondii* infection of southern sea otters (*Enhydra lutris nereis*). International Journal for Parasitology 32 (8), 997–1006.

Miller, D.L., Liggett, A., Radi, Z.A., Branch, L.O., 2003. Gastrointestinal cryptosporidiosis in a puppy. Veterinary Parasitology 115 (3), 199–204.

Miller, M.A., Grigg, M.E., Kreuder, C., James, E.R., Melli, A.C., Crosbie, P.R., Jessup, D.A., Boothroyd, J.C., Brownstein, D., Conrad, P.A., 2004. An unusual genotype of *Toxoplasma gondii* is common in California sea otters (*Enhydra lutris nereis*) and is a cause of mortality. International Journal for Parasitology 34 (3), 275–284.

Miller, W.A., Miller, M.A., Gardner, I.A., Atwill, E.R., Harris, M., Ames, J., Jessup, D., Melli, A., Paradies, D., Worcester, K., Olin, P., Barnes, N., Conrad, P.A., 2005. New genotypes and factors associated with *Cryptosporidium* detection in mussels (*Mytilus* spp.) along the California coast. International Journal for Parasitology 35 (10), 1103–1113.

Miller, M.A., Barr, B.C., Nordhausen, R., James, E.R., Magargal, S.L., Murray, M., Conrad, P.A., Toy-Choutka, S., Jessup, D.A., Grigg, M.E., 2009. Ultrastructural and molecular confirmation of the development of *Sarcocystis*

neurona tissue cysts in the central nervous system of southern sea otters (*Enhydra lutris nereis*). International Journal for Parasitology 39 (12), 1363–1372.

Milstein, T.C., Goldsmid, J.M., 1997. Parasites of feral cats from southern Tasmania and their potential significance. Australian Veterinary Journal 75 (3), 218–219.

Mimioğlu, M., Güralp, N., Sayin, F., 1960. Ankara köpeklerinde görülen parazit türleri ve bunlarin yayilis nisbeti, vol. 6. Veteriner Fakultesi (Ankara Universitesi), pp. 53–68 (in Turkish, English summary).

Mirza, M.Y., 1970. Incidence and Distribution of Coccidia (Sporozoa: Eimeriidae) in Mammals from Baghdad Area (M.S. thesis), Baghdad, Iraq. 195 p.

Mirzaei, M., 2012. Epidemiological survey of *Cryptosporidium* spp. in companion and stray dogs in Kerman, Iran. Veterinaria Italiana 48 (3), 291–296.

Mirzaei, M., Fooladi, M., 2013. Coproscopy survey on gastrointestinal parasites in owned dogs of Kerman city, Iran. Veterinaria Italiana 49 (3), 309–313.

Mirzaghavami, M., Sadraei, J., Forouzandeh, M., 2016. Detection of *Cryptosporidium* spp. in free ranging animals of Tehran, Iran. Journal of Parasitic Diseases: Official Organ of the Indian Society for Parasitology 40 (4), 1528–1531.

Mirzayans, A., Eslami, A.H., Anwar, M., Sanjar, M., 1972. Gastrointestinal parasites of dogs in Iran. Tropical Animal Health and Production 4 (1), 58–60.

Mitchell, S.M., Zajac, A.M., Lindsay, D.S., 2009. Development and ultrastructure of *Cystoisospora canis* Neméseri, 1959 (syn. *Isospora canis*) monozoic cysts in two noncanine cell lines. Journal of Parasitology 95 (4), 793–798.

Modrý, D., 2001. Case 3187. *Isospora* Schneider, 1881 (Protista, Apicomplexa): proposed designation of *I. suis* Biester, 1934 as the type species. Bulletin of Zoological Nomenclature 54, 272–273.

Mohammed, O.B., 2000. Prevalence, Identity and Phylogeny of Sarcocystis Parasites from Gazelles in Saudi Arabia (Ph.D. thesis) (#323554). Kingston University, London.

Mohammed, O.B., Davies, A.J., Hussein, H.S., Daszak, P., 2000. *Sarcocystis* infections in gazelles at the King Khalid wildlife research Center, Saudi Arabia. The Veterinary Record 146 (8), 218–221.

Mohammed, O.B., Davies, A.J., Hussein, H.S., Daszak, P., Ellis, J.T., 2003. *Hammondia heydorni* from the arabian mountain gazelle and red fox in Saudi Arabia. Journal of Parasitology 99 (3), 535–539.

Molloy, S.F., Smith, H.V., Kirwan, P., Nichols, R.A., Asaolu, S.O., Connelly, L., Holland, C.V., 2010. Identification of a high diversity of *Cryptosporidium* species genotypes and subtypes in a pediatric population in Nigeria. The American Journal of Tropical Medicine and Hygiene 82 (4), 608–613.

Montali, R.J., Bartz, C.R., Teare, J.A., Allen, J.T., Appel, M.J., Bush, M., 1983. Clinical trials with canine distemper vaccines in exotic carnivores. Journal of the American Veterinary Medical Association 183 (11), 1163–1167.

Monticello, T.M., Levy, M.G., Bunch, S.E., Fairley, R.A., 1987. Cryptosporidiosis in a feline leukemia virus-positive cat. Journal of the American Veterinary Medical Association 191 (6), 705–706.

Moore, C.E., Elwin, K., Phot, N., Seng, C., Mao, S., Suy, K., Kumar, V., Nader, J., Bousfield, R., Perera, S., Bailey, J.W., Beeching, N.J., Day, N.P., Parry, C.M., Chalmers, R.M., 2016. Molecular characterization of *Cryptosporidium* species and *Giardia duodenalis* from symptomatic Cambodian children. PLoS Neglected Tropical Diseases 10 (7), e0004822.

Moré, G., Pantchev, A., Skuballa, J., Langenmayer, M.C., Maksimov, P., Conraths, F.J., Venturini, M.C., Schares, G., 2014. *Sarcocystis sinensis* is the most prevalent thick-walled *Sarcocystis* in beef for consumers in Germany. Parasitology Research 113 (6), 2223–2230.

Morgan, U.M., Thompson, R.C., 1998. PCR detection of cryptosporidium: the way forward? Parasitology Today 14 (6), 241–245.

Morgan, B.B., Waller, E.F., 1940. Severe parasitism in a raccoon (*Procyon lotor lotor*, Linnaeus). Transactions of the American Microscopical Society 59, 523–527.

Morgan, U.M., Sargent, K.D., Elliot, A., Thompson, R.C.A., 1998. *Cryptosporidium* in cats – additional evidence for *C. felis*. Veterinary Journal (London, England: 1997) 156 (2), 159–161.

Morgan, U.M., Deplazes, P., Forbes, D.A., Spano, F., Hertzberg, H., Sargent, K.D., Elliot, A., Thompson, R.C.A., 1999a. Sequence and PCR-RFLP analysis of the internal transcribed spacers of the rDNA repeat unit in isolates of *Cryptosporidium* from different hosts. Parasitology 118 (1), 49–58.

Morgan, U.M., Morris, P.T., Fayer, R., Deplazes, P., Thompson, R.C.A., 1999b. Phylogenetic relationships among isolates of *Cryptosporidium*: evidence for several new species. Journal of Parasitology 85 (6), 1126–1133.

Morgan, U.M., Xiao, L., Fayer, R., Lai, A.A., Thompson, R.C.A., 1999c. Variation in *Cryptosporidium*: towards a taxonomic revision of the genus. International Journal for Parasitology 29 (11), 1733–1751.

Morgan, U.M., Weber, R., Xiao, L., Sulaiman, I., Thompson, R.C.A., Ndiritu, W., Lal, A., Moore, A., Deplazes, P., 2000a. Molecular characterization of *Cryptosporidium* isolates obtained from human immunodeficiency virus-infected individuals living in Switzerland, Kenya, and the United States. Journal of Clinical Microbiology 38 (3), 1180–1183.

Morgan, U.M., Xiao, L., Monis, P., Fall, A., Irwin, P.J., Fayer, R., Denholm, K.M., Limor, J., Lal, A., Thompson, R.C., 2000b. *Cryptosporidium* spp. in domestic dogs: the "dog" genotype. Applied and Environmental Microbiology 66 (5), 2220–2223.

Morgan-Ryan, U.M., Fall, A., Ward, L.A., Hijjawi, N., Sulaiman, I., Fayer, R., Thompson, R.C., Olson, M., Lal, A., Xiao, L., 2002. *Cryptosporidium hominis* n. sp. (Apicomplexa: Cryptosporidiidae) from *Homo sapiens*. Journal of Eukaryotic Microbiology 49 (6), 433–440.

Motamedi, G.R., Dalimi, A., Nouri, A., Aghaeipour, K., 2011. Ultrastructural and molecular characterization of *Sarcocystis* isolated from camel (*Camelus dromedarius*) in Iran. Parasitology Research 108 (4), 949–954.

Moudgil, A.D., 2015. Studies on the Prevalence and Management of Parasitic Infections in Zoo Animals (Ph.D. dissertation). Guru Angad Dev Veterinary and Animal Sciences University, Ludhiana, India. 144 p.

de Moura Costa, M.D., 1956. Isosporose do cão-dom a descrição do uma nova variedade (*Isospora bigemina* Stiles, 1891 *bahiensis* n. var.), vol. 3. Boletim do Instituto Biológico da Bahia (Salvador), pp. 107–112 (in Portuguese).

Mtambo, M.M., Nash, A.S., Blewett, D.A., Smith, H.V., Wright, S., 1991. *Cryptosporidium* infection in cats: prevalence of infection in domestic and feral cats in the Glasgow area. The Veterinary Record 129 (23), 502–504.

Mugridge, N.B., Morrison, D.A., Heckeroth, A.R., Johnson, A.M., Tenter, A.M., 1999. Phylogenetic analysis based on full-length large subunit ribosomal RNA gene sequence comparison reveals that *Neospora caninum* is more closely related to *Hammondia heydorni* than to *Toxoplasma gondii*. International Journal for Parasitology 29 (10), 1545–1556.

Mukherjee, A.K., Krassner, S.M., 1965. A new species of coccidia (Protozoa: Sporozoa) of the genus *Isospora* Schneider, 1881, from the jackal, *Canis aureus* Linnaeus. Proceedings of the Zoological Society of Calcutta 18 (1), 35–40.

Müller, J., Aguado-Martinez, A., Manser, V., Balmer, V., Winzer, P., Ritler, D., Hostettler, I., Arranz-Solís, D., Ortega-Mora, L., Hemphill, A., 2015. Buparvaquone is active against *Neospora caninum* in vitro and in experimentally infected mice. International Journal for Parasitology. Drugs and Drug Resistance 5 (1), 16–25.

Munday, B.L., Black, H., 1976. Suspected *Sarcocystis* infections of the bovine placenta and foetus. Parasitology Research 51 (1), 129–132.

Munday, B.L., Corbould, A., 1973. The possible role of the dog in the epidemiology of ovine sarcosporidiosis. British Veterinary Journal 130 (1), ix–xi.

Munday, B.L., Obendorf, D.L., 1984. Morphology of *Sarcocystis gigantea* in experimentally-infected sheep. Veterinary Parasitology 16 (3–4), 193–199.

Munday, B.L., Rickard, M.D., 1974. Is *Sarcocystis tenella* two species? Australian Veterinary Journal 50 (12), 558–559.

Munday, B.L., Barker, I.K., Rickard, M.O., 1975. The developmental cycle of a species of *Sarcocystis* occurring in dogs and sheep with observations on pathogenicity in the intermediate host. Parasitology Research 46 (2), 111–123.

Munday, B.L., Humphrey, J.D., Kila, V., 1977. Pathology produced by, prevalence of, and probable life cycle of species of *Sarcocystis* in the domestic fowl. Avian Diseases 21 (4), 697–703.

Munday, B.L., Mason, R.W., Hartley, W.J., Presidente, P.J.A., Obendorf, D., 1978. *Sarcocystis* and related organisms in Australian wildlife. I. Survey findings in mammals. Journal of Wildlife Diseases 14 (4), 417–433.

Mundim, M.J.S., Rosa, L.A.G., Hortêncio, S.M., Faria, E.S.M., Rodrigues, R.M., Cry, M.C., 2007. Prevalence of *Giardia duodenalis* and *Cryptosporidium* spp. in dogs from different living conditions in Uberlândia, Brazil. Veterinary Parasitology 144 (3), 356–359.

Munro, R., Synge, B., 1991. Coccidiosis in seals. The Veterinary Record 129 (8), 179–180.

Murasugi, E., Asano, R., Kawamura, T., Fukuda, Y., Yamamoto, Y., 1996. Anti-toxoplasma antibody levels in the main-land raccoon dog, *Nyctereutes procyonoides viverrinus*, in southeastern Kanagawa prefecture. Kansenshogaku Zasshi. The Journal of the Japanese Association for Infectious Diseases 70 (10), 168–171 (in Japanese, English summary).

Murata, T., Shiramizu, K., Hara, Y., Inque, M., Shimoda, K., Nakama, S., 1991. First case of *Hepatozoon canis* infection of a dog in Japan. Journal of Veterinary Medical Science 53 (6), 1097–1099.

Murphy, T.M., Walochnik, J., Hassl, A., Moriarty, J., Mooney, J., Toolan, D., Sanchez-Miguel, C., O'Loughlin, A.O., McAuliffe, A., 2007. Study on the prevalence of *Toxoplasma gondii* and *Neospora caninum* and molecular evidence of *Encephalitozoon cuniculi* and *Encephalitozoon (Septata) intestinalis* infections in red foxes (*Vulpes vulpes*) in rural Ireland. Science Digest 146 (3), 227–234.

Musaev, M.A., Veisov, A.M., 1983. New species of coccidia of the genera *Eimeria* and *Isospora* from weasel (*Mustela nivalis* Lennans (sic), 1766). Izvestia Akademii Nauk Azerbaijdzhanskoi SSR, Seria Biologicheskich Nauk 5, 64–70 (in Russian).

Muthusamy, D., Rao, S.S., Ramani, S., Monica, B., Banerjee, I., Abraham, O.C., Mathai, D.C., Primrose, B., Muliyil, J., Wanke, C.A., Ward, H.D., Kang, G., 2006. Multilocus genotyping of *Cryptosporidium* sp. isolates from human immunodeficiency virus-infected individuals in South India. Journal of Clinical Microbiology 44 (2), 632–634.

Myers, P., 2000a. Herpestidae. (On-line), Animal Diversity Web. http://animaldiversity.org/accounts/Herpestidae/.

Myers, P., 2000b. Phocidae. (On-line), Animal Diversity Web. http://animaldiversity.org/accounts/Phocidae/.

Myers, P., 2000c. Procyonidae. (On-line), Animal Diversity Web. http://animaldiversity.org/accounts/Procyonidae/.

Nagano, Y., Finn, M.B., Lowery, C.J., Murphy, T., Moriarty, J., Power, E., Toolan, D., O'Loughlin, A., Watabe, M., McCorry, K.A., Crothers, E., Dooley, J.S., Rao, J.R., Rooney, P.J., Millar, B.C., Matsuda, M., Elborn, J.S., Moore, J.E., 2007. Occurrence of *Cryptosporidium parvum* and bacterial pathogens in faecal material in the red fox (*Vulpes vulpes*) population. Veterinary Research Communications 31 (5), 559–564.

Nascimento, C.O.M., Silva, M.L.C.R., Kim, P.C.P., Gomes, A.A.B., Gomes, A.L.V., Maia, R.C.C., Almeida, J.C., Mota, R.A., 2015. Occurrence of *Neospora caninum* and *Toxoplasma gondii* DNA in brain tissue from hoary foxes (*Pseudalopex vetulus*) in Brazil. Acta Tropica 146 (1), 60–65.

Nash, A.S., Mtambo, M.M., Gibbs, H.A., 1993. *Cryptosporidium* infection in farm cats in the Glasgow area. The Veterinary Record 133 (23), 576–577.

Navarrete, I., Reina, D., Habela, M., Nieto, C.G., Serrano, F., Pérez, E., 1990. Parasites of roe deer (*Capreolus capreolus*) in Caceres province, Spain. In: Verhandlungsbericht Internationalen Symposiums über die Erkrankungen der Zoo-und Wildtiere, vol. 23, pp. 225–227.

Neal, E.G., 1977. Badgers. Blandord Publishing, Ltd., London, United Kingdom.

Neitz, W.O., 1965. A check-list and host-list of the zoonoses occurring in mammals and birds in South and South West Africa. Onderstepoort Journal of Veterinary Research 32 (2), 189–374 (*nos non videbo illum*).

Neméseri, L., 1959. Adatok a kutya coccidiosisákoz. I. *Isospora canis* (To the coccidiosis of dog. I. *Isospora canis*). Mágyar Állatorvosok Lapja (Budapest) 14, 91–92 (in Hungarian, Russian and English summaries).

Neméseri, L., 1960. Beiträge zur Äetiologie der Coccidiose der Hund. I. *Isospora canis* n. sp (Contributions to the etiology of coccidiosis in the dog. I. *Isospora canis* n. sp.). Acta Veterinaria Academy Science Hungary 10, 95–99 (in German).

Nery-Guimaraes, F., Lage, H.A., 1973. Prevalencia e ciclo evolutivo de *Isospora felis* Wenyon, 1923 e *I. rivolta* (Grassi, 1879) Wenyon, 1923 em gatos. Memorias do Instituto Oswaldo Cruz 71 (1), 43–66 (in Portuguese, English summary).

Neufeld, J.L., Brandt, R.W., 1974. Cholangiohepatitis in a cat associated with a coccidia-like organism. Canadian Veterinary Journal 15 (5), 156–159.

Neves, D., Lobo, L., Simões, P.B., Cardoso, L., 2014. Frequency of intestinal parasites in pet dogs from an urban area (Greater Oporto, northern Portugal). Veterinary Parasitology 200 (3), 295–298.

Newman, C., MacDonald, D.W., Anwar, M.A., 2001. Coccidiosis in the European badger, *Meles meles* in Wytham woods: infection and consequences for growth and survival. Parasitology 123 (Pt 2), 133–142.

Niak, A., 1972. The prevalence of *Toxocara cati* and other parasites in Liverpool cats. Veterinary Records 91 (22), 534–536.

Nichol, S., Ball, S.J., Snow, K.R., 1981a. Prevalence of intestinal parasites in feral cats in some urban areas of England. Veterinary Parasitology 9 (2), 107–110.

Nichol, S., Ball, S.J., Snow, K.R., 1981b. Prevalence of intestinal parasites in domestic cats from the London area. The Veterinary Record 109 (12), 252–253.

Nichols, R.A., Campbell, B.M., Smith, H.V., 2003. Identification of *Cryptosporidium* spp. oocysts in United Kingdom noncarbonated natural mineral waters and drinking waters by using a modified nested PCR-restriction fragment length polymorphism assay. Applied and Environmental Microbiology 69 (7), 4183–4189.

Nichols, R.A., Campbell, B.M., Smith, H.V., 2006. Molecular fingerprinting of *Cryptosporidium* oocysts isolated during water monitoring. Applied and Environmental Microbiology 72 (8), 5428–5435.

Nieschulz, O., 1924a. Ein weiterer Fall von *Eimeria canis* Wenyon (Another case of *Eimeria canis*). Berliner und Münchener Tierärztliche Wochenschrift 37, 220–221 (in German).

Nieschulz, O., 1924b. Over een geval van *Eimeria*-infectie bij een kat (*Eimeria felina* n. sp.) (About a case of *Eimeria* infection in a cat (*Eimeria felina* n. sp.)). Netherlands Journal of Veterinary Science 51, 129–131 (in Dutch).

Nieschulz, O., 1925. Zur Verbreitung von *Isospora*-Infektionem bei Hunden und Katzen in den Niederland (For the decomposition of *Isospora*-infections in dogs and cats in the Netherlands). Zentralblatt für Bakteriologie. I. Abteilung Originale 94, 137–141 (in German).

Nieschulz, O., Bos, A., 1933. Ueber die Coccidien der Silberfüchfe. Deutsche Tierärztliche Wochenschrift 52, 819–820 (in German).

Novilla, M.N., Carpenter, J.W., Kwapien, R.P., 1980. Dual infection of Siberian polecats with *Encephalitozoon cuniculi* and *Hepatozoon mustelis* n. sp. In: Montali, R.J. (Ed.), Symposium on the Comparative Pathology of Zoo Animals. National Zoological Park, Smithsonian Institution, 1978. Smithsonian Institution Press, Washington, DC, pp. 353–363.

Nowak, R.M., 1991. fifth ed. Walker's Mammals of the World, vol. 1. Johns Hopkins University Press, Baltimore, MD, USA. 642 p.

Nukerbaeva, K.K., 1981a. Coccidia of sables (*Martes zibellina*). Izvestia Akademii Nauk Kazakhskoi Sovetskoi Sotsialisticheskoi Respubliki, Seria Biologicheskich Nauk 1, 30–33 (in Russian, no English summary).

Nukerbaeva, K.K., 1981b. Protozoal Diseases of Farmed Fur Animals. Institute of Zoology, Kazakh Academy of Sciences, Nauka, Alma-Ata, pp. 30–152.

Nukerbaeva, K.K., Svanbaev, S.K., 1973. Koktsidii pushnykh zverei v Kazakhstane (Coccidia of fur-bearing mammals in Kazakhstan). Vestnik Sel'skokhoziaistvennoi Nauki Kazakhstana 12, 50–54 (in Russian).

Nukerbaeva, K.K., Svanbaev, S.K., 1974. K voprosu o spetsifichnosti koksidii plotoyadnykh. Izvestia Akademii Nauk Kazakhskoi Sovetskoi Sotsialisticheskoi Respubliki, Seria Biologicheskich Nauk 12 (2), 35–40 (in Russian).

Nukerbaeva, K.K., Svanbaev, S.K., 1977. Results from the study of coccidia in wild fur animals. Akademia Nauk Kazakhskoi SSR, Trudy Instituta Zoologii 37, 5–90 (in Russian).

Nunes, C.M., 1993. Freqüência de ocorrência de parasitas intestinais em cães (*Canis familiaris*) na grande São Paulo (dados parciais). In: Anais do VIII Seminário Brasileiro de Parasitologia Veterinária, Londrína – PR, 12 a 16 de Setembro.

Nutter, F.B., Levine, J.F., Stoskopf, M.K., Gamble, H.R., Dubey, J.P., 1998. Seroprevalence of *Toxoplasma gondii* and *Trichinella spiralis* in North Carolina black bears (*Ursus americanus*). Journal of Parasitology 84 (5), 1048–1050.

Nutter, F.B., Dubey, J.P., Levine, J.F., Breitschwerdt, E.B., Ford, R.B., Stoskopf, M.K., 2004. Seroprevalences of antibodies against *Bartonella henselae* and *Toxoplasma gondii* and fecal shedding of *Cryptosporidium* spp., *Giardia* spp., and *Toxocara cati* in feral and pet domestic animals. Journal of the American Veterinary Medical Association 225 (9), 1394–1398.

Nyakatura, K., Bininda-Emonds, O.R.P., 2012. Updating the evolutionary history of Carnivora (mammalia): a new species-level supertree complete with divergence time estimates. BioMed Central Biology 10 (12), 1–31.

Nyambura Njuguna, A., Maina Kagira, J., Muturi Karanja, S., Ngotho, M., Mutharia, L., Wangari Maina, N., 2017. Prevalence of *Toxoplasma gondii* and other gastrointestinal parasites in domestic cats from households in Thika Region, Kenya. BioMed Research International:7615810.

O'Brien, S., Nash, W., Wildt, D., Bush, M., Benveniste, R., 1985. Molecular solution to the riddle of the giant panda's phylogeny. Nature 317 (12), 140–144.

Ocholi, R.A., Kalejaiye, J.O., Okewole, P.A., 1989. Acute disseminated toxoplasmosis in two captive lions (*Panthera leo*) in Nigeria. The Veterinary Record 124 (19), 515–516.

Odening, K., 1983. Sarkozysten in eimer antarktischen Robbe. Angewandte Parasitologie 24, 197–200 (in German).

Odening, K., 1984. Oozysten neben Sarkozysten in der Muskulatur einer antarktischen Robbe. Angewandte Parasitologie 25, 214–216 (in German).

Odening, K., 1997. Die *Sarcocystis*-Infektion: Wechselbeziehungen zwischen freilebenden Wildtieren, Haustieren und Zootieren (*Sarcocystis* infection: interrelationships between wild animals, domestic animals and zoo animals). Der Zoologische Garten 67, 317–340 (in German).

Odening, K., 1998. The present state of species-systematics in *Sarcocystis* Lankester, 1882 (Protista, Sporozoa, Coccidia). Systematic Parasitology 41 (3), 209–233.

Odening, K., Stolte, M., Walter, G., Bockhardt, L., Jakob, W., 1994a. Sarcocysts (*Sarcocystis* sp.: Sporozoa) in the European Badger, *Meles meles*. Parasitology 108 (4), 421–424.

Odening, K., Stolte, M., Walter, G., Bockhardt, I., 1994b. The European badger (Carnivora: Mustelidae) as intermediate host of further three *Sarcocystis* species (Sporozoa). Parasite 1 (1), 23–30.

Odening, K., Wesemeier, H.-H., Pinkowski, M., Walter, G., Bockhardt, L., 1994c. European hare and European rabbit (Lagomorpha) as intermediate hosts of *Sarcocystis* species (Sporozoa) in central Europe. Acta Protozoologica 33 (1), 177–189.

Odening, K., Stolte, M., Walter, G., Bockhardt, I., 1995. Cyst wall ultrastructure of two *Sarcocystis* spp. from European mouflon (*Ovis ammon musimon*) in Germany compared with domestic sheep. Journal of Wildlife Diseases 31 (4), 550–554.

Odening, K., Stolte, M., Bockhardt, I., 1996a. On the diagnostics of *Sarcocystis* in cattle: sarcocysts of a species unusual for *Bos taurus* in a dwarf zebu. Veterinary Parasitology 66 (1–2), 19–24.

Odening, K., Wesemeier, H.-H., Bockhardt, L., 1996b. On the sarcocysts of two further *Sarcocystis* species being new for the European hare. Acta Protozoologica 35 (1), 69–72.

Odening, K., Stolte, M., Bockhardt, I., 1999. Einheimische *Sarcocystis*-Arten (Sporozoa) in exotischen Zoosäugetieren (Gayal, Cerviden, Cameliden, Ozelot) (Indigenous *Sarcocystis* species in exotic zoo mammals (Gayal, Cerviden, Cameliden, Ozelot)). Der Zoologische Garten 69, 109–125 (in German).

O'Dwyer, L.H., Massard, C.L., de Souza, J.C.P., 2001. *Hepatozoon canis* infection associated with dog ticks of rural areas of Rio de Janeiro State, Brazil. Veterinary Parasitology 94 (3), 143–150.

Oertly, K.D., Walls, K.W., 1980. Prevalence of antibodies to *Toxoplasma gondii* among bobcats of West Virginia and Georgia. Journal of the American Veterinary Medical Association 177 (9), 852–853.

Ogassawara, S., Benassi, S., Larsson, C.E., Hagiwara, M.K., 1986. Prevalęncia de endoparasitas em gatos na cidade de São Paulo. Revista da Faculdade de Medicina Veterinária e Zootecnia da Universidade de São Paulo 23 (1), 39–46 (in Portuguese, English summary).

Ohino, A., Shinzato, T., Sueyoshi, T., Tominaga, M., Arakaki, M., Shiroma, S., Ohshiri, K., Saito, M., Itagaki, H., 1993. Prevalence of *Sarcocystis* infection pigs in Okinawa Prefecture. Journal of the Japanese Veterinary Association 46, 979–982.

Ojo, K.K., Reid, M.C., Kallur Siddaramaiah, L., Müller, J., Winzer, P., Zhang, Z., Keyloun, K.R., Vidadala, R.S., Merritt, E.A., Hol, W.G., Maly, D.J., Fan, E., Barrett, L.K., Van Voorhis, W.C., Hemphill, A., 2014. *Neospora caninum* calcium-dependent protein kinase 1 is an effective drug target for neosporosis therapy. PLoS One 9 (3), e92929.

Oksanen, A., Åsbakk, K., Prestrud, K.W., Aars, J., Derocherr, A.E., Tryland, M., Wilg, Ø., Dubey, J.P., Sonne, C., Dietz, R., Anderesen, M., Born, E.W., 2009. Prevalence of antibodies against *Toxoplasma gondii* in polar bears (*Ursus maritimus*) from Svalbard and East Greenland. Journal of Parasitology 95 (1), 89–94.

Olcott, A.T., Speer, C.A., Hendricks, L.D., 1982. Endogenous development of *Isospora arctopitheci* Rodhain, 1933 in the marmoset *Sanguinus geoffroyi*. Proceedings of the Helminthological Society of Washington 49, 118–126.

O'Leary, M.A., Bloch, J.I., Flynn, J.J., Gaudin, T.J., Giallombardo, A., Giannini, N.P., Goldberg, S.L., Kraatz, B.P., Luo, Z.-X., Meng, J., Ni, X., Novacek, M.J., Perini, F.A., Randall, Z.S., Rougier, G.W., Sargis, E.J., Silcox, M.T., Simmons, N.B., Spaulding, M., Velazco, P.M., Weksler, M., Wible, J.R., Cirranello, A.L., 2013. The placental mammal ancestor and the post-K-Pg radiation of placentals. Science 339 (6120), 662–667.

Olias, P., Gruber, A.D., Heydorn, A.O., Kohls, A., Mehlhorn, H., Hafez, H.M., Lierz, M., 2009. A novel *Sarcocystis*-associated encephalitis and myositis in racing pigeons. Avian Pathology 38 (2), 121–128.

Oliveira, P.R., Silva, P.L., Parreira, Y.F., Ribeiro, S.C.A., Gomes, J.B., 1990. Prevalęncia de endoparasitos em cães da regïão de Uberlândia, Minas Gerais. Brazilian Journal of Veterinary Research and Animal Science, São Paulo 27 (2), 193–197 (in Portuguese, English summary).

de Oliveira, F.R., Da Stabenow, C., Massad, F.V., Lopes, C.W.G., 2007. Hypnozoites of *Cystoisospora* Frenkel, 1977 (Apicomplexa: Cystoisosporinae) in Mongolian gerbil lymph nodes and their transmission to cats free of coccidia. Revista Brasileira de Parasitologia Veterinaria 16 (2), 72–76.

de Oliveira Lemos, F., Almosny, N.P., Soares, A.M., Alencar, N.X., 2012. *Cryptosporidium* species screening using Kinyoun technique in domestic cats with diarrhea. Journal of Feline Medicine and Surgery 14 (2), 113–117.

Olson, M.E., Roach, P.D., Stabler, M., Chan, W., 1997. Giardiasis in ringed seals from the Western Arctic. Journal of Wildlife Diseases 33, 646–648.

Onuma, S.S.M., Melo, A.L.T., Kantek, D.L.Z., Crawshaw-Junior, P.G., Morato, R.G., May-Júnior, J.A., Pacheco, T.A., de Aguiar, D.M., 2014. Exposure of free-living jaguars to *Toxoplasma gondii*, *Neospora caninum* and *Sarcocystis neurona* in the Brazilian Pantanal. Brazilian Journal of Veterinary Parasitology 23 (4), 547–553.

Ordeix, L., Lloret, A., Fondevila, D., Dubey, J.B., Ferrer, J.B., Fondati, A., 2002. Cutaneous neosporosis during treatment of pemphigus foliaceus in a dog. Journal of the American Animal Hospital Association 38 (5), 415–419.

Oronan, R.B., Licuan, D.A., Licuan, D.A., Delos-Santos, J.P.S., Lastica, E.A., 2013. Detection of antibodies against *Toxoplasma gondii* and *Chlamydophila felis* in Malayan civets (*Viverra tangalunga*), Palawan bearcats (*Arctictis binturong whitei*) and Asian palm civets (*Paradoxurus hermaphroditus*) at a wildlife facility in Quezon City, Philippines. Philippines Journal of Veterinary Animal Science 39 (2), 287–292.

Ortuno, A., Castella, J., Almeria, S., 2002. Seroprevalence of antibodies to *Neospora caninum* in dogs from Spain. Journal of Parasitology 88 (6), 1263–1266.

Oryan, A., Ahmadi, N., Mousavi, S.M.M., 2010. Prevalence, biology, and distribution pattern of *Sarcocystis* infection in water buffalo (*Bubalus bubalis*) in Iran. Tropical Animal Health and Production 42 (7), 1513–1518.

Osman, M., Bories, J., El Safadi, D., Poirel, M.T., Gantois, N., Benamrouz-Vanneste, S., Delhaes, L., Hugonnard, M., Certad, G., Zenner, L., Viscogliosi, E., 2015. Prevalence and genetic diversity of the intestinal parasites *Blastocystis* sp. and *Cryptosporidium* spp. in household dogs in France and evaluation of zoonotic transmission risk. Veterinary Parasitology 214 (1–2), 167–170.

Osten-Sacken, N., Słodkowicz-Kowalska, A., Pacoń, J., Skrzypczak, Ł., Werner, A., 2017. Intestinal and external parasites of raccoon dogs (*Nyctereutes procyonoides*) in western Poland. Annals of Parasitology 63 (1), 37–44.

Overdulve, J.P., 1970a. The identity of *Toxoplasma* Nicolle & Manceaux, 1909 with *Isospora schneider*, 1881 (I). Proceedings of the Koninklijke Nederlandse Akademie van Wetenschappen. Series C 73 (1), 129–151.

Overdulve, J.P., 1970b. The probable identity of *Toxoplasma* and *Isospora* and the role of the cat in the transmission of toxoplasmosis. Tijdschrift voor Diergeneeskunde 95 (2), 149–155.

Overdulve, J.P., 1978. Prudish Parasites. The Discovery of Sexuality, and Studies on the Life Cycle, Particularly the Sexual Stages in Cats, of the Sporozoan Parasite *Isospora* (*Toxoplasma*) *gondii* (self-published). Drukkerig Elinkwijk BV, Utrecht, The Netherlands. 83 p.

Overgaauw, P.A., van Zutphen, L., Hoek, D., Yaya, F.O., Roelfsema, J., Pinelli, E., van Knapen, F., Kortbeek, L.M., 2009. Zoonotic parasites in fecal samples and fur from dogs and cats in the Netherlands. Veterinary Parasitology 163 (1–2), 115–122.

Pagès, M., Calvignac, S., Klein, C., Paris, M., Hughes, S., Hänni, C., 2008. Combined analysis of fourteen nuclear genes refines the Ursidae phylogeny. Molecular Phylogenetics and Evolution 47 (1), 73–83.

Pak, S.M., 1979. Occurrence of *Sarcocystis* in *Vulpes corsac*. In: X Vses. Konferenz Prirodnogo Ochagovost' Boleznei. 9–11 October, 1979. USSR, Dushanbe (*nos non videbo illum*).

Pak, S.M., Perminova, V.V., Eshtokina, N.V., 1979. *Sarcocystis citelli vulpes* n. sp. iz zheltykh suslikov (*Citellus fulvus*) (*Sarcocystis citellivulpes* n. sp. in the yellow suslik *Spermophilus fulvis*). In: Beyer, T.V., Bezukladnikova, N.A., Galuzo, I.G., Konovalova, S.I., Pak, S.M. (Eds.), Toksoplazmidy. Protozoologiya, Akademii Nauk Sovetskoi Sotsialisticheskoi Respubliki, pp. 111–114 (in Russian, no English summary). (*nos non videbo illum*, as cited in Levine and Ivens, 1981).

Pak, S.M., Sklyarova, O.N., Pak, L.S., 1989. *Sarcocystis alectorivulpes* and *Sarcocystis alectoributeonis* – new sarcosporidian species of *Alectoris chugar*. Izvestia Akademii Nauk Kazakhskoi Sovetskoi Sotsialisticheskoi Respubliki, Seria Biologicheskaia 6, 25–30 (in Russian). (*nos non videbo illum*).

Pak, S.M., Sklyarova, O.N., Dymkova, N.D., 1991. Sarcocysts (Sporozoa, Apicomplexa) of some species of wild mammals. Izvestia Akademii Nauk Kazakhskoi Sovetskoi Sotsialisticheskoi Respubliki, Seria Biologicheskaia 5, 35–40 (in Russian). (*nos non videbo illum*).

Palmer, C.S., Thompson, R.C.A., Traub, R.J., Rees, R., Robertson, I.D., 2008a. National study of the gastrointestinal parasites of dogs and cats in Australia. Veterinary Parasitology 151 (2–4), 181–190.

Palmer, C.S., Traub, R.J., Robertson, I.D., Devlin, G., Rees, R., Thompson, R.C.A., 2008b. Determining the zoonotic significance of *Giardia* and *Cryptosporidium* in Australian dogs and cats. Veterinary Parasitology 154 (1–2), 142–147.

Panciera, R.J., Mathew, J.S., Ewing, S.A., Cummings, C.A., Drost, W.T., Kocan, A.A., 2000. Skeletal lesions of canine hepatozoonosis caused by *Hepatozoon americanum*. Veterinary Pathology 37 (3), 225–230.

Pande, B.P., Bhatia, B.B., Chauhan, P.P.S., Garg, R.K., 1970. Species composition of coccidia of some of the mammals and birds at the Zoological Gardens, Lucknow (Uttar Pradesh). Indian Journal of Animal Science 40, 154–166.

Pande, B.P., Bhatia, B.B., Chauhan, P.P.S., 1972. A new genus and species of cryptosporidid coccidia from India. Acta Veterinaria Academiae Scientiarum Hungaricae 22 (3), 231–234.

Pantchev, N., Gassmann, D., Globokar-Vrhovec, M., 2011. Increasing numbers of *Giardia* (but not coccidian) infections in ferrets, 2002 to 2010. The Veterinary Record 168 (19), 519.

Paoletti, B., Otranto, D., Weigl, S., Giangaspero, A., Di Cesare, A., Traversa, D., 2011. Prevalence and genetic characterization of *Giardia* and *Cryptosporidium* in cats from Italy. Research in Veterinary Science 91 (3), 397–399.

Papazahariadou, M., Founta, A., Papadopoulos, E., Chliounakis, S., Antoniadou-Sotiriadou, K., Theodorides, Y., 2007. Gastrointestinal parasites of shepherd and hunting dogs in the Serres Prefecture, Northern Greece. Veterinary Parasitology 148 (2), 170–173.

Paré, J., Hietala, S.K., Thurmond, M.C., 1995. An enzyme-linked immunosorbent assay (ELISA) for serological diagnosis of *Neospora* sp. infection in cattle. Journal of Veterinary Diagnostic Investigation 7 (3), 352–359.

Paris, J.K., Wills, S., Balzer, H.J., Shaw, D.J., Gunn-Moore, D.A., 2014. Enteropathogen co-infection in UK cats with diarrhoea. BMC Veterinary Research 10, 13.

Pas, A., Dubey, J.P., 2008. Toxoplasmosis in sand fox (*Vulpes rueppelli*). Journal of Parasitology 94 (4), 976–977.

Pasa, S., Voyvoda, H., Karagenc, T., Atasoy, A., Gazyagci, S., 2011. Failure of combination therapy with imidocarb dipropionate and toltrazuril to clear *Hepatozoon canis* infection in dogs. Parasitology Research 109 (3), 919–926.

Patitucci, A.N., Pérez, M.J., Rozas, M.A., Israel, K.F., 2001. *Neosporosis canina*: presencia de anticuerpos séricos en poblaciones caninas Rurales y urbanas de Chile (*Neosporosis canine*: detection of sera antibodies in rural and urban canine population of Chile). Archivos de Medicina Veterinaria 33 (2), 227–232 (in Spanish).

Patnaik, M.M., 1966. Coccidian parasites of domestic animals in Orissa. Orissa Veterinary Journal 1, 25–28.

Patnaik, M.M., Acharjyo, L.N., 1970. *Eimeria nycticebi* n. sp. and *E. coucangi* n. sp. from Indian slowloris (*Nycticebus coucang*), and notes on *Isospora leonina* from an African lion (*Panthera leo leo*). Orissa Veterinary Journal 5, 13–14.

Patnaik, M.M., Acharjyo, L.N., 1971. Notes on the coccidian parasites of wild mammals in captivity at Nandankanan. Orissa Veterinary Journal 6 (3/4), 133–135.

Patnaik, M.M., Acharjyo, L.N., 1977. Remarks on *Isospora bengalensi* Patnaik and Acharjyo 1971, from leopard cat. Orissa Veterinary Journal 11 (1), 47.

Patnaik, M.M., Ray (sic), S.K., 1966. Letters to the editor. Indian Journal of Animal Health 5, 203.

Patnaik, M.M., Roy, S.K., 1965. Coccidia of Indian mongoose (*Herpestes edwardsii*). Indian Journal of Animal Health 4 (1), 33–36.

Patou, M.-L., McIenachan, P.A., Morley, C.G., Couloux, A., Jennings, A.P., Veron, G., 2009. Molecular phylogeny of the Herpestidae (Mammalia, Carnivora) with a special emphasis on the Asian *Herpestes*. Molecular Phylogenetics and Evolution 53 (1), 69–80.

Patterson, M., Fox, J.G., 2007. Parasites of ferrets. In: Baker, D.G. (Ed.), Flynn's Parasites of Laboratory Animals, second ed. Wiley Blackwell, pp. 501–508.

Patterson-Kane, J.C., Gibbons, L.M., Jefferies, R., Morgan, E.R., Wenzlow, N., Redrobe, S.P., 2009. Pneumonia from *Angiostrongylus vasorum* infection in a red panda (*Ailurus fulgens fulgens*). Journal of Veterinary Diagnostic Investigation 21 (2), 270–273.

Patton, W.S., 1908. The haemogregarines of mammals and reptiles. Parasitology 1, 318–321.

Patton, S., Rabinowitz, A.R., 1994. Parasites of wild Felidae in Thailand: a coprological survey. Journal of Wildlife Diseases 30 (3), 472–475.

Patton, S., Rabinowitz, A.R., Randolph, S., Johnson, S.S., 1986. A coprological survey of parasites of wild neotropical Felidae. Journal of Parasitology 72 (4), 517–520.

Pavlásek, I., 1983. Experimental infection of cat and chicken with *Cryptosporidium* sp. oocysts isolated from a calf. Folia Parasitologica (Praha) 30 (2), 121–122.

Pavlásek, I., Ryan, U., 2007. The first finding of a natural infection of *Cryptosporidium muris* in a cat. Veterinary Parasitology 144 (3–4), 349–352.

Pecka, Z., 1988. Parasitic protozoa of the genus *Sarcocystis* (Apicomplexa, Sarcocystidae) in pheasants, hens and some free-living birds in Czechoslovakia. Věstník Československé Společnosti Zoologické 52, 266–270.

Pecka, Z., 1990. Muscular sarcocystosis of fowls and pheasants in Czechoslovakia. Veterinářství 40, 314–315.

Pellérdy, L.P., 1955. Beiträge zur Kenntnis der Coccidien des Dachses (*Meles taxus*) (Contirbutions to the knowledge of the coccidia of the badger (*Meles taxus*)). Acta Veterinaria Academiae Scientiarum Hungaricae 5, 421–423 (in German).

Pellérdy, L.P., 1959. A note on R.S. Bray's article "On the parasitic Protozoa of Liberia. VI. A further note on the coccidia of the mongoose." Acta Veterinaria 9, 181–182.

Pellérdy, L.P., 1963. Catalogue of Eimeriidae (Protozoa: Sporozoa). Akademiai Kiado, Budapest, Hungary. 160 p.

Pellérdy, L.P., 1965. Coccidia and Coccidiosis. Akadémiai Kiadó, Budapest, Hungary. 657 p.

Pellérdy, L.P., 1974a. Coccidia and Coccidiosis, second ed. Verlag Paul Parey, Berlin and Hamburg, Germany, and Akadémiai Kiadó, Budapest, Hungary. 959 p.

Pellérdy, L.P., 1974b. Studies on the coccidia of the domestic cat, *Isospora novocati* sp. n. Acta Veterinaria Academiae Scientiarum Hungaricae 24 (1–2), 127–131.

Pelster, B., 1973. Vergleichende elektronenmikroskopische Untersuchungen an den Makrogamenten von *Isospora felis* und *I. rivolta* (Comparative electron microscopic investigations on the microgametes of *Isospora felis* and *I. rivolta*). Zeitschrift für Parasitenkunde 41 (1), 29–46 (in German, English summary).

Pelster, B., Piekarski, G., 1971. Elektroniumikroskopische Analyse der Mikrogametenentwicklung bei *Toxoplasma gondii* (Electron microscopic studies on the microgametogeny of *Toxoplasma gondii*). Zeitschrift für Parasitenkunde 37 (4), 267–277 (in German, English summary).

Penzhorn, B.L., De Cramer, K.G., Booth, L.M., 1992. Coccidial infection in German shepherd dog pus in a breeding unit. Journal of the South African Veterinary Association 63 (1), 27–29.

Penzhorn, B.L., Booth, L.M., Meltzer, D.G.A., 1994. *Isospora rivolta* recovered from cheetahs. Journal of the South African Veterinary Association 65 (1), 2.

Penzhorn, B.L., Durand, D.T., Lane, E., Ide, A., Hofmeyr, M.S., 1998. Recovery of Sarcocystis oocysts from a free-ranging wild dog (Lycaon pictus): to the editor. Journal of the South African Veterinary Association 69 (2), 42.

Pereira, M.J.S., Lopes, C.W.G., 1982. Crab-eating fox (*Cerdocyon thous*) as a final host for *Sarcocystis capracanis* (Apicomplexa: Sarcocystidae). Arquivos da Universidade Federal Rural do Rio de Janeiro 5, 233.

Perez, R.R., Rubini, A.S., O'Dwyer, L.H., 2004. The first report of *Hepatozoon* spp. (Apicomplexa, Hepatozoidae) in domestic cats from São Paulo state, Brazil. Parasitology Research 94 (2), 83–85.

Perez Tort, G., Petetta, L., Favre, M.E., Mas, J., Robles, A.M., 2007. First description of an outbreak of hepatozoonosis. Veterinaria Argentina 24, 399.

Perkins, F.O., Barta, J.R., Clopton, R.E., Peirce, M.A., Upton, S.J., 2000. Phylum Apicomplexa Levine, 1970. In: Lee, J.J., Leedale, G.F., Bradbury, P. (Eds.), An Illustrated Guide to the Protozoa, vol. 1. second ed. Society of Protozoologists, Lawrence, KS, pp. 190–369.

Perryman, L.E., Kapil, S.J., Jones, M.L., Hunt, E.L., 1999. Protection of calves against cryptosporidiosis with immune bovine colostrum induced by a *Cryptosporidium parvum* recombinant protein. Vaccine 17 (17), 2142–2149.

Perz, J.F., Le Blancq, S.M., 2001. *Cryptosporidium parvum* infection involving novel genotypes in wildlife from lower New York State. Applied and Environmental Microbiology 67 (3), 1154–1162.

Peteshev, V.M., Gauzo, I.G., Polomoshnov, A.P., 1974. Cats – definitive hosts of *Besnoitia* (*Besnoitia besnoiti*). Izvestia Akademii Nauk Kazakhskoi Sovetskoi Sotsialisticheskoi Respubliki, Seria Biologicheskaia 1, 33–38 (in Russian).

Pfefferkorn, E.R., Borotz, S.E., 1994. Comparison of mutants of *Toxoplasma gondii* selected for resistance to azithromycin, spiramycin, or clindamycin. Antimicrobial Agents and Chemotherapy 38 (1), 31–37.

Pfefferkorn, E.R., Nothnagel, R.F., Borotz, S.E., 1992. Parasiticidal effect of clindamycin on *Toxoplasma gondii* grown in cultured cells and selection of a drug-resistant mutant. Antimicrobial Agents and Chemotherapy 36 (5), 1091–1096.

Pieniazek, N.J., Bornay-Llinares, F.J., Slemenda, S.B., da Silva, A.J., Moura, I.N., Arrowood, M.J., Ditrich, O., Addiss, D.G., 1999. New *Cryptosporidium* genotypes in HIV-infected persons. Emerging Infectious Diseases 5 (3), 444–449.

Pizzi, H.L., Rico, C.M., Pessat, O.A.N., 1978. Hallazgo del ciclo ontogenico selvatico del *Toxoplasma gondii* en felidos salvajes (*Oncifelis geofroyi, Felis colocola y Felis eirá*) de la provincia de Cordoba. Revista Militar de Veterinaria 251 (17), 293–294.

Plutzer, J., Karanis, P., 2009. Genetic polymorphism in *Cryptosporidium* species: an update. Veterinary Parasitology 165 (3), 187–199.

Pocock, R.I., 1921. On the external characters and classification of the Mustelidae. Proceedings of the Zoological Society of London 1921, 803–837.

Poli, A., Mancianti, F., Carli, M.A., Stroscio, M.C., Kramer, L., 1998. *Neospora caninum* infection in a Bernese cattle dog from Italy. Veterinary Parasitology 78 (2), 79–85.

Polomoshnov, A.P., 1979. Final hosts of *Toxoplasma*. Voprosy Prirodnoi Ochagovosti Boleznei 10, 68–72 (in Russian).

Pomerantz, J., Rasambainarivo, F.T., Dollar, L., Rahajanirina, L.P., Andrianaivoarivelo, R., Parker, P., Dubovi, E., 2016. Prevalence of antibodies to selected viruses and parasites in introduced and endemic carnivores in western Madagascar. Journal of Wildlife Diseases 52 (3), 544–552.

Ponce-Macotela, M., Peralta-Abarca, G.E., Martínez-Gordillo, M.N., 2005. *Giardia intestinalis* and other zoonotic parasites: prevalence in adult dogs from the southern part of Mexico City. Veterinary Parasitology 131 (1–2), 1–4.

Poonacha, K.B., Pippin, C., 1982. Intestinal cryptosporidiosis in a cat. Veterinary Pathology 19, 708–710.

Porchet-Henneré, E., Ponchel, G., 1994. Ultrastructure of *Sarcocystis tenella* cyst architecture and aspect of endozoites in scanning electron microscopy. Comptes Rendus Hebdomadaires des Seances de l'Academie des Sciences. Serie D: Sciences Naturelles 294 (14), 1179–1181.

Poulin, R., 2007. Evolutionary Ecology of Parasites, second ed. Princeton University Press, Princeton, New Jersey, USA. 360 p.

Powell, E.C., McCarely, J.B., 1975. A murine *Sarcocystis* that causes an *Isospora*-like infection in cats. Journal of Parasitology 61 (5), 928–931.

Pozio, E., 2016. *Trichinella pseudospiralis* an elusive nematode. Veterinary Parasitology 231, 97–101.

Prakas, P., Oksanen, A., Butkauskas, D., Sruoga, A., Kutkienė, L., Švažas, S., Isomursu, M., Liaugaudaité, S., 2014. Identification and intraspecific genetic diversity of *Sarcocystis rileyi* from ducks, *Anas* spp., in Lithuania and Finland. Journal of Parasitology 100 (5), 657–661.

Prakas, P., Liaugaudaité, S., Kutkienė, L., Sruoga, A., Švažas, S., 2015. Molecular identification of *Sarcocystis rileyi* sporocysts in red foxes (*Vulpes vulpes*) and raccoon dogs (*Nyctereutes procyonoides*) in Lithuania. Parasitology Research 114 (5), 1671–1676.

Prasad, H., 1961a. A new species of *Isospora* from the fennec fox *Fennecus zerda* Zimmerman. Zeitschrift für Parasitenkunde 21 (2), 130–135.

Prasad, H., 1961b. The coccidia of the zorille *Ictonyx* (*Zorilla*) *capensis* Kaup. Journal of Protozoology 8, 55–58.

Prescott, J.F., 2000. Lincosamides, macrolides and pleuromutilins. In: Prescott, J.F., Baggot, J.D., Walker, R.D. (Eds.), Antimicrobial Therapy in Veterinary Medicine, third ed. Iowa State University Press, Ames, USA, pp. 229–262.

Presidente, P.J.A., Karsta, L.H., 1975. *Hepatozoon* sp. infection in mink from southwestern Ontario. Journal of Wildlife Diseases 11 (4), 479–481.

Prestrud, K.W., Åsbakk, K., Fuglei, E., Mørk, T., Stien, A., Ropstad, E., Tryland, M., Gabrielsen, G.W., Lydersen, C., Kovacs, K.M., Loonen, J.J.E., Sagerup, K., Oksanen, A., 2007. Serosurvey for *Toxoplasma gondii* in arctic foxes and possible sources of infection in the high Arctic of Svalbard. Veterinary Parasitology 150 (1), 6–12.

Priest, J.W., Bern, C., Xiao, L., Roberts, J.M., Kwon, J.P., Lescano, A.G., Checkley, W., Cabrera, L., Moss, D.M., Arrowood, M.J., Sterling, C.R., Gilman, R.H., Lammie, P.J., 2006. Longitudinal analysis of *Cryptosporidium* species-specific immunoglobulin G antibody responses in Peruvian children. Clinical and Vaccine Immunology 13 (1), 123–131.

Qian, W., Wang, H., Shan, D., Li, B., Liu, J., Liu, Q., 2015. Activity of several kinds of drugs against *Neospora caninum*. Parasitology International 64 (6), 597–602.

Qin Qin, M.S., Wei, F., Li, M., Dubovi, E.J., Loeffler, I.K., 2007. Serosurvey of infectious disease agents of carnivores in captive red pandas (*Ailurus fulgens*) in China. Journal of Zoo and Wildlife Medicine 38 (1), 42–50.

Queen, E.V., Marks, S.L., Farver, T.B., 2012. Prevalence of selected bacterial and parasitic agents in feces from diarrheic and healthy control cats from northern California. Journal of Veterinary Internal Medicine 26 (1), 54–60.

Quinn, P.J., Ramsden, R.O., Johnston, D.H., 1976. Toxoplasmosis: a serological survey in Ontario wildlife. Journal of Wildlife Diseases 12 (4), 504–510.

Quiroga, D.A., Lombardero, O.J., Zorrilla, R., 1969. *Sarcocystis tilopodi* n. sp. en guanacos (*Lama guanicoe*) de la Republica Argentina. Gaceta Veterinaria (Buenos Aires) 31, 67–70 (in Spanish).

Raccurt, C.P., 2007. Worldwide human zoonotic cryptosporidiosis caused by *Cryptosporidium felis*. Parasite 14 (1), 15–20 (in French).

Raccurt, C.P., Brasseur, P., Verdier, R.I., Li, X., Eyma, E., Stockman, C.P., Agnamey, P., Guyot, K., Totet, A., Liautaud, B., Nevez, G., Dei-Cas, E., Pape, J.W., 2006. Human cryptosporidiosis and *Cryptosporidium* spp. in Haiti. Tropical Medicine and International Health 11 (6), 929–934 (in French).

Rademacher, U., Jakob, W., Bockhardt, I., 1999. *Cryptosporidium* infection in beech martens (*Martes foina*). Journal of Zoo and Wildlife Medicine 30 (3), 421–422.

Rah, H., Chomel, B.B., Follmann, E.H., Kasten, R.W., Hew, C.H., Farver, T.B., Garner, G.W., Amstrup, S.C., 2005. Serosurvey of selected zoonotic agents in polar bears (*Ursus maritimus*). The Veterinary Record 156 (1), 7–13.

Railliet, A., 1886a. Comment on Moulé, M.: psorospermies du tissu musculaire de mouton (Psorospermia of sheep muscle tissue). Bulletin et Mémoires de la Societé Centrale do Médecine Vetérinaire 40, 130 (in French).

Railliet, A., 1886b. Psorospermies géants dans l'oesophage et les muscles du mouton (Giant psorospermia in the esophagus and sheep muscles). Bulletin et Mémoires de la Societé Centrale do Médecine Vetérinaire 40, 130–134 (in French).

Railliet, A., Lucet, A., 1890. Une nouvelle maladie parasitaire de l'oie domestique, détérminée par des coccidies (A new parasitic disease of domestic goose, determined by coccidia). Comptes Rendus des Seances Socété de Biologie (Paris) 42, 293–294 (in French).

Railliet, A., Lucet, A., 1891. Note sur quelques espèces de coccidies encore peu étudiées (Note on some species of coccidia still little studied). Bulletin de la Societe Zoologique de France 16, 246–250 (in French).

Rainwater, K.L., Marchese, K., Slavinski, S., Humberg, L.A., Dubovi, E.J., Jarvis, J.A., McAloose, D., Calle, P.P., 2017. Health survey of free-ranging raccoons (*Procyon lotor*) in Central Park, New York, New York, USA: implications for human and domestic animal health. Journal of Wildlife Diseases 53 (2), 272–284.

Rajasekariah, G.R., Hegde, K.S., Srinivasa Gowda, R.N., Abdul Rahman, S., Subbarao, H., 1971. A study of some parasites from panther cub (*Felis pardus*, Linn.) with the description of *Eimeria anekalensis* n. sp. Mysore Journal of Agricultural Sciences 54 (4), 404–409.

Rakich, P.M., Dubey, J.P., Contarino, J.K., 1992. Acute hepatic sarcocystosis in a chinchilla. Journal of Veterinary Diagnostic Investigation 4 (4), 484–486.

Rambozzi, L., Menzano, A., Mannelli, A., Romano, S., Isaia, M.C., 2007. Prevalence of cryptosporidian infection in cats in Turin and analysis of risk factors. Journal of Feline Medicine and Surgery 9 (5), 392–396.

Ramírez-Barrios, R.A., Barboza-Mena, G., Muñoz, J., Angulo-Cubillán, F., Hernández, E., González, F., Escalona, F., 2004. Prevalence of intestinal parasites in dogs under veterinary care in Maracaibo, Venezuela. Veterinary Parasitology 121 (1–2), 11–20.

Ramos-Vera, J.A., Dubey, J.P., Watson, G.L., Winn-Elliot, M., Patterson, J.S., Yamini, B., 1997. Sarcocystosis in mink (*Mustela vison*). Journal of Parasitology 83 (6), 1198–1201.

Rao, S.R., Bhatavdekar, M.Y., March, 1957. *Eimeria rayii* sp. nov. a new coccidium from a dog, belonging to the genus *Eimeria*. Bombay Veterinary College Magazine 6, 7–8.

Rastegaïeff, E.F., 1929a. Coccidie chez le tigre. Bulletin de la Societe de Pathologie Exotique 22, 640 (in French).

Rastegaïeff, E.F., 1929b. *Eimeria felina* Niesch. Chez la lionne. Bulletin de la Societe de Pathologie Exotique 22, 641 (in French).

Rastegaïeff, E.F., 1929c. *Eimeria mesnili* n. sp. chez *Canis lagopus*. Bulletin de la Societe de Pathologie Exotique 22, 640 (in French).

Rastegaïeff, E.F., 1930. Zur Frage über Coccidien wilder Tiere. Archiv für Protistenkunde 71, 377–404 (in German).

Ratcliffe, E.J., 1974. Through the Badger Gate. Bell Publishing Ltd., Kent, United Kingdom.

Ratcliffe, H.L., Worth, C.B., 1951. Toxoplasmosis of captive wild birds and mammals. American Journal of Pathology 27 (4), 655–667.

Rátz, I., 1908. Szakosztályunk ülései. Állattani Közlemények 7, 177–178 (in Hungarian).

Rátz, I., 1909. Az izmokban élösködö véglények és a magyar faunában elöforduló fajaik (The muscles parasitic protozoa and the Hungarian fauna species are occurring) (In Hungarian), or Die Sarcosporidien und ihre in Ungarn vorkommenden Arten (The Sarcosporidia and their species occurring in Hungary). Állattani Közlemények 8, 1–37 (in German).

Ravaszova, P., Halanova, M., Goldova, M., Valencakova, A., Malcekova, B., Hurníková, Z., Halan, M., 2012. Occurrence of *Cryptosporidium* spp. in red foxes and brown bear in the Slovak Republic. Parasitology Research 110 (1), 469–471.

Ravindran, R., Kumar, K.G.A., Gafoor, V.M.A., 2011. Parasitic infections in wild animals of Kerala. Zoos' Print Journal 26 (5), 34.

Rehg, J.E., Gigliotti, F., Stokes, D.C., 1988. Cryptosporidiosis in ferrets. Laboratory Animal Science 38 (2), 155–158.

Reichenow, F., 1921. 'Dei Coccidien' in Handbuch der Pathogenen Protozoen. In: von Prowazek, S., Nöller, W. (Eds.), Lief. VIII. Leipzig, Germany, p. 1136.

Reid, D.G., Jinchu, H., Yan, H., 1991. Ecology of the red panda *Ailurus fulgens* in the Wolong Reserve, China. Journal of Zoology 225, 347–364.

Rengifo-Herrera, C., Ortega-Mora, L.M., Gómez-Bautista, M., García-Moreno, F.T., García-Párraga, D., Castro-Urda, F.J., Pedraza-Díaz, S., 2011. Detection and characterization of a *Cryptosporidium* isolate from a southern elephant seal (*Mirounga leonina*) from the Antarctic peninsula. Applied and Environmental Microbiology 77 (4), 1524–1527.

Rengifo-Herrera, C., Ortega-Mora, L.M., Álvarez-Garcia, G., Gómez-Bautista, M., García-Párraga, D., García-Peña, F.J., Pedraza-Díaz, S., 2012. Detection of *Toxoplasma gondii* antibodies in Antarctic pinnipeds. Veterinary Parasitology 190 (1), 259–262.

Rengifo-Herrera, C., Ortega-Mora, L.M., Gómez-Bautista, M., García-Pena, F.J., García-Párraga, D., Pedraza-Díaz, S., 2013. Detection of a novel genotype of *Cryptosporidium* in Antarctic pinnipeds. Veterinary Parasitology 191 (1–2), 112–118.

Rewell, R.E., 1948. Report of the pathologist for the year 1947. Proceedings of the Zoological Society of London 118, 501–514.

Richards, C.S., 1961. *Hepatozoon procyonis*, n. sp., from the raccoon. Journal of Eukaryotic Microbiology 8 (4), 360–362.

Richini-Pereira, V.B., Marson, P.M., da Silva, R.C., Langoni, H., 2016. Genotyping of *Toxoplasma gondii* and *Sarcocystis* spp. in road-killed wild mammals from central western region of the State of São Paulo, Brazil. Revista da Sociedade Brasileira de Medicina Tropical 49 (5), 602–607.

Ridala, V., 1936. Hõberebaste koktsidioosist ja teistest tähtsamatest hõberebaste parasitaarhaigustest (Coccidiosis and some other important parasitic diseases of silver foxes). Eesti Loomaarstlik Ringvaade 12 (7), 241–256 (in Estonian, English summary).

Ride, W.D.L., Cogger, H.G., Dupuis, C., Kraus, O., Minelli, A., Thompson, F.C., Tubbs, P.K. (Eds.), 1999. International Code of Zoological Nomenclature, fourth ed. The International Trust for Zoological Nomenclature, The Natural History Museum. London SW7 5BD, United Kingdom. 306 p. (in English and French).

Riemann, H.P., Fowler, M.E., Schulz, T., Lock, A., Thilsted, J., Pulley, L.T., Henrickson, R.V., Henness, A.M., Franti, C.E., Behymer, D.E., 1974. *Toxoplasma* in Pallas cats. Journal of Wildlife Diseases 10 (4), 471–477.

Rinaldi, L., Biggeri, A., Carbone, S., Musella, V., Catelan, D., Veneziano, V., Cringoli, G., 2006. Canine faecal contamination and parasitic risk in the city of Naples (southern Italy). BMC Veterinary Research 2, 29.

Rinaldi, L., Maurelli, M.P., Musella, V., Veneziano, V., Carbone, S., di Sarno, A., Paone, M., Cringoli, G., 2008. *Giardia* and *Cryptosporidium* in canine faecal samples contaminating an urban area. Research in Veterinary Science 84 (3), 413–415.

Rivolta, S., 1873. Dei Parassiti Vegetali. Torino (*nos non videbo illum*, as cited by Wenyon, 1923).

Rivolta, S., 1874. Sopra alcune specie di Tenie delle pecore e sopra specials cellule oviformes dei villi del cane e del gatto (Above Some Species of Tenie of the Sheep and on Specials Oviformes Cells of the Villi of the Dog and the Cat). Pisa (*nos non videbo illum*, as cited by Wenyon, 1923).

Rivolta, S., 1878. Della gregarinosi dei polli e dell'ordinamento delle gregarine e dei psorospermi degli animali domestici (Of the gregarinosis of chickens and of the ordering of gregarines and psorosperms of domestic animals). Giornale di Anatomia, Fisiologia e Patologia degli Animali (Pisa) 4, 220–235 (in Italian, no English summary).

Robel, R.J., Barnes, N.A., Upton, S.J., 1989. Gastrointestinal helminths and protozoa from two raccoon populations in Kansas. Journal of Parasitology 75 (6), 1000–1003.

Roberts, M.S., Gittleman, J.L., 1984. *Ailurus fulgens*. Mammalian Species (American Society of Mammalogists) 222, 1–8.

Roberts, W.L., Mahrt, J.L., Hammond, D.M., 1972. The fine structure of the sporozoites of *Isospora canis*. Zeitschrift für Parasitenkunde 40 (3), 183–194.

Robertson, I.D., Thompson, R.C., 2002. Enteric parasitic zoonoses of domesticated dogs and cats. Microbes and Infection 4 (8), 867–873.

da Rocha, E.M., Lopes, C.W.G., 1971. Comportamento da *Isospora canis*, *Isospora felis* e *Isospora rivolta* em infecções experimentais en cães e gatos (Behavior of *Isospora canis*, *Isospora felis* and *Isospora rivolta* in experimental infections in dogs and cats). Arqivos da Universidade Federal Rural do Rio de Janeiro 1 (2), 65–70 (in Portuguese, English summary).

Rodhain, J., 1933. On a coccidia from the intestine of a titi monkey. Comptes Rendus des Seances Socété de Biologia (Paris) 114, 1357–1358.

Rodrigues, A.F.S.F., Fernandes, B.F., Lemos, M., Daemon, E., Fabrino, K.L., Melo, R.C.N., Massard, C.L., 2004. Caracterização morfológica de gametócitos de *Hepatozoon procyonis* (Apicomplexa: Hepatozoidae) em *Nasua nasua* (Carnivora, Procyonidae). Revista Brasileira de Parasitologia Veterinaria 13 (Suppl. 1), 241 (in Portuguese).

Rodrigues, A.F.S.F., Daemon, E., Massard, C.L., 2007. Morphological and morphometrical characterization of gametocytes of *Hepatozoon procyonis* Richards, 1961 (Protista, Apicomplexa) from a Brazilian wild procyonid *Nasua nasua* and *Procyon cancrivorus* (Carnivora, Procyonidae). Parasitology Research 100 (2), 347–350.

Rodriguez, A., Carbonell, E., 1998. Gastrointestinal parasites of the Iberian lynx and other wild carnivores from central Spain. Acta Parasitologica 43 (3), 128–136.

Roe, W.D., Michael, S., Fyfe, J., Burrows, E., Hunter, S.A., Howe, L., 2017. First report of systemic toxoplasmosis in a New Zealand sea lion (*Phocarctos hookeri*). New Zealand Veterinary Journal 65 (1), 46–50.

Romer, A.S., 1968. Notes and Comments on Vertebrate Paleontology. University of Chicago Press, Chicago, Illinois, USA. 304 p.

Romero, J.J., Pérez, E., Frankena, K., 2004. Effect of a killed whole *Neospora caninum* tachyzoite vaccine on the crude abortion rate of Costa Rican dairy cows under field conditions. Veterinary Parasitology 123 (3–4), 149–159.

Rommel, M., 1979. Das Frettchen (*Putorius putorius furo*) ein zusätzlicher Endwirt für *Sarcocystis muris*. Zeitschrift für Parasitenkunde 58 (2), 187–188 (in German).

Rommel, M., Geisel, O., 1975. Untersuchungen über die Verbreitung und den Lebenszyklus einer Sarkosporidienart des Pferdes (*Sarcocystis equicanis* n. spec.) Berliner und Münchener Tierärztliche Wochenschrift 88, 468–471 (in German).

Rommel, M., Krampitz, H.E., 1975. Beiträge zum Lebenszyklus der Frenkelien. I. Die identität von *Isospora buteonis* aus dem Mäusebussard mit eimer Frenkelienart (*F. clethrionomyobuteonis* spec. n.) aus der Rötelmaus. Berliner und Münchener Tierärztliche Wochenschrift 88, 338–340 (in German).

Rommel, M., Seyerl, F.V., 1976. Der erstmalige Nachweis von *Hammondia hammondi* (Frenkel und Dubey 1975) im Kot einer Katz in Deutschland (The first isolation of *Hammondia hammondi* from the faeces of a cat in Germany). Berliner und Münchener Tierärztliche Wochenschrift 89, 398–399 (in German, English summary).

Rommel, M., Zielasko, B., 1981. Untersuchungen uber den Lebenszyklus von *Isospora burrowsi* (Trayser und Todd, 1978) aus dem Hund. Berliner und Münchener Tierärztliche Wochenschrift 94, 87–90 (in German).

Rommel, M., Heydorn, A.-O., Gruber, F., 1972. Beiträge zum Lebenszyklus der Sarkosporidien. I. Die Sporozyte von *S. tenella* in den Fäzes der Katze. Berliner und Münchener Tierärztliche Wochenschrift 85, 101–105 (in German).

Rommel, M., Heydorn, A.-O., Fischle, B., Gestrich, R., 1974. Beiträge zum Lebenszyklus der Sarkosporidien. V. Weitere Endwirte der Sarkosporidien von Rind, Schaf und Schwein und die Bedeutung des Zwischenwirtes fur die Verbreitung diser Parasitose. Berliner undMünchener Tierärztliche Wochenschrift 85, 392–396 (in German).

Rommel, M., Schwerdtfeger, A., Blewaska, S., 1981. The *Sarcocystis muris*-infection as a model for research on the chemotherapy of acute sarcocystosis of domestic animals. Zentralblatt für Bakteriologie, Mikrobiologie und Hygiene. I. Abteilung Originale Reihe A: Medizinische Mikrobiologie, Infektionskrankheiten und Parasitologie 250 (1–2), 268–276.

Rooney, J.R., Prickett, M.E., Delaney, F.M., Crowe, M.W., 1970. Focal myelitis-encephalitis in horses. The Cornell Veterinarian 60 (3), 494–501.

Rooney, A.L., Limon, G., Vides, H., Cortez, A., Guitian, J., 2014. *Sarcocystis* spp. in llamas (*Lama glama*) in Southern Bolivia: a cross sectional study of the prevalence, risk factors and loss in income caused by carcass downgrades. Preventive Veterinary Medicine 116 (3), 296–304.

Rosonke, B.J., Brown, S.R., Tornquist, S.J., Snyder, S.P., Garner, M.M., Blythe, L.L., 1999. Encephalomyelitis associated with a *Sarcocystis neurona*-like organism in a sea otter. Journal of the American Veterinary Medical Association 215 (12), 1839–1842.

Roth, C., 1988. *Leptoplesictis* Major 1903 (Mammalia, Carnivora, Viverridae) aus dem Orleanium und Astaracium/Miozän von Frankreich und Deutschland. Paläontologische Zeitschrift 62, 333–343 (in German, English and French summary).

Ruecker, N.J., Hoffman, R.M., Chalmers, R.M., Neumann, N.F., 2011. Detection and resolution of *Cryptosporidium* species and species mixtures by genus-specific nested PCR-restriction fragment length polymorphism analysis, direct sequencing, and cloning. Applied and Environmental Microbiology 77 (12), 3998–4007.

Ruehlmann, D., Podell, M., Oglesbee, M., Dubey, J.P., 1995. Canine neosporosis: a case report and literature review. Journal of the American Animal Hospital Association 31 (2), 174–183.

Ruiz, A., Frenkel, J.K., 1976. Recognition of cyclic transmission of *Sarcocystis muris* by cats. Journal of Infections Diseases 133 (4), 409–418.

Ruiz, A., Frenkel, J.K., 1980. *Toxoplasma gondii* in Costa Rican cats. American Journal of Tropical Medicine and Hygiene 29 (6), 1150–1160.

Ruppanner, R., Jessup, D.A., Ohishi, I., Behymer, D.E., Franti, C.E., 1982. Serologic survey for certain zoonotic diseases in black bears. Journal of the American Veterinary Medical Association 181 (11), 1288–1291.

Ryan, U., Power, M., 2012. *Cryptosporidium* species in Australian wildlife and domestic animals. Parasitology 139 (13), 1673–1688.

Ryan, M.J., Wyand, D.S., Nielsen, S.W., 1982. A Hammondia-like coccidian with a mink- muskrat life cycle. Journal of Wildlife Diseases 18 (1), 29–35.

Ryan, U., Xiao, L., Read, C., Zhou, L., Lal, A.A., Pavlásek, I., 2003. Identification of novel *Cryptosporidium* genotypes from the Czech Republic. Applied and Environmental Microbiology 69 (7), 4302–4307.

Ryšavý, B., 1954. Příspěvek k poznání kokcidií našich i dovezených obratlovců (Contribution to the knowledge of our and imported vertebrates). Ceskoslovenska Parazitologie 1, 131–174.

Sabshin, S.J., Levy, J.K., Tupler, T., Tucker, S.J., Greiner, E.C., Leutenegger, C.M., 2012. Enteropathogens identified in cats entering a Florida animal shelter with normal feces or diarrhea. Journal of the American Veterinary Medical Association 241 (3), 331–337.

Sahasrabudhe, V.K., Shah, H.L., 1966. The occurrence of *Sarcocystis* sp. in the dog. Journal of Protozoology 13 (4), 531.

Saito, M., Itagaki, T., Shibata, Y., Itagaki, H., 1995. Morphology and experimental definitive hosts of *Sarcocystis* sp. from sika deer, *Cervus nippon centralis*, in Japan. Japanese Journal of Parasitology 44 (3), 218–221.

Saito, M., Shibata, Y., Kubo, M., Itagaki, H., 1997. *Sarcocystis mihoensis* n. sp. from sheep in Japan. Journal of Veterinary Medical Science 59 (2), 103–106.

Sakuma, M., Nishio, T., Nakanishi, N., Izawa, M., Asari, Y., Okamura, M., Shimokawa-Miyama, T., Setoguchi, A., Endo, Y., 2011. A case of Iriomote Cat (*Prionilurus bengalensis irionmotensis*) with *Hepatozoon felis* parasitemia. Journal of Veterinary Medical Science 73 (10), 1381–1384.

Salb, A.L., Barkema, H.W., Elkin, B.T., Thompson, R.C.A., Whiteside, D.P., Black, S.R., Dubey, J.P., Kutz, S.J., 2008. Dogs as sources and sentinels of parasites in humans and wildlife, Northern Canada. Emerging Infectious Diseases 14 (1), 60–63.

Samarasinghe, B., Johnson, J., Ryan, U., 2008. Phylogenetic analysis of *Cystoisospora* species at the rRNA ITA1 locus and development of a PCR-RFLP assay. Experimental Parasitology 118 (4), 592–595.

Samuel, W.M., Pybus, M.J., Kocan, A.A., 2001. Parasitic Diseases of Wild Mammals, second ed. Iowa State University Press, Ames, Iowa, USA. 559 p.

Sangster, L.T., Styer, E.L., Hall, G.A., 1985. Coccidia associated with cutaneous nodules in a dog. Veterinary Pathology 22 (2), 186–188.

Santín, M., Dixon, B.R., Fayer, R., 2005. Genetic characterization of *Cryptosporidium* isolates from ringed seals (*Phoca hispida*) in Northern Quebec, Canada. Journal of Parasitology 91 (3), 712–716.

Santín, M., Trout, J.M., Vecino, M.A., Dubey, J.P., Fayer, R., 2006. *Cryptosporidium*, *Giardia* and *Enterocytozoon bieneusi* in cats from Bogota (Colombia) and genotyping of isolates. Veterinary Parasitology 141 (3–4), 334–339.

de Santis-Kerr, A.C., Raghavan, M., Glickman, N.W., Caldanaro, R.J., Moore, G.E., Lewis, H.B., Schantz, P.M., Glickman, L.T., 2006. Prevalence and risk factors for *Giardia* and coccidia species of pet cats in 2003–2004. Journal of Feline Medicine and Surgery 8 (5), 292–301.

Santoro, M., D'Alessio, N., Cerrone, A., Lucibelli, M.G., Borriello, G., Aloise, G., Auriemma, C., Riccone, N., Galiero, G., 2017. The Eurasian otter (*Lutra lutra*) as a potential host for rickettsial pathogens in southern Italy. PLoS One 12, e0173556.

Sargent, K.D., Morgan, U.M., Elliot, A., Thompson, R.C.A., 1998. Morphological and genetic characterisation of *Cryptosporidium* oocysts from domestic cats. Veterinary Parasitology 77 (4), 221–227.

Sasanelli, M., Paradies, P., Greco, B., Eyal, O., Zaza, V., Baneth, G., 2010. Failure of imidocarb dipropionate to eliminate *Hepatozoon canis* in naturally infected dogs based on parasitological and molecular evaluation methods. Veterinary Parasitology 171 (3–4), 194–199.

Sato, H., 1976. Experimental studies on the large forms of canine and feline coccidia in Japan. Bulletin of Azabu Veterinary College 31, 255–286 (in Japanese, English summary).

Sato, J.J., Hosoda, T., Wolsan, M., Suzuki, H., 2004. Molecular phylogeny of arctoids (Mammalia: Carnivora) with emphasis on phylogenetic and taxonomic positions of ferret-badgers and skunks. Zoological Science 21 (1), 111–118.

Sato, S., Kabeya, H., Makino, T., Suzuki, K., Asano, M., Inoue, S., Sentsui, H., Nogami, S., Maruyama, S., 2011. Seroprevalence of *Toxoplasma gondii* infection in feral raccoons (*Procyon lotor*) in Japan. Journal of Parasitology 97 (5), 956–957.

Schares, G., Heydorn, A.O., Cüppers, A., Conraths, F.J., Mehlhorn, H., 2001a. *Hammondia heydorni*-like oocysts shed by a naturally infected dog and *Neospora caninum* NC-1 cannot be distinguished. Parasitology Research 87 (10), 808–816.

Schares, G., Wenzel, U., Müller, T., Conraths, F.J., 2001b. Serological evidence for naturally occurring transmission of *Neospora caninum* among foxes (*Vulpes vulpes*). International Journal for Parasitology 31 (4), 418–423.

Schares, G., Heydorn, A.O., Cüppers, A., Mehlhorn, H., Geue, L., Peters, M., Conraths, F.J., 2002. In contrast to dogs, red foxes (*Vulpes vulpes*) did not shed *Neospora caninum* upon feeding of intermediate host tissues. Parasitology Research 88 (1), 44–52.

Schares, G., Pantchev, N., Barutzki, D., Heydorn, A.O., Bauer, C., Conraths, F.J., 2005. Oocysts of *Neospora caninum*, *Hammondia heydorni*, *Toxoplasma gondii* and *Hammondia hammondi* in faeces collected from dogs in Germany. International Journal for Parasitology 35 (14), 1525–1537.

Schaumann, R., Ackermann, G., Pless, B., Claros, M.C., Goldstein, A.C., Rodloff, A.C., 2000. In vitro activities of fourteen antimicrobial agents against obligately anaerobic bacteria. International Journal of Antimicrobial Agents 16 (3), 225–232.

Schneideer, C.R., 1967a. *Besnoitia darlingi* (Brumpt, 1913) in Panama. Journal of Protozoology 14 (1), 78–82.

Schneideer, C.R., 1967b. Cross-immunity evidence of the identity of *Besnoitia panamensis* from lizards and *B. darlingi* from opossums. Journal of Parasitology 53 (4), 886.

Schneider, A., 1881. Sur les psorospermies oviformes ou coccidies. Especes nouvelles ou peu connues. Archives de Zoologie Expérimentale et Générale 9, 387–404 (in French).

Schneider, C.R., 1968. *Hepatozoon procyonis* Richards, 1961, in a Panamanian raccoon, *Procyon cancrivorus panamensis* (Goldman). Revista de Biologia Tropical 15 (1), 123–135.

Schneider, T., Kaup, F.-J., Drommer, W., Thiel, W., Rommel, M., 1984. Zur Feinstruktur und Entwicklung von *Sarcocystis aucheniae* beim *Lama* (Investigations on the fine structure and biology of *Sarcocystis aucheniae* of the llama). Zeitschrift für Parasitenkunde 70 (4), 451–458 (in German).

Schreck, W., Dürr, U., 1970. Excystations-und Infektionsversuche mit Kokzidienoocysten bei neugeborenen Tieren. Zentralblatt für Bakteriologie, Mikrobiologie und Hygiene. I. Abteilung Originale Reihe A: Medizinische Mikrobiologie, Infektionskrankheiten und Parasitologie 125, 252–258 (in German).

Scioscia, N.P., Olmos, L., Gorosábel, A., Bernad, L., Pedrana, J., Hecker, Y.P., Gual, I., Gos, M.L., Denegri, G.M., Moore, D.P., Moré, G., 2017. Pampas fox (*Lycalopex gymnocercus*) new intermediate host of *Sarcocystis svanai* (Apicomplexa: Sarcocystidae). Parasitology International 66 (3), 214–218.

Scorza, A.V., Lappin, M.R., 2017. Prevalence of selected zoonotic and vector-borne agents in dogs and cats on the Pine Ridge Reservation. Veterinary Sciences 4 (3) pii E43.

Scorza, A.V., Brewer, M.M., Lappin, M.R., 2003. Polymerase chain reaction for the detection of *Cryptosporidium* spp. in cat feces. Journal of Parasitology 89 (2), 423–426.

Scorza, A.V., Duncan, C., Miles, L., Lappin, M.R., 2011. Prevalence of selected zoonotic and vector-borne agents in dogs and cats in Costa Rica. Veterinary Parasitology 183 (1–2), 178–183.

Scorza, V., Willmott, A., Gunn-Moore, D., Lappin, M.R., 2014. *Cryptosporidium felis* in faeces from cats in the UK. The Veterinary Record 174 (24), 609.

Sealander, J.A., 1943. Notes on some parasites of the mink in southern Michigan. Journal of Parasitology 29, 361–362.

Sedlaczek, J., Wesemeier, H.-H., 1995. On the diagnostics and nomenclature of *Sarcocystis* species (Sporozoa) in roe deer (*Capreolus capreolus*). Applied Parasitology 36 (2), 73–82.

Sedlák, K., Bártová, E., 2006a. Seroprevalences of antibodies to *Neospora caninum* and *Toxoplasma gondii* in zoo animals. Veterinary Parasitology 136 (3–4), 223–231.

Sedlák, K., Bártová, E., 2006b. The prevalence of *Toxoplasma gondii* IgM and IgG antibodies in dogs and cats from the Czech Republic. Veterinární Medicína 51, 555–558.

Seneviratna, P., Edward, A.G., DeGiusti, D.L., 1975. Frequency of *Sarcocystis* spp. in Detroit metropolitan area, Michigan. American Journal of Veterinary Research 36 (3), 337–339.

Sepúlveda, M.A., Seguel, M., Alvarado-Rybak, M., Verdugo, C., Muñoz-Zanzi, C., Tamayo, R., 2015. Postmortem findings in four South American sea lions (*Otaria byronia*) from an urban colony in Valdivia, Chile. Journal of Wildlife Diseases 51 (1), 279–282.

Serra, C.M.B., Uchôa, C.M.A., Coimbra, R.A., 2003. Parasitological study with faecal samples of stray and domiciliated cats (*Felis catus domesticus*) from the Metropolitan Area of Rio de Janeiro, Brazil. Revista da Sociedade Brasileira de Medicina Tropical 36 (3), 331–334.

Sevá, A.P., Funada, M.R., Souza, S.O., Nava, A., Richtzenhain, L.J., Soares, R.M., 2010. Occurrence and molecular characterization of *Cryptosporidium* spp. isolated from domestic animals in a rural area surrounding Atlantic dry forest fragments in Teodoro Sampaio municipality, State of São Paulo, Brazil. Brazilian Journal of Veterinary Parasitology 19 (4), 249–253.

Shah, H.L., 1969. The Coccidia (Protozoa: Eimeriidae) of the Cat (Ph.D. dissertation). University of Illinois, Urbana, Illinois, USA. 148 p.

Shah, H.L., 1970a. *Isospora* species of the cat and attempted transmission of *I. felis* Wenyon, 1923 from the cat to the dog. Journal of Protozoology 17 (4), 603–609.

Shah, H.L., 1970b. Sporogony of the oocysts of *Isospora felis* Wenyon, 1923 from the cat. Journal of Protozoology 17 (4), 609–614.

Shah, H.L., 1971. The life cycle of *Isospora felis*, Wenyon, 1923, a coccidium of the cat. Journal of Protozoology 18 (1), 3–17.

Shanker, D., Bhatia, B.B., Saleque, A., 1991. *Hammondia heydorni* in experimental pup fed goat muscles. Bioved 1 (2), 151–152.

Shastri, U.V., 1990. Isolation of *Toxoplasma* oocysts from a cat (*Felis catus*) at Parbhani (Maharastra). Journal of Veterinary Parasitology 4, 45–46.

Sheffield, H.G., Melton, M.J., 1970. *Toxoplasma gondii*: the oocyst, sporozoite, and infection of cultured cells. Science 167 (3919), 892–893.

Shelton, G.C., Kintner, L.D., MacKintosh, D.O., 1968. A coccidia-like organism associated with subcutaneous granulomata in a dog. Journal of the American Veterinary Medical Association 152 (2), 263–267.

Shimura, K., Ito, S., 1986. Isolation of *Hammondia hammondi* in Japan. Japanese Journal of Veterinary Science 48 (5), 901–908.

Shukla, R., Giraldo, P., Kraliz, A., Finnigan, M., Sanchez, A.L., 2006. *Cryptosporidium* spp. and other zoonotic enteric parasites in a sample of domestic dogs and cats in the Niagara region of Ontario. The Canadian Veterinary Journal 47 (12), 1179–1184.

Siam, M.A., Salem, G.H., Ghoneim, N.H., Michael, S.A., El-Refay, M.A.H., 1994. Public health importance of enteric parasitosis in captive Carnivora. Assiut Veterinary Medical Journal 32 (63), 131–140.

Silva, S.O., Richtzenhain, L.J., Barros, I.N., Gomes, A.M., Silva, A.V., Kozerski, N.D., de Araújo Ceranto, J.B., Keid, L.B., Soares, R.M., 2013. A new set of primers directed to 18S rRNA gene for molecular identification of *Cryptosporidium* spp. and their performance in the detection and differentiation of oocysts shed by synanthropic rodents. Experimental Parasitology 135 (3), 551–557.

Simonato, G., di Regalbono, A.F., Cassini, R., Traversa, D., Beraldo, P., Tessarin, C., Pietrobelli, M., 2015. Copromicroscopic and molecular investigations on intestinal parasites in kenneled dogs. Parasitology Research 114 (5), 1963–1970.

Simonato, G., di Regalbono, A.F., Cassini, R., Traversa, D., Tessarin, C., di Cesare, A., Pietrobelli, M., 2017. Molecular detection of *Giardia duodenalis* and *Cryptosporidium* spp. in canine fecal samples contaminating public areas in Northern Italy. Parasitology Research 116 (12), 3411–3418.

Simpson, V.R., Monies, R.J., Riley, P., Cromey, D.S., 1997. Foxes and neosporosis. The Veterinary Record 141 (19), 503.

Šimůnek, J., Smola, J., 1998. Antibiotics, Sulfonamides and Quinolones in Veterinary Medicine. LAST Steinhauser, S.R.O, Tišnov, Czech Republic. 136 p. (in Czech).

Singh, N., 1962. (Unpublished M. V. Sci. thesis). Agra University. (cited in Patnai, and Roy, 1965).

Singh, P., Gupta, M.P., Singla, L.D., Singh, N., Sharma, D.R., 2006. Prevalence and chemotherapy of gastro-intestinal helminthic infections in wild carnivores in Mahendra Choudhury Zoological Park, Punjab. Journal of Veterinary Parasitology 20 (1), 17–23.

Singla, L.D., Aulakh, G.S., Sharma, R., Juyal, P.D., Singh, J., 2009. Concurrent infection of *Taenia taeniaeformis* and *Isospora felis* in a stray kitten: a case report. Veterinární Medicína 54 (2), 81–83.

Sisk, D.B., Gosser, M.S., Styer, E.L., 1984. Intestinal cryptosporidiosis in two pups. Journal of the American Veterinary Medical Association 184 (7), 835–836.

Skidmore, L.V., 1929. Note on a new species of coccidia from the pocket gopher *Geomys bursarius* Shaw. Journal of Parasitology 15, 183–184.

Skidmore, L.V., McGrath, C.B., 1933. Clinical and case reports: canine coccidiosis due to *Eimeria canis*. Journal of the American Veterinary Medical Association 32, 627–629.

SkírNisson, K., Pálmadóttir, G.L., 1993. Parasites of farm minks and farm foxes in Iceland. In: Proceedings of the XVI Symposium of the Scandinavian Society for Parasitology, Norway, 30 September – 2 October, 1993, vol. 3, No. 2.

Šlapeta, J.R., Modrý, D., Votýpka, J., Jirků, M., Koudela, B., Lukeš, J., 2001. Multiple origin of the dihomoxenous life cycle in sarcosporidia. International Journal for Parasitology 31 (4), 413–417.

Šlapeta, J.R., Koudela, B., Votýpka, J., Modrý, D., Hořejš, R., Lukeš, J., 2002a. Coprodiagnosis of *Hammondia heydorni* in dogs by PCR based amplification of ITS 1 rRNA: differentiation from morphologically indistinguishable oocysts of *Neospora caninum*. Veterinary Journal (London, England: 1997) 163 (2), 147–154.

Šlapeta, J.R., Modrý, D., Kyselová, I., Hořejš, R., Lukeš, J., Koudela, B., 2002b. Dog shedding oocysts of *Neospora caninum*: PCR diagnosis and molecular phylogenetic approach. Veterinary Parasitology 109 (3–4), 157–167.

Slattery, J.P., O'Brien, S.J., 1995. Molecular phylogeny of the red panda (*Ailurus fulgens*). Journal of Heredity 86 (6), 413–422.

Sledge, D.G., Bolin, S.R., Lim, A., Kaloustian, L.L., Heller, R.L., Carmona, F.M., Kiupel, M., 2011. Outbreaks of severe enteric disease associated with *Eimeria furonis* infection in ferrets (*Mustela putorius furo*) of 3 densely populated groups. Journal of the American Veterinary Medical Association 239 (12), 1584–1588.

Śmielewska-Loś, E., Pacoń, J., Jańczak, M., Phoneczka, K., 2003. Prevalence of antibodies to *Toxoplasma gondii* and *Neospora caninum* in wildlife and farmed foxes (*Vulpes vulpes*). Electronic Journal of Polish Agricultural Universities, Series Veterinary Medicine. 6 (2), 1–6. http://www.ejpau.media.pl/articles/volume6/issue2/veterinary/art-06.pdf.

Smith, T.G., 1996. The genus *Hepatozoon* (Apicomplexa: Adeleina). Journal of Parasitology 82 (4), 565–585.

Smith, D.D., Frenkel, J.K., 1977. *Besnoitia darlingi* (Protozoa: Toxoplasmatinae): Cyclic transmission by cats. Journal of Parasitology 63 (6), 1066–1071.

Smith, D.D., Frenkel, J.K., 1978. Cockroaches as vectors of *Sarcocystis muris* and other coccidia in the laboratory. Journal of Parasitology 64 (2), 315–319.

Snyder, D.E., 1984. *Eimeria* spp. In: Raccoons in Illinois. Annual Midwest Conference of Parasitologists Program Booklet. Abstract #12, p. 10.

Snyder, D.E., 1988. Indirect immunofluorescent detection of oocysts of *Cryptosporidium parvum* in the feces of naturally infected raccoons (*Procyon lotor*). Journal of Parasitology 74 (6), 1050–1052.

Snyder, D.E., Sanderson, G.C., Toivio-Kinnucan, M., Blagburn, B.L., 1990. *Sarcocystis kirkpatricki* n. sp. (Apicomplexa: Sarcocystidae) in muscles of raccoons (*Procyon lotor*) from Illinois. Journal of Parasitology 76 (4), 495–500.

Soares, R.M., Cortez, L.R.P.B., Gennari, S.M., Sercundes, M.K., Keid, L.B., Pena, H.F.J., 2009. Crab-eating fox (*Cerdocyon thous*), a South American canid, as definitive host for *Hammondia heydorni*. Veterinary Parasitology 162 (1), 46–50.

Soares, R.M., Lopes, E.G., Keid, L.B., Sercundes, M.K., Martins, J., Richtzenhain, L.J., 2011. Identification of *Hammondia heydorni* oocysts by a heminested-PCR (hnPCR-AP10) based on the *H. heydorni* RAPD fragment AP10. Veterinary Parasitology 175 (1–2), 168–172.

Sobrino, R., Cabezón, O., Millán, J., Pabón, M., Arnal, M.C., Luco, D.F., Gortázar, C., Dubey, J.P., Almería, S., 2007. Seroprevalence of *Toxoplasma gondii* antibodies in wild carnivores from Spain. Veterinary Parasitology 148 (3), 187–192.

Sobrino, R., Dubey, J.P., Pabón, M., Linarez, N., Kwok, O.C., Millán, J., Arnal, M.C., Luco, D.F., López-Gatius, F., Thulliez, P., Gortázar, C., Almería, S., 2008. *Neospora caninum* antibodies in wild carnivores from Spain. Veterinary Parasitology 155 (3), 190–197.

Somvanshi, R., Koul, G.L., Biswas, J.C., 1987. *Sarcocystis* in a leopard (*Panthera pardus*). Indian Veterinary Medicine Journal 11, 174–175.

Soriano, S.V., Pierangeli, N.B., Roccia, I., Bergagna, H.F.J., Lazzarini, L.E., Celescinco, A., Saiz, M.S., Kossman, A., Contreras, P.A., Arias, C., Basualdo, J.A., 2010. A wide diversity of zoonotic intestinal parasites infects urban and rural dogs in Neuquén, Patagonia, Argentina. Veterinary Parasitology 167 (1), 81–85.

Sorvillo, F., Ash, L.R., Berlin, O.G., Morse, S.A., 2002. *Baylisascaris procyonis*: an emerging helminthic zoonosis. Emerging Infectious Diseases 8 (4), 355–359.

Sotiriadou, I., Pantchev, N., Gassmann, D., Karanis, P., 2013. Molecular identification of *Giardia* and *Cryptosporidium* from dogs and cats. Parasite 20, 8.

Spada, E., Proverbio, D., Della Pepa, A., Domenichini, G., Bagnagatti De Giorgi, G., Traldi, G., Ferro, E., 2013. Prevalence of faecal-borne parasites in colony stray cats in northern Italy. Journal of Feline Medicine and Surgery 15 (8), 672–677.

Spain, C.V., Scarlett, J.M., Wade, S.E., McDonough, P., 2001. Prevalence of enteric zoonotic agents in cats less than 1 year old in central New York State. Journal of Veterinary Internal Medicine 15 (1), 33–38.

Speer, C.A., Dubey, J.P., 1982. *Sarcocystis wapiti* sp. nov. from the North American wapiti (*Cervus elaphus*). Canadian Journal of Zoology 60 (5), 881–888.

Speer, C.A., Hammond, D.M., Mahrt, J.L., Roberts, W.L., 1973. Structure of the oocyst and sporocyst walls and excystation of sporozoites of *Isospora canis*. Journal of Parasitology 59 (1), 35–40.

Speer, C.A., Pond, D.B., Ernst, J.V., 1980. Development of *Sarcocystis hemionilatrantis* Hudkins and Kistner, 1977 in the small intestine of coyotes. Proceedings of the Helminthological Society of Washington 47, 106–113.

Spencer, J.A., Higginbotham, M.J., Blagburn, B.L., 2003. Seroprevalence of *Neospora caninum* and *Toxoplasma gondii* in captive and free-ranging nondomestic felids in the United States. Journal of Zoo and Wildlife Medicine 34 (3), 246–249.

Sprehn, C., Gramer, J., 1931. Das Darmcoccid *Lucetina canivelocis* (Weidmann, 1915) in Silberfüchsen. Berliner Tierärztliche Wochenschrift 47, 261–263 (in German).

Springer, M.S., Meredith, R.W., Janecka, J.E., Murphy, W.J., 2011. The historical biogeography of Mammalia. Philosophical Transactions of the Royal Society B 366, 2478–2502.

Stafford, K.J., West, D.M., Vermunt, J.J., Pomroy, W., Adlington, B.A., Calder, S.M., 1994. The effect of repeated doses of toltrazuril on coccidial oocyst output and weight gain in infected lambs. New Zealand Veterinary Journal 42 (3), 117–119.

Stanek, J.F., Dubey, J.P., Oglesbee, M.J., Reed, S.M., Lindsay, D.S., Capitini, L.A., Njoku, C.J., Vittitow, K.L., Saville, W.J.A., 2002. Life cycle of *Sarcocystis neurona* in its natural intermediate host, the raccoon, *Procyon lotor*. Journal of Parasitology 88, 1151–1158.

Stehr-Green, J.K., Murray, G., Schantz, P.M., Wahlquist, S.P., 1987. Intestinal parasites in pet store puppies in Atlanta. American Journal of Public Health 77 (3), 345–346.

Steinman, A., Shpigel, N.Y., Mazar, S., King, R., Baneth, G., Savitsky, I., Shkap, V., 2006. Low seroprevalence of antibodies to *Neospora caninum* in wild canids in Israel. Veterinary Parasitology 137 (1–2), 155–158.

Stepanova, E.V., Kondrashin, A.V., Sergiev, V.P., Morozova, L.F., Turbabina, N.A., Maksimova, M.S., Brazhnikov, A.I., Shevchenko, S.B., Morozov, E.N., 2017. Significance of chronic toxoplasmosis in epidemiology of road traffic accidents in Russian Federation. PLoS One 12 (9), e0184930.

Stieve, E., Beckmen, K., Kania, S.A., Widner, A., Patton, S., 2010. *Neospora caninum* and *Toxoplasma gondii* antibody prevalence in Alaska wildlife. Journal of Wildlife Diseases 46 (2), 348–355.

Stiles, C.W., 1891. Note préliminaire sur quelques parasites. Bulletin de la Société de Zoologique de France 16, 163–164 (in French).

Stiles, C.W., 1892. Notes on parasites. No. II. Journal of Comparative Medicine and Veterinary Archives 13 (9), 517–526.

Stojecki, K., Karamon, J., Sroka, J., Ceneck, T., 2012. Molecular diagnostics of *Sarcocystis* spp. infections. Polish Journal of Veterinary Sciences 15 (3), 589–596.

Stolte, M., Bockhardt, I., Odening, K., 1996a. A comparative scanning electron microscopic study of the cyst wall in 11 *Sarcocystis* species of mammals. Journal of the Zoological Society of London 239 (4), 821–832.

Stolte, M., Odening, K., Walter, G., Bockhardt, I., 1996b. The raccoon as an intermediate host of three *Sarcocystis* species in Europe. Journal of the Helminthological Society of Washington 63 (1), 145–149.

Stolte, M., Bockhardt, I., Odening, K., 1998. Scanning electron microscopic identification of *Sarcocystis gracilis* from roe deer and cattle. Journal of Zoology 244 (2), 265–268.

Streitel, R.H., Dubey, J.P., 1976. Prevalence of *Sarcocystis* infection and other intestinal parasitisms in dogs from a humane shelter in Ohio. Journal of the American Medical Association 168 (5), 423–424.

Strickberger, M.W., 1996. Evolution, second ed. Jones and Barlett Publishers, Sudbury, Massachusetts, USA. 670 p.

Strohbusch, M., Müller, N., Hemphill, A., Krebber, R., Greif, G., Gottstein, B., 2009. Toltrazuril treatment of congenitally acquired *Neospora caninum* infection in newborn mice. Parasitology Research 104 (6), 1335–1343.

Stronen, A.V., Sallows, T., Forbes, G.J., Wagner, B., Paquet, P.C., 2011. Diseases and parasites in wolves of the Riding Mountain National Park region, Manitoba, Canada. Journal of Wildlife Diseases 47 (1), 222–227.

Stuart, P., Zintl, A., de Waal, T., Mulcahy, G., Hawkins, C., Lawton, C., 2012. Investigating the role of wild carnivores in the epidemiology of bovine neosporosis. Parasitology 140 (3), 296–302.

Stuart, P., Golden, O., Zintl, A., de Waal, T., Mulcahy, G., McCarthy, E., Lawton, C., 2013. A coprological survey of parasites of wild carnivores in Ireland. Parasitology Research 112 (10), 3587–3593.

Sturdee, A.P., Chalmers, R.M., Null, S.A., 1999. Detection of *Cryptosporidium* oocysts in wild mammals of mainland Britain. Veterinary Parasitology 80 (4), 273–280.

Su, B., Fu, Y., Wang, Y., Jin, L., Chakraborty, R., 2001. Genetic diversity and population history of the red panda (*Ailurus fulgens*) as inferred from mitochondrial DNA sequence variations. Molecular Biology and Evolution 18 (6), 1070–1076.

Sugár, L., 1980. *Isospora wetzeli* sp. n. (Protozoa: Coccidia) found in the common red fox (*Vulpes Vulpes* L.). Parasitologia Hungarica 13 (1), 5–6.

Sugár, L., Entzeroth, R., Chobotar, B., 1990. Ultrastructure of *Sarcocystis sibirica* (Matchulski, 1947) from the Siberian roe deer, *Capreolus pygargus*. Parasitologia Hungarica 23 (1), 13–17.

Sulaiman, I.M., Morgan, U.M., Thompson, R.C., Lal, A.A., Xiao, L., 2000. Phylogenetic relationships of *Cryptosporidium* parasites based on the 70-kilodalton heat shock protein (HSP70) gene. Applied and Environmental Microbiology 66 (6), 2385–2391.

Sulaiman, I.M., Lal, A.A., Xiao, L., 2002. Molecular phylogeny and evolutionary relationships of *Cryptosporidium* parasites at the actin locus. Journal of Parasitology 88 (2), 388–394.

Sundermann, C.A., 1988. Dermal coccidiosis in dogs. Journal of the Alabama Academy of Sciences 59 (3), 105 (Abstract).

Sundermann, C.A., Blagburn, B.L., Swango, L.J., Boosinger, T.R., 1990. Development of *Caryospora bigenetica* (Apicomplexa) in canines. Journal of Protozoology 37 (1), 5A (Abstract 27).

Suteu, E., Mircean, V., 1996. Semnalarea infestatiei cu *Sarcocystis porcifelis* la mistret (*Sus scrofa ferus*) (Report *Sarcocystis porcifelis* infestation in wild boar (*Sus scrofa ferus*)). Revista Română de Medicină Veterinară 6, 165–167 (in Romanian).

Suzán, G., Ceballos, G., 2005. The role of feral mammals on wildlife infectious disease prevalence in two nature reserves within Mexico City limits. Journal of Zoo and Wildlife Medicine 36 (3), 479–484.

Svanbaev, S.K., 1956. Materialy k faune koktsidii dikikh mlekopitayushchikh Zapodnogo Kazakhstana (Materials on the fauna of coccidia of wild mammals in western Kazakhstan). Akademia Nauk Kazakhskoi SSR, Alma-Ata Instituta Zoologii, Trudy 5, 180–191 (in Russian).

Svanbaev, S.K., 1960. Coccidia of silver-black foxes in the Alma-Atinskoi region. Trudy Instituta Zoologii, Akademia Nauk Kazakhskoi SSR 14, 34–36.

Svanbaev, S.K., Rachmatullina, N.K., 1971. The question on coccidia from fur-bearing animals in Kazakhstan. Akademia Nauk Kazakhskoi SSR, Trudy Instituta Zoologii 31, 165–170 (in Russian).

Svoboda, M., Svobodová, V., 1987. Effects of breed, sex, age, management and nutrition on the incidence of *Toxoplasma gondii* antibodies in dogs and cats. Acta Veterinaria Brno 56, 315–330.

Svobodová, V., Knotek, Z., Svoboda, M., 1998. Prevalence of IgG and IgM antibodies specific to *Toxoplasma gondii* in cats. Veterinary Parasitology 80 (2), 173–176.

Swellengrebel, N.H., 1914. Zur Kenntnis der Entwicklungsgeschichte von *Isospora bigemina* (Stiles) (To know the evolution of *Isospora bigemina* [Stiles]). Archiv für Protistenkunde 32, 379–392 (in German).

Sykes, J.E., Papich, M.G., 2014. Chapter 10-antiprotozoal drugs. In: Sykes, J.E. (Ed.), Canine and Feline Infectious Diseases. Elsevier, Inc., Saunders, pp. 97–104.

Sykes, J.E., Dubey, J.P., Lindsay, L.L., Prato, P., Lappin, M.R., Guo, L.T., Mizisin, A.P., Shelton, G.D., 2011. Severe myositis associated with *Sarcocystis* spp. infection in 2 dogs. Journal of Veterinary Internal Medicine 25 (6), 1277–1283.

Tadros, W., Laarman, J.J., 1975. The weasel, *Mustela nivalis* as the final host of a *Sarcocystis* of the common European vole, *Microtus arvalis*. Proceedings of the Koninklijke Nederlandse Akademic van Wetenschappen Series C-Biological and Medical Sciences 78 (3), 325–326.

Tadros, W., Laarman, J.J., 1976. *Sarcocystis* and related coccidian parasites: a brief general review, together with a discussion on some biological aspects of their life cycles and a new proposal for their classification. Acta Leidensia 44, 1–107.

Tadros, W., Laarman, J.J., 1977. The cat *Felis catus* as the final host of *Sarcocystis cuniculi* Brumpt, 1913 of the rabbit *Oryctolagus cuniculus*. Proceedings of the Koninklijke Nederlandse Akademic van Wetenschappen Series C-Biological and Medical Sciences 80, 351–352.

Tadros, W., Laarman, J.J., 1978a. Note on the specific designation of *Sarcocystis putorii* (Railliet and Lucet, 1891) comb. nov. of the common European vole, *Microtus arvalis*. Proceedings of the Koninklijke Nederlandse Akademic van Wetenschappen Series C-Biological and Medical Sciences 81, 466–468.

Tadros, W., Laarman, J.J., 1978b. A comparative study of the light and electron microscopic structure of the walls of the muscle cysts of several species of *Sarcocystid eimeriid* coccidia. Proceedings of the Koninklijke Nederlandse Akademic van Wetenschappen Series C-Biological and Medical Sciences 81 (4), 469–491.

Tadros, W., Laarman, J.J., 1979. Muscular sarcosporidiosis in the common European weasel, *Mustela nivalis*. Zeitschrift für Parasitenkunde 58 (3), 195–200.

Tadros, W., Laarman, J.J., 1980. Further investigations on the life history and transmission of *Sarcocystis sebeki* of *Apodemus sylvaticus*. Tropical Geographic Medicine 32 (4), 362.

Tadros, W., Laarman, J.J., 1982. Current concepts on the biology, evolution and taxonomy of tissue cyst-forming eimeriid Coccidia. Advances in Parasitology 20, 293–468.

Takács, A., Szabó, L., Juhász, L., Takács, A.A., Lanszki, J., Takás, P.T., Heltai, M., 2014. Data on the parasitological status of golden jackal (Canis aureus L., 1758) in Hungary. Acta Veterinaria Hungarica 62 (1), 33–41.

Takos, M.J., 1957. Sarcosystis in the kinkajou. Journal of Parasitology 43 (1), 8.

Tangtrongsup, S., Scorza, A.V., Reif, J.S., Ballweber, L.R., Lappin, M.R., Salman, M.D., 2017. Prevalence and multilocus genotyping analysis of Cryptosporidium and Giardia isolates from dogs in Chiang Mai, Thailand. Veterinary Sciences 4 (2) pii E26.

Tejero, F., Arcay-de-Peraza, L., 1982. Cystoisospora felis: initial penetrative ability into cell cultures from rat peritoneal exudate. Acta Cientifica Venezolana 33, 338–341.

Tenter, A.M., 1995. Current research on Sarcocystis species of domestic animals. International Journal for Parasitology 25 (11), 1311–1330.

Tenter, A.M., Johnson, A.M., 1997. Phylogeny of the tissue cyst-forming eimeriid coccidia. Advances in Parasitology 39, 69–139.

Tenter, A.M., Baverstock, P.R., Johnson, A.M., 1992. Phylogenetic relationships of Sarcocystis species from sheep, goats, cattle and mice based on ribosomal RNA sequences. International Journal for Parasitology 22 (4), 503–513.

Tenter, A.M., Vietmeyer, C., Johnson, A.M., Janitschke, K., Rommel, M., Lehmacher, W., 1994. ELISAs based on recombinant antigens for seroepidemiological studies on Toxoplasma gondii infections in cats. Parasitology 109 (1), 29–36.

Tenter, A.M., Barta, J.R., Beveridge, I., Duszynski, D.W., Mehlhorn, H., Morrison, D.A., Thompson, R.C.A., Conrad, P.A., 2002. The conceptual basis for a new classification of the coccidia. International Journal for Parasitology 32, 595–616.

Thiermann, E., 1962. Aislamiento de Toxoplasma gondii por inoculacion experimental de deganos de un zorro culpeo (Dusicyon culpaeus) (The isolation of Toxoplasma gondii by experimental inoculation of mascerated organs of a culpeo fox (Dusciyon culpaeus)). Boletin Chileno de Parasitologia 17 (2), 53 (in Spanish).

Thilsted, J.P., Dubey, J.P., 1989. Neosporosis-like abortions in a herd of dairy cattle. Journal of Veterinary Diagnostic Investigations 1 (3), 205–209.

de Thoisy, B., Demar, M., Aznar, C., Carme, B., 2003. Ecological correlates of Toxoplasma gondii exposure in free-ranging neotropical mammals. Journal of Wildlife Diseases 39 (2), 456–459.

Thomas, N.J., Cole, R.A., 1996. The risk of disease and threats to the wild population. Endangered Species Update (Special Issue: Conservation and Management of the Southern Sea Otter) 13 (12), 23–27.

Thomas, D.M., Stanton, N.L., 1994. Eimerian species (Apicomplexa: Eimeriina) in Gunnison's prairie dogs (Cynomys gunnisoni-zuniensis) and rock squirrels (Spermophius variegatus grammurus) from southeastern Utah. Journal of the Helminthological Society of Washington 61, 17–21.

Thomas, N.J., Dubey, J.P., Lindsay, D.S., Cole, R.A., Meteyer, C.U., 2007. Protozoal meningoencephalitis in sea otters (Enhydra lutris): a histopathological and immunohistochemical study of naturally occurring cases. Journal of Comparative Pathology 137 (2), 102–121.

Thomaz, A., Meireles, M.V., Soares, R.M., Pena, H.F.J., Gennari, S.M., 2007. Molecular identification of Cryptosporidium spp. from fecal samples of felines, canines and bovines in the state of São Paulo, Brazil. Veterinary Parasitology 150 (4), 291–296.

Thompson, R.C.A., Palmer, C.S., O'Handley, R., 2008. The public health and clinical significance of Giardia and Cryptosporidium in domestic animals. The Veterinary Journal 177 (1), 18–25.

Thompson, R.C.A., Colwell, D.D., Shury, T., Appelbee, A.J., Read, C., Njiru, Z., Olson, M.E., 2009. The molecular epidemiology of Cryptosporidium and Giardia infections in coyotes from Alberta, Canada, and observations on some cohabiting parasites. Veterinary Parasitology 159, 167–170.

Thornton, J.E., Bell, R.R., Reardon, M.J., 1974. Internal parasites of coyotes in southern Texas. Journal of Wildlife Diseases 10, 232–236.

Thulin, J.D., Granstrom, D.E., Gelberg, H.B., Morton, D.G., French, R.A., Giles, R.C., 1992. Concurrent protozoal encephalitis and canine distemper virus infection in a raccoon (Procyon lotor). The Veterinary Record 130 (8), 162–164.

Tiangtip, R., Jongwutiwes, S., 2002. Molecular analysis of Cryptosporidium species isolated from HIV-infected patients in Thailand. Tropical Medicine and International Health 7 (4), 357–364.

Tinar, R., 1985. Ankara'da iki çiftlikte Yetiştirilen vizonlarda (Mustela vison) görülen coccidiose etkenleri (The factors of coccidiosis grown in two mink (Mustela vison) farms in Ankara). Fakültesi Veteriner Medicin Universitesi Basimevi Ankara 23, 464–473 (in Turkish).

Tizard, I.R., Billett, J.B., Ramsden, R.O., 1976. The prevalence of antibodies against Toxoplasma gondii in some Ontario mammals. Journal of Wildlife Diseases 12 (3), 322–325.

Tomimura, T., 1957. Experimental studies on coccidiosis in dogs and cats (1) the morphology of oocysts and sporogony of Isospora felis and its artificial infection in cats. Japanese Journal of Parasitology 6 (1), 12–24.

de Tommasi, A.S., Giannelli, A., de Caprariis, D., Ramos, R.A., Di Paola, G., Crescenzo, G., Dantas-Torres, F., Baneth, G., Otranto, D., 2014. Failure of imidocarb dipropionate and toltrazuril/emodepside plus clindamycin in treating Hepatozoon canis infection. Veterinary Parasitology 200 (3–4), 242–245.

Torres, P., Hott, A., Boehmwald, H., 1972. Protozoos, helmintos y arthropodos en gatos de la ciudad de Valdivia y su importancia para el hombre. Archivos de Medicina Veterinaria (Chile) 4, 2–11 (in Spanish).

Torres, J., Modrý, D., Fernández, J., Šlapeta, J.R., Koudela, B., 2000. Isospora lutrae n. sp. (Apicomplexa: Eimeriidae), a new coccidium from the European otter Lutra lutra (L.) (Carnivora: Mustilidae) from Spain. Systematic Parasitology 47 (1), 59–63.

Torrey, E.F., Yolken, R.H., 2003. Toxoplasma gondii and Schizophrenia. Emerging Infectious Diseases 9 (11), 1375–1380.

Tosini, F., Drumo, R., Elwin, K., Chalmers, R.M., Pozio, E., Cacciò, S.M., 2010. The CpA135 gene as a marker to identify Cryptosporidium species infecting humans. Parasitology International 59 (4), 606–609.

Traldi, G., 1990. Report of Cryptosporidium in an adult dog. Atti della Società Italiana delle Scienze Veterinarie 44, 1293–1294.

Trayser, C.V., 1973. Life Cycle of Isospora Species (M.S. thesis). University of Illinois, Urbana, Illinois, USA. 46 p.

Trayser, C.V., Todd, K.S., 1978. Life cycle of Isospora burrowsi n. sp. (Protozoa: Eimeriidae) from the dog Canis familiaris. American Journal of Veterinary Research 39 (1), 95–98.

Triffitt, M.J., 1927. Observations on the oocysts of coccidia found in the faeces of carnivores. Protozoology 3 (1), 59–64.

Turnwald, G.H., Barta, O., Taylor, W.H., Kreeger, J., Coleman, S.U., Pourciau, S.S., 1988. Cryptosporidiosis associated with immunosuppression attributable to distemper in a pup. Journal of the American Veterinary Medical Association 192 (1), 79–81.

Tysnes, K., Gjerde, B., Nødtvedt, A., Skancke, E., 2011. A cross-sectional study of Tritrichomonas foetus infection among healthy cats at shows in Norway. Acta Veterinaria Scandinavica 53, 39.

Tzannes, S., Batchelor, D.J., Graham, P.A., Pinchbeck, G.L., Wastling, J., German, A.J., 2008. Prevalence of Cryptosporidium, Giardia and Isospora species infections in pet cats with clinical signs of gastrointestinal disease. Journal of Feline Medicine and Surgery 10 (1), 1–8.

Tzipori, S., Campbell, I., 1981. Prevalence of Cryptosporidium antibodies in 10 animal species. Journal of Clinical Microbiology 14 (4), 455–456.

Tzipori, S., Angus, K.W., Campbell, I., Gray, E.W., 1980. Cryptosporidium: evidence for a single-species genus. Infection and Immunity 30 (3), 884–886.

Uehlinger, F.D., Greenwood, S.J., McClure, J.T., Conboy, G., O'Handley, R., Barkema, H.W., 2013. Zoonotic potential of Giardia duodenalis and Cryptosporidium spp. and prevalence of intestinal parasites in young dogs from different populations on Prince Edward Island, Canada. Veterinary Parasitology 196 (3–4), 509–514.

Uga, S., Matsumura, T., Ishibashi, K., Yoda, Y., Yatomi, K., Kataoka, N., 1989. Cryptosporidiosis in dogs and cats in Hyogo Prefecture, Japan. Japanese Journal of Parasitology 38 (3), 139–143 (in Japanese, English summary).

Uggla, A., Mattson, S., Juntti, N., 1990. Prevalence of antibodies to Toxoplasma gondii in cats, dogs and horses in Sweden. Acta Veterinaria Scandinavica 31 (2), 219–222.

Ukwah, B.N., Ezeonu, I.M., Ezeonu, C.T., Roellig, D., Xiao, L., 2017. Cryptosporidium species and subtypes in diarrheal children and HIV-infected persons in Ebonyi and Nsukka, Nigeria. Journal of Infection in Developing Countries 11 (2), 173–179.

Umbetaliev, S.S., October 1979. Sarcosporidia of Marmota. In: X Vsesoyuznaya Konferentsiya po Prirodnoi Ochagovosti Boleznei, vol. 1. USSR, Dushanbe, pp. 148–149. from Dubey et al., 2015, nos non videbo illum.

Umurzakoff, M.D., Nukerbaeva, K.K., 1985. Life cycle of Eimeria vison in minks. Izvestia Akademii Nauk Kazakhskoi Sovetskoi Sotsialisticheskoi Respubliki, Seria Biologicheskikh Nauk 0 (2), 48–53 (in Russian).

Uni, S., Matsubayashi, M., Ikeda, E., Suzuki, Y., 2003. Characteristics of a hepatozoonosis in lungs of Japanese black bears (Ursus thibetanus japonicus). Journal of Veterinary Medical Science 65 (3), 385–388.

Upton, S.J., 2000. Suborder Eimeriorina, Léger, 1911. In: Lee, J.J., Leedale, G.F., Bradbury, P. (Eds.), An Illustrated Guide to the Protozoa, vol. 1. second ed. Society of Protozoologists, Lawrence, KS, pp. 318–339.

Upton, S.J., Barnard, S.M., 1988. Development of Caryospora bigenetica (Apicomplexa: Eimeriorina) in experimentally infected mice. International Journal for Parasitology 18 (1), 15–20.

Ushigome, N., Yoshino, T., Suzuki, Y., Kawajiri, M., Masaki, K., Endo, D., Asakawa, M., 2011. The parasitological survey on animals in Kawasaki Yumemigasaki Zoological Park. Japanese Journal of Zoological and Wildlife Medicine 16 (2), 133–137.

Van Bolhuis, G.H., Philippa, J.D.W., Gajadhar, A.A., Osterhaus, M.E., Kuiken, T., 2007. Fatal enterocolitis in harbour seals (Phoca vitulina) caused by infection with Eimeria phocae. The Veterinary Record 160 (9), 297–300.

Van Pelt, R.W., Dieterich, R.A., 1973. Staphylococcal infection and toxoplasmosis in a young harbor seal. Journal of Wildlife Diseases 9 (3), 258–261.

Van Rensburg, I.B.J., Silkstone, M.A., 1984. Concomitant feline infectious peritonitis and toxoplasmosis in a cheetah (Acinonyx jubatus). Journal of the South African Veterinary Association 55 (4), 205–207.

Varga, I., Dubos-Kováca, M., 1988. Hammondia heydorni-fertőzöttség kutyában; az első hazai eset megállapítása. Magyar Állatorvosok Lapja 43 (1), 27–30 (in Hungarian, English summary).

Vashisht, K., Lichtensteiger, C.A., Miller, L.A., Gondim, L.F.P., McAllister, M.M., 2005. Naturally occurring *Sarcocystis neurona*-like infection in a dog with myositis. Veterinary Parasitology 133 (1), 19–25.

Vaughn, T., Ryan, J., Czaplewski, N., 2011. Mammalogy, fifth ed. Jones and Bartlett Publishers, Sudbury, Massachusetts, USA. 747 p.

Venturini, L., Petrucelli, M., Piscopo, M., Ungaza, J.M., Venturini, M.C., Bacigalupe, D., Basso, W., Dubey, J.P., 2002. Natural *Besnoitia* sp. infection in rabbits from Argentina. Veterinary Parasitology 107 (4), 273–278.

Verdon, R., Polianski, J., Gaudebout, C., Marche, C., Garry, L., Pocidalo, J.J., 1994. Evaluation of curative anticryptosporidial activity of paromomycin in a dexamethasone-treated rat model. Antimicrobial Agents and Chemotherapy 38 (7), 1681–1682.

Vilhena, H., Martinez-Diaz, V.I., Cardoso, L., Vieira, L., Altet, L., Francino, O., Pastor, J., Silvestre-Ferreira, A.C., 2013. Feline vector-borne pathogens in the north and centre of Portugal. Parasites and Vectors 6, 99.

Vincent-Johnson, N.A., Macintire, D.K., Lindsay, D.S., Lenz, S.D., Baneth, G., Shkap, V., Blagburn, B.L., 1997. A new *Hepatozoon* species from dogs: description of the causative agent of canine hepatozoonosis in North America. Journal of Parasitology 83 (6), 1,165–1,172.

Visco, R.J., Caruin, R.M., Selby, L.A., 1977. Effect of sex and prevalence of intestinal parasitism in dogs. Journal of the American Veterinary Medical Association 170 (8), 835–837.

Visco, R.J., Caruin, R.M., Selby, L.A., 1978. Effect of sex and prevalence of intestinal parasitism in cats. Journal of the American Veterinary Medical Association 172 (7), 797–800.

Vitaliano, S.N., Silva, D.A.O., Mineo, T.W.P., Ferreira, R.A., Bevilacqua, E., Mineo, J.R., 2004. Seroprevalence of *Toxoplasma gondii* and *Neospora caninum* in captive maned wolves (*Chrysocyon brachyurus*) from southeastern and midwestern regions of Brazil. Veterinary Parasitology 122 (4), 253–260.

Vitaliano, S.N., Soares, H.S., Minervino, A.H.H., Santos, A.L.Q., Werther, K., Marvulo, M.F.V., Siqueira, D.B., Pena, H.F.J., Soares, R.M., Su, C., Gennari, S.M., 2014. Genetic characterization of *Toxoplasma gondii* from Brazilian wildlife revealed abundant new genotypes. International Journal for Parasitology. Parasites and Wildlife 3 (3), 276–283.

von Cord Gottschalk, H., 2000. Eine neue mustelidenkokzidie aus *Lutra lutra* (L.) (A new mustelid coccidia from *Lutra lutra* L.). Der Zoologische Garten 70 (6), 361–368 (in German, English summary).

von Gerhard Skofitsch, O.K., Schenn, G., 1983. *Eimeria canis* (Apicomplexa: Eimeriidae): eine seltene Sporozoeninfektion beim Hund. Mitteilungen des Naturwissenschaftlichen Vereines für Steiermark 113, 159–162 (In German, English summary).

von Hessling, T., 1854. Histologische Mitteilungen. Zeitschrift für Wissenschaftliche Zoologie 5, 189–199 (in German, no English summary). (*nos non videbo illum*, from Sedlaczek and Wesemeier, 1995).

Voyvoda, H., Pasa, S., Uner, A., 2004. Clinical *Hepatozoon canis* infection in a dog in Turkey. The Journal of Small Animal Practice 45 (12), 613–617.

Wacha, R.S., Christiansen, J.L., 1982. Development of *Caryospora bigenetica* n. sp. (Apicomplexa: Eimeriidae) in rattlesnakes and laboratory mice. Journal of Protozoology 29 (2), 272–278.

Wahlström, K., Nikkilä, T., Uggla, A., 1999. *Sarcocystis* species in skeletal muscle of otter (*Lutra lutra*). Parasitology 118 (1), 59–62.

Wait, L.F., Srour, A., Smith, L.G., Cassey, P., Sims, S.K., McAllister, M.M., 2015. A comparison of antiserum and protein A as secondary reagents to assess *Toxoplasma gondii* antibody titers in cats and spotted hyenas. Journal of Parasitology 102 (3), 390–392.

Walker, E.P., Warnick, F., Hamlet, S.E., Lange, K.I., Davis, M.A., Uible, H.E., Wright, P.F., Revised by Paradiso, J.L., 1975. Mammals of the World, third ed., 2 vols. Johns Hopkins University Press, Baltimore, MD, USA. 1549 p.

Wallace, G.D., 1971. Experimental transmission of *Toxoplasma gondii* by filth-flies. American Journal of Tropical Medicine and Hygiene 20 (3), 411–413.

Wallace, G.D., 1973a. Intermediate and transport hosts in the natural history of *Toxoplasma gondii*. American Journal of Tropical Medicine and Hygiene 22 (4), 456–464.

Wallace, G.D., 1973b. *Sarcocystis* in mice inoculated with *Toxoplasma*-like oocysts from cat feces. Science 180 (4093), 1375–1377.

Wallace, G.D., 1973c. The role of the cat in the natural history of *Toxoplasma gondii*. American Journal of Tropical Medicine and Hygiene 22 (3), 313–322.

Wallace, G.D., 1975. Observations on a feline coccidium with some characteristics of *Toxoplasma* and *Sarcocystis*. Zeitschrift für Parasitenkunde 46 (3), 167–178.

Wallace, G.D., Frenkel, J.K., 1975. *Besnoitia* species (Protozoa, Sporozoa, Toxoplasmatidae): recognition of cyclic transmission by cats. Science 188 (4186), 369–371.

Wang, J.S., Liew, C.T., 1990. Prevalence of *Cryptosporidium* spp. in birds in Taiwan. Taiwan Journal of Veterinary Medicine and Animal Husbandry 56, 45–57.

Wang, G.L., Wei, T., Wang, X.Y., Li, W.Y., Zhang, P.C., Dong, M.X., Xiao, H., 1988. The morphology and life cycle of *Sarcocystis micros* n. sp. Chinese Journal of Veterinary Science and Technology 6 (1), 9–11 (in Chinese).

Wang, R., Zhang, L., Feng, Y., Ning, C., Jian, F., Xiao, L., Zhao, J., Wang, Y., 2008. Molecular characterization of a new genotype of *Cryptosporidium* from American minks (*Mustela vison*) in China. Veterinary Parasitology 154 (1–2), 162–166.

Wang, R., Zhang, X., Zhu, H., Zhang, L., Feng, Y., Jian, F., Ning, C., Qi, M., Zhou, Y., Fu, K., Wang, Y., Sun, Y., Wang, Q., Xiao, L., 2011. Genetic characterizations of *Cryptosporidium* spp. and *Giardia duodenalis* in humans in Henan, China. Experimental Parasitology 127 (1), 42–45.

Wang, T., Chen, Z., Xie, Y., Hou, R., Wu, Q., Gu, X., Lai, W., Peng, X., Yang, G., 2015a. Prevalence and molecular characterization of *Cryptosporidium* in giant panda (*Ailuropoda melanoleuca*) in Sichuan province, China. Parasites and Vectors 8, 344.

Wang, T., Chen, Z., Yu, H., Xie, Y., Gu, X., Lai, W., Peng, X., Yang, G., 2015b. Prevalence of *Cryptosporidium* infection in captive lesser panda (*Ailurus fulgens*) in China. Parasitology Research 114 (2), 773–776.

Wanha, K., Edelhofer, R., Gabler-Eduardo, C., Prosl, H., 2005. Prevalence of antibodies against *Neospora caninum* and *Toxoplasma gondii* in dogs and foxes in Austria. Veterinary Parasitology 128 (3–4), 189–193.

Wapenaar, W., Jenkins, M.C., O'Handley, R.M., Barkema, H.W., 2006. *Neospora caninum*-like oocysts observed in feces of free-ranging red foxes (*Vulpes vulpes*) and coyotes (*Canis latrans*). Journal of Parasitology 92 (6), 1270–1274.

Wapenaar, W., Barkema, H.W., Schares, G., Rouvinen-Watt, K., Zeijlemaker, L., Poorter, B., O'Handley, R.M., Kwok, O.C.H., Dubey, J.P., 2007. Evaluation of four serological techniques to determine the seroprevalence of *Neospora caninum* in foxes (*Vulpes vulpes*) and coyotes (*Canis latrans*) on Prince Edward Island, Canada. Veterinary Parasitology 145 (1), 51–58.

Watkins, C.V., Harvey, L.A., 1942. On the parasites of silver foxes on some farms in the southwest. Parasitology 34, 155–179.

Wei, T., Chang, P.Z., Dong, M.X., Wang, X.Y., Xia, A.Q., 1985. Description of two new species of *Sarcocystis* from the yak (*Poeophagus grunniens*). Scientia Agricultura Sinica 4, 80–85.

Wei, T., Wang, X., Zhang, P., Dong, M., Li, W., 1989. Identification of *Sarcocystis* sp. in yak fetus tissue. Chinese Journal of Veterinary Science Techniques 11, 28–29.

Wei, T., Wang, X., Zhang, P., Dong, M., Wang, X., 1990. Host spectrum of two *Sarcocystis* species from yak. Journal of Chinese Traditional Medicine 5, 8–10.

Weidman, F.D., 1915. *Coccidium bigeminum* Stiles in swift-foxes (habitat western U.S.). Journal of Comparative Pathology 28, 320–323.

Weiss, L.M., Kim, K. (Eds.), 2007. *Toxoplasma gondii*. The Model Apicomplexan: Perspectives and Methods. Elsevier/Academic Press Inc., London, United Kingdom. 777 p.

Welsh, T., Burek-Huntington, K., Savage, K., Rosenthal, B., Dubey, J.P., 2014. *Sarcocystis canis* associated hepatitis in a Steller sea lion (*Eumetopias jubatus*) from Alaska. Journal of Wildlife Diseases 50 (2), 405–408.

Wenyon, C.M., 1923. Coccidiosis of cats and dogs and the status of *Isospora* of man. Annals of Tropical Medicine and Parasitology 17 (2), 231–289.

Wenyon, C.M., 1926a. Coccidia of the genus *Isospora* in cats, dogs, and man. Parasitology 18, 253–266.

Wenyon, C.M., 1926b. Protozoology: A Manual for Medical Men, Veterinarians and Zoologists, vol. II. Bailliere, Tindall and Cassel, Ltd., London, pp. 1085–1095.

Wenyon, C.M., 1926c. Protozoology, 2 vols. Wood, New York, NY, USA. 1579 p.

Wenyon, C.M., Sheather, L., 1925. Exhibition of specimens illustrating *Isospora* infections of dogs. In: Proceedings of a Laboratory Meeting of the Society [held at the Royal Army Medical College, Millibank, London, SW] Transactions of the Royal Society of Tropical Medicine and Hygiene 19 (Abstract No. 10), p. 321.

Wenzel, R., Erber, M., Boch, J., Schellner, H.P., 1982. Sarkosporidien-Infektion beim Haushuhn, Fasan und Bleßhuhn. Berliner und Münchener Tierärztliche Wochenschrift 95, 188–193 (in German).

Werner, A., Sulima, P., Majewska, A.C., 2004. Evaluation of usefulness of different methods for detection of *Cryptosporidium* in human and animal stool samples. Wiadomosci Parazytologiczne 50 (2), 209–220 (in Polish).

Wesemeier, H.-H., Sedlaczek, J., 1995a. One known *Sarcocystis* species and one found for the first time in fallow deer (*Dama dama*). Applied Parasitology 36 (4), 299–302.

Wesemeier, H.-H., Sedlaczek, J., 1995b. One known *Sarcocystis* species and two found for the first time in red deer and wapiti (*Cervus elaphus*) in Europe. Applied Parasitology 36 (4), 245–251.

Wesemeier, H.-H., Odening, K., Walter, G., Bockhardt, I., 1995. The black-backed jackal (Carnivora: Canidae) in Namibia as intermediate host of two *Sarcocystis* species (Protozoa: Sarcocystidae). Parasite 2 (4), 391–394.

Wetzel, R., 1938. Ein neues Coccid (*Cryptosporidium vulpis* sp. nov.) aus dem Rotfuchs. Archiv für Wissenschaftliche und Praktische Tierheilkunde 74 (1), 39–40 (in German).

White, A.C., Chappell, C.L., Hayat, C.S., Kimball, K.T., Flanigan, T.P., Goodgame, R.W., 1994. Paromomycin for cryptosporidiosis in AIDS: a prospective, double blinded trial. The Journal of Infectious Diseases 170 (2), 419–424.

Wicht, R.J., 1981. Transmission of *Sarcocystis rileyi* to the striped skunk (*Mephitis mephitis*). Journal of Wildlife Diseases 17 (3), 387–388.

Wielinga, P.R., de Vries, A., van der Goot, T.H., Mank, T., Mars, M.H., Kortbeek, L.M., van der Giessen, J.W., 2008. Molecular epidemiology of *Cryptosporidium* in humans and cattle in The Netherlands. Intermatinal Journal for Parasitology 38 (7), 809–817.

Wilber, P.G., Duszynski, D.W., Upton, S.J., Seville, R.S., Corliss, J.O., 1998. A revision of the taxonomy and nomenclature of the *Eimeria* (Apicomplexa: Eimeriidae) from rodents in the Tribe Marmotini (Sciuridae). Systematic Parasitology 39 (2), 113–135.

Wilkinson, G.T., 1977. Coccidial infection in a cat colony. The Veterinary Record 100 (8), 156–157.

Williams, E.S., Thorne, E.T., 1996. Infections and parasitic diseases of captive carnivores, with special emphasis on the black-footed ferret (*Mustela nigripes*). Revue Scientifique et Technique (International Office of Epizootics) 15 (1), 91–114.

Williams, E.S., Thorne, E.T., Kwiatkowski, D.R., Oakleaf, B., 1992. Overcoming disease problems in the black-footed ferret recovery program. Transactions of the North American Wildlife and Natural Resources Conference 57, 474–485.

Williams, B.H., Chimes, M.J., Gardner, C.H., 1996. Biliary coccidiosis in a ferret (*Mustela putorius furo*). Veterinary Pathology 33 (4), 437–439.

Willingham, A.L., Ockens, N.W., Kapel, C.M.O., Monrad, J., 1996. A helminthological survey of wild red foxes (*Vulpes vulpes*) from the metropolitan area of Copenhagen. Journal of Helminthology 70 (3), 259–263.

Wilson, R.B., Holscher, M.A., 1983. Cryptosporidiosis in a pup. Journal of the American Veterinary Medical Association 183 (9), 1005–1006.

Wilson, D.E., Reeder, D.M., 2005. third ed. Mammal Species of the World, vol. 1. Johns Hopkins University Press, Baltimore, MD, USA. 743 p.

Wilson, D.E., Reeder, D.M., 2017. http://vertebrates.si.edu/msw/mswCFApp/msw/index.cfm.

Wittner, M., Rowin, K.S., Tanowitz, H.B., Hobbs, J.F., Saltzman, S., Wenz, B., Hirsch, R., Chisholm, E., Healy, G.R., 1982. Successful chemotherapy of transfusion babesiosis. Annals of Internal Medicine 96 (5), 601–604.

Wobesser, G., Cawthorn, R.J., Gajadhar, A.A., 1983. Pathology of *Sarcocystis campestris* infection in Richardson's ground squirrels (*Spermophilus richardsoni*). Canadian Journal of Comparative Medicine 47 (2), 198–202.

Woke, P.A., Jacobs, L., Jones, F.E., Melton, M.L., 1953. Experimental results on possible arthropod transmission of toxoplasmosis. Journal of Parasitology 39 (5), 523–532.

Wolfe, A., Hogan, S., Maguire, D., Fitzpatrick, C., Vaughan, L., Wall, D., Hayden, T.J., Mulcahy, G., 2001. Red foxes (*Vulpes vulpes*) in Ireland as hosts for parasites of potential zoonotic and veterinary significance. The Veterinary Record 149 (25), 759–763.

Woodmansee, D.B., Powell, E.C., 1984. Cross-transmission and in vitro excystation experiments with *Sarcocystis muris*. Journal of Parasitology 70 (1), 182–183.

Woodroffe, R., 1999. Managing disease threats to wild mammals. Animal Conservation 2 (3), 185–193.

Wozencraft, W.C., 2005. Order carnivora. In: Wilson, D.E., Reeder, D.A. (Eds.), Mammal Species of the World. A Taxonomic and Geographic Reference, vol. 1. third ed. The Johns Hopkins University Press, Baltimore, MD, USA, pp. 532–628.

Wund, M., 2005. Mephitidae. (On-line), Animal Diversity Web http://animaldiversity.org/accounts/Mephitidae/.

Wund, M., Myers, P., 2005. Mammalia. (On-line), Animal Diversity Web http://animaldiversity.org/accounts/Mammalia/.

Xiao, L., Feng, Y., 2008. Zoonotic cryptosporidiosis. FEMS Immunology and Medical Microbiology 52 (3), 309–323.

Xiao, B.N., Zeng, D.L., Zhang, C.G., Wang, M., Li, Y., Gong, Z.F., 1993. Development of *Sarcocystis cruzi* in buffalo (*Bubalus bubalis*) and cattle (*Bos taurus*). Acta Veterinaria et Zootechnica Sinica 24, 185–192.

Xiao, L., Limor, J.R., Li, L., Morgan, U., Thompson, R.C., Lal, A.A., 1999a. Presence of heterogeneous copies of the small subunit rRNA gene in *Cryptosporidium parvum* human and marsupial genotypes and *Cryptosporidium felis*. Journal of Eukaryotic Microbiology 46 (5), 44S–45S.

Xiao, L., Morgan, U.M., Limor, J., Escalante, A., Arrowood, M., Shulaw, W., Thompson, R.C., Fayer, R., Lal, A.A., 1999b. Genetic diversity within *Cryptosporidium parvum* and related *Cryptosporidium* species. Applied and Environmental Microbiology 65 (8), 3386–3391.

Xiao, L., Limor, J.R., Sulaiman, I.M., Duncan, R.B., Lal, A.A., 2000. Molecular characterization of a *Cryptosporidium* isolate from a black bear. Journal of Parasitology 86 (5), 1166–1170.

Xiao, L., Bern, C., Limor, J., Sulaiman, I., Roberts, J., Checkley, W., Cabrera, L., Gilman, R.H., Lal, A.A., 2001. Identification of 5 types of *Cryptosporidium* parasites in children in Lima, Peru. The Journal of Infectious Diseases 183 (3), 492–497.

Xiao, L., Fayer, R., Ryan, U., Upton, S.J., 2004. *Cryptosporidium* taxonomy: recent advances and implications for public health. Clinical Microbiology Reviews 17 (1), 72–97.

Xie, Y., Zhang, Z., Wang, C., Lan, J., Li, Y., Chen, Z., Fu, Y., Nie, H., Yan, N., Gu, X., Wang, S., Peng, X., Yang, G., 2011. Complete mitochondrial genomes of *Baylisascaris schroederi*, *Baylisascaris ailuri* and *Baylisascaris transfuga* from giant panda, red panda and polar bear. Gene 482 (1–2), 59–67.

Xu, H., Jin, Y., Wu, W., Li, P., Wang, L., Li, N., Feng, Y., Xiao, L., 2016. Genotypes of *Cryptosporidium* spp., *Enterocytozoon bieneusi* and *Giardia duodenalis* in dogs and cats in Shanghai, China. Parasites and Vectors 9, 121.

Xue, I.B., Davey, P.G., Philips, G., 1996. Variation in post-antibiotic effect of clindamycin against clinical isolates of *Staphylococcus aureus* and implications for dosing of patients with osteomyelitis. Antimicrobial Agents and Chemotherapy 40 (6), 1403–1407.

Yai, L.E., Bauab, A.R., Hirschfeld, M.P., de Oliveira, M.L., Damaceno, J.T., 1997. The first two cases of *Cyclospora* in dogs, São Paulo, Brazil. Revista do Instituto de Medicina Tropical de São Paulo 39 (3), 177–179.

Yakimoff, W.L., 1932. On a new species of coccidium occurring in cat. Vestnik Mikrobiologii Epidemiologii I Parazitologii 11 (4), 309–310 (in Russian, English summary).

Yakimoff, W.L., 1933. Zur Frage der Eimeriose der Katzen (On the question of eimeriosis of cats). Archiv für Protistenkunde 80, 172–176 (in German).

Yakimoff, W.L., Gousseff, W.F., 1934. Coccidia of martins and sables. Journal of Parasitology 20 (4), 251–252.

Yakimoff, W.L., Gousseff, W.F., 1936. Zur Frage der Kokzidien der Füchse (On the question of coccidia of foxes). Wiener Tierärztliche Monatschrift 23, 359–361 (in German).

Yakimoff, W.L., Lewkowitsch, E.N., 1932. Isospora theileri n. sp., Coccidie der Schakale (Isospora theileri n. sp., coccidia of jackals). Archiv für Protistenkunde 77, 533–537 (in German).

Yakimoff, W.L., Matikaschwili, I.L., 1932. Coccidiosis of skunks. Annals of Tropical Medicine and Parasitology 25, 539–545.

Yakimoff, W.L., Matikaschwili, I.L., 1933. Coccidiosis in raccoons: Eimeria nuttalli n. sp., parasite of Procyon lotor. Parasitology 24, 574–575.

Yakimoff, W.L., Matschoulsky, S.N., 1935. As coccidioses dos ursos, lobos e cães selvagens. Archivos do Instituto Biologico 6, 171–177 (in Portuguese, English summary).

Yakimoff, W.L., Matschoulsky, S.N., 1940. Koktsidii zhivotnykh soologicheskogo sada v Tashkente (Coccidia of the animals in the Tashkent Zoological Garden). Magasin de parasitologie de l'Institut zoologique de l'Académie des Sciences de L'URSS 8, 236–248 (in Russian, no English summary).

Yakimoff, W.L., Sokoloff, I.I., 1934. Die Sarkozysten des Renntieres und des Maral (Sarcocystis gruneri n. sp.). Berliner Tierärztliche Wochenschrift 50, 772–774.

Yakimoff, W.L., Terwinsky, S.K., 1930. Coccidiosis of sables. Fur Animal Syndicate 2, 19–21 (in Russian).

Yakimoff, W.L., Terwinsky, S.K., 1931. Die coccidiose des Zobeltieres (The coccidiosis of the sable animal). Archiv für Protistenkunde 73, 56–59 (in German).

Yakimoff, W.L., Matikaschwili, I.L., Rastegaïeff, E.F., 1933a. Zur Frage über die Coccidien der Schakale, Eimeria (sic) dutoiti (n. sp.) (On the question about the coccidia of the jackals, Eimeria dutoit (n. sp.)). Archiv für Protistenkunde 80, 177–178 (in German).

Yakimoff, W.L., Matikaschwili, I.L., Rastegaïeff, E.F., Lewkowitsch, E.N., 1933b. Coccidia of the Felidae. Parasitology 25, 389–391.

Yamamoto, N., Kon, M., Saito, T., Maeno, N., Koyama, M., Sunaoshi, K., Yamaguchi, M., Morishima, Y., Kawanaka, M., 2009. Prevalence of intestinal canine and feline parasites in Saitama Prefecture, Japan. Kansenshogaku Zasshi (The Journal for the Japanese Association for Infectious Diseases) 83 (3), 223–228 (in Japanese, English summary).

Yanai, T., Tomita, A., Masegi, T., Ishikawa, K., Iwasaki, T., Yamazoa, K., Uede, K., 1995. Histopathologic features of naturally occurring hepatozoonosis in wild martens (Martes melampus) in Japan. Journal of Wildlife Diseases 31 (2), 233–237.

Yang, G.Y., Wang, C.D., 2000. Advances on parasites and parasitology of Ailurus fulgens. Chinese Journal of Veterinary Science 26, 36–38.

Yang, R., Ying, J.L., Monis, P., Ryan, U., 2015. Molecular characterisation of Cryptosporidium and Giardia in cats (Felis catus) in Western Australia. Experimental Parasitology 155, 13–18.

Yang, Z., Zhao, W., Wang, J., Ren, G., Zhang, W., Liu, A., 2017. Molecular detection and genetic characterizations of Cryptosporidium spp. in farmed foxes, minks, and raccoon dogs in northeastern China. Parasitology Research 117 (1), 169–175.

Yantis, D., Moeller, R., Braun, R., Gardiner, C.H., Aguirre, A., Dubey, J.P., 2003. Hepatitis associated with a Sarcocystis canis-like protozoan in a Hawaiian Monk Seal (Monachus schauinslandi). Journal of Parasitology 89 (6), 1258–1260.

Yi-Fan, C., Le, Y., Yin, D., Jiang-Hui, B., Duszynski, D.W., 2012. Emendation of 2 Isospora species (Apicomplexa: Eimeriidae) infecting the steppe polecat, Mustela eversmanii Lesson, 1827, in China, to the genus Cystoisospora (Apicomplexa: Sarcocystidae). Comparative Parasitology 79, 147–152.

Yonzon, P.B., Hunter, M.L., 1991. Conservation of the red panda Ailurus fulgens. Biological Conservation 5, 1–11.

Yoshiuchi, R., Matsubayashi, M., Kimata, I., Furuya, M., Tani, H., Sasai, K., 2010. Survey and molecular characterization of Cryptosporidium and Giardia spp. in owned companion animal, dogs and cats, in Japan. Veterinary Parasitology 174 (3–4), 313–316.

Yu, X.L., Chen, N.H., Hu, D.M., Zhang, W., Li, X.X., Wang, B.Y., Kang, L.P., Li, X.D., Liu, Q., Tian, K.G., 2009. Detection of Neospora caninum from farm-bred young blue foxes (Alopex lagopus) in China. Journal of Veterinary Medical Science 71 (1), 113–115.

Yu, L., Peng, D., Liu, J., Luan, P., Liang, L., Lee, H., Lee, M., Ryder, O.A., Zhang, Y., 2011. On the phylogeny of Mustelidae subfamilies: analysis of seventeen nuclear non-conding loci and mitochondrial complete genomes. BMC Evolutionary Biology 11, 92.

Yu, Z., Ruan, Y., Zhou, M., Chen, S., Zhang, Y., Wang, L., Zhu, G., Yu, Y., 2017. Prevalence of intestinal parasites in companion dogs with diarrhea in Beijing, China, and genetic characteristics of Giardia and Cryptosporidium species. Parasitology Research 117 (1), 35–43.

Zarnke, R.L., Dubey, J.P., Kwok, O.C.H., Ver Hoef, J.M., 1997. Serologic survey for Toxoplasma gondii in grizzly bears from Alaska. Journal of Wildlife Diseases 33 (2), 267–270.

Zeman, D.H., Dubey, J.P., Robison, D., 1993. Fatal hepatic sarcocystosis in an American black bear. Journal of Veterinary Diagnostic Investigation 5 (3), 480–483.

Zhang, Y.P., Ryder, O.A., 1993. Mitochondrial DNA sequence evolution in the Arctoidea. Proceeding of the National Academy of Sciences 90, 9557–9561.

Zhang, S.-Y., Wei, M.-X., Zhou, Z.-Y., Yu, J.-Y., Shi, X.-Q., 2000. Prevalence of antibodies to *Toxoplasma gondii* in the sera of rare wildlife in the Shanghai zoological Garden, People's republic of China. Parasitology International 49 (2), 171–174.

Zhang, H., Compaore, M.K.A., Lee, E.G., Liao, M., Zhang, G., Sugimoto, C., Fujisaki, K., Nishikawa, Y., Zuan, X., 2007. Apical membrane antigen 1 is a cross-reactive antigen between *Neospora caninum* and *Toxoplasma gondii*, and the anti-NcAMA1 antibody inhibits host cell invasion by both parasites. Molecular Biochemistry and Parasitology 151 (2), 205–212.

Zhang, X.X., Cong, W., Ma, J.G., Lou, Z.L., Zheng, W.B., Zhao, Q., Zhu, X.Q., 2016a. First report of *Cryptosporidium canis* in farmed Arctic foxes (*Vulpes lagopus*) in China. Parasites and Vectors 9, 126–130.

Zhang, S., Tao, W., Liu, C., Jiang, Y., Wan, Q., Li, Q., Yang, H., Lin, Y., Li, W., 2016b. First report of *Cryptosporidium canis* in foxes (*Vulpes vulpes*) and raccoon dogs (*Nyctereutes procyonoides*) and identification of several novel subtype families for *Cryptosporidium* mink genotype in minks (*Mustela vison*) in China. Infection, Genetics and Evolution 41, 21–25.

Zhou, L., Fayer, R., Trout, J.M., Ryan, U.M., Schaefer III, F.W., Xiao, L., 2004. Genotypes of *Cryptosporidium* species infecting fur-bearing mammals differ from those of species infecting humans. Applied and Environmental Microbiology 70 (12), 7574–7577.

Ziegler, P.E., Wade, S.E., Schaaf, S.L., Stern, D.A., Nadareski, C.A., Mohammed, H.O., 2007. Prevalence of *Cryptosporidium* species in wildlife populations within a watershed landscape in southeastern New York State. Veterinary Parasitology 177 (1–2), 176–184.

Zimmerman, H.S., 1959. Invasionkrankheiten bei Farmnerzen. Acta Parasitologica Polonica 7, 539–547 (in German).

Zoll, W.M., Needle, D.B., French, S.J., Lim, A., Bolin, S., Langohr, I., Agnew, D., 2015. *Sarcocystis* spp. infection in two red panda cubs (*Ailurus fulgens*). Journal of Comparative Pathology 153 (2–3), 185–189.

Zuo, Y.X., Chen, X.W., Li, Y.J., Ma, T.C., Tang, D.H., Fan, L.X., Zhao, M.L., 1995. Studies on *Sarcocystis* species of cattle and water buffalo with description of a new species of *Sarcocystis*. In: Proceedings of the 10th Anniversary of the Founding of Chinese Parasitological Society. Chinese Science and Technology Press, Beijing, PR China, pp. 20–24 (in Chinese).

Glossary and Abbreviations

18S rRNA A component of the small eukaryotic ribosomal subunit (40S). 18S rRNA is the structural RNA for the small component of eukaryotic cytoplasmic ribosomes, and thus one of the basic components of all eukaryotic cells.

28S rRNA The structural ribosomal RNA for the large component, or large subunit of eukaryotic cytoplasmic ribosomes, and thus one of the basic components of all eukaryotic cells.

Altricial Refers to an animal being born (mammal) or hatched (bird) being in an undeveloped state that requires care and feeding by its parents.

Aposematic coloration Warning coloration. Conspicuous, recognizable markings of an animal to warn potential predators of the harm or bad taste that will come from attacking or eating it.

Auctores (L. noun) of various authors.

Baculum A bone found in the penis of many placental mammals.

b.i.d To take a medication twice daily.

Bradyzoites (syn. cystozoites) Slowly multiplying zoites within tissue cysts that reproduce by endodyogeny and do not appear until the cysts become mature.

BW Body weight.

CAPC Companion Animal Parasite Council. An independent council of veterinarians, veterinary parasitologists, and other animal health care professionals established to create guidelines for the optimal control of internal and external parasites that threaten the health of pets and people.

Cardiomyocytes Myocytes (muscle cells) that make up the cardiac muscle (heart muscle).

Cathemeral An activity pattern in which an animal is neither prescriptively nocturnal, diurnal, or crepuscular, but irregularly active at any time of night or day, according to prevailing circumstances.

CI Continuous Integration CI is a development practice that requires integrating code into a shared repository several times a day. Each check-in is then verified by an automated build, allowing teams to detect problems early.

Clade(s) An according to the principles of cladistics, a group of organisms believed to have evolved from a common ancestor.

Colics Severe, often fluctuating abdominal pain caused by obstruction or intestinal gas in the intestines.

Convergent evolution The independent evolution of a feature in species of different lineages. For example, wings have evolved many times independently (flies, birds, bats); and Australian koalas have fingerprints that are indistinguishable from those of humans.

COWP *Cryptosporidium* oocyst wall protein gene.

Cox1 Cytochrome oxidase subunit 1 gene encodes a subunit of the cytochrome c oxidase that is part of the respiratory chain that catalyzes the reduction of oxygen to water in mitochondria. It is often used as a DNA barcode to identify animal species.

CPV Canine parvovirus. A type 2 contagious virus mainly affecting dogs, and thought to originate in cats. The current consensus is that the feline panleukopenia mutated into CPV2.

Crepuscular The behavior of appearing or being active in the twilight, such as just before dawn or just after sunset.

Cross-transmission An experimental procedure that attempts to transmit a parasite of one host species to a different host species that may, or may not, be related to the original host.

Definitive host A host in which a parasite achieves sexual maturity.

DFAT Direct fluorescence microscopy is a cell-imaging technique that relies on the use of antibodies to label a specific target antigen with a fluorescent dye (i.e., fluorophores or fluorochromes); the fluorophore allows visualization of the target distribution in the sample under a fluorescent microscope (e.g., epifluorescence and confocal microscopes). Direct fluorescent microscopy uses a single antibody directed against the target of interest. The primary antibody is directly conjugated to a fluorophore.

Diurnal During the day or daytime.

DPI (PI) Abbreviations used throughout this book to refer to post-inoculation, usually in days, meaning the time period between when a host is inoculated with a parasite and the day a particular stage of the parasite's life history is seen/discovered.

EIN Extraintestinal stages that occur in the tissues (mesenteric lymph nodes, liver, spleen, lungs, brain, musculature) of cats and dogs (definitive hosts) when fed sporulated oocysts of certain *Cystoisospora* species to which they are susceptible.

ELISA Enzyme-linked immunosorbent assay is a biochemical technique used mainly in immunology to detect the presence of an antibody or an antigen in a sample.

Endogenous stages Refers to the asexual (merogony) and sexual (gamogony) stages of the coccidian life cycle that take place within epithelial or endothelial cells of the gastrointestinal tract or associated organs (e.g., liver, bile ducts, etc.).

Endopolygeny Process in which the parasite nucleus becomes multilobed before formation of numerous merozoites. This occurs while still in the mother cell.

Encephalomyelitis (EPM) Inflammation of the brain and spinal cord, typically due to acute viral or protozoal infection. Mostly, EPM refers to equine protozoal myeloencephalitis, which remains an important neurologic disease of horses. There are no pathognomonic clinical signs for the disease, and infected horses can have focal or multifocal central nervous system (CNS) disease.

Exogenous stages Refers to the oocysts discharged into the environment in the feces from an infected animal; the oocysts form after fusion of the micro- and macrogametes, both produced intracellularly.

FeLV Refers to feline leukemia virus, a retrovirus that infects cats that can be transmitted from infected individuals via the transfer of saliva or nasal secretions. If not overcome by the infected animal's immune system, the virus can be lethal.

FIV Refers to feline immunodeficiency virus, a lentivirus that affects 2.5%–4% of cats worldwide and is related to human immunodeficiency virus. There are 5 subtypes of FIV based on nucleotide sequence differences coding for the viral envelope (env) or polymerase (pol). It is the only nonprimate lentivirus to cause an AIDS-like syndrome, but it is not typically fatal for cats.

Gametogony (Gamogony) The process of gamete formation.

Genotype Generally refers to the specific genetic makeup of a cell, organism, or individual. However, it is also used by researchers to distinguish genetically distinct populations of oocysts for which there is insufficient information to assign species status. In particular it is used for *Cryptosporidium* species where oocysts are especially small with virtually no structural differences between species.

gp60 60 kilodalton glycoprotein gene.

HCN An abbreviation used throughout this book to refer to the host cell nucleus.

Hepatosplenomegaly A disorder where both the liver and spleen swell beyond their normal size, usually due to an infection including with tissue infecting coccidia.

Heteroxenous A parasite life cycle where two or more hosts are involved; that is, there is a mandatory intermediate host within which biological development of the parasite must take place for the life cycle to be continued.

Homoxenous (monoxenous) A parasite life cycle where the parasite has only a single host.

HSP70 Heat shock protein 70 gene.

H&E Hematoxylin (haematoxylin) and eosin stain is one of the principal stains in histology.

IFA (IFAT) Immunofluorescence antibody technique is a traditional laboratory assay that utilizes fluorescent dyes to identify the presence of antibodies bound to specific antigens. The IFA is very useful to detect the serologic response of a host that has been exposed to certain coccidian species.

IHC Immunohistochemistry involves exploiting the process of antibodies binding to antigens in the cells of a tissue section to selectively image the antigens or proteins.

Intermediate host A host in which a parasite develops to some extent, but not to sexual maturity.

ITS-1/ ITS-2 DNA sequences that separate the eukaryotic 18S, 5.8S, and 26S rRNA genes that are found as repeat units arranged in tandem arrays in the nucleolar organizing regions. Both have been used as molecular characters to differentiate closely related species in taxonomic/systematic studies of coccidia with varying success.

I.V. (i.v.) Intravenous.

Karyology (Karyological) The minute cytological characteristics of the cell nucleus especially with regard to the chromosomes of a single cell or of the cells of an organism or group of organisms.

Karyorrhexis Fragmentation of the nucleus of a dying cell where the chromatin is distributed irregularly throughout the cytoplasm.

kg Kilogram = 1,000 g.

kGy Kilogray. A derived metric measurement unit of absorbed radiation dose of ionizing radiation (e.g., X-rays). The kilogray is equal to one thousand gray (1,000 Gy), and the gray is defined as the absorption of 1 J of ionizing radiation by 1 kg (1 J/kg) of matter (e.g., animal tissue).

Koch's Postulates Four conditions designed to establish a causal relationship between a microbe and a disease. These are: (1) The microbe must be found in all hosts suffering the disease. (2) The microbe must be isolated from the diseased organism in pure form or culture. (3) The microbe should cause the same disease/infection/condition when introduced into a healthy, noninfected host, generally of the same host species. (4) The microbe must be able to be reisolated from the inoculated experimental host and be identical in form and structure to the original causative agent.

KPg Cretaceous–Paleogene (KPg) extinction event, also known as the Cretaceous–Tertiary (K–T) extinction, was a mass extinction approximately 66 million years ago where three-quarters of the plant and animal species on Earth disappeared over a geologically short period of time.

Lapsus calami (L.) an unintentional mistake, a "slip of the pen."

LM Light microscope; refers to the study of a specimen using a light microscope.

M An abbreviation used throughout this book to refer to the micropyle, usually a circular opening at one end of the oocyst, usually the more pointed end.

MAT Modified agglutination test is one of the most commonly used tests for the detection of antibodies to *Toxoplasma gondii* in human and other animal sera.

Meningoencephalitis Inflammation of the brain and surrounding tissues, usually caused by infection.

Meningoencephalomyelitis Inflammation of the meninges, brain, and spinal cord.

Merogony The process of merozoite formation via asexual reproduction. Also called schizogony in the older literature.

Merozoite A daughter cell resulting from merogony.

Metrocytes Cells accumulating inside *Sarcocystis* species' tissue cyst wall and eventually giving rise to infective bradyzoites.

Microgranulate Salinopharm® 120 microGranulate is an anticoccidial feed additive for the prophylactic control of coccidiosis in chickens for fattening and chickens reared for laying. Salinopharm® 120 is produced by means of microgranulation, which combines inseparably the carrier and the active ingredient of the product.

Monophyly A group of organisms that forms a clade, which consists of all the descendants of a common ancestor.

Monotypic Having only one type or representative, (especially of a genus) containing only one species.

Monoxenous (homoxenous) A parasite life cycle where the parasite has only a single host.

Monozoic An oocyst or sporocyst of a coccidian developing into a single sporozoite without division.

MYA Million years ago.

Myocytes Dominant cell type found in muscle tissue.

MZTC Monozoic tissue cyst.

N An abbreviation used throughout this book to refer either to the nucleus (sing.) or nuclei (pl.) within various coccidian stages.

NAT *Neospora* antigen test.

Necrosis Death of most or all of the cells in an organ or tissue due to disease, injury, or failure of the blood supply.

Nocturnal Active, occurring, or when things are done at night.

Nomen nudum (L.) (plural *nomina nuda*) is a term used for a name that is unavailable because it does not have a description, reference, or indication.

Nos non videbo illum (L.) we did not see (*Non vidi*) this original paper.

Omnivore/omnivorous An organism that eats food of both plant and animal origin.

OR An abbreviation used throughout this book to refer to the oocyst residuum, a structure often found within the oocyst.

Paraphyletic When a group consists of the group's last common ancestor and all descendants of that ancestor excluding a few—typically only one or two—monophyletic subgroups. The group is said to be paraphyletic *with respect to* the excluded subgroups.

Parasitemia The demonstrable presence of parasites in the blood.

Parasitologist A curious person who seeks the truth in some very strange places; sometimes described as a person who sits on one stool, while examining another one. A rare and beautiful object scientifically and often slow in going to seed.

Parasitophorous vacuole (PV) A vacuolated space inside a host cell that surrounds a developing stage (e.g., meront, gamont) of an apicomplexan parasite.

Paratenic host (=Transport host) A host in which a parasite survives without undergoing any further biological development.

Pari passu (L.) hand-in-hand, side-by-side, equal footing; that is, all similar endogenous stages at the same time.

PCR/ PCR-RFLP Polymerase chain reaction/ restriction fragment length polymorphism. PCR is technique used in molecular biology to amplify a single copy or a few copies of a segment of DNA across several orders of magnitude, generating thousands to millions of copies of a particular DNA sequence. RFLP is a technique employed with PCR that exploits variations in homologous DNA sequences. In RFLP the DNA sample is broken into pieces (and digested) by restriction enzymes and the resulting *fragments* are separated according to their lengths by gel electrophoresis. RFLP is now largely obsolete due to the rise of inexpensive DNA sequencing technologies.

Per os (p.o.) By mouth, orally.

PG An abbreviation used throughout this book to refer to the polar granule, a small, usually refractile structure often found within the oocyst.

Phylogeny The evolution of a genetically related group of organisms as distinguished from the development of the individual organism.

Plantigrade Walking on the soles of the feet, like a human or a bear.

Plesiomorphic A primitive character trait that is shared with an ancestral clade.

PMN Polymorphonucleocyte is a category of white blood cells characterized by the presence of granules in their cytoplasm and the varying shapes of the nucleus, which is usually lobed into three segments.

Polymyositis One of the inflammatory myopathies, a group of muscle diseases that involves inflammation of the muscles or associated tissues.

Polyradiculoneuritis An inflammation that develops suddenly when the body's immune system attacks the nerves that results in generalized weakness and paralysis.

Pro parte (L.) Used in nomenclature to denote that a taxon includes more than one currently recognized entity, and that only one of those entities is being considered.

PSB An abbreviation used throughout this book to refer to the parastieda body, a structure of unknown composition that is found at the more rounded end of the sporocyst (SP), opposite the Stieda body (SB), which is located at its more pointed end.

Pseudoparasite An organism whose presence within another is interpreted as parasitic but which is only present by accident.

Pyknosis Prior to karyorrhexis, the irreversible condensation of chromatin in the nucleus of a cell undergoing necrosis or apoptosis.

Quaternary ammonium compounds Used as antimicrobials and disinfectants, especially those containing long alkyl chains.

RG An abbreviation used throughout this book to refer to the refractile granule or globule, a spheroidal to subspheroidal structure or structures often, but not always, found inside sporozoites (SZ).

Rhoptries Elongated, electron dense bodies extending within the polar rings of an apicomplexan.

SB An abbreviation used throughout this book to refer to the Stieda body, a nipple-like structure found at the more pointed end of the sporocyst (SP).

SCID mice Mice homozygous for the severe combined immune deficiency spontaneous mutation Prkdc^{scid}, commonly referred to as scid, are characterized by absence of functional T cells and B cells, lymphopenia, hypogammaglobulinemia, and a normal hematopoietic microenvironment.

SEM Scanning electron microscope.

Seroprevalence The number of individuals positive for a pathogen divided by the total number examined in a population, as measured in blood serum.

Serosurvey A test of blood serum from a group of individuals to determine seroprevalence.

Sibling species Any of two or more related species that are morphologically nearly identical but are incapable of producing fertile hybrids. The species can only be differentiated by genetic, biochemical, behavioral, or ecological factors, and likely diverged recently.

s.i.d Once daily; an abbreviation for how frequently to administer drug dosages.

SP An abbreviation used throughout this book to refer to the sporocyst, which encloses sporozoites (SZ).

SPF Specific pathogen free.

Sporogony The formation of spores; or in the case of eimeriid coccidia, it is the process by which the sporoplasm (inside the oocyst) gives rise to sporocysts, and these to sporozoites. This developmental process takes place inside the oocyst usually when it leaves the confines of the host's gastrointestinal tract. The availability of molecular O_2 seems critical for this process to continue successfully.

Spurious infection When a parasite invades a host but does not succeed in colonizing it, for example merely passing through the digestive tract.

SR An abbreviation used throughout this book to refer to the sporocyst residuum, a structure often found within a sporocyst (SP).

SSB An abbreviation used throughout this book to refer to the substieda body, a structure that lies immediately under the Stieda body (SB) at the more pointed end of the sporocyst (SP).

Synapsid reptiles Mammal-like reptiles, also called stem- or proto-mammals, that evolved from basal amniotes and is one of the two major groups of present day amniotes (the other, sauropsids, includes birds and reptiles).

Syzygy When the macro- and microgamete are attached or pressed against one another during development.

SZ An abbreviation used throughout this book to refer the sporozoites that are enclosed within the sporocyst (SP).

Tachyzoites Rapidly dividing tissue zoites, seen early in the infection, that infect and destroy cells in many tissues and organs; they reproduce asexually by endodyogeny in the intermediate host.

TEM Transmission electron microscope; refers to the use of this instrument to study the ultrastructural details of biological specimens at magnifications far exceeding those of the LM.

Theilierosis A disease of cattle and other ruminants caused by *Theileria parva*. It is called East Coast Fever in countries where it exists.

t.i.d. Abbreviation for "ter in die" (L.) meaning three times a day.

Trophozoite The activated, intracellular feeding stage in the apicomplexan life cycle.

Unsporulated Condition in which the oocyst(s) of species of coccidia has not undergone the process of development (sporulation) into a mature, infective form.

USNPC United States National Parasite Collection, now housed at the Smithsonian Institution, Washington, D.C., USA.

Vaccination Administration of antigenic material (in the form of a vaccine) to stimulate an individual's immune system to develop adaptive immunity to the pathogen being vaccinated against.

Visceral larval migrans A condition in humans caused by the migratory larvae of certain nematodes (i.e., *Toxocara canis*, *T. cati*, *Baylisascaris procyonis*) and for which humans are a dead-end host for the parasite.

Viverrids A group considered to be ancient inhabitants of Old World tropics. These are small to medium-sized carnivores with 15 genera and 35 species commonly called civets or genets and found throughout southern and southeast Asia, most of Africa and into southern Europe.

Xenodiagnosis Diagnostic method used to document the presence of an infectious agent by exposing possibly infected tissue to a vector and then examining the vector for the presence of the agent it may have ingested.

Zoonosis (sing.)/zoonoses (pl.) Disease agents of wild or domesticated animals that are transmissible to humans when they come in contact with each other.

Index